SHERLOCK'S DISEASES OF THE LIVER
AND BILIARY SYSTEM

Companion Website

This book has a companion website

www.wiley.com/go/sherlock/liver

with:

- All 700 figures and captions in the book as Powerpoints for downloading

Sherlock's Diseases of the Liver and Biliary System

EDITED BY

JAMES S. DOOLEY

Centre for Hepatology
University College London Medical School and
Royal Free Sheila Sherlock Liver Centre
Royal Free Hospital
London
UK

ANNA S. F. LOK

Division of Gastroenterology
University of Michigan Health System
Ann Arbor
USA

ANDREW K. BURROUGHS

Royal Free Sheila Sherlock Liver Centre
Royal Free Hospital;
University College London
London
UK

E. JENNY HEATHCOTE

Division of Gastroenterology
University Health Network
University of Toronto
Toronto
Ontario
Canada

12TH EDITION

WILEY-BLACKWELL

A John Wiley & Sons, Ltd., Publication

This edition first published 2011, © 1963, 1968, 1975, 1981, 1985, 1989, 1993, 1997, 2002, 2011 by Blackwell Publishing Ltd

Blackwell Publishing was acquired by John Wiley & Sons in February 2007. Blackwell's publishing program has been merged with Wiley's global Scientific, Technical and Medical business to form Wiley-Blackwell.

First published 1955
Second edition 1958
Third edition 1963
Fourth edition 1968
Fifth edition 1975
Sixth edition 1981
Seventh edition 1985
Eighth edition 1989
Ninth edition 1993
Tenth edition 1997
Eleventh edition 2002

Registered office: John Wiley & Sons Ltd, The Atrium, Southern Gate, Chichester, West Sussex, PO19 8SQ, UK

Editorial offices: 9600 Garsington Road, Oxford, OX4 2DQ, UK
The Atrium, Southern Gate, Chichester, West Sussex, PO19 8SQ, UK
111 River Street, Hoboken, NJ 07030-5774, USA

For details of our global editorial offices, for customer services and for information about how to apply for permission to reuse the copyright material in this book please see our website at www.wiley.com/wiley-blackwell

The right of the author to be identified as the author of this work has been asserted in accordance with the Copyright, Designs and Patents Act 1988.

Library of Congress Cataloging-in-Publication Data

Sherlock's diseases of the liver and biliary system / edited by James S. Dooley ... [et al.]. – 12th ed.
   p. ; cm.
  Diseases of the liver and biliary system
  Rev. ed. of: Diseases of the liver and biliary system / Sheila Sherlock. 11th ed. 2002.
  Includes bibliographical references and index.
  ISBN 978-1-4051-3489-7 (hardcover : alk. paper)
  1. Liver–Diseases. 2. Biliary tract–Diseases. I. Dooley, James (James S.) II. Sherlock, Sheila, Dame. Diseases of the liver and biliary system. III. Title: Diseases of the liver and biliary system.
  [DNLM: 1. Liver Diseases. 2. Biliary Tract Diseases. WI 700]
  RC845.S52 2011
  616.3'6–dc22

2010039149

A catalogue record for this book is available from the British Library.

This book is published in the following electronic formats: ePDF 9781444341263; Wiley Online Library 9781444341294; ePub 9781444341270; Mobi 9781444341287

Set in 9.5/12 pt Palatino by Toppan Best-set Premedia Limited
Printed and bound in Singapore by Markono Print Media Pte Ltd

01 2011

Contents

29 The Liver in the Neonate, in Infancy and Childhood, 568

Deirdre A. Kelly

30 The Liver in Pregnancy, 602

Andrew K. Burroughs & E. Jenny Heathcote

31 The Liver in Systemic Disease, 615

Humphrey J. F. Hodgson

32 The Liver in Infections, 632

Christopher C. Kibbler

33 Space-Occupying Lesions: the Diagnostic Approach, 660

Neil H. Davies & Dominic Yu

34 Benign Liver Tumours, 671

Ian R. Wanless

Companion Website

This book has a companion website

www.wiley.com/go/sherlock/liver

with:

- All 700 figures and captions in the book as Powerpoints for downloading

List of Contributors

Paul Adams MD
Professor of Medicine
Chief of Gastroenterology
University Hospital
University of Western Ontario
London, Ontario, Canada

Curtis K. Argo MD, MS
Assistant Professor of Medicine
Division of Gastroenterology and Hepatology
Department of Internal Medicine
University of Virginia Health System
Charlottesville, VA, USA

Meena B. Bansal MD
Assistant Professor of Medicine
Division of Liver Diseases
Mount Sinai School of Medicine
New York, NY, USA

Margaret F. Bassendine BSc, MBBS, FRCP, FRCP(E), DSc(Med)
Professor of Hepatology
Institute of Cellular Medicine
Medical School
Newcastle University
Newcastle upon Tyne, UK

Andrew K. Burroughs FRCP, FMedSci
Consultant Physician and Professor of Hepatology
Royal Free Sheila Sherlock Liver Centre
Royal Free Hospital
University College London
London,UK

Stephen H. Caldwell MD
Professor and Director of Hepatology
Division of Gastroenterology and Hepatology
Department of Internal Medicine
University of Virginia Health System
Charlottesville, VA, USA

Roger W. Chapman MD, FRCP
Consultant Hepatologist,
Department of Translational Gastroenterology,
John Radcliffe Hospital
Oxford, UK

Antonio Craxi MD
Professor of Internal Medicine and Gastroenterology
University of Palermo
Palermo, Italy

Brian R. Davidson MD, FRCS
Professor of Surgery
Academic Department of Surgery
University College London Medical School
Royal Free Hospital
London, UK

Neil H. Davies MB BS, FRCS, FRCR
Consultant Interventional Radiologist
Department of Radiology
Royal Free Hampstead NHS Trust
London, UK

Chris Day FMedSci
Pro-Vice Chancellor and Professor of Liver Medicine
Faculty of Medical Sciences
Newcastle University Medical School
Newcastle upon Tyne, UK

Amar Paul Dhillon MD, FRCP, FRCPath
Professor of Histopathology
Department of Cellular Pathology
University College London Medical School
Royal Free Campus
London, UK

Rosa Di Stefano PhD
Virologist
Department of Virology
University of Palermo
Palermo, Italy

James S. Dooley MD, FRCP
Reader and Honorary Consultant in Medicine
Centre for Hepatology
University College London Medical School;
Royal Free Sheila Sherlock Liver Centre
Royal Free Hospital
London, UK

Geoffrey Dusheiko FCP(SA), FRCP, FRCP(Edin)
Professor of Medicine
Centre for Hepatology
University College London Medical School;
Royal Free Sheila Sherlock Liver Centre
Royal Free Hospital
London, UK

Elwyn Elias MD, FRCP
Honorary Professor of Hepatology
University of Birmingham
Birmingham, UK

Patrizia Farci MD
Chief, Hepatic Pathogenesis Section
Laboratory of Infectious Diseases
National Institute of Allergy and Infectious Diseases
National Institutes of Health
Bethesda, MD, USA

Robert J. Fontana MD
Professor of Medicine
Division of Gastroenterology
Department of Internal Medicine
University of Michigan Medical School
Ann Arbor, MI, USA

Scott L. Friedman MD
Fishberg Professor of Medicine
Chief, Division of Liver Diseases
Mount Sinai School of Medicine
New York, NY, USA

Guadalupe Garcia-Tsao MD
Professor of Medicine
Section of Digestive Diseases
Yale School of Medicine
New Haven, Connecticut;
Veterans Affairs Connecticut Healthcare System
West Haven, Connecticut, USA

John L. Gollan MD, PhD, FRCP, FRACP
Dean and Stokes-Shackleford Professor of Medicine
University of Nebraska Medical Center
Omaha, NE, USA

Nedim Hadžić MD
Reader in Paediatric Hepatology
King's College London School of Medicine
King's College Hospital
London, UK

E. Jenny Heathcote MB BS, MD, FRCP, FRCP(C)
Frances Family Chair in Hepatology Research
Professor of Medicine
University of Toronto
Head, Patient Based Clinical Research
Toronto Western Hospital Research Institute
Toronto, Ontario, Canada

Gideon M. Hirschfield MBBChir, MRCP, PhD
Assistant Professor of Medicine
Liver Centre
Toronto Western Hospital
Toronto, Ontario, Canada

Humphrey J. F. Hodgson FRCP, DM, FMedSci
Sheila Sherlock Chair of Medicine
Centre for Hepatology
University College London School of Medicine;
Royal Free Sheila Sherlock Liver Centre
Royal Free Hospital
London, UK

Dhanpat Jain MD
Associate Professor of Pathology
Yale School of Medicine
New Haven, CT, USA

Peter Karayiannis BSc, PhD, FIBMS, FRCPath
Reader in Molecular Virology
Imperial College
London, UK

Deirdre A. Kelly MD, FRCP, FRCPI, FRCPCH
Professor of Paediatric Hepatology
Liver Unit
Birmingham Children's Hospital
University of Birmingham
Birmingham, UK

Christopher C. Kibbler MA, FRCP, FRCPath
Professor of Medical Microbiology
Centre for Clinical Microbiology
University College London Medical School;
Department of Medical Microbiology
Royal Free Hampstead NHS Trust
London, UK

Rahul S. Koti MD, FRCS
Honorary Lecturer in Surgery
Academic Department of Surgery
University College London Medical School
Royal Free Hospital
London, UK

William M. Lee MD, FACP
Professor of Internal Medicine
University of Texas
Southwestern Medical Center at Dallas
Dallas, TX, USA

Jay H. Lefkowitch MD
Professor of Clinical Pathology
College of Physicians and Surgeons
Columbia University
New York, NY, USA

Anna S. F. Lok MBBS, MD, FRCP
Alice Lohrman Andrews Research Professor in Hepatology
Director of Clinical Hepatology
Division of Gastroenterology
University of Michigan Health System
Ann Arbor, MI, USA

P. Aiden McCormick MD, FRCP, FRCPI
Consultant Hepatologist and Newman Clinical
Research Professor,
St Vincent's University Hospital and University
College Dublin,
Dublin
Ireland

Giorgina Mieli-Vergani MD, PhD
Alex Mowat Chair of Paediatric Hepatology
King's College London School of Medicine
King's College Hospital
London, UK

Pramod K. Mistry MD, PhD, FRCP
Professor of Pediatrics and Medicine
Chief, Pediatric Gastroenterology and Hepatology
Yale University School of Medicine
New Haven, CT, USA

Marsha Y. Morgan FRCP
Reader in Medicine and Honorary Consultant Physician
Centre for Hepatology
Royal Free Campus
University College London Medical School
London, UK

Sandeep Mukherjee MB BCh, MPH, FRCPC
Associate Professor of Internal Medicine
Nebraska Medical Center
Section of Gastroenterology and Hepatology
Omaha, NE, USA

James O'Beirne MB BS, MD, MRCP
Consultant Physician and Hepatologist
Royal Free Sheila Sherlock Liver Centre
Royal Free Hospital
London, UK

David Patch MB BS, FRCP
Hepatologist
Royal Free Sheila Sherlock Liver Centre
Royal Free Hospital
London, UK

Marion G. Peters MD, FRACP
John V. Carbone MD Endowed Chair in Medicine
Division of Gastroenterology
University of California, San Francisco
San Francisco, CA, USA

Eve A. Roberts MD, MA, FRCPC
Departments of Paediatrics, Medicine and Pharmacology
University of Toronto
Toronto, Ontario, Canada

Simon Rushbrook MD, MRCP
Consultant Gastroenterologist,
Department of Gastroenterology,
Norfolk and Norwich Hospital,
Norwich, UK

Leonard B. Seeff MD
Former Senior Scientific Officer
National Institute of Diabetes and Digestive and Kidney
Diseases
National Institutes of Health
Bethesda, MD, USA

Morris Sherman MB BCh, PhD, FRCP(C)
Associate Professor of Medicine
University of Toronto
Toronto, Ontario, Canada

Vincent Soriano MD, PhD
Assistant Director
Hospital Carlos III
Department of Infectious Diseases
Madrid, Spain

Stephen Stewart MBChB, PhD
Consultant Hepatologist and Director of Liver Centre
Mater Misericordiae University Hospital
Dublin

Norah Terrault MD, MPH
Professor of Medicine and Surgery
Division of Gastroenterology
University of California San Francisco
San Francisco, CA, USA

Howard C. Thomas BSc, PhD, FRCP, FRCPath, FMedSci
Liver Unit
Department of Hepatology and Gastroenterology
Imperial College London
London, UK

Shannan R. Tujios MD
Fellow, Division of Digestive Diseases
Department of Internal Medicine
Southwestern Medical Center at Dallas
Dallas, TX, USA

Ian R. Wanless MD, CM, FRCPC
Professor of Pathology
Department of Pathology
Dalhousie University
Queen Elizabeth II Health Services Centre
Halifax, Canada

Dominic Yu MB BS, MRCPI, FRCR
Consultant Radiologist
Department of Radiology
Royal Free Hampstead NHS Trust
London, UK

Preface to the Twelfth Edition

The 11th edition marked the end of an era. Professor Dame Sheila Sherlock died in December 2001, having a month before seen and enjoyed an advanced copy of her latest textbook. Her journey in Hepatology began in the 1940s, and she was instrumental in its development and recognition as a major specialty. In 1955 she published the first edition of what was to become a classic textbook. Single handed she updated the script on a regular basis and it became an influential instrument for the development of Hepatology. There were many translations of the editions over subsequent 50 years. Recognising the growth and complexity of the subject, she involved a co-author from 1993. Many attribute their career in liver disease to reading and enjoying her approach to Hepatology through her book.

The question of a 12th edition was raised on several occasions over the subsequent years. Although some wondered whether it should cease with her passing, many others constantly asked when the next edition would be—a reflection of the special content, presentation and readability—an accessible source to relevant information for student to specialist physician.

Continuing a two author book was not thought practicable. The growth of Hepatology as a speciality demanded a greater pool of expertise, in viral, immune and genetic diseases, as well as the management of the complications of acute and chronic liver disease, and of course, liver transplantation.

Dame Sheila always promoted the internationalism of Hepatology and therefore it was a short step to draw together editors and contributors from the UK, Europe and North America. The challenge—apart from updating the previous edition with pertinent data—was to keep the ethos of the book. The style of English, the lay out of text and the clarity of figures and tables were hallmarks. With this in mind contributors were approached with expertise in particular areas; most had trained or worked with Dame Sheila. It is a tribute to her influence that the resultant text comes from such an international community, many of whom had close links with her.

Apart from updating the previous chapters, there have been other changes. New chapters have been com-missioned including those on fibrogenesis, non alcoholic fatty liver disease, HIV and the liver, and transplantation in patients with hepatitis B, C or HIV infection. Some previous chapters, which have stood the test of time on their own, have been removed or combined with others. Thus Budd Chiari syndrome joins the portal hypertension chapter, and biliary imaging that on gallstones and benign bile duct diseases.

The 12th edition contains more than 2240 new references and over 130 new figures. Each chapter begins with learning points. The previous artwork has been reformatted, alongside the new figures and tables. As before the book is intended for a wide readership across students, trainees, general and specialist physicians.

We are most grateful to the production team at Wiley Blackwell, in particular Rebecca Huxley (whose 3rd edition this is). Anne Bassett and Annette Abel have enthusiastically taken on the challenge of collecting manuscripts and proofs and chasing the large number of contributors, working beyond the call of duty to produce the book rapidly. We are grateful to Jane Fallows for the new artwork and reworking of the old. As before the publishers have allowed the latest important publications to be included at the proofing stage.

We dedicate this edition to the memory of Sheila Sherlock and to Geraint James, her husband of 50 years who died in October 2010. He knew of the development of the new edition and took pleasure in its anticipation. We hope that their two daughters, Amanda and Auriole, always referenced in previous prefaces with their life stories, will take pleasure from seeing the legacy of their mother's exceptional life preserved in this textbook.

The science and practice of Hepatology continue to move on at breathtaking speed. This progress is reflected in the 12th edition of *Sherlock's Diseases of the Liver and Biliary System*, in a manner which we hope will continue to enthuse its readers.

James S. Dooley
Anna S.F. Lok
Andrew K. Burroughs
E. Jenny Heathcote
March 2011

Preface to the First Edition

My aim in writing this book has been to present a comprehensive and up-to-date account of diseases of the liver and biliary system, which I hope will be of value to physicians, surgeons and pathologists and also a reference book for the clinical student. The modern literature has been reviewed with special reference to articles of general interest. Many older more specialized classical contributions have therefore inevitably been excluded.

Disorders of the liver and biliary system may be classified under the traditional concept of individual diseases. Alternatively, as I have endeavoured in this book, they may be described by the functional and morphological changes which they produce. In the clinical management of a patient with liver disease, it is important to assess the degree of disturbance of four functional and morphological components of the liver—hepatic cells, vascular system (portal vein, hepatic artery and hepatic veins), bile ducts and reticulo-endothelial system. The typical reaction pattern is thus sought and recognized before attempting to diagnose the causative insult. Clinical and laboratory methods of assessing each of these components are therefore considered early in the book. Descriptions of individual diseases follow as illustrative examples. It will be seen that the features of hepatocellular failure and portal hypertension are described in general terms as a foundation for subsequent discussion of virus hepatitis, nutrition liver disease and the cirrhoses. Similarly blood diseases and infections of the liver are included with the reticulo-endothelial system, and disorders of the biliary tract follow descriptions of acute and chronic bile duct obstruction.

I would like to acknowledge my indebtedness to my teachers, the late Professor J. Henry Dible, the late Professor Sir James Learmonth and Professor Sir John McMichael, who stimulated my interest in hepatic disease, and to my colleagues at the Postgraduate Medical School and elsewhere who have generously invited me to see patients under their care. I am grateful to Dr A. G. Bearn for criticizing part of the typescript and to Dr A. Paton for his criticisms and careful proof reading. Miss D. F. Atkins gave much assistance with proof reading and with the bibliography. Mr Per Saugman and Mrs J. M. Green of Blackwell Scientific Publications have co-operated enthusiastically in the production of this book.

The photomicrographs were taken by Mr E. V. Willmott, FRPS, and Mr C. A. P. Graham from section prepared by Mr J. G. Griffin and the histology staff of the Postgraduate Medical School. Clinical photographs are the work of Mr C. R. Brecknell and his assistants. The black and white drawings were made by Mrs H. M. G. Wilson and Mr D. Simmonds. I am indebted to them all for their patience and skill.

The text includes part of unpublished material included in a thesis submitted in 1944 to the University of Edinburgh for the degree of MD, and part of an essay awarded the Buckston–Browne prize of the Harveian Society of London in 1953. Colleagues have allowed me to include published work of which they are jointly responsible. Dr Patricia P. Franklyn and Dr R. E. Steiner have kindly loaned me radiographs. Many authors have given me permission to reproduce illustrations and detailed acknowledgments are given in the text. I wish also to thank the editors of the following journals for permission to include illustrations: *American Journal of Medicine, Archives of Pathology, British Heart Journal, Circulation, Clinical Science, Edinburgh Medical Journal, Journal of Clinical Investigation, Journal of Laboratory and Clinical Investigation, Journal of Pathology and Bacteriology, Lancet, Postgraduate Medical Journal, Proceedings of the Staff Meetings of the Mayo Clinic, Quarterly Journal of Medicine, Thorax* and also the following publishers: Butterworth's Medical Publications, J. & A. Churchill Ltd, The Josiah Macy Junior Foundation and G. D. Searle & Co.

Finally I must thank my husband, Dr D. Geraint James, who, at considerable personal inconvenience, encouraged me to undertake the writing of this book and also criticized and rewrote most of it. He will not allow me to dedicate it to him.

SHEILA SHERLOCK
1955

CHAPTER 1
Anatomy and Function

Jay H. Lefkowitch

College of Physicians and Surgeons, Columbia University, New York, NY, USA

Learning points

- The liver is derived from a foregut endodermal bud which develops in the third week of gestation and divides into two parts: hepatic and biliary.

- The Couinaud classification subdivides the liver into eight segments (segments I–IV in the left lobe, segments V–VIII in the right lobe) based on vascular and biliary anatomical landmarks.

- The lobule described by Kiernan is the most widely used unit of liver microanatomy, consisting of a hexagon-like region of liver parenchyma with a central vein as its hub and portal tracts located in the periphery of the hexagon.

- Hepatocytes are functionally heterogeneous within the lobular parenchyma, whereby centrilobular cells subserve different functions (e.g. drug metabolism) from periportal cells (e.g. bile salt-dependent bile formation).

- Uncomplicated regeneration of hepatocytes and/or bile duct epithelium usually occurs by cell division of the indigenous cells; however, when normal regenerative capacity is overwhelmed there may be activation of progenitors cells located in the region of the canals of Hering.

Development of the liver and bile ducts

The liver begins as a hollow endodermal bud from the foregut (duodenum) during the third week of gestation. The bud separates into two parts—hepatic and biliary. The *hepatic* part contains bipotential progenitor cells that differentiate into hepatocytes or ductal cells, which form the early primitive bile duct structures (bile duct plates). Differentiation is accompanied by changes in cytokeratin type within the cell [1]. Normally, this collection of rapidly proliferating cells penetrates adjacent mesodermal tissue (the septum transversum) and is met by ingrowing capillary plexuses from the vitelline and umbilical veins, which will form the sinusoids. The connection between this proliferating mass of cells and the foregut, the *biliary* part of the endodermal bud, will form the gallbladder and extrahepatic bile ducts. Bile begins to flow at about the 12th week. Connective tissue cells of portal tracts are derived from the mesoderm of the septum transversum. Kupffer cells derive from circulating monocytes and possibly yolk sac macrophages. Hepatic stellate cells appear to be mesodermal derivatives from submesothelial cells located beneath the surface of the developing liver [2]. The fetal liver is the main site of haemopoiesis by the 12th week; this subsides in the fifth month coincident with the onset of bone marrow haemopoietic activity, so that only a few haemopoietic cells remain at birth.

Anatomy of the liver

The liver, the largest organ in the body, weighs 1200–1500 g and comprises one-fiftieth of the total adult body weight. It is relatively larger in infancy, comprising one-eighteenth of the birth weight. This is mainly due to a large left lobe.

Sheltered by the ribs in the right upper quadrant, the upper border lies approximately at the level of the nipples. There are two anatomical lobes, the right being about six times the size of the left (Figs 1.1–1.3). Lesser segments of the right lobe are the *caudate lobe* on the posterior surface and the *quadrate lobe* on the inferior surface. The right and left lobes are separated anteriorly by a fold of peritoneum called the falciform ligament, posteriorly by the fissure for the ligamentum venosum and inferiorly by the fissure for the ligamentum teres.

The liver has a double blood supply. The *portal vein* brings venous blood from the intestines and spleen and the *hepatic artery*, coming from the coeliac axis, supplies the liver with arterial blood. These vessels enter the liver through a fissure, the *porta hepatis*, which lies far back on the inferior surface of the right lobe. Inside the porta, the portal vein and hepatic artery divide into branches to the right and left lobes, and the right and left hepatic

Sherlock's Diseases of the Liver and Biliary System, Twelfth Edition. Edited by
James S. Dooley, Anna S.F. Lok, Andrew K. Burroughs, E. Jenny Heathcote.
© 2011 by Blackwell Publishing Ltd. Published 2011 by Blackwell Publishing Ltd.

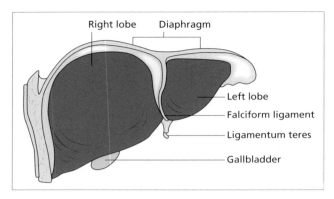

Fig. 1.1. Anterior view of the liver.

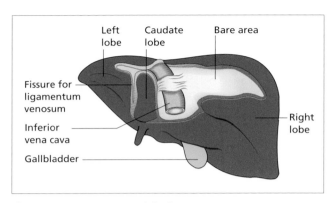

Fig. 1.2. Posterior view of the liver.

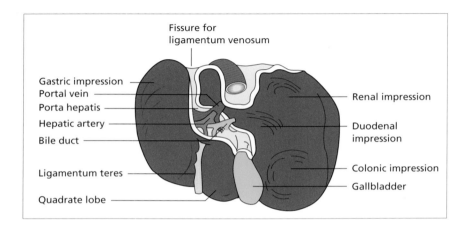

Fig. 1.3. Inferior view of the liver.

bile ducts join to form the common hepatic duct. The *hepatic nerve plexus* contains fibres from the sympathetic ganglia T7–T10, which synapse in the coeliac plexus, the right and left vagi and the right phrenic nerve. It accompanies the hepatic artery and bile ducts into their finest ramifications, even to the portal tracts and hepatic parenchyma [3].

The *ligamentum venosum*, a slender remnant of the ductus venosus of the fetus, arises from the left branch of the portal vein and fuses with the inferior vena cava at the entrance of the left hepatic vein. The *ligamentum teres*, a remnant of the umbilical vein of the fetus, runs in the free edge of the falciform ligament from the umbilicus to the inferior border of the liver and joins the left branch of the portal vein. Small veins accompanying it connect the portal vein with veins around the umbilicus. These become prominent when the portal venous system is obstructed inside the liver.

The venous drainage from the liver is into the *right* and *left hepatic veins* which emerge from the back of the liver and at once enter the inferior vena cava very near its point of entry into the right atrium.

Lymphatic vessels terminate in small groups of glands around the porta hepatis. Efferent vessels drain into glands around the coeliac axis. Some superficial hepatic lymphatics pass through the diaphragm in the falciform ligament and finally reach the mediastinal glands. Another group accompanies the inferior vena cava into the thorax and ends in a few small glands around the intrathoracic portion of the inferior vena cava.

The *inferior vena cava* makes a deep groove to the right of the caudate lobe about 2 cm from the midline.

The *gallbladder* lies in a fossa extending from the inferior border of the liver to the right end of the porta hepatis.

The liver is completely covered with peritoneum, except in three places. It comes into direct contact with the diaphragm through the bare area which lies to the right of the fossa for the inferior vena cava. The other areas without peritoneal covering are the fossae for the inferior vena cava and gallbladder.

The liver is kept in position by peritoneal ligaments and by the intra-abdominal pressure transmitted by the tone of the muscles of the abdominal wall.

Functional liver anatomy: sectors and segments

Based on the external appearances described above, the liver has a right and left lobe separated along the line of insertion of the falciform ligament. This separation, however, does not correlate with blood supply or biliary drainage. A *functional anatomy* is now recognized based upon vascular and biliary anatomy. The *Couinaud* classification [4] defines eight segments (segments I-IV in the left lobe, V-VIII in the right lobe), while the *Bismuth* classification [5] divides the liver into four sectors. These can be correlated with results seen with imaging techniques.

The main portal vein divides into right and left branches and each of these supplies two further subunits (variously called sectors). The sectors on the right side are anterior and posterior and, in the left lobe, medial and lateral—giving a total of four sectors (Fig. 1.4). Using this definition, the right and left side of the liver are divided not along the line of the falciform ligament, but along a slightly oblique line to the right of this, drawn from the inferior vena cava above to the gallbladder bed below. The right and left side are independent with regard to portal and arterial blood supply, and bile drainage. Three planes separate the four sectors and contain the three major hepatic vein branches.

Closer analysis of these four hepatic sectors produces a further subdivision into segments (Fig. 1.5). The right anterior sector contains segments V and VIII; right posterior sector, VI and VII; left medial sector, IV; left lateral sector, II and III. There is no vascular anastomosis between the macroscopic vessels of the segments but communications exist at the sinusoidal level. Segment I,

the equivalent of the caudate lobe, is separate from the other segments and does not derive blood directly from the major portal branches or drain by any of the three major hepatic veins.

This functional anatomical classification allows interpretation of radiological data and is of importance to the

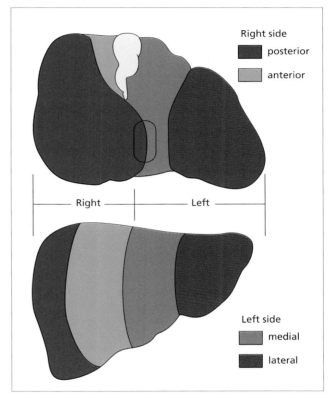

Fig. 1.4. The sectors of the human liver.

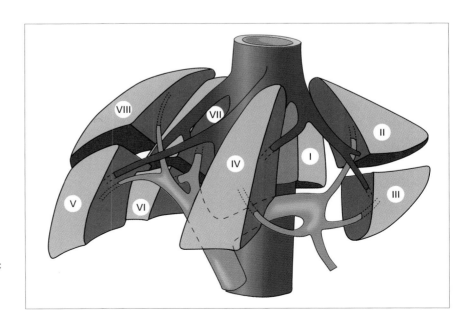

Fig. 1.5. Schematic representation of the functional anatomy of the liver. Three main hepatic veins (dark blue) divide the liver into four sectors, each of them receiving a portal pedicle; hepatic veins and portal veins are intertwined as the fingers of two hands [5].

surgeon planning a liver resection. There are wide variations in portal and hepatic vessel anatomy which can be demonstrated by spiral computed tomography (CT) and magnetic resonance imaging (MRI) reconstruction [6].

Anatomical abnormalities of the liver

These are being increasingly diagnosed with more widespread use of CT and ultrasound scanning.

Accessory lobes. The livers of the pig, dog and camel are divided into distinct and separate lobes by strands of connective tissue. Occasionally, the human liver may show this reversion and up to 16 lobes have been reported. This abnormality is rare and without clinical significance. The lobes are small and usually on the undersurface of the liver so that they are not detected clinically but are noted incidentally at scanning, operation or necropsy. Rarely they are intrathoracic [7]. An accessory lobe may have its own mesentery containing hepatic artery, portal vein, bile duct and hepatic vein. This may twist and demand surgical intervention.

Ectopic liver. Small nodules of normal liver derived from the embryologic hepatic bud may be found in less than 1% of laparoscopies and autopsies near the gallbladder, hepatic ligaments, gastrorenal ligament, omentum, retroperitorneum and thorax. These may give rise to hepatocellular carcinoma [8,9].

Riedel's lobe. This is fairly common and is a downward tongue-like projection of the right lobe of the liver [10]. It is a simple anatomical variation; it is not a true accessory lobe. The condition is more frequent in women. It is detected as a mobile tumour on the right side of the abdomen which descends with the diaphragm on inspiration. It may come down as low as the right iliac region. It is easily mistaken for other tumours in this area, especially a visceroptotic right kidney. It does not cause symptoms and treatment is not required. Rarely, it is a site for metastasis or primary hepatocellular carcinoma. Scanning may be used to identify Riedel's lobe and other anatomical abnormalities.

Cough furrows on the liver. These are vertical grooves on the convexity of the right lobe. They are one to six in number and run anteroposteriorly, being deeper posteriorly. These represent diaphragmatic sulci and fissures produced by pressure exerted by diaphragmatic muscle on peripheral structurally weak liver parenchymal zones associated with watershed vascular distribution [11]. Chronic cough produces such pressure.

Corset liver. This is a horizontal fibrotic furrow or pedicle on the anterior surface of one or both lobes of the liver just below the costal margin [12]. The mechanism is unknown, but it affects elderly women who have worn corsets for many years. It presents as an abdominal mass in front of and below the liver and is isodense with the liver. It may be confused with a hepatic tumour.

Lobar atrophy. Interference with the portal supply or biliary drainage of a lobe may cause atrophy. There is usually hypertrophy of the opposite lobe. Left lobe atrophy found at post-mortem or during scanning is not uncommon and is probably related to reduced blood supply via the left branch of the portal vein. The lobe is decreased in size with thickening of the capsule, fibrosis and prominent biliary and vascular markings. The vascular problem may date from the time of birth. Loss of left lobe parenchyma in this instance develops by the process of ischaemic extinction due to impaired flow from the affected large portal vein branch. Replacement fibrosis ensues. This large vessel extinction process should be distinguished from cirrhosis in which the entire liver is affected by numerous intrahepatic and discrete extinction lesions, which affect small hepatic veins and portal vein branches during the course of inflammation and fibrosis. Hence, in cirrhosis the entire liver surface is diffusely converted to regenerative parenchymal nodules surrounded by fibrosis.

Obstruction to the right or left hepatic bile duct by benign stricture or cholangiocarcinoma is now the most common cause of lobar atrophy [13]. The alkaline phosphatase is usually elevated. The bile duct may not be dilated within the atrophied lobe. Relief of obstruction may reverse the changes if cirrhosis has not developed. Distinction between a biliary and portal venous aetiology may be made using technetium-labelled iminodiacetic acid (IDA) and colloid scintiscans. A small lobe with normal uptake of IDA and colloid is compatible with a portal aetiology. Reduced or absent uptake of both isotopes favours biliary disease.

Agenesis of the right lobe [14]. This rare lesion may be an incidental finding associated, probably coincidentally, with biliary tract disease and also with other congenital abnormalities. It can cause presinusoidal portal hypertension. The other liver segments undergo compensatory hypertrophy. It must be distinguished from lobar atrophy due to cirrhosis or hilar cholangiocarcinoma.

Situs inversus (SI). In the exceedingly rare *SI totalis* or *abdominalis* the liver is located in the left hypochondrium and may be associated with other anomalies including biliary atresia, polysplenia syndrome, aberrant hepatic artery anatomy and absent portal vein. Hepatic surgery (partial hepatectomy, liver transplantation) is feasible, but complex. Other conditions associated with displacement of the liver from its location in

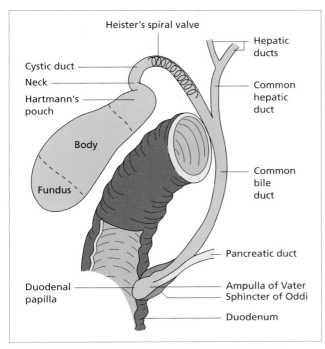

Heister's spiral valve

Cystic duct

Neck

Hartmann's pouch

Body

Fundus

Duodenal papilla

Hepatic ducts

Common hepatic duct

Common bile duct

Pancreatic duct

Ampulla of Vater

Sphincter of Oddi

Duodenum

Fig. 1.6. Gallbladder and biliary tract.

the right upper quadrant include *congenital diaphragmatic hernias, diaphragmatic eventration* and *omphalocoele.*

Anatomical abnormalities of the gallbladder and biliary tract are discussed in Chapter 12.

Anatomy of the biliary tract (Fig. 1.6)

The *right* and *left hepatic ducts* emerge from the liver and unite in the porta hepatis to form the *common hepatic duct.* This is soon joined by the *cystic duct* from the gall-bladder to form the common bile duct.

The *common bile duct* runs between the layers of the lesser omentum, lying anterior to the portal vein and to the right of the hepatic artery. Passing behind the first part of the duodenum in a groove on the back of the head of the pancreas, it enters the second part of the duodenum. The duct runs obliquely through the posteromedial wall, usually joining the main pancreatic duct to form the *ampulla of Vater* (c. 1720). The ampulla makes the mucous membrane bulge inwards to form an eminence, the *duodenal papilla.* In about 10–15% of subjects the bile and pancreatic ducts open separately into the duodenum.

The dimensions of the common bile duct depend on the technique used. At operation it is about 0.5–1.5 cm in diameter. Using ultrasound the values are less, the common bile duct being 2–7 mm, with values greater than 7 mm being regarded as abnormal. Using endoscopic cholangiography, the duct diameter is usually less than 11 mm, although after cholecystectomy it may be more in the absence of obstruction.

The duodenal portion of the common bile duct is surrounded by a thickening of both longitudinal and circular muscle fibres derived from the intestine. This is called the *sphincter of Oddi* (c. 1887).

The *gallbladder* is a pear-shaped bag 9 cm long with a capacity of about 50 mL. It always lies above the transverse colon, and is usually next to the duodenal cap overlying, but well anterior to, the right renal shadow. The fundus is the wider end and is directed anteriorly; this is the part palpated when the abdomen is examined. The body extends into a narrow neck which continues into the cystic duct. The *valves of Heister* are spiral folds of mucous membrane in the wall of the cystic duct and neck of the gallbladder. *Hartmann's pouch* is a sacculation at the neck of the gallbladder; this is a common site for a gallstone to lodge.

The mucosa is in delicate, closely woven folds; instead of glands there are indentations of mucosa which usually lie superficial to the muscle layer. Increased intraluminal pressure in chronic cholecystitis results in formation of branched, diverticula-like invaginations of the mucosa which reach into the muscular layer, termed *Rokitansky–Aschoff sinuses.* There is no submucosa or muscularis mucosae. The gallbladder wall consists of a loose connective tissue lamina propria and muscular layer containing circular, longitudinal and oblique muscle bundles without definite layers, the muscle being particularly well developed in the neck and fundus. The outer layers are the subserosa and serosa. The distensible normal gallbladder fills with bile and bile acids secreted by the liver, concentrates the bile through absorption of water and electrolytes and with meals contracts under the influence of cholecystokinin (acting through preganglionic cholinergic nerves) to empty bile into the duodenum.

Blood supply. The gallbladder receives blood from the *cystic artery.* This branch of the hepatic artery is large, tortuous and variable in its anatomical relationships. Smaller blood vessels enter from the liver through the gallbladder fossa. The venous drainage is into the *cystic vein* and thence into the portal venous system. Attention to the vascular-biliary anatomy in the reference area known as *Calot's triangle* (bordered by the cystic duct, common hepatic duct and lower edge of the liver) reduces the risk of vascular injuries and potential biliary strictures. Most bile duct injuries occur at cholecystectomy (incidence of <1.3% for either open or laparoscopic cholecystectomy). After liver transplantation 10–33% of patients may develop biliary complications, of which biliary stricture is the most important.

The arterial blood supply to the supraduodenal bile duct is generally by two main (axial) vessels which run beside the bile duct. These are supplied predominantly by the retroduodenal artery from below, and the right hepatic artery from above, although many other vessels contribute. This pattern of arterial supply would explain why vascular damage results in bile duct stricturing [15].

Lymphatics. There are many lymphatic vessels in the submucous and subperitoneal layers. These drain through the cystic gland at the neck of the gallbladder to glands along the common bile duct, where they anastomose with lymphatics from the head of the pancreas.

Nerve supply. The gallbladder and bile ducts are liberally supplied with nerves, from both the parasympathetic and the sympathetic system.

Surface marking (Figs 1.7, 1.8)

Liver. The upper border of the right lobe is on a level with the 5th rib at a point 2 cm medial to the right midclavicular line (1 cm below the right nipple). The upper border of the left lobe corresponds to the upper border of the 6th rib at a point in the left midclavicular line (2 cm below the left nipple). Here only the diaphragm separates the liver from the apex of the heart.

The lower border passes obliquely upwards from the 9th right to the 8th left costal cartilage. In the right nipple line it lies between a point just under to 2 cm below the costal margin. It crosses the midline about midway between the base of the xiphoid and the umbilicus and the left lobe extends only 5 cm to the left of the sternum.

Gallbladder. Usually the fundus lies at the outer border of the right rectus abdominis muscle at its junction with the right costal margin (9th costal cartilage) (Fig. 1.8). In

an obese subject it may be difficult to identify the outer border of the rectus sheath and the gallbladder may then be located by the Grey–Turner method. A line is drawn from the left anterior superior iliac spine through the umbilicus; its intersection with the right costal margin indicates the position of the gallbladder. These guidelines depend upon the individual's build. The fundus may occasionally be found below the iliac crest.

Methods of examination

Liver. The lower edge should be determined by palpation just lateral to the right rectus muscle. This avoids mistaking the upper intersection of the rectus sheath for the liver edge.

The liver edge moves 1–3 cm downwards with deep inspiration. It is usually palpable in normal subjects

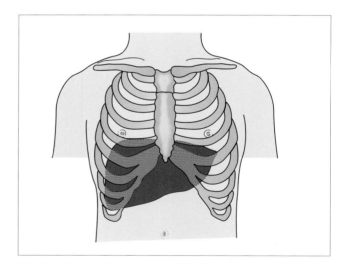

Fig. 1.7. The surface marking of the liver.

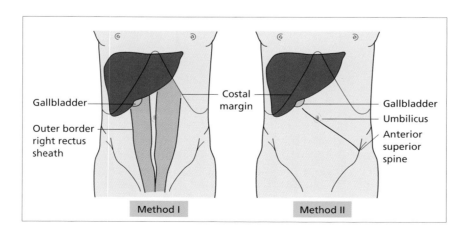

Fig. 1.8. Surface markings of the gallbladder. Method I: the gallbladder is found where the outer border of the right rectus abdominis muscle intersects the 9th costal cartilage. Method II: a line drawn from the left anterior superior iliac spine through the umbilicus intersects the costal margin at the site of the gallbladder.

inspiring deeply. The edge may be tender, regular or irregular, firm or soft, thickened or sharp. The lower edge may be displaced downwards by a low diaphragm, for instance in emphysema. Movements may be particularly great in athletes or singers. Some patients with practice become very efficient at 'pushing down' the liver. The normal spleen can become palpable in similar fashion. Common causes of a liver palpable below the umbilicus are malignant deposits, polycystic or Hodgkin's disease, amyloidosis, congestive cardiac failure and gross fatty change. Rapid change in liver size may occur when congestive cardiac failure is corrected, cholestatic jaundice relieved, or when severe diabetes is controlled. The surface can be palpated in the epigastrium and any irregularity or tenderness noted. An enlarged caudate lobe, as in the Budd–Chiari syndrome or with some cases of cirrhosis, may be palpated as an epigastric mass.

Pulsation of the liver, usually associated with tricuspid valvular incompetence, is felt by manual palpation with one hand behind the right lower ribs posteriorly and the other anteriorly on the abdominal wall.

The upper edge is determined by fairly heavy percussion passing downwards from the nipple line. The lower edge is recognized by very light percussion passing upwards from the umbilicus towards the costal margin. Percussion is a valuable method of determining liver size and is the only clinical method of determining a small liver.

The anterior liver span is obtained by measuring the vertical distance between the uppermost and lowermost points of hepatic dullness by percussion in the right midclavicular line. This is usually 12–15 cm. Direct percussion is as accurate as ultrasound in estimating liver span [16].

Friction may be palpable and audible, usually due to recent biopsy, tumour or perihepatitis. The venous hum of portal hypertension is audible between the umbilicus and the xiphisternum. An arterial murmur over the liver may indicate a primary liver cancer or acute alcoholic hepatitis.

Gallbladder. The gallbladder is palpable only when it is distended. It is felt as a pear-shaped cystic mass usually about 7 cm long. In a thin person, the swelling can sometimes be seen through the anterior abdominal wall. It moves downwards on inspiration and is mobile laterally but not downwards. The swelling is dull to percussion and directly impinges on the parietal peritoneum, so that the colon is rarely in front of it. Gallbladder dullness is continuous with that of the liver.

Abdominal tenderness should be noted. Inflammation of the gallbladder causes a positive *Murphy's sign*. This is the inability to take a deep breath when the examining fingers are hooked up below the liver edge. The inflamed gallbladder is then driven against the fingers and the pain causes the patient to catch their breath.

The enlarged gallbladder must be distinguished from a *visceroptotic right kidney*. This, however, is more mobile, can be displaced towards the pelvis and has the resonant colon anteriorly. A *regenerative* or *malignant nodule* feels much firmer.

Imaging. A plain film of the abdomen, including the diaphragms, may be used to assess liver size and in particular to decide whether a palpable liver is due to actual enlargement or to downward displacement. On moderate inspiration the normal level of the diaphragm, on the right side, is opposite the 11th rib posteriorly and the 6th rib anteriorly.

Ultrasound, CT or MRI can be used to study liver size, shape and content.

Microanatomy of the liver

For over a century, many models of liver substructure have been proposed [17]. The most popular of these is the *lobule* introduced by Kiernan in 1833 as the basic architectural unit, based on pig dissections [18]. He described circumscribed, hexagonal lobules consisting of a central tributary of the hepatic vein (central vein) and at the periphery a portal tract containing the bile duct, portal vein radicle and hepatic artery branch. Cords (plates) of liver cells and blood-containing sinusoids extend between these two systems. The lobule has foundations in pig, camel, raccoon and polar bear livers, in which such hexagonal units are surrounded by interlobular connective tissue septa [19]. Such septa have no counterparts in human liver.

Stereoscopic reconstructions and scanning electron microscopy have shown the human liver as cords of liver cells radiating from a central vein, and interlaced in orderly fashion by sinusoids (Figs 1.9, 1.10). The terminal branches of the portal vein discharge their blood into the sinusoids and the direction of flow is determined by the higher pressure in the portal vein than in the central vein (or terminal hepatic venule)—see below.

The *portal tracts* are small connective tissue islands containing triads composed of the portal vein radicle, the hepatic arteriole and bile duct (Fig. 1.11). Portal tracts are surrounded by a limiting plate of liver cells. Histological sections of normal liver show portal tracts containing dyads as frequently as triads, with the portal vein being the most frequently absent element. Within each linear centimetre of liver tissue obtained at biopsy there are usually two interlobular bile ducts, two hepatic arteries and one portal vein per portal tract, with six full portal triads [20].

The liver has to be divided *functionally*. Traditionally, the unit is based on a central hepatic vein and its

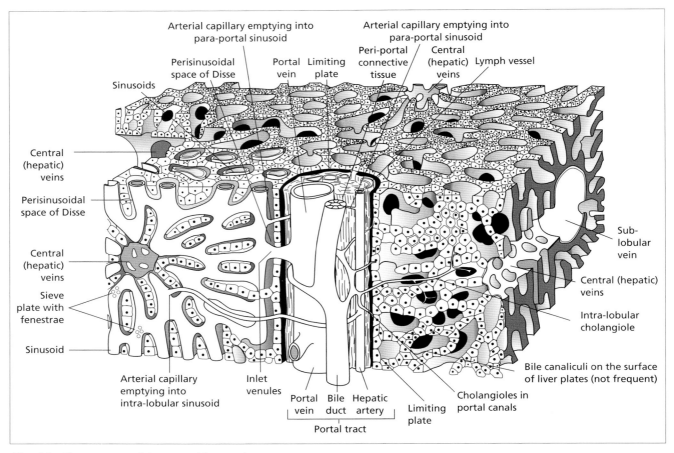

Fig. 1.9. The structure of the normal human liver.

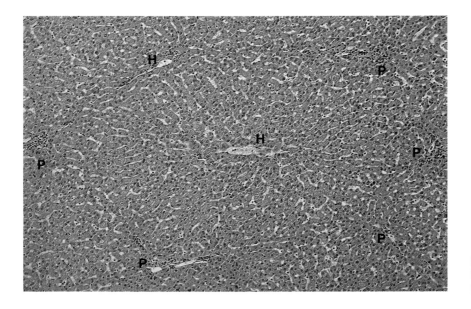

Fig. 1.10. Normal hepatic histology. H, terminal hepatic vein; P, portal tract. (H & E, ×60.)

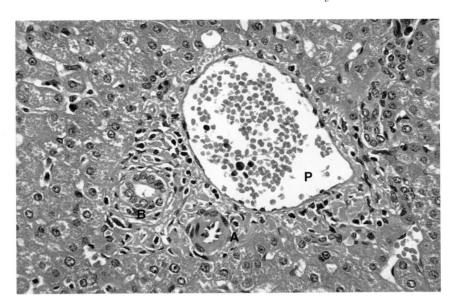

Fig. 1.11. Normal portal tract. A, hepatic artery; B, bile duct; P, portal vein. (H & E.)

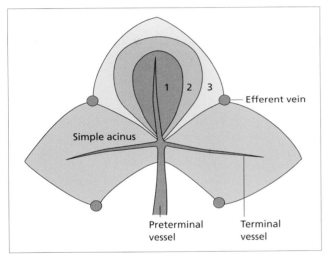

Fig. 1.12. The complex acinus according to Rappaport. Zone 1 is adjacent to the entry (portal venous) system. Zone 3 is adjacent to the exit (hepatic venous) system.

surrounding liver cells. However, Rappaport [21] envisages a series of functional *acini*, each centred on the portal tract with its terminal branch of portal vein, hepatic artery and bile duct (zone 1) (Figs 1.12, 1.13). These interdigitate, mainly perpendicularly, with terminal hepatic veins of adjacent acini. The circulatory peripheries of acini (adjacent to terminal hepatic veins) (zone 3) suffer most from injury, whether viral, toxic or anoxic. Bridging necrosis may extend from the periphery (acinar zone 1) to zone 3. The regions closer to the axis formed by afferent vessels and bile ducts survive longer and may later form the core from which regeneration will proceed. The contribution of each acinar zone to liver cell regeneration depends on the acinar location of damage [21].

The liver cells (*hepatocytes*) comprise about 60% of the liver. They are polygonal and approximately 30 μm in diameter. The nucleus is single or, less often, multiple and divides by mitosis. The lifespan of liver cells is about 150 days in experimental animals. The hepatocyte has three surfaces: one facing the sinusoid and space of Disse, the second facing the canaliculus and the third facing neighbouring hepatocytes (Fig. 1.14). There is no basement membrane.

The sinusoids are lined by endothelial cells with small pores (fenestrae) for macromolecule diffusion from blood to hepatocytes. On the vascular side of the sinusoids are the phagocytic cells of the reticuloendothelial system (Kupffer cells) and pit cells with natural killer function.

There are approximately 202×10^3 cells in each milligram of normal human liver, of which 171×10^3 are parenchymal and 31×10^3 littoral (sinusoidal, including Kupffer cells).

The *space of Disse* between hepatocytes and sinusoidal endothelial cells contains a few collagen fibrils and the hepatic stellate cells, which have also been called fat-storing cells, Ito cells and lipocytes. These cells store vitamin A and when activated in disease become collagen-synthesizing myofibroblasts. The *hepatic lymphatics* are found in the periportal connective tissue and are lined throughout by endothelium. Tissue fluid seeps through the endothelium into the lymph vessels.

The branch of the *hepatic arteriole* forms a plexus around the bile ducts and supplies the structures in the portal tracts. It empties into the sinusoidal network at different levels. There are no direct hepatic arteriolar–portal venous anastomoses.

The excretory system of the liver begins with the *bile canaliculi* (Figs 1.14, 1.15). These are formed by

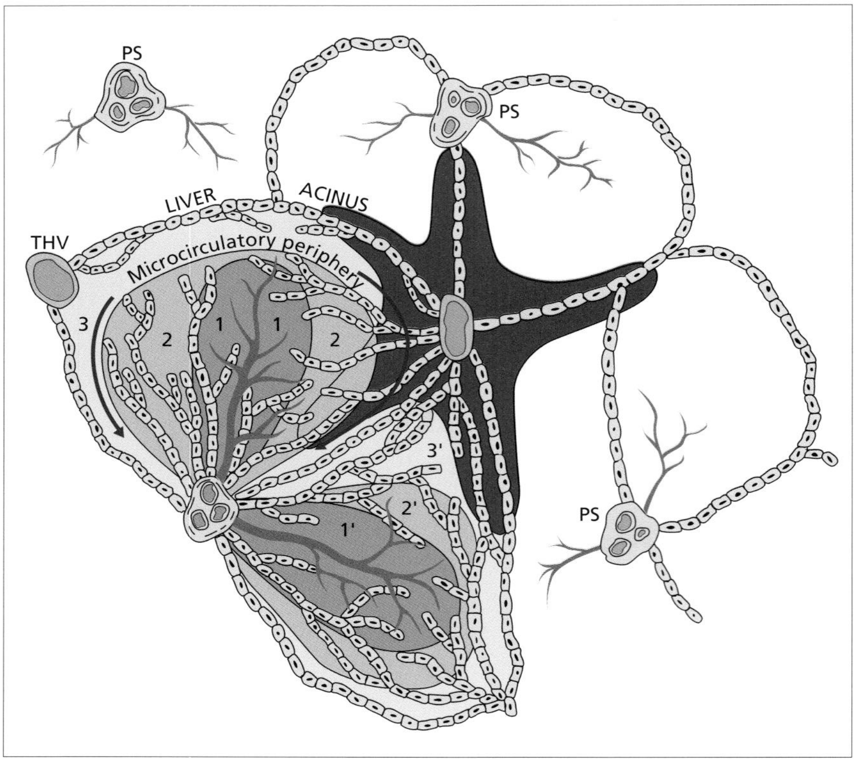

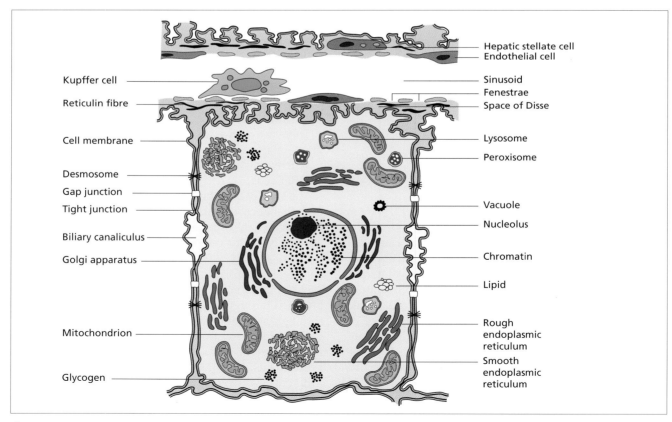

Fig. 1.13. Blood supply of the simple liver acinus, zonal arrangements of cells and the microcirculatory periphery. The acinus occupies adjacent sectors of the neighbouring hexagonal fields. Zones 1, 2 and 3, respectively, represent areas supplied with blood of first, second and third quality with regard to oxygen and nutrient content. These zones centre on the terminal afferent vascular branches, bile ductules, lymph vessels and nerves (PS) and extend into the triangular portal field from which these branches crop out. Zone 3 is the microcirculatory periphery of the acinus since its cells are as remote from their own afferent vessels as from those of adjacent acini. The *perivenular* area is formed by the most peripheral portions of zone 3 of several adjacent acini. In injury progressing along this zone, the damaged area assumes the shape of a starfish (darker tint around a terminal hepatic venule, THV, in the centre). 1–3, microcirculatory zones; 1′–3′, zones of neighbouring acinus [21].

Fig. 1.14. The organelles of the liver cell.

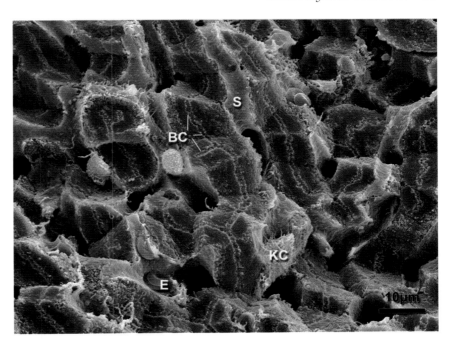

Fig. 1.15. Colourized scanning electron micrograph of liver showing hepatocytes in green, sinusoids (S) in light pink, erythrocytes (E), Kupffer cells (K) and bile canaliculi (BC). (Courtesy of Ms Jackie Lewin, UCL Medical School, London.)

modifications of the contact surfaces of liver cells and are covered by microvilli. The plasma membrane is reinforced by microfilaments forming a supportive cytoskeleton. The canalicular surface is sealed from the rest of the intercellular surface by junctional complexes including tight junctions, gap junctions and desmosomes. The intralobular canalicular network drains into the canals of Hering lined by low cuboidal epithelium which connect via short bile ductules to the larger terminal bile ducts within the portal tracts. Bile ducts are classified into small (less than 100 μm in diameter), medium (about 100 μm) and large (more than 100 μm) calibre types.

Hepatic ultrastructure (electron microscopy) and organelle functions

Hepatocytes (Figs 1.14–1.17)

The liver cell margin is straight except for a few anchoring pegs (desmosomes). From it, equally sized and spaced microvilli project into the lumen of the bile canaliculi. Along the sinusoidal border, irregularly sized and spaced microvilli project into the perisinusoidal tissue space. The microvillous structure indicates active secretion or absorption, mainly of fluid.

The *nucleus* has a double contour with pores allowing interchange with the surrounding cytoplasm. Human liver after puberty contains tetraploid nuclei and, at about age 20, in addition, octoploid nuclei are found. Increased polyploidy has been regarded as precancerous. In the chromatin network one or more nucleoli are embedded.

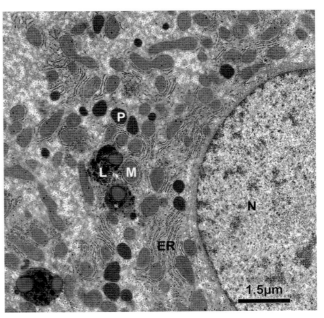

Fig. 1.16. Electron microscopic appearances of part of a normal human liver cell. N, nucleus; M, mitochondrion; P, peroxisome; L, lysosome; ER, rough endoplasmic reticulum. (Courtesy of Ms. Jackie Lewin, UCL Medical School, London).

The *mitochondria* also have a double membrane, the inner being invaginated to form grooves or cristae. An enormous number of energy-providing processes take place within them, particularly those involving oxidative phosphorylation. They contain many enzymes,

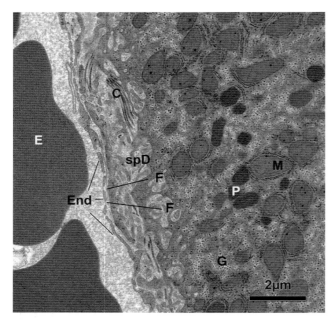

Fig. 1.17. Transmission electron micrograph showing an hepatocyte (right) with its microvillus membrane surface facing onto the space of Disse (spD) and the overlying endothelium (End). The endothelium has fenestrations (F) and there are a few collagen bundles (C) in the space of Disse. Erythrocytes (E) are present within the sinusoidal lumen. M, mitochondrion; P, peroxisome; G, glycogen granules. (Courtesy of Ms Jackie Lewin, UCL Medical School, London.)

particularly those of the citric acid cycle and those involved in β-oxidation of fatty acids. They can transform energy so released into adenosine diphosphate (ADP). Haem synthesis occurs here.

The *rough endoplasmic reticulum* (RER) is seen as lamellar structures lined by ribosomes. These are responsible for basophilia under light microscopy. They synthesize specific proteins, particularly albumin, those used in blood coagulation and enzymes. They may adopt a helix arrangement, as polysomes, for co-ordination of this function. Glucose-6-phosphatase is synthesized. Triglycerides are synthesized from free fatty acids and complexed with protein to be secreted by exocytosis as lipoprotein. The RER may participate in glycogenesis.

The *smooth endoplasmic reticulum* (SER) forms tubules and vesicles. It contains the microsomes. It is the site of bilirubin conjugation and the detoxification of many drugs and other foreign compounds (P450 systems). Steroids are synthesized, including cholesterol and the primary bile acids, which are conjugated with the amino acids glycine and taurine. The SER is increased by enzyme inducers such as phenobarbital.

Peroxisomes are versatile organelles, which have complex catabolic and biosynthetic roles, and are distributed near the SER and glycogen granules. Peroxisomal enzymes include simple oxidases, β-oxidation cycles, the glyoxalate cycle, ether lipid synthesis, and cholesterol and dolichol biosynthesis. Several disorders of peroxisomal function are recognized of which Zellweger syndrome is one [22]. Endotoxin severely damages peroxisomes [23].

The *lysosomes* are membrane-bound, electron-dense bodies adjacent to the bile canaliculi. They contain many hydrolytic enzymes which, if released, could destroy the cell. They are the site of deposition of ferritin, lipofuscin, bile pigment, copper and senescent organelles.

The *Golgi apparatus* consists of a system of particles and vesicles, again lying near the canaliculus. It may be regarded as a 'packaging' site before excretion into the bile. This entire group of lysosomes, microbodies and Golgi apparatus is a means of sequestering any material which is ingested and has to be excreted, secreted or stored for metabolic processes in the cytoplasm. The Golgi apparatus, lysosomes and canaliculi are concerned in cholestasis (Chapter 11).

The intervening cytoplasm contains granules of glycogen, lipid and ferritin.

The *cytoskeleton* supporting the hepatocyte consists of microtubules, microfilaments and intermediate filaments [24]. Microtubules contain tubulin and control subcellular mobility, vesicle movement and plasma protein secretion. Microfilaments are made up of actin, are contractile and are important for the integrity and motility of the canaliculus and for bile flow. Intermediate filaments are elongated branched filaments comprising cytokeratins [1]. They extend from the plasma membrane to the perinuclear area and are fundamental for the stability and spatial organization of the hepatocyte. They become disrupted or lost with hepatocellular injury by alcohol, lipid peroxidation by-products and ischaemia [25].

Sinusoidal cells

The sinusoidal cells (endothelial cells, Kupffer cells, hepatic stellate cells and pit cells) form a functional and histological unit together with the sinusoidal aspect of the hepatocyte [26]. These cells interact via cytokines and other signalling mechanisms [27,28]. The close structural relationship of sinusoidal cells to hepatic cords is evident on transmission (Fig. 1.17) and scanning electron microscopy (Fig. 1.15).

Endothelial cells line the sinusoids and have fenestrae, which provide a graded barrier between the sinusoid and space of Disse (Fig. 1.18). The Kupffer cells anchor on the endothelium by their cytoplasmic projections.

The hepatic stellate cells lie in the space of Disse between the hepatocytes and the endothelial cells (Fig. 1.19). *Disse's space* contains tissue fluid which flows outwards into lymphatics in the portal zones. When sinu-

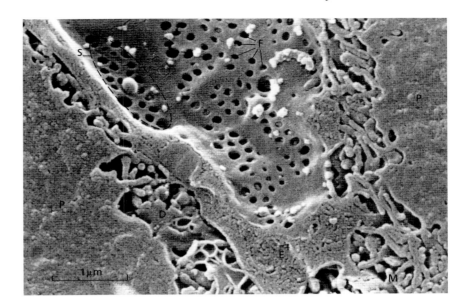

Fig. 1.18. Scanning electron micrograph of sinusoid showing fenestrae (F) grouped into sieve plates (S). D, space of Disse; E, endothelial cell; M, microvilli; P, parenchymal cell. (Courtesy of Professor E. Wisse.)

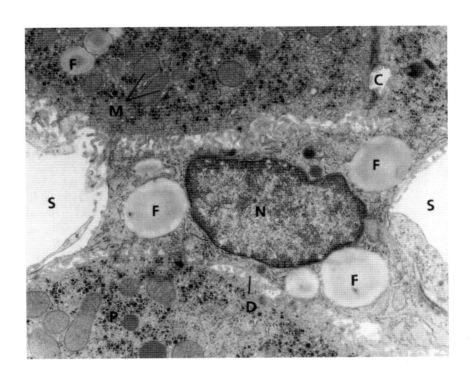

Fig. 1.19. Transmission electron micrograph of an hepatic stellate cell. Note the characteristic fat droplets (F). C, bile canaliculus; D, space of Disse; M, mitochondria; N, nucleus; P, parenchymal cell; S, lumen of sinusoid. (×12 000) (Courtesy of Professor E. Wisse.)

soidal pressure rises, lymph production in Disse's space increases and this plays a part in ascites formation where there is hepatic venous outflow obstruction.

Endothelial cells. These cells form a continuous lining to the sinusoids. They differ from endothelial cells elsewhere in not having a regular basement membrane. The endothelial cells act as a sieve between the sinusoid and space of Disse, have specific and non-specific endocytotic activity and have a variety of receptors. Their capacity to act as a sieve is due to fenestrae, around 0.15 μm in diameter (Fig. 1.18). These make up 6–8% of the total endothelial cell surface, and there are more in the centrilobular zone of the sinusoid than the periportal area. Extracellular matrix affects their function.

Fenestrae are clustered into sieve plates, and act as biofilters and transport pores between sinusoidal blood and the plasma within the space of Disse. They have a dynamic cytoskeleton [29]. This maintains and regulates their size, which can be changed by many influences including alcohol, nicotine, serotonin, endotoxin and partial hepatectomy. The fenestrae filter macromolecules of differing size. Particles greater than 0.2 μm in diameter, which includes large triglyceride-rich parent chylomicrons, will not pass. Smaller triglyceride-depleted, cholesterol-rich and retinol-rich remnants can enter the space of Disse [30]. In this way the fenestrae have an important role in chylomicron and lipoprotein metabolism. Open fenestrae are located in the thin cytoplasmic periphery of the endothelial cells while close to the endothelial nuclei fenestrae are multifolded and labyrinth-like [31].

Endothelial cells have a high capacity for endocytosis (accounting for 45% of all pinocytotic vesicles in the liver) and are active in clearing macromolecules and small particles from the circulation [32]. Coated and uncoated membrane-bound vesicles on endothelium are present near their nuclei or on non-fenestrated portions of their cytoplasm [31]; these are involved in various endocytic functions. There is receptor-mediated endocytosis for several molecules including transferrin, caeruloplasmin, modified high density lipoprotein (HDL) and low density lipoprotein (LDL), hepatic lipase and very low density lipoprotein (VLDL). Hyaluronan (a major polysaccharide from connective tissue) is taken up and this provides a method for assessing hepatic endothelial cell capacity. Endothelial cells can also clear small particles (<0.1 μm) from the circulation, as well as denatured collagen. Scanning electron microscopy has shown a striking reduction in the number of fenestrae, particularly in zone 3 in alcoholic patients, with formation of a basal lamina, which is also termed capillarization of the sinusoid [33].

Kupffer cells. These are highly mobile macrophages attached to the endothelial lining of the sinusoid, in greater numbers in the periportal areas [34]. They have microvilli and intracytoplasmic-coated vesicles and dense bodies which make up the lysosomal apparatus. They proliferate locally but under certain circumstances macrophages can immigrate from an extrahepatic site. They are responsible for removing old and damaged blood cells or cellular debris, also bacteria, viruses, parasites and tumour cells. They do this by endocytosis (phagocytosis, pinocytosis), including absorptive (receptor-mediated) and fluid phase (non-receptor-mediated) mechanisms [35]. Several processes aid this, including cell surface Fc and complement receptors. Coating of the particle with plasma fibronectin or opsonin also facilitates phagocytosis, since Kupffer cells have specific binding sites for fibronectin on the cell surface. These cells also take up and process oxidized LDL (thought to be atherogenic), and remove fibrin in disseminated intravascular coagulation. Alcohol reduces the phagocytic capacity.

Kupffer cells are activated by a wide range of agents, including endotoxin, sepsis, shock, interferon-γ, arachidonic acid and tumour necrosis factor (TNF). The result of activation is the production of an equally wide range of products: cytokines, hydrogen peroxide, nitric oxide, TNF, interleukin (IL) 1, IL6 and IL10, interferon-α and -β, transforming growth factor (TGF-β) and various prostanoids [36]. This whole array acts alone or in combination to stimulate other events in the cytokine cascade, but also increases discomfort and sickness. The Kupffer cell products may be toxic to parenchymal cells and endothelial cells. Kupffer cell-conditioned medium inhibits albumin synthesis in parenchymal cells, as do IL1, IL6 and TNF-α. The toxicity of endotoxin is caused by the secretory products of Kupffer cells since endotoxin itself is not directly toxic.

Hepatic stellate cells (fat-storing cells, lipocytes, Ito cells). These cells lie within the subendothelial space of Disse. They have long cytoplasmic extensions, some giving close contact with parenchymal cells, and others reaching several sinusoids, where they may regulate blood flow and hence influence portal hypertension [37]. In normal liver they are the major storage site of retinoids, giving the morphological characteristic of cytoplasmic lipid droplets. When empty of these droplets, they resemble fibroblasts. They contain actin and myosin and contract in response to endothelin-1 and substance P [38]. With hepatocyte injury, hepatic stellate cells lose their lipid droplets, proliferate, migrate to zone 3 of the acinus, change to a myofibroblast-like phenotype, and produce collagen type I, III and IV and laminin [39]. Stellate cells also release matrix proteinases and inhibitory molecules of matrix proteinases [40] (tissue inhibitor of metalloproteinases, TIMP) (Chapter 6). Collagenization of the space of Disse results in decreased access of protein-bound substrates to the hepatocyte.

Pit cells. These are highly mobile, liver-specific, natural killer lymphocytes attached to the sinusoidal surface of the endothelium [36,41]. They are short-lived cells and are renewed from circulating large granular lymphocytes, which differentiate within the sinusoids. They have characteristic granules and rod-cored vesicles. Pit cells show spontaneous cytotoxicity against tumour- and virus-infected hepatocytes.

There are complex interactions between Kupffer and endothelial cells, as well as sinusoidal cells and hepatocytes [27]. Kupffer cell activation by lipopolysaccharide suppresses hyaluronan uptake by endothelial cells, an effect probably mediated by leukotrienes [42]. Cytokines produced by sinusoidal cells can both stimulate and inhibit hepatocyte proliferation [28].

In or around the space of Disse, all major constituents of a basement membrane can be found including type

IV collagen, laminin, heparan sulphate, protoglycan and fibronectin. All cells impinging on the sinusoid can contribute to this matrix. The matrix within Disse's space influences hepatocellular function [27], affecting expression of tissue-specific genes such as albumin as well as the number and porosity of sinusoidal fenestrations [43]. It may be important in liver regeneration.

In liver disease, particularly in the alcoholic, the liver microcirculation may be altered by collagenization of the space of Disse—formation of a basement membrane beneath the endothelium and modification of the endothelial fenestrations [33]. All these processes are maximal in zone 3. They contribute to deprivation of nutrients intended for the hepatocyte and to the development of portal hypertension.

Bile duct epithelial cells

Bile duct epithelial cells [44] (cholangiocytes) line the extrahepatic and intrahepatic bile ducts, and modify the bile derived from the canaliculi of the hepatocytes. Cholangiocytes have both secretory (bicarbonate) and reabsorptive processes, which are under the control of hormones (e.g. secretin), peptides (endothelin-1) and cholinergic innervation. Cholangiocytes derived from different levels of the bile duct have different properties— as is true for hepatocytes from different areas of the acinus. This heterogeneity may explain in part the distribution of different diseases across specific areas of the biliary tree. Primary cilia on cholangiocytes [45] serve as mechano- and chemosensors and express polycystin

proteins which, if mutated, lead to fibropolycystic diseases [46] (Chapter 14).

Functional heterogeneity of the liver
(Fig. 1.20)

Hepatocytes show different structural and functional characteristics depending on their acinar location [47]. The relative functions of cells in the circulatory periphery of acini (zone 3) adjacent to terminal hepatic veins are different from those in the circulatory area adjacent to terminal hepatic arteries and portal veins (zone 1). This zonation is related to the lobular/acinar oxygen gradient [48] and to signalling via the Wnt/β-catenin pathway [49].

Krebs' cycle enzymes (urea synthesis and glutaminase) are found in the highest concentration in zone 1, whereas glutamine synthetase is perivenular (Fig. 1.20). Cells in zone 3 receive their oxygen supply last and are particularly prone to anoxic liver injury.

The drug-metabolizing P450 enzymes are present in greater amounts in zone 3. This is particularly so after enzyme induction, for instance with phenobarbital. Hepatocytes in zone 3 receive a higher concentration of any toxic product of drug metabolism. They also have a reduced glutathione concentration. This makes them particularly susceptible to hepatic drug reactions as exemplified by the centrilobular necrosis produced by 'predictable' or 'direct' hepatotoxins such as paracetamol (acetaminophen, Tylenol) and carbon tetrachloride.

Fig. 1.20. The functional heterogeneity of hepatocytes in perivenular (acinar zones 3) versus periportal (acinar zones 1) regions affects many synthetic and metabolic processes. Below, a portion of a lobule immunostained with antibody to glutamine synthetase shows localization of the enzyme to several layers of hepatocytes surrounding the central vein (CV). Negative staining is present elsewhere. PT, portal tract.

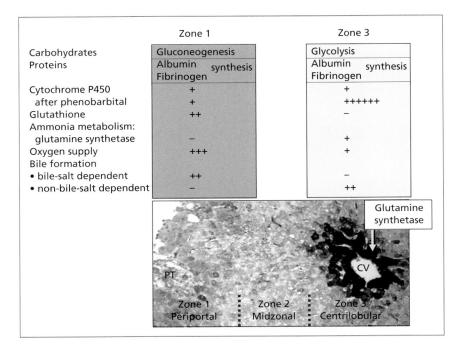

	Zone 1	Zone 3
Carbohydrates	Gluconeogenesis	Glycolysis
Proteins	Albumin synthesis Fibrinogen	Albumin synthesis Fibrinogen
Cytochrome P450	+	+
after phenobarbital	+	++++++
Glutathione	++	–
Ammonia metabolism: glutamine synthetase	–	+
Oxygen supply	+++	+
Bile formation		
• bile-salt dependent	++	–
• non-bile-salt dependent	–	++

Glutamine synthetase

PT

CV

Zone 1
Periportal

Zone 2
Midzonal

Zone 3
Centrilobular

Hepatocytes in zone 1 receive blood with a high bile salt concentration and, therefore, are particularly important in bile-salt-dependent bile formation. Hepatocytes in zone 3 are important in non-bile-salt-dependent bile formation. There are also zonal differences in the hepatic transport rate of substances from the sinusoid to canaliculus.

The cause of the metabolic difference between the zones varies. For some functions (gluconeogenesis, glycolysis, ketogenesis) it appears to be dependent upon the direction of blood flow along the sinusoid. For others (cytochrome P450) the gene transcription rate differs between perivenular and periportal hepatocytes. The differential expression of glutamine synthetase across the acinus is already established in fetal liver.

Dynamics of the hepatic microenvironment in physiology and disease (Fig. 1.21)

The sinusoidal plasma membrane of the hepatocyte is a receptor-rich and metabolically dynamic domain which is separated from the bile canaliculus by a lateral domain which participates in cell–cell interactions. Toll-like receptors on the hepatocyte surface react with microbial substances such as lipopolysaccharide (LPS) of Gram-negative bacteria resulting in a wave of intracellular signalling [50]. Receptor-mediated endocytosis is responsible for the transfer of large molecules such as glycoproteins, growth factors and carrier proteins (transferrin [51]). These ligands bind to receptors on the sinusoidal membrane, the occupied receptors cluster into a coated (clathrin) pit and endocytosis proceeds. The fate of the ligand within the cell varies according to the molecule involved, and the pathways are complex. Certain ligands, once bound to cell surface receptors, are then transferred for further interaction with claudin and occluden proteins located in tight junctions prior to clathrin-pit endocytosis. This is true of hepatitis C virus entry into liver cells [52]. Many ligands terminate in lysosomes where they are broken down while the receptor returns to the sinusoidal plasma membrane to perform again. Some ligands such as copper pass by vesicular transport across the cell to be discharged into the bile canaliculus.

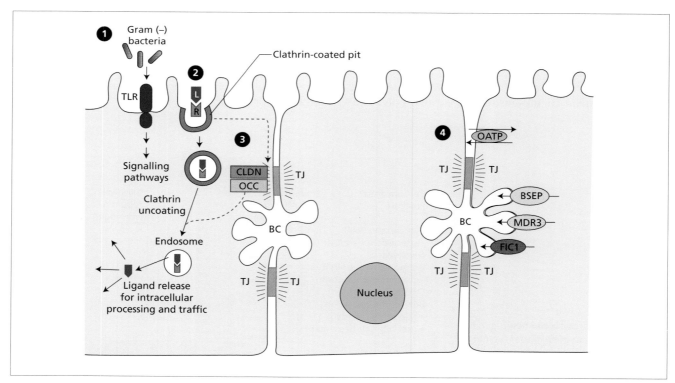

Fig. 1.21. Hepatocellular uptake and transport processes include: (1) surface Toll-like receptors (TLRs) for binding microbes and their constituent products; (2) endocytosis into clathrin-coated pits of ligands bound to cell surface receptors results in clathrin uncoating, ligand release from the endosome and further intracellular trafficking of the ligand; (3) certain receptor-ligand moieties (e.g. HCV entry into cells) require further interaction with claudins and occluden in tight junctions; and (4) bile transport proteins on the bile canalicular membrane (see text for further detail). CLDN, claudin; OCC, occluden; BC, bile canaliculus; L, ligand; R, cell surface receptor; TJ, tight junction; OATP, organic anion transport protein; BSEP, bile salt export pump; MDR3, multidrug resistance protein 3; FIC1, familial intrahepatic cholestasis 1.

Transport proteins are present on hepatocyte basolateral and apical (canalicular) membranes for uptake of organic acids and bile salt export [53] (see Chapter 11). Organic acid transport protein (OATP), bile salt export pump (BSEP), familial intrahepatic cholestasis 1 (FIC1) and multidrug resistance protein 3 (MDR3) are examples (Fig. 1.21). Jaundice and histological cholestasis may result from inhibition (e.g. BSEP by drugs and LPS) or mutation (e.g. FIC1 in Byler's disease; MDR3 in intrahepatic cholestasis of pregnancy) of transport proteins.

Hepatocyte death and regeneration
(Fig. 1.22)

Normal liver structure and function depends upon a balance between cell death and regeneration [54,55].

Cell death

Hepatocytes die as a result of either necrosis or apoptosis. The characteristic of *necrosis* is loss of plasma membrane integrity with release of the cellular contents locally which elicit an inflammatory response. This may potentiate the disease process and lead to further cell death. Ischaemia results in necrosis.

Apoptosis is the mechanism by which cells, damaged, senescent or excess to requirement, self-destruct with the least production of inflammatory products [56]. There is DNA fragmentation; organelles remain viable. Thus in comparison with necrotic cells, there is minimal release of injurious products, although there may still be a fibrotic reaction. Equilibrium within normal tissue depends upon the mitotic rate equalling the rate of apoptosis. Cytokine release from lymphocytes and other immune cells also causes apoptosis [57]. The classical example of immunologically-mediated apoptosis is the apoptotic body (apoptotic hepatocyte) found in periportal regions of interface hepatitis (piecemeal necrosis) in chronic hepatitis [58].

Pathological processes can alter the cellular mechanisms involved in apoptosis, leading to disease [56,57]. Increased apoptosis affecting cholangiocytes may lead to ductopenia. Apoptosis is increased in alcoholic and non-alcoholic fatty liver disease [59–61]. If cells containing a mutation predisposing to malignant change do not undergo apoptosis, malignant transformation is enhanced.

The pathway to apoptotic cellular destruction is complex, and can be described in morphological and biochemical terms. Once the process is initiated a cascade of changes occurs, which may be irreversible after a particular stage is reached. There is great interest in the development of agents that interfere with the apoptotic process, since these may have a therapeutic place in diseases where apoptosis is increased or decreased.

Regeneration

When there is a need for additional hepatocytes, patches of quiescent cells [62] are stimulated by mediators (primers), including cytokines, to move into a primed state ($G_0 \rightarrow G_1$), when growth factors can stimulate DNA synthesis and cellular replication (Fig. 1.22). Priming activates transcription factors including NFκB and STAT 3. Regeneration may be rapid, as seen after partial hepatectomy.

If hepatocytes are damaged so that this response is impaired, hepatocytes may be derived from progenitor/ stem cells ('oval cells' in rodents) located in the vicinity of the canals of Hering and nearby small bile ductules [63]. In the fetus such stem cells are near ductal plates [64]. Hepatocytes may also be derived from extrahepatic stem cells, probably of bone marrow origin [65,66]. The specificity of hepatocellular or bile duct epithelial differentiation by progenitor cells is encoded by progenitor cell transcription factors, which can be reprogrammed according to the cell type required. Hepatocyte nuclear

Fig. 1.22. Liver cell death and regeneration. Hepatocytes are lost either through apoptosis or necrosis. The liver normally regenerates through cellular replication. Priming is necessary for hepatocytes to respond to growth factors. If hepatocyte loss is massive or the toxic attack persists, cellular replication may not be possible. Liver cells may then be derived from progenitor/ stem cells either from within the liver or from the bone marrow.

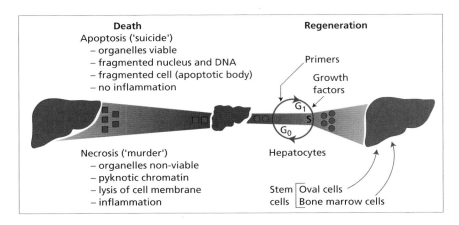

factor 1α (HNF1α) and HNF4α regulate gene transcription for hepatocyte lineage, while HNF1β and HNF6 mediate development of the gallbladder and bile ducts [67]. NOTCH signalling in cooperation with the transforming growth factor-β (TGF-β)/activin pathway further specifies bile duct tubulogenesis [68].

References

1 van Eyken P, Desmet VJ. Cytokeratins and the liver. *Liver* 1993; **13**: 113–122.

2 Asahina K, Tsai SY, Li P *et al.* Mesenchymal origin of hepatic stellate cells, submesothelial cells, and perivascular mesenchymal cells during mouse development. *Hepatology* 2009; **49**: 998–1011.

3 Bioulac-Sage P, Lafon ME, Saric J *et al.* Nerves and perisinusoidal cells in human liver. *J. Hepatol.* 1990; **10**: 105–112.

4 Couinaud C. *Le Foie. Etudes Anatomiques et Chirurgicales.* Paris: Masson, 1957.

5 Bismuth H. Surgical anatomy and anatomical surgery of the liver. *World J. Surg.* 1982; **6**: 3–9.

6 van Leeuwen MS, Noordzij J, Fernandez MA *et al.* Portal venous and segmental anatomy of the right hemiliver: observations based on three-dimensional spiral CT renderings. *Am. J. Roentgenol.* 1994; **163**: 1395–1404.

7 Han S, Soylu L. Accessory liver lobe in the left thoracic cavity. *Ann. Thorac. Surg.* 2009; **87**: 1933–1934.

8 Le Bail B, Carles J, Saric J *et al.* Ectopic liver and hepatocarcinogenesis. *Hepatology* 1999; **30**: 585–586.

9 Seo U-H, Lee H-J, Ryu W-S *et al.* Laparoscopic resection of a hepatocellular carcinoma arising from an ectopic liver. *Surg. Laparosc. Endosc. Percutan. Tech.* 2008; **18**: 508–510.

10 Kudo M. Riedel's lobe of the liver and its clinical implication. *Intern. Med.* 2000; **39**: 87–88.

11 Macchi V, Feltrin G, Parenti A *et al.* Diaphragmatic sulci and portal fissures. *J. Anat.* 2003; **202**: 303–308.

12 Philips DM, LaBrecque DR, Shirazi SS. Corset liver. *J. Clin. Gastroenterol.* 1985; **7**: 361–368.

13 Hadjis NS, Blumgart LH. Clinical aspects of liver atrophy. *J. Clin. Gastroenterol.* 1989; **11**: 3–7.

14 Radin DR, Colletti PM, Ralls PW *et al.* Agenesis of the right lobe of the liver. *Radiology* 1987; **164**: 639–642.

15 Northover JMA, Terblanche J. A new look at the arterial supply of the bile duct in man and its surgical implications. *Br. J. Surg.* 1979; **66**: 379–384.

16 Skrainka B, Stahlhut J, Fullbeck CL *et al.* Measuring liver span. Bedside examination vs. ultrasound and scintiscan. *J. Clin. Gastroenterol.* 1986; **8**: 267–270.

17 Roskams T, Desmet VJ, Verslype C. Development, structure and function of the liver. In: Burt A D, Portmann BC, Ferrell LD, eds. *MacSween's Pathology of the Liver*, 5th edn. Edinburgh: Churchill Livingstone Elsevier, 2007, p. 1.

18 Kiernan F. The anatomy and physiology of the liver. *Phil. Trans. R. Soc. Lond.* 1833; **123**: 711–770.

19 Beresford WA, Henninger JM. A tabular comparative histology of the liver. *Arch. Histol. Jpn.* 1986; **49**: 267–281.

20 Crawford AR, Lin X-Z, Crawford JM. The normal adult human liver biopsy: a quantitative reference standard. *Hepatology* 1998; **28**: 323–331.

21 Rappaport AM. The microcirculatory acinar concept of normal and pathologic hepatic structure. *Beitr. Pathol.* 1976; **157**: 215–243.

22 Shimozawa N. Molecular and clinical aspects of peroxisomal diseases. *J. Inherit. Metab. Dis.* 2007; **30**: 193–197.

23 Contreras MA, Khan M, Smith BT *et al.* Endotoxin induces structure-function alterations of rat liver peroxisomes: Kupffer cells released factors as possible modulators. *Hepatology* 2000; **31**: 446–455.

24 Feldmann G. The cytoskeleton of the hepatocyte. Structure and functions. *J. Hepatol.* 1989; **8**: 380–386.

25 Lackner C, Gogg-Kamerer M, Zatloukal K *et al.* Ballooned hepatocytes in steatohepatitis: the value of keratin immunohistochemistry for diagnosis. *J. Hepatol.* 2008; **48**: 821–828.

26 Smedsrod B, De Bleser PJ, Braet F *et al.* Cell biology of liver endothelial and Kupffer cells. *Gut* 1994; **35**: 1509–1516.

27 Selden C, Khalil M, Hodgson HJF *et al.* What keeps hepatocytes on the straight and narrow? Maintaining differentiated function in the liver. *Gut* 1999; **44**: 443–446.

28 Maher JJ, Friedman SL. Parenchymal and nonparenchymal cell interactions in the liver. *Semin. Liver Dis.* 1993; **13**: 13–20.

29 Braet F, De Zanger R, Baekeland M *et al.* Structure and dynamics of the fenestrae-associated cytoskeleton of rat liver sinusoidal endothelial cells. *Hepatology* 1995; **21**: 180–189.

30 Fraser R, Dobbs BR, Rogers GWT. Lipoproteins and the liver sieve: the role of the fenestrated sinusoidal endothelium in lipoprotein metabolism, atherosclerosis and cirrhosis. *Hepatology* 1995; **21**: 863–874.

31 Braet F, Riches J, Geerts W *et al.* Three-dimensional organization of fenestrae labyrinths in liver sinusoidal endothelial cells. *Liver Int.* 2009; **29**: 603–613.

32 Smedsrod B, Pertoft H, Gustafson S *et al.* Scavenger functions of the liver endothelial cell. *Biochem. J.* 1990; **266**: 313–327.

33 Horn T, Christoffersen P, Henriksen JH. Alcoholic liver injury: defenestration in noncirrhotic livers. A scanning microscopic study. *Hepatology* 1987; **7**: 77–82.

34 Kolios G, Valatas V, Kouroumalis E. Role of Kupffer cells in the pathogenesis of liver disease. *World J. Gastroenterol.* 2006; **14**: 7413–7420.

35 Toth CA, Thomas P. Liver endocytosis and Kupffer cells. *Hepatology* 1992; **16**: 255–266.

36 Smedsrod B, LeCouteur D, Ikejima K *et al.* Hepatic sinusoidal cells in health and disease: update from the 14th International Symposium. *Liver Int.* 2009; **29**: 490–499.

37 Rockey DC, Weisiger RA. Endothelin induced contractility of stellate cells from normal and cirrhotic rat liver: implications for regulation of portal pressure and resistance. *Hepatology* 1996; **24**: 233–240.

38 Sakamoto M, Ueno T, Kin M *et al.* Ito cell contraction in response to endothelin-1 and substance P. *Hepatology* 1993; **18**: 973–983.

39 Friedman SL. Mechanisms of hepatic fibrogenesis. *Gastroenterology* 2008; **134**: 1655–1669.

40 Arthur MJP, Mann DA, Iredale JP. Tissue inhibitors of metalloproteinases, hepatic stellate cells and liver fibrosis. *J. Gastroenterol. Hepatol.* 1998; **13**: S33–S38.

41 Wisse E, Luo D, Vermijlen D *et al.* On the function of pit cells, the liver-specific natural killer cells. *Semin. Liver Dis.* 1997; **17**: 265–286.

42 Deaciuc IV, Bagby GJ, Niesman MR *et al.* Modulation of hepatic sinusoidal endothelial cell function by Kupffer cells: an example of intercellular communication in the liver. *Hepatology* 1994; **19**: 464–470.

43 McGuire RF, Bissell DM, Boyles J *et al.* Role of extracellular matrix in regulating fenestrations of sinusoidal endothelial cells isolated from normal rat liver. *Hepatology* 1992; **15**: 989–997.

44 Kanno N, LeSage G, Glaser S *et al.* Functional heterogeneity of the intrahepatic biliary epithelium. *Hepatology* 2000; **31**: 555–561.

45 Masyuk AI, Masyuk T, LaRusso NF. Cholangiocyte primary cilia in liver health and disease. *Dev. Dyn.* 2008; **237**: 2007–2012.

46 Everson GT, Taylor MRG, Doctor RB. Polycystic disease of the liver. *Hepatology* 2004; **40**: 774–782.

47 Gebhardt R. Metabolic zonation of the liver: regulation and implications for liver function. *Pharmacol. Ther.* 1992; **33**: 275–354.

48 Jungermann K, Kietzmann T. Oxygen: modulator of metabolic zonation and disease of the liver. *Hepatology* 2000; **31**: 255–260.

49 Burke ZD, Reed KR, Phesse TJ *et al.* Liver zonation occurs through a β-catenin-dependent, c-Myc-independent mechanism. *Gastroenterology* 2009; **136**: 2316–2324.

50 Seki E, Brenner DA. Toll-like receptors and adaptor molecules in liver disease: update. *Hepatology* 2008; **48**: 322–335.

51 Anderson GJ, Frazer DM. Hepatic iron metabolism. *Semin. Liver Dis.* 2005; **25**: 420–432.

52 Burlone ME, Budkowska A. Hepatitis C virus cell entry: role of lipoproteins and cellular receptors. *J. Gen. Virol.* 2009; **90**: 1055–1070.

53 Kullak-Ublick GA, Stieger B, Meier PJ. Enterohepatic bile salt transporters in normal physiology and liver disease. *Gastroenterology* 2004; **126**: 322–342.

54 Fausto N. Liver regeneration and repair: hepatocytes, progenitor cells, and stem cells. *Hepatology* 2004; **39**: 1477–1487.

55 Kaplowitz N. Mechansim of liver cell injury. *J. Hepatol.* 2000; **32** (Suppl. 1): 39–47.

56 Jaeschke H, Gujral JS, Bajt ML. Apoptosis and necrosis in liver disease. *Liver Int.* 2004; **24**: 85–89.

57 Lemasters JJ. Dying a thousand deaths: redundant pathways from different organelles to apoptosis and necrosis. *Gastroenterology* 2005; **129**: 351–360.

58 Kerr JFR, Searle J, Halliday WJ *et al.* The nature of piecemeal necrosis in chronic active hepatitis. *Lancet* 1979; **ii**: 827–828.

59 Natori S, Rust C, Stadheim LM *et al.* Hepatocyte apoptosis is a pathologic feature of human alcoholic hepatitis. *J. Hepatol.* 2001; **34**: 248–253.

60 Ziol M, Tepper M, Lohez M *et al.* Clinical and biological relevance of hepatocyte apoptosis in alcoholic hepatitis. *J. Hepatol.* 2001; **34**: 254–260.

61 Feldstein AE, Canbay A, Angulo P *et al.* Hepatocyte apoptosis and Fas expression are prominent features of human nonalcoholic steatohepatitis. *Gastroenterology* 2003; **125**: 437–443.

62 Grisham JW. Hepatocyte lineages: of clones, streams, patches, and nodules in the liver. *Hepatology* 1997; **25**: 250–252.

63 Kuwahara R, Kofman AV, Landis CS *et al.* The hepatic stem cell niche: identification by label-retaining cell assay. *Hepatoloy* 2008; **47**: 1994–2002.

64 Zhang L, Theise N, Chua M *et al.* The stem cell niche of human livers: symmetry between development and regeneration. *Hepatology* 2008; **48**: 1598–1607.

65 Crosbie OM, Reynolds M, McEntee G *et al. In vitro* evidence for the presence of haematopoietic stem cells in the adult human liver. *Hepatology* 1999; **29**: 1193–1198.

66 Theise ND, Badve S, Saxena R *et al.* Derivation of hepatocytes from bone marrow cells in mice after radiation-induced myeloablation. *Hepatology* 2000; **31**: 235–240.

67 Limaye PB, Alarcón G, Walls AL *et al.* Expression of specific hepatocyte and cholangiocyte transcription factors in human liver disease and embryonic development. *Lab. Invest.* 2008; **88**: 865–872.

68 Zong Y, Panikkar A, Xu J *et al.* Notch signaling controls liver development by regulating biliary differentiation. *Development* 2009; **136**: 1727–1739.

CHAPTER 2
Assessment of Liver Function

Sandeep Mukherjee & John L. Gollan
Nebraska Medical Center, Omaha, NE, USA

Learning points

- No one single test can be used to assess liver function.
- 'Liver function tests' is a misleading term as this includes several biochemical tests that reflect liver injury and not liver function.
- Childs–Pugh score and Model for Endstage Liver Disease are used to estimate severity and prognosis of liver disease and candidacy for liver transplantation, respectively.
- The liver plays a central role in the metabolism of carbohydrates, lipids and proteins.
- As people age, liver blood flow and first-pass metabolism of drugs is reduced but hepatic microsomal monooxygenase activity is preserved.

Selection of biochemical tests

Liver function tests (LFTs) or liver biochemical tests can be used to screen for liver disease, direct diagnostic work-up, and assess severity, prognosis and response to treatment (Table 2.1). Although the term LFT is firmly entrenched in the medical literature, this term is frankly erroneous as these investigations provide indirect evidence of hepatobiliary disease. LFTs that more accurately reflect liver function are serum albumin, serum bilirubin and prothrombin time, which is standardized to the international normalized ratio (INR). As the prevalence of liver disease is only between 2 and 4% in the general population (higher for fatty liver disease and viral hepatitis), the more investigations are multiplied, the greater chance there is of a biochemical abnormality being demonstrated. A few simple tests of established value should be used and if an abnormality is found it should be repeated to confirm it is real.

LFT abnormalities may be classified into the following categories: hepatocellular (elevations predominantly in aspartate aminotransferase (AST) and alanine aminotransferase (ALT)); cholestatic (increases predominantly in alkaline phosphatase (ALP), γ-glutamyl transpeptidase (γ-GT) and bilirubin); and infiltrative (increases in ALP, γ-GT and occasionally bilirubin).

The tests most useful in the *diagnostic work-up of jaundice* (Chapter 11) are the ALP, aminotransferase and bilirubin tests. An isolated rise in serum unconjugated bilirubin suggests Gilbert's syndrome, haemolysis, ineffective erythropoiesis or use of medications such as bunamiodyl (cholecystographic agent) flavaspidic acid, probenicid and rifampicin.

The *severity of liver cell damage* is assessed by serial measurement of total bilirubin, albumin and prothrombin time after vitamin K. This is reflected by their incorporation into the Childs–Pugh (CP) score and Model for Endstage Liver Disease (MELD), which are used to estimate severity and prognosis of liver disease and assess candidacy for liver transplantation, respectively [1,2]. Rising arterial ammonia levels also reflect severe hepatic dysfunction in patients with acute liver failure (ALF) whereas hyperammonaemia in decompensated cirrhosis does not always correlate with hepatic encephalopathy or progression of liver disease (Chapter 8).

The diagnosis of *minimal hepatocellular damage* may be suspected by noting minimally elevated aminotransferases and sometimes serum bilirubin. Patients who are heavy drinkers of alcohol with or without liver disease (ALD) may have just a raised γ-GT with or without biochemical evidence of liver damage (Chapter 25). However, this degree of biochemical abnormality also occurs in well-compensated cirrhosis, heart failure and fever, reflecting the lack of sensitivity and specificity of these investigations for diagnosing and assessing severity of liver disease.

Hepatic infiltrations from cancer, granulomatous disease, amyloidosis or Hodgkin's disease are suggested by ALP and γ-GT levels increased disproportionately to bilirubin. Sarcoidosis and tuberculosis are the two most

Sherlock's Diseases of the Liver and Biliary System, Twelfth Edition. Edited by
James S. Dooley, Anna S.F. Lok, Andrew K. Burroughs, E. Jenny Heathcote.
© 2011 by Blackwell Publishing Ltd. Published 2011 by Blackwell Publishing Ltd.

Table 2.1. Essential serum methods in hepatobiliary disease

Test	Normal range	Value
Bilirubin		
total	5–17 μmol/L*	Diagnosis of jaundice; assess severity
conjugated	<5 μmol/L	Gilbert's disease, haemolysis
Alkaline phosphatase	35–130 iu/L	Diagnosis of cholestasis, hepatic infiltrations
Aspartate transaminase (AST/SGOT)	5–40 iu/L	Early diagnosis of hepatocellular disease; follow progress
Alanine transaminase (ALT/SGPT)	5–35 iu/L	ALT relatively lower than AST in alcoholism
γ-glutamyl transpeptidase (γ-GT)	10–48 iu/L	Diagnosis of alcohol abuse, marker biliary cholestasis
Albumin	35–50 g/L	Assess severity
γ-globulin	5–15 g/L	Diagnosis chronic hepatitis and cirrhosis; follow course
Prothrombin time (PT) (after vitamin K)	12–16 s	Assess severity

*0.3–1.0 mg/dL.

Table 2.2. Quantitative hepatic function tests

Site	Substrate	Function
Cytosol	Galactose*	Galactokinase (phosphorylation)
Microsome (cytochrome P450 system)	Aminopyrine	N-demethylation
	Caffeine	N-demethylation
	Lignocaine	N-deethylation
	Antipyrine	Hydroxylation/demethylation
Sinusoidal receptor membrane	Galactose-terminated glycoprotein	Asialoglycoprotein receptor

*Low dose assesses hepatic perfusion.

common granulomatous diseases that may produce jaundice whereas jaundice from amyloidosis is extremely rare.

Fibrosis may be assessed by serum markers, including hyaluronate, procollagen type III peptide, matrix metalloproteins and their inhibitors, multiparameter biochemical panels and transient liver elastography (Chapter 6).

Quantitative methods of assessment of liver function provide a better measure of hepatic function than injury (Table 2.2). However, with few exceptions, these investigations are infrequently performed due to their cost and complexity.

The liver is central to the metabolism of protein, carbohydrate and fat (Fig. 2.1) as well as being important in drug metabolism (Chapter 24).

Bile pigments

Bilirubin

Bilirubin metabolism is described in detail in Chapter 11.

Total bilirubin is increased in cholestatic and hepatocellular liver disease more commonly than infiltrative disease. It is often associated with a rise in liver enzymes. Bilirubin is predominantly conjugated and water soluble. Patients with marked hyperbilirubinaemia (bilirubin > 425 μmol/L) often have severe liver disease coexisiting with renal dysfunction or another cause of unconjugated hyperbilirubinaemia, such as haemolysis [3]. An isolated rise in bilirubin without enzyme elevation should first be fractionated to determine if the aetiology is familial or due to haemolysis (Fig. 2.2).

Serum bilirubin estimations are based on the van den Bergh diazo reaction, which involves the spectrophotometric detection of azo derivatives derived by the reaction of plasma with the diazonium ion of sulphanilic acid [4]. This reaction separates bilirubin into a water-soluble direct form representing conjugated bilirubin and an indirect, lipid-soluble form representing unconjugated bilirubin. These diazo reactions are subject to error, particularly at low total serum bilirubin concentrations. More accurate methods for estimation include alkaline methanolysis with chloroform extraction, high performance gas liquid chromatography (HPGLC), thin layer chromatography (TLC) and spectrophotometric determination, but are too elaborate to be clinically useful [5].

Faecal inspections are an important investigation in jaundice. Clay-coloured stools indicate cholestatic jaundice but may also occur in hepatocellular jaundice. The colour will be normal in haemolytic jaundice. Rarely, pale stools occur in very severe bilirubin glucuronyl transferase deficiency.

Bilirubin cannot be detected in the *urine* of normal subjects as bilirubin is predominantly unconjugated, insoluble in water and bound to albumin. In contrast, bilirubin glucuronides, the products of bilirubin conjugation, are water soluble. They appear in the urine even when serum total bilirubin is normal as the renal threshold for glomerular filtration of conjugated bilirubin is

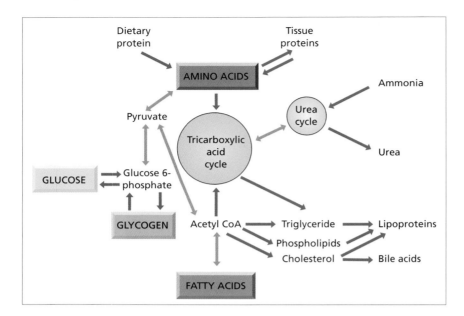

Fig. 2.1. The important metabolic pathways of protein, carbohydrate and fat in the liver.

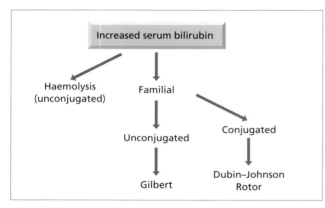

Fig. 2.2. Algorithm for managing a patient with an isolated increase in serum total bilirubin.

low. Conjugated bilirubin, however, will bind covalently to albumin when jaundice is prolonged and severe, giving rise to a complex called δ bilirubin (or biliprotein) [6]. δ bilirubin has a long half-life, cannot be renally cleared and accounts for the absence of bilirubinuria and slow resolution of jaundice in patients recovering from severe hepatobiliary disease.

Urobilinogen

Bacterial β-glucuronidases convert bilirubin in the colon to a series of colourless tetrapyrroles collectively called urobilinogen of which 80–90% is normally excreted in the faeces either unchanged or as oxidized orange derivatives called urobilins. The remaining 10–20% is absorbed and undergoes an enteric circulation with re-excretion into bile by the liver while a small proportion

is excreted in the urine. This complex process depends on several factors such as urine flow rate and pH. Spot urinary urobilinogen is a poor predictor of hepatic disease with a high proportion of false-negative results [7].

Bromsulphalein

The intravenous dye bromsulphalein (BSP) is rapidly removed by the liver with a first-pass clearance between 50 and 80%. Its removal is related to hepatic blood flow and is excreted into the biliary canaliculus by an ATP-dependent export pump (MRP2, ABCC2), a member of the ATP-binding cassette protein family [8]. This test is rarely performed now due to the cost, occasional side-effects such as anaphylaxis, lack of specificity and inconvenience. However, it does have a role in the diagnosis of Dubin–Johnson syndrome and its differentiation from Rotor's syndrome [9]. A blood sample is taken 45 min and 2 h after injection. A higher level of BSP at 2 h rather than at 45 min is diagnostic of Dubin–Johnson syndrome and reflects release of conjugated BSP into the blood stream after normal initial uptake. In Rotor's syndrome, BSP clearance is slow with no secondary rise.

Serum enzyme tests

These tests usually indicate the type of liver injury, whether hepatocellular, cholestatic or infiltrative but cannot differentiate one form of hepatitis from another or determine whether cholestasis is intra- or extra-hepatic. They are valuable in directing specific serological tests, imaging or liver biopsy to reach the diagnosis. Only a few tests are necessary and the combination of

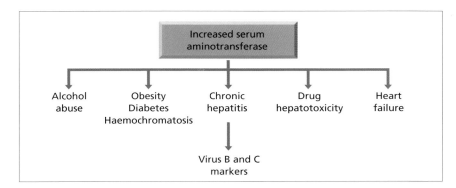

Fig. 2.3. Algorithm for managing a patient with an isolated increase in serum aminotransferase on routine screening.

AST, ALT, ALP and bilirubin is usually adequate. Ideally, normal ALT values should be adjusted for body mass index and sex [10]. During pregnancy, ALT, AST and γ-GT levels, as well as bile acid and bilirubin concentrations remain within the normal range, whereas an elevated alkaline phosphatase is of placental origin during the third trimester [11].

Aminotransferases

The aminotransferases (previously called aminotransaminases) catalyse transfer of amino groups from either aspartate or alanine to the keto group of α-ketoglutaric acid forming oxaloacetic acid (OAA) and pyruvic acid, respectively. These enzymes are important in gluconeogenesis as they catalyse glucose synthesis from non-carbohydrate sources. Enzymatic reduction of oxaloacetic acid and pyruvic acid to malate and lactate, respectively, is coupled with oxidation of the reduced form of nicotinamide dinucleotide (NADH) to nicotinamide dinucleotide (NAD). As only NADH absorbs light at 340 nm, this reaction can be followed spectrophotometrically to accurately assay these enzymes.

Aspartate aminotransferase (AST; serum glutamic oxaloacetic transaminase or SGOT) is an isoenzyme located in the cytoplasm and mitochondria of many tissues. Although normal AST serum activity is cytosolic in origin, 80% of AST activity within the liver is mitochondrial and predominates in periportal hepatocytes. In decreasing order of concentration AST is present in large quantities in liver, heart, skeletal muscle, kidneys, brain, pancreas, lungs, leucocytes and erythrocytes. Macro-AST is a rare condition characterized by isolated AST elevation due to binding of AST with an immunoglobulin which is not cleared by the blood or kidneys [12]. It is a benign condition and is not reflective of liver disease. Markedly low AST levels have been reported in patients on chronic haemodialysis, possibly due to dialysis or pyridoxine deficiency [13,14].

Alanine aminotransferase (ALT; serum glutamic pyruvic transaminase or SGPT) is a cytosolic enzyme also present in liver. Although the absolute amount is less than AST, a greater proportion is present in liver compared with kidney, heart and skeletal muscles. A serum increase is therefore more specific for liver damage than AST.

Transferase determinations with viral serologies are useful in the early diagnosis of viral hepatitis, but there is no correlation between transferase level with either the degree of hepatocyte necrosis or prognosis. Measurements should be performed promptly as these enzymes have short half-lives (AST 12–22 h; ALT 37–47 h) [15]. Patients may develop fatal acute hepatic necrosis despite falling transaminase values.

Routine screening may show unexpectedly raised aminotransferase levels (Fig. 2.3). These are often due to non-alcoholic fatty liver disease (NAFLD), alcohol abuse, viral hepatitis and haemochromatosis. Less common causes include autoimmune hepatitis, α1-antitrypsin deficiency, Wilson's disease, drug-induced liver disease and non-hepatic disorders such as Addison's disease [16], anorexia nervosa [17], coeliac disease [18] and hyperthyroidism [19]. Important causes of markedly elevated transaminases are viral hepatitis (including herpes simplex hepatitis), paracetamol (acetaminophen) or other drug-induced hepatotoxicity, ischaemic hepatitis and severe autoimmune hepatitis [20]. Calculous biliary obstruction with cholangitis is an important but frequently under appreciated cause of AST elevation greater than 10 times the upper limit of normal, which may improve with antibiotics over 48–72 h despite unresolved obstruction.

Very high levels are unusual in ALD and suggest a coexisting disorder such as paracetamol toxicity or acute viral hepatitis. A ratio of AST to ALT greater than two may be useful in diagnosing ALD. This occurs because damage is primarily mitochondrial (thus more AST is released systemically) and ALT synthesis is more sensitive than AST to pyridoxal 5-phosphate deficiency, leading to lower serum ALT levels [21]. An elevated AST to ALT ratio has also been described as a specific but non-sensitive marker of advanced fibrosis or cirrhosis in NAFLD [22] and chronic hepatitis C [23].

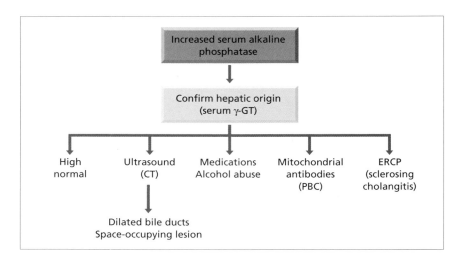

Fig. 2.4. Algorithm for managing a patient with an isolated increase in serum alkaline phosphatase or serum γ-glutamyl transpeptidase (γ-GT). CT, computed tomography; ERCP, endoscopic retrograde cholangiopancreatography; PBC, primary biliary cirrhosis.

Alkaline phosphatase

The alkaline phosphatases (ALP) are a group of enzymes that catalyse hydrolysis of phosphate esters at neutral pH. Magnesium and zinc are important co-factors. ALP in the liver is cytosolic, associated with sinusoidal and canalicular membranes and rises in cholestasis and to a lesser extent when liver cells are damaged (Fig. 2.4). ALP is present, in decreasing order of quantity, in placenta, ileal mucosa, kidney, bone and liver but more than 80% of serum ALP is from the liver or bone. ALP half-life is 3 days. Bone, liver and kidney ALP are coded by the same gene and share a common protein structure but differ in their carbohydrate content [24]. Mechanisms of the increase are believed to be related to increased hepatobiliary synthesis from enhanced translation of messenger ribonucleic acid of ALP and serum secretion through canalicular leakage into the sinusoid rather than failure to excrete ALP. Due to *de novo* ALP synthesis in acute biliary obstruction, serum levels are initially normal in contrast to marked transferase elevations. Serum hepatic ALP may be distinguished from bone ALP by isoenzyme fractionation but this is not routinely carried out as a concomitant rise in γ-GT confirms a hepatobiliary source.

An isolated rise in ALP may also be of intestinal origin, as observed in patients with blood groups O and B who secrete intestinal ALP postprandially. As these enzymes may remain elevated for up to 12 h, levels must be determined under fasting conditions [25]. Up to 52% of patients with mild isolated ALP elevations (less than twofold elevation) will have enzyme normalization within 1–3 months although in hospitalized patients, sepsis in the absence of jaundice may account for up to 32% of cases [26].

Raised ALP levels are sometimes observed with primary or secondary hepatic tumours, even without jaundice or involvement of bone. Increased values without jaundice are also found with other space-occupying lesions or infiltrative disease such as amyloid, abscess, lymphoma or granulomas. Non-specific mild elevations are seen in a variety of conditions including Hodgkin's disease, heart failure, hyperthyroidism and up to 15% of patients with renal cell carcinoma in the absence of involvement of the hepatobiliary system or bone (Stauffer's syndrome). Low ALP levels are associated with hypothyroidism, Wilson's disease with haemolysis, congenital hypophosphatasia, pernicious anaemia, zinc deficiency, severe hepatic insufficiency and in children recovering from severe enteritis.

Gamma glutamyl transpeptidase or transferase

Gamma glutamyl transpeptidase (γ-GT) is a membrane-bound enzyme that catalyses transfer of γ glutamyl groups of peptides such as glutathione to other amino acids. Levels are increased in cholestasis and hepatocellular disease and occur in the same spectrum of hepatobiliary diseases as elevated ALP. γ-GT is ubiquitous but in decreasing order of abundance is present in proximal renal tubule, liver, pancreas (acinar cells and ductules) and intestine. Serum γ-GT activity arises primarily from the liver and, within the hepatobiliary system, is present in highest concentration in the epithelium lining of fine biliary ducts. The main role of this test is to confirm a raised ALP is of hepatobiliary origin.

An isolated rise in γ-GT is seen in patients with alcohol abuse, even without liver disease, due to microsomal enzyme induction and impaired clearance (half-life of 7–10 days increases to 28 days). Screening for γ-GT may have led to more alcohol abusers being identified although levels do not rise in one-third of individuals.

There also is no correlation between alcohol consumption and elevated serum γ-GT levels with hepatic γ-GT in patients with biopsy-proven alcoholic liver disease. An increased level can lead to over-investigation in an individual who has never taken alcohol or a social drinker who has never abused alcohol.

Unfortunately, many factors influence the level so that increases are non-disease-specific. Disorders include hepatobiliary disease, alcoholism, chronic obstructive airways disease, diabetes mellitus, hyperthyroidism, rheumatoid arthritis and several medications such as barbiturates, carbamazepine, cimetidine, furosemide, heparin, isotretinoin, methotrexate, oral contraceptives, phenytoin and valproate. On the other hand, it has excellent sensitivity and a high predictive value for screening for biliary tract disease such that levels are rarely normal in intrahepatic cholestasis. Exceptions are subtypes of progressive familial intrahepatic cholestasis (type 1 or Byler's disease and type 2) and benign recurrent intrahepatic cholestasis type 1 (or Summerskill's syndrome) [27].

Lactic dehydrogenase

Lactic dehydrogenase (LDH) is a cytoplasmic enzyme with five isoenzymes present in serum. Marked increases are found in patients with neoplasms and hepatic involvement and ischaemic hepatitis. The ALT:LDH ratio has been reported to discriminate between acute viral hepatitis (greater than 1.5) from ischaemic hepatitis and paracetamol toxicity (less than 1.5), with excellent sensitivity and specificity [28].

Quantitative assessment of hepatic function (Table 2.2)

Chronic liver diseases pass through a long period of minimum non-specific symptoms ('compensated') until the final stage of ascites, jaundice, variceal bleeding, encephalopathy and precoma ('decompensated'). Serum albumin and prothrombin time give some indication of the synthetic function of the liver, but this is usually maintained until late disease. Serial estimates of *quantitative liver function* in the early stages may be helpful for monitoring treatment and assessing prognosis but have no diagnostic role. Such tests suffer from the drawback of their complexity (multiple blood samples or measurement of isotopes). The lack of a major impact above routine laboratory tests and CP score or MELD is reflected in their present role in clinical research rather than the routine management of patients. These investigations have been reviewed elsewhere [29] and will not be discussed.

Lipid and lipoprotein metabolism

Lipids

The liver is central to lipid (cholesterol, phospholipid, triglyceride) and lipoprotein metabolism. Lipoproteins, hydrophobic within and hydrophilic on the outside, allow lipid transport in the plasma.

Cholesterol (from the Greek words *chole*, bile, and *stereos*, solid) is found in cell membranes and is a precursor of bile acids and steroid hormones. It is synthesized in all tissues, but the most active site of synthesis is the liver. Cholesterol derived from intestinal absorption reaches the liver in chylomicron remnants. Cholesterol synthesis takes place mainly from acetyl coenzyme A (CoA) in the microsomal fraction and in cytosol (Fig. 2.5). The rate-limiting step of cholesterol synthesis is the conversion of 3-hydroxy-3-methylglutaryl-CoA (HMG-CoA) to mevalonate by the enzyme HMG-CoA reductase which is located almost exclusively in periportal cells. Synthesis is increased in biliary duct obstruction, terminal ileal resection, biliary or intestinal lymph fistula and medications such as cholestyramine, corticosteroids and thyroid hormones. Cholesterol synthesis is inhibited by bile acids, cholesterol feeding, fasting and medications such as clofibrate, nicotinic acid and statins.

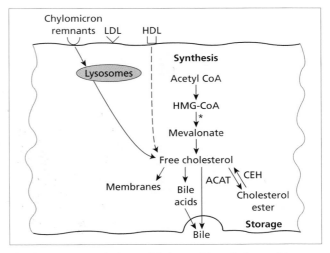

Fig. 2.5. Hepatic cholesterol balance. Free cholesterol is derived from intracellular synthesis, and from the uptake of chylomicron remnants and lipoproteins from the circulation. Storage is as cholesterol ester: ACAT (acyl CoA-cholesterol ester transferase, which esterifies free cholesterol to fatty acids) and CEH (cholesteryl ester hydrolase, which hydrolyses the ester linkage). Bile acids are synthesized from free cholesterol, and both are secreted into bile. 3-hydroxy-3-methylglutaryl coenzyme A (HMG-CoA) reductase is the rate-limiting step. HDL, high density lipoprotein; LDL, low density lipoprotein.

Cholesterol in membranes and in bile is present almost exclusively as free cholesterol. Bile provides the only significant route for cholesterol excretion. In plasma and tissues such as liver, adrenal and skin, cholesterol esters are also found, which are more non-polar and metabolically inactive than free cholesterol. Esterification is carried out by plasma lecithin cholesterolacyl transferase (LCAT) [30].

Phospholipids contain one or more phosphoric acid groups and another polar group such as a heterogeneous base, for example choline or ethanolamine with long-chain fatty acid residues. Phospolipids are important constituents of cell membranes and participate in many reactions. The most abundant phospholipid in plasma and most cellular membranes is phosphatidyl choline (lecithin) which accounts for 66% of all phospholipids. Phosphatidyl secretion into bile (22%) is also greater than cholesterol secretion (4%), and is promoted by bile salts secretion into the canalicular lumen via canalicular bile acid transporter. This induces vesiculation of the outer, canalicular membrane leading to increased supply of phospholipids to the inner, cytoplasmic membrane by phosphatidylcholine transfer protein and sterol carrier protein 2 [31]. Phospholipid translocation from inner to outer membrane occurs via the multidrug resistance protein 2 (MDR2) pathway which combine with bile salts to form vesicles [32].

Triglycerides are simpler compounds than the phospholipids. They have a backbone of glycerol, the hydroxy groups of which have been esterified with fatty acids. Naturally occurring triglycerides contain a variety of fatty acids; they act as a store of energy and also a method of transport of energy from the small intestine and liver to peripheral tissues.

Lipoproteins

These are essential for the circulation and metabolism of lipids. They are separated by their differing density on ultracentrifugation, which explains their nomenclature. Their surface comprises apolipoprotein, of several different types (Table 2.3), free cholesterol and phospholipids. Inside there is cholesterol ester, triglycerides and fat-soluble vitamins. There are two prominent metabolic cycles for lipoproteins: one is involved in fat absorbed from the intestine, and the other is responsible for the handling of endogenously synthesized lipid (Fig. 2.6).

Dietary fat is absorbed from the small intestine and incorporated into chylomicrons [33,34]. These enter the circulation via the thoracic duct where triglyceride is removed by lipoprotein lipases and utilized or stored in tissue. The chylomicron remnant is taken up by the liver by the low density lipoprotein (LDL) receptor-related protein [34]. The cholesterol enters metabolic pathways or plasma membranes, or is excreted in bile.

Table 2.3. Properties of lipoproteins

Lipoproteins	Apolipoprotein	Source	Carries
Chylomicrons	B48, AI, C-II, E	Intestine	Dietary fat
VLDL	B100, C-II, E	Liver	Hepatic triglyceride and cholesterol
LDL	B100	From VLDL	Cholesterol
HDL	A-I, A-II	Peripheral tissue	Cholesterol ester

HDL, high density lipoprotein; LDL, low density lipoprotein; VLDL, very low density lipoprotein.

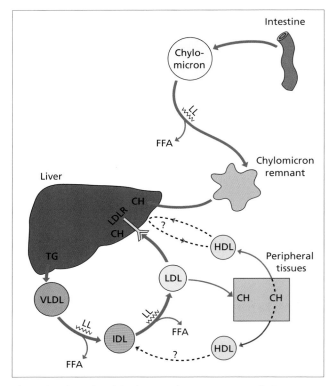

Fig. 2.6. The role of the liver in lipoprotein metabolism. CH, cholesterol; FFA, free fatty acid; LDLR, LDL receptor; LL, lipoprotein lipase; TG, triglyceride. (For lipoproteins see Table 2.3.)

In the endogenous pathway, cholesterol and triglyceride leave the liver in very low density lipoprotein (VLDL), which is synthesized predominantly in the mitochondria of perivenous hepatocytes. In the circulation, triglyceride is removed by lipoprotein lipase. As a result, VLDL particles become smaller, forming intermediate density lipoprotein (IDL), and then LDL, the major carrier for cholesterol. The predominant route for removal of LDL is by LDL receptors on the liver surface, but receptors on other cells are also important in atheromatous plaques formation. High density lipoprotein (HDL) facilitates cholesterol removal from peripheral tissues. Cholesterol is transported out of the cell by the cholesterol-efflux regulatory protein, expressed from the adenosine triphosphate (ATP) binding cassette transporter 1 gene (*ABC1*) [35]. HDL is either taken up by the liver, or is incorporated into IDL, resulting in the mature LDL. This removal of peripheral cholesterol is an important pathway, as reflected in the protective effect of a high HDL–cholesterol level against coronary artery disease. HDL metabolism is still unclear. Most apolipoproteins are made by the liver, some by the intestines. Apart from being components of lipoproteins, some have other functions: Apo A-1 activates plasma LCAT; C-11 activates lipoprotein lipase.

Changes in liver disease

Cholestasis. Total and free cholesterol are increased. This is not due simply to the retention of cholesterol normally excreted in bile. The mechanism is uncertain but four factors have been implicated: (1) regurgitation of biliary cholesterol into the circulation; (2) increased hepatic synthesis of cholesterol; (3) reduced plasma LCAT activity; and (4) regurgitation of biliary lecithin, which produces a shift of cholesterol from pre-existing tissue cholesterol into the plasma. Whereas slight increases to 1.5–2 times normal are sometimes seen in acute cholestasis, very high values are found in chronic conditions, especially postoperative stricture and cholestatic liver diseases, such as primary biliary cirrhosis. Studies in primary biliary cirrhosis patients with hypercholesterolàemia do not show an increased risk of coronary artery disease [36]. Values over five times the upper limit of normal are associated with skin xanthomas. Malnutrition lowers the serum cholesterol so values may be normal in carcinomatous biliary obstruction.

The level of cholesterol ester is decreased due to LCAT deficiency. Triglycerides tend to be increased. An abnormal lipoprotein, lipoprotein X, very rich in free cholesterol and lecithin, is found, which appears on electron microscopy as bilamellar discs [37]. Red cell changes in cholestasis are related to abnormalities in cholesterol and lipoprotein.

Parenchymal injury. Triglycerides tend to be increased relating to an accumulation of LDL. Cholesterol ester is reduced due to a low LCAT. In cirrhosis, total serum cholesterol values are usually normal. Low results indicate malnutrition or decompensation. In the fatty liver due to alcohol, VLDL and triglycerides are increased. Triglyceride incorporation into VLDL requires microsomal triglyceride transfer protein (MTTP)—genetic defects in MTTP or the effect of HCV or alcohol on MTTP will also prevent VLDL export and cause hepatic steatosis [37,38]. Drug toxicity can affect apolipoprotein synthesis and lead to difficulty in triglyceride export as VLDL, and hence fatty liver [39]. Apoprotein B-100, which is associated with VLDL, can be absent due to genetic reasons, deficiencies in amino acids such as threonine or as part of generalized protein malnutrition or kwashiorkor. Low levels of Apo A-1 have been described in Tangier's disease, a rare condition characterized by low levels of HDL and accelerated atherosclerosis due to a defect in the cell membrane protein ABCA1, a mediator of cholesterol secretion [40]. Serum cholesterol esters, lipoproteins, LCAT and lipoprotein X have no value in the diagnosis or assessment of liver function.

Bile acids

Bile acids are synthesized in a variety of tissues but predominantly in the liver [41], between 250 and 500 mg being produced and lost in the faeces daily, and maximal daily rates up to 4–6 g. Bile acids are stored in the gall bladder. Synthesis is under negative feedback control. The primary bile acids, cholic acid and chenodeoxycholic acid, are formed from cholesterol (Fig. 2.7). There are two different metabolic pathways for bile acid synthesis. The classical, well-established pathway is 7α-hydroxylation of cholesterol in the liver by CYP7A1, which synthesizes cholic acid (trihydroxy bile salt). The alternate pathway begins with 27α-hydroxylation of cholesterol in various tissues, including endothelium. It is mediated by CYP27 and synthesizes chenodeoxycholic acid (dihydroxy bile salt). Both enzymes belong to the cytochrome P450 group but differ in their substrate specificity, subcellular localization and tissue distribution [42]. The C-7α-hydroxylase is found in the endoplasmic reticulum while the C-27α-hydroxylating enzyme is found in mitochondria. The interplay between these two synthetic pathways in maintaining bile salt pool size and cellular cholesterol levels is under study. Hepatic synthesis is controlled by the amount of bile acid returning to the liver in the enterohepatic circulation. When exposed to colonic bacteria the primary bile acids undergo 7α-dehydroxylation with the production of the secondary bile acids, deoxycholic acid (most potent detergent properties of all bile acids) and very little lithocholic acid (monohydroxy bile salt). Ursodeoxycholic is a dihydroxy bile acid formed by the epimerization of other secondary bile acids and normally represents less than 3% of the bile acid pool [43]. Ursodeoxycholic acid differs from chenodeoxycholic acid by the orientation of a single hydroxyl group. It does not solubilize cholesterol well. In human bile, the

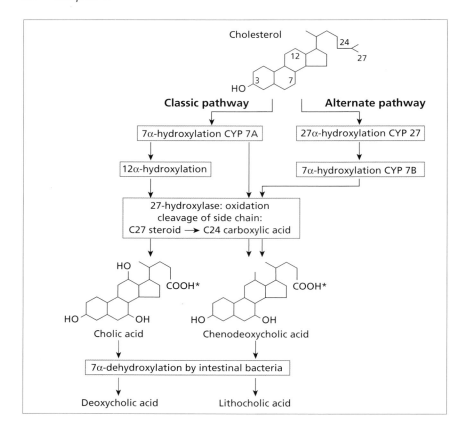

Fig. 2.7. Bile salt synthesis. There are two pathways: classic (neutral) and alternate (acidic). Classic pathway: 7α-hydroxylation is the initial, rate-limiting step, converting cholesterol to 7α-hydroxycholesterol. The cytochrome P450 enzyme responsible (CYP 7A) is restricted to hepatic microsomes. After further modifications, including 12α-hydroxylation for precursors of cholic acid, the mitochondrial enzyme sterol 27-hydroxylase cleaves the side chain, with the formation of chenodeoxycholate or cholate. The asterisks (*) indicate the site of conjugation with glycine and taurine. Alternate pathway: cholesterol is transported to mitochondria. CYP 27 catalyses 27-hydroxylation. This reaction can occur in many tissues. 7α-hydroxylation follows—by an oxysterol 7α-hydroxylase distinct from CYP 7A in the classic pathway. The alternate pathway leads to the predominant formation of chenodeoxycholic acid.

amount of cholic acid roughly equals the sum of the chenodeoxycholic and deoxycholic acid.

Bile acids are conjugated in the liver with the amino acids glycine or taurine in a ratio of approximately 3:1. The net effect of conjugation is to permit bile acids to achieve a sufficiently high intraluminal concentration in the small intestine to facilitate fat digestion and absorption. Conjugation also prevents precipitation at physiological pH and absorption in the biliary tree and small intestine. Sulphation and glucuronidation (as a detoxifying mechanism) may be increased with cirrhosis or cholestasis when these conjugates are found in excess. Bacteria can hydrolyse bile salts to bile acid and glycine or taurine.

Bile salts are excreted into the biliary canaliculus against an enormous concentration gradient between liver and bile. This depends in part on the intracellular negative potential of approximately $-35\,mV$, which provides potential-dependent facilitated diffusion, ATP-stimulated transporters and extent of conjugation. For example unconjugated bile acids are secreted via the bile salt export protein (BSEP, ABCB11), a member of the ATP-binding cassette family whereas glucuronated and sulphated bile salts are excreted by the canalicular multispecific organic anion transporter MRP2.

Bile salts enter into micellar and vesicular association with cholesterol and phospholipids. In the upper small intestine, the bile salt micelles are too large and too polar (hydrophilic) to be absorbed. They are intimately concerned with the digestion and absorption of lipids. When the terminal ileum and proximal colon are reached, absorption of 95% of bile acid takes place by an active transport process found only in the ileum, the apical sodium-dependent bile aid transporter (SLC10A2). Non-ionic, passive diffusion occurs throughout the whole intestine and is most efficient for unconjugated, dihydroxy bile acid. Oral administration of ursodeoxycholic acid interferes with the small intestinal absorption of both chenodeoxycholic and cholic acid [44].

The absorbed bile salts enter the portal venous system and reach the liver where they are taken up by the hepatocyte basolateral membrane; 90% of trihydroxy bile acids and 70–80% of dihydroxy bile acids undergo first-pass extraction from portal blood. This depends upon a sodium-taurocholate co-transport system (NTCP, SLC10A1) using the sodium gradient across the sinusoidal membrane as a driving force and multiple, sodium-independent, multispecific, organic anion transporters (OATP-A, OATP-C, SLC21A3, SLC21A6) for unconjugated bile acids. Chloride ions may also be involved. The most hydrophobic bile acids (unconjugated mono- and dihydroxy bile acids) probably enter the hepatocyte by simple diffusion ('flip-flop') across the lipid membrane. The mechanism of bile acid passage across the

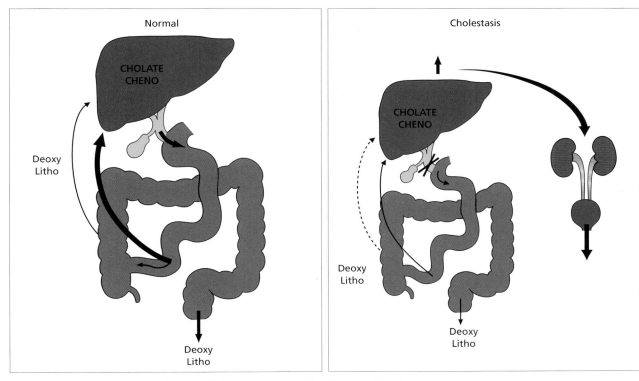

Fig. 2.8. The enterohepatic circulation of bile acids in normal subjects and in cholestasis.

liver cell from sinusoid to bile canaliculus is not as well understood, but may involve cytosolic bile acid-binding proteins such as 3α-hydroxysteroid dehydrogenase and microtubules [45]. Vesicles seem to play a role but only at higher bile acid concentrations [46]. The bile acids are reconjugated and re-excreted into bile. Lithocholic acid is not re-excreted but is rendered non-toxic by undergoing sulphation in the liver. This enterohepatic circulation of bile salts takes place 2–15 times daily (Fig. 2.8). Because absorption efficiency varies among the individual bile acids they have different synthesis and fractional turnover rates. In cholestasis, bile acids are excreted in the urine by active transport and passive diffusion. They tend to be sulphated and these conjugates are actively secreted by the renal tubule [47].

Changes in disease

Normal serum bile salt concentrations depend on normal hepatic blood flow, hepatic uptake and secretion and intestinal motility. Dysfunction in any of these areas can affect serum bile acid levels. Bile salts increase the biliary excretion of water, lecithin, cholesterol and conjugated bilirubin. Ursodeoxycholic acid produces a much greater choleresis than chenodeoxycholic or cholic acid [48]. Altered biliary excretion of bile salts with defective biliary micelle formation is important in the pathogenesis of gallstones (Chapter 12). It also leads to

the steatorrhoea of cholestasis. Bile salts form simple and mixed micelles with phospholipid and cholesterol to emulsify dietary fat, assist pancreatic lipolysis and release gastrointestinal hormones and play a part in the mucosal phase of absorption. Diminished secretion leads to steatorrhoea (Fig. 2.9).

Disordered intrahepatic metabolism of bile salts may be important in the pathogenesis of cholestasis (Chapter 11). They used to be thought to have a role in the pruritus of cholestasis but data now suggest that other substances are responsible (Chapter 11).

Bile salts may be responsible for target cells in the peripheral blood of jaundiced patients (Chapter 4) and for the secretion of conjugated bilirubin in urine. If bile acids are deconjugated by small intestinal bacteria, the resulting free bile acids are absorbed. Micelle formation and absorption of fat are then impaired. This may partly explain the malabsorption complicating diseases with bacterial overgrowth in the small intestine. Terminal ileum resection interrupts the enterohepatic circulation and allows large amounts of primary bile acids to reach the colon and to be dehydroxylated by bacteria, thereby reducing the body's bile salt pool. The altered bile salts in the colon cause a secretory pattern of diarrhoea by stimulating profound electrolyte and water secretion [49]. Lithocholic acid is mostly excreted in the faeces and only slightly absorbed. It is cirrhotogenic to experimental animals and can be used to produce experimental

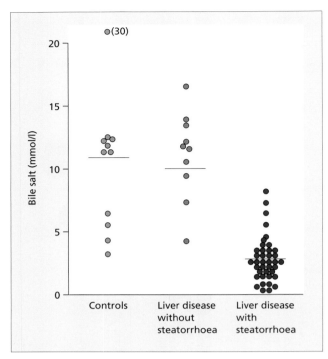

Fig. 2.9. Patients with chronic, non-alcoholic liver disease and steatorrhoea show a reduced bile salt concentration in their aspirated contents compared with control subjects and patients with chronic liver disease.

gallstones. Taurolithocholic acid can also cause intrahepatic cholestasis, perhaps by interfering with the bile-salt-independent fraction of bile flow. The importance of bile acids in health is illustrated by the consequences of a cessation in synthesis: inability to excrete cholesterol, arrest of bile acid-dependent bile flow, malabsorption of fat-soluble vitamins and irreversible faecal loss.

Serum bile acids

Enzymatic assays are based on the use of bacterial 3-hydroxysteroid dehydrogenase. The use of a bioluminescence assay has improved the sensitivity of this enzymatic technique up to that of radioimmunoassay. Radioimmunoassay techniques can also measure individual bile acids. The serum concentration of total bile acids reflects the extent to which bile acids reabsorbed from the intestine have escaped extraction on their first passage through the liver. Raised levels of serum bile acids are specific for hepatobiliary disease. Sensitivity of serum bile acid estimations is less than originally thought and are not performed routinely.

Amino acid metabolism

Amino acids derived from the diet and from tissue breakdown reach the liver via the portal vein. Specific Na$^+$-independent and Na$^+$-dependent systems mediate the transport of free amino acids across the sinusoidal membrane of the hepatocyte [50]. Some are transaminated or deaminated to keto acids, which are then metabolized by many pathways including the tricarboxylic acid cycle (Krebs–citric acid cycle).

Ammonia concentrations can be high in portal venous blood and are often intestinal in origin. Ammonia normally undergoes a high degree of hepatic extraction. It is viewed as an important factor in the development of hepatic encephalopathy (Chapter 8). It is metabolized to urea in the Krebs–Henseleit cycle of the mitochondrial matrix of periportal hepatocytes (high extraction, low affinity system). Excess ammonia which escapes ureagenesis is synthesized into glutamine in pericentral hepatocytes via glutamine synthetase (low extraction, high affinity system).

Experimentally, at least 85% of liver must be removed before this mechanism fails significantly and before blood and urinary amino acid levels increase. In ALF, an elevated arterial ammonia and low blood urea level may be observed, reflecting dysfunction of the Krebs urea cycle in a failing liver but in decompensated cirrhosis, hyperammonaemia is related to the dysfunction of the glutamine synthesis and portosystemic shunting of ammonia from the small and large intestine.

Clinical significance

Despite preservation of amino acid conjugation in advanced hepatocellular damage, generalized or selective amino aciduria is common in hepatocellular disease. In severe liver disease, the usual picture is an increase in the plasma concentration of one or both of the aromatic amino acids, tyrosine and phenylalanine, together with methionine, and a reduction in the branched-chain amino acids valine, leucine and isoleucine (Fig. 2.10) [51]. The changes are explained by impaired hepatic function, portosystemic shunting of blood, hyperinsulinaemia and hyperglucagonaemia. Patients with minimal liver disease also show changes, particularly a reduction in plasma proline, perhaps reflecting increased collagen production. There is no difference in the ratio between branched-chain and aromatic amino acids whether or not the patients show hepatic encephalopathy. In ALF, generalized aminoaciduria involving particularly cysteine and tyrosine carries a poor prognosis as do arterial ammonia concentrations greater than 200 μg/dl, which correlate strongly with cerebral oedema (Chapter 5) [52].

Plasma proteins

The plasma proteins produced by the hepatocyte are synthesized on polyribosomes bound to the rough endoplasmic reticulum before secretion into plasma

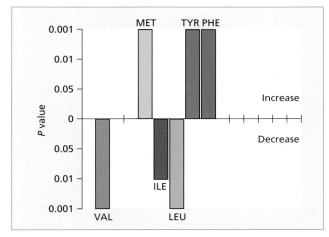

Fig. 2.10. The plasma amino acid pattern in cryptogenic cirrhosis (mean of 11 patients) compared with normal individuals. The aromatic amino acids and methionine are increased while the branched-chain amino acids are decreased. ILE, isoleucine; MET, methionine; PHE, phenylalanine; TYR, tyrosine; VAL, valine [51].

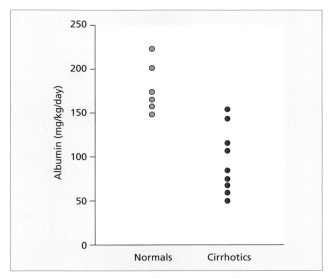

Fig. 2.11. The absolute synthesis of serum albumin (^{14}C carbonate method) in cirrhosis is reduced [56].

Table 2.4. Serum (plasma) proteins synthesized by the liver

	Normal concentration
Albumin	40–50 g/L
α_1-antitrypsin*	2–4 g/L
α-fetoprotein	<10 KU/L
α_2-macroglobulin	2.2–3.8 g/L
Caeruloplasmin*	0.2–0.4 g/L
Complement components (C_3, C_6 and C_1)	
Fibrinogen*	2–6 g/L
Haemopexin	0.8–1.0 g/L
Prothrombin (factor II)†	
Transferrin*, ferritin*	

*Acute phase proteins.
†Vitamin K dependent; also factors VII and X.

[53]. Falls in concentration usually reflect decreased hepatic synthesis although changes in plasma volume and losses, for instance into gut or urine, may contribute. The hepatocyte makes albumin, fibrinogen, α_1-antitrypsin, haptoglobin, caeruloplasmin, transferrin and several coagulation factors (Table 2.4). Some liver-produced proteins are acute phase reactors and rise in response to tissue injury such as inflammation (Table 2.4). These include fibrinogen, haptoglobin, α_1-antitrypsin, C_3 component of complement ferritin and caeruloplasmin. An acute phase response may contribute to well-maintained or increased serum concentrations of these proteins, even with hepatocellular disease. The mechanism is complex, but cytokines (interleukin (IL) 1, IL6, TNF-α) play a role [54]. IL6 binds to the cell-surface receptor and this stimulates a message from the hepatocyte membrane to the nucleus where there is induction of specific nuclear factors, which interact with promoter elements at the 5′ end of several acute phase plasma protein genes. There are also post-transcriptional as well as transcriptional mechanisms. Cytokines not only stimulate production of acute phase proteins but also inhibit the synthesis of albumin, transferrin and a range of other proteins [55].

Immunoglobulins IgG, IgM and IgA are synthesized by the B cells of the lymphoid system. Their levels are elevated in all cirrhotics as a non-specific response to bacteremia.

Albumin is quantitatively the most important plasma protein synthesized by the liver. The average size of the albumin pool in adults is 500 g. Between 12 and 15 g is synthesized daily by the normal liver (Figs 2.11, 2.12). Cirrhotic patients can only synthesize about 4 g (35 mg/kg per day in Child C cirrhosis) [57,58]. The fractional synthetic rate of albumin is approximately 6% per day compared with 25% for total liver protein. In liver disease, the fall in serum albumin concentration is slow as the half-life of albumin is about 22 days. Thus a patient with acute hepatitis may have a virtually normal serum albumin value while lower levels would be expected in decompensated cirrhotic patients.

The prothrombin time measures the time required for plasma to clot after addition of tissue factor and phospholipid (Chapter 4) [59].

α_1-Antitrypsin deficiency is inherited (Chapter 29).

Haptoglobin is a glycoprotein composed of two types of polypeptide chains, α and β, covalently associated by disulphide bonds. Haptoglobin is largely synthesized by hepatocytes. Hereditary deficiencies are frequent in

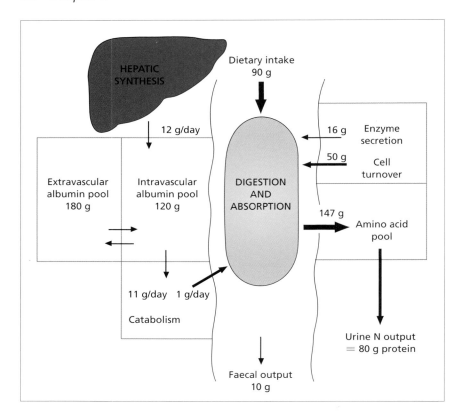

Fig. 2.12. The turnover of plasma albumin in a 70-kg adult seen in the context of the daily protein economy of the gastrointestinal tract and overall nitrogen balance. The total exchangeable albumin pool of about 300 g is distributed between the intravascular and extravascular compartments in a ratio of approximately 2:3. In this simplified schema the balance sheet is expressed in terms of grams of protein (6.25 × grams of nitrogen). Losses do not include relatively minor routes, e.g. 2 g/day from the skin [53].

American black people. Low values are found in severe, chronic hepatocellular disease, megaloblastic anaemia and haemolytic crises.

Caeruloplasmin is a serum glycoprotein which contains six copper atoms per molecule and is present in human fetal serum by the fifth week of gestation. It is the major copper-binding protein in plasma and has oxidase activity. A low concentration is found in 95% of those who are homozygous and about 10% of those heterozygous for Wilson's disease (Chapter 27). Caeruloplasmin increases to normal in patients with Wilson's disease who have a liver transplant. Caeruloplasmin should be measured in all patients with chronic hepatitis, even if over the age of 50 years. Low values are also found in severe, decompensated cirrhosis not due to Wilson's disease. High values are found in pregnancy, following oestrogen therapy and large bile duct obstruction.

Transferrin is the iron transport protein and consists of a single polypeptide chain arranged in two lobes with greater than 40% amino acid homology between them. Although many cells can synthesize transferrin, the hepatocyte is the most important source. Hepatic synthesis of transferrin is inversely proportional to iron status such that transferrin synthesis is greatest during iron deficiency and reduced during iron overload. Two important functions of transferrin are transporting iron in the ferric state and delivering iron to cell-surface transferrin receptors [60]. Plasma transferrin is more than 90% saturated with iron in patients with untreated idiopathic haemochromatosis (Chapter 26). Reduced values may be found with cirrhosis. Serum ferritin see Chapter 26.

The *C_3 component of complement* tends to be reduced in cirrhosis, normal in chronic hepatitis and increased in compensated primary biliary cirrhosis. Low values in ALF and alcoholic cirrhosis with or without hepatitis reflect reduced hepatic synthesis. There is a correlation with prolonged prothrombin time and hypoalbuminaemia [61]. There is also a contribution from increased consumption due to activation of the complement system. Transient reductions are found in the early 'immune complex' stage of acute hepatitis B.

α-fetoprotein is a 70-kDa glycoprotein, which is a normal component of plasma protein in human foetuses older than 6 weeks. It reaches maximum concentration between 12 and 16 weeks of fetal life. It disappears from the circulation soon after birth but reappears in patients with primary liver cancer (Chapter 35). It is not specific for hepatocellular carcinoma as raised values have been reported with chronic viral hepatitis, embryonic tumours of the ovary and testis, embryonic hepatoblastoma, gastrointestinal tract carcinomas with hepatic secondaries and ataxia telangectasia. Although values greater than 400 ng/mL are virtually confined to primary liver cancer, levels are not elevated in most cases of hepatocellular carcinomas [62].

Electrophoretic pattern of serum proteins

Electrophoresis is used to determine the proportions of the various serum proteins. In cirrhosis, albumin is reduced.

The α_1-globulins contain glycoproteins and hormone-binding globulins. They tend to be low in hepatocellular disease, falling in parallel with the serum albumin. An increase accompanies acute febrile illnesses and malignant disease. Ninety per cent of α_1-globulin consists of α_1-antitrypsin, and an absent α_1-globulin may indicate α_1-antitrypsin deficiency.

The α_2- and β-globulins include lipoproteins. In cholestasis, the increase in α_2- and β-globulin components correlates with height of serum lipids.

The γ-globulins rise in hepatic cirrhosis due to increased production. The increased numbers of plasma cells in marrow, and even in the liver itself, may be the source. The γ-globulin peak in hepatocellular disease shows a wide base (*polyclonal gammopathy*). *Monoclonal gammopathy* is rare and may be age-related rather than related to chronic liver disease. The dip between β- and γ-globulins tends to be bridged.

Immunoglobulins. IgG is markedly increased in autoimmune hepatitis, less so in cryptogenic cirrhosis. In autoimmune hepatitis the raised level of IgG falls during treatment with corticosteroids. There is a slow and sustained increase in viral hepatitis and it is also increased in alcoholic cirrhosis.

IgM is markedly increased in primary biliary cirrhosis and to a lesser extent in viral hepatitis and cirrhosis.

IgA is markedly increased in cirrhosis of the alcoholic but also in primary biliary and cryptogenic cirrhosis. The increase in serum secretory IgA, the predominant immunoglobulin in bile, may be related to communication of the bile canaliculus with the space of Disse and/or through the bile duct into the portal blood vessels [63].

In chronic hepatitis with active inflammation and cryptogenic cirrhosis the pattern is surprisingly similar, with increases in IgG, IgM and to a lesser extent IgA. About 10% of patients with chronic cholestasis due to large bile duct obstruction show increases in all three main immunoglobulins. Patterns are not diagnostic of any one disease but together with other data add support to considering a particular diagnosis.

Carbohydrate metabolism

The liver occupies a key position in carbohydrate metabolism (Fig. 2.1) [64]. In the fed state, glycogen synthesis occurs preferentially in the perivenous hepatocytes whereas in the fasting or postabsorptive state,

glucose release via glycogenolysis and gluconeogenesis initially occur in periportal hepatocytes. Once glycogen stores are replenished, glucose may be metabolized to fat or lactate. Lactate is released into the systemic circulation and taken up by periportal cells as a substrate for gluconeogenesis.

In ALF the blood glucose level may be low but this is uncommon in chronic liver disease. In addition to glucose, the liver also metabolizes fructose and galactose.

In fasted patients with cirrhosis the contribution of carbohydrates to energy production is reduced (2 vs. 38% in normal controls) with the contribution from fat increasing (86 vs. 45%) [65]. This may be caused by impaired release of hepatic glucose or a reduced reserve of glycogen in the liver. After eating a meal, however, cirrhotic patients, like control subjects, make immediate use of dietary carbohydrate, indeed perhaps to a greater degree, because of a reduced ability to store and then mobilize energy as triglyceride.

The oral and intravenous glucose tolerance tests may show impairment in cirrhosis and there is relative insulin resistance (Chapter 28).

Galactose tolerance is also impaired in hepatocellular disease and oral and intravenous tests have been devised. Results are independent of insulin secretion. Galactose removal by the liver has been used to measure hepatic blood flow.

Effects of ageing on the liver

Although there are many studies of hepatic function and ageing, results have been conflicting or unsubstantiated. However, liver weight and volume decrease with age, and liver blood flow is reduced [66]. There is compensatory hypertrophy of hepatocytes.

In animals, the rate of hepatic regeneration declines with increasing age but whether this is related to lower circulating levels of hepatotrophic factors is not clear. Somatic mutations, including gene rearrangements, increase with age and are more frequent in the liver than the brain in experimental models [67].

Structural changes in the hepatocyte include an increase in secondary lysosomes and residual bodies, with a concomitant accumulation of lipofuscin. There are conflicting data on structural changes in mitochondria. However, impaired mitochondrial enzyme activity and defects in the respiratory chain are reported. No consistent mitochondrial DNA mutations are seen.

In animals, protein synthesis by the liver falls with age. Since the total protein content of cells remains relatively constant it is thought that protein turnover is also reduced. Hepatic nitrogen clearance (conversion of α-amino nitrogen into urea nitrogen) is impaired with advancing age [68].

First-pass metabolism of drugs is reduced and this may be due to reduced liver mass and hepatic blood flow rather than to alterations in the relevant enzyme systems [69]. It has been suggested that increased hepatocyte volume extends the path for oxygen diffusion (the 'oxygen diffusion barrier' hypothesis) which might affect cell function [70]. Hepatic microsomal mono-oxygenase enzyme activity does not appear to decline with age [71]. Fatal reactions to halothane and drugs such as benoxyprofen are more frequent in the elderly, but the overall increase in adverse reactions observed may be related to the multiplicity of drugs that these patients receive.

Cholesterol saturation of bile increases with age due to enhanced hepatic secretion of cholesterol and decreased bile acid synthesis. This may explain age as a risk factor for cholesterol gallstones.

References

1 Pugh RN, Murray-Lyon IM, Dawson JL et al. Transection of the esophagus for bleeding esophageal varices. Br. J. Surg. 1973; **60**: 646–649.

2 Kamath PS, Wiesner RH, Malinchoc M et al. A model to predict survival in patients with end-stage liver disease. Hepatology 2001; **33**: 464–70.

3 Imperial JC, Keeffe EB. Laboratory tests. In: Bacon BR, O'Grady JG, Di Bisceglie AM, Lake JR, eds. Comprehensive Clinical Hepatology, 2nd edn. Philadelphia: Elsevier Mosby, 2006, p.79.

4 den Bergh AAH, Muller P. Uber eine und eine indirekte Diazoreaktion auf Bilirubin. Biochem. Z. 1916; **77**: 90.

5 Tiribelli C, Ostrow JD. New concepts in bilirubin and jaundice: report of the Third International Bilirubin Workshop, April 6–8, 1995, Trieste, Italy. Hepatology 1996; **24**: 1296–1311.

6 Fevery J, Blanckaert N. What can we learn from analysis of serum bilirubin? J. Hepatol. 1986; **2**: 113–121.

7 Binder L, Smith D, Kupka T et al. Failure of prediction of liver function test abnormalities with the urine urobilinogen and urine bilirubin assays. Arch. Pathol. Lab. Med. 1989; **113**: 73–76.

8 Kubitz R, Wettstein M, Warskulat U et al. Regulation of the multidrug resistance protein 2 in the rat liver by lipopolysaccharide and dexamethasone. Gastroenterology 1999; **116**: 401–410.

9 Mandema E, DeFraiture WH, Niewig HO et al. Familial chronic idiopathic jaundice (Dubin–Sprinz disease) with a note on bromsulphalein metabolism in this disease. Am. J. Med. 1960; **28**: 42–50.

10 Prati D, Taioli E, Zanella A et al. Updated definitions of healthy ranges for serum alanine aminotransferase levels. Ann. Intern. Med. 2002; **137**: 1–10.

11 Jamjute P, Ahmad A, Ghosh T et al. Liver function test and pregnancy. J. Matern. Fetal Neonatal Med. 2009; **22**: 274–283.

12 Caropreso M, Fortunato G, Lenta S et al. Prevalence and long-term course of macro-aspartate aminotransferase in children. J. Pediatr. 2009; **154**: 744–748.

13 Fabrizi F, Lunghi G, Finazzi S et al. Decreased serum aminotransferase activity in patients with chronic renal failure: impact on the detection of viral hepatitis. Am. J. Kidney Dis. 2001; **38**: 1009–1015.

14 Allman MA, Pang E, Yau DF et al. Elevated plasma vitamers of vitamin B6 in patients with chronic renal failure in regular hemodialysis. Eur. J. Clin. Nutr. 1992; **46**: 679–683.

15 Price CP, Alberti KGMM. Biochemical assessment of liver function. In: Wright R, Alberti KGMM, Karran S, Millward-Sadler GH, eds. Liver and Biliary Disease-Pathophysiology, Diagnosis and Managemement. London: W.B.Saunders, 1979, p. 381–416.

16 Rizvi AA, Kerrick JG. Liver involvement and abnormal iron variables in undiagnosed Addison's disease. Endocr. Pract. 2001; **7**: 184–188.

17 Fong HF, Divasta AD, Difabio D et al. Prevalence and predictors of abnormal liver enzymes in young women with anorexia nervosa. J. Pediatr. 2008; **153**: 247–253.

18 Volta U, Granito A, De Franceschi L et al. Anti-tissue transglutaminase antibodies as predictors of silent coeliac disease in patients with hypertransaminasaemia of unknown origin. Dig. Liver Dis. 2001; **33**: 420–425.

19 Kubota S, Amino N, Matsumoto Y et al. Serial changes in liver function tests in patients with thyrotoxicosis induced by Graves' disease and painless thyroiditis. Thyroid 2008; **18**: 283–287.

20 Whitehead MW, Hawkes ND, Hainsworth I et al. A prospective study of the causes of notably raised aspartate aminotransferase of liver origin. Gut 1999; **45**: 129–133.

21 Ludwig S, Kaplowitz N. Effect of serum pyridoxine deficiency on serum and liver transaminases in experimental liver injury in the rat. Gastroenterology 1980; **79**: 545–549.

22 Angulo P, Keach JC, Batts KP et al. Independent predictors of liver fibrosis in patients with nonalcoholic steatohepatitis. Hepatology 1999; **30**: 1356–1362.

23 Giannini E, Risso D, Botta F et al. Validity and clinical utility of the aspartate aminotransferase-alanine aminotransferase ratio in assessing disease severity and prognosis in patients with hepatitis C virus-related chronic liver disease. Arch. Intern. Med. 2003; **163**: 218–224.

24 Weiss MJ, Ray K, Henthorn PS et al. Structure of the human liver/bone/kidney alkaline phosphatase gene. J. Biol. Chem. 1988; **263**: 12002–12010.

25 Nakano T, Shimanuki T, Matsushita M et al. Involvement of intestinal alkaline phosphatase in serum apolipoprotein B-48 level and its association with ABO and secretor blood group types. Biochem. Biophys. Res. Commun. 2006; **341**: 33–38.

26 Maldonado O, Demasi R, Maldonado Y et al. Extremely high levels of alkaline phosphatase in hospitalized patients. J. Clin. Gastroenterol. 1998; **27**: 342–345.

27 O'Leary JG, Pratt DS. Cholestasis and cholestatic syndromes. Curr. Opin. Gastroenterol. 2007; **23**: 232–236.

28 Cassidy WM, Reynolds TB. Serum lactic acid dehydrogenase in the differential diagnosis of acute hepatocellular injury. J. Clin. Gastroenterol. 1994; **19**: 118–121.

29 Zucker SD, Gollan JL. Physiology of the liver. In: Haubrich WS, Schaffner F, Berk JE, eds. Bockus Gastroenterology, 5th edn. Philadelphia: Wiley Saunders, 1995, p. 1858–1905.

30 Jonas A. Lecithin cholesterol acyl transferase. Biochim. Biophys. Acta. 2000 ; **1529**: 245–256.

31 Oude Elferink RP, Groen AK. Mechanisms of biliary lipid secretion and their role in lipid homeostasis. *Semin. Liv. Dis.* 2002; **20**: 293–305.

32 Crawford JM, Mockel GM, Crawford AR *et al.* Imaging biliary lipid secretion in the rat: ultrastructural evidence for vesiculation of the hepatocyte canalicular membrane. *J. Lipid Res.* 1995; **36**: 2147–2163.

33 Mansbach CM 2nd, Gorelick F. Dietary lipid absorption, complex lipid synthesis and intracellular packaging and secretion of chylomicrons. *Am. J. Physiol. Gastrointest. Liver Physiol.* 2007; **293**: G645–650.

34 Williams KJ. Molecular processes that handle- and mishandle- dietary lipids. *J. Clin. Invest.* 2008; **118**: 3247–3259.

35 Wade DP, Owen JS. Regulation of the cholesterol efflux gene, ABCA1. *Lancet* 2001; **357**: 161–163.

36 Solaymani-Dodaran M, Aithal GP, Card T *et al.* Risk of cardiovascular and cerebrovascular events in primary biliary cirrhosis: a population-based cohort study. *Am. J. Gastroenterol.* 2008; **103**: 2784–2788.

37 Mirandola S, Realdon S, Iqbal J *et al.* Liver microsomal triglyceride transfer protein is involved in hepatitis C liver steatosis. *Gastroenterology* 2006; **130**: 1661–1669.

38 Wilfred de Alwis NM, Day CP. Genetics of alcoholic liver disease and nonalcoholic fatty liver disease. *Semin. Liver Dis.* 2007; **27**: 44–54.

39 Sacks FM. The apolipoprotein story. *Atherosclerosis* 2006; **7** (*Suppl.*): 23–27.

40 Nofer JR, Remaley AT. Tangier disease: still more questions than answers. *Cell. Mol. Life Sci.* 2005; **62**: 2150–2156.

41 Hofmann AF. Bile acids-trying to understand their chemistry and biology with the hope of helping patients. *Hepatology* 2009; **49**: 1403–1418.

42 Pikuleva IA. Cytochrome P450s and cholesterol homeostasis. *Pharmacol. Ther.* 2006; **112**: 761–773.

43 Beuers U. Drug insight: mechanisms and sites of action of ursodeoxycholic acid in cholestasis. *Nat. Clin. Pract. Gastroenterol. Hepatol.* 2006; **3**: 318–328.

44 Stiehl A, Raedsch R, Rudolph G. Acute effects of ursodeoxycholic and chenodeoxycholic acid on the small intestinal absorption of bile acids. *Gastroenterology* 1990; **98**: 424–428.

45 Wolkoff AW, Cohen DE. Bile acid regulation of hepatic physiology: I. Hepatocyte transport of bile acids. *Am. J. Physiol. Gastrointest. Liver Physiol.* 2003; **284**: G175–179.

46 Takikawa H. Hepatobiliary transport of bile acids and organic anions. *J. Hepatobiliary Pancreat. Surg.* 2002; **9**: 443–447.

47 Sturm E, Wagner M, Trauner M. Nuclear receptor ligands in therapy of cholestatic liver disease. *Front. Biosci.* 2009; **14**: 4299–4325.

48 Carulli N, Bertolotti M, Carubbi F *et al.* Review article: effect of bile salt pool composition on hepatic and biliary functions. *Aliment. Pharmacol. Ther.* 2000; **14**: 14–18.

49 Robb BW, Matthews JB. Bile salt diarrhea. *Curr. Gastroenterol. Rep.* 2005; **7**: 379–383.

50 Moseley RH. Hepatic amino acid transport. *Semin. Liver Dis.* 1996; **16**: 137–145.

51 Morgan MY, Marshall AW, Milsom JP *et al.* Plasma amino-acid patterns in liver disease. *Gut* 1982; **23**: 362–370.

52 Clemmesen JO, Larsen FS, Kondrup J *et al.* Cerebral herniation in patients with acute liver failure is correlated with arterial ammonia concentration. *Hepatology* 1994; **29**: 648–653.

53 Tavill AS. The synthesis and degradation of liver-produced proteins. *Gut* 1972; **13**: 225–241.

54 Sehgal PB. Interleukin-6: a regulator of plasma protein gene expression in hepatic and nonhepatic tissues. *Mol. Biol. Med.* 1990; **7**: 117–130.

55 Andus T, Bauer J, Gerok W. Effects of cytokines on the liver. *Hepatology* 1991; **13**: 364–375.

56 Tavill AS, Craigie A, Rosenoer VM. The measurement of the synthetic rate of albumin in man. *Clin. Sci.* 1968; **34**: 1–28.

57 Ballmer PE, Reichen J, McNurlan MA *et al.* Albumin but not fibrinogen synthesis correlates with galactose elimination capacity in patients with cirrhosis of the liver. *Hepatology* 1996; **24**: 53–59.

58 Barle H, Nyberg B, Essen P *et al.* The synthesis rates of total liver protein and plasma albumin determined simultaneously *in vivo* in humans. *Hepatology* 1997; **25**: 154–158.

59 Robert A, Chazouillères O. Prothrombin time in liver failure: time, ratio, activity percentage or International Normalized Ratio. *Hepatology* 1996; **24**: 1392–1394.

60 Pietrangelo A. Physiology of iron transport and the hemochromatosis gene. *Am. J. Physiol. Gastrointest. Liver Physiol.* 2002; **282**: 403–414.

61 Ellison RT, Horsburgh CR Jr, Curd J. Complement levels in patients with hepatic dysfunction. *Dig. Dis. Sci.* 1990; **35**: 231–235.

62 Nguyen MH, Garcia RT, Simpson PW *et al.* Racial differences in effectiveness of alpha-feto protein for diagnosis of hepaticellular carcinoma in hepatitis C virus cirrhosis. *Hepatology* 2002; **36**: 410–417.

63 Fukuda Y, Nagura H, Asai J *et al.* Possible mechanisms of elevation of serum secretory immunoglobulin A in liver disease. *Am. J. Gastroenterol.* 1986; **81**: 315–324.

64 Boden G, Cox Jr C. Carbohydrate metabolism. In: Rodes J, Benhamou JP, Blei A, Reichen J, Rizzetto M, eds. *Oxford Textbook of Clinical Hepatology*, 3rd edn. London: Wiley Blackwell, 2007, p. 129–133.

65 Schneeweiss B, Graninger W, Ferenci P *et al.* Energy metabolism in patients with acute and chronic liver disease. *Hepatology* 1990; **11**: 387–393.

66 Zoli M, Magalotti D, Bianchi G *et al.* Total and functional hepatic blood flow decrease in parallel with ageing. *Age Ageing* 1999; **28**: 29–33.

67 Dolle ME, Vijg J. Genome dynamics in aging mice. *Genome Research* 2002; **11**: 1732–1738.

68 Fabbri A, Marchesini G, Bianchi G *et al.* Kinetics of hepatic amino-nitrogen conversion in ageing man. *Liver* 1994; **14**: 288–294.

69 Schmucker DL. Age-related changes in liver structure and function: implications for disease? *Exp. Gerontol.* 2005; **40**: 650–659.

70 Le Couteur DG, Warren A, Cogger VC *et al.* Old age and the hepatic sinusoid. *Anat. Rec.* 2008; **291**: 672–683.

71 Parkinson A, Mudra DR, Johnson C *et al.* The effects of gender, ethnicity and liver cirrhosis on cytochrome P450 enzyme activity in human liver microsomes and inducibilty in cultured human hepatocytes. *Liver Toxicol. Appl. Pharmacol.* 2004; **199**: 193–209.

CHAPTER 3
Biopsy of the Liver

David Patch[1] & Amar Paul Dhillon[2]

[1] Liver Transplantation and Hepatobiliary Unit, Royal Free Hospital and University College London, London, UK
[2] Department of Cellular Pathology, University College London Medical School, London, UK

> **Learning points**
>
> - Liver biopsy can be used to: confirm or refute the clinical diagnosis; identify additional clinically unsuspected conditions; assess severity, progression and complications of disease; and evaluate response to and complications of treatment.
>
> - Reliable liver biopsy interpretation requires knowledge of the clinical context, an experienced hepatopathologist and an adequate liver biopsy sample.
>
> - The distribution of a particular disease throughout the liver determines the chance of a non-directed liver biopsy adequately representing the disease in question.
>
> - Focal diseases are particularly prone to error in random samples.
>
> - A liver biopsy sample containing at least 11 complete portal tracts is necessary for the proper evaluation of chronic viral hepatitis (i.e. approximately 20 mm of a biopsy taken with a 1.4 mm internal diameter (16 gauge) needle, and progressively longer samples of thinner biopsies).
>
> - The 'stage score' of liver disease is not the same as collagen quantification.

A needle biopsy of the liver was said to have been first performed by Paul Ehrlich in 1883 (Table 3.1). The first published series was by Schüpfer [1] in France, where the technique was used for the diagnosis of cirrhosis and hepatic tumours. However, the method only achieved popularity in the 1930s when it was used by Huard and co-workers in France, and by Baron in the USA. The Second World War saw a rapid increase in the use of liver biopsy, largely to investigate the many cases of non-fatal viral hepatitis which were affecting the armed forces of both sides [2–4].

It is hard, if not impossible, to envisage management of patients without recourse to liver biopsy, and yet it is a procedure that is often feared by patients, and when done incorrectly can have devastating complications. There is, however, a significant body of evidence to guide the clinician with respect to technique, complications and contraindications.

Selection and preparation of the patient

Most biopsies are performed as day case procedures because of patient preference and reduction of costs. The majority of complications occur within 3 h of biopsy, but may occur up to 24 h after the procedure. In 1989, the American Gastroenterological Association and subsequently the British Society of Gastroenterology [5] published consensus statements on out-patient percutaneous liver biopsy, recommending that patients undergoing this procedure should have no conditions that might increase the risk of the biopsy including: encephalopathy, ascites, hepatic failure with severe jaundice or evidence of significant extrahepatic biliary obstruction, significant coagulopathies or serious diseases involving other organs such as severe congestive heart failure or advanced age.

The consensus statements also recommended that the place where the biopsy is performed should have easy access to a laboratory, blood bank and in-patient facilities should the need arise, and there should be staff to observe the patients for 6 h. The patient should be hospitalized if there is any significant complication, including pain requiring more than one dose of analgesic in the 4 h following liver biopsy. The patient should also be able to return easily to the hospital where the biopsy was undertaken within 30 min, and should have a reliable individual to stay with them on the first postbiopsy night. These recommendations are eminently sensible and should form the backbone of any local biopsy policy. Out-patient biopsies should ideally be performed

---

Sherlock's Diseases of the Liver and Biliary System, Twelfth Edition. Edited by James S. Dooley, Anna S.F. Lok, Andrew K. Burroughs, E. Jenny Heathcote.
© 2011 by Blackwell Publishing Ltd. Published 2011 by Blackwell Publishing Ltd.

Table 3.1. History of liver biopsies

Author	Date	Country	Purpose
Ehrlich	1883	Germany	Glycogen
Lucatello	1895	Italy	Tropical
Schüpfer	1907	France	Cirrhosis
Huard *et al.*	1935	France	General
Baron	1939	USA	General
Iversen & Roholm	1939	Denmark	Hepatitis
Axenfeld & Brass	1942	Germany	Hepatitis
Dible *et al.*	1943	UK	Hepatitis

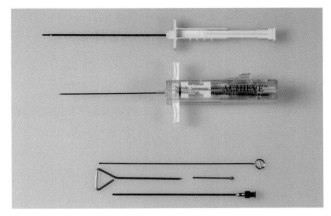

Fig. 3.1. Three biopsy devices—a standard Trucut needle, an automated Trucut device and a Menghini needle.

in the early morning so that, should complications occur, the vast majority of patients will be still in hospital.

The method of biopsy is dictated by coagulation indices and indication. Percutaneous biopsies should not be performed if the one-stage prothrombin time is more than 3 s prolonged over control values. Whilst fresh frozen plasma is frequently used to correct coagulation indices, there is little evidence it reduces the risk of haemorrhage [5]. Again, although recombinant factor VIIa can correct prothrombin time, a reduced risk of bleeding has not been shown—in addition, its major drawback is expense.

Evidence-based guidelines on safe platelet thresholds do not exist [5]; in thrombocytopenic patients the risk of haemorrhage depends on the function of the platelets rather than on their numbers. A patient with 'hypersplenism' and a platelet count of less than 50 000 is much less likely to bleed than one with leukaemia, who may have a higher platelet count. This distinction particularly arises in patients with haematological problems or after organ transplants where the effects on the bone marrow of cytotoxic therapy, viruses and other infective agents and of possible graft-versus-host reaction may lead to significant abnormalities of platelet function. Alternative techniques to percutaneous biopsy are often used in patients with a platelet count less than 80 000, and some centres 50 000 [5].

Additional risk factors have identified patients with an increased incidence of complications following standard percutaneous biopsy (the alternative techniques are in parentheses): the unco-operative patient (sedation, transvenous or real-time ultrasound-guided), extrahepatic biliary obstruction (real-time ultrasound-guided), ascites (transvenous), cystic lesions (real-time ultrasound-guided), hepatic amyloidosis (transvenous), obesity (transvenous or real-time ultrasound-guided), sickle hepatopathy (transvenous), chronic renal failure (transvenous), and valvular heart disease (consider antibiotic prophylaxis). There is an increased risk of bleeding in patients with malignancy but often these biopsies

are real-time ultrasound-guided using thinner needles, with less risk of complications.

All patients being considered for liver biopsy should undergo a prebiopsy ultrasound in order to exclude anatomical variation associated with increased risk of visceral perforation—such as the presence of small bowel between a shrunken liver and the abdominal wall (Chilaiditi's syndrome), or an intrahepatic gall bladder. Ultrasound also permits the detection of focal lesions such as haemangioma, which may be asymptomatic and may not have been suspected.

Informed consent

Informed consent should be obtained in writing prior to the biopsy procedure in accordance with individual hospital policies. The consent form should clearly document the morbidity and mortality associated with the route of biopsy, and preferably this should also be documented in the patients notes when the biopsy is initially being discussed, so that the patient can be given sufficient time to refuse the procedure.

Techniques

The Menghini needle obtains a specimen by aspiration [6], whilst the sheathed 'Trucut' uses a cutting technique (Figs 3.1, 3.2) [7]. Fragmentation of the biopsy is greater with the Menghini method, but the procedure is quicker, easier, has fewer complications [8] and can provide longer specimens in comparison with the standard Trucut specimen [9]. Furthermore, the Menghini needle is cheaper. Pain associated with the procedure is often due to the operator applying insufficient local anaesthetic in the skin, and none in the capsule/parenchyma. Sufficient 1–2% lignocaine solution should be used.

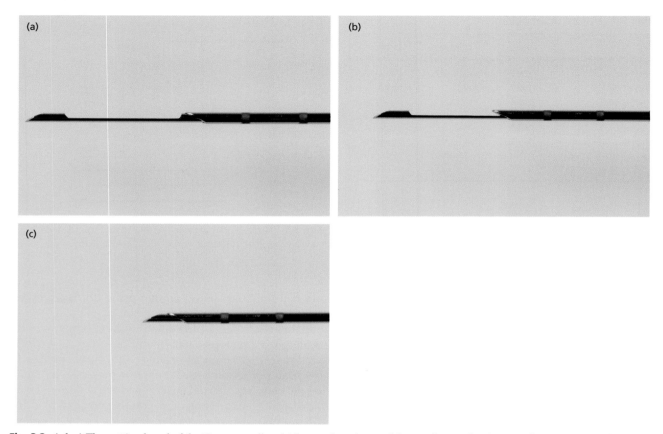

(a)

(b)

(c)

Fig. 3.2. (a,b,c) The cutting bevel of the Trucut needle which must be advanced forward, over the tissue in the recession in the needle.

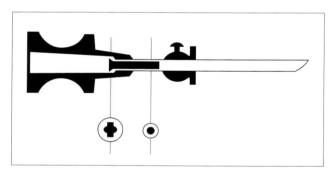

Fig. 3.3. Longitudinal section of the Menghini liver biopsy needle. Note the nail in the shaft of the needle.

Menghini 'one second' needle biopsy (Fig. 3.3). The 1.4-mm diameter needle is used routinely. A shorter needle is available for paediatric use. The tip of the needle is oblique and slightly convex towards the outside. The needle is fitted within its shaft with a blunt nail. This internal block prevents the biopsy from being fragmented or distorted by violent aspiration into the syringe. The original publication [6] documented a width measured on the slide (fixed tissue) of 0.75 mm using a 15 G needle.

Sterile saline (5 mL or more) is drawn into the syringe, which is inserted through the anaesthetized track down to, but not through, the intercostal space. To clear the needle of any skin fragments, 1 to 2 mL of solution are injected. Aspiration is now commenced and maintained. This is the slow part of the procedure. With the patient holding their breath in expiration, the needle is rapidly introduced perpendicularly to the skin into the liver substance and extracted. This is the quick part of the procedure. The tip of the needle is now placed on sterile paper and some of the remaining saline flushed through the needle to deposit the biopsy gently onto the paper. The tissue is transferred into fixative.

Trucut needle. This involves a three-stage process, requiring greater operator skill and patient compliance. The patient holds their breath in expiration whilst the needle is advanced along the anaesthetized tract into the parenchyma. The needle tip is then extended, followed by the cutting bevel. To avoid a scissoring action, there needs to be a slight forward force, so that the cutting bevel actually moves forward, slicing liver, as opposed to pulling the needle tip back. This needle results in less fragmentation, and a more reliable specimen in fibrotic livers.

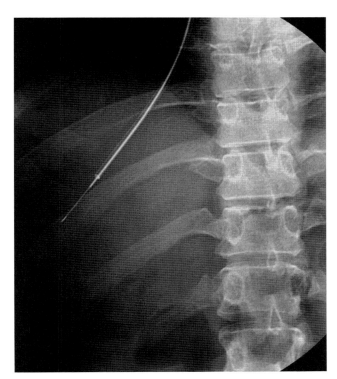

Fig. 3.4. Transvenous liver biopsy. Transvenous liver biopsy. The catheter is in the hepatic vein and the Quick-Core needle is taking the liver biopsy.

Newer generations of narrower gauge (18 or 20 G) spring loaded Trucut needles require less skill, but are more expensive. The maximum length is determined by the fixed length of the trough in the needle (2 cm) [9].

The intercostal approach is the most frequently used method [8]. Care must be taken to assess the borders of the liver either by percussion or by ultrasound. The liver may be higher than expected (particularly in transplant patients) or lower, such as in patients with chronic lung disease. If there is any doubt with respect to percussion, ultrasound should be used. Some centres use ultrasound at the time of the biopsy in all patients. It does minimize the likelihood of obtaining inadequate specimens, but has not been shown conclusively to reduce major complications [10]. New generation, portable ultrasound equipment is becoming less expensive and the better performance of a liver biopsy can make this cost-effective [11]. In any case, many biopsies are being performed by radiologists who routinely use ultrasound.

If an epigastric mass is present or imaging indicates left lobe disease, an anterior approach is used.

Transjugular (transvenous liver biopsy) [12]. A special Trucut needle (18 or 19 G, Quickcore) is inserted through a catheter placed in the hepatic vein via the jugular vein under fluoroscopic guidance. The needle is then introduced into the liver tissue by transfixing the hepatic

Table 3.2. Indications for transjugular liver biopsy

Coagulation defects and congenital clotting disorders
Acute liver failure pre-transplant
Massive ascites
Small liver
Measurement of hepatic venous pressure gradient
Unco-operative patient
Severe obesity

venous wall (Fig. 3.4). In patients with advanced liver disease, it has the advantage of facilitating measurement of wedged and free hepatic venous pressure and of opacifying the hepatic vein (Table 3.2). A review of 7000 biopsies [12] indicated that the transjugular technique provided samples of similar quality to those from the percutaneous approach. Biopsies are thinner than with the intercostal technique. Providing four passes are performed, biopsies are adequate to stage chronic viral hepatitis [13,14].

Directed (guided biopsy). This involves simultaneous imaging of the lesion in the liver and the advancing biopsy needle tip. Ultrasound is commonly employed, but computed tomography (CT) may be required if the lesion is not visible on ultrasound. Spring-loaded Trucut needles are preferred, and, in patients with poor coagulation, a gel foam plug may be injected through the outer cannula of the Trucut needle after the inner cutting needle, once its contained specimen has been removed [15]. This can be effective in preventing major bleeding.

In chronic liver disease, the blind technique yields sufficient diagnostic material 81% of the time, but this can be raised to 95% if a laparoscopic directed liver biopsy is used [16].

Fine-needle guided biopsy. Using a 22 G (0.7 mm) needle adds to the safety. It is particularly useful for the diagnosis of focal lesions, although diagnostic accuracy may not be improved [17]. Because of the size, fine-needle biopsy is not so useful in generalized disease such as chronic hepatitis or cirrhosis. Cytological examination of the aspirate is useful for tumour typing [18] and this technique will allow introduction of local therapies such as ethanol or acetic acid.

After care

Observations should be frequent (quarter hourly for 2 h, half hourly for 2 h and hourly for 2 h) and analgesia should be prescribed [5]. During the puncture the patient may complain of a drawing feeling across the epigastrium. Afterwards some patients have a slight ache in the right side for about 24 h and some complain

Table 3.3. Fatalities from needle liver biopsy

Source	Date	Reference	Biopsies	Mortality (%)
USA	1953	1,2	20 016	0.17
Europe combined	1964	3	23 382	0.01
Germany	1967	4	80 000	0.015
Italy	1986	5	68 276	0.009
USA	1990	6	9 212	0.11

1 Zamcheck. *N. Engl. J. Med.* 1953; **249**: 1020.
2 Zamcheck. *N. Engl. J. Med.* 1953; **249**: 1062.
3 Thaler. *Wien. Klin. Wchschr.* 1964; **29**: 533.
4 Lindner. *Dtsch. Med. Wschr.* 1967; **92**: 1751.
5 Piccinino. *J. Hepatol.* 1986; **2**: 165 [8].
6 McGill. *Gastroenterology* 1990; **99**: 1396 [20].

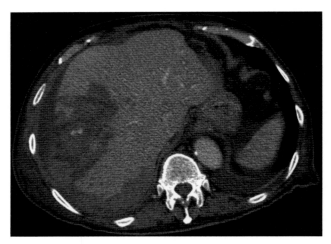

Fig. 3.5. A CT scan showing a bleed following a biopsy. A sharp, white area of contrast is present within the parenchyma of the pseudoaneurysm.

of pain referred from the diaphragm to the right shoulder—this often indicates a capsular haematoma.

Number of passes

It has been demonstrated that taking more than one core of liver at biopsy can increase the diagnostic yield [19], but more passes increase the incidence of complications of percutaneous biopsy [8,20,21]. If an adequate specimen is not obtained after two passes, an alternative approach should be employed after a suitable period of observation.

Risks and complications

Major and minor complications occur in up to 6% of patients and can be fatal in 0.04 to 0.11% [8,20] (Table 3.3). Major complications of transjugular liver biopsy are reported in 0.6%, with intraperitoneal bleeding in 0.2% due to capsular perforation; mortality is 0.09% [12]. Paediatric cases have higher complication rates with transjugular biopsy [12].

Prospective evaluation does not show differences in bleeding between Menghini and Trucut needles [22], but retrospective studies suggest more complications with Trucut needles [8]. No studies have compared the newer (but more expensive) spring loaded Trucut needles (e.g. Temno, Quikcore) with the Menghini needle.

The usual indicators of complications following biopsy are severe pain (either shoulder tip or abdominal) unrelieved by a single injection of pethidine, hypotension and tachycardia. The presence of all or some of the signs should prompt the physician to recommend the patient is observed overnight and if ongoing, investigate and treat. Bleeding may be a life-threatening event, particularly if not detected immediately, so that prompt recognition is essential (see below).

Pleurisy and perihepatitis

A friction rub caused by fibrinous perihepatitis or pleurisy may be heard on the next day. It is of little consequence and pain subsides with analgesics. A chest X-ray may show a small pneumothorax.

Haemorrhage (Fig. 3.5)

In a series of 9212 biopsies, there were 10 (0.11%) fatal and 22 (0.24%) non-fatal haemorrhages [20]. Malignancy, age, female sex and number of passes were the only predictable factors for bleeding. Bleeding might be related to factors other than clotting diathesis, such as the failure of mechanical compression of the needle tract by elastic tissue [23].

Bleeding from the puncture wound usually consists of a thin trickle lasting 10–60 s and the total blood loss is only 5–10 mL. Serious haemorrhage is usually intraperitoneal but may be intrathoracic from an intercostal artery. The bleeding results from perforation of distended portal or hepatic veins or aberrant arteries. The occasional laceration of a major intrahepatic vessel cannot be avoided. In some cases, a tear of the liver follows deep breathing *during* the intercostal procedure.

Perforation of the capsule with intraperitoneal haemorrhage may rarely follow transvenous biopsy, but this should be apparent at the time of biopsy [12].

Spontaneous cessation of bleeding can occur, but otherwise angiography followed by transcatheter embolization is usually successful. Laparotomy is indicated if bleeding continues despite embolization, or when a large haematoma requires evacuation. The threshold for laparotomy may be lower in the transplant patient, in whom arterial embolization carries the risk of major bile duct injury.

Severe haemothorax usually responds to blood transfusion and chest aspiration.

Intrahepatic haematomas

At 2–4h post-biopsy, intrahepatic haematomas are detected by ultrasound in only about 2% [24]. This is probably an underestimate as the haematomas remain isoechoic for the first 24–48h and are not detectable by ultrasound. The day after biopsy, haematomas, usually asymptomatic, are detected in 23% [25]. They can cause fever, rises in serum transaminases, a fall in haematocrit and, if large, right upper quadrant tenderness and an enlarging liver. They may be seen in the arterial phase of a dynamic CT scan as triangular hyperdense segments. Occasionally, haematomas are followed by delayed haemorrhage.

Haemobilia

Haemobilia follows bleeding from a damaged hepatic vessel, artery or vein, into the bile duct (Fig. 3.6). It is marked by biliary colic with enlargement and tenderness of the liver and sometimes the gallbladder. The diagnosis is confirmed by ultrasound, magnetic resonance (MR) cholangiography or endoscopic retrograde cholangiopancreatography (ERCP). It may be treated by hepatic arterial embolization. However, spontaneous recovery is usual. Endoscopic drainage/ sphincterotomy may be required to remove clotted blood from the biliary tree.

Arteriovenous fistula

An arteriovenous fistula may be shown by contrast enhanced CT and/or by hepatic arteriography (Figs 3.7, 3.8). The fistula may close spontaneously, otherwise it can be treated by direct hepatic arterial catheterization and embolization of the feeding artery.

Biliary peritonitis

This is the second commonest complication after haemorrhage. It was seen 49 times after 123 000 biopsies, with 12 deaths. The bile usually comes from the gallbladder, which may be in an unusual position, or from dilated bile ducts. Biliary scintigraphy demonstrates the leak [26]. Surgical management is usually necessary, although ERCP and nasobiliary drainage/ stenting may be used for biliary leak and localized peritonitis.

Puncture of other organs

Puncture of organs such as the kidney or colon are a recognized, but fortunately rare, complication, and often are asymptomatic.

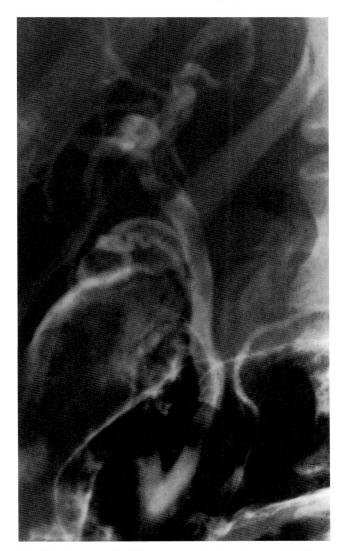

Fig. 3.6. Haemobilia following needle liver biopsy. ERCP shows linear filling defects in the common bile duct.

Infection

Transient bacteraemia is relatively common, particularly in patients with cholangitis. Septicaemia is rarer. Patients with mechanical heart valves should be given antibacterial prophylaxis. Blood cultures are usually positive for *Escherichia coli*.

Carcinoid crisis

This can follow percutaneous biopsy [27].

Sampling variability

Liver biopsy histopathology is only a part of formulating a diagnosis in liver disease. Together with the other

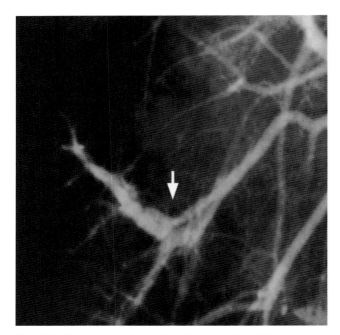

Fig. 3.7. Hepatic arteriography taken post liver biopsy shows an arteriovenous fistula (arrow).

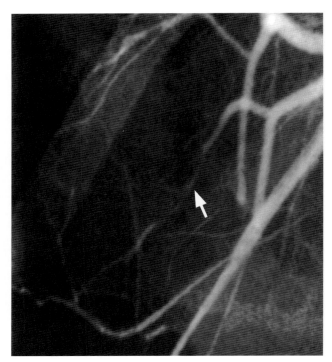

Fig. 3.8. Same patient as in Fig. 3.7. The arteriovenous fistula has been successfully embolized (arrow).

investigations, it can be an important part of the overall picture. By itself, it can be irrelevant or confusing. Given the risks of liver biopsy to the patient, the information available in the biopsy should be maximized by insisting upon close clinicopathological correlation.

Although a biopsy sample is such a small fraction (approx 1/50000th) of the liver it is often sufficiently representative to be of diagnostic value [28]. Some histopathological features, such as cholestasis, steatosis, inflammation and fibrosis related to chronic viral hepatitis, are usually diffuse enough for reliable assessment provided that minimum standards of biopsy adequacy are recognized. When the biopsy is inadequate for the clinical question being considered, it is incumbent on the histopathologist to state this in the biopsy assessment. Therefore it is essential that the histopathologist is informed properly about the clinical context of the biopsy. Poor clinical information and statements such as 'abnormal LFTs' or 'database negative' or 'the pathologist should be blinded' are not appropriate to the diagnostic situation and can be misleading and dangerous. Traditionally, a biopsy containing six portal tracts has been considered adequate for diagnosis [28]. Recently, a reproducible assessment of chronic viral hepatitis (the relevant studies have mostly been concerned with HCV) has been considered as needing a sample containing at least 11 complete portal tracts (i.e. ~20 mm of a biopsy taken with a 1.4 mm internal diameter (16 G) needle, and progressively longer samples of thinner biopsies) [29]. Small, inadequate samples underestimate the severity of

the disease. However, specific studies are needed to establish the adequacy of sample size for each individual disease, and thus to establish the degree of confidence that can be placed on the particular sample that happens to be available.

Focal diseases are particularly prone to sampling error. Granulomas, tumour deposits and abscesses may be missed. When the diameter of the needle is less than that of cirrhotic nodules, nodularity will not be evident and cirrhosis will be underdiagnosed. Macronodular cirrhosis, and the increasing use of thinner needles are especially problematic. Misdiagnosis is often due to smallness of the sample, especially failure to obtain portal tracts, or the focal nature of the disease process, or in particular the inexperience of the interpreter.

Interobserver variation is lessened by improving the adequacy of liver biopsy specimens [30]. Using the 1.6 G Menghini needle, a liver biopsy from a normal adult contains six portal tracts per linear centimetre of tissue [31]. The diagnostic yield may be improved if three consecutive samples could be obtained by redirecting the biopsy needle through a single percutaneous entry site, but this unacceptably increases the complication rate [21]. Multiple passes are more safely performed with the transjugular route and indeed four passes provide very adequate specimens [13,14]. Fibrous tissue is increased under the capsule in operative biopsies and this may give a false impression of the liver as a whole. Operative biopsies may also show artefactual change such as patchy loss of glycogen, haemorrhage, polymorph infiltration and even focal necrosis. These are presumably related to the effects of trauma, circulatory changes and hypoxia.

Naked-eye appearances

A satisfactory biopsy is 2–4 cm long and weighs 20–40 mg.

The cirrhotic liver tends to crumble into fragments of irregular contour. The fatty liver has a pale greasy look and floats in the formol–saline fixative. The liver containing malignant deposits is often dull white in colour. The liver from a patient with Dubin–Johnson hyperbilirubinaemia is diffusely chocolate coloured.

In cholestatic jaundice, the green central areas contrast with the less green periportal areas. The vascular centres of lobules in hepatic congestion may be obvious, and pathologists sometimes compare this mottled appearance with the cut surface of a nutmeg. The liver after paracetamol (acetaminophen) poisoning has a similar macroscopical appearance.

Preparation of the specimen

The biopsy is usually fixed in 10% formol–saline. The time taken to fix a small piece of tissue such as a liver biopsy sample is less than for a larger surgical resection specimen. Fixation at room temperature, and routine tissue processing takes about 12 h, and special histotechnical methods can be used to achieve faster fixation, and processing. Routine stains include haematoxylin and eosin and stains for connective tissue (for example reticulin, Masson's trichrome, chromotrope aniline blue, picroSirius red). Liver biopsy specimens are frequently stained for iron (Perls) and by the diastase/PAS (periodic acid–Schiff) methods. Orcein staining is also useful. This demonstrates: dark brown elastic fibres; hepatitis B surface antigen in the hepatocyte cytoplasm as a uniform, finely brown material; and copper-associated protein in lysosomes as black–brown granules in the periportal area in chronic cholestasis and more irregularly in Wilson's disease.

Biopsy material (at least 3 mm in length) can be removed from paraffin blocks and analysed retrospectively for iron and copper content by atomic absorption spectrophotometry [32]. If iron overload is suspected, the unfixed specimen must not be placed in saline as this leads to rapid loss of iron.

Frozen sections are needed to demonstrate lipids. These are stained with fat stains such as Oil Red O.

Small samples for electron microscopy are rapidly fixed in glutaraldehyde and preserved at 4°C until processed. Electron microscopy can be valuable for diagnosis of tumours of uncertain origin and storage disorders, including Wilson's disease, Niemann–Pick disease and Dubin–Johnson syndrome.

Cytological preparations are made by smearing the aspirated material on a slide.

Interpretation

The normal liver architecture is based on an ordered, repeating lobular structural unit which is about 1 mm in diameter. Portal tracts have a regular relationship to centrilobular outflow venules. The blood feeding into the sinusoids comes from both the hepatic artery and the portal vein branches, and the drainage is via the terminal hepatic venules, which are tributaries of the hepatic vein. Hepatocytes are polygonal cells arranged in one cell thick liver cell plates. They are stable cells, with a remarkable ability to divide and regenerate in response to a stimulus, such as surgical resection. Bile drainage begins with the bile canaliculi (formed by the contact surfaces of hepatocytes) which drain into thin-walled channels (canals of Hering and bile ductules), and then into interlobular bile ducts in portal tracts. These drain into larger septal ducts, segmental ducts, and main right and left hepatic ducts. Portal tracts contain branches of the hepatic artery, portal vein and bile duct (the portal triad), set in fibroelastic connective tissue. The meeting of the portal tract with the limiting plate of hepatocytes is called the interface, and this is one of the special sites of inflammatory activity in hepatitis. This structural organization is essential to normal liver function, as well as being a morphological first step to the recognition of liver disease.

Cells other than hepatocytes and biliary cells reside in the liver, including: Kupffer cells (macrophages attached to the endoluminal surface of the sinusoidal endothelium, which have a mainly phagocytic function); lymphocytes such as pit cells (natural killer lymphocytes—also attached to the endoluminal surface of the endothelium—which have a cytotoxic function, e.g. against virus infected hepatocytes); and hepatic stellate cells (also known as Ito cells, which lie in the space of Disse, and in their quiescent state are involved with the storage of vitamin A, but when activated in response to hepatic injury they can transform into myofibroblast-like cells and make collagen). Detailed liver biopsy appearances of specific hepatic diseases are described in individual chapters, and detailed histology can be found in Klatskin and Conn [33], Scheuer and Lefkowitch [34] and Burt *et al.* [35].

Indications (Table 3.4) [5]

Liver biopsy can be used to: confirm or refute the clinical diagnosis; identify additional clinically unsuspected

Table 3.4. Indications for liver biopsy

Drug-related hepatitis
Chronic hepatitis
Cirrhosis
Liver disease in the alcoholic
Intrahepatic (ductopenic) cholestasis
Infective conditions
Storage diseases
Posthepatic transplantation
Complications of renal transplantation
Space-occupying lesions
Unexplained hepatomegaly or enzyme elevations

conditions; assess severity, progression and complications of disease; and evaluate response to and complications of treatment.

The numbers of liver biopsies are said to be falling due to increasing use of cholangiography, imaging, virological and immunological diagnostic tools, but there are few reliable data to support this contention. As the so-called 'non-invasive' technologies answer some of the clinical questions for which liver biopsy was necessary previously, other clinical questions and indications for biopsy are emerging. Liver biopsy can be considered a part of the general assessment of patients with liver disease. A recent position paper has stated [36]: 'The use of liver biopsy to obtain tissue for histological interpretation is a long-standing pillar of the practice and science of hepatology and remains a standard for diagnosis and treatment'.

Currently, liver biopsies are rarely performed in patients with typical acute jaundice. The possibility of tumour seeding, which is about 2.3% (without ablative techniques) [37], has to be taken into account when biopsy of patients with malignant tumours is being considered. Patients with typical primary biliary cirrhosis and positive serum mitochondrial antibodies may not need a biopsy for diagnosis. Neither may patients with genotype 2 chronic hepatitis C without other risk factors for chronic liver disease. Formerly, biopsy was not required for patients with fatty liver secondary to obesity but, currently, biopsy is used to distinguish between simple fatty liver and steatohepatitis. The management of patients following hepatic transplantation nowadays often includes liver biopsy.

Drug-related liver disease. This can be difficult to identify histopathologically and the history is essential. Sometimes the histopathological distinction from acute viral hepatitis is impossible.

Chronic hepatitis. This remains an important indication. Biopsy is needed for diagnosis and to follow the progress of disease and the effects of treatment [38]. Formal sys-

tematic assessment can be made of chronic viral hepatitis related inflammation (grading) and fibrosis/architectural damage (staging) [39]. Different histopathological 'scoring' systems for these formal assessments have been proposed [40]. Such histopathological assessment systems are often misunderstood, and it is important to appreciate that the 'scores' generated are neither numbers nor measurements, but descriptions [41] (Fig. 3.9). At best the scores are ordered categorical assignments, and appropriate statistical methodology must be used to analyse the scores [41].

Alcohol-related disease. Liver biopsy is used for diagnosis, management (identification of active steatohepatitis) and prognosis (disease stage).

Cholestasis. Extra-hepatic cholestasis can usually be diagnosed by cholangiography with imaging and without the need for liver biopsy. Biopsy is particularly useful in characterizing small duct disease when the biopsy shows ductopenia in the absence of any radiological changes.

Infections. These include tuberculosis, brucellosis, syphilis, histoplasmosis, coccidioidomycosis, pyogenic infection, leptospirosis, amoebiasis and opportunistic infections such as herpes, cytomegalovirus and cryptosporidiosis. When indicated, the appropriate stains for the causative organism should be performed and a portion of the biopsy cultured.

Fever. Liver biopsy is useful in elucidating the cause of fever of unknown origin [16].

Storage diseases. These include amyloidosis and glycogen disease. Haemochromatosis and Wilson's disease can be diagnosed and the effect of therapy is assessed by serial biopsies.

Liver transplant. Liver biopsy is useful in the pretransplant work-up. Post-transplant problems include rejection [42], recurrent or *de novo* hepatitis, including autoimmune hepatitis, ductopenic rejection, infections and biliary problems. Liver biopsy is essential to unravel these complications.

Renal transplants. Liver biopsy is useful in evaluating the chronic liver disease in recipients of kidney transplants [43].

Space-occupying lesions. These are diagnosed by direct biopsy under imaging control.

Other indications. These include obscure hepatomegaly or splenomegaly, and abnormal biochemical tests of

Appearance	Ishak stage: Categorical description	Ishak stage: Categorical assignment	Fibrosis measurement*
	No fibrosis (normal)	0	1.9%
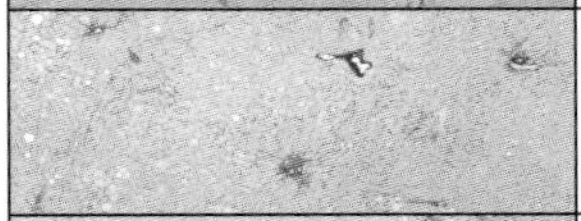	Fibrous expansion of some portal areas ± short fibrous septa	1	3.0%
	Fibrous expansion of most portal areas ± short fibrous septa	2	3.6%
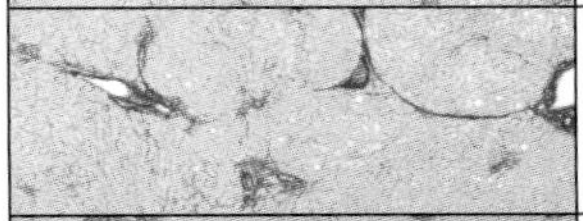	Fibrous expansion of most portal areas with occasional portal to portal (P-P) bridging	3	6.5%
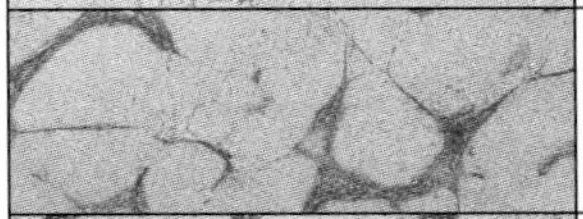	Fibrous expansion of portal areas with marked bridging (portal to portal (P-P) as well as portal to central (P-C))	4	13.7%
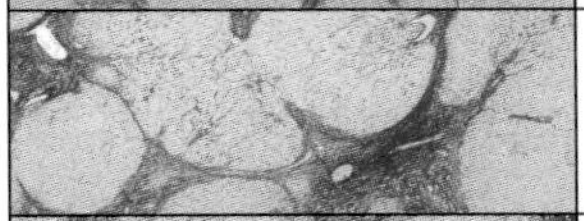	Marked bridging (P-P and/or P-C), with occasional nodules (incomplete cirrhosis)	5	24.3%
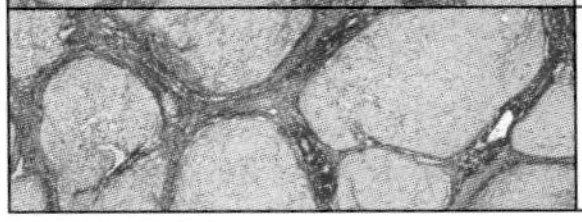	Cirrhosis, probable or definite	6	27.8%

Fig. 3.9. Stage components of the Ishak system. * Proportion (%) of area of illustrated section showing Sirius red staining for collagen (collagen proportionate area). Histopathological chronic liver disease stage 'scores' are descriptive categorical assignments which are different from liver fibrosis measurements. (From [41].)

uncertain cause, particularly where fatty liver is suspected.

Special methods [34]

The new disciplines of genomics, and proteomics and other molecular techniques require well-characterized patient and tissue databases, and archived tissue with appropriate patient consent and ethical approval to achieve their potential. Detailed description of all of the ways in which liver tissue can be explored in the laboratory is not possible in this chapter, and the established diagnostic special tissue investigations are described in other chapters. However, the most important point is to realize is that liver tissue is an extremely valuable resource and its uses are limited only by current knowledge and our ability to formulate the right questions [44]. Hepatopathology is not merely the provision of representational images of liver disease at the microscopic level, but the biopsy itself or a tissue archive with application of appropriate molecular techniques is a very valuable resource.

Bile canaliculi may be shown by staining for adenosine triphosphatase (ATPase) and glucose-6-phosphatase. Electron microscopy may be combined with histochemistry. ATPase is localized to the microvilli of the canaliculi and 5-nucleotidase to the microvilli of the sinusoidal border. Acid phosphatase is found in Kupffer cells, degenerating foci and regenerating nodules; alkaline phosphatase defines cholangioles.

Immunohistochemical stains may be used to demonstrate antigens of viral hepatitis A, B, C, D and E, as well as herpes and adenovirus. Immunohistochemistry is also used to diagnose amyloid disease, α_1-antitrypsin deficiency, and IgG4-related autoimmune hepatitis.

Markers for bile duct epithelial cells such as cytokeratins 7 and 19 are useful in cholestatic disorders and especially for ductular reactions and ductopenia. Immunostaining for specific tumour markers may be useful in detecting the origin of tumour metastases and distinguishing hepatocellular carcinoma from cholangiocarcinoma. Immunostaining for CD34 (which reveals the capillarized sinusoids of hepatocellular carcinomas [45]), glypican-3 and HSP-70 can help to identify hepatocellular carcinomas. Immunostaining for β-catenin, L-FABP, GS, SAA and CRP help to characterize the newly described variants of liver cell adenoma [46].

In situ hybridization techniques, using complementary DNA or RNA sequences, are being increasingly used to assess viral infection, for instance cytomegalovirus, Epstein–Barr virus (EBV), herpes virus and hepatitis B or C viruses (HBV or HCV).

Polymerase chain reaction (PCR) is useful in human immunodeficiency virus (HIV), HBV and HCV infections, but the whole biopsy is required for the analysis. Tissue retrieved from the paraffin block can be used for mycobacterial PCR after histopathological sections have been cut.

Mononuclear cells in liver biopsies may be studied by histochemistry using monoclonal antibodies specific for various antigens [47]. Flow cytometry is used to immunotype lymphocytes from fresh liver tissue.

Polarized light is useful for showing: malarial and schistosomal pigment; amyloid after Congo red staining; and protoporphyrin crystals in protoporphyria.

Ultraviolet light may help to identify porphyrins in fresh frozen sections from patients with porphyria cutanea tarda.

Quantitative analysis of liver biopsy specimens has been plagued by sampling and methodological difficulties. The possibility of a simple, practical quantitative assessment (collagen proportionate area) of liver biopsy fibrosis using image analysis of picroSirius red stained histological sections, and which does not compromise routine diagnostic histopathology, has been described recently. This type of measurement is essential if the emerging antifibrosis therapies are to be evaluated properly [48].

References

1 Schüpfer F. De la possibilité de faire 'intra vitam' un diagnostic histo-pathologique précis des maladies du foie et de la rate. *Sem. Méd.* 1907; **27**: 229.
2 Axenfeld H, Brass K. Klinische und bioptische Untersuchungen über den sogenannten Icterus catarrhalis. *Frankfurt Z. Pathol.* 1942; **57**: 147.
3 Iversen P, Roholm K. On aspiration biopsy of the liver, with remarks on its diagnostic significance. *Acta. Med. Scand.* 1939; **102**: 1.
4 Sherlock S. Aspiration liver biopsy, technique and diagnostic application. *Lancet* 1945; **ii**: 397.
5 Grant A, Neuberger J. Guidelines of the use of liver biopsy in clinical practice. British Society of Gastroenterology. *Gut* 1999; **45** (Suppl. 4): iIVI–1IVII.
6 Menghini G. One-second needle biopsy of the liver. *Gastroenterology* 1958; **35**: 190–199.
7 Colombo M, del Ninno E, de Franchis R *et al.* Ultrasound assisted percutaneous liver biopsy: superiority of the Trucut over the Menghini needle for diagnosis of cirrhosis. *Gastroenterology* 1988; **95**: 487–489.
8 Piccinino F, Sagnelli E, Pasquale G *et al.* Complications following percutaneous liver biopsy. A multicentre retrospective study on 68276 biopsies. *J. Hepatol.* 1986; **2**: 165–173.
9 Cholongitas E, Senzolo M, Standish R *et al.* A systematic review of the quality of liver biopsy specimens. *Am. J. Clin. Pathol.* 2006; **125**: 710–721.
10 Papini E, Pacella CM, Rozzi Z *et al.* A randomized trial of ultra sound guided anterior subcostal liver biopsy versus the conventional Menghini technique. *J. Hepatol.* 1991; **13**: 291–297.
11 Pisha T, Gabriel S, Therneau T *et al.* Cost-effectiveness of ultrasound-guided liver biopsy. *Hepatology* 1998; **27**: 1220.
12 Kalambokis G, Manousou P, Vibhakorn S *et al.* Transjugular liver biopsy—indications, adequacy, quality of specimens and complications—a systematic review. *J. Hepatol.* 2007; **47**: 284–294.
13 Cholongitas E, Quaglia A, Samonakis D *et al.* Transjugular liver biopsy in patients with diffuse liver disease: comparison of 3 cores with 1 or 2 cores for accurate histological interpretation. *Liver Int.* 2007; **27**: 646–653.
14 Vibhakorn S, Cholongitas E, Kalambokis G *et al.* A comparison of four versus three pass transjugular biopsy using a 19G Tru-Cut needle and a randomised study using a cassette to prevent biopsy fragmentation. *Cardiovasc. Intervent. Radiol.* 2009; **32**: 508–513.
15 Sawyerr AM, McCormick PA, Tennyson GS *et al.* A comparison of transjugular and plugged percutaneous liver biopsy in patients with impaired coagulation. *J. Hepatol.* 1993; **17**: 81–85.
16 Pagliaro L, Rinaldi F, Craxi A *et al.* Percutaneous blind biopsy vs. laparoscopy with guided biopsy in diagnosis of cirrhosis: a prospective, randomised trial. *Dig. Dis. Sci.* 1983; **28**: 39–43.
17 Buscarini L, Fornari F, Bolondi L *et al.* Ultrasound-guided fine-needle biopsy of focal liver lesions: techniques, diagnostic accuracy and complications. *J. Hepatol.* 1990; **11**: 344–348.
18 Glenthoj A, Sehested M, Torp-Pedersen S. Diagnostic reliability of histological and cytological fine needle biopsies from focal liver lesions. *Histopathology* 1989; **15**: 435–439.
19 Holtz T, Moseley RH, Scheiman JM. Liver biopsy in fever of unknown origin: a reappraisal. *J. Clin. Gastroenterol.* 1993; **17**: 29–32.
20 McGill DB, Rakela J, Zinsmeister AR *et al.* A 21-year experience with major haemorrhage after percutaneous liver biopsy. *Gastroenterology* 1990; **99**: 1396–1400.
21 Maharaj B, Bhoora IG. Complications associated with percutaneous needle biopsy of the liver when one, two or three specimens are taken. *Postgrad. Med. J.* 1992; **68**: 964–967.
22 Forssell P, Bonkowsky H, Anderson P, Howell D. Intrahepatic haematoma after aspiration liver biopsy. A prospective randomized trial using two different needles. *Dig. Dis. Sci.* 1981; **26**: 631–635.
23 Ewe K. Bleeding after liver biopsy does not correlate with indices of peripheral coagulation. *Dig. Dis. Sci.* 1981; **26**: 388–393.
24 Hederstrom E, Forsberg L, Floren C-H *et al.* Liver biopsy complications monitored by ultrasound. *J. Hepatol.* 1989; **8**: 94–98.
25 Minuk GY, Sutherland LR, Wiseman DA *et al.* Prospective study of the incidence of ultrasound-detected intrahepatic and subcapsular haematomas in patients randomized to 6

or 24h of bed rest after percutaneous liver biopsy. *Gastroenterology* 1987; **92**: 290–293.

26 Veneri RJ, Gordon SC, Fink-Bennett D. Scintigraphic and culdoscopic diagnosis of bile peritonitis complicating liver biopsy. *J. Clin. Gastroenterol.* 1989; **11**: 571–573.

27 Bissonnette RT, Gibney RG, Berry BR *et al*. Fatal carcinoid crisis after percutaneous fine-needle biopsy of hepatic metastasis: case report and literature review. *Radiology* 1990; **174**: 751–752.

28 Bravo AA, Sheth SG, Chopra S. Liver biopsy. *N. Engl. J. Med.* 2001; **344**: 495–500.

29 Guido M, Rugge M. Liver biopsy sampling in chronic viral hepatitis. *Semin. Liver Dis.* 2004; **24**: 89–97.

30 Rousselet MC, Michalak S, Dupre F *et al*. Sources of variability in histological scoring of chornic viral hepatitis. *Hepatology* 2005; **41**: 257–264.

31 Crawford AR, Lin X-Z, Crawford JM. The normal adult human liver biopsy: a quantitative reference standard. *Hepatology* 1998; **28**: 323–331.

32 Olynyk JK, O'Neill R, Britton RS *et al*. Determination of hepatic iron concentration in fresh and paraffin-embedded tissue: diagnostic implications. *Gastroenterology* 1994; **106**: 674–677.

33 Klatskin G, Conn HO. *Histopathology of the Liver*, Vols 1 and 2. New York: Oxford University Press, 1993.

34 Scheuer PJ, Lefkowitch JH. *Liver Biopsy Interpretation*, 7th edn. Elsevier Saunders, Philadelphia, 2006.

35 Burt AD, Portmann BC, Ferrell LD, eds. *MacSween's Pathology of the Liver*, 5th edn. Churchill Livingstone Elsevier, 2007.

36 Rockey DC, Caldwell SH, Goodman ZD *et al*; American Association for the Study of Liver Diseases Position Paper. Liver biopsy. *Hepatology* 2009; **49**: 1017–1044.

37 Stigliano R, Marelli L, Yu D *et al*. Seeding following percutaneous diagnostic and therapeutic approaches for hepatocellular carcinoma. What is the risk and the outcome? Seeding risk for percutaneous approach of HCC. *Cancer Treat. Rev.* 2007; **33**: 437–447.

38 Bedossa P, Carrat F. Liver biopsy: The best, not the gold standard. *J. Hepatol.* 2009; **50**: 1–3.

39 Desmet VJ, Gerber M, Hoofnagle JH *et al*. Classification of chronic hepatitis: diagnosis, grading and staging. *Hepatology* 1994; **19**: 1513–1520.

40 Goodman ZD. Grading and staging systems for inflammation and fibrosis in chronic liver diseases. *J. Hepatol.* 2007; **47**: 598–607.

41 Standish R, Cholongitas E, Dhillon A *et al*. An appraisal of the histopathological assessment of liver fibrosis. *Gut* 2006; **55**: 569–578.

42 Datta-Gupta S, Hudson A, Burroughs AK *et al*. Grading of cellular rejection after orthotopic liver transplantation. *Hepatology* 1995; **21**: 46–57.

43 Rao KV, Anderson WR, Kasiske BL *et al*. Value of liver biopsy in the evaluation and management of chronic liver disease in renal transplant recipients. *Am. J. Med.* 1993; **94**: 241–250.

44 Desmet VJ. The amazing universe of hepatic microstructure. *Hepatology* 2009; **50**: 333–344.

45 Dhillon AP, Colombari R, Savage K, Scheuer PJ. An immunohistochemical study of the blood vessels within primary hepatocellular tumours. *Liver* 1992; **12**: 311–318.

46 Bioulac-Sage P, Rebouissou S, Thomas C *et al*. Hepatocellular adenoma subtype classification using molecular markers and immunohistochemistry. *Hepatology* 2007; **46**: 740–748.

47 Hata K, Van Thiel DH, Herberman RB *et al*. Phenotypic and functional characteristics of lymphocytes isolated from liver biopsy specimens from patients with active liver disease. *Hepatology* 1992; **15**: 816–823.

48 Calvaruso V, Burroughs AK *et al*. Computer-assisted image analysis of liver collagen: relationship to Ishak scoring and hepatic venous pressure gradient. *Hepatology* 2009; **49**: 1236–1244.

CHAPTER 4
Haematological Disorders of the Liver

Pramod K. Mistry & Dhanpat Jain
Yale School of Medicine, New Haven, CT, USA

Learning points

- Coagulopathy complicates acute and chronic liver diseases.
- Platelet and erythrocyte abnormalities in chronic liver disease lead to bleeding tendency and haemolytic anaemia, respectively.
- Aplastic anaemia may complicate non-A to E hepatitis.
- The liver is involved prominently in myelo- and lymphoproliferative disorders.
- Significant hepatic morbidity may arise due to haemoglobinopathies.
- Lysosomal storage diseases commonly involve the liver resulting in a spectrum of disease ranging from benign hepatomegaly to advanced liver disease.

General features

Hepatocellular failure, portal hypertension and jaundice may affect the blood picture. Chronic liver disease is usually accompanied by 'hypersplenism'. Diminished erythrocyte survival is frequent. In addition, both parenchymal hepatic disease and cholestatic jaundice may produce blood coagulation defects. Dietary deficiencies, alcoholism, bleeding and difficulties in hepatic synthesis of proteins used in blood formation or coagulation add to the complexity of the problem.

Spontaneous bleeding, bruising and purpura, together with a history of bleeding after minimal trauma such as venepuncture, are more important indications of a bleeding tendency in patients with liver disease than laboratory tests.

Blood volume

Plasma volume is frequently increased in patients with cirrhosis, especially with ascites and also with long-standing obstructive jaundice or with hepatitis. This hypervolaemia may partially, and sometimes totally, account for a low peripheral haemoglobin or erythrocyte level. Total circulating haemoglobin is reduced in only about half the patients.

Erythrocyte changes

The red cells may be *hypochromic*. This is often due to gastrointestinal bleeding, leading to iron deficiency. In portal hypertension, anaemia follows gastro-oesophageal bleeding and is enhanced by thrombocytopenia and disturbed blood coagulation. In cholestasis or cirrhosis of the alcoholic, haemorrhage may be from an ulcer or gastritis. Epistaxis, bruising and bleeding gums add to the anaemia.

The erythrocytes are usually *normocytic*. This is a combination of the microcytosis of chronic blood loss and the macrocytosis inherent in patients with liver disease. Thus the red cell membrane cholesterol and phospholipid content and/or ratio is changed and this results in various morphological abnormalities, including thin macrocytes and target cells.

Thin macrocytes are frequent and are associated with a normoblastic marrow. These resolve when liver function improves.

Target cells are also thin macrocytes. They are found in both hepatocellular and cholestatic jaundice. They are flat, macrocytic and have an increased surface area and increased resistance to osmotic lysis. They are particularly prominent in cholestasis where a rise in bile acids may contribute by inhibiting lecithin cholesterol acyl transferase (LCAT) activity [1]. The red cell membrane LCAT is decreased, resulting in loading of the membrane with both cholesterol and lecithin. Membrane fluidity is unchanged.

Spur cells are cells with unusual, thorny projections. They are also termed *acanthocytes* (Fig. 4.1). They are

Sherlock's Diseases of the Liver and Biliary System, Twelfth Edition. Edited by James S. Dooley, Anna S.F. Lok, Andrew K. Burroughs, E. Jenny Heathcote.
© 2011 by Blackwell Publishing Ltd. Published 2011 by Blackwell Publishing Ltd.

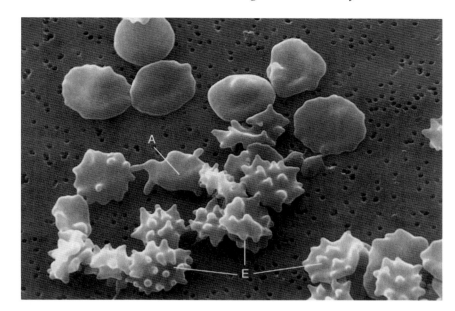

Fig. 4.1. Scanning electron micrograph of abnormal red cells from a patient with alcoholic hepatitis, showing echinocytes (E) at various stages of development, and an acanthocyte (A). (Courtesy of Dr J. Owen and Ms J. Lewin.)

associated with far advanced liver disease, usually in alcoholics. Severe anaemia and haemolysis are also found. Their appearance is a bad prognostic sign. They disappear after liver transplantation [2]. The mechanism of their formation is unclear but they may be derived from *echinocytes*, which are also called burr cells [3]. These spiculated cells are not usually seen on dry blood films but are present on wet films or scanning electron microscopy in many patients with liver disease. They form because of an interaction with the abnormal HDL found in liver disease [3]. There is excess accumulation of unesterified cholesterol compared with phospholipid, with resultant reduced membrane fluidity and the formation of thorny projections. Reticuloendothelial cells in the spleen modify these rigid cells with removal of membrane.

Alcoholics show genuine *thick macrocytes*, which are probably related to the toxic effect of alcohol on the bone marrow. Folic acid and vitamin B_{12} deficiency may contribute.

Bone marrow of chronic hepatocellular failure is hyperplastic and normoblastic. In spite of this, erythrocyte volume is depressed and the marrow therefore does not seem able to compensate completely for the anaemia (*relative marrow failure*).

Folate and vitamin B_{12} metabolism

The liver stores folate and converts it to its active storage form, tetrahydrofolate. Folate deficiency may accompany chronic liver disease, usually in the alcoholic. This is largely due to dietary deficiency. Serum folate levels are low. Folate therapy is useful. The liver also stores vitamin B_{12} [4]. Hepatic levels are reduced in liver

disease. When hepatocytes become necrotic the vitamin is released into the blood and high serum B_{12} levels are recorded. This is shown in hepatitis, active cirrhosis and with primary liver cancer. Values in cholestatic jaundice are normal.

Megaloblastic anaemia is rare with chronic liver disease and vitamin B_{12} therapy is rarely needed.

Erythrocyte survival and haemolytic anaemia

Increased red cell destruction is almost constant in hepatocellular failure and jaundice of all types [5]. This is reflected in erythrocyte polychromasia and reticulocytosis. The mechanism is extremely complex. The major factor is hypersplenism with destruction of red blood cells in the spleen. Also, spur cells have membrane defects, particularly decreased fluidity, and this, with the altered architecture, exacerbates splenic destruction. In some instances, however, the spleen is not the site of erythrocyte destruction. Splenectomy or corticosteroid therapy have little effect [5].

Haemolysis may occur in Wilson's disease (Chapter 27), and this diagnosis is likely in the young patient presenting with haemolysis and liver dysfunction.

Haemolysis may be acute in patients with alcoholic hepatitis who also have hypercholesterolaemia (*Zieve's syndrome*) [6].

Rarely, an autoimmune haemolytic anaemia with a positive Coombs' test is seen in chronic hepatitis, primary biliary cirrhosis and primary sclerosing cholangitis. Haemolytic anaemia may also follow liver transplantation due to 'passenger lymphocytes' in a mismatch donor organ [7] or a delayed transfusion reaction. A syndrome of haemolysis, elevated liver enzymes and a low platelet count (the HELLP syndrome) is a rare complication of the third trimester of pregnancy (Chapter 30) [8]. Haemolysis is a complication of ribavirin therapy due to oxidative damage to the red cell membrane with binding of specific IgG [9].

Aplastic anaemia is a rare complication of acute viral hepatitis, usually type non-A to E hepatitis. It may be fatal but response to intensive immunosuppressive treatment is reported [10]. It may follow liver transplantation [11].

Changes in the leucocytes and platelets

Leucopenia and thrombocytopenia are commonly found in patients with cirrhosis, usually with a mild anaemia ('*hypersplenism*').

Leucocytes

The leucopenia is of the order of $1.5–3.0 \times 10^9/L$, with the depression mainly affecting polymorphs. Occasionally it may be more severe.

Leucocytosis accompanies cholangitis, fulminant hepatitis, alcoholic hepatitis, hepatic abscess and malignant disease. Atypical lymphocytes are found in the peripheral blood in viral infections such as infectious mononucleosis and viral hepatitis.

Platelets

Abnormalities in platelet count and function are common in patients with all forms of liver disease.

Platelet count. In patients with chronic liver disease and portal hypertension, a low platelet count is due in part to increased splenic sequestration and to low thrombopoietin levels. Thus, although platelet counts rise after the insertion of a transjugular intrahepatic portosystemic shunt, they do not return to normal [12]. Plasma concentration of thrombopoietin, the key regulator of platelet function produced mainly by the liver, is reduced in patients with cirrhosis, correlates with platelet count and rises after liver transplantation [13–15].

In chronic liver disease, increased destruction of platelets is minimal and their half-life is normal, calling into question whether there is any biological effect of the IgG and IgM antibodies detected in patients with chronic hepatitis [16,17]. Decreased production of platelets from the bone marrow follows alcohol excess, folic acid deficiency and viral hepatitis.

Platelet function. In particular, aggregation is impaired in patients with cirrhosis, particularly Child's grade C, due to an intrinsic defect and circulating serum factors [18]. There is reduced availability of arachidonic acid for prostaglandin production, and also a reduction in platelet adenosine triphosphate and 5-hydroxytryptamine [19]. Abnormal platelet aggregation due to disseminated intravascular coagulation may be an additional important factor in severe liver failure.

The thrombocytopenia of chronic liver disease (usually $60–90 \times 10^9/L$) is extremely frequent and is largely due to hypersplenism. It is very rarely of clinical significance. Unless the patient is actually suffering from the leucopenia or thrombocytopenia the spleen should not be removed; mere demonstration of a low platelet or leucocyte count is not sufficient. The circulating platelets and leucocytes, although in short supply, are functioning well, in contrast to those of leukaemia. Splenectomy is contraindicated. The mortality in patients with liver disease is high and the operation is liable to be followed by splenic and portal vein thrombosis, which preclude later operations on the portal vein and may make hepatic transplantation more difficult.

The liver and blood coagulation [20–22]

Disturbed blood coagulation in patients with hepatobiliary disease is particularly complex [23]. This is due to the many changes in pathways that lead to fibrin production occurring at the same time as changes in the fibrinolytic process (Fig. 4.2, Table 4.1). Changes in platelet number and function are discussed in the previous section. Despite the complexity of the changes, the end result is abnormal coagulation, which needs therapeutic intervention if there is bleeding or if a procedure is planned that risks haemorrhage. However, there is little relationship between abnormal clotting tests and risk of bleeding [24]. Platelet number and function may be more important than the degree of abnormality of the prothrombin time for risk of bleeding with invasive procedures [25].

The hepatocyte is the principal site of synthesis of all the *coagulation proteins* with the exception of von Willebrand factor and factor VIIIC. The proteins include the vitamin K-dependent factors II, VII, IX and X, also labile factor V, factor VIII, contact factors XI and XII, fibrinogen and fibrin-stabilizing factor XIII. The half-life of all these clotting proteins is very short and hence reductions can rapidly follow acute hepatocellular necrosis. Factor VII is particularly affected with a half-life of 100–300 min.

Vitamin K is a fat-soluble vitamin produced by intestinal bacteria. Deficiency occurs most commonly due to cholestasis, intra- and extrahepatic, but may also follow treatment with bile acid chelators (cholestyramine) or oral antibiotics. The vitamin K-dependent proteins are made in the rough endoplasmic reticulum. They all have a number of glutamic acid residues in their aminoterminal region that must be converted, postribos-

skeleton, is usually a harmless trait, the haemolysis being compensated. It may occasionally develop into active decompensated haemolytic anaemia.

Various enzyme defects

Many of the hereditary non-spherocytic anaemias are now known to be due to various defects in the metabolism of the red cells. They include deficiency of pyruvate kinase or triose phosphate isomerase, or deficiency in the pentose phosphate pathway such as glucose-6-phosphate dehydrogenase (G6PD). These conditions may be of particular importance in the aetiology of neonatal jaundice. The gene responsible for G6PD deficiency has now been cloned and a wide range of mutations recognized. These are beginning to explain the wide spectrum of clinical pictures seen in this condition ranging from haemolysis during the neonatal period, after infection or after the ingestion of certain drugs, to chronic anaemia irrespective of any of these factors. Variants of the gene are now recognized where there is no significant reduction in enzyme activity in red cells [55].

Viral hepatitis can precipitate destruction of G6PD-deficient cells and so cause acute haemolytic anaemia and very high serum bilirubin concentrations.

Sickle cell disease [56,57]

The abnormal haemoglobin crystallizes in the erythrocytes when the oxygen tension is reduced. There are crises of blood destruction with acute attacks of pain. The liver may be affected acutely by sickling crises. There is right upper quadrant pain, fever and increased jaundice, associated with systemic and haematological features of sickling. This should help to differentiate the clinical picture from a common bile duct stone. Fulminant liver failure is rare [58]. A distinct clinical picture of intrahepatic cholestasis is also recognized but is unusual [59]. Histologically there is intracanalicular cholestasis, sinusoidal dilatation, packing of the sinuses by sickled erythrocytes, Kupffer cell hyperplasia and erythrophagocytosis.

There may be chronic elevation of transaminases and/or alkaline phosphatase with hepatic scarring. Several factors have been implicated including microvascular stasis, with recurrent ischaemic episodes, and transfusion-related disease (haemosiderosis and viral hepatitis).

Jaundice accompanying sickle cell disease is always particularly deep, the high serum bilirubin levels being related to the combination of haemolysis and impaired hepatocellular function. Depth of jaundice *per se* should not be regarded as an indication of severity. Concomitant viral hepatitis or obstructed bile ducts lead to exceptionally high serum bilirubin values.

Gallstones are found in 25% of children and 50–70% of adults with homozygous sickle cell disease. They are usually in the gallbladder; duct calculi are rare. In two-thirds of adults the stones are asymptomatic. The high frequency of gallbladder stones may be due in part to changes in gallbladder volume and motility. Elective cholecystectomy may be hazardous and precipitate a sickle crisis [56].

Hepatic histology

Active and healed areas of necrosis may have followed anoxia due to vascular obstruction by impacted sickle cells or by Kupffer cells swollen with phagocytosed erythrocytes following intrahepatic sickling. The widened sinusoids show a foam-like fibrin reticulum within their lumen. This intrasinusoidal fibrin may later result in fibre deposition in the space of Disse and narrowed sinusoids. Bile plugs are prominent. Fatty change is related to anaemia. Multiple transfusions lead to hepatic siderosis which is not accurately reflected by the serum ferritin [60].

The classic findings are of intrasinusoidal sickling, Kupffer cell erythrophagocytosis and ischaemic necrosis. It is difficult to explain the severe liver dysfunction on these histological findings, which have been reported largely on autopsy specimens. Superimposed complications such as septicaemia or viral hepatitis complicate the histological findings [61].

Electron microscopy

The changes are those of hypoxia. There are sinusoidal aggregates of sickled erythrocytes, fibrin and platelets, with increased collagen and occasional basement membrane-like material in the space of Disse.

Clinical features

Asymptomatic patients commonly have raised serum transaminases and hepatomegaly. Hepatitis B and C and iron overload may have complicated transfusions.

In about 10%, the crisis selectively affects the liver. It lasts 2–3 weeks. It is marked by abdominal pain, fever, jaundice, an enlarged tender liver and a rise in serum transaminases. In some patients the crisis is precipitated by *Salmonella* infection or by folic acid deficiency.

Acute liver failure, usually with cholestasis, is rare. Jaundice is very deep with a markedly increased PT and encephalopathy but with only modestly increased serum transaminases. Liver biopsy shows the changes of sickle cell disease with marked zone 2 necrosis and cholestasis. The diagnosis of hepatic sickle crisis from viral hepatitis is difficult. In general, in viral hepatitis pain is less, jaundice deeper and transaminase elevations more prolonged. Liver biopsy and hepatitis viral markers usually help to make the distinction. Exchange transfusion has been successful [58]. Liver transplantation has been attempted successfully in carefully selected patients [62].

Prolonged intrahepatic cholestasis associated with sickle cell anaemia has also responded to exchange transfusion [59].

Acute cholecystitis and choledocholithiasis may simulate hepatic crisis or viral hepatitis. Magnetic resonance, endoscopic or percutaneous cholangiography are important investigations in excluding biliary obstruction. Complications after cholecystectomy are common, and this is indicated only if there is great difficulty in making a distinction from abdominal crisis or where symptoms are clearly related to gallbladder disease. Preoperative exchange transfusion may lessen later complications.

General features include leg ulcers, which are frequent. The upper jaw is protuberant and hypertrophied. The fingers are clubbed. Bone deformities seen radiologically include rarefaction and narrowing of the cortex of the long bones and a 'hair-on-end' appearance in the skull.

Thalassaemia

Crises of red cell destruction and fever and the reactionary changes in bone are similar to those seen in sickle cell disease. The liver shows siderosis and sometimes fibrosis. The haemosiderosis may progress to an actual haemochromatosis and require chelation therapy using desferrioxamine or other chelator therapy (Chapter 26). The stainable iron in the liver cells may be greater in those who have undergone splenectomy (usually performed to reduce blood transfusion requirements) as a storage organ for iron.

Transfusion-acquired hepatitis B and C may lead to chronic liver disease.

Episodes of intrahepatic cholestasis of uncertain nature can also develop. Gallstones may be a complication.

Previously, the commonest cause of death in thalassaemia major was heart failure but the clinical course of the disease is changing with improved therapy including, in particular, iron chelation.

Treatment

This may include folic acid, blood transfusion, iron chelation therapy, antiviral treatment and occasionally splenectomy with pneumococcal vaccination. Bone marrow transplantation may be considered but the survival is worse in those with liver disease [63].

Paroxysmal nocturnal haemoglobinuria [64]

In this rare acquired disease, there is intravascular, complement-mediated haemolysis. The defect is due to mutation of the *PIG-A* gene on chromosome X which results in deficient biosynthesis of the glycosylphosphatidylinositol (GPI) anchor. This leads to an absence of certain proteins on the red cell surface. The cells are sensitive to lysis when the pH of the blood becomes more acid during sleep. During an episode of haemolysis the urine passed in the morning may be brown or reddish-brown due to haemoglobinuria. Diagnosis is made by flow cytometry [65].

Acutely, the patients show a dusky, reddish jaundice and the liver enlarges. Aspartate transaminase may be increased (due to haemolysis) and serum studies show iron deficiency (due to urinary loss of haemoglobin). Liver histology shows some centrizonal necrosis and siderosis.

Hepatic vein thrombosis presenting as Budd–Chiari syndrome may be a complication. Liver histology shows centrizonal haemorrhagic necrosis and some siderosis. Bile duct changes similar to primary sclerosing cholangitis, perhaps due to ischaemia, have also been reported [66].Treatment is with eculizumab which is a monoclonal antibody to the C5 complement protein [67].

Acquired haemolytic anaemia

The haemolysis is due to extracorpuscular causes. Spherocytosis is slight and osmotic fragility only mildly impaired.

The patient is moderately jaundiced. The increased bilirubin is unconjugated, but in severe cases conjugated bilirubin increases and appears in the urine. This may be related to bilirubin overload in the presence of liver damage. Blood transfusion accentuates the jaundice, for transfused cells survive poorly.

The haemolysis may be *idiopathic*. The increased haemolysis is then due to autoimmunization. The Coombs' test is positive.

The *acquired* type may complicate other diseases, especially those involving the reticuloendothelial system. These include Hodgkin's disease, the leukaemias, reticulosarcoma, carcinomatosis and uraemia. The anaemia of hepatocellular jaundice is also partially haemolytic. The Coombs' test is usually negative.

Autoimmune haemolytic anaemia is a rare complication of autoimmune chronic hepatitis and primary biliary cirrhosis.

Wilson's disease may present as a haemolytic crisis (Chapter 27).

Haemolytic disease of the newborn

See Chapter 29.

Incompatible blood transfusion

Chills, fever and backache are followed by jaundice. Urobilinogen is present in the urine. Liver function tests give normal results. In severe cases free haemoglobin is detected in blood and urine. Diagnostic difficulties arise when a patient suffering from a disease that may be complicated by hepatocellular failure or biliary obstruction becomes jaundiced soon after a blood transfusion.

The liver in myelo- and lymphoproliferative disease [68]

The liver contains multipotential cells that can differentiate into reticuloendothelial, myeloid and lymphoid cells. These can be affected by malignant disease (leukaemia, lymphoma), usually in association with systemic disease, but rarely occur as a primary hepatic disease. Reduced haemopoietic activity in the marrow is followed by extramedullary haemopoiesis in the liver. Reticuloendothelial storage diseases affect the liver as well as other organs. This section outlines the involvement of the liver in this broad group of diseases.

The liver is involved to a variable extent, usually with no functional effect, but with mildly abnormal liver function tests. However, liver biopsies are helpful for diagnosis. The infiltrates can be diffuse or focal, and may localize to portal areas, sinusoids, or both. Staining of sections with monoclonal antibodies may be necessary to define the cell type or disease. Involvement in a biopsy may be very focal, so that serial sections may be required. If scanning shows a focal lesion, guided biopsy is worthwhile.

Rarely, fulminant liver failure complicates the primary disease, due to replacement of hepatocytes with malignant cells. This is reported in acute lymphoblastic leukaemia [69] and non-Hodgkin's lymphoma [70]. It is important to differentiate these from liver failure due to viral or drug hepatitis, since liver transplantation is contraindicated when there is underlying haematological malignancy, although one successful case with combination chemotherapy has been reported [70,71].

Acute and chronic abnormalities of liver function tests may be due to treatment. Drugs given should be reviewed. More aggressive chemotherapy has increased hepatotoxic drug reactions. Multiple blood transfusions are a frequent cause of viral hepatitis, particularly hepatitis C and non-A, non-B, non-C, and to a lesser extent type B. This is usually mild in the immunocompromised host. Hepatitis B may be reactivated during cytotoxic or immunosuppressive therapy, and there may be a fulminant hepatitis-like episode following withdrawal of treatment. This is thought to be due to a rebound effect with the return of immunity, and clearance of a large number of hepatocytes containing the virus [72,73].

Appropriate antiviral prophylaxis with entecavir or tenofovir must be given to prevent this, and monitoring for viral resistance instituted.

Gastrointestinal haemorrhage may complicate myeloproliferative diseases, leukaemia or lymphoma. In some this is caused by peptic ulceration or erosions. There may be portal hypertension due to hepatic, portal or splenic vein thrombosis related to a hypercoagulable state. Evidence for a myeloproliferative disorder was found in 14 of 33 patients with non-tumour-related portal vein thrombosis [74].

Occasionally, the portal hypertension is presinusoidal and seems to be secondary to infiltrative lesions in the portal zones and sinusoids. In others, increased blood flow due to splenomegaly may be important. Portal and central zone fibrosis can be related to cytotoxic therapy.

Leukaemia

Myeloid [68]

The enlarged liver is smooth and firm, and the cut section shows small, pale nodules.

Microscopically both portal tracts and sinusoids are infiltrated with immature and mature cells of the myeloid series. The immature cells lie outside the sinusoidal wall.

The portal tracts are enlarged with myelocytes and polymorphs, both neutrophil and eosinophil; round cells are also conspicuous. The liver cell cords are compressed by the leukaemic deposits.

Lymphoid

Macroscopically, the liver is moderately enlarged, with pale areas on section.

Microscopically, the leukaemic infiltration involves mostly the portal tracts, but may also involve the sinusoids. The portal areas are enlarged and contain both mature and immature cells of the lymphatic series. The sinusoids are not affected. The liver cells are normal.

Hairy cell leukaemia

The liver is usually involved although specific clinical and biochemical features are rare. Sinusoidal and portal infiltration with mononuclear 'clear' cells similar to those in spleen and bone marrow is seen with sinusoidal congestion and beading. Angiomatous lesions, usually periportal, consist of blood spaces lined by hairy cells.

Bone marrow transplantation

Liver abnormalities occur at some time in the majority of patients within 12 months of bone marrow

Table 4.3. Hepatobiliary disease and bone marrow transplantation

Problem	Related to
Pre-existing	
Fungal	Granulocytopenia
Viral (hepatitis type B, C)	Blood products
Drug	Medication
Biliary	Stones
Post-transplantation	
Early neutropenic phase (up to 4 weeks)	
acute graft-versus-host disease	Donor marrow
veno-occlusive disease	Cytoreductive therapy
nodular regenerative hyperplasia	
drug induced	Including TPN
Extra-hepatic bacterial sepsis	Bacteria/ endotoxin
fungal	
biliary disease	Sludge
Intermediate (4–15 weeks)*	
Viral	Cytomegalovirus
	Hepatitis type B, C
Late (>15 weeks)	
chronic graft-versus-host disease	Multiorgan disease
chronic viral infection	
fungal	Immunosuppression
tumour recurrence	

*As well as continuing early problems.

transplantation [75]. The changes range from abnormal liver function tests alone, to coagulation abnormalities, ascites and hepatorenal failure. There are many possible causes (Table 4.3); more than one may be responsible at any one time. Pre-existing liver disease increases the risk.

In the first 15 weeks, the most common causes of liver abnormality are acute graft-versus-host disease (GVHD), intrahepatic veno-occlusive disease, drug-induced reactions and infection.

Jaundice and abnormal liver enzyme tests accompany the systemic manifestations of *acute GVHD*—rash and diarrhoea. This usually begins 3–8 weeks post-transplant. The hepatic changes may persist to give cholestatic chronic GVHD with intrahepatic bile duct damage. Chronic GVHD may also develop *de novo*.

The development of jaundice, painful hepatomegaly, weight gain and ascites in the first weeks after bone marrow transplantation suggests a diagnosis of *veno-occlusive disease*. This is due to high-dose cytoreductive therapy given 5–10 days before the marrow infusion. The incidence varies from one report to another, ranging from less than 5% to over 60%, probably reflecting different patient groups, conditioning regimens and diagnostic criteria. Mortality in severely affected individuals is high, around 50%. There is controversy whether histological evidence of venular occlusion is needed for diagnosis. A percutaneous liver biopsy is often contraindicated by a low platelet count, prolonged coagulation tests and ascites. A transjugular liver biopsy should be used [76,77], with a low bleeding risk. This route also allows the wedged hepatic venous pressure to be measured [76],which helps to evaluate prognosis; when the hepatic venous pressure gradient is 20 mmHg or more the prognosis is grave. The histological changes include marked centrizonal haemorrhagic necrosis and obliteration of the central venules, often by fibrin thrombi. It has now been shown that the primary abnormality is the injury to the perivenular sinusoidal endothelium and injury to the central vein is not an essential component; hence the new name for the disease is 'sinusoidal obstruction syndrome'. Four histological abnormalities correlate with the clinical severity of disease: occluded hepatic venules, eccentric luminal narrowing/phlebosclerosis, hepatocyte necrosis and sinusoidal fibrosis [78]. Studies suggest that ursodeoxycholic acid [79], defibrotide [80] and tissue plasminogen activator [81] may be useful in the prevention or treatment of veno-occlusive disease [82].

Opportunistic *fungal* and *bacterial infections* occur during neutropenic periods and may cause abnormal liver function; *viral infections* occur later.

Helpful data to identify the cause of the hepatic abnormality include: (1) timing of the changes related to drugs, chemotherapy, radiation and bone marrow infusion; (2) the dose of cytoreductive (conditioning) therapy; (3) the source of donor marrow; (4) pretreatment viral serology; (5) the degree of immunosuppression; and (6) evidence of systemic disease. Bacteriological and virological data are important. Often more than one process is involved. In one series transvenous liver biopsy provided useful data for patient management in over 80% of cases [76,82].

After bone marrow transplantation, hepatobiliary scintiscanning and ultrasound commonly show abnormalities of questionable clinical significance. Doppler ultrasonography is not reliable for the diagnosis of veno-occlusive disease [83].

Lymphoma

In *Hodgkin's disease*, the infiltrate composed of mature lymphocytes, large pale epithelioid cells, eosinophils,

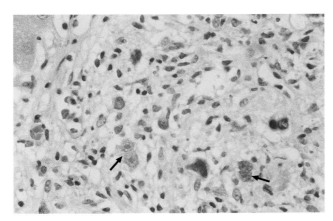

Fig. 4.4. Infiltration of portal zones by Hodgkin's cells including large Reed–Sternberg like cells (arrow) (H & E).

plasma cells and classic Reed–Sternberg cells is seen spreading out from the portal tracts (Fig. 4.4). The classic Reed–Sternberg cells are less often seen on liver biopsies; however, their identification is facilitated by use of immunohistochemical markers (CD30 and CD15).

In patients with known extrahepatic Hodgkin's disease but without obvious Reed–Sternberg cells in sections of the liver, hepatic involvement is suggested by portal infiltrates larger than 1 mm in diameter, changes of acute cholangitis, portal oedema and portal infiltrates with predominance of plasma cells, eosinophils and a few atypical mononuclear Hodgkin's cells. These changes should stimulate a wider search for the diagnostic Reed–Sternberg cell in further sections or application of immunohistochemical markers [84].

Liver can be secondarily involved in virtually all types of *non-Hodgkin's lymphoma* and most often the portal areas show the infiltrate. In small lymphocytic lymphoma (SLL/CLL), a dense, monotonous proliferation of normal-appearing lymphocytes is seen, which may also be seen in the sinusoids. The more aggressive lymphomas tend to form tumour masses with destruction of underlying hepatic parenchyma. The liver may also be involved in angioimmunoblastic T-cell lymphoma (formerly called angioimmunblastic lymphadenopathy), which resembles Hodgkin's disease without the presence of Reed–Sternberg cells.

Liver granulomas with or without tumorous infiltrate can be found in some lymphomas. Caseation without evidence of tuberculosis has also been reported [85].

Paraproteinaemia and amyloidosis may be complications.

Diagnosis of hepatic involvement

Hepatic involvement occurs in about 70% of cases and immediately puts the patient into stage IV [86]. Detection

of hepatic involvement can be extremely difficult. While hepatomegaly suggests liver involvement, its absence does not exclude it. Fever, jaundice and splenomegaly increase the likelihood. Increases in serum γ-glutamyl transpeptidase (γ-GT) and transaminase values are suggestive, although often non-specific.

Focal defects may be shown by ultrasound, CT and MRI scanning. Enlarged abdominal lymph nodes may also be seen.

Needle liver biopsy rarely reveals Hodgkin's tissue if the CT scan is normal. Ultrasound or CT-guided liver biopsy add to the chances of obtaining Hodgkin's tissue. Laparoscopy with liver biopsy may establish the diagnosis in the absence of positive CT scans [87]. A negative needle biopsy does not exclude hepatic involvement, especially if an epithelioid histiocyte reaction is seen. Sinusoidal dilatation in zone 2 and 3 is found in 50% and may be a subtle clue to the diagnosis [88]. Diffuse infiltrates, focal tumour-like masses, increased portal tract cellularity (Fig. 4.5), sinusoidal infiltrates, granulomatous reaction or simply lymphoid aggregates can all be seen [86].

Presentation as jaundice may provide great diagnostic difficulties (Table 4.4). Lymphoma should always be considered in patients with jaundice, fever and weight loss. Rarely, lymphomatous infiltration presents as acute liver failure [70,89].

Jaundice in lymphoma (Table 4.4)

Hepatic infiltrates may be massive or present as space-occupying lesions. Large intrahepatic deposits are the commonest cause of deep jaundice. Histological evidence is essential for diagnosis.

Biliary obstruction is more frequent with non-Hodgkin's lymphoma than with Hodgkin's disease [90]. It is usually due to hilar lymph nodes which are less mobile than those along the common bile duct, which can be pushed aside. Occasionally, the obstructing glands are periampullary. Primary lymphoma of the bile duct itself is reported [91]. Investigations include endoscopic or percutaneous cholangiography and brush cytology. Known lymphoma elsewhere draws attention to this as a possible cause of bile duct obstruction. Differentiation from other causes of extrahepatic biliary obstruction is difficult, and depends on the appearances on imaging and at cholangiography, and the results of cytology and biopsy.

Rarely, an idiopathic intrahepatic, usually cholestatic, jaundice may be seen in Hodgkin's [92] and non-Hodgkin's lymphoma [93]. It is unrelated to deposits in the liver or bile duct compression. Hepatic histology shows canalicular cholestasis. These changes are unrelated to therapy. The diagnosis is difficult and is

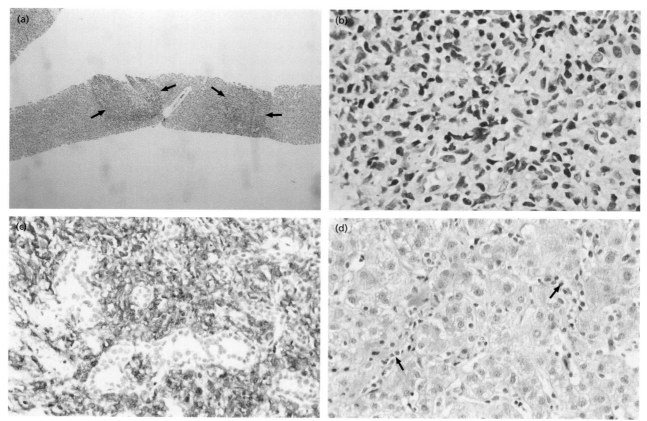

Fig. 4.5. Patterns of hepatic histology in lymphoma. (a) Low power showing dense portal cellular infiltrates (arrows) (H & E). (b) Higher power of portal area showing intermediate and large mononuclear cells. (c) Immunohistochemistry showing that the cells have a B cell phenotype (stained brown with antibody to CD20). Bile ducts are not stained. (d) Sinusoidal pattern of infiltration by lymphoma cells. Occasional atypical mononuclear cells are seen within the hepatic sinusoids (arrows).

made after full investigation. Liver histology may show loss of intrahepatic bile ducts [92].

Rarely, haemolysis causes deep jaundice. It may be due to Coombs' positive autoimmune haemolytic anaemia. Jaundice is exacerbated by bilirubin overload following blood transfusion.

Chemotherapy may cause jaundice. Almost all the cytotoxic drugs can be incriminated if given in sufficient dose. Common culprits include methotrexate, 6-mercaptopurine, cytosine arabinoside, procarbazine and vincristine. Hepatic irradiation in a dose usually exceeding 35 Gy (3500 rad) may cause jaundice.

Post-transfusion viral hepatitis B, C or non-A, non-B, non-C, may affect the immunocompromised patient. Opportunist infections are also encountered.

Primary hepatic lymphoma [94]

Primary hepatic lymphoma is rare and virtually all histological types have been reported. It may present as a solitary mass in 60%, multiple masses in 35% and diffuse disease in 5% [95]. Most are B-cell lymphomas, and less frequently of T-cell type. Amongst primary B-cell lymphoma, low-grade mucosa-associated lymphoid tissue (MALT) have also been reported [96,97]. Another unique primary hepatic lymphoma is hepatosplenic γδ T-cell lymphoma, which is very aggressive, and clinically and histologically mimics acute hepatitis. Presentation of hepatic lymphomas otherwise is mainly with pain, hepatomegaly, a palpable mass and elevated alkaline phosphatase and bilirubin. Fever, night sweats and weight loss occur in 50% of cases. There is no lymphadenopathy. Ultrasound and CT show a non-specific space-occupying lesion in the liver in the majority but there may be diffuse hepatomegaly without tumour. Diagnosis is by liver biopsy. Sometimes histology may initially be confusing suggesting poorly differentiated carcinoma or hepatitis, or showing extensive haemorrhagic necrosis suggesting Budd–Chiari syndrome. Application of immunohistochemical markers and molecular tests to identify the clonal B- or T-cell nature of the infiltrate helps establish the diagnosis.

Table 4.4. Features of jaundice in lymphoma

Feature	Comment
Related to lymphoma	
Hepatic infiltrates	
massive	Scans
tumour mass	Liver biopsy
Biliary obstruction	Usually hilar
	Investigate endoscopic or percutaneous cholangiography
	Non-Hodgkin's usually
Intrahepatic cholestasis	Rare
	Liver biopsy
	'pure' cholestasis
	loss of bile ducts
	Usually Hodgkin's
Haemolysis	Autoimmune haemolytic anaemia
	Positive Coombs' test
Related to therapy	
Chemotherapy	High dose can cause fulminant liver failure (Chapter 24)
Hepatic irradiation	More than 35 Gy (3500 rad) (Chapter 24)
Post-transfusion (hepatitis C)	(Chapter 20)
Hepatitis B reactivation	(Chapter 18)
Opportunist infections	(Chapter 32)

Primary lymphoma of the liver may be found incidentally or complicating acquired immune deficiency syndrome (AIDS) or other immunosuppressed states, for example organ transplantation [98]. Patients with preexisting cirrhosis have a poor prognosis. Negative α-fetoprotein and carcinoembryonic antigen with a high LDH level in a patient with a liver mass should raise the possibility of lymphoma.

Treatment of hepatic involvement

The treatment depends on the histological type of lymphoma. Aggressive combination chemotherapy has considerably improved the prognosis of intrahepatic Hodgkin's deposits causing jaundice. Use of targeted therapy with rituximab in CD20 positive B-cell lymphomas has been a significant advance in recent years. Treatment of hepatic lymphomas is the same as for other stage IV nodal lymphoma patients regardless of the jaundice. Similarly, those with 'idiopathic' cholestasis should receive the therapy appropriate for their lymphoma. If MOPP (mechlorethamine, Oncovin, procarbazine and prednisone) has failed, ABVD (Adriamycin, bleomycin, vinblastine and dacarbazine) should be tried. If jaundice is persistent, some palliation may be achieved by moderate local irradiation.

Extrahepatic biliary obstruction is treated by external radiation and, if necessary, the insertion of temporary internal stents by the endoscopic or percutaneous route.

If drug toxicity is the cause, treatment may have to be changed or doses reduced.

Treatment for non-Hodgkin's lymphoma causing jaundice is the same as that for Hodgkin's disease.

Primary hepatic lymphoma is treated by chemotherapy or occasionally by lobectomy [94].

Lymphosarcoma

Nodules of lymphosarcomatous tissue may be found in the liver, especially in the portal tracts. Macroscopically they resemble metastatic carcinoma. The liver may also be involved in giant follicular lymphoma.

Multiple myeloma

The liver may be involved in plasma cell myeloma, the portal tracts and sinusoids being filled with plasma cells. Solitary primary hepatic plasmacytoma has also been reported. Associated amyloidosis may involve the hepatic arterioles.

Angioimmunoblastic lymphadenopathy

This resembles Hodgkin's disease. The liver shows a pleomorphic portal zone infiltrate (lymphocytes, plasma cells and blast cells) without histiocytes or Reed–Sternberg cells.

Extramedullary haemopoiesis

The pluripotent haematopoetic stem cells or endothelial derived stem cells in the liver are capable of giving rise to mature adult erythrocytes, leucocytes or platelets. If the stimulus for blood regeneration is sufficiently strong, this function can be resumed. This is rare in the adult although myeloid metaplasia in the liver of the anaemic infant is not unusual. In the adult, it occurs with bone marrow replacement or infiltration, and especially in association with secondary carcinoma of bone, myelofibrosis, myelosclerosis, multiple myeloma and the marble bone disease of Albers-Schoenberg. It complicates all conditions associated with a leucoerythroblastic anaemia.

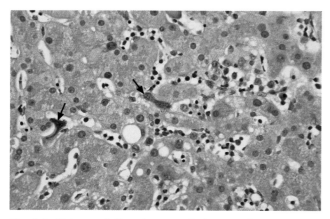

Fig. 4.6. Extra-medullary haemopoiesis—megakaryocytes (arrows), erythroblasts, normoblasts and polymorphs are seen in the hepatic sinusoids (H & E).

The condition is well exemplified by myelofibrosis and myelosclerosis, where the liver is enlarged, with a smooth firm edge. The spleen is enormous, and its removal results in even greater enlargement of the liver with increased liver enzymes. The mortality after splenectomy is 10–20%, some caused by hepatic dysfunction due to the increase in extramedullary haemopoiesis.

Ascites occurs in a low percentage of patients with extramedullary haemopoiesis, and may be due to portal hypertension, or, after splenectomy, peritoneal deposits of extramedullary haemopoiesis.

Microscopic features

The conspicuous abnormality is a great increase in the cellular content, both in the portal tracts and in the distended sinusoids (Fig. 4.6). The cells are of all types and varying maturity. The haemopoietic tissue may form discrete foci in the sinusoids. Rarely, larger foci may be seen on CT or MRI scanning [99].

Electron microscopy shows haematological cells in the sinusoids with transformation of perisinusoidal cells into fibroblasts and myofibroblast-like cells.

Portal hypertension. This may be due to portal vein thrombosis or, rarely, extensive sinusoidal infiltration with haemopoietic cells. Disse's space fibrosis contributes. Nodular regenerative hyperplasia may also cause portal hypertension (Chapter 9).

Systemic mastocytosis

This is a group of diseases characterized by extensive infiltration by mast cells that may affect several organ systems. The exact nature of the disorder remains unclear, although many of them have been shown to be clonal proliferations and have an aggressive behaviour. It can present with hepatomegaly as well as lymphadenopathy and skin lesions. Liver biopsy, stained with haematoxylin and eosin, shows polygonal cells with eosinophilic granules predominantly in portal tracts, with fewer in the sinusoids [100]. While staining with Giemsa and toluidine blue shows the typical metachromatic cytoplasmic granules, these days more specific immunohistochemical markers (c-Kit, CD25 and tryptase) are used to identify mast cells [101]. Presence of mast cells is not uncommon in various inflammatory liver disorders, but severe liver disease is unusual except in those with aggressive mastocytosis. Nodular regenerative hyperplasia, portal venopathy and veno-occlusive disease are reported [102] and may be responsible for portal hypertension and ascites. The latter carries a poor prognosis. Cirrhosis occurs in up to 5% of patients [100].

Langerhans' cell histiocytosis (histiocytosis X)

The underlying pathology of this rare condition is proliferation of Langerhans' cells and constitutes a spectrum of disorders comprising several entities (which overlap), including eosinophilic granuloma (bone lesions), Hand–Schüller–Christian disease (endocrine lesions; skin) and Letterer–Siwe disease (disseminated type; lungs, bone marrow, skin, lymph nodes, spleen, liver). The mechanism of liver injury is not known. Cholestasis is due to sclerosing cholangitis affecting intrahepatic ducts or proliferating histiocytic cells in periportal areas [103]. Liver disease is present in one-third of patients. Portal hypertension and variceal haemorrhage may develop. Liver failure due to biliary cirrhosis is unusual. The Langerhans' cell can easily be identified in the polymorphic infiltrate by their expression of CD1a and S100. Electron microscopy shows trilamellar rod-shaped structures (Birbeck granules) within the cells, but is seldom required for diagnostic purposes. Transplantation has been successful with no evidence of recurrent disease up to 7 years later [104].

Haemophagocytic lymphohistiocytosis [105]

This a rare and often fatal disease of overactive histiocytes and lymphocytes, usually presenting in children under 2 years of age but also in adults. The liver is affected by infiltration of both lymphocytes and histiocytes, biochemically mimicking a hepatitis, with haemophagocytosis, which is a hall mark of the disease. Cholestasis and bile duct injury are reported.

Lipid storage diseases

The lipidoses are disorders in which abnormal amounts of lipids are stored in the cells of the reticuloendothelial system. They may be classified according to the lipid stored: xanthomatosis (cholesterol); Gaucher's disease (glucocerebroside); Niemann–Pick disease type A and B (sphingomyelin) or Niemann–Pick disease type C (lysosomal cholesterol).

Primary and secondary xanthomatosis

Cholesterol is stored mainly in the skin, tendon sheaths, bone and blood vessels. The liver is rarely involved but there may be isolated nests of cholesterol-containing foamy histiocytes in the liver. Investigation of the liver is of little diagnostic value.

Cholesteryl ester storage disease [106]

This rare, autosomal recessive, relatively benign disease is due to a deficiency of lysosomal acid lipase/ cholesteryl ester hydrolase. It presents with symptomless hepatomegaly. The liver is orange in colour and hepatocytes contain excess cholesteryl ester and triglyceride. A septate fibrosis may lead to cirrhosis and patients may have early vascular disease. Complete enzyme deficiency (Wolman's disease) results in death in early infancy due to involvement of the liver, adrenals and histiocytes.

Gaucher's disease [107]

This rare, autosomal recessive disease was first described in 1882. It is the commonest lysosomal storage disorder. It is due to a deficiency of lysosomal acid β-glucosidase so that glucosylceramide, derived from membrane glycosphingolipids of time-expired white and red blood cells, accumulates in the reticuloendothelial system throughout the body, particularly in the liver, bone marrow and spleen. Three types are recognized:
• Type 1 (adult, chronic, non-neuronopathic) is the mildest and most common form of Gaucher's disease. It occurs rarely in all ethnic groups (non-Jewish: 1 in 40 000) but is most common in Ashkenazi Jews (1 in 850). The central nervous system is spared.
• Type 2 (infantile, acute, neuronopathic) is rare. In addition to the visceral involvement there is massive, fatal neurological involvement, with death in infancy.
• Type 3 (juvenile, subacute, neuronopathic) is also rare. There is gradual and heterogeneous neurological involvement.

The various forms represent different mutations in the structural gene for acid β-glucosidase on chromosome 1, although there is a variability in severity of disease within a specific genotype [108]. Four mutations account for over 95% of disease alleles in Ashkenazi patients, but only 75% of non-Jewish patients. Patients homozygous for the L444P mutation are at high risk of

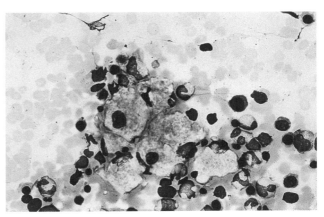

Fig. 4.7. Gaucher's disease. Smears of sternal bone marrow show large pale Gaucher cells with fibrillary cytoplasm and eccentric hyperchromatic nuclei. (Courtesy of Dr Atul Mehta.)

neurological disease, whereas the presence of at least one allele with N370S precludes this form of disease [108]. Variation in tissue damage within each genotype is probably due to individual differences in the macrophage response to glucosylceramide accumulation, but the mechanisms are unknown.

The characteristic Gaucher cell is approximately 70–80 μm in diameter, oval or polygonal in shape and with pale cytoplasm. It contains two or more peripherally placed hyperchromatic nuclei between which fibrils pass parallel to each other (Fig. 4.7). These cells accumulate in the perisinusoidal space and can form large aggregates. Associated fibrosis is variable and can be severe to resemble cirrhosis. The Gaucher cell is quite different from the foamy cell of xanthomatosis or Niemann–Pick disease.

Electron microscopy. The accumulated glycolipid formed from degraded cell membranes precipitates within the lysosomes and forms long (20–40 nm), rod-like tubules. These are seen by light microscopy. A somewhat similar cell is seen in chronic myeloid leukaemia and in multiple myeloma due to increased turnover of β-glucocerebroside.

Chronic adult form (type 1)

This is the most common type. It is of variable severity and age of onset but usually commences insidiously before the age of 30 years. It is chronic and may be recognized in quite old people.

The mode of presentation is variable, with unexplained hepatosplenomegaly (especially in children), avascular osteonecrosis, fragility fractures or bone pain. Additionally there may be a bleeding diathesis, with non-specific anaemia.

The clinical features include pigmentation which may be generalized or a patchy, brownish tan. The lower legs may have a symmetrical pigmentation, leaden grey in colour and containing melanin. The eyes show yellow pingueculae.

The spleen is enormous and the liver is moderately enlarged, smooth and firm. Superficial lymph glands are not usually involved.

Hepatic involvement is often associated with fibrosis and abnormal liver function tests. Serum alkaline phosphatase is usually increased, sometimes with a rise in transaminase. Severe fibrosis may develop but life-threatening liver disease affects only a small minority. Ascites and portal hypertension with variceal bleeding are associated with large areas of confluent fibrosis with a characteristic MRI appearance [21]. Other hepatic manifestations include high incidence of cholesterol gallstone disease and hyperferritinaemia associated with iron overload in some patients [109,110].

Bone X-rays. The long bones exhibit failure of bone remodelling, reflected by expansion of the lower ends of the femora, so that the waist normally seen above the condyles disappears. The appearance has been likened to that of an Erlenmeyer flask.

Sternal marrow shows the diagnostic Gaucher cells (Fig. 4.7).

Biopsy. Aspiration liver biopsy should be performed if sternal puncture has yielded negative results. The liver is diffusely involved (Fig. 4.8)

Peripheral blood changes. With diffuse bone marrow involvement, a leucoerythroblastic picture may be seen. Alternatively, leucopenia and thrombocytopenia with prolonged bleeding time may be associated with only a moderate hypochromic microcytic anaemia [111].

Gold standard for diagnosis is the measurement of acid β-glucosidase activity in peripheral blood leucocytes; screening for common *GBA1* (the gene that encodes acid β-glucosidase) mutations may be helpful.

Biochemical changes. Serum alkaline phosphatase is usually increased, sometimes with a rise in transaminase. Serum ferritin is elevated usually with normal transferrin saturation; in approximately 3% of patients there is evidence of iron overload [110]. Serum cholesterol tends to low due to low HDL cholesterol [109].

Treatment

The standard of care is enzyme replacement therapy [112]. The acid β-glucosidase was first prepared from pooled human placentae, though most patients now receive enzyme made by recombinant technology. It is given by intravenous infusion. Several treatment regimens have been shown to be effective. After endogenous enzymatic deglycosylation, exogenous enzyme is taken up by mannose receptors on macrophages, in the liver, spleen and skeleton, where it is highly effective in reversing the haematological and visceral (liver, spleen) features. Skeletal disease is slow to respond [112].

Splenectomy, partial or total, has been done for the very large spleen causing abdominal discomfort, and occasionally for thrombocytopenia or an acquired haemolytic anaemia. Total splenectomy is followed by more aggressive bone disease and preplanned enzyme therapy is needed to prevent this.

Liver transplantation for decompensated cirrhosis has been done [113,114]. This does not correct the metabolic defect, and enzyme replacement therapy remains necessary. Bone marrow transplantation has been performed, but while curative, the risks are considered prohibitive in comparison with enzyme replacement therapy.

Substrate reduction therapy via inhibitors of glucosylceramide synthase are showing promising results [115].

Acute infantile Gaucher's disease (type 2)

This acute form of the disease presents within the first 6 months of life and is usually fatal before 2 years. The child appears normal at birth. There is cerebral involvement, progressive cachexia and mental deterioration. The liver and spleen are enlarged and superficial lymph nodes may also be palpable.

Autopsy shows Gaucher cells throughout the reticuloendothelial system. They are, however, not found in the brain. The pathogenesis of the cerebral disease is not understood but probably involves direct toxicity of accumulating lipids on the neuronal cells.

Niemann–Pick diseases [116–118]

Niemann–Pick disease type A and type B are inherited as autosomal recessive deficiency of the enzyme sphingomyelinase, in the lysosomes of the reticuloendothelial system. This results in the lysosomal storage of sphingomyelin. The liver and spleen are predominantly involved.

The characteristic cell is pale, ovoid or round, 20–40 μm in diameter. In the unfixed state it is loaded with granules; when fixed in fat solvents the granules are dissolved, giving a vacuolated and foamy appearance. There are usually only one or two nuclei. Electron microscopy shows lysosomes as laminated myelin-like figures. These contain the abnormal lipid.

Niemann–Pick disease *type A* (acute, neuronopathic form) occurs in infants, who die before the age of 2 years. The condition starts in the first 3 months, with

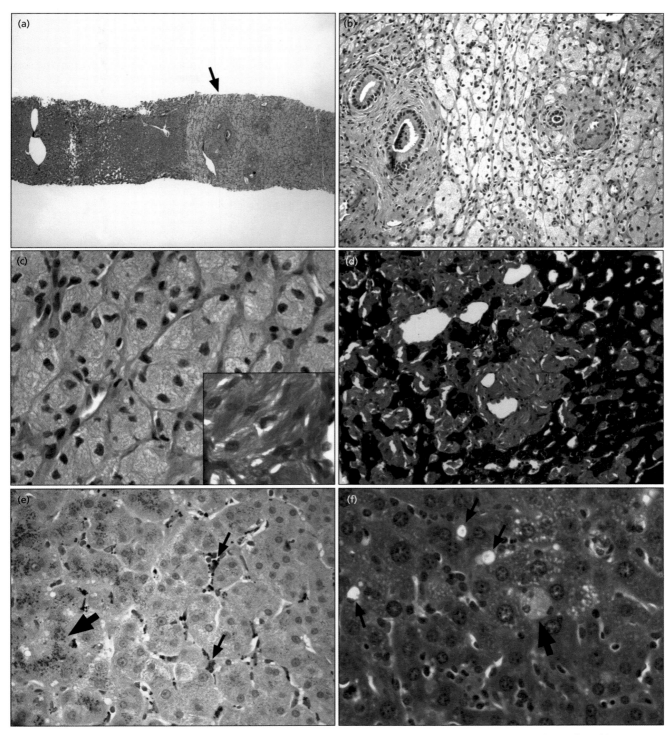

Fig. 4.8. Gaucher's disease. (a) Liver biopsy (H & E) shows aggregates of Gaucher cells replacing chunks of hepatic parenchyma (arrows). (b) & (c) Higher magnification showing morphology of Gaucher cells with pale eosinophilic cytoplasm producing a 'wrinkled tissue paper' appearance (H & E). Inset shows periodic acid–Schiff (PAS) stain highlighting the cytoplasm of these cells. (d) PAS stain showing clusters of pink-staining Gaucher cells infiltrating into the hepatic sinusoids. (e) Increased haemosiderin deposition in Kupffer cells (thin arrows) and hepatocytes (thick arrows) in Gaucher's disease patient (Perl's stain). (f) Liver biopsy showing prominence of lipdotic stellate cells (thin arrows) in the perisinusoidal space (H & E). A small aggregate of Gaucher cells (thick arrow) can also be seen.

anorexia, weight loss and retardation of growth. The liver and spleen enlarge, the skin becomes waxy and acquires a yellowish-brown coloration on exposed parts. The superficial lymph nodes are enlarged. There are pulmonary infiltrates. The patient is blind, deaf and mentally retarded.

The fundus may show a cherry-red spot due to retinal degeneration at the macula.

The peripheral blood shows a microcytic anaemia and in the later stages the foamy Niemann–Pick cell may be found.

The disease may present as *neonatal cholestatic jaundice* which remits. Progressive neurological deterioration appears in late childhood.

Type B (chronic, non-neuronopathic form) is associated with neonatal cholestasis which resolves. Cirrhosis develops slowly and may lead to portal hypertension, ascites and liver failure [119]. Liver transplantation for hepatic failure has been successful [114]. Although hepatic lipid accumulation was not seen at 10 months, longer follow-up is needed to assess the metabolic outcome.

Diagnosis is made by marrow puncture, which reveals characteristic Niemann–Pick cells, or by finding a low level of sphingomyelinase in leucocytes.

Bone marrow transplant has been done for patients with early severe liver disease [120]. Preliminary reports were promising with reduction of sphingomyelin from liver, spleen and bone marrow, but longer follow-up is needed.

Niemann–Pick type C disease is due to genetic mutations in NPC1 protein, a transporter of cholesterol in lysosomal membrane. Thus cholesterol-laden lysosomes accumulate with secondary accumulation of other lipids [118]. Affected infants may present with neonatal cholestasis and severe liver involvement and there is progressive neurodegenerative disease. Occasionally, adults may present with hepatomegaly and neurodegenerative disease. Other than cholesterol, glycosphingolipids accumulate which forms the rational for use of substrate inhibitors of glucocerebroside synthesis. One such inhibitor, miglustat, has shown promising results in a randomized controlled trial [117].

Sea-blue histiocyte syndrome

This rare condition is characterized by histiocytes staining a sea-blue colour with Wright or Giemsa stain in bone marrow and in reticuloendothelial cells of the liver. The cells contain deposits of phosphosphingolipid and glucosphingolipid. Clinically, the liver and spleen are enlarged. The prognosis is usually good although thrombocytopenia and hepatic cirrhosis have been reported. Other sphingolipidosis should be excluded such as Niemann–Pick disease [121].

Coagulation and fibrosis

Prothrombotic mechanisms contribute to hepatic fibrosis in rat models, as anticoagulants act on hepatic stellate cells to prevent fibrosis [122], and may do so in humans [123]. As stable cirrhosis is a prothrombotic state [29,39], and cirrhosis may be worsened by intrahepatic intravascular thromboses [124], anticoagulant therapy might have a therapeutic role in chronic liver disease.

References

1 Cooper RA, Arner EC, Wiley JS *et al.* Modification of red cell membrane structure by cholesterol-rich lipid dispersions. A model for the primary spur cell defect. *J. Clin. Invest.* 1975; **55**: 115–126.
2 Chitale AA, Sterling RK, Post AB *et al.* Resolution of spur cell anemia with liver transplantation: a case report and review of the literature. *Transplantation* 1998; **65**: 993–995.
3 Owen JS, Brown DJ, Harry DS *et al.* Erythrocyte echinocytosis in liver disease. Role of abnormal plasma high density lipoproteins. *J. Clin. Invest.* 1985; **76**: 2275–2285.
4 Okuda K. Discovery of vitamin B12 in the liver and its absorption factor in the stomach: a historical review. *J. Gastroenterol. Hepatol.* 1999; **14**: 301–308.
5 Pitcher CS, Williams R. Reduced red cell survival in jaundice and its relation to abnormal glutathione metabolism. *Clin. Sci.* 1963; **24**: 239–252.
6 Zieve L. Hemolytic anemia in liver disease. *Medicine* (Baltimore) 1966; **45**: 497–505.
7 Dzik WH, Mondor LA, Maillet SM *et al.* ABO and Lewis blood group antigens of donor origin in the bile of patients after liver transplantation. *Transfusion* 1987; **27**: 384–387.
8 Pereira SP, O'Donohue J, Wendon J *et al.* Maternal and perinatal outcome in severe pregnancy-related liver disease. *Hepatology* 1997; **26**: 1258–1262.
9 De Franceschi L, Fattovich G, Turrini F *et al.* Hemolytic anemia induced by ribavirin therapy in patients with chronic hepatitis C virus infection: role of membrane oxidative damage. *Hepatology* 2000; **31**: 997–1004.
10 Brown KE, Tisdale J, Barrett AJ *et al.* Hepatitis-associated aplastic anemia. *N. Engl. J. Med.* 1997; **336**: 1059–1064.
11 Goss JA, Schiller GJ, Martin P *et al.* Aplastic anemia complicating orthotopic liver transplantation. *Hepatology* 1997; **26**: 865–869.
12 Gschwantler M, Vavrik J, Gebauer A *et al.* Course of platelet counts in cirrhotic patients after implantation of a transjugular intrahepatic portosystemic shunt—a prospective, controlled study. *J. Hepatol.* 1999; **30**: 254–259.
13 Goulis J, Chau TN, Jordan S *et al.* Thrombopoietin concentrations are low in patients with cirrhosis and thrombocytopenia and are restored after orthotopic liver transplantation. *Gut* 1999; **44**: 754–758.
14 Peck-Radosavljevic M, Zacherl J, Wichlas M *et al.* Thrombopoietic cytokines and reversal of thrombocytopenia after liver transplantation. *Eur. J. Gastroenterol. Hepatol.* 1999; **11**: 151–156.
15 Roberts LN, Patel RK, Arya R. Haemostasis and thrombosis in liver disease. *Br. J. Haematol.* 2010; **148**: 507–521.

16 Kosugi S, Imai Y, Kurata Y *et al.* Platelet-associated IgM elevated in patients with chronic hepatitis C contains no anti-platelet autoantibodies. *Liver* 1997; **17**: 230–237.

17 Nagamine T, Ohtuka T, Takehara K *et al.* Thrombocytopenia associated with hepatitis C viral infection. *J. Hepatol.* 1996; **24**: 135–140.

18 Violi F, Ferro D, Basili S *et al.* Hyperfibrinolysis resulting from clotting activation in patients with different degrees of cirrhosis. The CALC Group. Coagulation Abnormalities in Liver Cirrhosis. *Hepatology* 1993; **17**: 78–83.

19 Laffi G, Marra F, Gresele P *et al.* Evidence for a storage pool defect in platelets from cirrhotic patients with defective aggregation. *Gastroenterology* 1992; **103**: 641–646.

20 Castelino DJ, Salem HH. Natural anticoagulants and the liver. *J. Gastroenterol. Hepatol.* 1997; **12**: 77–83.

21 Paramo JA, Rocha E. Hemostasis in advanced liver disease. *Semin. Thromb. Hemost.* 1993; **19**: 184–190.

22 Quintarelli C, Ferro D, Valesini G *et al.* Prevalence of lupus anticoagulant in patients with cirrhosis: relationship with beta-2-glycoprotein I plasma levels. *J. Hepatol.* 1994; **21**: 1086–1091.

23 Lisman T, Caldwell SH, Burroughs AK *et al.* Haemostasis and thrombosis in patients with liver disease: the ups and downs. *J. Hepatol.* 2010; **53**: 362–371.

24 Mannucci PM. Abnormal haemostasis tests and bleeding in chronic liver disease: are they related? No. *J. Throm. Haemost.* 2006; **4**: 712–713.

25 Giannini EG, Greco A, Marenco S *et al.* Incidence of bleeding following invasive procedures in patients with thrombocytopenia and advanced liver disease. *Clin. Gastroenterol. Hepatol.* 2010; **8**: 899–902.

26 Furie B, Furie BC. Molecular basis of vitamin K-dependent gamma-carboxylation. *Blood* 1990; **75**: 1753–1762.

27 Langley PG, Williams R. Physiological inhibitors of coagulation in fulminant hepatic failure. *Blood Coagul. Fibrinolysis* 1992; **3**: 243–247.

28 Bell H, Odegaard OR, Andersson T *et al.* Protein C in patients with alcoholic cirrhosis and other liver diseases. *J. Hepatol.* 1992; **14**: 163–167.

29 Tripodi A, Primignani M, Chantarangkul V *et al.* An imbalance of pro- vs. anti-coagulation factors in plasma from patients with cirrhosis. *Gastroenterology* 2009; **137**: 2105–2111.

30 Casella JF, Lewis JH, Bontempo FA *et al.* Successful treatment of homozygous protein C deficiency by hepatic transplantation. *Lancet* 1988; **1**: 435–438.

31 Hayashi T, Kamogawa A, Ro S *et al.* Plasma from patients with cirrhosis increases tissue plasminogen activator release from vascular endothelial cells in vitro. *Liver* 1998; **18**: 186–190.

32 Leebeek FW, Kluft C, Knot EA *et al.* A shift in balance between profibrinolytic and antifibrinolytic factors causes enhanced fibrinolysis in cirrhosis. *Gastroenterology* 1991; **101**: 1382–1390.

33 Lisman T, Leebeek FW, Mosnier LO *et al.* Thrombin-activatable fibrinolysis inhibitor deficiency in cirrhosis is not associated with increased plasma fibrinolysis. *Gastroenterology* 2001; **121**: 131–139.

34 Violi F, Ferro D, Basili S *et al.* Hyperfibrinolysis increases the risk of gastrointestinal hemorrhage in patients with advanced cirrhosis. *Hepatology* 1992; **15**: 672–676.

35 Ben-Ari Z, Osman E, Hutton RA *et al.* Disseminated intravascular coagulation in liver cirrhosis: fact or fiction? *Am. J. Gastroenterol.* 1999; **94**: 2977–2982.

36 Bakker CM, Knot EA, Stibbe J *et al.* Disseminated intravascular coagulation in liver cirrhosis. *J. Hepatol.* 1992; **15**: 330–335.

37 Violi F, Ferro D, Basili S *et al.* Association between low-grade disseminated intravascular coagulation and endotoxemia in patients with liver cirrhosis. *Gastroenterology* 1995; **109**: 531–539.

38 Sogaard KK, Horváth-Puhó E, Grønbaek H *et al.* Risk of thromboembolism in patients with liver disease: a nationwide population-based case-control study. *Am. J. Gastroenterol.* 2009; **104**: 96–101.

39 Gatt A, Riddell A, Calvaruso V *et al.* Enhanced thrombin generation in patients with cirrhosis induced coagulopathy. *J. Thromb. Haemost.* 2010; **8**: 1994–2000.

40 Northup PG, McMahon MM, Ruhl AP *et al.* Coagulopathy does not fully protect hospitalised cirrhosis patients from peripheral venous thromboembolism. *Am. J. Gastroenterol.* 2006; **101**: 1524–1528.

41 Pereira LM, Langley PG, Hayllar KM *et al.* Coagulation factor V and VIII/V ratio as predictors of outcome in paracetamol induced fulminant hepatic failure: relation to other prognostic indicators. *Gut* 1992; **33**: 98–102.

42 Blake JC, Sprengers D, Grech P *et al.* Bleeding time in patients with hepatic cirrhosis. *BMJ* 1990; **301**: 12–15.

43 Papatheodoridis GV, Patch D, Webster GJ *et al.* Infection and hemostasis in decompensated cirrhosis: a prospective study using thrombelastography. *Hepatology* 1999; **29**: 1085–1090.

44 Chau TN, Chan YW, Patch D *et al.* Thrombelastographic changes and early rebleeding in cirrhotic patients with variceal bleeding. *Gut* 1998; **43**: 267–271.

45 Bernstein DE, Jeffers L, Erhardtsen E *et al.* Recombinant factor VIIa corrects prothrombin time in cirrhotic patients: a preliminary study. *Gastroenterology* 1997; **113**: 1930–1937.

46 Papatheodoridis GV, Chung S, Keshav S *et al.* Correction of both prothrombin time and primary haemostasis by recombinant factor VII during therapeutic alcohol injection of hepatocellular cancer in liver cirrhosis. *J. Hepatol.* 1999; **31**: 747–750.

47 Bechstein WO, Neuhaus P. A surgeon's perspective on the management of coagulation disorders before liver transplantation. *Liver Transpl. Surg.* 1997; **3**: 653–655.

48 Mor E, Jennings L, Gonwa TA *et al.* The impact of operative bleeding on outcome in transplantation of the liver. *Surg. Gynecol. Obstet.* 1993; **176**: 219–227.

49 Porte RJ, Molenaar IQ, Begliomini B *et al.* Aprotinin and transfusion requirements in orthotopic liver transplantation: a multicentre randomised double-blind study. EMSALT Study Group. *Lancet* 2000; **355**: 1303–1309.

50 Boylan JF, Klinck JR, Sandler AN *et al.* Tranexamic acid reduces blood loss, transfusion requirements, and coagulation factor use in primary orthotopic liver transplantation. *Anesthesiology* 1996; **85**: 1043–8; discussion 30A–31A.

51 Warnaar N, Mallett SV, Klinck JR *et al.* Aprotinin and the risk of thrombotic complications after liver transplantation: an analysis of 1492 patients. *Liver Transpl.* 2009; **15**: 747–753.

52 Zanella A, Berzuini A, Colombo MB *et al.* Iron status in red cell pyruvate kinase deficiency: study of Italian cases. *Br. J. Haematol.* 1993; **83**: 485–490.

53 Hoblinger A, Erdmann C, Strassburg CP *et al.* Coinheritance of hereditary spherocytosis and reversibility of cirrhosis in a young female patient with hereditary hemochromatosis. *Eur. J. Med. Res.* 2009; **14**: 182–184.

54 Iolascon A, Miraglia del Giudice E, Perrotta S *et al.* Hereditary spherocytosis: from clinical to molecular defects. *Haematologica* 1998; **83**: 240–257.

55 Beutler E. G6PD: population genetics and clinical manifestations. *Blood Rev.* 1996; **10**: 45–52.

56 Banerjee S, Owen C, Chopra S. Sickle cell hepatopathy. *Hepatology* 2001; **33**: 1021–1028.

57 Ebert EC, Nagar M, Hagspiel KD. Gastrointestinal and hepatic complications of sickle cell disease. *Clin. Gastroenterol. Hepatol.* 2010; **8**: 483–489.

58 Stephan JL, Merpit-Gonon E, Richard O *et al.* Fulminant liver failure in a 12-year-old girl with sickle cell anaemia: favourable outcome after exchange transfusions. *Eur. J. Pediatr.* 1995; **154**: 469–471.

59 O'Callaghan A, O'Brien SG, Ninkovic M *et al.* Chronic intrahepatic cholestasis in sickle cell disease requiring exchange transfusion. *Gut* 1995; **37**: 144–147.

60 Olivieri NF. Progression of iron overload in sickle cell disease. *Semin. Hematol.* 2001; **38** (Suppl. 1): 57–62.

61 Omata M, Johnson CS, Tong M *et al.* Pathological spectrum of liver diseases in sickle cell disease. *Dig. Dis. Sci.* 1986; **31**: 247–256.

62 Mekeel KL, Langham MR Jr, Gonzalez-Peralta R *et al.* Liver transplantation in children with sickle-cell disease. *Liver Transpl.* 2007; **13**: 505–508.

63 Lucarelli G, Galimberti M, Polchi P *et al.* Marrow transplantation in patients with thalassemia responsive to iron chelation therapy. *N. Engl. J. Med.* 1993; **329**: 840–844.

64 Young NS, Meyers G, Schrezenmeier H *et al.* The management of paroxysmal nocturnal hemoglobinuria: recent advances in diagnosis and treatment and new hope for patients. *Semin. Hematol.* 2009; **46** (Suppl. 1): S1–S16.

65 Madkaikar M, Gupta M, Jijina F, Ghosh K. Paroxysmal nocturnal haemoglobinuria: diagnostic tests, advantages and limitations. *Eur. J. Haematol.* 2009; **83**: 503–511.

66 Le Thi Huong D, Valla D, Franco D *et al.* Cholangitis associated with paroxysmal nocturnal hemoglobinuria: another instance of ischemic cholangiopathy? *Gastroenterology* 1995; **109**: 1338–1343.

67 Zareba KM. Eculizumab: a novel therapy for paroxysmal nocturnal hemoglobinuria. *Drugs Today* 2007; **43**: 539–546.

68 Walz-Mattmuller R, Horny HP, Ruck P *et al.* Incidence and pattern of liver involvement in haematological malignancies. *Pathol. Res. Pract.* 1998; **194**: 781–789.

69 Souto P, Romãozinho JM, Figueiredo P *et al.* Severe acute liver failure as the initial manifestation of haematological malignancy. *Eur. J. Gastroenterol. Hepatol.* 1997; **9**: 1113–1115.

70 Woolf GM, Petrovic LM, Rojter SE *et al.* Acute liver failure due to lymphoma. A diagnostic concern when considering liver transplantation. *Dig. Dis. Sci.* 1994; **39**: 1351–1358.

71 Doi H, Horiike N, Hiraoka A *et al.* Primary hepatic marginal zone B cell lymphoma of mucosa-associated lymphoid tissue type: case report and review of the literature. *Int. J. Hematol.* 2008; **88**: 418–423.

72 Bird GL, Smith H, Portmann B *et al.* Acute liver decompensation on withdrawal of cytotoxic chemotherapy and immunosuppressive therapy in hepatitis B carriers. *Q. J. Med.* 1989; **73**: 895–902.

73 Lau JY, Lai CL, Lin HJ *et al.* Fatal reactivation of chronic hepatitis B virus infection following withdrawal of chemotherapy in lymphoma patients. *Q. J. Med.* 1989; **73**: 911–917.

74 Valla D, Lai CL, Lin HJ *et al.* Etiology of portal vein thrombosis in adults. A prospective evaluation of primary myeloproliferative disorders. *Gastroenterology* 1988; **94**: 1063–1069.

75 Forbes GM, Davies JM, Herrmann RP *et al.* Liver disease complicating bone marrow transplantation: a clinical audit. *J. Gastroenterol. Hepatol.* 1995; **10**: 1–7.

76 Shulman HM, Gooley T, Dudley MD *et al.* Utility of transvenous liver biopsies and wedged hepatic venous pressure measurements in sixty marrow transplant recipients. *Transplantation* 1995; **59**: 1015–1022.

77 Kalambokis G, Manousou P, Vibhakorn S *et al.* Transjugular liver biopsy— indications, adequacy, quality of specimens, and complications—a systematic review. *J. Hepatol.* 2007; **47**: 284–294.

78 Shulman HM, Fisher LB, Schoch HG *et al.* Veno-occlusive disease of the liver after marrow transplantation: histological correlates of clinical signs and symptoms. *Hepatology* 1994; **19**: 1171–1181.

79 Essell JH, Schroeder MT, Harman GS *et al.* Ursodiol prophylaxis against hepatic complications of allogeneic bone marrow transplantation. A randomized, double-blind, placebo-controlled trial. *Ann. Intern. Med.* 1998; **128**: 975–981.

80 Richardson PG, Soiffer RJ, Antin JH *et al.* Defibrotide for the treatment of severe hepatic veno-occlusive disease and multi-organ failure post stem cell transplantation: a multicenter, randomized, dose-finding trial. *Biol. Blood Marrow Transplant.* 2010; **16**: 1005–1017.

81 Terra SG, Spitzer TR, Tsunoda SM. A review of tissue plasminogen activator in the treatment of veno-occlusive liver disease after bone marrow transplantation. *Pharmacotherapy* 1997; **17**: 929–937.

82 Senzolo M, Germani G, Cholongitas E *et al.* Veno -occlusive disease: update on clinical management. *World J. Gastroenterol.* 2007; **13**: 2918–2924.

83 Sharafuddin MJ, Foshager MC, Steinbuch M *et al.* Sonographic findings in bone marrow transplant patients with symptomatic hepatic venoocclusive disease. *J. Ultrasound Med.* 1997; **16**: 575–586.

84 Dich NH, Goodman ZD, Klein MA. Hepatic involvement in Hodgkin's disease. Clues to histologic diagnosis. *Cancer* 1989; **64**: 2121–2126.

85 Johnson LN, Iseri O, Knodell RG. Caseating hepatic granulomas in Hodgkin's lymphoma. *Gastroenterology* 1990; **99**: 1837–1840.

86 Jaffe ES. Malignant lymphomas: pathology of hepatic involvement. *Semin. Liver Dis.* 1987; **7**: 257–268.

87 Sans M, Andreu V, Bordas JM *et al.* Usefulness of laparoscopy with liver biopsy in the assessment of liver involvement at diagnosis of Hodgkin's and non-Hodgkin's lymphomas. *Gastrointest. Endosc.* 1998; **47**: 391–395.

88 Bruguera M, Caballero T, Carreras E *et al.* Hepatic sinusoidal dilatation in Hodgkin's disease. *Liver* 1987; **7**: 76–80.

89 Cameron AM, Truty J, Truell J *et al.* Fulminant hepatic failure from primary hepatic lymphoma: successful treatment with orthotopic liver transplantation and chemotherapy. *Transplantation* 2005; **80**: 993–996.

90 Feller E, Schiffman FJ. Extrahepatic biliary obstruction by lymphoma. *Arch. Surg.* 1990; **125**: 1507–1509.

91 Maymind M, Mergelas JE, Seibert DG *et al.* Primary non-Hodgkin's lymphoma of the common bile duct. *Am. J. Gastroenterol.* 1997; **92**: 1543–1546.

92 Hubscher SG, Lumley MA, Elias E. Vanishing bile duct syndrome: a possible mechanism for intrahepatic cholestasis in Hodgkin's lymphoma. *Hepatology* 1993; **17**: 70–77.

93 Watterson J, Priest JR. Jaundice as a paraneoplastic phenomenon in a T-cell lymphoma. *Gastroenterology* 1989; **97**: 1319–1322.

94 Zafrani ES, Gaulard P. Primary lymphoma of the liver. *Liver* 1993; **13**: 57–61.

95 Ohsawa M, Aozasa K, Horiuchi K *et al.* Malignant lymphoma of the liver. Report of five cases and review of the literature. *Dig. Dis. Sci.* 1992; **37**: 1105–1109.

96 Belhadj K, Reyes F, Farcet JP *et al.* Hepatosplenic gammadelta T-cell lymphoma is a rare clinicopathologic entity with poor outcome: report on a series of 21 patients. *Blood* 2003; **102**: 4261–4269.

97 Chim CS, Choy C, Ooi GC *et al.* Primary hepatic lymphoma. *Leuk. Lymphoma* 2001; **40**: 667–670.

98 Scoazec JY, Degott C, Brousse N *et al.* Non-Hodgkin's lymphoma presenting as a primary tumor of the liver: presentation, diagnosis and outcome in eight patients. *Hepatology* 1991; **13**: 870–875.

99 Wong Y, Chen F, Tai KS *et al.* Imaging features of focal intrahepatic extramedullary haematopoiesis. *Br. J. Radiol.* 1999; **72**: 906–910.

100 Horny HP, Kaiserling E, Campbell M *et al.* Liver findings in generalized mastocytosis. A clinicopathologic study. *Cancer* 1989; **63**: 532–538.

101 Kupfer SS, Hart J, Mohanty JR. Aggressive systemic mastocytosis presenting with hepatic cholestasis. *Eur. J. Gastroenterol. Hepatol.* 2007; **19**: 901–905.

102 Mican JM, Di Bisceglie AM, Fong TL *et al.* Hepatic involvement in mastocytosis: clinicopathologic correlations in 41 cases. *Hepatology* 1995; **22**: 1163–1170.

103 Iwai M, Kashiwadani M, Okuno T *et al.* Cholestatic liver disease in a 20-yr-old woman with histiocytosis X. *Am. J. Gastroenterol.* 1988; **83**: 164–168.

104 Zandi P, Panis Y, Debray D *et al.* Pediatric liver transplantation for Langerhans' cell histiocytosis. *Hepatology* 1995; **21**: 129–133.

105 Gupta S, Weitzman S. Primary and secondary hemophagocytic lymphohistiocytosis: clinical features, pathogenesis, and therapy. *Expert. Rev. Clin. Immunol.* 2010; **6**: 137–154.

106 Elleder M, Chlumská A, Hyánek J *et al.* Subclinical course of cholesteryl ester storage disease in an adult with hypercholesterolemia, accelerated atherosclerosis, and liver cancer. *J. Hepatol.* 2000; **32**: 528–534.

107 Mistry PK. Gaucher's disease: a model for modern management of a genetic disease. *J. Hepatol.* 1999; **30** (Suppl. 1): 1–5.

108 Mistry PK. Genotype/ phenotype correlations in Gaucher's disease. *Lancet* 1995; **346**: 982–983.

109 Taddei TH, Dziura J, Chen S *et al.* High incidence of cholesterol gallstone disease in type 1 Gaucher disease: characterizing the biliary phenotype of type 1 Gaucher disease. *J. Inherit Metab. Dis.* 2010; **33**: 291–300.

110 Stein P, Yu H, Jain D *et al.* Hyperferrtiniemia and iron overload in Gaucher disease. *Am. J. Hematol.* 2010; **85**: 472–476.

111 Sherlock S, Learmonth J. Aneurysm of the splenic artery; with an account of an example complicating Gaucher's disease. *Br. J. Surg.* 1942; **30**: 151.

112 Andersson HC, Charrow J, Kaplan P *et al.* Individualization of long-term enzyme replacement therapy for Gaucher disease. *Genet. Med.* 2005; **7**: 105–110.

113 Ayto R, Hughes DA, Jeevaratnam P *et al.* Long term outcomes of liver transplantation in type 1 Gaucher disease. *Am. J. Transplant.* 2010; **10**: 1934–1939.

114 Smanik EJ, Tavill AS, Jacobs GH *et al.* Orthotopic liver transplantation in two adults with Niemann-Pick and Gaucher's diseases: implications for the treatment of inherited metabolic disease. *Hepatology* 1993; **17**: 42–49.

115 Lukina E, Watman N, Avila Arreguin E *et al.* A Phase 2 study of eliglustat tartrate (Genz-112638), an oral substrate reduction therapy for Gaucher disease type 1. *Blood* 2010; **116**: 893–899.

116 Schuchman EH. The pathogenesis and treatment of acid sphingomyelinase-deficient Niemann-Pick disease. *Int. J. Clin. Pharmacol. Ther.* 2009; **47** (Suppl. 1): S48–57.

117 Patterson MC, Vecchio D, Prady H *et al.* Miglustat for treatment of Niemann-Pick C disease: a randomised controlled study. *Lancet Neurol.* 2007; **6**: 765–772.

118 Wraith JE, Levade T, Mengel E *et al.* Recommendations on the diagnosis and management of Niemann-Pick disease type C. *Mol. Genet. Metab.* 2009; **98**: 152–165.

119 Putterman C, Zelingher J, Shouval D. Liver failure and the sea-blue histiocyte/ adult Niemann-Pick disease. Case report and review of the literature. *J. Clin. Gastroenterol.* 1992; **15**: 146–149.

120 Vellodi A, Hobbs JR, O'Donnell NM *et al.* Treatment of Niemann-Pick disease type B by allogenic bone marrow transplantation. *Br. Med. J. Clin. Res. Ed.* 1987; **295**: 1375–1376.

121 Long RG, Lake BD, Pettit JE *et al.* Adult Niemann-Pick disease: its relationship to the syndrome of the sea-blue histiocyte. *Am. J. Med.* 1977; **62**: 627–635.

122 Abe W, Ikejima K, Lang T. Low molecular weight heparin prevents hepatic fibrinogenesis caused by carbon tetrachloride in the rat. *J. Hepatol.* 2007; **46**: 286–294.

123 Calvaruso V, Maimone S, Gatt A *et al.* Coagulation and fibrosis in chronic liver disease. *Gut* 2008; **57**: 1722–1727.

124 Wanless IR, Wong F, Blendis LM *et al.* Hepatic and portal vein thrombosis in cirrhosis: role in development of parenchymal extinction and portal hypertension. *Hepatology* 1995; **21**: 1238–1247.

CHAPTER 5
Acute Liver Failure

Shannan R. Tujios & William M. Lee
University of Texas Southwestern Medical Center, Dallas, TX, USA

Learning points

- Acute liver failure is the clinical syndrome of liver dysfunction, coagulopathy, and encephalopathy developing within 26 weeks of onset of symptoms in patients without pre-existing liver disease.

- Viral hepatitis is the most common cause worldwide while paracetamol overdose prevails in Western countries.

- Survival depends on the underlying aetiology, early treatment, and the diligent care of complications.

- Cerebral oedema and intracranial hypertension are unique complications of acute liver failure.

- Transplantation can provide rescue for patients with advanced coma grades. Those with milder degrees of encephalopathy may recover fully without need of a graft.

Acute liver failure describes the clinical syndrome of severe impairment of liver function (encephalopathy, coagulopathy and jaundice) within 6 months of the onset of symptoms [1]. Although usually due to an acute insult (most frequently virus or drug) in a previously healthy person, acute liver failure may occasionally result from chronic liver disease, in particular Wilson's disease or autoimmune chronic hepatitis. Other less common aetiologies include ischaemia, Budd–Chiari syndrome, acute fatty liver of pregnancy and malignancy. A cause for acute liver failure cannot be identified in as many as 15% of cases [2]. The best predictor of spontaneous survival and need for liver transplantation is the underlying aetiology. Determining the aetiology is essential to management of acute liver failure [3].

Acute liver failure developing in less than a week after onset of illness is associated with the highest incidence of cerebral oedema, a frequent cause of death in this setting. Other complications that may lead to death include sepsis with increased susceptibility to bacterial

and fungal infections, multiple organ dysfunction with circulatory instability, renal and pulmonary failure, acid–base and electrolyte disturbances and coagulopathy [4]. These make intensive care, referral to a specialist unit, the availability of liver transplantation and temporary hepatic support vitally important.

The survival of patients has improved with intensive care and the advent of transplantation, rising from less than 20% in the early 1970s to current survival of near 70%. Changing patterns in aetiology have impacted outcomes as well, with paracetamol (acetaminophen) accounting for nearly half of acute liver failure cases in the USA and UK. Paracetamol, shock and hepatitis A have favourable outcomes with spontaneous recovery of 58 to 64% compared to drug-induced, autoimmune and indeterminate causes, where spontaneous survival is less than 30% [2]. Patients transplanted for acute liver failure have 1-year survival rates at greater than 70% [5].

The key to optimal treatment is early recognition of acute liver failure, determining the aetiology, estimating the severity and, if appropriate, transfer to a facility capable of liver transplantation.

Definition

The original definition of fulminant hepatic failure by Trey and Davidson in 1959 stipulated an onset of hepatic encephalopathy within 8 weeks of the first symptoms of illness, in patients without pre-existing liver disease [1]. A broader definition includes patients with onset of disease to encephalopathy of as long as 26 weeks, although the majority of cases are of much shorter duration. One widely used classification separates acute liver failure into hyperacute, acute and subacute, based on the time interval between the development of jaundice and encephalopathy (Table 5.1) [6].

An alternative classification groups liver failure into fulminant, subfulminant and late-onset hepatic failure. Fulminant hepatic failure is when time from jaundice to

---

Sherlock's Diseases of the Liver and Biliary System, Twelfth Edition. Edited by
James S. Dooley, Anna S.F. Lok, Andrew K. Burroughs, E. Jenny Heathcote.
© 2011 by Blackwell Publishing Ltd. Published 2011 by Blackwell Publishing Ltd.

Table 5.1. Classification of acute liver failure [6]

Liver failure subcategory	Jaundice to encephalopathy	Clinical presentation	Common aetiologies	Prognosis
Hyperacute	0–7 days	Cerebral oedema common	Paracetamol, hepatitis A, ischaemia	Fair
Acute	8–28 days	Cerebral oedema less common	Hepatitis B, drugs	Poor
Subacute	29 days to 12 weeks	Cerebral oedema rare; ascites, peripheral oedema and renal failure more common	Drugs, indeterminate	Very poor

encephalopathy is less than 2 weeks and subfulminant hepatic failure when time is greater than 2 weeks [7]. Late-onset liver failure describes encephalopathy developing more than 8 weeks (but less than 24 weeks) after the first symptoms [8].

Epidemiology and aetiologies
(Fig. 5.1, Table 5.2)

The most common cause of acute liver failure worldwide is viral hepatitis. Asia and the developing world contribute the most cases, probably because of higher prevalence of viral hepatitis and less exposure to drugs. Most Western countries have shown a decline in viral aetiologies during the last decade and an increase in paracetamol and idiosyncratic drug-induced cases of liver failure [9]. The exception to this pattern is Spain, where paracetamol is not readily available and hepatitis B remains the most common identifiable cause [10]. In the USA and UK, paracetamol self-poisoning accounts for 45–60% of acute liver failure with idiosyncratic drug reactions accounting for 12% of cases [11].

Viral hepatitis

The hepatitis virus responsible varies from one geographical location to another. In the USA, only 11% of acute liver failure is viral, with 2.5% being from hepatitis A, 7.7% from hepatitis B and the remainder from other viruses [12]. In India, over 95% of acute liver failure is due to viruses, with 40% secondary to hepatitis E and 25–30% to hepatitis B [13]. Even with the development of the hepatitis B vaccine, over half of acute liver failure cases in Greece are due to hepatitis B, though this has decreased from over 70% in the 1980s [14]. Hepatitis B accounts for almost 80% of acute liver failure cases and represents two-thirds of liver transplants [15]. Although these cases are designated as acute, many probably represent flares of chronic hepatitis B, that arises from changes in balance between immune response and virus replication.

Although hepatitis A has a broad distribution, it remains a rare cause of acute liver failure and is declining rapidly in the USA. Indicators of poor prognosis include creatinine above 2.0 mg/dL, alanine aminotransferase less than 2600 IU/mL, and need for ventilatory or pressor support [16]. Those with chronic liver disease may be more susceptible, with liver failure occurring in up to 41% of patients with underlying chronic hepatitis C who contract hepatitis A [17]. Vaccination against hepatitis A as well as hepatitis B is recommended for those with chronic liver disease due to hepatitis C as well as other causes [18].

Liver failure occurs in approximately 1% of patients with acute hepatitis B and jaundice [19]. IgM hepatitis B core antibody (anti-HBc) will be positive in fulminant hepatitis B. However, diagnosis may be obscured since one-third to one-half of patients become seronegative for hepatitis B surface antigen (HBsAg) after a few days [20,21]. Early studies suggested that core promoter and precore variants may increase the risk of acute liver failure but this has not been validated in later studies [22–24]. Superinfection with hepatitis D virus precipitates 4% of acute liver failure in hepatitis B endemic areas but is uncommon in the USA [25]. Reactivation of viral replication in inactive carriers of hepatitis B can trigger acute liver failure, either spontaneously or due to chemotherapy or immunosuppression for organ transplantation [26].

Hepatitis C as a cause of acute liver failure appears to be extremely rare in the USA and Europe but may be more common in the East. In some series, HCV RNA was detected in up to half of patients with non-A, non-B fulminant hepatitis. However, markers of chronic hepatitis B infection can be suppressed by acute HCV infection, resulting in erroneous attribution of the liver damage to hepatitis C alone [15].

Hepatitis E, like hepatitis A, is spread primarily through contaminated water supplies. While rare in the West, it is a leading cause of acute liver failure in endemic areas such as India, Central and Southeast Asia, Mexico and North Africa [13]. Pregnant women are particularly at risk for acute liver failure but pregnancy itself does

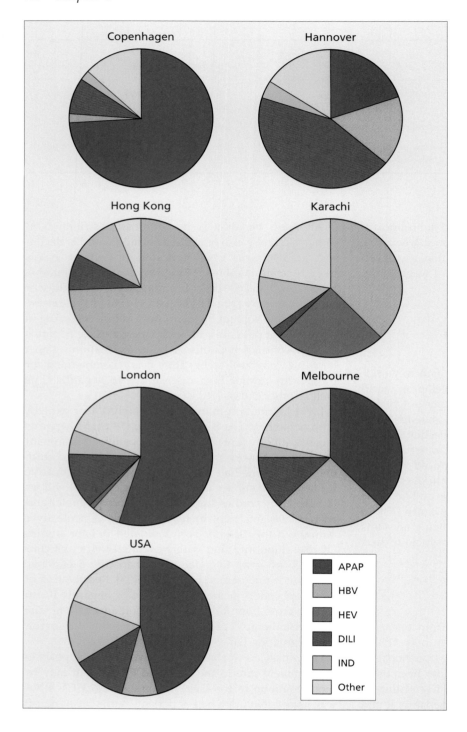

Fig. 5.1. Differences of aetiologies of acute liver failure worldwide (unpublished data, WM Lee).

not appear to impart a worse prognosis once liver failure is present [27].

Other viruses can cause a fatal hepatic necrosis especially in immunocompromised individuals. These include herpes simplex, varicella zoster, cytomegalovirus, adenoviruses, Epstein–Barr, dengue fever and parvovirus B19 [28–32]. In a survey of indeterminate acute liver failure patients in the US, no instance of hepatitis E or parvovirus B19 was identified [33].

Paracetamol

Paracetamol is a dose-related toxin, the most common suicidal agent in the UK (Chapter 24). In 1998, legisla-

Table 5.2. Causes of acute liver failure

Infections Hepatitis A, B, C, D, E Herpes simplex Epstein–Barr virus Cytomegalovirus Transfusion-transmitted virus (TTV) Dengue fever ***Drugs and toxins*** Paracetamol Carbon tetrachloride Idiosyncratic drug reactions* Mushroom poisoning Sea anemone sting ***Ischaemic*** Cardiogenic shock Hypotension Heat stroke Cocaine, methamphetamines, ephedrine ***Vascular*** Acute Budd–Chiari syndrome Sinusoidal obstruction syndrome ***Miscellaneous*** Wilson's disease Acute fatty liver of pregnancy Eclampsia/ HELLP syndrome Malignancy Primary graft non-function after liver transplantation

*See Table 5.3.

Table 5.3. Some drugs that may cause idiosyncratic liver failure

Injury leading to acute liver failure [38]:

Isoniazid	Isoflurane
Sulfonamides	Lisinopril
Phenytoin	Nicotinic acid
Nitrofurantoin	Imipramine
Propylthiouracil	Gemtuzumab
Halothane	Amphetamines/ ecstasy
Disulfiram	Labetalol
Valproic acid	Etoposide
Amiodarone	Flutamide
Dapsone	Tolcapone
Herbals*	Quetiapine
Didanosine	Nefazodone
Efavirenz	Allopurinol
Metformin	Methyldopa
Ofloxacin	Ketoconazole
Ciproflixacin	
Pyrazinamide	
Troglitazone	
Diclofenac	

Combination agents with enhanced toxicity:

Trimethoprim–sulfamethoxazole
Rifampin–isoniazid
Amoxicillin–clavulanate

*Some herbal products/ dietary supplements that have been associated with hepatotoxicity include: kava kava, chaparral, skullcap, germander, pennyroyal, jin bu huan, heliotrope, rattleweed, comfrey, sunnhemp, senecio, impila, greater celandine, gum thistle, he shon wu, ma huang, lipokinetix, bai-fang herbs, Hydroxycut®.

tion enacted in the UK mandated that paracetamol be sold in blister packs with a limit on the number of tablets obtainable without prescription. Since then, there has been a reduction in the frequency of severe paracetamol-related hepatotoxicity, the number listed for transplant and deaths [34]. However, in the USA paracetamol remains the leading cause of acute liver failure, comprising 46% of cases in the US Acute Liver Failure Study Group (ALFSG) database. In contrast to the UK, nearly half of the paracetamol acute liver failure cases were considered unintentional and strongly related to over use and abuse of narcotic-containing compounds [35].

The characteristic picture of paracetamol toxicity includes very high serum aspartate or alanine aminotransferase levels (reported up to 48 000 IU/L) accompanied by relatively low bilirubin levels (4–6 mg/dL), exemplifying the acuity of the injury [36]. Patients in the USA with acetaminophen-related acute liver failure are equally divided between those who are suicidal and those who are considered to be unintentional overdoses. The unintentional patient typically will have taken medication above the daily recommended dose for several days for a specific cause of pain, denies suicidal intent and fails to recognize the risk of toxicity [37]. Alcohol may be an important cofactor in the non-suicidal patient. Among patients who developed liver failure and reported taking <4 gm/day, alcohol abuse was present in 65% [35].

Other aetiologies

Idiosyncratic drug reactions may cause acute liver failure in up to 12% of cases in Western countries and much fewer in developing nations (Table 5.3). Cases are typically subacute with moderately elevated aminotransferases and high bilirubin levels and poor survival without transplantation (approximately 25% in most series) [38]. The most frequent culprits are antituberculosis medications, non-steroidal anti-inflammatory drugs, anaesthetic agents and antiseizure medications [39]. Acute liver failure is also reported with the recreational drug 'ecstasy' (3,4-methylene dioxymetamphetamine) [40]. Herbal remedies, especially those containing green tea extract, have been implicated in acute liver failure [41].

Mushroom poisoning, usually *Amanita phalloides*, can cause acute liver failure; it is preceded by muscarinic effects, such as profuse sweating, vomiting and diarrhoea within hours to a day of ingestion. Mortality approaches 30%. Early recognition is important to optimize supportive measures and to be alerted to the possibility of liver failure [42].

Pregnant women may develop hepatic necrosis during the third trimester, due to eclampsia and/or fatty liver (Chapter 30).

Vascular causes of ischaemic hepatitis include low cardiac output in a patient with underlying cardiac disease, systemic hypotension as seen with sepsis or cardiac events, acute Budd–Chiari syndrome, and sinusoidal-obstruction syndrome occurring after bone marrow transplantation. 'Shock liver' is rarely fatal and prognosis depends on the patient's underlying medical condition, whereas Budd–Chiari and sinusoidal-obstruction syndrome have poorer outcomes [43,44].

Massive infiltration of the liver with tumour such as in lymphoma can lead to acute liver failure. Such a cause should be considered in the differential diagnosis since liver transplantation is contraindicated, and specific therapy may be life saving [45].

Wilson's disease may present with liver failure associated with profound haemolytic anaemia and renal failure. Patients are usually diagnosed between the ages of 5 and 40 years. Fulminant hepatic failure due to Wilson's disease is universally fatal without liver transplantation [46].

Autoimmune hepatitis may rarely present as acute liver failure and may be the underlying cause in patients with indeterminate disease [47].

Clinical features

The patient with acute liver failure typically develops non-specific symptoms such as nausea, vomiting, and malaise, jaundice and signs of hepatic encephalopathy, evolving relatively quickly. The liver is often shrunken due to loss of hepatic mass and may be as small as 600 g in size (normal approximately 1600 g). Declining hepatocellular function impairs synthesis of clotting factors and glucose leading to coagulopathy and hypoglycaemia. Metabolic acidosis results from reduced clearance and increased production of lactate. Tachycardia, hypotension, hyperventilation and fever may occur and signs of the systemic inflammatory response may be present. Transfer of the patient to a specialist liver centre with a transplantation service should be done earlier rather than later. The presence of any degree of encephalopathy necessitates an immediate transfer to a transplant facility unless contraindications are present.

Patients with a more gradual onset of hepatic insufficiency (over weeks rather than days, and variously called subfulminant, subacute or late onset) infrequently develop cerebral oedema. Ascites, oedema and renal failure are more likely in this slowly evolving setting; outcome depends on the underlying aetiology (Fig. 5.2) [3]. Those patients that survive without transplant usually have a complete recovery [48].

Distinction from chronic liver disease

A note should be made of any history of liver disease, the duration of symptoms and the presence of a hard liver, marked splenomegaly and vascular spiders on the skin. In patients with evidence of chronic liver disease, perform a full evaluation for potential causes of decompensation. Infection, gastrointestinal bleeding, dehydration, sedatives and alcohol are common culprits. In the alcoholic, recent heavy drinking can add acute hepatitis to underlying chronic liver disease. In these circum-

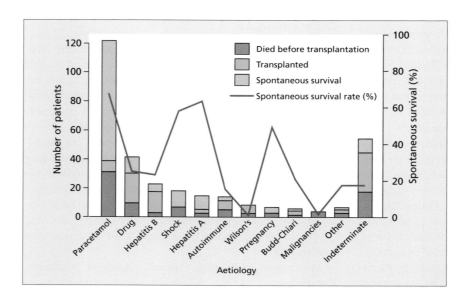

Fig. 5.2. Outcomes in acute liver failure in the USA by aetiology [3].

stances the liver is large. Acute alcoholic hepatitis is potentially reversible and merits aggressive supportive effort.

Initial investigations

Laboratory (Table 5.4)

A broad array of blood tests must be ordered initially to establish the aetiology and severity of the injury. Assessing prognosis is central to management. Despite some drawbacks, the prothrombin time/ international normalized ratio (INR) reflects the liver's synthetic function and is central to the assessment of the severity, absent plasma replacement. Elevated white blood cell count may signify an underlying infection. Low haemoglobin level may be a sign of haemolysis, often seen in Wilson's disease [49] or indicate gastrointestinal blood loss. The platelet count is low in nearly 80% for unclear reasons [3].

Serum chemistries including glucose, electrolytes, urea and creatinine are measured. Hypoglycaemia can be severe, contributing to altered mental status. Sodium, potassium and phosphorus are commonly low as is carbon dioxide in the setting of hyperventilation. Liver function tests including bilirubin, aminotransferases, alkaline phosphatase, total protein and albumin are routinely done and are usually markedly abnormal. The aminotransferases have little prognostic value since levels can fall as the patient's condition worsens or improves. Acidosis is common in paracetamol-related liver failure and is a sign of poor prognosis.

Viral serologies may identify potential aetiologies; the appropriate IgM antibodies are useful in identifying hepatitis A and B. HBsAg may have been cleared but hepatitis B surface antibody (anti-HBs) will generally not be present. Serum HBV DNA usually falls quickly and may be undetectable. In those positive for HBV, serum hepatitis D antibody should be sought. Antihepatitis C virus antibody (anti-HCV) and PCR for HCV RNA are required for diagnosis of HCV-related acute hepatic failure (Chapter 20). Hepatitis E serology IgM should be done if other aetiologies are excluded since HEV can be seen in non-endemic areas and in persons who have not travelled.

Herpes simplex virus and varicella zoster virus serologies and PCR should be checked, especially in immunosuppressed or pregnant patients, as these require specific treatment [50,51]. Liver biopsy, if performed, will show specific viral inclusions, but the presence of skin lesions merit initiation of acyclovir therapy.

Paracetamol level and toxicology screen should be obtained. However, paracetamol levels are often undetectable in the setting of unintentional cases if symptoms have already developed. Hepatotoxicity cannot be

Table 5.4. Investigations of acute liver failure

Haematology
Complete blood count: white blood cells, haemoglobin, haematocrit, anti-hepatitis B core
Coagulation panel: prothrombin time/INR, factor V
Blood group

Biochemical
Serum chemistries: sodium, potassium, bicarbonate, chloride, urea, creatinine, calcium, magnesium, phosphate, glucose
Hepatic panel: aspartate aminotransferase (AST), alanine aminotransferase (ALT), alkaline phosphatase, albumin, total protein, total bilirubin

Arterial blood gas
pH, $PaCO_2$, PaO_2, lactate, ammonia

Virology
Hepatitis B surface antigen and IgM anticore
Hepatitis A (IgM) antibody
Hepatitis C antibody (for underlying chronic infection)
HCV RNA
IgM hepatitis E antibody (in endemic areas)
Hepatitis D antibody if hepatitis B positive
HSV, CMV, EBV PCR (if history of immunosuppression)
Human immunodeficiency virus (if considering transplantation)

Autoimmune markers
Antinuclear antibody (ANA)
Antismooth-muscle antibody (SMA)
Antiliver/ kidney microsome 1 (ALKM1)
Immunoglobulins

Toxicology
Paracetamol level
Blood alcohol
Urine drug screen

Miscellaneous
Urine copper
Pregnancy test

Microbiology
Blood culture, aerobic and anaerobic
Urine culture and microscopy
Sputum culture and microscopy

Other studies
Chest X-ray, electrocardiogram
Liver ultrasound with Dopplers
Electroencephalogram (EEG), non-contrast head CT (in some cases)
Liver biopsy

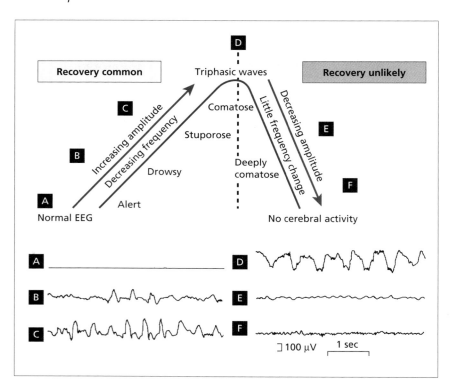

Fig. 5.3. Evolution of the EEG in liver failure. The progression from grade A to D is marked by increasing amplitude, decreasing frequency and increasing drowsiness. At D, triphasic waves appear and the interrupted line indicates the limit beyond which recovery is unlikely. From E to F amplitude decreases with little frequency change and at F there is no cerebral activity.

accurately predicted using the standard Rumack–Matthew nomogram if the precise time of ingestion is unknown, if the patient took multiple overdoses over time or if the patient had been taking extended-release preparations [52–55]. Paracetamol levels may be falsely elevated with bilirubin concentrations more than 10 mg/dL depending on the assay [56]. Markedly elevated aminotransferases, often more than 3500 IU/L, are strongly suggestive of paracetamol toxicity [36]. Paracetamol protein adducts correlate with hepatotoxicity and remain detectable for up to 12 days after ingestion. The detection of adducts, currently a research-only assay, may provide an important clinical tool when it becomes more widely available [57].

Antinuclear antibodies, smooth muscle antibodies, antibodies to liver/kidney microsomes type 1 and immunoglobulin levels should be checked for possible autoimmune hepatitis; liver biopsy may help to establish the diagnosis and is encouraged in indeterminate case settings [58].

Serum ceruloplasmin is unhelpful in fulminant Wilson's disease since levels are low in nearly 50% of all forms of acute liver failure [59]. Measurement of the ratio of alkaline phosphatase to bilirubin of less than 4 and aspartate aminotransferase to alanine aminotransferase greater than 2.2 is highly accurate in diagnosing Wilson's disease and can be obtained more rapidly than tests such as urine copper [60].

Electroencephalogram (EEG)

Continuous EEG recording shows slowing of cortical activity and up to 50% of patients with acute liver failure to have subclinical seizure/epileptiform activity (Fig. 5.3). This is not recognized clinically without EEG because the patient is usually paralysed and ventilated. EEG monitoring is controversial since prophylactic phenytoin is of unproven value [61,62].

Computed tomography (CT)

Non-contrast computed tomography of the brain is insensitive for detecting intracranial hypertension (Fig. 5.4) but may help rule out other pathology, such as haemorrhage. The yield of such studies is low and may not justify the risk of moving a critically ill patient [63–65].

Abdominal imaging and liver biopsy

Abdominal ultrasound is used to assess for vasculature patency and mass lesions. Hepatic nodularity is commonly seen in the acute setting, reflecting regenerative nodules rather than cirrhosis [66]. CT scanning will show a reduction in liver size but correlation of liver size with survival is imprecise.

Liver histology can show considerable variability of necrosis that may be prognostically misleading [67].

(a) (b)

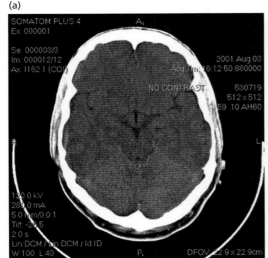

Fig. 5.4. Cerebral oedema on CT scanning in a patient with acute liver failure. (a) Head CT at presentation showing clear demarcation between white and gray matter. (b) Head CT 48 h later demonstrating loss of demarcation between white and gray matter and effacement of sulci.

Sampling error precludes use of liver biopsy for prognosis. Transjugular liver biopsy should be performed if there is any suspicion of malignancy or autoimmune hepatitis [38]. It may aid in diagnosis (Fig. 5.5). In a retrospective study a liver volume of less than 1000 mL and/or hepatic parenchymal necrosis of greater than 50% indicated a poor prognosis, but findings above these two thresholds did not necessarily indicate a good outcome [68].

Complications and management of acute liver failure

Acute liver failure represents a syndrome precipitated by various causes rather than a single disease. In addition to the defining hepatic encephalopathy and coagulopathy, significant hepatocyte death incites a cytokine storm which may result in systemic inflammatory response syndrome (SIRS), multiple system organ failure and ultimately death [69,70]. Treatment has focused on the management of complications except for a few aetiology specific therapies (Table 5.5). However, a recent double-blind placebo controlled trial of intravenous *N*-acetylcysteine (NAC) demonstrated improved transplant-free survival in non-paracetamol acute liver failure patients with early stage encephalopathy, perhaps offering a common therapy for fulminant hepatic failure [71].

Hepatic encephalopathy

Hepatic encephalopathy and cerebral oedema with raised intracranial pressure (ICP) are hallmarks of acute liver failure (Fig. 5.6). Once stupor develops with or without decerebrate posturing (stage 3–4 encephalopathy), cerebral oedema is likely.

The pathogenesis of hepatic encephalopathy is multifactorial (Chapter 8) and centres on failure of the liver to remove toxic, mainly gut-derived, substances from the circulation. Arterial ammonia levels rise and appear to contribute to astrocyte swelling. Levels greater than 150 to 200 mmol/L have been shown to correlate with cerebral oedema and herniation [73–75]. In contrast to the coma of cirrhotic patients, portal–systemic encephalopathy due to shunting of blood past the liver is of minor importance.

The onset of encephalopathy is often sudden, may precede jaundice, and, unlike chronic liver disease, may be associated with agitation, changes in personality, delusions and restlessness. Asterixis may be transient. Fetor hepaticus is usually present.

Management of the portosystemic encephalopathy of cirrhosis has centred on lactulose and non-absorbable antibiotics. However, lactulose has shown no benefit in acute liver failure and may increase aspiration risk and bowel distension, which complicates transplantation [76]. There is not enough evidence to recommend non-absorbable antibiotics in acute liver failure. In cirrhosis, L-ornithine L-aspartate (LOLA) treats encephalopathy by increasing muscle metabolism of ammonia but a recent randomized controlled trial showed no benefit in acute liver failure [77].

The prognosis for patients with stage 1 or 2 encephalopathy (confused or drowsy) is good. For stage 3 or 4 it is much poorer. Obtunded patients should be electively intubated for airway protection. Sedation with propofol is preferred as it may lower intracranial

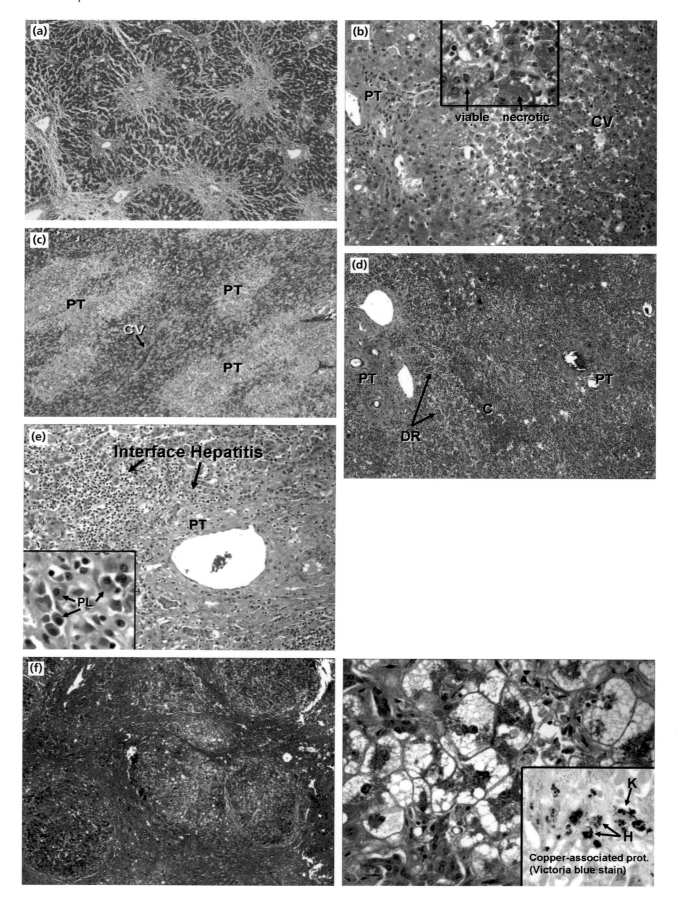

Fig. 5.5. Histological features of acute liver failure. (a) Autopsy specimen from a patient who died of cerebral oedema following paracetamol ingestion. Haematoxylin and eosin slide demonstrates centrilobular necrosis with surviving periportal hepatocytes. (b) Explanted liver in a case of paracetamol toxicity. Necrotic hepatocytes with eosinophilic cytoplasm around the central vein (CV) with viable hepatocytes surrounding the portal tracts (PT). (c) Explanted liver of a patient with fulminant acute hepatitis B. Multilobular hepatic necrosis centred around the central vein (CV) with inflammatory infiltration of the portal tracts (PT). (d) Explanted liver of a patient with acute liver failure following black cohosh ingestion. Massive hepatic necrosis with minimal centrilobular (C) parenchyma remaining. Portal tracts (PT) expanded by inflammatory cells and bile duct reaction (DR). (e) Higher magnification demonstrating features of autoimmune hepatitis with interface hepatitis and multiple plasma cells (PL). (f) Explanted liver of a 20-year-old patient with Wilson's disease. Trichrome stain shows cirrhosis with bands of fibrosis surrounding regenerative nodules. Haematoxylin and eosin slide (right) shows severe hepatocyte injury with ballooning degeneration, microsteatosis and cholestasis. Victoria blue stain highlights copper pigment within the hepatocytes (H) and Kupffer cells (K). Histology courtesy of Jay Lefkowitch, MD, Columbia University College of Physicians and Surgeons, New York, NY.

pressure [78]. Progression of encephalopathy is often triggered by infection and empiric antibiotics should be administered to these patients [79].

Cerebral oedema and intracranial hypertension

Acute liver failure is uniquely associated with cerebral oedema, which can lead to an increase in intracerebral pressure. This is uncommon in patients with stage 1 or 2 encephalopathy, but develops in the majority with stage 4. Raised intracerebral pressure can lead to brainstem herniation, which remains a leading cause of death [80]. The cause is not fully understood and is probably multifactorial, influenced by altered brain osmolality, cellular metabolism and cerebral blood flow (Fig. 5.7) [81–83].

The rapid rise of ammonia appears critical for the development of cerebral oedema [84]. Ammonia crosses the blood–brain barrier to be taken up by the astrocytes, where it is converted to the osmotically active glutamine. Water passively diffuses into the astrocyte, causing swelling [85]. In addition, inflammatory cytokines exacerbate vasodilation, resulting in increased cerebral blood flow, vasogenic oedema and increased intracranial pressure [86].

The net blood supply to the brain depends on the balance between carotid arterial pressure and intracerebral pressure (cerebral perfusion pressure = mean arterial pressure – intracranial pressure). Cerebral blood flow autoregulation (maintained blood flow despite falling or rising blood pressure) is lost in patients with fulminant hepatic failure [87]. This can lead to relative intracranial hypertension due to increasing cerebral blood flow and interstitial water, as well as cerebral hypoperfusion and hypoxia due to systemic hypotension.

Clinically, raised intracerebral pressure is suggested by systolic hypertension (sustained or intermittent), increased muscle tone and myoclonus, which progress to extension and hyperpronation of the arms and extension of the legs (decerebrate posturing). Dysconjugate eye movements and skewed positions of the eyes may be seen. If not controlled by treatment, this clinical picture progresses to loss of pupillary reflexes and respiratory arrest from brainstem herniation.

The most accurate method of diagnosing intracranial hypertension is insertion of an ICP monitor. Many centres rely on ICP monitors once patients reach stage 3 to 4 encephalopathy to guide management despite evidence showing no benefit in survival and 4 to 20% risk of complications [88]. Other centres use non-invasive monitors such as infrared spectroscopy, transcranial Doppler, or jugular venous oximetry unless signs of progressive cerebral oedema [89]. If an ICP monitor is inserted, the goal of cerebral perfusion pressure is above 50 mmHg and intracranial pressure below 25 mmHg [90].

General management of cerebral oedema includes limiting stimulation, elevating the head to 30 degrees, and correction of acidosis and electrolytes. Additional therapies focus on decreasing cerebral oedema by increasing intravascular osmotic gradient (hypertonic saline, mannitol) or by reducing cerebral blood flow (hyperventilation, barbiturates, indomethacin and hypothermia) [91].

Prophylactic infusion of 30% hypertonic saline to keep serum sodium 145–155 mmol/L in patients with severe encephalopathy is associated with fewer episodes of intracranial hypertension [92]. Trials are needed to test its efficacy in established intracranial hypertension.

Once obvious neurological signs develop or ICP is above 25 mmHg for over 10 min, a bolus of intravenous mannitol (0.25–1 g/kg, 20% solution) is recommended. This can be repeated if serum osmolality is less than 320 mOsm/L. Volume overload can develop and ultrafiltration may be necessary in the setting of renal impairment. Nearly 60% of intracranial hypertension cases respond and mannitol has been shown to improve survival [93].

Hyperventilation, to induce cerebral vasoconstriction and reduce cerebral blood volume, has an effect that is

Table 5.5. Intensive care of acute liver failure

Cerebral oedema/ intracranial hypertension

Grade 1/2 encephalopathy

Consider transfer to liver transplant facility and listing for transplantation
Head CT: rule out other causes of decreased mental status; little utility to identify cerebral oedema
Avoid stimulation, avoid sedation if possible
Antibiotics: surveillance and treatment of infection required; prophylaxis possibly helpful for unexplained deterioration
Lactulose: possibly helpful

Grade 3/4 encephalopathy

Continue management strategies listed above
Intubate trachea (may require sedation)
Elevate head of bed
Consider placement of ICP monitoring device
Immediate treatment of seizures required; prophylaxis of unclear value
Mannitol (0.25–1 g/kg i.v. bolus): use for severe elevation of ICP or first clinical signs of herniation, monitor urine output and serum osmolarity
Hypertonic saline (30% 5–10 mL/h): goal serum sodium 145–155 mmol/L, avoid rapid correction
Hyperventilation: effects short-lived; may use for impending herniation
Barbiturate coma (pentobarbital 3–5 mg/kg i.v. bolus then 1–3 mg/kg/h or thiopental 5–10 mg/kg i.v. bolus then 3–5 mg/kg/h): watch for hypotension
Continuous renal replacement, hypothermia (32–35°C), i.v. indomethacin (25 mg bolus) may have some benefit in very refractory cases

Infection
Aseptic techniques
Surveillance for and prompt antimicrobial treatment of infection required
Antifungal coverage for patients not responding to broad spectrum antibiotics
Antibiotic prophylaxis possibly helpful but not proven

Coagulopathy
Vitamin K (10 mg i.v. or subcutaneous)
FFP: give only for invasive procedures or active bleeding
Platelets: give for platelet counts <10000/mm^3 or invasive procedures
Recombinant activated factor VII (40 µg/kg bolus): give 30 min before procedure if coagulopathy refractory to FFP
Cryoprecipitate: for fibrinogen <100 mg/dL and bleeding
Exchange plasmapheresis: allows transfusion of large amount of FFP
Prophylaxis for stress ulceration: give H2 blocker or PPI

Haemodynamics/ renal failure
Arterial line
Pulmonary artery catheterization
Volume replacement
Check cortisol and cosyntropin stimulation test; hydrocortisone 200–300 mg/day for adrenal insufficiency
Pressor support (noradrenaline preferred over dopamine or adrenaline) as needed to maintain adequate mean arterial pressure
Avoid nephrotoxic agents
Continuous modes of haemodialysis if needed, such as venovenous haemodialysis
Vasopressin: potentially harmful

Pulmonary
Sedation for endotracheal intubation and suctioning to prevent increased ICP
Ventilator management: tidal volumes 6 mL/kg, low PEEP, aim for $Paco_2$ 30–40 mmHg

Metabolic concerns
Follow closely: glucose, potassium, magnesium, phosphate
Consider nutrition: enteral feedings preferred over total parenteral nutrition

---

ICP, intracranial pressure; FFP, fresh frozen plasma; PEEP, positive end-expiratory pressure.

not sustained. In the case of impending herniation, it may be used temporally [94,95]. Thiopental (5–10 mg/kg load followed by 3–5 mg/kg per h) or pentobarbital (3–5 mg/kg load followed by 1–3 mg/kg per h) infusion induces a barbiturate coma that is effective in some patients where mannitol has failed. Significant hypotension complicates its use [96]. Corticosteroids are not effective in controlling cerebral oedema or improving survival in acute liver failure [93]. Intravenous indomethacin in 25-mg boluses is given in refractory cases of intracranial hypertension to cause vasoconstriction and reduce cerebral blood flow. The risk of causing cerebral ischaemia as well as the renal and gastric toxicities limits its use [97].

Hypothermia (32 to 35°C) prevents brain oedema by decreasing arterial ammonia and brain uptake of ammonia, reducing cerebral blood flow and re-establishing cerebral autoregulation [98,99]. Preliminary studies in patients with acute liver failure showed decreased intracranial pressure and stabilization until transplant [100]. However, hypothermia increases the risk of sepsis, clotting problems and cardiac arrhythmias [101,102]. Randomized controlled trials are needed to determine its potential impact on mortality in acute liver failure [103]. Based on current clinical data, hypothermia cannot be recommended but these results emphasize that hyperthermia should be avoided [104].

Coagulopathy

The liver synthesizes all the coagulation factors (except factor VIII), inhibitors of coagulation and proteins

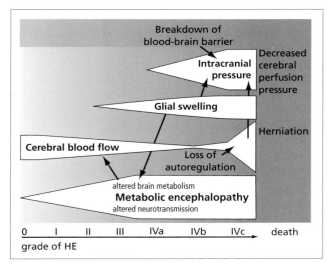

Fig. 5.6. Brain dysfunction in acute liver failure. Proposed interrelation of metabolic encephalopathy, intracranial pressure and changes in cerebral blood flow during the progression of the disease. HE, hepatic encephalopathy [72].

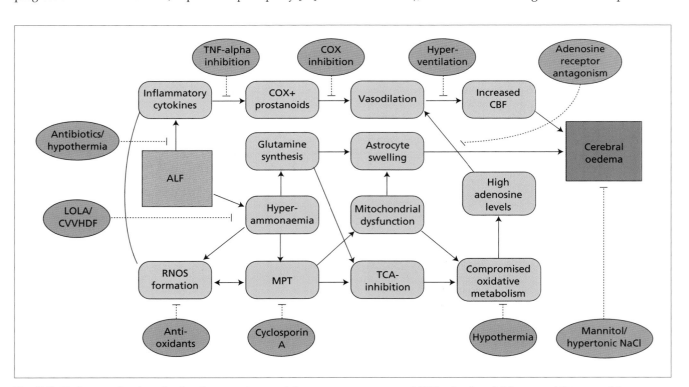

Fig. 5.7. Pathogenesis of cerebral oedema and potential targets for therapy. ALF, acute liver failure; CBF, cerebral blood flow; COX, cyclo-oxygenase; CVVHDF, continuous venovenous haemodiafiltration; LOLA, L-ornithine L-aspartate; MPT, mitochondrial permeability transition; NaCl, saline; RNOS, reactive nitrogen and oxygen species; TCA, tricarboxylic acid; TNF, tumour necrosis factor [84].

involved in the fibrinolytic system (Chapter 4). It is also involved in the clearance of activated clotting factors. The coagulopathy of fulminant hepatic failure is thus complex and due not only to factor deficiency, but also to enhanced fibrinolytic activity and decreased platelet number and function. The failing liver's inability to remove activated clotting factors may precipitate disseminated intravascular coagulation [105].

The resulting coagulopathy predisposes to bleeding. This is a potential cause of death; it may be spontaneous, from the mucous membranes, the gastrointestinal tract or into the brain. Clinically significant spontaneous bleeding occurs in approximately 5% of acute liver failure patients. Bleeding after invasive procedures poses a more significant problem, with fatal haemorrhage occurring in 1 to 4% after ICP monitor insertion [106].

The prothrombin time and its associated INR is a widely used guide to prognosis and is one of the criteria used in deciding whether transplantation should be done (Table 5.6). However, the high INR levels seen in acute liver failure may overestimate the risk of bleeding and values vary among different laboratories [108,109]. Factor V levels and fibrinogen levels should also be serially monitored; declining factor V levels portend a poor prognosis.

Coagulopathy is managed by routine intravenous or subcutaneous vitamin K [110]. Fresh frozen plasma, cryoprecipitate and platelets are given for INR at or above 1.5, fibrinogen less than 100 mg/dL and platelets less than 50 000/mm^3 but only if there is active bleeding or prior to invasive procedures. Prophylactic blood products are not advised, as they do not decrease the risk of bleeding, result in volume overload and obscure the trend of INR as a prognostic value [111]. Recombinant activated factor VII can correct coagulopathy non-responsive to plasma but has a risk of thrombosis [112]. Use of recombinant factor VIIa is controversial in this setting, but it is often given prior to invasive procedures if fresh frozen plasma alone fails to correct the coagulopathy.

Metabolic derangements

Hypoglycaemia is found in 40% of patients with acute liver failure. It may be persistent and intractable. Plasma insulin levels are high due to reduced hepatic uptake; gluconeogenesis is reduced in the failing liver. Hypoglycaemia can cause rapid neurological deterioration and death. Blood glucose levels less than 60 mg/dL should be treated with a continuous infusion of 5 or 10% dextrose. Enteral feedings should be initiated early unless contraindicated. Liver failure is a catabolic state; there is no need to restrict protein.

Hypokalaemia is common and due in part to urinary losses with inadequate replacement, and administration of glucose. Hyponatraemia frequently worsens cerebral oedema. Other electrolyte changes include hypophosphataemia, hypocalcaemia and hypomagnesaemia. Electrolytes and glucose should be monitored twice daily and promptly corrected.

Acid–base changes are common. Respiratory alkalosis is due to hyperventilation, probably related to direct stimulation of the respiratory centre by unknown toxic substances. Respiratory acidosis can be caused by elevated ICP and respiratory depression, or pulmonary complications. Lactic acidosis develops in about half of the patients reaching stage 3 coma. It is related to inadequate tissue perfusion due to hypotension and hypoxaemia. Metabolic acidosis is more frequent in paracetamol-induced acute liver failure. Fall in pH is one of the criteria used in transplant decisions.

Infection

Infection affects up to 90% of patients with acute liver failure and stage 2 or more encephalopathy and is one

Table 5.6. King's College Hospital criteria for liver transplantation in acute liver failure [107]

Paracetamol
pH <7.30 (irrespective of grade of encephalopathy)
or
Prothrombin time >100 s (INR >7) and serum creatinine >300 mmol/L (>3.4 mg/dL) in patients with grade 3 or 4 encephalopathy

Non-paracetamol patients
Prothrombin time >100 s (INR >7) (irrespective of grade of encephalopathy)
or
Any three of the following variables (irrespective of grade of encephalopathy)
age <10 or >40 years
aetiology: non-A–E hepatitis, 'viral' hepatitis no agent identified, halothane hepatitis, idiosyncratic drug reaction
duration of jaundice before onset of encephalopathy >7 days
prothrombin time >50 s (INR >3.5)
serum bilirubin >300 mmol/L (17.4 mg/dL)

of the main causes of death. The majority of infections are pulmonary followed by urinary tract and blood. More than two-thirds of infections are due to Gram-positive organisms, usually staphylococci, but streptococci and Gram-negative bacilli are also found [113]. Fungal infections occur in about one-third of patients, often unrecognized and ominous [114]. The typical manifestations of sepsis such as fever and leucocytosis may be absent [113,115].

The high rate of infection can be related to poor host defences with impaired Kupffer cell function and to the reduction of factors such as fibronectin, opsonins and chemoattractants, including components of the complement system. Poor respiratory effort and cough reflex and the presence of endotracheal tubes, venous lines and urinary catheters place the patient at increased risk. To pre-empt septic complications, sputum and urine should be sent for culture daily. Venous and arterial line sites should be inspected regularly; cannulas should be replaced if inflamed, if fever develops or otherwise routinely every 3–5 days. The tip of the catheter is sent for culture.

Studies of prophylactic systemic antibiotics and intestinal decontamination have shown benefit both individually and in combination. Their use is, however, controversial. Prophylactic intravenous antibiotics reduce infection by 80% but do not improve outcome or reduce the length of stay. Selective enteric decontamination adds no benefits to parenteral antibiotics [116]. In this study multiresistant bacteria were found, possibly secondary to the third-generation cephalosporin used.

The most appropriate antibiotic regimen will depend on the incidence, type and sensitivity of bacteria in each hospital but usually includes a third generation cephalosporin or fluoroquinolone. Vancomycin is indicated if there is concern for line sepsis. Fungal coverage should be added for those that fail to improve with antibacterial medications. Blanket use of broad-spectrum antibiotics should be narrowed down to a specific choice once positive cultures are available. Antibiotics should be given to patients that have positive cultures, signs of infection, are hypotensive, progress to stage 3 coma or are listed for liver transplant.

Renal

Renal failure, which develops in 30–70% of patients, negatively impacts survival [117]. It may be related to liver cell failure itself (hepatorenal syndrome), to acute tubular necrosis secondary to complications of acute liver failure (sepsis, bleeding, hypotension), or direct nephrotoxicity of the drug or other insult responsible for the hepatic damage (e.g. paracetamol overdose) [118]. The hepatorenal syndrome (Chapter 10) results from a combination of factors including a hyperdynamic circulation with lowered renal perfusion pressure, activation of the sympathetic nervous system and increased synthesis of vasoactive mediators which decrease glomerular capillary ultrafiltration [119]. Urinalysis helps distinguish the cause, with urine sodium more than 10 mEq/L with active sediment more consistent with acute tubular necrosis and urine sodium less than 10 mEq/L seen in prerenal azotaemia and hepatorenal syndrome.

When renal failure develops, monitoring of fluid balance becomes even more critical. Intravenous fluid challenge of 1 to 1.5 L of crystalloid and colloid should be attempted first to treat any prerenal azotaemia. Low-dose dopamine has no proven benefit in renal failure over other vasopressors and is not routinely recommended [120]. Continuous renal replacement therapy (CRRT) with bicarbonate buffer is indicated over intermittent haemodialysis even in haemodynamically stable acute liver failure patients to prevent fluctuations in intracranial pressure. In addition to correcting uraemia, fluid overload, acidosis and hyperkalaemia, CRRT may decrease cerebral oedema by removing ammonia and cooling the patient [121].

Haemodynamic changes

Hypotension with a low peripheral vascular resistance and increased cardiac output are features of liver failure. Possible mediators include prostaglandins and nitric oxide. Tissue hypoxia at the microcirculatory level is frequent with consequent lactic acidosis. When crystalloid or albumin infusions do not correct the fall in blood pressure, vasopressors are frequently needed to maintain mean arterial pressure above 60 mmHg or cerebral perfusion pressure below 50 mmHg. Noradrenaline (norepinepherine) is preferred. Vasopressin should be used cautiously as it causes cerebral vasodilation and might increase intracranial pressure [122,123].

Persistent hypotension should prompt evaluation for adrenal insufficiency. Hydrocortisone (200–300 mg/day) has been shown to be beneficial in septic patients with inadequate adrenal response. A retrospective review of acute liver failure patients showed that those receiving hydrocortisone required less vasopressor support but there was no benefit in survival [124,125].

Cardiac dysrhythmias of most types are noted in the later stages and relate to electrolyte abnormalities, acidosis, hypoxia and the insertion of catheters into the pulmonary artery. Depression of brainstem function due to cerebral oedema and herniation eventually leads to circulatory failure.

Gastrointestinal bleeding

Critically ill patients, including those with acute liver failure, are at risk for gastrointestinal haemorrhage.

Intravenous infusion of histamine-2 receptor blockers has been shown to decrease bleeding gastroduodenal erosions in this population [126]. Proton pump inhibitors and sulcralfate are used for prophylaxis but have not been proven effective in controlled trials.

Pulmonary complications

Patients often need endotracheal intubation and mechanical ventilation to prevent aspiration in the later stages of encephalopathy. Coma and respiratory depression can manifest as hypoxemia. Intrapulmonary arteriovenous shunting adds to the hypoxia. Primary lung injury is rare but can occur and may be more common in paracetamol-induced acute liver failure [127]. Intravenous fluids can contribute to pulmonary oedema. Adult respiratory distress syndrome (ARDS) develops late in the course.

Respiratory status is monitored using continuous pulse oximetry. Daily chest X-rays are obtained to monitor for infection and are abnormal in over half of patients. Once mechanical ventilation is needed, low tidal volume (6 mL/kg ideal body weight) and positive end-expiratory pressure levels are used to minimize barotrauma and worsening of intracranial pressure.

Acute pancreatitis

Acute haemorrhagic and necrotizing pancreatitis has been reported in 44% of patients dying with acute liver failure [128]. More recently, a study reported hyperamylasaemia in 12% of acute liver failure patients, only 9% of whom had clinical pancreatitis. An elevated serum amylase level is not an independent predictor of survival and appears to be influenced by renal and multi-organ failure [129]. Pancreatitis is difficult to recognize in the comatose patient but, rarely, it may be the cause of death.

Specific therapies

Over the years survival of patients with acute liver failure has improved due to meticulous attention to the detail of good supportive care combined with better knowledge of the most important functions lost when the liver cell fails. However, outcome is still largely dependent on the underlying cause. In order to optimize survival, one must establish the diagnosis of acute liver failure quickly, evaluate the potential aetiologies and therapies, and estimate the severity to appropriately identify those that will need transplantation (Fig. 5.8).

Paracetamol hepatotoxicity

Acute liver failure due to paracetamol should be suspected based on history of suicidal attempt or ingestion of compound pain medications. Doses exceeding 10 g/day are usually needed but severe hepatic injury can occasionally occur with as little as 4 g/day in susceptible patients. Even if history is negative, aminotransferases over 3500 IU/L with low bilirubin levels are usually indicative of paracetamol toxicity [36].

NAC is the antidote for paracetamol poisoning, repleting glutathione that detoxifies the harmful metabolite, *N*-aminoparaquinoneimine (NAPQI). While it is most effective when given within 10 h of paracetamol overdose, NAC may be of benefit 48 h or more after ingestion and should be administered even if acute liver failure has developed [130]. NAC may be given orally (140 mg/kg followed by 70 mg/kg every 4 h for 17 doses) but intravenous administration (150 mg/kg in 5% dextrose over 15 min then 50 mg/kg over 4 h followed by 100 mg/kg over 16 h) is recommended if encephalopathy is present. Anaphylactoid reactions occur rarely and can be managed by discontinuation, antihistamines and adrenaline [131].

Mushroom poisoning

Amanita phalloides is responsible for most of the deaths due to mushroom poisoning. It is toxic in small amounts (0.1–0.3 mg/kg), even after cooking. History of recent mushroom ingestion followed by nausea, vomiting and diarrhoea should prompt treatment with gastric lavage and activated charcoal. Intravenous penicillin G (300 000 to 1 million units/kg per day) is the most common antidote used in the USA but silibinin (30–40 mg/kg/day oral or i.v.) with or without NAC may be more effective [132].

Hepatitis B

Acute liver failure may occur in acute hepatitis B infection or with reactivation of chronic infection either spontaneously or with immunosuppression. In a small prospective study of patients with severe acute hepatitis B, lamivudine therapy (100–150 mg/day) was associated with decreased need for transplant and decreased the risk of re-infection after transplantation [133]. Other antivirals are also used in this setting, particularly when long-term viral suppression is indicated (Chapter 18) (e.g. after liver transplantation). Prophylactic antiviral therapy should be initiated in patients who are HBsAg positive and should also be considered in HBsAg-negative anti-HBc positive patients prior to chemotherapy or organ transplantation to prevent reactivation [26].

Herpes simplex virus

Herpes hepatitis is a rare cause of acute liver failure, usually in immunosuppressed or pregnant patients.

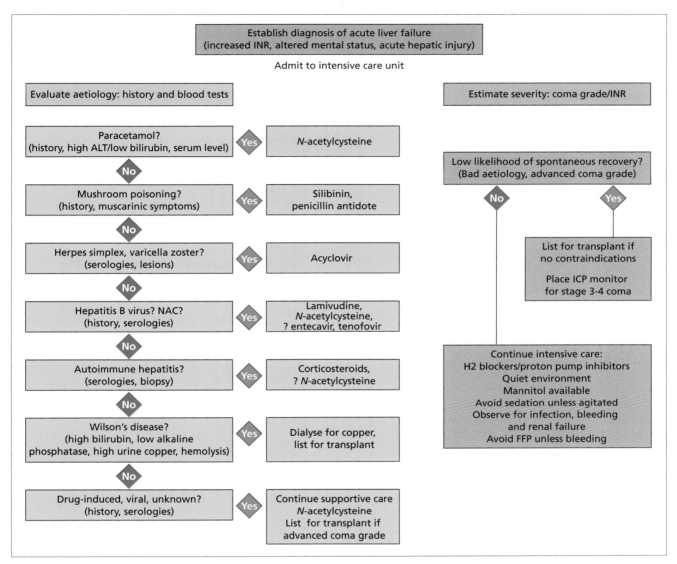

Fig. 5.8. Suggested algorithm for triage, diagnosis and treatment of the patient with acute liver failure. ALT, alanine aminotransferase; INR, international normalized ratio; ICP, intracranial pressure; FFP, fresh frozen plasma.

Diagnosis can be difficult. Skin lesions are absent in over half. Infection is confirmed by detectable HSV DNA or liver biopsy. Presence of a vesicular rash and/or immunosuppression and high aminotransferases should trigger HSV testing and consideration of liver biopsy and initiation of treatment. Despite treatment with intravenous acyclovir (30 mg/kg daily), prognosis is poor [134,135].

Autoimmune hepatitis

Fulminant liver failure is an uncommon presentation of autoimmune hepatitis. Autoantibodies may be absent. Liver biopsy demonstrating plasma cell rich interface hepatitis (frequently extending throughout the lobule)

may be required for definitive diagnosis. Patients are treated with prednisone or prednisolone 60 mg/day. Biopsies that show multilobar collapse, persistently elevated bilirubin and failure to respond to steroids within 2 weeks impart a dismal prognosis and these patients should be listed for transplantation [136].

Pregnancy

Acute liver failure may occur in the setting of acute fatty liver of pregnancy or severe pre-eclampsia (Chapter 30). Acute fatty liver of pregnancy usually presents in first-time mothers during their third trimester with symptoms of malaise, right upper quadrant pain, hypoglycaemia and jaundice. Hypertension and proteinuria are common. HELLP (haemolysis, elevated liver enzymes, low platelets) syndrome is also a complication of pre-eclampsia that can result in acute liver failure. Prompt delivery of the fetus usually results in recovery, though postpartum liver transplantation is occasionally needed [137].

Wilson's disease

Fulminant Wilson's disease is 100% fatal without liver transplantation. As mentioned previously, high bilirubin and low alkaline phosphatase levels suggest Wilson's disease and high urine copper levels confirm the diagnosis. The usual therapies of penicillamine or trientine are ineffective in acute liver failure and are not recommended. Albumin dialysis, CRRT, plasmapheresis or plasma exchange can be initiated to remove copper and alleviate renal tubular damage until a graft becomes available [46].

Prognosis

A number of factors influence survival and have prognostic value. One of the most important predictors of outcome is the underlying aetiology. Transplant-free survival is over 50% for acute liver failure due to paracetamol, hepatitis A, ischaemia and pregnancy, compared to less than 25% for other causes [3]. The severity of encephalopathy also impacts survival. The overall survival for those reaching grade 3 or 4 encephalopathy is 20% without transplantation. If only grade 1 or 2 coma is reached, survival is around 65%. Those who survive rarely if ever develop cirrhosis.

The advent of successful liver transplantation for acute liver failure has made prediction of survival particularly important. Indications, whether clinical or laboratory, that spontaneous recovery is unlikely are therefore of vital importance. Several prognostic systems have been developed in order to determine which patients will survive without transplantation but all lack sufficient sensitivity.

The most widely used prognostic tool is the King's College Criteria for paracetamol and non-paracetamol acute liver failure (Table 5.6). Predictive accuracies were initially reported to be 85% for paracetamol and 95% for non-paracetamol. Studies since have confirmed that King's criteria have a reasonable positive predictive value (80% for paracetamol, 70–90% in non-paracetamol) but negative predictive values range from 25 to 90%. Therefore a substantial number of patients that do not fulfil the King's criteria will eventually die without transplantation [138]. Arterial lactate above 3.5 mmol/L portends a poor prognosis and may increase the predictive accuracy of the King's criteria [139].

The Clichy criteria for fulminant viral hepatitis has shown that a factor V level less than 20% in patients younger than 30 years of age and less than 30% in those with grade 3 or 4 encephalopathy is associated with mortality [140]. Additional proposed prognostic models include factor VIII and factor V ratios, serial prothrombin times, α fetoprotein, hyperphosphataemia, Gc-globulin levels, the Acute Physiology and Chronic Health Evaluation (APACHE II) scores, and change in the Model for End-stage Liver Disease (MELD) scores to name a few [141]. Although some show promise, none reach the ideal of recognizing only those who would benefit from transplantation; the King's College Criteria remains the most widely utilized prognostic score.

Liver transplantation (Chapter 36)

Hepatic transplantation has to be considered for patients reaching grade 3 and 4 coma due to acute liver failure. Survival without transplantation is less than 20% rising to 60–80% with transplantation. However, it is frequently difficult to judge both the right time and the necessity for transplant. If too early, the operation may be unnecessary and the patient will be committed to lifetime immunosuppression; if too late, the chances of successful transplantation are reduced.

Indications

The decision to select an individual for potential transplant is based on validated criteria, including pH, age, aetiology, time between onset of jaundice and encephalopathy, prothrombin time and serum bilirubin level, or a plasma factor V level of less than 20% of normal. In the original studies, use of these criteria identified about 95% of fatal cases. Knowing the aetiology can help determine when transplant evaluation should be performed; paracetamol patients do relatively well, while Wilson's disease and drug-induced liver injury patients are unlikely to survive without grafting.

Acute liver failure is universally regarded as an urgent indication for liver transplantation. However, there is a delay on average of about 2 days in obtaining an acceptable donor liver after putting out the request. Although the majority will survive the waiting time and still require a transplant, 9% will improve and be removed from the list while 10% will have died. Up to 22% develop contraindications while waiting for a graft [3]. This has led to the suggestion that all patients with hyperacute liver failure should be listed for transplantation on admission to hospital, or when they reach grade 3 encephalopathy, and that the decision as to whether or not transplantation is necessary should be reviewed when the donor liver becomes available.

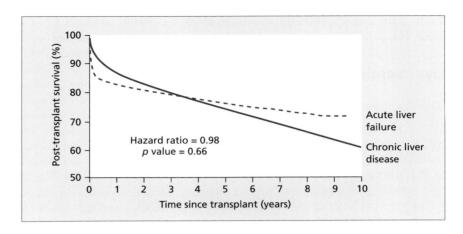

Fig. 5.9. Adjusted survival after liver transplant for acute liver failure versus cirrhosis. Data adjusted for recipient age, gender, race, body mass index, medical condition, dialysis, diabetes, life support, previous abdominal surgery, HCV-positivity, portal vein thrombosis, as well as donor factors including age, race, cause of death, donation after cardiac death, cold ischaemia time, partial or split liver and living donor [2].

Contraindications

Absolute contraindications are severe infection, malignancy outside the liver, brain death, severe cardiac or pulmonary disease and multiorgan system failure. Fixed dilated pupils for prolonged periods of time (1 h or more) and cerebral perfusion pressure less than 40 mmHg or ICP more than 35 mmHg for longer than 1–2 h suggest serious neurological compromise. Relative contraindications are age over 70, a rapidly increasing requirement for vasopressor support, infection under treatment and a history of psychiatric problems [5].

Intraoperative and postoperative care

During dissection of the native liver and reperfusion of the graft, intracranial pressure can increase. Some surgeons use venovenous bypass during the operation to prevent cerebral perfusion fluctuations but this is not routine procedure. If an ICP monitor is in place prior to transplant, it should be utilized for the first 10–12 h post-transplant and then removed. Significant intracranial hypertension (ICP >25 mmHg) should be treated [5,65].

Graft selection

The survival of patients that have reached stage 4 encephalopathy is dismal and a donor liver may be difficult to find. Therefore it may be necessary to use an organ with incompatible blood group or significant steatosis. ABO-identical grafts are optimal but ABO-compatible grafts have comparable 1-year outcomes. However, older donor age, steatosis and ABO-incompatibility can contribute to primary graft nonfunction, acute cellular rejection and intrahepatic biliary strictures. All have been linked to decreased graft and patient survival [5].

Outcomes

Technically, the transplant operation is less difficult than that for chronic liver disease as cachexia, portal venous collaterals and adhesions generally are not present. Coagulation defects can be controlled with plasma derivatives and platelets. Most deaths occur within the first 3 months after surgery due to sepsis or neurological complications. Initial survival is less than that seen overall when transplantation is done for cirrhosis but 5-year survival rates are actually better for acute liver failure (Fig. 5.9) [2]. There are several factors that influence transplant survival in acute liver failure. Pretransplant multiple organ system failure, which often complicates acute liver failure, strongly predicts post-transplant mortality [142]. The urgency of the situation leads to the use of more marginal grafts. One single-centre review found that age over 45 years, vasopressor requirement, use of high-risk grafts and transplantation prior to 2000 were associated with the poorest outcomes [143].

Living donor liver transplantation (LDLT)

This is a well-established procedure of liver transplantation for children using a left or left lateral lobe from a living donor. Paediatric acute liver failure patients that receive a LDLT have the same outcome as those that receive a whole graft. LDLT is more complicated for adults who typically require a right lobe. This poses more risk to the donor with complications in up to 25% and a mortality rate of 0.2%. Concerns with this approach for acute liver failure include issues of informed consent under the pressure of an emergency situation, which may interfere with a potential donor's ability to make a well-considered decision. Full donor evaluation may not be completed if the patient is rapidly deteriorating, placing the donor at increased risk. Additionally, the graft must be large enough for recovery while leaving sufficient residual hepatocyte mass for the donor [5].

Liver support systems

Auxiliary liver transplantation

In auxiliary transplants, the native liver is left in place and the donor liver graft either placed in the right upper quadrant alongside the native liver (heterotopic), or part of the native liver is resected and replaced with a reduced size graft (orthotopic). Studies suggest a similar 1-year survival without the need for life long immunosuppression in most patients [144].

Artificial and bioartificial liver support

Liver assist devices aim to provide support until the native liver recovers its function spontaneously, or until a donor liver is available. They are generally either artificial detoxification systems or cell-based systems designed to provide metabolic and synthetic function as well. Much research has focused on the use of columns or membranes that would allow removal of toxic metabolites. Charcoal haemoperfusion, despite early promise, has not shown benefit in controlled trials [145]. More recent artificial liver support systems (MARS, Molecular Absorbent Recirculating System (Gambro®, Canada), and FPAD, Fractionated Plasma Separation, Adsorption, and Dialysis system (Prometheus®, Fresenius Medical Care, Germany)) attempt to remove tightly protein-bound toxins by perfusion over resins or albumin. The MARS system uses an albumin-impregnated dialysis membrane and a dialysate containing 5% human albumin. The dialysate is perfused over charcoal and resin adsorbents and finally dialysed to remove water-soluble toxins including ammonia. In FPAD, a membrane separates out the patient's albumin and passes it through columns of adsorbents and water-soluble toxins are removed by haemodialysis.

Meta-analysis of six studies including four randomized controlled trials showed no mortality benefit in acute and acute on chronic liver failure with MARS [146]. Improved transplant-free survival has been reported with MARS in paracetamol acute liver failure. When MARS is compared to FPAD, it appears to have more effect on circulatory dysfunction while FPAD removes bilirubin and urea more efficaciously. Preliminary experience with both of these artificial liver support systems have shown some benefit but more evaluation is needed before wide spread implementation in acute liver failure can be recommended.

Bioartificial liver support systems use bioreactors containing viable hepatocytes in culture. Five systems have reached an advanced stage of clinical assessment: Bio-

artificial Liver (AMC BAL; Hep-Art Medical Devices, Netherlands), HepatAssist® (Arbios, USA), Extra-corporeal Liver Assist Device (ELAD; Vital Therapies, Inc., USA), Bioartificial Liver Support System (BLSS; Excorp Medical Inc., USA) and Molecular Extra-corporeal Liver support System (MELS; Virchow Clinic in Berlin, Germany). Most systems use porcine hepatocytes, while the ELAD system uses a hepatoblastoma cell line. Anticoagulated plasma or whole blood is passed through a device allowing metabolic transfer between cells and perfusate (Fig. 5.10). Protocols differ as to whether the plasma or blood is first passed over a charcoal column or other device [147]. These devices have shown improved clinical and biochemical measure and safety in phase I and II clinical trials, but have failed to show improvement in 30-day mortality [148]. These techniques hold promise for the future but whether the results will ever regularly lead to a recovery of the native liver rather than bridge the gap to successful transplantation remains to be seen. None are in use routinely at this time.

Hepatocyte transplantation

In experimental animals with acute liver failure, hepatocyte transplantation may improve survival. Only 0.5 to 3% of the normal hepatocyte mass is necessary. A limited number of studies have been done in patients with acute liver failure who were not candidates for liver transplantation. There was an improvement in encephalopathy score, arterial ammonia, prothrombin time, and aminopyrine and caffeine clearances. No clinical improvement was seen in the first 24 h after hepatocyte transplantation. None of the patients survived. Immunosuppression is necessary for the survival of the transplanted cells. Complications include hypoxaemia and infiltrates on chest X-ray after intraportal hepatocyte transplantation [149]. No randomized, controlled data are available. Developments are needed in the method of delivery of hepatocytes, the prophylaxis of infections and strategies for preventing rejection without the need for immunosuppressive drugs.

Conclusion

Acute liver failure is a rare but devastating condition caused by a wide range of insults. Advances have been made in recent years in understanding the pathophysiology yet an ideal prognostic model is still out of reach. Early referral of patients to a specialist centre must be emphasized since rapid deterioration is the rule. Delayed action closes the window of opportunity for safe transfer and successful transplantation. While improvements in intensive care and liver transplantation have improved survival, morbidity and mortality remain unacceptably

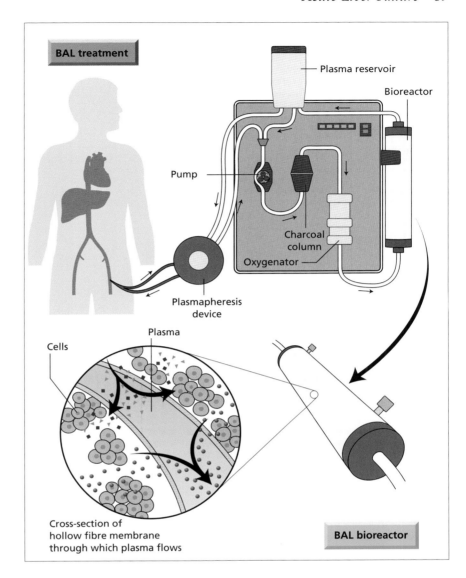

Fig. 5.10. Schematic of bioartificial liver support system with a bioreactor containing porcine hepatocytes [148].

high. Donor grafts are a limited resource and liver transplantation cannot be accepted as the perfect treatment, especially when the liver fully recovers if the patient can be supported. Liver assist devices show promise but need further evaluation.

References

1 Trey C, Davidson C. The management of fulminant hepatic failure. *Prog. Liver Dis.* 1970; **3**: 282–298.
2 Lee WM, Squires RH, Nyberg SL *et al*. Acute liver failure: summary of a workshop. *Hepatology* 2008; **47**: 1401–1415.
3 Ostapowicz GA, Fontana RJ, Schiodt FV. Results of a prospective study of acute liver failure at 17 tertiary care centers in the United States. *Ann. Intern. Med.* 2002; **137**: 947–954.
4 Lee WM. Medical progress: acute liver failure. *N. Engl. J. Med.* 1993; **329**: 1862–1874.
5 Liou IW, Larson AM. Role of liver transplantation in acute liver failure. *Semin. Liver Dis.* 2008; **28**: 201–209.
6 O'Grady JG, Schalm SW. Acute liver failure: redefining the syndromes. *Lancet* 1993; **342**: 273–276.
7 Bernuau J, Rueff B, Benhamou JP. Fulminant and subfulminant liver failure: definitions and causes. *Semin. Liver Dis.*1986; **6**: 97–106.
8 Ellis AJ, Saleh M, Smith H. Late-onset hepatic failure: clinical features, serology and outcome following transplantation. *J. Hepatol.* 1995; **23**: 363.
9 Polson J, Lee WM. Etiologies of acute liver failure. location, location, location! *Liver Transpl.* 2007; **13**: 1362–1363.
10 Escorsell A, Mas A, Mata M. Acute liver failure in Spain: analysis of 267 cases. *Liver Transpl.* 2007; **13**: 1389–1395.
11 Ichal P, Samuel D. Etiology and prognosis of fulminant hepatitis in adults. *Liver Transpl.* 2008; **14**: S67–S79.
12 Lee WM. Acute liver failure in the United States. *Semin. Liver Dis.*2003; **23**: 217–226.

13 Acharya SK, Panda SK, Saxena A *et al.* Acute hepatic failure in India: a perspective from the East. *J. Gastroenterol. Hepatol.* 2000; **15**: 473–479.

14 Koskinas J, Deutsch M, Kountouras D *et al.* Aetiology and outcome of acute hepatic failure in Greece: experience of two academic hosptital centres. *Liver Int.* 2008; **28**: 821–827.

15 Cheng V, Lo C-M, Lau GK. Current issues and treatment of fulminant hepatic failure including transplantation in Hong Kong the Far East. *Semin. Liver Dis.* 2003; **23**: 239–250.

16 Taylor RM, Davern T, Munoz S *et al.* Fulminant hepatitis A virus infection in the United States: incidence, prognosis, and outcomes. *Hepatology* 2006; **44**: 1589–1597.

17 Vento S, Garofano T, Renzini C *et al.* Fulminant hepatitis associated with hepatitis A virus superinfection in patients with chronic hepatitis C. *N. Engl. J. Med.* 1996; **338**: 286–290.

18 Jacobs RJ, Koff RS, Meyerhoff AS. The cost-effectiveness of vaccinating chronic hepatitis C patients against hepatitis A. *Am. J. Gastroenterol.* 2002; **97**: 427–434.

19 Berk PD, Popper H. Fulminant hepatic failure. *Am. J. Gastroenterol.* 1978; **69**: 349–400.

20 Saracco G, Macagno S, Rosina F *et al.* Serologic markers with fulminant hepatitis in persons positive for hepatitis B surface antigen: a worldwide epidemiologic and clinical survey. *Ann. Intern. Med.* 1988; **108**: 380–383.

21 Fagan EA, Williams R. Fulminant viral hepatitis. *Br. Med. Bull.* 1990; **46**: 462–480.

22 Sato S, Suzuki K, Akahane Y *et al.* Hepatitis B virus strains with mutations in the core promoter in patients with fulminant hepatitis. *Ann. Intern. Med.* 1995; **122**: 241–248.

23 Wai CT, Fontana RJ. Clinical significance of hepatitis B virus genotypes, variants, and mutants. *Clin. Liver Dis.* 2004; **8**: 321–352.

24 Chu CM, Yeh CT, Chiu CT *et al.* Precore mutant of hepatitis B virus prevails in acute and chronic infections in an area in which hepatitis B is endemic. *J. Clin. Microbiol.* 1996; **34**: 1815–1818.

25 Feray C, Chitnis DS, Artwani KK. Prevalence of anti-delta antibodies in central India. *Trop. Gastroenterol.* 1999; **20**: 29.

26 Hoofnagle JH. Reactivation of hepatitis B. *Hepatology* 2009; **49**: S156–S165.

27 Bhatia V, Singhal A, Panda SK *et al.* A 20 year single center experience with acute liver failure during pregnancy: is the prognosis really worse? *Hepatology* 2008; **48**: 1577–1585.

28 Ling LM, Wilder-Smith A, Leo YS. Fulminant hepatitis in dengue haemorrhagic fever. *J. Clin. Virol.* 2006; **38**: 265–268.

29 Norvell JP, Blei AT, Jovanovic BD *et al.* Herpes simplex virus hepatitis: an analysis of the published literature and institutional cases. *Liver Transpl.* 2007; **10**: 1428–1434.

30 Pishvaian AC, Bahrain M, Lewis JH. Fatal varicella-zoster hepatitis presenting with severe abdominal pain: a case report and review of the literature. *Dig. Dis. Sci.* 2006; **7**: 1221–1225.

31 Wang WH, Wang HL. Fulminant adenovirus hepatitis following bone marrow transplantion. A case report and brief review of the literature. *Arch. Pathol. Lab. Med.* 2003; **127**: 246–248.

32 Pardi DS, Romero Y, Mertz LE *et al.* Hepatitis-associated aplastic anemia and acute parvovirus B19 infection: a report of two cases and a review of the literature. *Am. J. Gastroenterol.* 1998; **93**: 468–470.

33 Lee WM, Brown KE, Young NS *et al.* Brief report: no evidence for parvovirus B19 or hepatitis E virus as a cause of acute liver failure. *Dig. Dis. Sci.* 2006; **51**: 1712–1715.

34 Bernal W. Changing patterns of causation and the use of transplantation in the United Kingdom. *Semin. Liver Dis.* 2003; **23**: 227–237.

35 Larson AM, Polson J, Fontana RJ *et al.* Acetaminophen-induced acute liver failure: results of a United States multicenter, prospective study. *Hepatology* 2005; **42**: 1364–1372.

36 Zimmerman HJ, Maddrey WC. Acetaminophen (paracetamol) hepatotoxicity with regular intake of alcohol: analysis of instances of therapeutic misadventure. *Hepatology* 1995; **22**: 767–773.

37 Schiodt FV, Rochling FA, Casey DL *et al.* Acetaminophen toxicity in an urban county hospital. *N. Engl. J. Med.* 1997; **337**: 1112–1117.

38 Polson J, Lee WM. AASLD position paper: the management of acute liver failure. *Hepatology* 2005; **41**: 1179–1197.

39 Lee WM. Drug-induced hepatotoxicity. *N. Engl. J. Med.* 2003; **349**: 474–485.

40 Andreu V, Mas A, Bruguera M. Ecstasy: a common cause of severe acute hepatotoxicity. *J. Hepatol.* 1998; **29**: 394–397.

41 Chalasani N, Fontana RJ, Bonkovsky HL *et al.* Causes, clinical features, and outcomes from a prospective study of drug-induced liver injury in the United States. *Gastroenterology* 2008; **135**: 1924–1934.

42 Escudie L, Francoz C, Vinel J-P *et al.* Amanita phalloides poisoning: reassessment of prognostic factors and indications for emergency liver transplantation. *J. Hepatol.* 2007; **46**: 466–473.

43 Ebert EC. Hypoxic liver injury. *Mayo Clin. Proc.* 2006; **81**: 1232–1236.

44 Birrer R, Takuda Y, Takara T. Hypoxic hepatopathy: pathophysiology and prognosis. *Intern. Med.* 2007; **46**: 1063–1070.

45 Lettieri CJ, Berg BW. Clinical features of non-hodgkins lymphoma presenting with acute liver failure: a report of five cases and review of published experience. *Am. J. Gastroenterol.* 2003; **98**: 1641–1646.

46 Roberts EA, Schilsky ML. Diagnosis and treatment of Wilson disease: an update. *Hepatology* 2008; **47**: 2089–2111.

47 Kessler WR, Cummings OW, Eckert G *et al.* Fulminant hepatic failure as the initial presentation of acute autoimmune hepatitis. *Clin. Gastroenterol. Hepatol.* 2004; **2**: 625–631.

48 Karvountzis GG, Redeker AG, Peters RL. Long term follow-up studies of patients surviving fulminant hepatitis. *Gastroenterology* 1974; **67**: 870–877.

49 McCullough AJ, Fleming CR, Thistle JL *et al.* Diagnosis of Wilson's disease presenting as fulminant hepatic failure. *Gastroenterology* 1983; **84**: 161–167.

50 Abbo L, Alcaide ML, Plano JR *et al.* Fulminant hepatitis from herpes simplex type 2 in an immunocompetent adult. *Transpl. Infect. Dis.* 2007; **4**: 323–326.

51 Roque-Afonso AM, Bralet MP, Ichai P *et al*. Chickenpox-associated fulminant hepatitis that led to liver transplantation in a 63-year-old woman. *Liver Transpl.* 2008; **14**: 1309–1312.
52 Rumack BH, Matthew H. Acetaminophen poisoning and toxicity. *Pediatrics* 1975; **55**: 871–876.
53 Rumack BH. Acetaminophen hepatotoxicity: the first 35 years. *J. Toxicol. Clin. Toxicol.* 2002; **40**: 3–20.
54 Rumack BH. Acetaminophen misconceptions. *Hepatology* 2004; **40**: 10–15.
55 Tan C, Graudins A. Comparative pharmokinetics of panadol extend and immediate-release paracetamol in a stimulated overdose model. *Emerg. Med. Australas.* 2006; **18**: 398–403.
56 Polson J, Wians FH, Orsulak P *et al*. False positive acetaminophen concentrations in patients with liver injury. *Clinica Chimica Acta* 2008; **391**: 24–30.
57 James LP, Letzig LG, Simpson PM *et al*. Pharmacokinetics of acetaminophen protein adducts in adults with acetaminophen overdose and acute liver failure. *Drug. Metab. Dispos.* 2009; **37**: 1779–1784.
58 Czaja AJ, Freese DK. Diagnosis and treatment of autoimmune hepatitis. *Hepatology* 2002; **36**: 479–497.
59 Eisenbach C, Sieg O, Stremmel W *et al*. Diagnostic criteria for acute liver failure due to Wilson disease. *World J. Gastroenterol.* 2007; **11**: 1711–1714.
60 Korman JD, Volenberg I, Balko J *et al*. Screening for Wilson disease in acute liver failure: a comparison of currently available diagnostic tests. *Hepatology* 2008; **48**: 1167–1174.
61 Ellis AJ, Wendon JA, Williams R. Subclinical seizure activity and prophylactic phenytoin infusion in acute liver failure: a controlled clinical trial. *Hepatology* 2000; **32**: 536–541.
62 Bhatia V, Batra Y, Acharya SK. Prophylactic phenytoin does not improve cerebral edema or survival in acute liver failure—a controlled clinical trial. *J. Hepatol.* 2004; **41**: 89–96.
63 Munoz SJ, Robinson M, Northrup B *et al*. Elevated intracranial pressure and computed tomography of the brain in fulminant hepatocellular failure. *Hepatology* 1991; **13**: 209–212.
64 Wijdicks EF, Plevak DJ, Rakela J *et al*. Clinical and radiologic features of cerebral edema in fulminant hepatic failure. *Mayo Clin. Proc.* 1995; **70**: 119–124.
65 Stravitz RT, Kramer AH, Davern T *et al*. Intensive care of patients with acute liver failure: recommendations of the U.S. Acute Liver Failure Study Group. *Crit. Care Med.* 2007; **35**: 2498–2508.
66 Poff JA, Coakley FV, Qayyum A *et al*. Frequency and histopathologic basis of hepatic surface nodularity in patients with fulminant hepatic failure. *Radiology* 2008; **249**: 518–523.
67 Hanau C, Munoz SJ, Rubin R. Histopathological heterogeneity in fulminant hepatic failure. *Hepatology* 1995; **21**: 345–351.
68 Shakil AO, Jones BC, Lee RG *et al*. Prognostic value of abdominal CT scanning and hepatic histopathology in patients with acute liver failure. *Dig. Dis. Sci.* 2000; **45**: 334–339.
69 Rolando N, Wade J, Davalos M *et al*. The systemic inflammatory response syndrome in acute liver failure. *Hepatology* 2000; **32**: 734–739.
70 Antoniades CG, Berry PA, Wendon JA *et al*. The importance of immune dysfunction in determining outcome in acute liver failure. *J. Hepatol.* 2008; **49**: 845–861.
71 Lee WM, Hynan LS, Rossaro L *et al*. Intravenous N-acetylcysteine improves transplant-free survival in early stage non-acetaminophen acute liver failure. *Gastroenterology* 2009; **137**: 856–864.
72 Ferenci P. Brain dysfunction in fulminant hepatic failure. *J. Hepatol.* 1994; **21**: 487–490.
73 Bernal W, Hall C, Karvellas CJ *et al*. Arterial ammonia and clinical risk factors for encephalopathy and intracranial hypertension in acute liver failure. *Hepatology* 2007; **46**: 1844–1852.
74 Bhatia V, Singh R, Acharya SK. Predictive value of arterial ammonia for complications and outcome in acute liver failure. *Gut* 2006; **55**: 98–104.
75 Clemmesen JO, Larsen FS, Kondrup J *et al*. Cerebral herniation in patients with acute liver failure is correlated with arterial ammonia concentration. *Hepatology* 1999; **29**: 648–653.
76 Alba L, Hay JE, Angulo P. Lactulose therapy in acute liver failure. *J. Hepatol.* 2002; **36**: 33A.
77 Acharya SK, Bhatia V, Sreenivas V *et al*. Efficacy of L-ornithine L-aspartate in acute liver failure: a double-blind, randomized, placebo-controlled study. *Gastroenterology* 2009; **136**: 2159–2168.
78 Wijdicks EF, Nyberg SL. Propofol to control intracranial pressure in fulminant hepatic failure. *Transpl. Proc.* 2002; **34**: 1220–1222.
79 Vaquero J, Polson J, Chung C *et al*. Infection and the progression of hepatic encephalopathy in acute liver failure. *Gastroenterology* 2003; **125**: 755–764.
80 Ware AJ, D'Agostino AN, Combes B. Cerebral edema: a major complication of massive hepatic necrosis. *Gastroenterology* 1971; **61**: 877–884.
81 Blei AT. The pathophysiology of brain edema in acute liver failure. *Neurochem. Int.* 2005; **47**: 71–77.
82 Vaquero J, Chung C, Blei AT. Brain edema in acute liver failure. A window to the pathogenesis of hepatic encephalopathy. *Ann. Hepatol.* 2003; **2**: 12–22.
83 Jalan R. Intracranial hypertension in acute liver failure: pathophysiological basis of rational management. *Semin. Liver Dis.* 2003; **23**: 271–282.
84 Bjerring PN, Eefsen M, Hansen BA *et al*. The brain in acute liver failure. A tortuous path from hyperammonemia to cerebral edema. *Metab. Brain Dis.* 2009; **24**: 5–14.
85 Blei AT, Larsen FS. Pathophysiology of cerebral edema in fulminant hepatic failure. *J. Hepatol.* 1999; **31**: 771–776.
86 Jalan R, Olde Damink SW, Hayes PC *et al*. Pathogenesis of intracranial hypertension in acute liver failure: inflammation, ammonia and cerebral blood flow. *J. Hepatol.* 2004; **41**: 613–620.
87 Larsen FS, Ejlersen E, Clemmesen JO *et al*. Preservation of cerebral oxidative metabolism in fulminant hepatic failure: an autoregulation study. *Liver Transpl. Surg.* 1996; **2**: 348–353.
88 Vaquero J, Fontana RJ, Larson AM *et al*. Complications and use of intracranial pressure monitoring in patients with acute liver failure and severe encephalopathy. *Liver Transpl.* 2005; **11**: 1581–1589.
89 Bernal W, Auzinger G, Sizer E *et al*. Intensive care management of acute liver failure. *Semin. Liver Dis.* 2008; **28**: 188–200.

90 Lidofsky SD, Bass NM, Prager MC *et al*. Intracranial pressure monitoring and liver transplantation for fulminant hepatic failure. *Hepatology* 1992; **16**: 1–7.

91 Raghavan M, Marik PE. Therapy of intracranial hypertension in patients with fulminant hepatic failure. *Neurocrit. Care* 2006; **4**: 179–189.

92 Murphy N, Auzinger G, Bernel W *et al*. The effect of hypertonic sodium chloride on intracranial pressure in patients with acute liver failure. *Hepatology* 2004; **39**: 464–470.

93 Canalese J, Gimson AE, Davis C *et al*. Controlled trial of dexamethasone and mannitol for the cerebral oedema of fulminant hepatic failure. *Gut* 1982; **23**: 625–629.

94 Strauss G, Hansen BA, Knudsen GM *et al*. Hyperventilation restores cerebral blood flow autoregulation in patients with acute liver failure. *J. Hepatol.* 1998; **28**: 199–203.

95 Ede RJ, Gimson AE, Bihari D *et al*. Controlled hyperventilation in the prevention of cerebral oedema in fulminant hepatic failure. *J. Hepatol.* 1986; **2**: 43–51.

96 Forbes A, Alexander GJ, O'Grady JG *et al*. Thiopental infusion in the treatment of intracranial hypertension complicating fulminant hepatic failure. *Hepatology* 1989; **10**: 306–310.

97 Tofteng F, Larsen FS. The effect of indomethacin on intracranial pressure, cerebral perfusion and extracellular lactate and glutamate concentrations in patients with fulminant hepatic failure. *J. Cereb. Blood Flow Metab.* 2004; **24**: 798–804.

98 Rose C, Michalak A, Pannunzio M *et al*. Mild hypothermia delays the onset of coma and prevents brain edema and extracellular brain glutamate accumulation in rats with acute liver failure. *Hepatology* 2000; **31**: 872–877.

99 Jalan R, Olde Damink SW, Deutz NE *et al*. Restoration of cerebral blood flow autoregulation and reactivity to carbon dioxide in acute liver failure by moderate hypothermia. *Hepatology* 2001; **34**: 50–54.

100 Jalan R, Damink SW, Deutz NE *et al*. Moderate hypothermia for uncontrolled intracranial hypertension in acute liver failure. *Lancet* 1999; **354**: 1164–1168.

101 Schubert A. Side effects of mild hypothermia. *J. Neurosurg. Anesthesiol.* 1995; **7**: 139–147.

102 Polderman KH. Application of therapeutic hypothermia in the intensive care unit. Opportunities and pitfalls of a promising treatment modality—Part 2: Practical aspects and side effects. *Intensive Care Med.* 2004; **30**: 757–769.

103 Stravitz RT, Lee WM, Kramer AH *et al*. Therapeutic hypothermia for acute liver failure: toward a randomized, controlled trial in patients with advanced hepatic encephalopathy. *Neurocrit. Care* 2008; **9**: 90–96.

104 Wendon J, Lee WM. Encephalopathy and cerebral edema in the setting of acute liver failure: pathogenesis and management. *Neurocrit. Care* 2008; **9**: 97–102.

105 Munoz SJ, Stravitz RT, Gabriel DA. Coagulopathy of acute liver failure. *Clin. Liver Dis.* 2009; **13**: 95–107.

106 Blei AT, Olafsson S, Webster S *et al*. Complications of intracranial pressure monitoring in fulminant hepatic failure. *Lancet* 1993; **341**: 157–158.

107 O'Grady JG, Alexander GJ, Hayllar KM *et al*. Early indicators of prognosis in fulminant hepatic failure. *Gastroenterology* 1989; **97**: 439–445.

108 Trotter JF, Olson J, Lefkowitz J *et al*. Changes in international normalized ratio (INR) and model for endstage liver disease (MELD) based on selection of clinical laboratory. *Am. J. Transpl.* 2007; **7**: 1624–1628.

109 Tripodi A, Salerno F, Chantarangkul V *et al*. Evidence of normal thrombin generation in cirrhosis despite abnormal conventional coagulation tests. *Hepatology* 2005; **41**: 553–558.

110 Pereira SP, Rowbotham D, Fitt S *et al*. Pharmacokinetics and efficacy of oral versus intravenous mixed-micellar phylloquinone (vitamin K1) in severe acute liver disease. *J. Hepatol.* 2005; **42**: 365–370.

111 Gazzard BG, Henderson JM, Williams R. Early changes in coagulation following a paracetamol overdose and a controlled trial of fresh frozen plasma therapy. *Gut* 1975; **16**: 617–620.

112 Shami VM, Caldwell SH, Hespenheide EE *et al*. Recombinant activated factor VII for coagulopathy in fulminant hepatic failure compared with conventional therapy. *Liver Transpl.* 2003; **9**: 138–143.

113 Rolando N, Harvey F, Brahm J *et al*. Prospective study of bacterial infection in acute liver failure: an analysis of fifty patients. *Hepatology* 1990; **11**: 49–53.

114 Rolando N, Harvey F, Brahm J *et al*. Fungal infection: a common, unrecognised complication of acute liver failure. *J. Hepatol.* 1991; **12**: 1–9.

115 Rolando N, Philpott-Howard J, Williams R. Bacterial and fungal infection in acute liver failure. *Semin. Liver Dis.*1996; **16**: 389–402.

116 Rolando N, Wade JJ, Stangou A *et al*. Prospective study comparing the efficacy of prophylactic parenteral antimicrobials, with or without enteral decontamination, in patients with acute liver failure. *Liver Transpl. Surg.* 1996; **2**: 8–13.

117 Jain S, Pendyala P, Varma S *et al*. Effect of renal dysfunction in fulminant hepatic failure. *Trop. Gastroenterol.* 2000; **21**: 118–120.

118 Wilkinson SP, Moodie H, Arroyo VA *et al*. Frequency of renal impairment in paracetamol overdose compared with other causes of acute liver damage. *J. Clin. Pathol.* 1977; **30**: 141–143.

119 Moore K. Renal failure in acute liver failure. *Eur. J. Gastroenterol. Hepatol.* 1999; **11**: 967–975.

120 Bellomo R, Wan L, May C. Vasoactive drugs and acute kidney injury. *Crit. Care Med.* 2008; **36**: S179–186.

121 Davenport A. Continuous renal replacement therapies in patients with liver disease. *Semin. Dial.* 2009; **22**: 169–172.

122 Shawcross DL, Davies NA, Mookerjee RP *et al*. Worsening of cerebral hyperemia by the administration of terlipressin in acute liver failure with severe encephalopathy. *Hepatology* 2004; **39**: 471–475.

123 Eefsen M, Dethloff T, Frederiksen HJ *et al*. Comparison of terlipressin and noradrenalin on cerebral perfusion, intracranial pressure and cerebral extracellular concentrations of lactate and pyruvate in patients with acute liver failure in need of inotropic support. *J. Hepatol.* 2007; **47**: 381–386.

124 Harry R, Auzinger G, Wendon J. The clinical importance of adrenal insufficiency in acute hepatic dysfunction. *Hepatology* 2002; **36**: 395–402.

125 Harry R, Auzinger G, Wendon J. The effects of supraphysiological doses of corticosteroids in hypotensive liver failure. *Liver Int.* 2003; **23**: 71–77.

126 MacDougall BR, Williams R. H2-receptor antagonist in the prevention of acute upper gastrointestinal hemorrhage in fulminant hepatic failure: a controlled trial. *Gastroenterology* 1978; **74**: 464–465.

127 Baudouin SV, Howdle P, O'Grady JG *et al.* Acute lung injury in fulminant hepatic failure following paracetamol poisoning. *Thorax* 1995; **50**: 399–402.

128 Parbhoo SP, Welch J, Sherlock S. Acute pancreatitis in patients with fulminant hepatic failure. *Gut* 1973; **14**: 428.

129 Cote GA, Gottstein JH, Daud A *et al.* The role of etiology in the hyperamylasemia of acute liver failure. *Am. J. Gastroenterol.* 2009; **104**: 592–597.

130 Harrison PM, Keays R, Bray GP *et al.* Improved outcome of paracetamol-induced fulminant hepatic failure by late administration of acetylcysteine. *Lancet* 1990; **335**: 1572–1573.

131 Vale JA, Proudfoot AT. Paracetamol (acetaminophen) poisoning. *Lancet* 1995; **346**: 547–552.

132 Enjalbert F, Rapior S, Nouguier-Soule J *et al.* Treatment of amatoxin poisoning: 20-year retrospective analysis. *J. Toxicol. Clin. Toxicol.* 2002; **40**: 715–757.

133 Degertekin B, Lok AS. Indications for therapy in hepatitis B. *Hepatology* 2009; **49**: S129–137.

134 Levitsky J, Duddempudi AT, Lakeman FD *et al.* Detection and diagnosis of herpes simplex virus infection in adults with acute liver failure. *Liver Transpl.* 2008; **14**: 1498–1504.

135 Peters DJ, Greene WH, Ruggiero F *et al.* Herpes simplex-induced fulminant hepatitis in adults: a call for empiric therapy. *Dig. Dis. Sci.* 2000; **45**: 2399–2404.

136 Czaja AJ. Corticosteroids or not in severe acute or fulminant autoimmune hepatitis: therapeutic brinksmanship and the point beyond salvation. *Liver Transpl.* 2007; **13**: 953–955.

137 Hay JE. Liver disease in pregnancy. *Hepatology* 2008; **47**: 1067–1076.

138 Riordan SM, Williams R. Mechanisms of hepatocyte injury, multiorgan failure, and prognostic criteria in acute liver failure. *Semin. Liver Dis.* 2003; **23**: 203–215.

139 Bernal W, Donaldson N, Wyncoll D *et al.* Blood lactate as an early predictor of outcome in paracetamol-induced acute liver failure: a cohort study. *Lancet* 2002; **359**: 558–563.

140 Bismuth H, Samuel D, Castaing D *et al.* Orthotopic liver transplantation in fulminant and subfulminant hepatitis. The Paul Brousse experience. *Ann. Surg.* 1995; **222**: 109–119.

141 Polson J. Assessment of prognosis in acute liver failure. *Semin. Liver Dis.* 2008; **28**: 218–225.

142 Devlin J, Wendon J, Heaton N *et al.* Pretransplantation clinical status and outcome of emergency transplantation for acute liver failure. *Hepatology* 1995; **21**: 1018–1024.

143 Bernal W, Cross TJ, Auzinger G *et al.* Outcome after wait-listing for emergency liver transplantation in acute liver failure: a single centre experience. *J. Hepatol.* 2009; **50**: 306–313.

144 van Hoek B, de Boer J, Boudjema K *et al.* Auxiliary versus orthotopic liver transplantation for acute liver failure. EURALT Study Group. European Auxiliary Liver Transplant Registry. *J. Hepatol.* 1999; **30**: 699–705.

145 O'Grady JG, Gimson AE, O'Brien CJ *et al.* Controlled trials of charcoal hemoperfusion and prognostic factors in fulminant hepatic failure. *Gastroenterology* 1988; **94**: 1186–1192.

146 Khuroo MS, Farahat KL. Molecular adsorbent recirculating system for acute and acute-on-chronic liver failure: a meta-analysis. *Liver Transpl.* 2004; **10**: 1099–1106.

147 Stadlbauer V, Jalan R. Acute liver failure: liver support therapies. *Curr. Opin. Crit. Care* 2007; **13**: 215–221.

148 Demetriou AA, Brown RS, Busuttl RW *et al.* Prospective, randomized, multicenter, controlled trial of bioartificial liver in treating acute liver failure. *Ann. Surg.* 2004; **239**: 660–670.

149 Riordan SM, Williams R. Acute liver failure: targeted artificial and hepatocyte-based support of liver regeneration and reversal of multiorgan failure. *J. Hepatol.* 2000; **32**: 63–76.

CHAPTER 6
Hepatic Fibrogenesis

Meena B. Bansal & Scott L. Friedman
Division of Liver Diseases, Mount Sinai School of Medicine, New York, NY, USA

Learning points

- Fibrogenesis is the natural wound healing response to chronic liver injury.

- The activated hepatic stellate cell is the principal cell involved in fibrogenesis through its role in matrix production, secretion of proinflammatory and profibrogenic cytokines, and interactions with cells of the immune system.

- Matrix accumulation results from an imbalance where matrix synthesis exceeds degradation.

- Progression of fibrosis is influenced by modifiable factors such as body mass index (BMI) and alcohol intake, and non-modifiable factors, specifically genetic determinants.

- Non-invasive markers can distinguish between minimal fibrosis and cirrhosis but do not yet reliably distinguish between intermediate stages of fibrosis in individual patients.

Introduction

Fibrogenesis is the natural wound healing response to tissue injury. Scar tissue is produced in an effort to limit and encapsulate the area of damage. While acute hepatocellular injury activates fibrogenic pathways, it is when this is persistent that significant fibrosis accumulates ultimately leading to the development of cirrhosis. The transformation of normal to fibrotic liver and then cirrhosis is a complex process involving key components, including both hepatic parenchymal and non-parenchymal cells, the immune system, cytokines, proteinases and their inhibitors. This chapter is an overview of our current understanding of hepatic fibrogenesis and provides a framework to understand non-invasive markers of fibrogenesis and potential antifibrotic strategies.

Natural history of hepatic fibrosis

While fibrosis accumulates with time, the process is not linear and can differ significantly between individuals. The variable progression of fibrosis was first highlighted in patients with hepatitis C (Fig. 6.1) [1]. This study emphasized the influence of both modifiable and non-modifiable factors. Rapid progression of fibrosis correlated with greater age at the time of infection, male gender and alcohol consumption. One-third of patients had an expected median time to cirrhosis of 13 years while another third would never develop cirrhosis or would have a median time to cirrhosis of 50 years. This study led to the concept of 'rapid fibrosers' and 'slow fibrosers'.

Genetic determinants are thought to play a role. Data from non-alcoholic steatohepatitis (NASH) support this concept. Thus the prevalence of cryptogenic cirrhosis (generally thought to reflect end-stage NASH) is 3.1 fold higher among Hispanic American patients (and 3.9 fold lower in African Americans) compared with the prevalence in Europeans and other Americans. This is despite a similar prevalence of diabetes mellitus, a known risk factor for NASH [2]. Recently, specific single nucleotide polymorphisms (SNPs), which are a stable single base substitution found in more than 1% of the population, have been associated with different rates of fibrosis progression [3,4].

While fibrosis progression rates are useful to predict outcomes in patients with chronic liver disease, they accelerate in HCV as the disease advances [5]. A recent meta analysis examining stage-specific transition probabilities suggested that the probability of transition to a higher stage of fibrosis is greatest between F2 and F3 (4 stage system; Metavir) [6].

Therefore clinicians must make treatment decisions based on host, genetic and environmental factors that may impact on an individual's risk of disease. In addition, identification of relevant SNPs and gene signatures

Sherlock's Diseases of the Liver and Biliary System, Twelfth Edition. Edited by James S. Dooley, Anna S.F. Lok, Andrew K. Burroughs, E. Jenny Heathcote.
© 2011 by Blackwell Publishing Ltd. Published 2011 by Blackwell Publishing Ltd.

may not only help tailor therapy for individual patients, but also identify those patients who would benefit most from specific antifibrotic strategies when they become available.

Cellular and molecular features of hepatic fibrosis (Fig. 6.2)

Cellular anatomy of sinusoids

Between the sinusoid and hepatocytes, fenestrated endothelial cells line a basement membrane which separates the sinusoidal lumen from the space of Disse. Stellate cells lie in the space of Disse attached to the

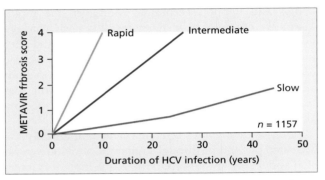

Fig. 6.1. Analysis of fibrosis progression in patients with chronic hepatitis C. Longitudinal studies allowed separation into rapid, intermediate and slow fibrosers based on Metavir scoring of fibrosis in liver biopsies. From [1] with permission.

basement membrane. Kupffer cells adhere to the sinusoidal surface of the fenestrated endothelium. Nutrients and other molecules reach the basal surface of the hepatocyte by passing through the fenestrae of the sinusoidal wall and across the space of Disse. This process is impaired by the cellular and matrix changes seen in liver injury.

Extracellular matrix composition in normal liver and hepatic scar tissue

Normal liver has a connective tissue matrix which includes type IV (non-fibrillary) collagen, glycoproteins (including fibronectin and laminin) and proteoglycans (including heparan sulphate). These constituents comprise the low-density basement membrane in the space of Disse, which separates the hepatocytes from the sinusoidal endothelium. This lattice-like matrix provides not only cellular support but also molecular signals that maintain the differentiated functions of cells. The basement membrane allows unimpeded transport of solutes and growth factors between sinusoid and hepatocytes.

After hepatic injury there is a three- to eightfold increase in extracellular matrix, composed predominantly of high-density interstitial fibril-forming collagens (types I and III, rather than type IV) as well as cellular fibronectin, hyaluronic acid and other matrix proteoglycans and glycoconjugates. In addition, there is loss of endothelial cell fenestrations and hepatocyte microvilli associated with this 'capillarization' of sinusoids, which impedes the metabolic exchange between blood and liver cells. The gradual accumulation of type

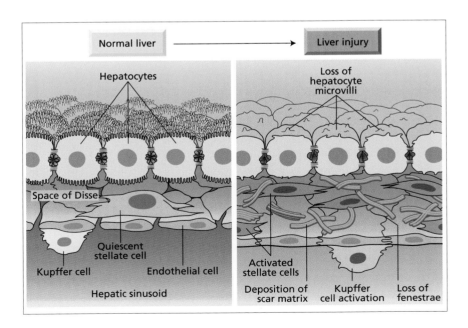

Fig. 6.2. Normal cellular and matrix relationship between sinusoid and hepatocyte, and changes after injury.

Day 3
(Quiescent)

Day 21
(Moderately Activated)

Passage 3
(Fully Activated)

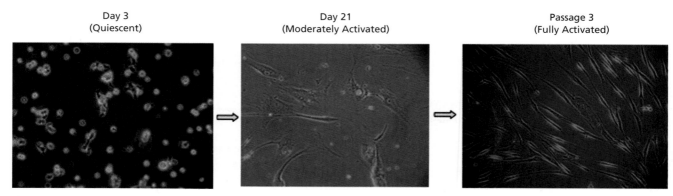

Fig. 6.3. Morphological changes in human hepatic stellate cells (HSCs) during culture-induced activation [11]. HSCs are isolated by density centrifugation from normal liver. Plated on plastic they are initially vitamin A-rich cells, exhibiting autofluorescence. Subsequently, they lose their vitamin A droplets, becoming more proliferative and spindle shaped. Culture-induced activation is a model system used to study *in vivo* activation. (Phase-contrast microscopy, ×200.)

I collagen results from both increased synthesis and reduced degradation, and is the hallmark of fibrogenesis.

Stellate cell activation: a central feature of hepatic fibrosis

The *hepatic stellate cell* (HSC) (also called lipocyte, fat-storing cell, Ito cell, pericyte) is the principal cell involved in fibrogenesis. It lies within the space of Disse and in direct contact with hepatocytes, endothelial cells, inflammatory cells and nerve fibres (Fig. 6.2). In the normal liver, these cells have intracellular droplets containing vitamin A. They contain 40–70% of the body stores of retinoids.

In its quiescent state the HSC produces predominantly type IV collagen, the collagen characteristic of a normal basement membrane. With injury, it undergoes phenotypic changes referred to as 'activation', characterized by loss of retinoid droplets, cellular proliferation, increased endoplasmic reticulum, increased contractility with expression of smooth muscle specific α-actin, and secretion of cytokines/ chemokines (Fig. 6.3). This phenotypic switch is also characterized by production of type I collagen, the high-density interstitial collagen characteristic of the cirrhotic liver, as well as matrix-degrading enzymes.

Stellate cell activation is a central event in hepatic fibrosis and can be conceptualized as occurring in at least two stages: (1) initiation and (2) perpetuation (Fig. 6.4).

Initiation refers to early events, including rapid changes in gene expression and a cellular phenotype that renders HSCs responsive to cytokines and other stimuli. Initiation is provoked by different factors depending on disease aetiology. Stimuli include oxidant stress signals (reactive oxygen intermediates), apoptotic bodies and lipopolysaccharide. Moreover, the rapid, disruptive effects of liver injury result in early changes in the extracellular matrix (ECM) composition and alter the homeostasis of neighbouring cells such as hepatic macrophages (Kupffer cells), sinusoidal endothelium and hepatocytes, resulting in paracrine stimuli that 'prime' the HSC to respond to a host of growth factors and cytokines.

Perpetuation involves cellular events that amplify the activated phenotype through enhanced cytokine expression and responsiveness, and the acquisition of features critical to the development of fibrosis.

These signals provide the impetus for scar formation through:

- enhanced HSC proliferation, contractility and fibrogenesis;
- altered matrix degradation;
- HSC chemotaxis;
- direct interactions between HSCs and the immune system;
- secretion of proinflammatory mediators.

Once the initiating injury signal is eliminated (i.e. treatment of underlying disease, discontinuation of hepatotoxins such as ethanol), HSCs either revert to the quiescent phenotype or are removed from the liver through programmed cell death, or apoptosis. This paradigm has provided the framework for the development of numerous antifibrotic approaches (see below).

Proliferation

With activation, HSCs proliferate rapidly. Platelet derived growth factor (PDGF-β) is the most potent mitogenic factor for HSCs by acting through its receptor, β-PDGFR [7]. Both the PDGF ligand and receptor are rapidly induced *in vivo* and in culture as HSCs activate [8,9]. Other stellate cell mitogens include vascular

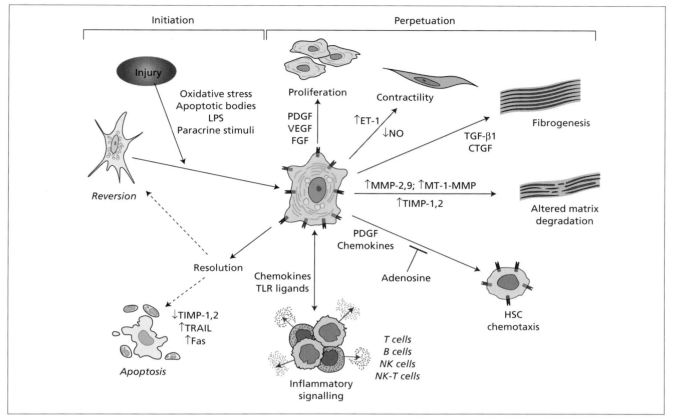

Fig. 6.4. Pathways of stellate cell (HSC) activation. Stellate cell activation can be divided into two phases: initiation and activation. Initiation is provoked by soluble stimuli that include oxidant stress signals (reactive oxygen intermediates), apoptotic bodies, lipopolysaccharide (LPS) and paracrine stimuli from neighbouring cell types including hepatic macrophages (Kupffer cells), sinusoidal endothelium and hepatocytes. Perpetuation follows, characterized by a number of specific phenotypic changes including proliferation, contractility, fibrogenesis, altered matrix degradation, chemotaxis, and inflammatory signalling. PDGF, platelet derived growth factor; VEGF, vascular endothelial growth factor; FGF, fibroblast growth factor; ET-1, endothelin-1; NO, nitric oxide; TGFβ1, transforming growth factor-β1; CTGF, connective tissue growth factor; MMP, matrix metalloproteinase; MT-MMP, membrane type matrix metalloproteinase; TRAIL, TNF-related apoptosis-inducing ligand; TIMP, tissue inhibitor of metalloproteinase; TLR, toll like receptor. Modified from [7], with permission.

endothelial growth factor (VEGF), thrombin, endothelial growth factor (EGF), transforming growth factor-α (TGF-α), keratinocyte growth factor, fibroblast growth factor (FGF), insulin-like growth factor IGF-1 and CXCL12 [10,11].

Contractility

During liver injury, the normally quiescent HSC also acquires 'myogenic' features including expression of alpha smooth muscle actin [12] and myosin [13], which confer contractile properties. Given their location within the space of Disse, HSC contractility contributes to increased portal resistance even with early fibrosis. This may be more reversible than when portal pressure is increased as a result of thickened septae and lobular distortion characteristic of advanced fibrosis.

Endothelin-1 and nitric oxide are key regulators that control HSC contractility through their mutually antagonistic activities. Contractility is also effected by many other factors including angiotensin II, eicosanoids, atrial naturetic peptide, somatostatin and carbon monoxide, among others [14,15].

Fibrogenesis

The production of type I collagen is the cardinal feature of the activated stellate cell. While other cytokines are important for the induction of HSC-derived collagen I, TGF-β1 remains the most potent fibrogenic cytokine. Cellular sources of TGF-β1 in chronic liver injury include sinusoidal endothelial cells, Kupffer cells and HSCs. Therefore, both autocrine and paracrine loops contribute to the development of liver fibrosis [16]. Other profibrogenic cytokines include CTGF, FGF and VEGF. Angiotensin II, the main effector of the renin–angiotensin system, is a functional cytokine that is a potential activator of collagen production in HSCs and a target of antifibrotic therapies [17].

Chemotaxis

Since fibrosis is a normal wound-healing response to encapsulate injury, it is not surprising that the HSCs migrate towards sites of injury driven by chemoattractants, which include PDGF [18], monocyte chemotactic protein-1 (MCP-1) [19] and CXCR3 ligands [20]. This ability to migrate to sites of injury may also be important for interactions with the immune system.

Inflammatory signalling

HSCs are also effectors in the liver's immune response to injury. HSCs secrete proinflammatory cytokines/chemokines such as MCP-1, underscoring their ability to promote inflammation rather than simply serving as a passive target of inflammatory cytokines. HSCs, like dendritic cells, can also function as professional antigen presenting cells by efficiently presenting antigen to MHC-I and MHC-II-restricted T cells *in vitro* and stimulating lymphocyte proliferation [21,22]. In addition, signalling by TLR4 (toll-like receptor 4) in HSCs in response to bacterial lipopolysaccharide further implicates this cell type in the liver's innate immune response to injury [23]. Interestingly, specific TLR4 SNPs contribute to fibrosis progression in HCV infection, providing a direct link between genetic risk and disease pathogenesis [4].

Other collagen-producing cells

While stellate cell activation is clearly central to most fibrosing chronic liver injury, other collagen-producing cells may also contribute to ECM accumulation in the liver. The relative contribution to fibrogenesis by different cell types may vary according to the aetiology of the liver disease. Within the liver, portal myofibroblasts are particularly important in biliary fibrosis [24]. Conversion, or 'transdifferentiation', of epithelial cells of the liver, hepatocytes and biliary epithelial cells, to become mesenchymal cells, a process referred to as epithelial–mesencyhmal transition (EMT), has been demonstrated in animal models but the contribution of EMT to human liver disease is not clear [25].

Liver sinusoidal endothelial cells also make collagen I. However these cells are particularly important in initiating the fibrogenic process through production of a splice variant of cellular fibronectin, called fibronectin extracellular domain A. Fibronectin extracellular domain A is produced early in animal models, and along with TGF-β1 contributes to myofibroblast differentiation [26].

While the majority of fibrogenic cells arise from resident hepatic populations, circulating cells derived from the bone marrow may migrate to the liver in the setting of chronic liver injury and contribute to fibrogenesis [27]. It is not certain, however, how much they contribute to the total fibrogenic population in human liver disease.

Local interactions influencing fibrogenesis

Cell–matrix, cell–cell, cytokine and immune interactions

Fibrosis is the net result of a complex interplay between resident hepatic cells, infiltrating inflammatory cells, several locally acting peptides called cytokines, and interactions between the ECM and cells.

Cell–matrix and cell–cell interactions

The ECM is not simply an inert scaffold for hepatocytes. Rather, individual ECM proteins contain domains that interact with HSCs and other cells through membrane receptors including integrins, thereby transducing their effects through cytoplasmic signalling pathways that regulate collagen synthesis and metalloproteinase activity [28]. For example, fibrillar collagen binds the tyrosine kinase receptor, discoidin domain receptor 2, on HSCs and stimulates the expression of matrix metalloproteinase-2 (MMP-2) [29]. In addition, proliferation of hepatocytes is regulated by the content/structure of the ECM [30]. Conversely, the proliferative capacity of hepatocytes may also directly affect fibrogenesis. In experimental studies of rats genetically lacking telomerase, there is shortening of chromosomal telomeres, and acceleration of progression to cirrhosis following CCl$_4$ injury [31]. Maintenance of chromosomal telomeres is vital for hepatocytes to proliferate normally. Therefore, not surprisingly, an inverse relationship between liver regeneration and liver fibrosis appears to exist.

Cytokine signalling

Cytokines are a family of proteins that function as mediators of cell communication. They include chemokines, interleukins, interferons, growth factors, angiogenic factors, soluble receptors and soluble proteases [17]. The cellular sources of cytokines depend on the underlying aetiology of liver disease. Regardless of the cellular source, however, unregulated cytokine synthesis and release are important for injury, inflammation and ultimately fibrosis. While an exhaustive characterization of these mediators is beyond the scope of this chapter (see review [17]), cytokines regulate fibrosis through either direct effects on HSCs (reviewed above) or by promoting inflammation.

Chronic inflammation and fibrosis are intricately linked. Interactions between HSCs and infiltrating leucocytes are critical in determining the outcome of liver injury. Not only do leucocyte-derived cytokines influence stellate cell activation and fibrogenesis, but HSC-derived cytokines/ chemokines are important for the recruitment and retention of inflammatory cells [32]. Their location within the space of Disse behind fenestrated endothelial cells position them to efficiently promote leucocyte infiltration into the liver.

Immune interactions

The immune interactions in the development of liver fibrosis are complex and differ based on disease aetiology and context [32]. Macrophages play divergent roles in liver fibrosis progression and regression. For example, depletion of macrophages during the induction of fibrosis results in decreased fibrosis progression, yet when macrophages are depleted during recovery, fibrosis regression is prolonged due to loss of macrophage-derived matrix proteases [33]. Natural killer (NK) cells, which contribute to immediate innate responses, may suppress fibrosis by killing activated myofibroblasts [34,35], while NKT cells can express profibrotic activity [36]. Adoptive transfer experiments in animals suggest that CD8 cells are more profibrogenic than CD4 cells [37], which could contribute to the increased rate of fibrosis observed in patients coinfected with HIV and HCV, where the CD4/CD8 ratio is typically reduced [38]. B cells may also contribute to matrix degradation but studies in humans are lacking [39].

Matrix production (fibrogenesis) and degradation (fibrinolysis) (Fig. 6.5)

The extracellular matrix during fibrogenesis consists of fibrillar collagen and matrix glycoproteins such as fibronectin, laminin, and hyaluronic acid. TGF-β1 is the most profibrogenic cytokine in chronic liver injury. During fibrinolysis, a net increase in interstitial collagenase activity occurs as a result of both increased MMPs and decreased tissue inhibitors of MMPs (TIMPS) (Fig. 6.5) and changes in converting enzymes (MT1-MMP and stromelysin). TIMP-1 plays a central role in fibrosis progression and regression. During fibrogenesis, TIMP-1 levels are increased resulting in both decreased degradation of type I collagen as well as persistence of activated stellate cells. Once injury ceases, TIMP-1 levels decline allowing for the degradation of scar matrix and apoptosis of activated stellate cells.

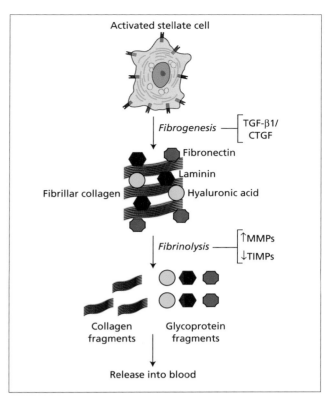

Fig. 6.5. Pathway of extracellular matrix production and degradation. Individual extracellular matrix components are cleaved and released into the blood (e.g. tissue inhibitor of metalloproteinase (TIMPs), matrix metalloproteinases (MMPs), transforming growth factor-β1(TGF-β1), connective tissue growth factor (CTGF)). These have been included in various serum biomarker panels.

The imbalance between matrix synthesis and degradation plays a major role in ECM accumulation during hepatic fibrogenesis [40]. While key sources of matrix-degrading activity are uncertain, both scar-associated macrophages and HSCs are potential sources of interstitial collagenases. Activated HSCs are the main source of MMP-2 [41], MMP-3 (stromelysin) [42] and MMP-13, the rodent equivalent of the human interstitial collagenase MMP-1 [43]. In addition, HSCs express RNA for TIMP-1 and TIMP-2, and produce TIMP-1 and MT1-MMP [44]. In contrast, Kupffer cells secrete type IV collagenase (MMP-9). The net result of the changes during hepatic injury is increased degradation of the normal basement membrane collagen, and reduced degradation of interstitial-type collagen. The latter may be explained by increased TIMP-1 and TIMP-2 expression relative to MMP-1 (interstitial collagenase).

The importance of TIMP-1 to matrix accumulation is illustrated by a model in which transgenic overexpression of human TIMP-1 in mice increased CCl$_4$-induced hepatic fibrosis sevenfold [45]. During the resolution of experimental liver injury, expression of

TIMP-1 and TIMP-2 is reduced, and net collagenase activity is increased, leading to removal of fibrotic matrix [46].

Because fibrolysis plays a critical role in fibrosis regression, breakdown components of the ECM, MMPs and TIMPs are often components of non-invasive fibrosis panels (see below and Fig. 6.5).

Clinical aspects of hepatic fibrosis

Invasive methods of diagnosis

Liver biopsy has been traditionally useful to determine the aetiology of liver disease, severity of inflammation and the amount of fibrosis. Several fibrosis staging systems have been developed, employing either a four-stage (IASL, Metavir, modified Scheuer; Batts-Ludwig) or six-stage system (Ishak). These grading and staging systems are useful for individual patients, whereas more complex systems such as Knodell are optimal for large cohort studies where statistical analyses are required [47].

While liver biopsy remains the current standard for the staging of fibrosis, limitations to liver biopsy include risks due to its invasive nature and associated stress for patients and physicians, and sampling error, even in diseases that affect the liver uniformly [48]. Because a single liver biopsy represents only 1/50 000 of the total organ volume, a small change in the angle of the biopsy needle could yield different results. Moreover, sampling error is an even greater concern in cases where the injury is heterogeneous. In a study of 124 patients with chronic HCV infection who underwent laparoscopic-guided biopsy of both the right and left hepatic lobes, the results were discordant in 33% of cases by at least one histological stage (modified Scheuer system) [49]. Therefore, managing patients by relying upon changes in fibrosis stage through sequential liver biopsies may be misleading. Increasing the length and width of a liver biopsy decreases, but does not eliminate, the possibility of sampling error [50–52]. There is therefore an increasing need for non-invasive markers of liver fibrosis in order to track progression or regression of disease following therapy.

Non-invasive methods of diagnosis

Current non-invasive markers rely on two distinct approaches: serum markers and imaging modalities [48].

Serum markers

These may involve direct or indirect components. Direct components include specific structural elements of fibrotic matrix, or inflammatory mediators implicated in either the production (fibrogenesis) or degradation (fibrolysis) of scar. Examples of direct components include, MMPs, TIMPs, TGF-β1 or ECM fragments released by fibrinolysis (Fig. 6.5). Indirect components are those laboratory investigations that may correlate with progression of fibrosis but are not directly responsible for fibrogenesis, for example platelet count. Current panels all include multiple rather than single markers to increase diagnostic accuracy.

The inclusion of routine laboratory tests in fibrosis marker panels is attractive, based on their ready availability and lower cost. Examples of such panels include AAR (aspartate aminotransferase (AST)/ alanine aminotransferase (ALT) ratio), APRI (AST/ platelet ratio), FIB-4 (platelets, AST, ALT and age), and Forns index (age, serum concentrations of total cholesterol, γ-glutamyl transpeptidase and platelet count). In patients with HCV, an AAR above 1, or APRI above 2.0, have been proposed as a test for cirrhosis, but an inadequate sensitivity and negative predictive value limit their widespread use [48]. In a study of 194 patients with HCV, APRI was superior to the AAR for predicting significant fibrosis but neither test reliably circumvented the need for liver biopsy [53].

A variety of proprietary panels have also emerged which include tests that are not part of routine investigation [54]. Examples are ELF (European/ Enhanced Liver Fibrosis test), Fibrotest, Fibrosure and Fibrospect. The ELF test combines three serum biomarkers which correlate with the level of liver fibrosis as assessed by liver biopsy [55]. These biomarkers are hyaluronic acid, procollagen III amino terminal peptide and TIMP-1. The pretest probability of disease within a specific population greatly influences the predictive value of the test, and this must be considered when screening patients using non-invasive markers.

Non-invasive serum markers clearly distinguish F0/ F1 from F4, but are less useful in differentiating between intermediate stages of fibrosis.

Imaging

Standard imaging techniques such as ultrasound, CT and MRI are able to detect advanced fibrosis when signs of portal hypertension are evident, but they cannot yet detect milder disease.

Liver stiffness, as assessed by ultrasound (Fibroscan, Echosens, France), and more recently by magnetic resonance elastography, is quantified by measuring how fast a mechanical pulse travels within the liver tissue—the stiffer the liver, the faster the wave velocity. Accumulating data indicate that elasticity parallels the stage of fibrosis at precirrhotic or cirrhotic stages. Fibroscan can reliably establish the diagnosis of cirrhosis in a patient with chronic liver disease [54]. However, whether it can differentiate between intermediate stages of fibrosis remains uncertain. Nonetheless, the large dynamic range provided by Fibroscan facilitates longitudinal follow-up of patients by assessing the change in stiffness over time. This approach has an advantage over liver biopsy because it is a direct measure of fibrosis (i.e. stiffness), whereas liver biopsy stages fibrosis based on the pattern but not the absolute amount of scar.

Contrast-enhanced ultrasonographic imaging (CEUS) uses intravenous administration of gas-filled microbubbles to enhance vascular signals and measure blood flow transit. Diminished hepatic vein transit time correlates with worsening liver disease [56]. However, CEUS is less attractive than other strategies because of its inability to differentiate between intermediate stages of fibrosis, the need for contrast reagents and high operator skill necessary. Other imaging techniques are under development and remain investigational, including MR spectroscopy and PET imaging [57].

Emerging antifibrotic targets and strategies

The improved understanding of the mechanisms underlying hepatic fibrogenesis make the development of antifibrotic therapies an emerging reality. While numerous targets demonstrate promise in animal models, currently no drugs have been approved as antifibrotic agents for clinical use. Therapies will need to be well-tolerated over decades and must be effective in reversing already established liver disease. The paradigm of stellate cell activation (Fig. 6.4) provides a framework to classify antifibrotic approaches. Where the primary disease cannot be cured, potential approaches will be to:

- reduce inflammation and/or modify the host response in order to avoid stimulating stellate cell activation;
- directly down-regulate stellate cell activation;
- neutralize proliferative, fibrogenic, contractile or proinflammatory responses of HSCs;
- stimulate apoptosis or senescence of HSCs;
- increase the degradation of scar matrix, by stimulating cells to produce matrix proteases, down-regulating their inhibitors, or directly administering matrix proteases.

Although there is clear progress towards antifibrotic therapies in humans, key questions remain:

- Will patients need life-long treatment?
- Will reversal of fibrosis reverse portal hypertension due to the architectural changes?
- Will reversing fibrosis reduce the risk of hepatocellular carcinoma?

Despite these uncertainties, tremendous advances in our understanding of the molecular mechanisms of fibrogenesis will ultimately lead to therapies that will alter the natural history of chronic liver disease.

References

1 Poynard T, Bedossa P, Opolon P. Natural history of liver fibrosis progression in patients with chronic hepatitis C. The OBSVIRC, METAVIR, CLINIVIR, and DOSVIRC groups. *Lancet* 1997; **349**: 825–832.

2 Browning J, Kumar K, Saboorian M *et al.* Ethnic differences in the prevalence of cryptogenic cirrhosis. *Am. J. Gastroenterol.* 2004; **99**: 292–298.

3 Bataller R, North KE, Brenner DA. Genetic polymorphisms and the progression of liver fibrosis: a critical appraisal. *Hepatology* 2003; **37**: 493–503.

4 Huang H, Shiffman M, Friedman S. A 7 gene signature identifies the risk of developing cirrhosis in patients with chronic hepatitis C. *Hepatology* 2007; **46**: 297–306.

5 Yi Q, Wang P, Krahn M. Improving the accuracy of long-term prognostic estimates in hepatitis C infection. *J. Viral. Hepatitis* 2004; **11**: 166–174.

6 Thein H, Yi Q, Dore G *et al.* Estimation of stage-specific fibrosis progression rates in chronic hepatitis C infection: a meta-analysis and meta-regression. *Hepatology* 2008; **48**: 418–431.

7 Pinzani M, Gesualdo L, Sabbah GM *et al.* Effects of platelet-derived growth factor and other polypeptide mitogens on DNA synthesis and growth of cultured rat liver fat-storing cells. *J. Clin. Invest.* 1989; **84**: 1786–1793.

8 Wong L, Yamasaki G, Johnson RJ *et al.* Induction of beta-platelet-derived growth factor receptor in rat hepatic lipocytes during cellular activation in vivo and in culture. *J. Clin. Invest.* 1994; **94**: 1563–1569.

9 Pinzani M, Milani S, Grappone C *et al.* Expression of platelet-derived growth factor in a model of acute liver injury. *Hepatology* 1994; **19**: 701–707.

10 Friedman SL. Mechanisms of hepatic fibrogenesis. *Gastroenterology* 2008; **134**: 1655–1669.

11 Hong F, Tuyama A, Lee T *et al.* Hepatic HSCs express functional CXCR4: role in stromal cell-derived factor -1α mediated stellate cell activation. *Hepatology* 2009: **49**: 2055–2067.

12 Rockey DC, Boyles JK, Gabbiani G *et al.* Rat hepatic lipocytes express smooth muscle actin upon activation in vivo and in culture. *J. Submicrosc. Cytol. Pathol.* 1992; **24**: 193–203.

13 Saab S, Tam SP, Tran BN *et al.* Myosin mediates contractile force generation by hepatic HSCs in response to endothelin-1. *J. Biomed Sci.* 2002; **9**: 607–612.

14 Rockey DC. Vascular mediators in the injured liver. *Hepatology* 2003; **37**: 4–12.

15 Reynaert H, Thompson MG, Thomas T *et al.* Hepatic HSCs: role in microcirculation and pathophysiology of portal hypertension. *Gut* 2002; **50**: 571–581.

16 Inagaki Y, Okazaki I. Emerging insights into transforming growth factor beta SMAD signal in hepatic fibrogenesis. *Gut* 2007; **56**: 284–292.

17 Moreno M, Bataller R. Cytokines and renin-angiotensin system signaling in hepatic fibrosis. *Clin. Liver Dis.* 2008; **12**: 825–852.

18 Melton A, Yee H. Hepatic stellate cell protrusions couple platelet-derived growth factor-BB to chemotaxis. *Hepatology* 2007; **45**: 1446–1453.

19 Marra F, Romanelli RG, Giannini C *et al.* Monocyte chemotactic protein-1 as a chemoattractant for human hepatic HSCs. *Hepatology* 1999; **29**: 140–148.

20 Bonacchi A, Romagnani P, Romanelli RG *et al.* Signal transduction by the chemokine receptor CXCR3: activation of Ras/ERK, Src, and phosphatidylinositol 3-kinase/ Akt controls cell migration and proliferation in human vascular pericytes. *J. Biol. Chem.* 2001; **276**: 9945–9954.

21 Vinas O, Bataller R, Sancho-Bru P *et al.* Human hepatic HSCs show features of antigen-presenting cells and stimulate lymphocyte proliferation. *Hepatology* 2003; **38**: 919–929.

22 Winau F, Hegasy G, Weiskirchen R *et al.* Ito cells are liver-resident antigen-presenting cells for activating T-cell responses. *Immunity* 2007; **26**: 117–129.

23 Seki E, De Minicis S, Osterreicher C *et al.* TLR4 enhances TGF-beta signaling and hepatic fibrosis. *Nat. Med.* 2007; **13**: 1324–1326.

24 Kinnman N, Housset C. Peribiliary myofibroblasts in biliary type liver fibrosis. *Front. Biosci.* 2002; **7**: D496–503.

25 Wells R. Cellular sources of extracellular matrix. *Clin. Liver Dis.* 2008; **12**: 759–768.

26 George J, Wang SS, Sevcsik AM *et al.* Transforming growth factor-beta initiates wound repair in rat liver through induction of the EIIIA-fibronectin splice isoform. *Am. J. Pathol.* 2000; **156**: 115–124.

27 Forbes SJ, Russo FP, Rey V *et al.* A significant proportion of myofibroblasts are of bone marrow origin in human liver fibrosis. *Gastroenterology* 2004; **126**: 955–963.

28 Friedman S, Maher J, Bissell D. Mechanisms and therapy of hepatic fibrosis: report of the AASLD single topic basic research conference. *Hepatology* 2000; **32**: 1401–1408.

29 Olaso E, Ikeda K, Eng F *et al.* DDR2 receptor promotes MMP-2 mediated proliferation and invasion by hepatic HSCs. *J. Clin. Invest.* 2001; **108**: 1369–1378.

30 Issa R, Zhou X, Trim N *et al.* Mutation in collagen-1 that confers resistance to the action of collagenase results in failure of recovery from CCl4-induced liver fibrosis, persistence of activated hepatic HSCs, and diminished hepatocyte regeneration. *FASEB J* 2003; **17**: 47–49.

31 Rudolph KL, Chang S, Millard M *et al.* Inhibition of experimental liver cirrhosis in mice by telomerase gene delivery *Science* 2000; **287**: 1253–1258.

32 Holt A, Salmon M, Buckley C *et al.* Immune interactions in hepatic fibrosis. *Clin. Liver Dis.* 2008; **12**: 861–882.

33 Duffield JS, Forbes SJ, Constandinou CM *et al.* Selective depletion of macrophages reveals distinct, opposing roles during liver injury and repair. *J. Clin. Invest.* 2005; **115**: 56–65.

34 Melhem A, Muhanna N, Bishara A *et al.* Anti-fibrotic activity of NK cells in experimental liver injury through killing of activated HSC. *J. Hepatol.* 2006; **45**: 60–71.

35 Radaeva S, Sun R, Jaruga B *et al.* Natural killer cells ameliorate liver fibrosis by killing activated HSCs in NJG2D-dependent and tumor necrosis factor-related apoptosis-inducing ligand-dependent manners. *Gastroenterology* 2006; **130**: 435–452.

36 Chuang Y, Lian Z, Yang G *et al.* Natural killer T cells exacerbate liver injury in a transforming growth factor beta receptor II dominant-negative mouse model of primary biliary cirrhosis. *Hepatology* 2007; **47**: 571–580.

37 Safadi R, Ohta M, Alvarez CE *et al.* Immune stimulation of hepatic fibrogenesis by CD8 cells and attenuation by transgenic interleukin-10 from hepatocytes. *Gastroenterology* 2004; **127**: 870–882.

38 Benhamou Y, Bochet M, Di Martino V *et al.* Liver fibrosis progression in human immunodeficiency virus and hepa-titis C virus coinfected patients. The Multivirc Group. *Hepatology* 1999; **30**: 1054–1058.

39 Novobrantseva T, Majeau G, Amatucci A *et al.* Attenuated liver fibrosis in the absence of B cells. *J. Clin. Invest.* 2005; **115**: 3072–3078.

40 Benyon D, Arthur MJP. Extracellular matrix degradation and the role of HSCs. *Sem. Liver Dis.* 2001; **21**: 373–384.

41 Arthur MJ, Stanley A, Iredale JP *et al.* Secretion of 72 kDa type IV collagenase/ gelatinase by cultured human lipocytes. Analysis of gene expression, protein synthesis and proteinase activity. *Biochem. J.* 1992; **287**: 701–707.

42 Vyas SK, Leyland H, Gentry J *et al.* Rat hepatic lipocytes synthesize and secrete transin (stromelysin) in early primary culture. *Gastroenterology* 1995; **109**: 889–898.

43 Schaefer B, Rivas-Estilla AM, Meraz-Cruz N *et al.* Reciprocal modulation of matrix metalloproteinase-13 and type I collagen genes in rat hepatic HSCs. *Am. J. Pathol.* 2003; **162**: 1771–1780.

44 Li D, Friedman SL. Liver fibrogenesis and the role of hepatic HSCs: new insights and prospects for therapy. *J. Gastroenterol. Hepatol.* 1999; **14**: 618–633.

45 Yoshiji H, Kuriyama S, Miyamoto Y *et al.* Tissue inhibitor of metalloproteinases-1 promotes liver fibrosis development in a transgenic mouse model. *Hepatology* 2000; **32**: 1248–1254.

46 Iredale JP, Benyon RC, Pickering J *et al.* Mechanisms of spontaneous resolution of rat liver fibrosis. Hepatic stellate cell apoptosis and reduced hepatic expression of metalloproteinase inhibitors. *J. Clin. Invest.* 1998; **102**: 538–549.

47 Goodman Z. Grading and staging systems for inflammation and fibrosis in chronic liver diseases. *J. Hepatol.* 2007; **47**: 598–607.

48 Rockey D, Bissell D. Noninvasive measures of liver fibrosis. *Hepatology* 2006; **43**: S113–S20.

49 Regev A, Berho M, Jeffers LJ *et al.* Sampling error and intraobserver variation in liver biopsy in patients with chronic HCV infection. *Am. J. Gastroenterol.* 2002; **97**: 2614–2618.

50 Guido M, Rugge M. Liver biopsy sampling in chronic viral hepatitis. *Sem. Liver Dis.* 2004; **24**: 89–97.

51 Bedossa P, Dargere D, Paradis V. Sampling variability of liver fibrosis in chronic hepatitis C. *Hepatology* 2003; **38**: 1449–1457.

52 Colloredo G, Guido M, Sonzogni A. Impact of liver biopsy size on histological evaluation of chronic viral hepatitis: the smaller the sample, the milder the disease. *J. Hepatol.* 2003; **39**: 239–244.

53 Lackner C, Struber G, Liegl B *et al.* Comparison and validation of simple noninvasive tests for prediction of fibrosis in chronic hepatitis C. *Hepatology* 2005; **41**: 1376–1382.

54 Guha I, Rosenberg W. Noninvasive assessment of liver fibrosis: serum markers, imaging, and other modalities. *Clin. Liver Dis.* 2008; **12**: 883–900.

55 Rosenberg WM, Voelker M, Thiel R *et al.* Serum markers detect the presence of liver fibrosis: a cohort study. *Gastroenterology* 2004; **127**: 1704–1713.

56 Blomley M, Lim A, Harvey C *et al.* Liver microbubble transit time compared with histology and Child-Pugh score in diffuse liver disease. A cross sectional study. *Gut* 2003; **52**: 1188–1193.

57 Bonekamp S, Kamel I, Solga S *et al.* Can imaging modalities diagnose and stage hepatic fibrosis and cirrhosis accurately? *J. Hepatol.* 2009; **50**: 17–35.

CHAPTER 7
Hepatic Cirrhosis

P Aiden McCormick

St Vincent's University Hospital and University College, Dublin, Ireland

Learning points

- Many of the complications of cirrhosis are due to the hyperdynamic circulation and haemodynamic changes in the splanchnic and systemic circulations.

- Patients with decompensated cirrhosis have a poor prognosis in comparison to patients with compensated cirrhosis.

- Precipitants of decompensation should be identified and treated even if the underlying cause of cirrhosis is not amenable to treatment.

- Screening, prevention and early treatment are important for some complications such as hepatocellular carcinoma, oesophageal varices, bone disease and malnutrition.

Definition

Cirrhosis is defined anatomically as a diffuse process with fibrosis and nodule formation. It is the end result of the fibrogenesis that occurs with chronic liver injury. This process is described in Chapter 6. Although the causes are many, without successful treatment or removal of the agent responsible, the end result of fibrogenesis is the same.

Fibrosis is not synonymous with cirrhosis. Fibrosis may be in acinar zone 3 in heart failure, or in zone 1 in bile duct obstruction and congenital hepatic fibrosis (Fig. 7.1), or interlobular in granulomatous liver disease, but without a true cirrhosis. In schistosomiasis, the ova excite a fibrous tissue reaction in the portal zones but this does not usually evolve into cirrhosis.

Nodule formation without fibrosis, as in partial nodular transformation (Fig. 7.1), is not cirrhosis.

Causes of cirrhosis (Table 7.1)

In Western countries the prevalence of alcoholic cirrhosis, NASH cirrhosis (non-alcoholic steatohepatitis) and viral cirrhosis, in particular hepatitis C, are all increasing. In developing countries, the predominant causes are hepatitis virus B and C, but alcohol and autoimmune conditions may be increasing.

Cirrhosis where the aetiology cannot be determined is termed cryptogenic. This is a diagnosis of exclusion. With improving diagnostic techniques the proportion of patients labelled cryptogenic is falling. In some cases it may be difficult to determine the aetiology as specific histological features may disappear with burnt out cirrhosis, for example autoimmune hepatitis, non-alcoholic steatohepatitis or sarcoidosis.

Cirrhosis and co-factors (Fig. 7.2)

In some forms of liver disease there is a single cause, for example in hepatitis B and C, primary biliary cirrhosis and primary sclerosing cholangitis. However, in many cases co-factors may be important. Thus the prevalence of subjects homozygous for the C282Y mutation for haemochromatosis is between 1/100 and 1/200 in the UK and Ireland. However, only a small fraction of these subjects ever manifest signs of cirrhosis due to haemochromatosis. Suggested co-factors include age, sex, obesity, alcohol, iron intake and other genetic factors as yet unknown. Similarly, many subjects drink excessive quantities of alcohol but only a small proportion ever develop cirrhosis. NASH cirrhosis only develops in a small proportion of obese diabetics.

Causes of liver disease also interact. Progressive disease is more likely in patients with hepatitis B or C who drink excess alcohol. Patients heterozygous for α-1-antitrypsin deficiency who are obese are more likely to manifest cirrhosis.

The risk of developing cirrhosis may also depend on the age and sex of the patient, duration of the disease and immunological status. For patients infected with hepatitis C, fibrosis progression is more rapid in patients infected at an older age and increases with duration of

Sherlock's Diseases of the Liver and Biliary System, Twelfth Edition. Edited by James S. Dooley, Anna S.F. Lok, Andrew K. Burroughs, E. Jenny Heathcote.
© 2011 by Blackwell Publishing Ltd. Published 2011 by Blackwell Publishing Ltd.

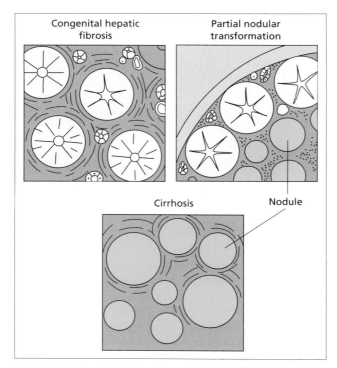

Fig. 7.1. Cirrhosis is defined as widespread fibrosis and nodule formation. Congenital hepatic fibrosis consists of fibrosis without nodules. Partial nodular transformation consists of nodules without fibrosis.

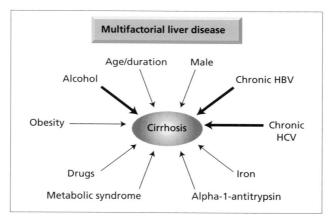

Fig. 7.2. Many liver diseases have a major initiating factor and a number of co-factors contributing to the development of cirrhosis.

infection [1]. Patients with insulin resistance or diabetes mellitus, or who are immunosuppressed, are at higher risk for developing cirrhosis from several aetiologies.

Thus in many cases there can be a principal factor and interacting co-factors which cause a patient to develop cirrhosis (Fig. 7.2). The relative importance of these co-factors may vary from patient to patient.

Table 7.1. Aetiology and definitive treatment of cirrhosis

Aetiology	Treatment
Viral hepatitis (B, C and D)	Antivirals
Alcohol	Abstention
NASH	Weight loss
Metabolic	
iron overload (HFE haemochromatosis)	Venesection
copper overload (Wilson's disease)	Copper chelator
α_1-antitrypsin deficiency	? Transplant
type IV glycogenesis	? Transplant
galactosaemia	Withdraw milk and milk products
tyrosinaemia	Withdraw dietary tyrosine. ? Transplant
Primary biliary cirrhosis	? Transplant
Primary sclerosing cholangitis	? Transplant
Hepatic venous outflow block	
Budd–Chiari syndrome	Relieve main vein block. ? Transplant
heart failure	Treat cardiac cause
Autoimmune hepatitis	Immunosuppression
Toxins and drugs, e.g. methotrexate, amiodarone	Identify and stop

NASH, non-alcoholic steatohepatitis.

Anatomical diagnosis

The diagnosis of cirrhosis depends on demonstrating widespread nodules in the liver combined with fibrosis. Cirrhosis may be classified as micronodular (Fig. 7.3), macronodular (Fig. 7.4) or mixed.

Liver biopsy is the gold standard for diagnosis [2]. Interpretation may be limited by small size and sampling error. This is particularly true if a suction needle rather than a cutting needle is employed to obtain the biopsy, resulting in many instances in fragmented liver tissue. Specialist liver histopathology is essential. Even with small biopsies the expert histopathologist may be able to make a diagnosis of cirrhosis in conjunction with the clinical situation or imaging findings, by recognizing a rim of fibrosis at the periphery of the fragments (Fig. 7.5), and the lack of normally related portal tracts and hepatic venules in the parenchyma, often with a widened reticulin pattern or architectural disruption. Conversely, a non-fragmented core of liver without definite nodules may be obtained from a macronodular cirrhotic liver.

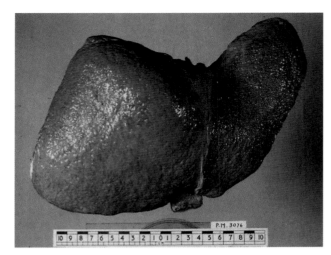

Fig. 7.3. The small finely nodular liver of micronodular cirrhosis.

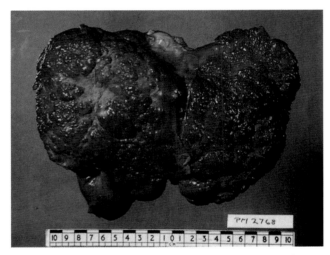

Fig. 7.4. The grossly distorted coarsely nodular liver of macronodular cirrhosis.

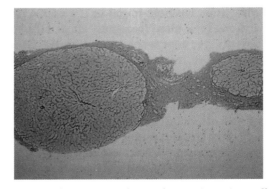

Fig. 7.5. Liver biopsy in cirrhosis: the specimen is small but nodules are shown outlined by reticulin. (Reticulin stain, ×40.)

Helpful diagnostic points in these circumstances include absence of portal tracts, abnormal vascular arrangements, hepatic arterioles not accompanied by portal veins, the presence of nodules with fibrous septa and variability in cell size and appearance in different areas of the biopsy [3].

Liver biopsy contributes to the diagnosis of the aetiology of cirrhosis by identifying features such as alpha-1 antitrypsin globules. The biopsy may help in the reclassification of cryptogenic cirrhosis by identifying histological markers of aetiology, such as steatosis indicating NASH, or inflammation suggesting autoimmune hepatitis (Table 7.2).

Liver biopsy is not without risk (see Chapter 3). If there are contraindications, such as ascites or a coagulation defect, the transjugular approach should be used. In many cases a diagnosis of cirrhosis can be made on the basis of a combination of clinical features and liver imaging. Ultrasound, CT or MRI may identify cirrhosis if nodular change or alterations to the shape and size of the liver can be appreciated. Imaging may miss early cirrhosis. Non-invasive fibroscanning is increasingly being used to assess liver fibrosis, as are combinations of serum markers (see Chapter 6).

Transient elastography (fibroscan) is a non-invasive method of evaluating liver fibrosis/ cirrhosis. It appears to be particularly useful in patients with chronic hepatitis C and is superior to laboratory based tests [4]. Fibroscan is technically difficult in obese subjects and this may limit its usefulness in the diagnosis of NASH cirrhosis.

Ultrasound is not reliable for the diagnosis of cirrhosis but is useful for screening for hepatocellular carcinoma in patients with known cirrhosis, and for evaluating patency of the portal vein and the presence of ascites. Contrast-enhanced ultrasound is helpful in distinguishing benign and malignant liver nodules.

CT scan can assess liver size and shape and identify liver nodules (Fig. 7.6). It provides an objective, permanent record for evaluating changes over time. Fatty change and space-occupying lesions can be recognized. After intravenous contrast, the portal vein and hepatic veins can be identified, and a collateral circulation with splenomegaly may confirm the diagnosis of portal hypertension. Ascites can be seen. Multiphase CT is useful in the evaluation of focal liver lesions and directed biopsy of a selected area can be performed safely. However the radiation dose with repeated multislice CT scans is substantial and may be an issue, particularly in younger patients.

MRI may identify cirrhosis of the liver but is expensive and many patients find the procedure claustrophobic. It is most useful for evaluating the biliary tree (MR cholangiography) or for evaluating possible malignancy in liver nodules (contrast enhanced MRI) (see Chapter 33).

Table 7.2. Histopathology and aetiology of cirrhosis

Aetiology	Morphological pattern	Fat	Cholestasis	Iron	Copper	Acidophilic bodies	PAS-positive globules	Mallory's hyalin	Ground-glass hepatocytes
Viral hepatitis B	Macro- or micronodular	−	−	−	−	+	−	−	+
Viral hepatitis C	Macro- or micronodular	+	−	±	−	+	−	−	−
Alcohol	Micro- or macronodular	+	±	±	−	±	−	+	−
Haemochromatosis	Micronodular	±	−	+	−	−	−	−	−
Wilson's disease	Macronodular	±	±	−	±	+	−	+	−
α_1-antitrypsin deficiency	Micro- or macronodular	±	±	−	±	±	+	±	−
Primary biliary	Biliary	−	+	−	+	−	−	±	−
Venous outflow obstruction	Reversed	−	−	−	−	−	−	−	−
Intestinal bypass operation	Micronodular	+	−	−	−	±	−	±	−
Indian childhood cirrhosis	Micronodular	−	±	−	+	−	−	+	−

− Usually absent; ± may be present; + usually present.

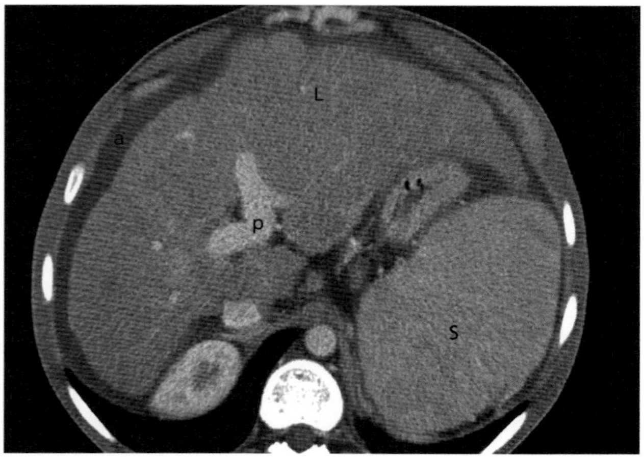

Fig. 7.6. CT scan, after intravenous contrast, in cirrhosis shows ascites (a), liver with irregular surface (L), patent portal vein (p) and splenomegaly (S).

Reversible cirrhosis

Cirrhosis is usually believed to be irreversible. However fibrosis may regress if the initiating insult is removed, for example hepatitis C, biliary obstruction, obesity or iron overload. Reversal of cirrhosis has been demonstrated in some patients [5–7]. In most cases repeat liver biopsies have shown a lesser degree of fibrosis rather than a reversion to normal liver. Nevertheless, they support the concept that irreversibility is not an absolute rule.

Clinical cirrhosis: compensated versus decompensated

Patients may present with complications of liver disease or the presence of liver disease may be picked up when they are seen for other reasons. Cirrhosis can be symptomatic or asymptomatic. Many patients are found to have abnormal liver tests during routine medical or preoperative examinations. These liver test abnormalities may be relatively minor. On physical examination the detection of unexpected hepatomegaly or splenomegaly may trigger further investigation. The finding of an enlarged, smooth, palpable left lobe in the epigastrium is a particularly useful clinical sign [8]. Investigations useful in the work up of a patient with suspected cirrhosis are summarized in Table 7.3.

In clinical terms, cirrhosis is described as are either 'compensated' or 'decompensated'. Decompensation means cirrhosis complicated by one or more of the following features: jaundice, ascites, hepatic encephalopathy or bleeding varices. Ascites is the usual first sign. Hepatorenal syndrome, hyponatraemia and spontaneous bacterial peritonitis are also features of decompensation but in these patients ascites invariably occurs

Table 7.3. General investigations in the patient with cirrhosis (see also Table 9.1)

Occupation, age, sex, domicile

Clinical history

    Fatigue and weight loss

    Anorexia and flatulent dyspepsia

    Abdominal pain

    Jaundice. Itching. Colour of urine and faeces

    Swelling of legs or abdomen

    Haemorrhage—nose, gums, skin, alimentary tract

    Loss of libido; menstrual history

    Past health: jaundice, hepatitis, drugs ingested, blood transfusion

    Social: alcohol consumption

    Family history: liver disease, autoimmune disease

Examination

    Nutrition, fever, fetor hepaticus, jaundice, pigmentation, purpura, finger clubbing, white nails, vascular spiders, palmar erythema, gynaecomastia, testicular atrophy, distribution of body hair, parotid enlargement, Dupuytren's contracture, blood pressure

    Abdomen: ascites, abdominal wall veins, liver, spleen

    Peripheral oedema

    Neurological changes: mental functions, stupor, tremor

Investigations

    Haematology

        haemoglobin, leucocyte and platelet count, prothrombin time (INR)

    Serum biochemistry

        bilirubin

        transaminase

        alkaline phosphatase

        γ-glutamyl-transpeptidase

        albumin and globulin

        immunoglobulins

        transferrin saturation and serum ferritin

        serum caeruloplasmin and copper

        α-1-antitrypsin phenotype

    If ascites present

        serum sodium, potassium, bicarbonate, chloride, urea and creatinine levels

        weigh daily

        24-h urine volume and sodium excretion

    Serum immunological

        smooth muscle, mitochondrial, nuclear, LKM1 antibodies, and ANCA

        hepatitis B antigen (HBsAg), anti-HCV (other markers of hepatitis, see Chapters 18 and 20)

        α-fetoprotein

    Endoscopy

    Hepatic ultrasound, CT or MRI scan

    Needle liver biopsy if blood coagulation permits

    EEG if neuropsychiatric changes

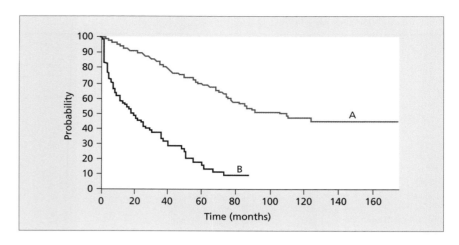

Fig. 7.7. Patients with decompensated cirrhosis (B) have much reduced probability of survival compared to patients with compensated cirrhosis (A). Reprinted with permission of John Wiley and Sons Inc. [9].

first. Compensated cirrhotic patients have none of these features.

This is a very important clinical distinction and has major implications for prognosis and treatment. Compensated cirrhotic patients have a 50% 10-year survival as compared to 50% survival at 18 months for decompensated patients [9] (Fig. 7.7). Cirrhotic patients become decompensated at the rate of approximately 10% per year. Decompensated patients can improve and become compensated with an associated improvement in prognosis. In general, patients with decompensated cirrhosis should be considered for liver transplantation.

Compensated cirrhosis

The disease may be discovered at a routine examination or biochemical screen, or at operation undertaken for some other condition. Cirrhosis may be suspected if the patient has vascular spiders, palmar erythema, unexplained epistaxis or oedema of the ankles. Firm enlargement of the liver, particularly in the epigastrium, and splenomegaly are helpful diagnostic signs. Confirmation should be sought by biochemical tests, scanning and, if necessary, liver biopsy.

Biochemical tests may be quite normal in this group. The most frequent changes are a slight increase in the serum transaminase or γ-glutamyl transpeptidase concentration. Portal hypertension may be present even with normal liver function tests. Diagnosis is confirmed by *liver imaging* or *needle liver biopsy*.

These patients may remain compensated until they die from another cause. Hepatocellular carcinoma occurs at a rate of 1–3% per year and appropriate screening is recommended (see Chapter 35). Decompensation may be precipitated by bacterial infection, surgery, trauma or medication.

Decompensated cirrhosis

The patient usually seeks medical advice because of ascites, jaundice or gastrointestinal bleeding. General health fails with weakness, muscle wasting and weight loss. Continuous mild fever (37.5–38°C) is often due to Gram-negative bacteraemia, to continuing hepatic cell necrosis, ongoing alcoholic hepatitis or to a complicating hepatocellular carcinoma. A liver flap may be present. Cirrhosis is the commonest cause of hepatic encephalopathy.

Jaundice implies that liver cell destruction exceeds the capacity for regeneration and is always serious. The deeper the jaundice the greater the inadequacy of liver cell function.

The skin may be pigmented. Clubbing of the fingers is occasionally seen. Purpura over the arms, shoulders and shins may be associated with a low platelet count. The circulation is over-active. The blood pressure is low. Sparse body hair, vascular spiders, palmar erythema, white nails and gonadal atrophy are common.

Ascites is usually preceded by abdominal distension. Oedema of the legs is frequently associated.

The liver may be enlarged, with a firm regular edge, or contracted and impalpable. The spleen may be palpable.

Vasodilatation and hyperdynamic circulation

Many of the complications seen in decompensated cirrhotic patients are believed to be due to vasodilatation and the hyperdynamic circulation (Fig. 7.8). Decompensated cirrhosis can be viewed as a circulatory or a haemodynamic disease. Vasodilatation is shown by flushed extremities, bounding pulses, capillary pulsations and relative arterial hypotension. Peripheral

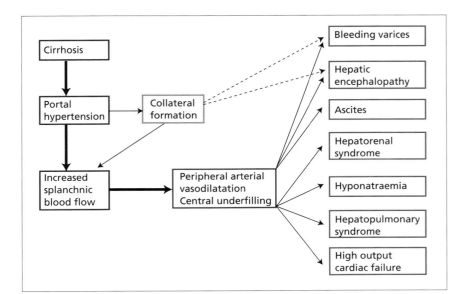

Fig. 7.8. Many of the complications of cirrhosis are due to arterial dilatation and the hyperdynamic circulation. Reprinted with permission of Elsevier from McCormick PA, Donnelly C. *Pharmacol. Ther.* 2008; **119**: 106.

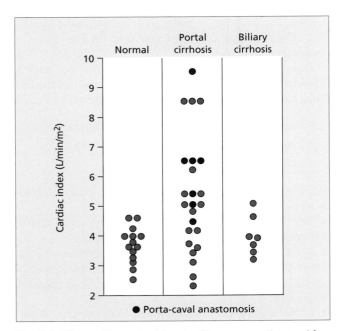

Fig. 7.9. The cardiac output is raised in many patients with hepatic cirrhosis but within normal limits in biliary cirrhosis. Mean normal cardiac index is 3.68 ± 0.60 L/min per m^2. Mean in hepatic cirrhosis is 5.36 ± 1.98 L/min per m^2. From Lunzer MR *et al.* [11].

Systemic vascular peripheral resistance is reduced as is the arteriovenous oxygen difference. In patients with cirrhosis, whole body oxygen consumption is decreased and tissue oxidation is abnormal. This has been related to the hyperdynamic circulation and to arteriovenous shunting. Thus, the vasodilator state of liver failure may contribute to general tissue hypoxia.

Vasomotor tone is decreased as shown by reduced vasoconstriction in response to mental exercise, the Valsalva manoeuvre and tilting from horizontal to vertical [11,12]. The cirrhotic patient shows arterial hyperactivity to endogenous vasoconstrictors. Autonomic neuropathy is a poor prognostic indicator [13]. The effective arterial blood volume falls as a consequence of an increase in the arterial vascular compartment induced by arterial vasodilatation. This activates the sympathetic and renin–angiotensin systems and is important in sodium and water retention and ascites formation. The hyperdynamic splanchnic circulation is related to portal hypertension.

A large number of arteriovenous anastomoses, which are normally present but functionally closed, may have opened under the influence of a vasodilator. The nature of the vasodilators concerned—there are likely to be many—remains speculative. They might be formed by the sick hepatocyte, fail to be inactivated by hepatocytes or bypass the liver through intra- or extrahepatic portal–systemic shunts. The vasodilators are likely to be of intestinal origin. In cirrhosis, increased permeability of the intestinal mucosa and portosystemic shunting allow endotoxin and cytokines to reach the systemic circulation and these could contribute [14,15].

arterial blood flow and portal venous blood flow are increased. Cardiac output is raised [10] (Fig. 7.9) and evidenced by tachycardia, an active precordial impulse and frequently an ejection systolic murmur. Renal blood flow, and particularly cortical perfusion, is reduced.

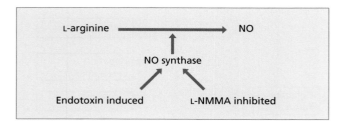

Fig. 7.10. Nitric oxide (NO) is a general vasodilator. It is produced from L-arginine, NO synthase being the responsible enzyme. This is induced by endotoxin and inhibited by L-NMMA.

Nitric oxide (NO), a potent endothelium-derived vasodilator, may be involved in the hyperdynamic circulation [16]. It is released from L-arginine by a family of NO synthase enzymes encoded by different genes (Fig. 7.10). The endothelial constituent, NO synthase (NOS3), plays an important part in regulating normal vasoconstrictor tone [17].

L-arginine analogues such as NG-monomethyl-L-arginine (L-NMMA) inhibit NO release. Inhibitors have been shown to reverse the hyperdynamic circulation in portal-hypertensive rats [18]. Cirrhotic rats show increased sensitivity to the pressor effect of NO inhibition and portal pressure rises [19]. NO synthase is inducible after stimulation with bacterial endotoxin or cytokines.

Various gastrointestinal peptides, such as vasoactive intestinal polypeptide (VIP) type II, have little effect on the portal circulation. Glucagon is unlikely to be the sole vasodilator responsible.

Prostaglandins (E_1, E_2 and E_{12}) have vasodilatory actions and prostanoids are released into the portal vein in patients with chronic liver disease [20]. They may play a part in vasodilatation.

After hepatic transplantation, portal pressure becomes normal. The cardiac index and splanchnic flow remain high due to the persistence of portal–systemic collateral flow [21]. These gradually return to normal over time.

Prognosis (Child–Pugh score, MELD, UKELD)

Poor prognosis is associated with a prolonged prothrombin time, marked ascites, gastrointestinal bleeding, advanced age, high daily alcohol consumption, high serum bilirubin and alkaline phosphatase, low albumin values and poor nutrition. The availability of liver transplantation has emphasized the need for an accurate prognosis so that surgery may be performed at the right time.

Child's classification (grades A–C)—which depends on jaundice, ascites, encephalopathy, serum albumin concentration and nutrition (see Table 9.4)—gives a good short-term prognostic guide. Prothrombin time can be used rather than nutritional status (Child–Pugh modification) and individual features scored by severity. The total score classifies patients into grade A, B or C [22], although published studies often differ in their choice of numerical boundary between one grade and another.

The MELD score was developed to determine prognosis in patients undergoing TIPS insertion. MELD stands for Model for End-stage Liver Disease. It is calculated from serum creatinine, prothrombin time (INR) and serum bilirubin. MELD was applied to liver transplantation and found to accurately predict waiting list mortality in cirrhotic patients. It is now widely used as a criterion for liver transplant listing and to determine priority for organ allocation. Use of the MELD score for organ allocation appears to have reduced mortality on the waiting list in the USA [23]. The addition of serum sodium to the calculation may further improve its predictive ability—MELD-Na [24]. A similar scoring system has been developed in the UK (UKELD). This also uses INR, serum creatinine, serum bilirubin and serum sodium and has similar predictive abilities to the MELD-Na. These scores can be calculated on-line using a number of websites.

Disease-specific scoring systems may be useful. Maddrey's discriminant function (DF) is helpful in alcoholic hepatitis [25]. It is calculated as follows:

$$DF = \text{serum bilirubin } (\mu mol/L)/17 + \text{prolongation of}$$
$$\text{prothrombin time in seconds compared to}$$
$$\text{controls} \times 4.6$$

A DF greater than 32 is associated with a very high in-hospital mortality (30–50%).

The following clinical points may be useful prognostically:

1 *Aetiology:* if the initiating factor can be removed the prognosis is better. Thus abstinence in alcoholic cirrhosis and antiviral treatment in viral cirrhosis may improve prognosis.

2 If decompensation has followed haemorrhage, infection or alcoholism, the prognosis is better than if it is spontaneous, because the *precipitating factor* is correctable.

3 The *response to therapy*: if the patient has failed to improve within 1 month of starting hospital treatment, the outlook is poor.

4 *Jaundice*, especially if persistent, is a serious sign.

5 *Neurological complications*: spontaneous or chronic hepatic encephalopathy carry a poor prognosis [26]. Autonomic neuropathy is also a poor prognostic indicator [13].

6 *Ascites* worsens the prognosis, particularly if resistant to diuretic therapy.

7 *Liver size*: a large liver carries a better prognosis than a small one because it is likely to contain more functioning cells.

8 *Portal venous pressure*: in many studies, prediction of survival by the Child–Pugh score is improved by adding portal pressure, derived from the hepatic venous pressure gradient [27].

9 *Haemorrhage from oesophageal varices*: portal hypertension must be considered together with the state of the liver cells. If function is good, haemorrhage may be tolerated; if poor, hepatic coma and death are probable.

10 *Biochemical tests*: if the serum albumin is less than 25 g/L the outlook is poor. Hyponatraemia (serum sodium <120 mmol/L), if unrelated to diuretic therapy, is grave. Serum transaminase and globulin levels give no guide to prognosis.

11 Persistent *hypotension* (systolic BP <100 mmHg) is a major concern, and remediable causes, for example sepsis, should be sought and treated.

Clinical and pathological associations

Gastrointestinal

Splenomegaly and abdominal wall venous collaterals usually indicate portal hypertension. Varices are visualized by endoscopy.

Peptic ulceration has been found in 11% of 324 patients with cirrhosis [28]. Seventy per cent were asymptomatic. Duodenal ulcers were more frequent than gastric ulcers. The prevalence of *Helicobacter pylori* based on serology is significantly greater in patients with cirrhosis than those without liver disease (76 vs. 42%) [29].

Small bowel bacterial overgrowth occurs in 30% of patients with alcoholic cirrhosis, being more frequent in those with than without ascites (37 vs. 5%) [30]. It is associated with older age and the administration of H₂-receptor antagonists or proton pump inhibitors. The hydrogen breath test correlates poorly with the results of microbiological culture from jejunal fluid [31].

Abdominal herniae are common with ascites. They should not be repaired unless endangering life or unless the cirrhosis is very well compensated.

Ultrasound shows that 18.5% of males and 31.2% of females with chronic liver disease have gallstones, usually of pigment type [32]. Surgery should be avoided unless the clinical indication is clearly strong, and transplantation not imminent, for the patient is a poor operative risk.

Chronic relapsing pancreatitis and pancreatic calcification are often associated with alcoholic liver disease.

Parotid gland enlargement may be seen in alcoholic cirrhotic patients or occasionally in sarcoidosis.

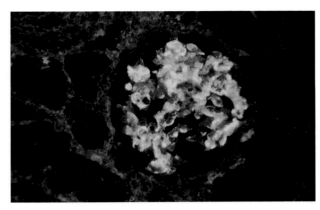

Fig. 7.11. IgA nephropathy: renal biopsy showing IgA deposition in glomerulus of cirrhotic patient (alcohol-related) with creatinine clearance of 20 mL/min and proteinuria (immunostaining with FITC rabbit antihuman IgA).

Renal

Changes in intrarenal circulation, and particularly a redistribution of blood flow away from the cortex, are found in all forms of cirrhosis. This predisposes to the *hepatorenal syndrome*. Intrinsic renal failure follows periods of hypotension and shock.

Glomerular changes include a thickening of the mesangial stalk and to a lesser degree of the capillary walls (*cirrhotic glomerular sclerosis*). Deposits of IgA are most frequent (Fig. 7.11) [33,34]. These are particularly found with alcoholic liver disease. The changes are usually latent, but occasionally are associated with proliferative changes and the clinical manifestations of glomerular involvement. Chronic hepatitis C infection is associated with cryoglobulinaemia and membranoproliferative glomerulonephritis [35].

Foetor hepaticus

This is a sweetish, slightly faecal smell of the breath which has been likened to that of a freshly opened corpse or mice. It complicates severe hepatocellular disease, especially with an extensive collateral circulation. It is presumably of intestinal origin, for it becomes less intense after defecation or when the gut flora is changed by wide-spectrum antibiotics. Gas chromatography suggests that it is due to dimethyl sulphide and ketones in alveolar air [36]. Foetor may be a useful diagnostic sign in patients seen for the first time in coma.

Skin changes

> An older Miss Muffett
> Decided to rough it
> And lived upon whisky and gin.
> Red hands and a spider
> Developed outside her—
> Such are the wages of sin [37].

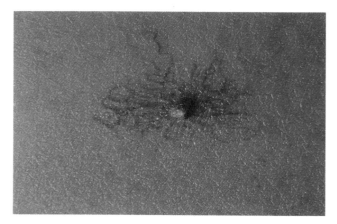

Fig. 7.12. A vascular spider. Note the elevated centre and radiating branches.

Vascular spiders [37] (Fig. 7.12)

Synonyms: *arterial spider, spider naevi, spider telangiectasis, spider angioma*

Arterial spiders are found in the vascular territory of the superior vena cava and very rarely below a line joining the nipples. Common sites are the necklace area, the face, forearms and dorsum of the hand (Fig. 7.12). The selective distribution of vascular spiders is not understood.

An arterial spider consists of a central arteriole, radiating from which are numerous small vessels resembling a spider's legs. It ranges in size from a pinhead to 0.5 cm in diameter. When sufficiently large it can be seen or felt to pulsate, and this effect is enhanced by pressing on it with a glass slide. Pressure on the central prominence with a pinhead causes blanching of the whole lesion, as would be expected from an arterial lesion.

Arterial spiders may disappear with improving hepatic function, whereas the appearance of fresh spiders is suggestive of progression. Multiple spiders and finger clubbing may suggest hepatopulmonary syndrome (HPS) [38]. Spiders can bleed profusely.

In association with vascular spiders, and having a similar distribution, numerous small vessels may be scattered in random fashion through the skin, usually on the upper arms. These resemble the silk threads in American dollar bills and the condition is called *paper money skin*.

A further association is the appearance of *white spots* on the arms and buttocks on cooling the skin [39]. Examination with a lens shows that the centre of each spot represents the beginnings of a spider.

Vascular spiders are most frequently associated with cirrhosis, especially of the alcoholic. They may appear transiently with viral hepatitis. Rarely they are found in normal adults. Up to 38% of children without liver disease may have at least one spider naevus [40]. During pregnancy, they appear between the second and fifth months, disappearing within 2 months of delivery. A few spiders are not sufficient to diagnose liver disease, but many new ones, with increasing size of old ones, should arouse suspicion.

Differential diagnosis

Hereditary haemorrhagic telangiectasis (HHT) lesions are usually on the upper body. Mucosal ones are common inside the nose, on the tongue, lips and palate, and in the pharynx, oesophagus and stomach. The nail beds, palmar surfaces and fingers are frequently involved. HHT with large hepatic angiomas can cause high output cardiac failure requiring liver transplantation.

Telangiectasia may be associated with cirrhosis. Calcinosis, Raynaud's phenomenon, sclerodactyly and telangiectasia (*CRST syndrome*) may be found in patients with primary biliary cirrhosis.

Campbell de Morgan's spots are very common, increasing in size and number with age. They are bright red, flat or slightly elevated and occur especially on the front of the chest and the abdomen.

The venous star is found with elevation of venous pressure. It usually overlies the main tributary to a vein of large size. It is 2–3 cm in diameter and is not obliterated by pressure. Venous stars are seen on the dorsum of the foot, legs, back and on the lower border of the ribs.

Palmar erythema (liver palms) (Fig. 7.13)

The hands are warm and the palms bright red in colour, especially the hypothenar and thenar eminences and pulps of the fingers. The soles of the feet may be similarly affected. The mottling blanches on pressure and the colour rapidly returns. When a glass slide is pressed on the palm it flushes synchronously with the pulse rate. The patient may complain of throbbing, tingling palms. Palmar erythema is not so frequently seen in cirrhosis as are vascular spiders.

Many normal people have *familial* palmar flushing, unassociated with liver disease. A similar appearance may be seen in prolonged rheumatoid arthritis, in pregnancy, with chronic febrile diseases, leukaemia and thyrotoxicosis.

Mechanism of skin changes

The vascular spiders and palmar erythema have been traditionally attributed to oestrogen excess. They are also seen in pregnancy when circulating oestrogens are increased. Oestrogens have an enlarging, dilating effect

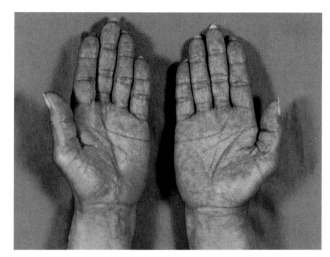

Fig. 7.13. Palmar erythema ('liver palms') in a patient with hepatic cirrhosis.

on the spiral arterioles of the endometrium, and such a mechanism may explain the closely similar cutaneous spiders. Oestrogens have induced cutaneous spiders in men, although this is not usual when such therapy is given for prostatic carcinoma. The liver certainly inactivates oestrogens, although oestradiol levels in cirrhosis are often normal. The ratio between oestrogens and androgens may be more important [41]. In male cirrhotic patients, although the serum oestradiol was normal, free serum testosterone was reduced. The oestradiol/free testosterone ratio was highest in male cirrhotic patients with spiders. The aetiology of the other skin lesions remains unknown.

Leuconychia

White finger nails are related to hypoalbuminaemia. They may be seen in patients with severe liver disease and/or associated malnutrition.

Clubbing

Digital clubbing and *hypertrophic osteoarthropathy* may complicate cirrhosis especially in patients with cystic fibrosis or HPS. These changes may be due to aggregated platelets, passing peripherally through pulmonary arteriovenous shunts, plugging capillaries and releasing PDGF [42].

Dupuytren's contracture

Dupuytren's contracture is a thickening of the palmar fascia in the hands. It may be seen in alcoholic cirrhosis but may also be idiopathic.

Nutrition

Protein–calorie malnutrition is a common complication of chronic liver disease and predicts shortened survival [43]. The cause appears to be multifactorial, but inadequate intake of protein and energy-producing food and an increased resting energy expenditure (REE) contribute. Dental and peridontal disease are common and reflect poor oral hygiene and dental care rather than cirrhosis *per se*. Fat stores and muscle mass are reduced in many cirrhotic patients, particularly the alcoholic and those who are Child's grade C (see Table 9.4). Alcoholic cirrhotic patients have muscle weakness which appears to be related to the severity of malnutrition rather than the severity of liver disease [44]. Muscle wasting is related to reduced muscle protein synthesis.

Steatorrhoea is frequent even in the absence of pancreatitis or alcoholism. It can be related to reduced hepatic bile salt secretion.

Nutritional status can be estimated at the bedside using anthropometric measurement of body mass index, mid arm muscle circumference, triceps skin fold thickness, subjective global assessment or a combination of these measures [43].

Endocrine changes

Hyperglycaemia

While up to 80% of cirrhotic patients are glucose intolerant, only 10–20% are truly diabetic. The prevalence of diabetes is greater among those with non-alcoholic liver disease-related cirrhosis, hepatitis C or alcohol-related cirrhosis compared with those with cholestatic cirrhosis [45].

Hypogonadism

Diminished libido and potency are frequent in men, particularly in alcoholic cirrhosis. The testes are soft and small. Secondary sexual hair is lost and men shave less often. Prostatic hypertrophy has a lower incidence in men with cirrhosis [46].

The female has ovulatory failure. The premenopausal patient loses feminine characteristics, particularly breast and pelvic fat. She is usually infertile; menstruation is erratic, diminished or absent, but rarely excessive.

In women with non-alcoholic liver disease, sexual behaviour, desire, frequency and performance are not impaired [47].

Gynaecomastia is often seen in patients receiving spironolactone. This decreases serum testosterone levels and reduces hepatic androgen-receptor activity [48] (Fig. 7.14). The breasts may be tender. Enlargement is caused by hyperplasia of the glandular elements. Young

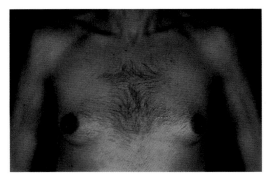

Fig. 7.14. Gynaecomastia in a patient with cirrhosis.

men with chronic autoimmune hepatitis may develop gynaecomastia but alcoholic liver disease is the commonest association.

Mechanism

The human liver has both androgen and oestrogen receptors which render it sensitive to androgens and oestrogens [49]. In cirrhosis, the end organ sensitivities to sex hormones may be changed. Hepatic androgen receptors fall and hepatic oestrogen receptor concentrations increase.

Feminization may be related to hepatic regeneration [50]. Partial hepatic resection or liver transplantation are associated with increases in serum oestrogens and reductions in testosterone, while oestrogen receptors increase.

Primary liver cancer occasionally presents with feminization [51]. Serum oestrone levels are high and can return to normal when the tumour is removed. The tumour can be shown to function as trophoblastic tissue.

Hypothalamic–pituitary function

Plasma gonadotrophins are usually normal although a minority of cirrhotic patients have high values. These normal levels, in spite of testicular failure, suggest either a primary testicular defect or a failure of the pituitary–hypothalamus. Impaired release of luteinizing hormone suggests a possible hypothalamic defect, at least in those with alcoholic liver disease [52].

Hypothalamic–pituitary dysfunction in some women with non-alcoholic liver disease may lead to amenorrhoea and oestrogen deficiency and also to osteoporosis [53].

Metabolism of hormones

Steroid hormones are conjugated in the liver. There seems to be little difficulty in the conjugation process even in the presence of hepatocellular disease. Conjugated hormones excreted in the bile undergo an enterohepatic circulation. In cholestasis the biliary excretion of oestrogens, and especially of polar conjugates, is greatly reduced. Any failure of hormone metabolism results in a rise in blood hormone levels. However feedback mechanisms between plasma hormone levels and hormone secretion prevent any but temporary rises in circulating levels. This may explain some of the difficulty in relating plasma hormone levels to clinical features.

Eye signs

Lid retraction and lid lag is significantly increased in patients with cirrhosis compared with a control population [54]. There is no evidence of thyroid disease. Serum free thyroxine is not increased.

Muscle cramps

Muscle cramps occur significantly more frequently in cirrhotic patients than in patients without liver disease, and correlate with the presence of ascites, low mean arterial pressure and plasma renin activity [55]. Cramps often respond to oral quinine sulphate.

Drug metabolism

In cirrhotic patients the effect of drugs is generally increased due to reduced elimination [56]. There are two particular causes: reduced hepatocyte mass rather than enzyme activity [57], and the shunting of blood past the liver. For drugs with a high hepatic extraction ratio (high first-pass effect) predicting the therapeutic effect after oral administration is difficult, due to the variation in the degree of shunting (both portosystemic and intrahepatic) between patients. The clinical effect of low extraction drugs in cirrhotic patients is more dependent on hepatocellular function and therefore more predictable. Overall drug dosage should be reduced according to the severity of liver disease.

Other components of the metabolic pathway may alter drug handling in cirrhosis including absorption, tissue distribution, protein binding, biliary secretion, enterohepatic circulation and target-organ responsiveness.

Laboratory findings

Haematology. There is usually a mild normocytic, normochromic anaemia; it is often macrocytic in the alcoholic. Gastrointestinal bleeding leads to hypochromic anaemia. The leucocyte and platelet counts are reduced ('hypersplenism'). The prothrombin time is prolonged and does not return to normal with vitamin K therapy. The bone marrow is macronormoblastic. Plasma cells are increased in proportion to the hyperglobulinaemia.

Serum biochemical changes. In addition to the raised serum bilirubin level, albumin is depressed and γ-globulin raised. The serum alkaline phosphatase is usually raised to about twice normal; very high readings are occasionally found, particularly with alcoholic cirrhosis. Serum transaminase values may be increased.

Urine. Urobilinogen is present in excess; bilirubin is also present if the patient is jaundiced. The urinary sodium excretion is diminished in the presence of ascites, and in a severe case less than 5 mmol is passed daily.

Elevation of the total serum globulin, and particularly gamma level, is a well-known accompaniment of chronic liver disease. Electrophoresis shows a polyclonal gamma response, but rarely a monoclonal picture may be seen. The increased γ-globulin values may be related in part to increased tissue autoantibodies, such as smooth muscle antibody. However, the major factor seems to be failure of the damaged liver to clear intestinal antigens. Patients with cirrhosis show increased serum antibodies to gastrointestinal tract antigens, particularly *Escherichia coli*. Such antigens bypass the liver through portal–systemic channels or through the internal shunts developing around the cirrhotic nodules. Once in the systemic circulation they provoke an increased antibody response from such organs as the spleen. Systemic endotoxaemia may arise similarly. Polymeric IgA and IgA–antigen complexes of gut origin can also reach the systemic circulation. Suppressor T-lymphocyte function is depressed in chronic liver disease and this would reduce the suppression of B lymphocytes and so favour antibody production.

Infections

Bacteraemia, pneumonia and urinary tract infections are common in cirrhotic patients. The human liver is bacteriologically sterile and the portal venous blood only rarely contains organisms. However, in the cirrhotic patient, bacteria, particularly intestinal, could reach the general circulation either by passing through a faulty hepatic filter or through portosystemic collaterals [58]. Patients with ascites are prone to spontaneous bacterial peritonitis, present in 10–20% of patients with ascites admitted to hospital [59]. Spontaneous bacterial empyema in a pre-existing hydrothorax may occur in the absence of spontaneous bacterial peritonitis. In the cirrhotic with febrile coma, bacterial meningitis should be considered. Nasal carriage of *Staphylococcus aureus* is increased in cirrhotic patients.

Sepsis should always be suspected in cirrhotic patients with unexplained pyrexia or deterioration. Empirical treatment with a broad-spectrum antibiotic is often necessary after appropriate specimens have been taken for microbiological culture. After gastrointestinal haemorrhage, the risk of sepsis is greater in Child C rather than Child A/B grade cirrhotic patients (53 vs. 18%). Prophylactic antibiotics significantly reduce the incidence and significantly increases short-term survival rates [60]. Antibiotic prophylaxis is now the standard of care in this situation.

Septicaemia is frequent in terminal hepatocellular failure. Multiple factors contribute. Kupffer cell and polymorphonuclear function are impaired [61]. Serum shows a reduction in factors such as fibronectin, opsonins and chemoattractants, including members of the complement cascade. Systemic toxaemia of intestinal origin results in deterioration of the scavenger functions of the reticuloendothelial system and also to renal damage [62]. These factors contribute to blood culture positive episodes. Urinary tract infections are particularly common in cirrhotic patients and are usually Gram-negative. Indwelling urinary catheters play a part.

Pneumonia especially affects alcoholics. Other infections include lymphangitis and endocarditis. Clinical features may be atypical with inconspicuous fever, no rigors and only slight leucocytosis.

Over half the infections in hospitalized cirrhotic patients are due to Gram-positive organisms [63]. With invasive investigations and treatment nosocomial infections are common and resistant organisms such as methicillin resistant *Staphylococcus aureus* (MRSA) and vancomycin-resistant enterococci (VRE) increasingly a problem. Community acquired infections are associated with lower mortality than nosocomial (15% vs. 31%) [63]. Prophylaxis for spontaneous bacterial peritonitis is associated with increased quinolone resistance.

Bad prognostic features are an absence of fever, elevated serum creatinine and marked leucocytosis. Bacterial infections increase the risk of mortality and rebleeding in patients with variceal haemorrhage [64]. Recurrent infections are ominous and sufferers should be considered for liver transplant.

Patients with liver failure should receive prophylactic antibiotics during invasive practical procedures and after gastrointestinal bleeding. Parenteral broad-spectrum antibiotics should be started when infection is suspected. Relative renal insufficiency may occur in cirrhotic patients with septic shock and these patients may benefit from intravenous hydrocortisone (50 mg 6 hourly) [65].

There has been a resurgence of tuberculosis, and tuberculous peritonitis is therefore still encountered but often not suspected.

Table 7.4. Pulmonary changes complicating chronic hepatocellular disease

Hypoxia
Intrapulmonary shunting
Ventilation–perfusion mismatch
Reduced transfer factor
Pleural effusion
Raised diaphragms
Basal atelectasis
Primary pulmonary hypertension
Portopulmonary shunting
Chest X-ray mottling

Table 7.5. Hepatopulmonary syndrome

Advanced chronic liver disease
Arterial hypoxaemia
Intrapulmonary vascular dilatation
No primary cardiopulmonary disease

Cardiopulmonary conditions

Hepatopulmonary syndrome

About a third of patients with decompensated cirrhosis have reduced arterial oxygen saturation and are sometimes cyanosed (Table 7.4). Causes include HPS (Table 7.5). This is defined as a clinical disorder associated with advanced liver disease, pulmonary vascular dilatation and a defect in oxygenation in the absence of detectable primary cardiopulmonary disease [66]. Po_2 is less than 80 mmHg (10.6 kPa) and the alveolar–arterial oxygen gradient exceeds 15 mmHg (2 kPa) breathing room air. Platypnoea (shortness of breath relieved by lying down) and orthodeoxia (fall in the arterial Po_2 in the upright position) are usual. The intrapulmonary shunting is due to marked dilatation of precapillary and capillary vessels. This results in diffusion limitation of capillary oxygenation and ventilation–perfusion mismatch (Fig. 7.15).

HPS is not related to type or severity of liver disease or portal hypertension. Patients with HPS have poorer quality of life and twice the mortality rate of cirrhotic patients without HPS [67].

The vasoactive substances that could induce pulmonary vasodilatation in cirrhosis are unknown. Candidates include NO, endothelin-1 and tumour necrosis factor α.

Diagnosis demands demonstration of pulmonary vasodilatation and an increased alveolar–arterial oxygen gradient on breathing room air. Contrast-enhanced echocardiography can demonstrate abnormal passage of microbubbles through the pulmonary circulation into the left side of the lung. Technetium 99m (^{99m}Tc) macro-aggregated albumin lung scanning is less sensitive.

Pulmonary angiography may show large pulmonary arteriovenous shunts and transoesophageal contrast echocardiography may be useful to exclude intracardiac shunts.

No pharmacological therapy is effective.

Progressive and severe hypoxaemia are an indication for liver transplant and this is currently the only effective treatment. Hypoxemia may take weeks or months to resolve following transplantation. Reversal is not always the case when pulmonary arteriovenous shunts are large and these may require coil embolotherapy, which should precede transplant.

Transjugular intrahepatic portosystemic shunt (TIPS) has improved arterial oxygen saturation in some patients but the results are unpredictable.

Portopulmonary hypertension

Portopulmonary hypertension is defined as portal hypertension and a mean pulmonary artery pressure above 25 mmHg and pulmonary vascular resistance above 240 dynes/s/cm^5, in the absence of other diseases associated with pulmonary hypertension [68]. It can occur with hepatic or prehepatic portal hypertension. Approximately 5% of transplant candidates have portopulmonary hypertension. Patients may be asymptomatic or complain of non-specific chest discomfort or dyspnoea on exertion. Physical examination may reveal a right ventricular heave or a loud second heart sound. Histometric study of the muscular pulmonary arteries shows dilatation and thickening of the wall and, rarely, thrombi. Plexogenic pulmonary arteriopathy, involving arteries 10–200 mm in diameter and once thought to be diagnostic of primary pulmonary hypertension, has been found at autopsy.

Significant pulmonary hypertension (mean pulmonary artery pressure >35 mmHg) is a relative contraindication to liver transplant, which can result in perioperative deaths from acute right ventricular failure. All liver transplant candidates should be screened using echocardiography. If right ventricular systolic pressure is above 50 mmHg, right heart catherization should be performed to confirm the diagnosis [68].

Portopulmonary hypertension can now be treated with prolonged oral sildenafil [69]. Many patients may respond with a reduction in pulmonary vascular resistance and pulmonary artery pressure and may proceed to liver transplantation. Bosentan is an alternative treatment but is not recommended for patients with moderate to severe hepatic impairment.

Cirrhotic cardiomyopathy

Cirrhotic patients, with the exception of NASH cirrhosis, are less liable to coronary and aortic atheroma than

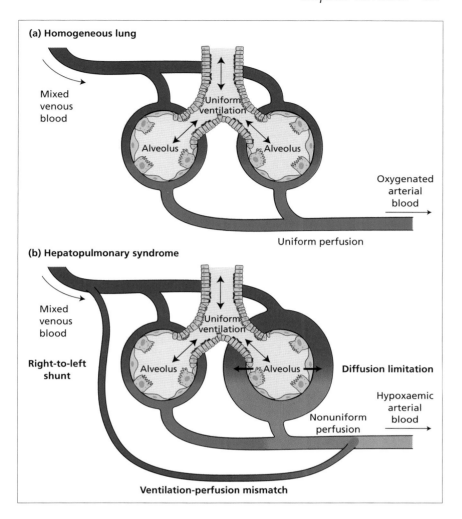

Fig. 7.15. Mechanisms of arterial hypoxemia in the hepatopulmonary syndrome in a two-compartment model of gas exchange in the lung. In a homogeneous lung with uniform alveolar ventilation and pulmonary blood flow in a healthy person (a), the diameter of the capillary ranges between 8 and 15 μm, oxygen diffuses properly into the vessel, and ventilation-perfusion is well balanced. In patients with the hepatopulmonary syndrome (b), many capillaries are dilated, and blood flow is not uniform. Ventilation–perfusion mismatch emerges as the predominant mechanism, irrespective of the degree of clinical severity, either with or without intrapulmonary shunt, and coexists with restricted oxygen diffusion into the centre of the dilated capillaries in the most advanced stages (bold arrows). From Rodriguez-Roisin R, Krowka MJ [66]. Copyright (2008) Massachussets Medical Society. All rights reserved.

the rest of the population. At autopsy, the incidence of coronary artery disease is about a quarter of that among total cases examined without cirrhosis. Cardiac abnormalities in cirrhosis are frequently attributed to the toxic effect of alcohol on the heart. However, it is increasingly recognized that cirrhosis *per se* can cause cardiac dysfunction.

A suggested definition of cirrhotic cardiomyopathy is the presence of one or more of the following:
1 baseline increased cardiac output but blunted ventricular response to stimuli;
2 systolic and/or diastolic dysfunction;
3 absence of overt left ventricular failure at rest;
4 electrophysiological abnormalities including prolonged Q–T interval on electrocardiography and chronotropic incompetence [70].

Major stresses such as TIPS, liver transplantation or sepsis may precipitate overt cardiac failure. The inability to increase cardiac output under stress may contribute to the development of hepatorenal syndrome [71]. Suggested pathogenic mechanisms include defects in the cardiomyocyte β-adrenergic signalling pathway, changes in the lipid composition causing decreased fluidity of the cardiomyocyte plasma membrane and the negative effects of substances such as nitric oxide, carbon monoxide and endocannabinoids on heart muscle.

There are few studies on the treatment of cirrhotic cardiomyopathy. Diuretics and beta-blockers may be helpful. Vasodilators and digitalis should probably be avoided. Cardiac function frequently improves following successful liver transplantation. Treatment with long-term aldosterone antagonists may be beneficial [72].

Management

General

Once the liver is disorganized, as in cirrhosis, it will never regain normal structure. Much can be achieved by symptomatic measures. The liver cells retain such an enormous regenerative capacity that, even though liver structure may not return to normal, functional compensation may be achieved.

The management of the *compensated* cirrhotic is directed towards maintenance of an adequate balanced diet, avoidance of alcohol and obesity, early detection of hepatocellular carcinoma, fluid retention and encephalopathy, maintenance of renal function and prevention of variceal haemorrhage. Treatment in the decompensated cirrhotic is directed towards the specific form of decompensation, for example hepatic encephalopathy, ascites, variceal bleeding. In many cases, the episode of decompensation is precipitated by an event such as sepsis, hypotension or injudicious administration of a medication. Identification and treatment of these precipitating causes may help to return the patient to a compensated state.

Specific

If the cause of cirrhosis is known then specific treatment should be given. Antiviral treatment is useful for hepatitis B and C. Steroids and immunosuppressive drugs may be used in autoimmune hepatitis. Ursodeoxycholic acid should be given early in the course of primary biliary cirrhosis and continued long term. Wilson's disease is treated with chelation therapy and haemochromatosis with venesection. In alcoholic cirrhosis, abstinence is essential. Weight loss may be beneficial in NASH cirrhosis.

Precipitating factors

In many patients with decompensated cirrhosis specific therapies may not be available or may take some time to show clinical effect. In this situation treatment is directed at the presenting complaints, usually bleeding varices, ascites, encephalopathy or sepsis. Precipitating factors may be important and amenable to treatment. A precipitating factor is something that depresses hepatocellular function and throws the patient with hitherto compensated liver disease into failure. Gastrointestinal haemorrhage or the fall in blood pressure following surgical operation may necessitate blood transfusion. An acute infection must be treated. If failure has followed an alcoholic episode, the patient is denied alcohol. Electrolyte disturbances, whether diuretic-induced or due to some other factor such as vomiting or diarrhoea, must be corrected.

Nutrition

Abnormal fuel metabolism and malnutrition is common in cirrhotic patients. They become catabolic after short periods of fasting. A diet containing 35–40 kcal and 1.2–1.5 g of protein/kg body weight per day is recommended [73]. Oral or enteral feeding is preferable to parenteral nutrition. Avoidance of fatty foods is not of any therapeutic value. Protein restriction is not recommended for hepatic encephalopathy and if used should be very short term. Late evening or nocturnal feeding appears beneficial. In a randomized controlled trial an oral nutritional supplement given at night (710 kcal between 21.00 and 07.00) was superior to the same supplement given during the day. Over a year the nocturnal feeding group gained the equivalent of 2 kg lean body mass [74]. Ascitic patients may require salt restriction but caloric and protein intake should be maintained.

Surgical procedures [75]

All operations in cirrhotic patients carry a high risk and a high mortality. Abdominal surgery in non-bleeding cirrhotic patients has an operative mortality of 30% and an additional morbidity rate of 30%. These are related to Child's grade—mortality being 10% in grade A, 31% in grade B and 76% in grade C patients. Operations on the biliary tract, for peptic ulcer disease or for colon resection, have a particularly bad prognosis. Predictive features of a poor outcome include a low serum albumin, the presence of infection and a prolonged prothrombin time. The surgical risk in patients with chronic liver disease emphasizes the need for a careful preoperative evaluation.

Upper abdominal surgery increases the difficulty, and should be avoided in potential candidates for liver transplantation.

References

1 Poynard T, Bedossa T, Opolon P. natural history of liver fibrosis progression in patients with chronic hepatitis C. The OBSVIRC, METAVIR, CLINIVIR and DOSVIRC groups. *Lancet* 1987; **349**: 825–832.

2 Rockey DC, Caldwell SH, Goodman ZD *et al*. Liver Biopsy: AASLD position paper. *Hepatology* 2009; **49**: 1017–1044.

3 Scheuer PJ, Lefkowitch JH. *Liver Biopsy Interpretation*, 7th edn. Elsevier Saunders, 2006, p. 171.

4 Castera L, Le Bail B, Roudot-Thoraval F *et al*. Early detection in routine clinical practice of cirrhosis and oesophageal varices in chronic hepatitis C: Comparison of transient elastography (FibroScan) with standard laboratory tests and non-invasive scores. *J. Hepatol.* 2009; **50**: 59–68.

5 Hammel P CA, O'Toole D, Ratouis A *et al*. Regression of liver fibrosis after biliary drainage in patients with chronic pancreatitis and stenosis of the common bile duct. *N. Eng. J. Med.* 2001; **344**: 418–423.

6 Dixon JB, Bhathal PS, Hughes NR *et al*. Nonalcoholic fatty liver disease: improvement in liver histological analysis with weight loss. *Hepatology* 2004; **39**: 1647–1654.

7 George SL, Bacon BR, Kusal L *et al*. Clinical, virologic, histologic, and biochemical outcomes after successful HCV therapy: a 5-year follow-up of 150 patients. *Hepatology* 2009; **49**: 729–738.

8 McCormick PA, Nolan N. Palpable epigastric liver as a sign of cirrhosis. A prospective study. *Eur. J. Gastro. Hepatol.* 2004; **16**: 1331–1334.

9 Gines P, Quintero E, Arroyo V *et al.* Compensated cirrhosis: natural history and prognostic factors. *Hepatology* 1987; **7**: 122–128.

10 Murray JF, Dawson AM, Sherlock S. Circulatory changes in chronic liver disease. *Am. J. Med.* 1958; **24**: 358–367.

11 Lunzer MR, Manghani KK, Newman SP *et al.* Impaired cardiovascular responsiveness in liver disease. *Lancet* 1975; **ii**: 382–385.

12 Lunzer M, Newman SP, Sherlock S. Skeletal muscle blood flow and neurovascular reactivity in liver disease. *Gut* 1973; **14**: 354–359.

13 Fleckenstein JF, Frank SM, Thuluvath PJ. Presence of autonomic neuropathy is a poor prognostic indicator in patients with advanced liver disease. *Hepatology* 1996; **23**: 471–475.

14 Lin R-S, Lee F-Y, Lee S-D *et al.* Endotoxemia in patients with chronic liver disease: relationship to severity of liver diseases, presence of esophageal varices, and hyperdynamic circulation. *J. Hepatol.* 1995; **22**: 165–172.

15 Lopez-Talavera JC, Merrill WW, Groszmann RJ. Tumor necrosis factor alpha: a major contributor to the hyperdynamic circulation in prehepatic portal-hypertensive rats. *Gastroenterology* 1995; **108**: 761–767.

16 Niederberger M, Martin PY, Gines P *et al.* Normalization of nitric oxide production corrects arterial vasodilation and hyperdynamic circulation in cirrhotic rats. *Gastroenterology* 1995; **109**: 1624–1630.

17 Clemens MG. Nitric oxide in liver injury. *Hepatology* 1999; **30**: 1–5.

18 Lee F-Y, Colombato LA, Albillos A *et al.* N-omega-nitro-L-arginine administration corrects peripheral vasodilation and systemic capillary hypotension and ameliorates plasma volume expansion and sodium retention in portal hypertensive rats. *Hepatology* 1993; **17**: 84–90.

19 Niederberger M, Gines P, Tsai P *et al.* Increased aortic cyclic guanosine monophosphate concentration in experimental cirrhosis in rats: evidence for a role of nitric oxide in the pathogenesis of arterial vasodilation in cirrhosis. *Hepatology* 1995; **21**: 1625–1631.

20 Wernze H, Tittor W, Goerig M. Release of prostanoids into the portal and hepatic vein in patients with chronic liver disease. *Hepatology* 1986; **6**: 911–916.

21 Henderson JM. Abnormal splanchnic and systemic haemodynamics of end-stage liver disease: what happens after liver transplantation? *Hepatology* 1993; **17**: 514–516.

22 Infante-Rivard C, Esnaola S, Villeneuve J-P *et al.* Clinical and statistical validity of conventional prognostic factors in predicting short-term survival among cirrhotics. *Hepatology* 1987; **7**: 660–664.

23 Olthoff KM, Brown RS, Delmonico FL *et al.* Summary report of a national conference: evolving concepts in liver allocation in the MELD and PELD era. *Liver Transpl.* 2004; **10**: A6–A22.

24 Kim WR, Biggins SW, Kremers WK *et al.* Hyponatremia and mortality among patients on the liver transplant waiting list. *N. Engl. J. Med.* 2008; **359**: 1018–1026.

25 Carithers RL, Herlong HF, Diehl AM *et al.* Methylprednisolone therapy in patients with severe alcoholic hepatitis. A randomized multicenter trial. *Ann. Intern. Med.* 1989; **110**: 685–690.

26 Bustamante J, Rimola A, Ventura P-J *et al.* Prognostic significance of hepatic encephalopathy in patients with cirrhosis. *J. Hepatol.* 1999; **30**: 890–895.

27 Armonis A, Patch D, Burroughs A. Hepatic venous pressure measurement: an old test as a new prognostic marker in cirrhosis? *Hepatology* 1997; **25**: 245–248.

28 Siringo S, Burroughs AK, Bolondi L *et al.* Peptic ulcer and its course in cirrhosis: an endoscopic and clinical prospective study. *J. Hepatol.* 1995; **22**: 633–641.

29 Siringo S, Vaira D, Menegatti M *et al.* High prevalence of *Helicobacter pylori* in liver cirrhosis. Relationship with clinical and endoscopic features and the risk of peptic ulcer. *Dig. Dis. Sci.* 1997; **42**: 2024–2030.

30 Morencos FC, De Las Heras Castano G, Ramos LM *et al.* Small bowel bacterial overgrowth in patients with alcoholic cirrhosis. *Dig. Dis. Sci.* 1995; **41**: 1252–1256.

31 Bauer TM, Schwacha H, Steinbrückner B *et al.* Diagnosis of small intestinal bacterial overgrowth in patients with cirrhosis of the liver: poor performance of the glucose breath hydrogen test. *J. Hepatol.* 2000; **33**: 382–386.

32 Sheen I-S, Liaw Y-F. The prevalence and incidence of cholecystolithiasis in patients with chronic liver diseases: a prospective study. *Hepatology* 1989; **9**: 538–540.

33 Newell GC. Cirrhotic glomerulonephritis: incidence, morphology, clinical features, and pathogenesis. *Am. J. Kidney Dis.* 1987; **9**: 183–190.

34 Noble-Jamieson G, Thiru S, Johnston P *et al.* Glomerulonephritis with end-stage liver disease in childhood. *Lancet* 1992; **339**: 706–707.

35 Jefferson JA, Johnson RJ. Treatment of hepatitis C-associated glomerular disease. *Semin. Nephrol.* 2000; **20**: 286–292.

36 Van den Velde S, Nevens F, Van Hee P *et al.* GC-MS analysis of breath odor compounds in liver patients. *J. Chromatogr. B Analyt. Technol. Biomed. Life Sci.* 2008; **875**: 344–348.

37 Bean WB. *Vascular Spiders and Related Lesions of the Skin*. Oxford: Blackwell Scientific Publications, 1959.

38 Martinez GP, Barbera JA, Visa J *et al.* Hepatopulmonary syndrome in candidates for liver transplantation. *J. Hepatol.* 2001; **34**: 756–758.

39 Martini GA. Über Gefässveränderungen der Haut bei Leberkranken. *Z. Klin. Med.* 1955; **150**: 470–526.

40 Finn SM, Rowland M, Lawlor F *et al.* The significance of cutaneous spider naevi in children. *Arch. Dis. Child.* 2006; **91**: 604–605.

41 Pirovino M, Linder R, Boss C *et al.* Cutaneous spider nevi in liver cirrhosis: capillary microscopical and hormonal investigations. *Klin. Wochenschr.* 1988; **66**: 298–302.

42 Dickinson CJ. The aetiology of clubbing and hypertrophic osteoarthropathy. *Eur. J. Clin. Invest.* 1993; **23**: 330–338.

43 Morgan MY, Madden AM, Soulsby CT *et al.* Derivation and validation of a new global method for assessing nutritional status in patients with cirrhosis. *Hepatology* 2006; **44**: 823–835.

44 Andersen H, Borre M, Jakobsen J *et al.* Decreased muscle strength in patients with alcoholic liver cirrhosis in relation to nutritional status, alcohol abstinence, liver function, and neuropathy. *Hepatology* 1998; **27**: 1200–1206.

45 Zein NN, Abdulkarim AS, Wiesner RH *et al.* Prevalence of diabetes mellitus in patients with end-stage liver cirrhosis due to hepatitis C, alcohol, or cholestatic disease. *J. Hepatol.* 2000; **32**: 209–217.

46 Bennett HS, Baggenstoss AH, Butt HR. The testis, breast and prostate of men who die of cirrhosis of the liver. *Am. J. Clin. Pathol.* 1950; **20**: 814–828.

47 Bach N, Schaffner F, Kapelman B. Sexual behaviour in women with nonalcoholic liver disease. *Hepatology* 1989; **9**: 698–703.

48 Francavilla A, Di Leo A, Eagon PK *et al.* Effect of spironol-actone and potassium canrenoate on cytosolic and nuclear androgen and oestrogen receptors of rat liver. *Gastroenterology* 1987; **93**: 681–686.

49 Eagon PK, Elm MS, Stafford EA *et al.* Androgen receptor in human liver: characterization and quantification in normal and diseased liver. *Hepatology* 1994; **19**: 92–100.

50 Van Thiel DH, Stauber RE, Gavaler JS *et al.* Evidence for modulation of hepatic mass by oestrogens and hepatic 'feminization'. *Hepatology* 1990; **12**: 547–552.

51 Kew MC, Kirschner MA, Abrahams GE *et al.* Mechanism of feminization in primary liver cancer. *N. Engl. J. Med.* 1977; **296**: 1084–1088.

52 Bannister P, Handley T, Chapman C *et al.* Hypogonadism in chronic liver disease: impaired release of luteinizing hormone. *Br. Med. J.* 1986; **293**: 1191–1193.

53 Cundy TF, Butler J, Pope RM *et al.* Amenorrhoea in women with nonalcoholic chronic liver disease. *Gut* 1991; **32**: 202–206.

54 Summerskill WHJ, Molnar GD. Eye signs in hepatic cirrhosis. *N. Engl. J. Med.* 1962; **266**: 1244–1248.

55 Angeli P, Albino G, Carraro P *et al.* Cirrhosis and muscle cramps: evidence of a causal relationship. *Hepatology* 1996; **23**: 264–273.

56 Huet P-M, Villeneuve J-P, Fenyves D. Drug elimination in chronic liver diseases. *J. Hepatol.* 1997; **26** (Suppl. 2): 63–72.

57 Meyer B, Luo H, Bargetzi M *et al.* Quantification of intrinsic drug-metabolizing capacity in human liver biopsy specimens: support for the intact-hepatocyte theory. *Hepatology* 1991; **13**: 475–481.

58 Caroli J, Platteborse R. Septicémie porto-cave. Cirrhosis du foie et septicémie à colibacille. *Sem. Hôp. Paris* 1958; **34**: 472–487.

59 Navasa M, Rimola A, Rods J. Bacterial infections in liver disease. *Semin. Liver Dis.* 1997; **17**: 323–333.

60 Bernard B, Grange JD, Khac EN *et al.* Antibiotic prophylaxis for the prevention of bacterial infections in cirrhotic patients with gastrointestinal bleeding: a meta-analysis. *Hepatology* 1999; **29**: 1655–1661.

61 Rajkovic IA, Williams R. Abnormalities of neutrophil phagocytosis, intracellular killing, and metabolic activity in alcoholic cirrhosis and hepatitis. *Hepatology* 1986; **6**: 252–262.

62 Rimola A, Soto R, Bory F *et al.* Reticuloendothelial system phagocytic activity in cirrhosis and its relation to bacterial infections and prognosis. *Hepatology* 1984; **4**: 53–58.

63 Fernandez J, Navasa M, Gomez J *et al.* Bacterial infections in cirrhosis: epidemiological changes with invasive procedures and norfloxacin prophylaxis. *Hepatology* 2002; **35**: 140–148.

64 Thalheimer U, Triantos CK, Samonakis DN *et al.* Infection, coagulation and variceal bleeding in cirrhosis. *Gut* 2005; **54**: 556–563.

65 Fernandez J, Escorsell A, Zabalza M *et al.* Adrenal insufficiency in patients with cirrhosis and septic shock: effect of treatment with hydrocortisone on survival. *Hepatology* 2006; **44**: 1288–1295.

66 Rodriguez-Roisin R, Krowka MJ. Hepatopulmonary syndrome—a liver-induced lung vascular disorder. *New Engl. J. Med.* 2008; **358**: 2378–2387.

67 Lallon MB, Krowka MJ, Brown RS *et al.* Impact of hepatopulmonary syndrome on quality of life and survival in liver transplant candidates. *Gastroenterology* 2008; **135**: 1168–1175.

68 Krowka MJ, Swanson KJ, Frantz RP *et al.* Portopulmonary hypertension: results from a 10-year screening algorithm. *Hepatology* 2006; **44**: 1502–1510.

69 Gough MS, White RJ. Sildenafil therapy is associated with improved hemodynamics in liver transplantation candidates with pulmonary arterial hypertension. *Liver Transpl.* 2009; **15**: 30–36.

70 Alqahtani SA, Fouad TR, Lee SS. Cirrhotic cardiomyopathy. *Semin. Liver Dis.* 2008; **28**: 59–69.

71 Ruiz-del-Arbor L, Urman J, Fernandez J *et al.* Systemic, renal and hepatic hemodynamic derangement in cirrhotic patients with spontaneous bacterial peritonitis. *Hepatology* 2003; **38**: 1210–1218.

72 Pozzi M, Grassi G, Ratti L *et al.* Cardiac, neuroadrenergic, and portal hemodynamic effects of prolonged aldosterone blockade in postviral child A cirrhosis. *Am. J. Gastroenterol.* 2005; **100**: 1110–1116.

73 Plauth M, Cabre E, Riggio O *et al.* ESPEN guidelines on enteral nutrition: liver disease. *Clin. Nutr.* 2006; **25**: 285–294.

74 Plank LD, Gane EJ, Peng S *et al.* Nocturnal nutritional supplementation improves total body protein status of patients with liver cirrhosis: a randomized 12-month trial. *Hepatology* 2008; **48**: 557–566.

75 Friedman LS. The risk of surgery in patients with liver disease. *Hepatology* 1999; **29**: 1617–1623.

CHAPTER 8
Hepatic Encephalopathy in Patients with Cirrhosis

Marsha Y. Morgan

Centre for Hepatology, Royal Free Campus, University College London Medical School, London, UK

Learning points

- Hepatic encephalopathy is the commonest complication of cirrhosis; it has a detrimental effect on health-related quality of life and on survival.

- Ammonia plays a key role in the pathogenesis of the syndrome via the induction of astrocyte swelling and the development of low-grade cerebral oedema; oxidative stress, disrupted glial–neuronal communication and neuronal dysfunction follow.

- There is no diagnostic gold standard; a combination of clinical examination, psychometric testing and electroencephalography is recommended. Nevertheless, the condition is often undiagnosed and so untreated.

- Therapy is directed at reducing circulating ammonia by use of non-absorbable disaccharides and non-absorbable antibiotics. It is generally effective.

- Newer diagnostic approaches have been proposed but need validation; newer treatment approaches, based on recent insights into the pathogenesis of the syndrome, need careful appraisal.

Hepatic encephalopathy is the term used to describe the complex and variable changes in neuropsychiatric status that complicate liver disease. This syndrome is the defining feature of fulminant hepatic failure and, in this setting, it is only one of a multitude of metabolic abnormalities caused by loss of functioning hepatocyte mass (see Chapter 5).

In patients with cirrhosis, a spectrum of neuropsychiatric abnormalities exists, ranging from clinically *indiscernible* changes in cognition to clinically *obvious* changes in intellect, behaviour, motor function and consciousness. Hepatic encephalopathy has a detrimental effect on health-related quality of life and on survival.

The pathogenesis of this syndrome remains unclear. Both hepatocellular failure and portal–systemic shunting are key elements in its development. Gut-derived toxins, predominantly ammonia, escape hepatic detoxification and impinge on the brain. There ammonia is detoxified by astrocytes. This process results in the development of low-grade cerebral oedema, which ultimately impacts on neuronal function.

The diagnosis remains difficult because the clinical signs, which are often subtle, are easily missed. There are a number of surrogate diagnostic techniques but these are used infrequently, except in specialist centres. This means that the condition is generally under-diagnosed. There is no specific treatment. A variety of approaches, based largely on reducing the production and increasing the elimination of ammonia, have been adopted and are effective. Recent insights into the pathogenesis of the syndrome have produced a number of newer treatment targets.

Classification

Overt hepatic encephalopathy

Clinically apparent or *overt* hepatic encephalopathy manifests as a neuropsychiatric syndrome encompassing a wide spectrum of mental and motor disorders [1,2]. It may arise over a period of hours or days in patients who have previously been stable. This so-called *episodic* overt encephalopathy may occur intermittently or more frequently. Between episodes patients may apparently return to normal although some degree of impairment may remain. Less frequently, patients present with *persistent* neuropsychiatric abnormalities which remain stable over time. These two forms of overt hepatic encephalopathy share a number of features and so a general description of their main characteristics is

Sherlock's Diseases of the Liver and Biliary System, Twelfth Edition. Edited by
James S. Dooley, Anna S.F. Lok, Andrew K. Burroughs, E. Jenny Heathcote.
© 2011 by Blackwell Publishing Ltd. Published 2011 by Blackwell Publishing Ltd.

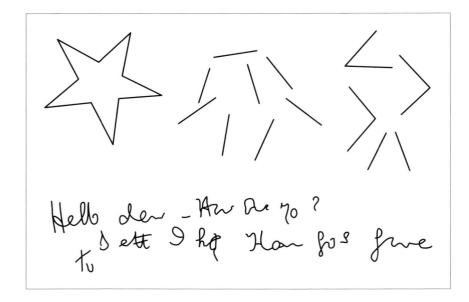

Fig. 8.1. Deficits commonly encountered in patient with cirrhosis with minimal evidence of cognitive dysfunction and in the absence of gross tremor or visual disturbance. *Above:* inability to copy the five-pointed star drawn by the examiner on the left side of the page. This constructional apraxia, or inability to draw or construct simple configurations, is very frequently encountered and is useful for monitoring progress.
Below: writing difficulties are common. The patient is attempting to write: 'Hello dear. How are you? Better I hope. That goes for me too'.

appropriate. It will be followed by a more detailed description of the differential features.

The changes in *mental state* range from subtle alterations in personality, intellectual capacity and cognitive function to more profound alterations in consciousness leading to deep coma with decerebrate posturing.

Personality changes include childishness, irritability and loss of concern for family and friends.

Intellectual deterioration varies from slight impairment of mental function to gross confusion. Isolated abnormalities appearing in a setting of clear consciousness relate to disturbances in visual spatial gnosis. These are most easily elicited as constructional apraxia, shown by an inability to reproduce simple designs with blocks or matches (Fig. 8.1). Writing is indistinct and oblivious of ruled lines (Fig. 8.1). Failure to distinguish objects of similar size, shape, function and position may lead to inappropriate behaviour. Insight into such behavioural anomalies is frequently preserved.

Early signs of *disturbed consciousness* include a reduction of spontaneous movement, a fixed stare, apathy, and slowness and brevity of responses. Day-time sleepiness may be a feature but the disturbances in night-time sleep behaviour, commonly observed in this population, are not, as generally believed, related to the presence of hepatic encephalopathy [3]. Coma at first resembles normal sleep, but further deterioration results in reaction only to intense or noxious stimuli progressing to complete unresponsiveness. Rapid changes in the level of consciousness are accompanied by delirium.

Foetor hepaticus, a sour, musty, faeculent smell, can be detected on the breath of some patients; it is attributed to the presence of mercaptans [4]. Its presence does not correlate with the degree or duration of encephalopathy and its absence does not exclude this condition.

The changes in *motor function* include rigidity, disorders of speech production, resting- and movement-induced tremor, asterixis, delayed diadochokinetic movements, hyper- or hyporeflexia, choreoathetoid movements, Babinsky's sign and transient focal symptoms [1,5–8]. Severe motor abnormalities are easily detected but subtle motor abnormalities, particularly mild extrapyramidal symptoms such as bradykinesia, rigidity and resting tremor, are less easily recognized [8].

Asterixis (flapping tremor) is the best known motor abnormality. It is caused by impaired inflow of joint and other afferent information to the brainstem reticular formation, resulting in arrhythmic lapses in posture. The tremor is absent at rest, less marked on movement and maximum on sustained posture. It is best demonstrated by asking the patient to stretch out their arms and hyperextend the wrists with separated digits and their forearm fixed (Fig. 8.2). The rapid flexion–extension movements at the metacarpophalangeal and wrist joints are often accompanied by lateral movements of the digits. The tremor is usually bilateral, although not bilaterally synchronous with one side affected more than the other. It may also be appreciated by asking the patient to tightly grip the examiner's hand. Similar changes may be observed in the arms, neck, jaw, protruded tongue, and tightly closed eyelids and the gait may be ataxic. A 'flapping' tremor is not specific for hepatic encephalopathy; it can also be observed in renal failure, respiratory failure, severe heart failure, hypomagnesaemia, and diphenylhydantoin intoxication.

Speech is slow and slurred and the voice is monotonous. In deep stupor, dysphasia becomes marked and is always combined with perseveration.

Deep tendon reflexes are usually exaggerated. Increased muscle tone is present at some stage and sustained ankle

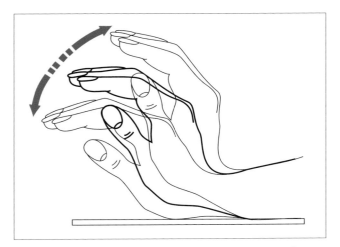

Fig. 8.2. 'Flapping' tremor elicited by attempted dorsiflexion of the wrist with the forearm fixed.

Table 8.1. Precipitants of hepatic encephalopathy in patients with cirrhosis

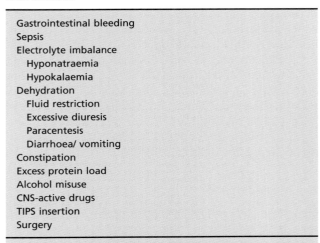

Gastrointestinal bleeding
Sepsis
Electrolyte imbalance
   Hyponatraemia
   Hypokalaemia
Dehydration
   Fluid restriction
   Excessive diuresis
   Paracentesis
   Diarrhoea/ vomiting
Constipation
Excess protein load
Alcohol misuse
CNS-active drugs
TIPS insertion
Surgery

TIPS, transjugular intrahepatic portal–systemic shunt.

clonus is often associated with rigidity. During coma, patients become flaccid and lose their reflexes. The plantar responses are usually flexor becoming extensor in the deepest stages of coma.

Excessive appetite, muscle twitching, grasping and sucking reflexes may also be seen. Visual disturbances, including reversible cortical blindness [9] and alternating gaze deviation [10], have been reported.

These individuals also show a wide spectrum of other abnormalities, including impaired psychomotor performance [11,12], disturbed neurophysiological function [13–17], altered cerebral neurochemical/ neurotransmitter homeostasis [18,19], reductions in global and regional cerebral blood flow and metabolism [20,21], and changes in cerebral fluid homeostasis [22].

The abnormalities observed in psychometric, neurophysiological and neural imaging studies, in patients with overt hepatic encephalopathy, do not necessarily correlate with one another or with the degree of impairment observed clinically, although, in general, the abnormalites increase as the clinical condition worsens.

Episodic hepatic encephalopathy

Episodic hepatic encephalopathy arises in patients who have previously been clinically stable. In approximately 50% of such individuals an obvious precipitant can be identified (Table 8.1). These precipitating factors compromise the patient by: (i) further depressing hepatic or cerebral function; (ii) increasing the nitrogenous load; or (iii) stimulating an inflammatory response. Hepatic function may be depressed by fluid loss and a reduction in hepatic perfusion following gastrointestinal bleeding, diuretic over-usage, large paracenteses and diarrhoea/ vomiting, or during an episode of sepsis. Gastrointestinal

bleeding will also substantially increase the intestinal nitrogen load as will dietary protein excess and constipation. Cerebral function may be compromised by infection and inflammation and following ingestion of alcohol, which is poorly tolerated. Excessive sensitivity to the cerebral effects of a number of psychoactive drugs, especially opiates and benzodiazepines, is often observed [23]. Surgical procedures are tolerated extremely poorly. The creation of surgical or transjugular intrahepatic portal–systemic shunts (TIPS) may precipitate or worsen hepatic encephalopathy by increasing the amount of toxin-laden blood that impinges on the brain.

Patients may return to normal following an episode of overt hepatic encephalopathy; the improvement in their clinical state is usually apparent before improvements in psychometric tests or the electroencephalogram (EEG). However, many will retain some degree of clinical, neuropsychometric or neurophysiological impairment in the longer term [24], particularly those with severely decompensated liver disease or those with large spontaneous or surgically created portal-systemic shunts.

Persistent hepatic encephalopathy

A small number of patients show persistent but stable evidence of hepatic encephalopathy. Many of these have extensive portal–systemic shunting, either multiple anastomotic channels or, more often, one major collateral shunt. In some the shunt may be surgically created or inserted as a TIPS. Some fluctuation in the clinical picture may be observed in relation to various precipitant, which usually manifests as a worsening of the predominant clinical features rather than by changes in conscious level. Parkinsonian features may be prominent with a fine tremor unaffected by intention, pronounced rigidity, staccato speech and a shuffling gait. Cerebellar features are often encountered, manifesting as gait disturbance, truncal ataxia, an intention tremor and dysarthria. Involuntary choreoathetoid movements may be observed. Clinical and biochemical evidence of liver disease may be equivocal or absent, and the neuropsychiatric disorder may dominate the picture. In consequence, the diagnosis is often missed.

Hepatic myelopathy

Hepatic myelopathy develops predominantly in men who have undergone surgical portal–systemic shunting and is far less common, and less well-defined, than hepatic encephalopathy. It presents as a progressive, spastic paraparesis without sensory impairment or sphincter dysfunction [25,26]; the clinical syndrome is accompanied by degenerative changes in the spinal cord.

Minimal hepatic encephalopathy

The term *minimal* hepatic encephalopathy is used to describe patients with cirrhosis who are 'clinically normal' but who show abnormalities of cognition and/or neurophysiological variables [12,27]. Use of this term has the advantage that it allows hepatic encephalopathy to be considered as a single syndrome with *quantitatively* distinct features relating to severity but it also has the disadvantage that it might not adequately convey the fact that its presence is not without consequence. It has a detrimental effect on health-related quality of life [28,29] and the ability to perform complex tasks, such as driving [30,31]; it also increases the risk of developing overt hepatic encephalopathy [16,32–34].

Diagnosis

The diagnosis may be easy—for example in a patient with known cirrhosis and gastrointestinal haemorrhage or sepsis, who, on admission, is confused and has a 'flapping' tremor. However, without the clinical background data, and an obvious precipitating event, hepatic encephalopathy may go unrecognized, and thus untreated.

There is no gold standard for diagnosing hepatic encephalopathy in patients with cirrhosis. There are a number of individual techniques that access different aspects of cerebral function, which can be used, singly or in combination, to provide diagnostic information. These include mental state assessment, psychometric

testing, electroencephalography, sensory and cognitive evoked potentials, and neuroimaging. In practice, any measure that has a proven relationship with the behavioural, prognostic and, possibly, pathophysiological features of this syndrome can be used as a surrogate marker.

Neurological examination including mental state assessment [35]

In patients with cirrhosis, the diagnosis or exclusion of overt, or clinically apparent, hepatic encephalopathy should be based on:

1 a careful and detailed neuropsychiatric history and examination, with particular attention paid to changes in mental state, for example memory, concentration, cognition and consciousness, and to changes in energy and activity levels, and overall health-related quality of life;

2 use of two-grading systems to assess mental status: the West Haven criteria [36] (Table 8.2), based on changes in consciousness, intellectual function and behaviour, and the Glasgow Coma Scale [39] (Table 8.3). Additional instruments such as the Hodkinson Mental State Test [40] or the Mini Mental Score Test [41], which have been widely applied in this patient population, can also be used;

3 a comprehensive neurological examination looking particularly for evidence of subtle motor abnormalities, including: hypomimia, dysarthria, increased tone,

Table 8.2. West Haven Criteria for grading mental state in patients with cirrhosis*

Grade	Features
0	No abnormalities detected
I	Trivial lack of awareness
	Euphoria or anxiety
	Shortened attention span
	Impairment of addition or subtraction
II	Lethargy or apathy
	Disorientation for time
	Obvious personality change
	Inappropriate behaviour
III	Somnolence to semi-stupor
	Responsive to stimuli
	Confused
	Gross disorientation
	Bizarre behaviour
IV	Coma, unable to test mental state

*The descriptions of the mental state alterations in hepatic encephalopathy are those originally proposed by Conn *et al.* [36] as a modification of Parsons-Smith criteria [13]. Alternative formulations have been proposed by Blei and Córdoba [37], Ferenci *et al.* [2] and Amodio *et al.* [38].

Table 8.3. The Glasgow Coma Score [39]

Variable	Score
Eye open	
Spontaneously	4
To command	3
To pain	2
No response	1
Best motor response	
Obeys verbal commands	6
Painful stimulus, localizes pain	5
Painful stimulus, flexion/ withdrawal response	4
Painful stimulus, abnormal flexion	3
Painful stimulus, extension	2
No response	1
Best verbal response	
Orientated and conversant	5
Disorientated and conversant	4
Inappropriate words	3
Incomprehensible sounds	2
No response	1
Total score	3 (Worst) to 15 (Best)

reduced speed or difficulty executing rapid, alternating movements, ataxia, increased deep tendon reflexes, impaired postural reflexes and abnormal movements such as tremors, particularly asterixis; the presence of sensory change and/or focal features would suggest an alternative or additional diagnosis;

4 the exclusion of other potential causes of neuropsychiatric abnormalities, for example concomitant neurological disorders such as subdural haematoma and Wernicke's encephalopathy, other metabolic abnormalities such as those associated with diabetes and renal failure, and intoxication with alcohol or drugs.

It would clearly be sensible to obtain corroborative reports from relatives or friends, particularly in relation to observed rather than subjective changes in behaviour and mental state.

Psychometric performance [35,42]

Impaired psychometric performance defines the presence of minimal hepatic encephalopathy in patients with cirrhosis who appear clinically unimpaired. It also provides an objective measure of severity in those with obvious clinical impairment. Patients with minimal hepatic encephalopathy show deficits in attention, visuospatial abilities, fine motor skills and working memory while other cognitive abilities are relatively preserved. Patients with overt hepatic encephalopathy show additional disturbances in psychomotor speed, executive function and concentration [43,44].

Attempts have been made to develop a simple but comprehensive diagnostic test battery based on the deficits in psychomotor function identified in this patient population. Test batteries are generally more reliable than single tests, and tend to be more strongly correlated with functional status. Promising results have been obtained using five paper and pencil tests, namely Number Connection Tests A and B, and the line tracing, serial dotting and digit symbol tests [12,44] (Fig. 8.3). This battery, which has been called the Psychometric Hepatic Encephalopathy Score (PHES), assesses the required domains of attention, visual perception and visuoconstructive abilities; it is easily applied and has been shown to have a high specificity for the diagnosis of hepatic encephalopathy. However, test scores have to be normalized for a number of confounding variables and at present normative databases are only available for German, Italian, Spanish and British populations.

Computer-based psychometric tests may allow a more precise quantification of reaction times and more refined testing. Instruments such as the Scan test, based on the Sternberg paradigm, tend to explore better-defined cognitive functions and to isolate subtle attention or memory defects [45].

Neurophysiology [35,46]

Electroencephalography (EEG)

The EEG primarily reflects cortical neuronal activity. Hepatic encephalopathy is characterized by a progressive slowing of the normal *alpha* frequency of 8 to13 Hz. Bursts of slow activity are observed in the *theta* (4–8 Hz) range, initially in the temporal areas, and then more diffusely over the scalp; further slowing into the *delta* (1–4 Hz) range may then occur. Triphasic waves or arrhythmic delta activity occur with more severe grades of encephalopathy; coma is characterized by slow, low-voltage delta activity with sequences of electric silence (Fig. 8.4).

The generalized slowing of the background EEG activity and the development of triphasic waves is not specific for hepatic encephalopathy; these changes are also observed in other metabolic encephalopathies (uraemia, hypocapnia and hyponatraemia) and in drug-induced encephalopathies (lithium, valproate and

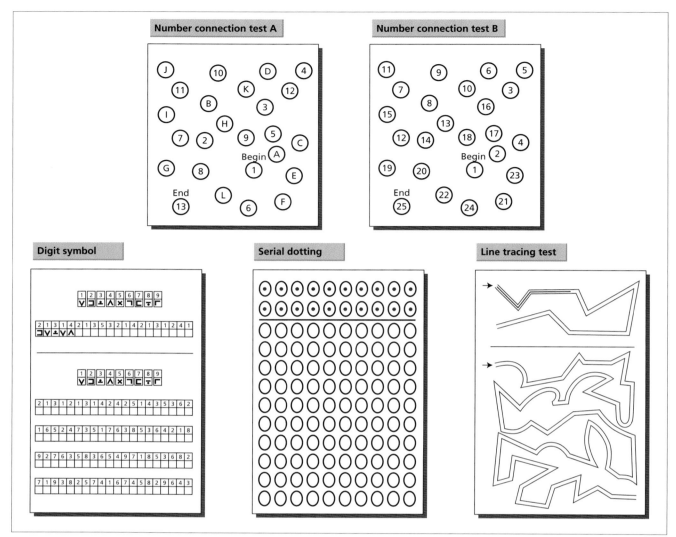

Fig. 8.3. The five paper and pencil tests that make up the Psychometric Hepatic Encephalopathy Score (PHES), which assesses attention, visual perception and visuoconstructive abilities [12,44]. Number Connection Tests A and B: subjects are asked to join the numbers or numbers and letters in sequence as quickly as possible. The time taken to complete the task is recorded. Digit Symbol Test: subjects are asked to insert symbols in the blank squares below the numbers using the key provided. The exercise is timed and the number correctly completed in 90 seconds recorded. Serial Dotting: subjects are asked to place a dot in the centre of each circle and to complete the page as quickly as possible. The time taken to complete the task is recorded. Line Tracing: subjects are asked to trace a line between the two guidelines as quickly and accurately as possible without moving the paper. The time taken to complete the task and the number of errors made are recorded.

baclofen) [47]. However, these conditions are usually easily distinguished on clinical grounds.

The sensitivity of the EEG for the diagnosis of hepatic encephalopathy varies. The best results are probably obtained using spectral analysis-based techniques [48]. Abnormalities of the EEG are reported in 43 to 100% of patients with overt hepatic encephalopathy and in 8 to 40% of clinically unimpaired patients with cirrhosis [35,49].

Recent advances in EEG analysis, such as fully automatic evaluation based on artificial neural networks [50], and techniques for providing spatial as well as temporal information [17], should provide better quantifiable and more informative data.

Evoked potentials

Sensory or exogenous evoked potentials (EPs) are generated by the passive reception of sensory stimuli triggered by visual, auditory or peripheral nerve (somatosensory) stimulation. They provide information on both cortical and brainstem activity. Abnormalities of

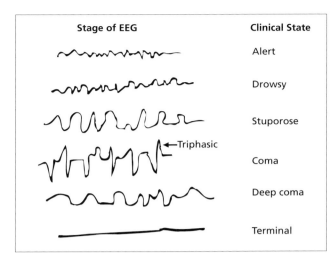

Stage of EEG	Clinical State
	Alert
	Drowsy
	Stuporose
	Coma ←Triphasic
	Deep coma
	Terminal

Fig. 8.4. EEG changes in patients with cirrhosis with increasing deterioration in neuropsychiatric status. There is an initial slowing in frequency with increasing amplitude. The amplitude then decreases. Finally there is an absence of rhythmic activity.

exogenous EPs which reflect cortical function have been described in patients with both minimal and overt hepatic encephalopathy. However, the data available are inconsistent; methodologies and data interpretation need to be standardized before recommendations can be made.

Cognitive or endogenous EPs are triggered by cognitive activity. The best known is P300 which is triggered when the subject receives an infrequent visual or auditory stimulus embedded in a series of otherwise irrelevant, frequent stimuli. The potential occurs about 300 ms after exposure to the rare stimulus, hence its name. Assessment of P300 latency has diagnostic potential for detecting the presence of minimal hepatic encephalopathy and for monitoring the status of patients with mild to moderate hepatic encephalopathy over time [34]. The techniques currently employed are not suitable for use in patients with higher grades of encephalopathy because of the need for patient cooperation.

Critical flicker fusion frequency

Critical flicker fusion frequency (CFF) is a technique that centres on the perception of light as flickering or fused as its frequency changes. In one study a threshold of 39 Hz in the flicker frequency completely separated patients with overt hepatic encephalopathy from their unimpaired counterparts; it separated cirrhotic patients with minimal hepatic encephalopathy from unimpaired individuals with a sensitivity of 55% and a specificity of 100% [51]. The utility of CFF for the diagnosis and monitoring of hepatic encephalopathy has been confirmed by others [52–55]. However, the technique requires patient

cooperation and is not sufficiently sensitive enough to be used as a stand alone technique for the detection of minimal hepatic encephalopathy.

Smooth pursuit eye movements

Smooth pursuit eye movements (SPEM) are the conjugate movements used to track, or pursue, the smooth trajectory of small targets. SPEM recordings show clear disruption of smooth pursuit in patients with minimal hepatic encephalopathy, and more pronounced disruption, if not complete loss of smooth pursuit, in patients with overt hepatic encephalopathy [56] (Fig. 8.5). The abnormalities in pursuit behaviour mirror the changes observed in clinical status and psychometric performance over time and following treatment. The technique requires patient cooperation and can not, therefore, be used across the whole spectrum of neuropsychiatric impairment. It does, however, provide insights into motor function which are not otherwise easy to access.

Functional and structural cerebral imaging [57,58]

The development of computed X-ray tomography (CT), magnetic resonance imaging (MRI), magnetic resonance spectroscopy (MRS), single photon emission tomography (SPET) and positron emission tomography (PET), and their functional imaging counterparts, has enabled rapid and non-invasive assessments of cerebral structure and metabolism to be made.

Cerebral CT and MR imaging [59,60]

Conventional cerebral CT and MR imaging may show evidence of cerebral and sometimes cerebellar atrophy in patients with cirrhosis. These changes are related to the severity of the liver dysfunction and do not relate to changes in cerebral function. They are most prominent in patients with a history of alcohol abuse. Hyperintensity in the basal ganglia on MRI T_1-weighted images may also be observed but does not correlate with either the presence or severity of hepatic encephalopathy (Fig. 8.6). These changes probably reflect pallidal deposition of manganese. Total body manganese is increased in patients with cirrhosis most likely reflecting the combined effects of hepatocellular failure, impaired biliary excretion and the presence of portal–systemic shunting of blood [61–65]. It is not clear whether the manganese deposits in the globus pallidus reflect intoxication or the presence of an adaptive process designed to improve the efficacy of ammonia detoxification by astrocytes. However, manganese accumulation may be responsible, at least in part, for up-regulation in the cerebral peripheral benzodiazepine receptors which play a role in the

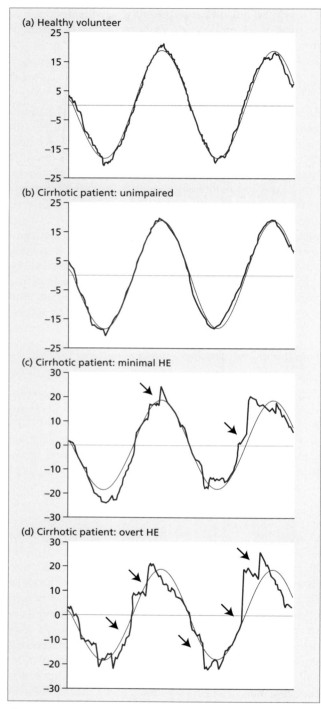

Fig. 8.5. Smooth pursuit movements in a healthy volunteer and in three individual patients with cirrhosis, by degree of neuropsychiatric impairment. The dot position is denoted in light gray, and the eye position in red. In the healthy volunteer (a) and in the unimpaired cirrhotic patient (b), pursuit is smooth. In the patient with minimal hepatic encephalopathy (c), pursuit is smooth but interspersed with corrective catch-up saccades (arrowed). In the patient with overt hepatic encephalopathy (d), pursuit is no longer smooth but accomplished by a series of corrective catch-up saccades (arrowed) producing a jerky or cogwheel pattern. HE: hepatic encephalopathy (Adapted from [56], with permission).

pathogenesis of hepatic encephalopathy (see below) [66,67].

Cerebral imaging, using these modalities, does not provide information of diagnostic importance in patients with cirrhosis and hepatic encephalopathy except to exclude other causes of cerebral dysfunction. However, newer MRI techniques may prove more informative. Magnetization transfer and diffusion-weighted imaging allow indirect assessment of changes in cerebral water content and distribution. Volumetric MRI provides precise measurements of whole or regional brain volumes and allows small difference in brain size to be monitored (co-registered MRI). Functional MRI provides measurements of the haemodynamic responses related to neural activity in the brain.

Cerebral MRS [68]

In vivo MRS can provide localized biochemical information on cerebral metabolic processes. Characteristic alterations have been observed in cerebral ^{1}H MRS in patients with cirrhosis, which correlate with the degree of neuropsychiatric impairment. These alterations, which are typified by relative reductions in the myo-inositol and choline resonances and a relative increase in the composite glutamine/ glutamate resonance, are thought to reflect changes in astrocyte volume homeostasis (Fig. 8.7). Possible advances in the field, including two-dimensional spectroscopy, spectral editing and the use of higher magnetic field strengths, may help resolve some of the current technical difficulties.

Radiotracer imaging [58]

Radiotracer imaging with SPECT and PET allows access to metabolic processes, neuronal activity and neurotransmitter systems. However, these are expensive and generally inaccessible techniques. They provide considerable insights into the pathophysiology of hepatic encephalopathy but currently have no place in the management of patients.

Blood ammonia

Measurement of blood ammonia may be of value in the differential diagnosis of hepatic encephalopathy. It can be particularly useful when a patient not known to have cirrhosis presents with fluctuating neurological symptoms and signs of seemingly unknown origin. The signs of chronic liver disease are likely to be minimal and the liver function tests are unlikely to be severely disturbed. In this instance measurement of blood ammonia may provide a vital clue. The pH-dependent partial pressure of gaseous ammonia in arterial blood correlates more closely with the clinical and neurophysiological changes observed than plasma ammonia concentrations [69].

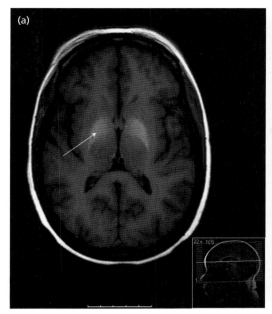

Fig. 8.6. T_1- and T_2-weighted MR images of the brain of a 53-year-old individual with cirrhosis and overt hepatic encephalopathy. (a) The T_1-weighted MR image shows bilateral, symmetrical hyperintensity of the globus pallidus (arrowed). (b) No corresponding changes are observed in the T_2-weighted MR image.

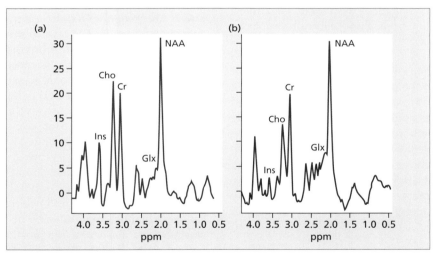

Fig. 8.7. ^{1}H-MR-spectroscopy water-suppressed spectra in a healthy individual (a) and in a patient with cirrhosis and hepatic encephalopathy (b) recorded with a stimulated echo acquisition mode pulse sequence (TR/TE, 1600/20 ms; acquisitions, 256). The main resonances correspond to *N*-acetylaspartate (NAA: 2.0 ppm), glutamine/ glutamate (Glx, 2.1–2.5 ppm), creatine/ phosphocreatine (Cr: 3.02 ppm), choline-containing compounds (Cho: 3.2 ppm) and myoinositol (Ins: 3.55 ppm). The presence of hepatic encephalopathy is characterized by a relative increase in the glutamate/ glutamine resonance and relative reductions in the myoinositol and choline resonances.

Cerebrospinal fluid

The cerebrospinal fluid (CSF) is usually clear and under normal pressure. Patients with severe Grade III/IV encephalopathy may have increased CSF protein concentrations, but the cell counts are normal. CSF glutamine concentrations may be increased and correlate significantly with both the presence and the degree of hepatic encephalopathy [70].

Neuropathological changes [71,72]

Examination of brain tissue is rarely, if ever, undertaken during life. Microscopically the most striking feature is proliferation of the astrocytes with development of enlarged nuclei, prominent nucleoli, margination of chromatin and accumulation of glycogen—changes referred to as Alzheimer type II astrocytosis. These changes are found particularly in the cerebral cortex, basal ganglia and cerebellum. Microglial changes may also be observed; neurones show only minor, if any, alterations.

More significant changes are seen in patients with persistent hepatic encephalopathy including: patchy cortical laminar or pseudolaminar necrosis with poly-microcavitation at the corticomedullary junctions and in the striatum and uneven degeneration of neurones and medullated fibres in the cerebral cortex, cerebellum and lenticular nuclei.

Demyelination in the pyramidal tracts is observed in patients with hepatic myelopathy.

Choice of diagnostic variables [58]

There are a number of techniques which provide information useful for the diagnosis and monitoring of hepatic encephalopathy in patients with cirrhosis. Ideally, the methods used should: (1) access variables germane to the pathophysiology of the syndrome; (2) have predictive validity; and (3) not expose the patient to unnecessary risk or harm. In practice, the selection of diagnostic tools will be determined by factors such as simplicity of use, accessibility and cost.

Current guidelines suggest: (1) a detailed clinical assessment to identify or exclude clinically apparent change; (2) an assessment of psychometric performance using the PHES battery or a validated computer-based system; (3) an electrophysiological assessment, for example an EEG or somatosensory/ cognitive EPs, if accessible; and (4) an assessment of health-related quality of life [2]. It is unlikely that these guidelines are followed, except perhaps in centres with on-going research interests. Most patients are probably suboptimally assessed by clinical examination alone or, at best, with the addition of a few simple psychometric tests. This is not a satisfactory situation but one which may improve if simpler tools, such as CFF, can be further validated.

Differential diagnosis

Neuropsychiatric abnormalities may arise in patients with cirrhosis that do not relate to the presence of hepatic encephalopathy. The clinician should be alert to the possibility of intracranial haemorrhage, cerebral trauma, infection or tumour, as well as possible drug-induced or other metabolic encephalopathies. Particular difficulties arise when faced with the occurrence of one or more confounding or competing events. The diagnosis is even more difficult to make if the patient is not known to have cirrhosis; then the origin of the neuropsychiatric abnormalities can not be appreciated and may prove elusive to the detriment of the patient.

Hyponatraemia, defined as a serum sodium of less than 136 mmol/L, can result in cerebral over-hydration and a metabolic encephalopathy [73]. Nausea and malaise are the earliest findings. Headache, lethargy and eventually seizures, coma and respiratory arrest will follow if the plasma sodium concentration continues to fall. Hyponatraemia is frequent among cirrhotic patients primarily as a result of fluid retention, although dietary sodium restriction, diuretic over-usage and paracentesis may play a role. Patients with cirrhosis may, therefore, manifest features of both hyponatraemic and hepatic encephalopathy [73]. Moreover, hyponatraemia may precipitate or worsen existing hepatic encephalopathy [74]. Hyponatraemia is a risk factor for the subsequent development of overt hepatic encephalopathy in patients undergoing TIPS [75].

The features of *alcohol withdrawal* may confound the clinical picture. Delirium tremens is distinguished by continuous motor and autonomic over-activity, profound insomnia, terrifying hallucinations and a finer, more rapid tremor. The patient is flushed, agitated, inattentive and perfunctory in their replies. Tremor, absent at rest, becomes coarse and irregular on activity. Treatment of alcohol withdrawal in a patient with cirrhosis is difficult and patients must be closely monitored. The sedation required may precipitate hepatic encephalopathy so it is best to start prophylactic anti-encephalopathy treatment from the outset.

Wernicke's encephalopathy is caused by thiamine deficiency and is most commonly seen in patient with a long history of alcohol misuse and a degree of malnutrition. It presents as an acute neuropsychiatric condition characterized by global confusion, eye signs and ataxia. The confusional state is accompanied by apathy, disorientation and disturbed memory, but drowsiness and stupor are uncommon. The ocular abnormalities include nystagmus, gaze palsies and ophthalmoplegia, while the ataxia affects the trunk and lower extremities. The clinical abnormalities may develop acutely or evolve over several days. Particular diagnostic difficulties arise in patient with alcoholic cirrhosis who are actively withdrawing from alcohol and who may in addition develop hepatic encephalopathy. Prophylactic parenteral thiamine should be given over several days to patients in this situation.

Wilson's disease, a condition of disordered copper metabolism, can cause both cirrhosis and neuropsychiatric abnormalities. Patients tend to present in early life but some may present later. Initially, they may exhibit mild cognitive deterioration and clumsiness, as well as changes in behaviour. Specific neurological symptoms then follow, including parkinsonism with or without a typical hand tremor, masked facial expressions, slurred speech, ataxia or dystonia. These neurological features may be accompanied by depression, anxiety and psychosis. However, the symptoms do not fluctuate; Kayser–Fleischer rings and disturbances in copper metabolism can usually be demonstrated and serve to differentiate.

Latent *functional psychoses*, such as bipolar disorder, may be precipitated by the onset of hepatic encephalopathy. Conversely, major psychoses may develop in patients with chronic liver disease independently of the presence of hepatic encephalopathy. The diagnosis is difficult; a previous history of mental health disorder and the response to anti-encephalopathy treatment may help clarify. The medical management of these patients can be difficult, particularly if major anti-psychotic medication is required.

Hepatic encephalopathy and liver transplantation

Significant difficulties arise in assessing patients for liver transplant when the only indication appears to be cognitive decline or the relatively fixed neurological abnormalities characteristic of persistent hepatic encephalopathy. In these instances attempts must be made to distinguish these changes from other causes of neurocognitive/ neurological impairment.

It might be imagined that abnormalities on cerebral imaging would favour an alternative pathology but this can not be relied upon with certainty. Mild to moderate *brain atrophy* is found in the majority of patients with long-standing hepatic encephalopathy, particularly those with alcohol-related cirrhosis, and does not necessarily indicate progressive dementia. Brain size may further decreases after liver transplantation due to the resolution of low-grade brain oedema but improvements are still seen in cognitive function [76].

Focal white matter lesions are a feature of several types of small-vessel cerebrovascular disease and are strongly associated with advanced age, high blood pressure, diabetes, stroke and myocardial infarction. They remain permanently visible on cerebral MR images and do not resolve. Their presence is associated with cognitive impairment, depression and gait abnormalities. Focal white matter lesions, radiologically indistinguishable from those associated with small vessel disease, are seen in the brains of patients with cirrhosis. However, they can markedly decrease in volume after liver transplantation. Thus, their presence, even if extensive, does not necessarily indicate that the patient's cognitive impairment is of vascular origin [76,77]. These lesions most probably reflect changes associated with the presence of low-grade brain oedema.

Advances in functional MR imaging and more widespread application of MRS may help resolve some of these issues. Currently, the best approach is to assess the degree of reversibility of the neuropsychiatric symptoms by maximizing treatment, if necessary in hospital so that compliance can be assured. Objective measures should be used to monitor improvement, preferably a combination of neuropsychometric and neurophysiological variables.

Prognosis

The presence of hepatic encephalopathy is associated with significant impairment in the ability to perform complex tasks, such as driving [30,31], a detrimental effect on health-related quality of life [28,29] and a substantial financial burden on health-care systems [78]. Its presence, in patients with cirrhosis, is also associated with a significant reduction in survival. Thus, the survival probability, after a first episode of an acute hepatic encephalopathy, is 42% at 1 year and 23% at 3 years [79].

Pathogenesis

The pathogenesis of hepatic encephalopathy has caused more controversy and division over the years than almost any other topic in hepatology. Many hypotheses have been proposed; most have been hotly contested and several, for example the false neurotransmitter theory and the gut–derived γ-aminobutyric acid (GABA) theory, have been abandoned. Any hypothesis regarding the pathogenesis of this syndrome must adequately explain the following:

1 the broad spectrum of clinical findings which appear to reflect dysfunction of multiple cerebral systems;
2 the fluctuant nature of the clinical picture, in particular its rapid evolution and its complete reversibility;
3 the mechanisms by which a variety of diverse condition precipitate deterioration in the clinical picture;
4 the mechanisms that result in alleviation of the clinical symptoms in response to treatment.

Recent advances in cellular and molecular biology, and in human non-invasive brain imaging/ quantification, have resulted in considerable progress in understanding the pathogenesis of this syndrome. In consequence, although there are still uncertainties, the emerging picture allows a number of individual findings, none of which explain the syndrome in its entirety, to be subtly integrated into a synergistic whole.

Key concepts and contributors

The two key players in the development of hepatic encephalopathy, in patients with cirrhosis, are hepatocellular failure and portal–systemic shunting. Portal–systemic shunting, in the absence of liver disease, for example following portal vein thrombosis, is not usually accompanied by the development of significant hepatic encephalopathy. However, creation of a surgical shunt or TIPS insertion in patients with chronic liver disease

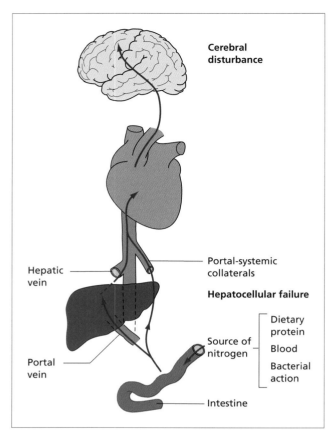

Fig. 8.8. Hepatocellular failure and portal–systemic shunting are key players in the development of hepatic encephalopathy in patients with cirrhosis. In the presence of these complications the hepatic clearance of gut-derived neurotoxic material is impaired. The neurotoxic material impinges on the brain, resulting in both direct and indirect impairment of astrocyte function. Complex changes then follow, which ultimately disrupt glioneuronal communication and neuronal function.

can precipitate or worsen existing neuropsychiatric change. Likewise, the presence of extensive portal–systemic shunting in the presence of well-preserved liver function, as in patients with schistosomal liver injury, is not usually associated with the development of major neuropsychiatric impairment.

In the presence of hepatocellular failure and portal–systemic shunting, the hepatic clearance of gut-derived neurotoxic material is impaired. This material impinges on the brain, resulting in both direct and indirect impairment of astrocyte function (Fig. 8.8). Complex changes then follow which involve brain water homeostasis, oxidative and nitrosative stress, cerebral neurotransmitters and possibly inflammation; the net effect is disruption of glioneuronal communication and neuronal function.

Thus, there are a number of key factors that determine the development of hepatic encephalopathy (Table 8.4).

Table 8.4. Key factors in the pathogenesis of hepatic encephalopathy

Gut-derived neurotoxins
Brain water homeostasis
Oxidative/ nitrosative stress
Astrocyte dysfunction
Neurotransmitter dysfunction
Infection and inflammation

These will be discussed individually. An attempt will then be made to integrate them into a cohesive model.

Gut-derived neurotoxins

Several gut-derived neurotoxins have been implicated in the pathogenesis of hepatic encephalopathy; by far the most important is ammonia.

Ammonia is produced in the intestine from dietary protein, deamination of glutamine via glutaminase and bacterial action in the colon. It is absorbed by non–ionic diffusion; concentrations in the portal vein are tenfold higher than in arterial blood. The hepatic extraction rate is high. The ammonia in portal blood, together with the ammonia derived from hepatic amino acid metabolism, is taken up by periportal hepatocytes and metabolized to urea via the urea cycle. Some ammonia is taken up by perivenous hepatocytes where it is converted to glutamine via glutamine synthetase. These two systems, working in concert, tightly control blood ammonia concentrations in the hepatic veins.

Blood ammonia levels may be increased in patients with cirrhosis for a number of reasons: (1) small bowel colonization with urease-containing bacteria; (2) enhanced intestinal absorption of ammonia secondary to the increased splanchnic blood flow associated with portal hypertension; (3) intra- and extra-hepatic portal systemic shunting; (4) reduction in functioning hepatocyte mass; (5) decreased ammonia metabolism in muscle as a result of loss of muscle mass; and (6) increased renal production of ammonia secondary to the respiratory alkalosis commonly seen in these patients, which is the result of primary hyperventilation [80] and hypokalaemia [81].

Cerebral uptake of ammonia is increased in patient with cirrhosis [82]. The blood–brain barrier remains anatomically intact in these patients but $^{13}NH_3$ PET studies have shown that the permeability surface area to ammonia is increased [82].

There is no urea cycle in the brain. Ammonia is detoxified, in astrocytes, by the synthesis of glutamine through amidation of glutamate via glutamine synthetase. Once inside the brain ammonia exerts deleterious effects at many levels but particularly on astrocytes. These cells proliferate and exhibit significant changes in morphology, characterized by development of enlarged pale nuclei, prominent nucleoli, peripheral margination of chromatin and accumulation of glycogen. These changes, which are referred to as Alzheimer type II astrocytosis, are most prominent in the cerebral cortex, basal ganglia and cerebellum. Ammonia also has direct effects on cortical neurones, which affect postsynaptic inhibitory potentials [83], and the activity of the tricarboxylic acid cycle [84].

Nevertheless, despite the obvious importance of ammonia in the pathogenesis of hepatic encephalopathy, the correlation between circulating blood ammonia concentrations and neuropsychiatric status is poor. This reflects, at least in part, the technical difficulties associated with its measurement, and the differences in blood and brain ammonia concentrations which can be explained by variation in the compartmental pH. Indeed, the pH-dependent partial pressure of gaseous ammonia in arterial blood correlates more closely with the clinical and neurophysiological changes observed than plasma ammonia concentrations [69]. The correlation between neuropsychiatric status and glutamine is better. CSF levels of glutamine increase as the degree of neuropsychiatric impairment increases [70], as does the height of the glutamine/ glutamate signal observed on cerebral ^{1}H-MRS [19].

Patients with congenital defects of one or more of the urea cycle enzymes may develop hyperammonaemia, and many features suggestive of hepatic encephalopathy including disturbed consciousness and Alzheimer type II astrocytosis [85]. However, they also develop seizures, which are rarely observed in patients with hepatic encephalopathy. Heterozygotes may develop hyperammonaemic coma following medication with sodium valproate.

Treatment that reduces the production and absorption of ammonia has a beneficial effect on patients with hepatic encephalopathy and is accompanied by reversal in the abnormalities observed on cerebral ^{1}H-MRS [86].

Other gut-derived toxins implicated in the pathogenesis of hepatic encephalopathy include:
(1) *indoles,* produced by bacterial degradation of tryptophan [87]; (2) *mercaptans,* the sulphur-containing compounds responsible for foetor hepaticus [4]; (3) *phenols,* produced by bacterial degradation of phenylalanine and tyrosine; and (4) *short-* and *medium-chain fatty acids.* These compounds may have direct and independent effects on cerebral function or, more likely, act synergistically with ammonia.

Brain water homeostasis

The influx of excess ammonia into the brain results in accumulation of osmotically active glutamine within astrocytes. This results in astrocyte swelling. This is countered by efflux from the cell of other osmotically active compounds, principally myoinositol, but also taurine and α-glycerophosphorylcholine. The net result is the development of low-grade cerebral oedema. *In vivo* cerebral ^{1}H-MRS studies in patients with cirrhosis and hepatic encephalopathy show a decrease in the myoinositol peak and an increase in the glutamine/ glutamate peak, supporting the concept of a disturbance in astrocytic volume homeostasis [88] (Fig. 8.7). The existence of low-grade cerebral oedema has also been demonstrated using cerebral magnetization and diffusion transfer MR imaging techniques [89,90] and by quantitative cerebral water mapping [91]. In addition, there is a good correlation between the changes observed on cerebral ^{1}H-MRS and the severity of hepatic encephalopathy in patients with cirrhosis [88,92]; the changes are aggravated after TIPS insertion [88] and largely resolve following successful treatment [90] and liver transplantation [89] (Fig. 8.9).

The small increases in astrocyte water content may have important functional consequences despite the absence of a clinically overt increase in intracranial pressure [93] (Table 8.5).

Ammonia-induced glutamine accumulation is not the only mechanism that triggers low-grade cerebral oedema. Hyponatraemia, inflammatory cytokines and benzodiazepines also promote astrocyte swelling, most probably in synergy with ammonia.

Oxidative/ nitrosative stress [94]

There is substantial evidence from studies in experimental animal models and from astrocytic cell culture for involvement of oxidative/ nitrosative stress in the pathogenesis of hepatic encephalopathy. However, few, if any, data are available in man.

Oxidative/ nitrosative stress arises when there is an imbalance between the production of reactive oxygen/ reactive nitric oxide species and their rate of removal by endogenous mechanisms. Sustained oxidative/ nitrosative stress may trigger cell damage and death.

Ammonia, hypo-osmotic swelling, inflammatory cytokines and benzodiazepines induce an oxidative/ nitrosative stress response in astrocytes with rapid formation of reactive oxygen (ROS) and nitric oxide (NOS) species. This stress response is mediated by *N*-methyl D-aspartate (NMDA) glutamate receptors but the mechanisms underlying this activation are unclear. The most likely cause for the formation of ROS is activation of nicotinamide adenine dinucleotide phosphate (NADPH) oxidase isoforms, while the formation of NOS is probably dependent on activation of Ca^{++}/calmodulin isoforms of nitric oxide synthase.

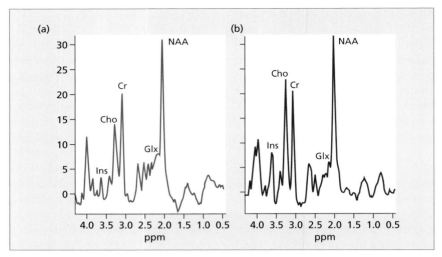

Fig. 8.9. ¹H-MR-spectroscopy water-suppressed spectra of an 8-mL voxel located in the parietal region in a patient with cirrhosis before (a) and after (b) liver transplantation, recorded with a stimulated echo acquisition mode pulse sequence (TR/TE, 1600/20 ms; acquisitions, 256). The main resonances correspond to *N*-acetylaspartate (NAA: 2.0 ppm), glutamine/ glutamate (Glx, 2.1–2.5 ppm), creatine/ phosphocreatine (Cr: 3.02 ppm), choline-containing compounds (Cho: 3.2 ppm), and myoinositol (Ins: 3.55 ppm). The initial spectrum shows an increase in the glutamate/ glutamine region and a decrease in the myoinositol and choline resonances. These abnormalities normalized after liver transplantation. The NAA indices are normal in both examinations. (Adapted from [68] with permission.)

Table 8.5. The consequences of astrocytic swelling

Activation of extracellularly regulated protein kinases
Up-regulation of peripheral benzodiazepine receptors
Modulation of amino acid transport
Elevation of intracellular calcium concentrations
Release of cellular taurine → affects synaptic plasticity and GABAergic tone
Modulation of multiple ion channels
Increased pH in endocytotic vesicles → affects receptor/ ligand sorting and neurotransmitter processing
Stimulation of glycogen synthesis
Activation of NMDA glutamate receptor
Induction of oxidative/ nitrosative stress
Predisposes to neuronal dysfunction

NMDA, *N*-methyl D-aspartate.

There is a close relationship between astrocyte swelling, NMDA receptor activation and oxidative stress. Astrocyte swelling induces oxidative stress through activation of the NMDA receptor and Ca⁺⁺-dependent mechanisms; NMDA activation and oxidative stress trigger astrocyte swelling. This indicates the presence of a signalling loop which allows mutual amplification of both the astrocyte swelling and oxidative stress.

Astrocytic dysfunction

Astrocytic function is disturbed in hepatic encephalopathy. Astrocyte swelling and oxidative/ nitrosative stress are major contributors (see below).

Oxidative/ nitrosative stress can promote covalent modification of tyrosine residues in astrocytic proteins. This process, which is known as protein tyrosine nitration, interferes with protein function and intracellular signal transduction. Astrocytes located near the blood–brain barrier are particularly affected; the process may, therefore, influence trans-astrocytic substrate transport. Not all proteins undergo tyrosine nitration, which may explain the selective alterations in blood–brain permeability observed in this condition.

Oxidative stress can induce RNA oxidation, which compromises translational accuracy/ efficacy and results in the formation of defective or unstable proteins. This may, in turn, result in multiple alterations in neurotransmitter receptor systems.

Nitrosative stress promotes mobilization of zinc from metallothionein and other proteins. Zn⁺⁺ may affect the activities of multiple enzymes and transcription factors and may augment GABAergic neurotransmission and decrease glutamate uptake (see below).

Ammonia also has a number of *direct* effects on astrocytic function, including alterations in gene expression [95], intracellular signal transduction, transport, metabolism and neurotransmitter processing, and the synthesis of neurosteroids.

These changes in astrocyte function result in disruption of glioneuronal communication, impairment of synaptic plasticity and slowing of oscillatory neuronal activity.

Alterations in cerebral neurotransmission

Hepatic encephalopathy is associated with changes in multiple neurotransmitter systems. However, there is still relatively little information as to which excitatory, inhibitory and modulatory systems are involved in the actual genesis of the syndrome. Difficulties arise because the functions of one system can be influenced both directly and indirectly by the activities of another. Overall, however, hepatic encephalopathy is associated with a shift in balance between inhibitory and excitatory neurotransmission favouring inhibition. This has been attributed to either alteration in the glutamatergic system or to an increase in GABAergic tone. However, alterations in other neurotransmitter systems and in the neuromodulators, adenosine and acetylcholine may also play a role.

Glutamate

Glutamate is the principle excitatory neurotransmitter in the brain. It is synthesized in presynaptic nerve terminals and stored in vesicles. After release and activation at various postsynaptic receptors it is removed from the synaptic cleft by astrocytic transporters. Within the astrocyte glutamate is converted to glutamine, by addition of ammonia, via glutamine synthetase. The glutamine is then transported into presynaptic neurones where it is transformed into glutamate (Fig. 8.10).

Total brain levels of glutamate are decreased in patients with cirrhosis dying in hepatic coma [96], most probably reflecting its consumption in the formation of glutamine in the presence of hyperammonaemia. However, glutamate concentrations in the extracellular spaces and in the CSF are increased, at least in experimental animals. This may reflect increased release from astrocytes in response to cell swelling and/or a defect in glial reuptake most probably mediated by ammonia-induced down regulation of astrocytic and neuronal glutamate transporters [97,98]. The increase in extracellular glutamate concentrations may result in NMDA receptor activation in astrocytes, which is a key factor in the development of the oxidative stress response (see below).

γ-Aminobutyric acid and the neurosteroid system [68]

GABA is the principal inhibitory neurotransmitter in the brain. It is usually synthesized from glutamate by gluta-

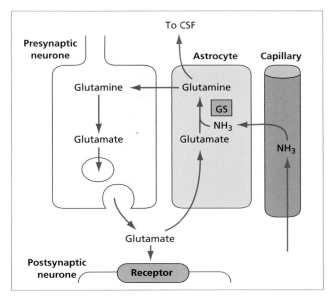

Fig. 8.10. Key steps in glutamatergic synaptic regulation and removal of ammonia by the brain. Glutamate is synthesized from its precursor glutamine in the presynaptic nerve terminal and is then stored in synaptic vesicles until ultimately released, via a calcium-dependent mechanism, into the synapse. Once released glutamate can act on glutamate receptors found in the synaptic cleft. Glutamate is taken up by the astrocyte and converted to glutamine via glutamine synthetase (GS) using ammonia.

mate dehydrogenase in presynaptic nerves and stored in vesicles. It binds to a specific receptor which is embedded in the postsynaptic neural membrane. This receptor is part of a larger GABA-A receptor complex which also has binding sites for benzodiazepines, barbiturates and neurosteroids (Fig. 8.11). The binding of any of these ligands opens a chloride channel; the influx of chloride ions results in hyperpolarization of the postsynaptic membrane and neuroinhibition.

Hepatic encephalopathy is associated with an increase in 'GABA-ergic tone'. Many neurotoxic and neuroactive compounds implicated in the pathogenesis of this syndrome, including ammonia, benzodiazepine-like ligands, proinflammatory cytokines and neurosteroids, were thought to produce their effects by modulating the function of the GABA-A receptor complex. However, studies have shown no alteration in the benzodiazepine, GABA or neurosteroid recognition sites on the GABA-A receptor complex in the brains of patients dying in hepatic coma [68]. The changes in GABA-ergic tone are now thought to be mediated by neurosteroids.

Neurosteroids are synthesized in the brain, primarily in astrocytes, independently of peripheral steroidogenesis in gonads and the adrenal. Neurosteroid synthesis is mediated via activation of the 'peripheral-type' benzodiazepine receptor (PTBR). Neurosteroids such as 3α-5α-tetrahydroprogesterone (allopregnanolone)

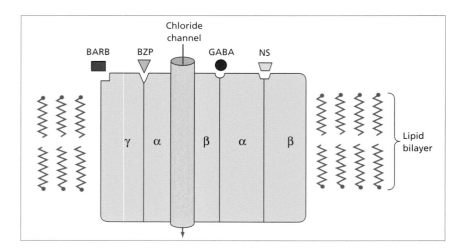

Fig. 8.11. Simplified model of the unfolded pentameric GABA-receptor/ ionophore complex embedded in a postsynaptic neural membrane. The receptor complex is made up of 2α, 2β and 1γ subunits. Binding of any of the depicted ligands, γ-aminobutyric acid (GABA), barbiturates (BARB), benzodiazepines (BZP) or neurosteroids (NS), to its specific binding site increases chloride ion conductance through the membrane with resultant hyperpolarization and neuroinhibition.

are potent, endogenous, positive allosteric modulators of both the GABA and benzodiazepine sites on the GABA-A receptor complex.

PTBA is located at the inner/outer mitochondrial membrane. It is independent of the central benzodiazepine receptors, which is part of the neuronal GABA-A complex. Autopsy and imaging studies in patients with hepatic encephalopathy show consistent up-regulation of components of the PTBR. This up-regulation is most probably mediated by ammonia and manganese [67], both of which accumulate as a result of hepatocellular failure and portal–systemic shunting of blood and, in the case of the later, impaired biliary excretion [62–66]. In addition, the function of PTBR is modulated by agonist ligands such as diazepam binding inhibitor (DBI) and octadecaneuropeptide (ODN), which are found in increased concentrations in the CSF and autopsied brains of patients with hepatic encephalopathy [68] (Fig. 8.12).

Allopregnanolone is increased in the brains of patients who have died in hepatic coma in concentrations sufficient to modulate components of the GABA-A receptors. The neurosteroids may also act synergistically with other potential neurotoxins such as ammonia and benzodiazepine-like compounds to further modulate GABA-A receptor function. The net effect is an increase in GABAergic tone and neural inhibition.

Neurosteroids are also synthesized in the kidney, adrenals and gonads. In patients with liver failure, circulating concentrations of neurosteroids and their precursors are increased. They are lipophilic and easily cross the blood–brain barrier and contribute to the changes described above.

Neurosteroids can affect the function not only of the GABA-A receptor in patients with hepatic dysfunction, but also the function of serotonin (5-HT$_3$), NMDA, glycine and opioid receptors and others. They can also

influence neuronal function by binding to intracellular receptors that can act as transcription factors, thus regulating gene expression.

Thus, neurosteroid accumulation in patients with liver failure has consequences for both cerebral neurotransmission and the expression of key genes encoding for brain proteins.

Involvement of the GABA-ergic system in the pathogenesis of hepatic encephalopathy is consistent with the increased sensitivity to benzodiazepines observed in these patients [23], and the short-term improvement in neuropsychiatric status seen in some patients with cirrhosis treated with the benzodiazepine antagonist, flumazenil [99].

Serotonin

The neurotransmitter serotonin (5-hydroxytryptamine; 5-HT) is involved in the control of cortical arousal and thus the conscious state. In patients with cirrhosis dying in hepatic coma, increases are seen in: (1) the activity of brain monoamine oxidase A, the enzyme responsible for metabolizing serotonin [100]; (2) in cerebral concentrations of the 5-HT metabolite, 5-hydroxyindole acetic acid (5-HIAA) [101]; and (3) in the number of HT$_2$ receptors [102]. These changes, together with the appearance of encephalopathy in patients with cirrhosis treated with the 5-HT blocker ketanserin for portal hypertension [103], implicate the serotonin system in hepatic encephalopathy. Where the dysfunction in this system primarily lies awaits further study.

Dopamine

Dopamine is a catecholamine neurotransmitter which has important roles in behaviour and cognition, motivation, mood, attention, working memory, learning and

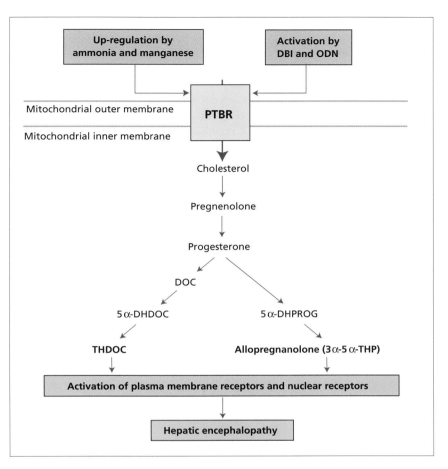

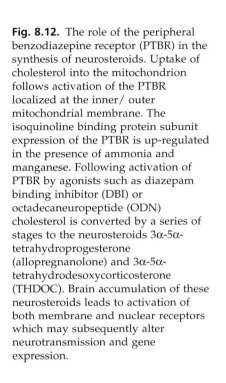

Fig. 8.12. The role of the peripheral benzodiazepine receptor (PTBR) in the synthesis of neurosteroids. Uptake of cholesterol into the mitochondrion follows activation of the PTBR localized at the inner/outer mitochondrial membrane. The isoquinoline binding protein subunit expression of the PTBR is up-regulated in the presence of ammonia and manganese. Following activation of PTBR by agonists such as diazepam binding inhibitor (DBI) or octadecaneuropeptide (ODN) cholesterol is converted by a series of stages to the neurosteroids 3α-5α-tetrahydroprogesterone (allopregnanolone) and 3α-5α-tetrahydrodesoxycorticosterone (THDOC). Brain accumulation of these neurosteroids leads to activation of both membrane and nuclear receptors which may subsequently alter neurotransmission and gene expression.

voluntary movement. In patients with cirrhosis dying in hepatic coma the activity of brain monoamine oxidase A, the enzyme responsible for dopamine degradation [104], and the cerebral concentrations of the dopamine metabolite homovanillic acid [101] are increased, while the number of D_2 dopamine receptors is decreased [105]. Dopamine depletion is the hallmark of Parkinson's disease. Manganese toxicity is characterized by its accumulation in the globus pallidus; subsequent neurodegenerative change results in reduction in the number of D_2 receptors and, in some patients, the development of extrapyramidal changes [106]. Extrapyramidal features are common in hepatic encephalopathy. In some patients these symptoms, together with the more general aspects of the syndrome, respond well to treatment with the dopamine agonist bromocriptine [107], further implicating the dopamine system in this condition.

Other neurotransmitter systems

Alterations have also been described in histaminergic and opioidergic neurotransmission but their role in the genesis of hepatic encephalopathy is uncertain.

Neuromodulatory systems

Alterations have also been reported in the activities of the neuromodulators acetylcholine [108] and adenosine [109].

Acetylcholine levels are considerably reduced in the brains of patients with cirrhosis dying in hepatic coma because of an increase in the activity of the acetylcholine-hydrolysing enzyme, acetylcholinesterase. Acetylcholine modulates release of other neurotransmitters through activation of both nicotinic and muscarinic receptors. Activation of nicotinic receptors mediates neuronal excitation while activation of muscarinic receptors suppresses GABAergic synaptic transmission. Nicotinic receptor density is significantly lower in the brains of these patients while the affinity of acetylcholine for the muscarinic receptor is reduced. These changes result in a net increase in inhibitory neurotransmission. Rivastigmine, a reversible cholinesterase inhibitor, improves psychometric performance in patient with hepatic encephalopathy when used in conjunction with lactulose [110].

Alterations in adenosinergic neuromodulation may further aggravate the excitatory/inhibitory imbalance.

Activation of the high-affinity A_1 and A_{2A} receptors results in modulation of neurotransmission at both pre- and postsynaptic levels. Activation of A_1 receptors results in a decrease in neurotransmitter release, while activation of A_{2A} receptors facilitates acetylcholine, glutamate and GABA release and activation of NMDA receptors. In addition, adenosine receptors play a crucial role in the control of dopamine D_2 receptor function in the basal ganglia. The adenosinergic receptors interact with one another; A_{2A} receptors can either inhibit or neutralize the consequences of A_1 receptor activation at the presynaptic level, thus conferring a degree of neural protection. Both A_1 and A_{2A} binding are reduced in the brains of patients with cirrhosis dying in hepatic coma possibly as a result of a compensatory neuroprotective mechanism [111].

Inflammation and infection [112]

Patients with cirrhosis have impaired host defence mechanisms; their neutrophils and macrophages have a reduced capacity to phagacytose and eliminate microbes. In addition, bacterial translocation from the gut results in chronic endotoxaemia. These patients are at increased risk of infection; infection frequently precipitates hepatic encephalopathy.

Recent interest has focused on the possible synergistic roles of inflammation and infection in modulating the cerebral effects of ammonia. The terms infection and inflammation are often used synonymously, but this is incorrect. Infection is caused by an exogenous pathogen; inflammation is the complex biological response of tissues to harmful stimuli which results in the release and circulation of proinflammatory cytokines and mediators. Infection and inflammation can coexist.

Astrocytes and endothelial cells are key components of the blood–brain barrier. They both respond to systemic inflammatory stimuli and play a role in eliciting an inflammatory response involving a number of pro-inflammatory and neurotransmitter pathways.

Ammonia also induces neutrophil dysfunction with release of reactive oxygen species which contribute to oxidative stress and systemic inflammation. This may further exacerbate the cerebral effects of ammonia while potentially reducing the efficacy of the neutrophil to deal with infection. However, neutrophil dysfunction may also play a more direct role in the pathogenesis of hepatic encephalopathy. Thus, endothelial–neutrophil interaction within the cerebral microcirculation, which is enhanced in the presence of hyperammonaemia and chronic endotoxaemia, may result in increase neutrophil migration across the blood–brain barrier. This will lead to the production of chemokines, proinflammatory cytokines and ROS, which will contribute to astrocyte oxidative stress.

Modulation of the intestinal microbiota by use of probiotics can reduce bacterial translocation and prevent the development of infection and hepatic encephalopathy in patients with cirrhosis [113].

A unified hypothesis (Fig. 8.13)

In patient with cirrhosis, ammonia escapes hepatic detoxificatiol and impinges on the brain. There it induces astrocyte swelling via its effects on glutamine/ glutamate synthesis, resulting in the development of low-grade cerebral oedema. Astrocyte swelling triggers NMDA activation and generates oxidative/ nitrosative stress. Astrocyte function is compromised both as a result of these indirect effects of ammonia and its more direct neurotoxic effects, which are independent of the changes in brain water homeostasis. Astrocyte dysfunction results in alterations in gene expression, modification of proteins and RNA, and disturbances in intracellular signal transduction and neurotransmission. As a result, glial–neuronal communication is disrupted and this impacts on synaptic plasticity and oscillatory electric networks. Slowed oscillatory communication may ultimately prove responsible for the cerebral dysfunction in hepatic encephalopathy.

Events such as gastrointestinal bleeding, constipation and dietary indiscretion can precipitate an episode of hepatic encephalopathy, in patients with cirrhosis, because they increase the circulating ammonia load. However, ammonia is not the only agent that causes astrocyte swelling in this setting. Inflammatory cytokines, hyponatraemia and benzodiazepines can all produce the same effect. Thus, hepatic encephalopathy can be precipitated by a variety of conditions that do not necessarily increase the circulating ammonia load, for example infection, electrolyte disturbances and drugs. The common pathway is astrocyte swelling. Treatment of the factor(s) responsible for precipitating an episode of hepatic encephalopathy can result in rapid amelioration of the symptoms. Agents that reduce the production and absorption of gut-derived neurotoxins, principally ammonia, are the mainstay of treatment.

In patients with cirrhosis, the astroglial osmolyte pool is significantly depleted as organic osmolytes, such as myoinositol and taurine, shift compartments to offset glutamine-induced osmotic stress. In consequence, there may be very little reserve available within the system to deal with additional osmotic shifts. This provides an explanation for the rapid changes sometimes observed in patient's neuropsychiatric status following apparently minor changes in their clinical condition.

This hypothesis is based largely on findings in experimental animals and in cell culture [93]. Thus, although

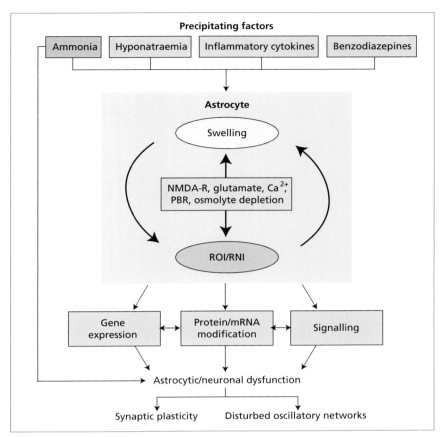

Fig. 8.13. A possible unifying hypothesis for the pathogenesis of hepatic encephalopathy. In patients with cirrhosis ammonia escapes hepatic detoxification and impinges on the brain where it has both direct and indirect neurotoxic effects on astrocyte function. Ammonia induces astrocytic swelling via its effects on glutamine/ glutamate synthesis, resulting in the development of low-grade cerebral oedema. This, in turn, results in activation of the *N*-methyl-D-aspartate (NMDA) receptor and the generation of reactive nitrogen/ oxygen species. Astrocyte function is compromised as a result of both the effects of cell swelling and oxidative/ nitrosative stress and as a result of the direct neurotoxic effects of ammonia. The resultant dysfunction causes alterations in gene expression, modification of proteins and RNA, and disturbances in intracellular signal transduction and neurotransmission. Glial–neuronal communication and neuronal function may be compromised as a consequence, resulting in disruption of multiple neurotransmitter systems, synaptic plasticity and oscillatory networks. These cerebral changes are the basis of the abnormalities observed in hepatic encephalopathy. Events such as gastrointestinal bleeding and constipation can precipitate hepatic encephalopathy because they increase the circulating ammonia load. Other agents such as inflammatory cytokines, benzodiazepines and hyponatraemia can also precipitate hepatic encephalopathy because they induce astrocyte swelling. PBR; peripheral benzodiazepine receptor, RNI; reactive nitrogen intermediates, ROI; reactive oxygen intermediates. (Adapted from Häussinger and Schliess [93], with permission.)

it explains many of the features of this syndrome, this caveat remains.

Management of hepatic encephalopathy [114,115]

Hepatic encephalopathy should be treated. A variety of treatment options are available but not all are suitable, or appropriate, for every patient. The management of episodic or recurrent encephalopathy, in patients with cirrhosis, centres initially on identification and treat-ment of any underlying or precipitating factors, although these may only be apparent in 50% of patients (Table 8.1). Once the episode has resolved it is important to instigate long-term treatment for any residual deficits. The management of chronic persistent encephalopathy is challenging and requires a different, multidimensional approach. Patients with minimal hepatic encephalopathy should also be treated, although many escape as their condition goes unrecognized.

The treatment options are described individually but are often used in combination. Guidelines are provided (Tables 8.6–8.8).

Table 8.6. Management of recurrent or episodic hepatic encephalopathy

Acute events:
General supportive measures
Identify and treat precipitating factors
Enemata 6–12 hourly for 48–72 h
Maintain adequate protein and energy intakes
Non-absorbable disaccharides:
    lactulose 40–120 mL daily or
    lactitol 20–40 g daily
If response inadequate, add:
Non-absorbable antibiotic for 5–7 days
    neomycin 4–6 g daily
    rifaxamin 400 mg three times daily
Between episodes (if necessary):
Avoid precipitating factors
Maintain adequate protein and energy intakes
Non-absorbable disaccharides
    lactulose 20–60 mL daily or
    lactitol 20–40 g daily and/or
Non-absorbable antibiotics
    rifaxamin 400 mg three times daily

Table 8.7. Management of persistent hepatic encephalopathy

General
Avoid precipitating factors
Maintain adequate protein and energy intakes
Increase protein from vegetable sources
Consider probiotics
Non-absorbable disaccharides
    lactulose 40–120 mL daily or
    lactitol 20–40 g daily
If response incomplete, add:
Rifaxamin 1.2 g daily
Bromocriptine 7.5 mg daily (if no fluid retention)
LOLA 6 g three times daily
Sodium benzoate 2 g twice daily (if no fluid retention)
Daily enemata
Continuing poor response, consider:
BCAA supplements
Revision of surgical shunts or TIPS
Blockage of large spontaneous shunts
If situation unresolved:
Hepatic transplantation, if other indications present
Colonic exclusion/ excision (if not transplantable)

TIPS, transjugular intrahepatic portal–systemic shunt; LOLA, L-ornithine-L-aspartate; BCAA, branched chain amino acids.

General supportive measures

In patients with minimal or stable persistent hepatic encephalopathy, management of the hepatic encephalopathy *per se* is usually all that is required. In patients with episodic/ recurrent hepatic encephalopathy, management is generally more problematic as precipitating

Table 8.8. Management of minimal hepatic encephalopathy

Avoid constipation
Avoid other precipitating factors
Maintain adequate protein and energy intakes
Non-absorbable disaccharides:
    lactulose 20–40 mL daily
    lactitol 10–20 g daily

factors, such as variceal haemorrhage or sepsis, may also require attention; some may need to be managed in an intensive care setting, at least initially.

Management of precipitating factors. The identification and correction of any precipitating events is of paramount importance. If symptoms do not improve then a search for a second complication, most often occult infection, needs to be made. Gastrointestinal haemorrhage should be managed vigorously with antibiotics, vasoactive drugs and endoscopic therapy; anaemia should be corrected early and blood pressure maintained to prevent further hepatic and renal insults. Infections, most commonly pulmonary, urinary or peritoneal, should be treated promptly using appropriate antibiotics. Electrolyte abnormalities should be managed by discontinuing diuretics and correcting the deficits, as appropriate. Deterioration in renal function should be corrected, if possible, by stopping diuretics, increasing the circulating volume to maintain renal perfusion and discontinuing any potentially nephrotoxic drugs. Sedatives should be stopped and their effects reversed, if possible.

Measures should be taken to: avoid falls and injuries; maintain intravenous lines; monitor vital signs, fluid balance and nutritional intake; and to avoid the development of aspiration pneumonia.

Diet. Patients with cirrhosis are unable to effectively store glycogen and rely on gluconeogenesis, an energy expensive process which utilizes amino acids, to maintain adequate glucose levels. This increases their daily energy and protein requirement. Guidelines recommend daily energy intakes of 35 to 45 kcal/kg and daily protein intakes of 1.2 to 1.5 g/kg [116]. Vegetable protein is better tolerated than animal protein; the benefits relate to the effects of dietary fibre on colonic function which include decreases in the transit time and intraluminal pH and an increase in faecal ammonia excretion [117]. The acceptability of vegetable protein diets varies considerably, reflecting the nature of the original diet. It is also important that food intake is spread evenly throughout the waking day to avoid protein loading; six snack-type meals are preferable to three main meals [116].

It may be difficult to maintain oral intake in patients presenting with gastrointestinal bleeding and in those with severe encephalopathy. It may be necessary, under these circumstances, to restrict dietary intake. A short period of dietary deprivation of up to 24 to 36h may not be harmful but prolonged restriction should be avoided. If intake has been restricted then some would council reintroducing protein incrementally. However, there is no evidence that restricting protein has any benefit on overall outcome [118].

Enemata. Enemata should be used in the acute situation. It is not sufficient to simply cleanse the bowel; tap water and saline enemata are ineffective [119]. The vehicle needs to be hyperosmolar to encourage ammonia extraction; both neutral phosphate and lactulose enemata are efficacious. In patients with chronic persistent encephalopathy daily enemata may provide a useful adjuvant to oral therapy.

Specific treatment

At present, treatment is directed primarily at reducing the production and absorption of gut-derived neurotoxins, particularly ammonia, mainly through dietary manipulation, bowel cleansing, non-absorbable disac-

charides and non-absorbable antibiotics. However, interest in the interorgan trafficking of ammonia has highlighted other potential targets for reducing circulating ammonia concentrations and other pathophysiological mechanisms have been identified, for example systemic inflammation, which may provide additional treatment targets. Management is, therefore, based on several, non-mutually exclusive treatment options.

Non-absorbable disaccharides

The non-absorbable disaccharide lactulose was first introduced into clinical practice in 1966. Lactitol was introduced in the mid-1980s.

The human small intestinal mucosa does not have enzymes to split these synthetic disaccharides. They are not absorbed in the small intestine but pass unchanged into the large intestine. There they are extensively metabolized by colonic bacteria to their constituent monosaccharides and then to volatile fatty acids and hydrogen ± methane (Fig. 8.14). Their beneficial effects reflect their ability to reduce the intestinal production/ absorption of ammonia. This is achieved in three ways:

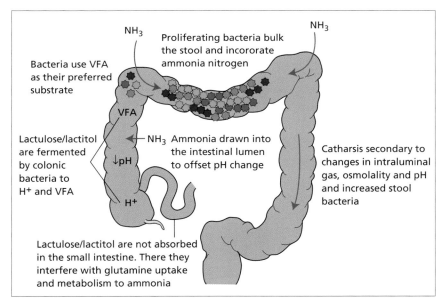

Fig. 8.14. Lactulose and lactitol are not absorbed in the small intestine because of the absence of the relevant disaccharidases. They pass unchanged into the colon where they are extensively metabolized by colonic bacteria, to produce volatile fatty acids (VFA), hydrogen ± methane. VFA are the preferred substrate for the intestinal bacteria; their presence in excess results in rapid bacterial growth which not only bulks the stool but results in utilization of ammonia nitrogen as it is incorporated into bacterial protein. The beneficial effects of the non-absorbed disaccharides in

patient with hepatic encephalopathy arise from: (1) a cathartic effect secondary to changes in intestinal gas formation, intraluminal pH and the intraluminal osmolality, and the bulking effect of the proliferating intestinal bacteria; and (2) more direct effects on ammonia metabolism viz interference with the uptake of glutamine and its metabolism in the small intestine and hence a reduction in small intestinal ammonia production and the incorporation of ammonia nitrogen into colonic bacterial protein.

1 A laxative effect: the colonic metabolism of these sugars results in an increase in intraluminal gas formation, an increase in intraluminal osmolality, a reduction in intraluminal pH and an overall decrease in transit time.

2 Uptake of ammonia by bacteria: the intraluminal changes in pH result in a leaching of ammonia from the circulation into the colon. The colonic bacteria use the released volatile fatty acids as substrate and proliferate. In doing so they use the trapped colonic ammonia as a nitrogen source for protein synthesis. The increase in bacterial numbers additionally 'bulks' the stool and contributes to the cathartic effect [117].

3 Reduction in intestinal ammonia production: non-absorbable disaccharides inhibit glutaminase activity and interfere with the uptake of glutamine by the intestinal wall and its subsequent metabolism to ammonia [120].

Lactulose (β-galactosidofructose) is generally prescribed as a syrup. The dose is adjusted to ensure passage of two semisoft stools/day; typical doses range from 15 to 30 mL two to four times a day. Approximately 30% of patients develop an aversion to its taste and may develop anorexia, flatulence and abdominal discomfort in the early weeks of treatment; however, tolerance improves over time. Over-enthusiastic use can result in profuse diarrhoea, dehydration and even renal failure, and should be avoided. The side effects most probably relate to the contamination of lactulose with other sugars; the crystalline preparation produces less side effects. Improvements in neuropsychiatric status are observed in approximately 80% of patients with hepatic encephalopathy, treated acutely; the most severely decompensated patients are less likely to respond [121]. Lactulose is efficacious in the longer-term but compliance with treatment is a potential issue [122]. Lactulose is also effective when delivered rectally (250 mL lactulose in 750 mL water) [119].

Lactitol (β-galactosidosorbitol) is a second-generation disaccharide, which is easily produced in a chemically pure crystalline form and can be dispensed as a powder. It is as efficacious, if not more efficacious, than lactulose [123,124]. It is also better tolerated with fewer side effects [123,125]. The dosage required to ensure passage of two semisoft stools/day ranges from 10 to 90 g.

The non-absorbable disaccharides are used widely as first line therapy for hepatic encephalopathy. However, a recent systematic review concluded that 'there is insufficient evidence at present to recommend or refute the use of non-absorbable disaccharides for hepatic encephalopathy' [126]. This review has itself been severely criticized [114]. Many physicians are convinced, through long and successful use, that these agents are effective [127] and more recent controlled trials provide further evidence of their efficacy [128].

Antibiotics

Antibiotics can be used to selectively eliminate urease-producing organisms from the intestinal tract. This reduces the production of ammonia.

Neomycin, is a poorly absorbed aminoglycoside antibiotic. It is prescribed in a dose of 4 to 6 g/day and was the standard treatment for hepatic encephalopathy from 1957 until the introduction of lactulose in 1966. Although generally considered efficacious, recent studies have shed doubt on its effectiveness [129,130]. Small quantities are absorbed and long-term use is associated with the development of nephrotoxicity and of irreversible ototoxicity. It should not be used for more than a week. Its use may be superseded by less toxic antibiotics.

Rifaximin, a synthetic antibiotic structurally related to rifamycin, has a very low rate of systemic absorption (0.4%). It is at least as effective, for the treatment of hepatic encephalopathy, as lactulose/ lactitol and other non-absorbable antibiotics, for example neomycin and paromomycin [131,132]. Rifaximin has an excellent safety profile. It is better tolerated than the non-absorbable disaccharides and hence compliance is likely to be better in the longer term [133].

One of the major risks associated with the long-term use of antibiotics, even those that are not absorbed, is the emergence of multiresistant organisms. One solution might be to use them intermittently with perhaps the addition of probiotics during the 'off treatment' periods [134].

Non-absorbable disaccharides and antibiotics combined

The therapeutic effects of non-absorbable disaccharides depend on their metabolism by colonic bacteria. The beneficial effects of the non-absorbable antibiotics depend on inhibition of bacterial activity in the colon. However, the non-absorbable disaccharides can be metabolized by a wide variety of bacterial species. Thus, while in theory there would appear to be little point in combining the two therapies, in practice they may have an additive effect. This may result in an enhanced clinical response in individuals who do not respond adequately to either agent alone [122,135].

Bromocriptine

Deficits in dopaminergic neurotransmission have been identified in cirrhotic patient with hepatic encephalopathy. Patients with stable, chronic, persistent hepatic encephalopathy with prominent extrapyramidal features, resistant to treatment with other agents, may benefit significantly from treatment with the specific dopamine agonist bromocriptine [107]. The dose is gradually increased from 2.5 mg once daily to a maximum of 5 mg twice daily. Ototoxicity has been reported [136], and treated patients should be monitored with audiograms 6-monthly. Treatment should be reserved for patients with well-compensated liver disease as use in patients with ascites has been associated with the syndrome of inappropriate ADH secretion [137].

L-*ornithine*-L-*aspartate*

L-ornithine-L-aspartate (LOLA) treatment promotes hepatic removal of ammonia by stimulating residual hepatic urea cycle activity and promoting glutamine synthesis, particularly in skeletal muscle [138]. Controlled studies show that *intravenous* LOLA administration reduces ammonia levels and improves mental state and psychometric performance in cirrhotic patients with overt hepatic encephalopathy [139,140]. Treatment with *oral* LOLA, in a dose of 6 g three times per day, confers some benefit but only in patients with at least Grade II encephalopathy [141]. This difference in the apparent efficacy of LOLA depending on its route of administration may be explained by the fact that most of the aspartate undergoes transamination in the intestinal mucosa so its efficacy when given orally depends largely on the effects of the ornithine moiety alone. Overall, however, the evidence for a beneficial effect of oral LOLA is not strong [142].

Branched-chain amino acids

Plasma branched chain amino acids (BCAA) are reduced in patients with cirrhosis while plasma aromatic amino acids are increased. These disturbances have been linked to the changes in cerebral neurotransmitter balance observed in hepatic encephalopathy and thus attempts have been made to treat the syndrome with BCAA. Significant increases in cerebral perfusion were observed, in several brain areas, following both intravenous and oral BCAA, suggesting a direct effect on cerebral function [143,144]. However, the results of the clinical trials are conflicting although there is a general consensus that BCAA supplementation is not an effective treatment for hepatic encephalopathy *per se* [145]. Nevertheless, there is evidence, from two long-term studies, that BCAA supplementation may have beneficial effects on nutrition and progression-free survival [146,147]. The mechanism of these beneficial effects is unknown. Leucine is a potent stimulator of the production of hepatocyte growth factor by stellate cells [148] so it might stimulate liver regeneration, thereby compensating for progressive liver cell death.

Probiotics

The first attempts to treat hepatic encephalopathy by populating the colonic lumen with non-urease-producing bacteria, so called probiotics, were first undertaken more than 30 years ago [149,150]. Subsequently, a number of studies have been undertaken using a variety of probiotic and symbiotic (probiotic plus fermentable fibre) preparations. The studies are very heterogeneous and not easily compared [113,151–153]. However, patients treated with these preparations generally show improvement in their neuropsychiatric status comparable to that achieved with lactulose [152,153]. Treatment adherence is excellent and few adverse effects have been reported.

Sodium benzoate

Sodium benzoate is used to treat individuals with urea cycle enzyme deficiencies because it metabolically fixes ammonia by utilizing alternative pathways for waste nitrogen excretion; it conjugates with glycine and the excess nitrogen is excreted in the urine as hippurate. In the only large, randomized, controlled trial, available to date, this compound was equally as efficacious as lactulose for the treatment of hepatic encephalopathy but possibly less well tolerated [154]. The recommended dose is 5 g twice daily but patients rarely tolerate more than 2 g twice daily, because of the gastrointestinal side effects. The sodium content is also a concern.

Zinc

Zinc is an essential trace element and is a component of many metalloenzymes and metal–protein complexes such as metallothionine. Poor zinc status impairs nitrogen metabolism by reducing the activity of urea cycle enzymes in the liver and of glutamine synthetase in muscle. Zinc deficiency may play a role in the pathogenesis of hepatic encephalopathy; serum zinc concentrations are reduced in these patients and correlate inversely with blood ammonia concentrations [155].

A small number of controlled studies have been undertaken [114] but do not provide clear evidence for a beneficial effect of zinc supplementation in this condition. There are also questions about the long-term safety of zinc supplementation, which need to be resolved.

Flumazenil

Deficits in GABAergic neurotransmission and increases in circulating benzodiazepine-like ligands have been identified in patient with hepatic encephalopathy. Flumazenil is a selective benzodiazepine-receptor antagonist which, when infused intravenously, can induce transient, variable but sometimes significant, short-term improvement in hepatic encephalopathy in some patient with cirrhosis [156]. However, it has no significant effect on overall recovery or survival. It is not recommended for routine clinical use.

Shunt occlusion

Many patients with persistent hepatic encephalopathy have evidence of significant spontaneous portal–systemic shunting [157]. These patients often have well-preserved liver function but respond poorly, if at all, to standard treatment. Interventional radiological techniques can be used to close the shunts. Options include: vascular embolization [158], vascular plugging with an Amplatzer device [159], and balloon occlusion [160]. Laparoscopic disconnection, which is particularly suitable for paraumbilical vein shunts, is also an option [161].

TIPS insertion is complicated, in a minority of patients, by the development of persistent, disabling hepatic encephalopathy, which is difficult to treat. Reduction or even occlusion of the TIPS may be required [162]. Patients with surgically created shunts can develop debilitating hepatic encephalopathy. Attempts can be made to block these non-invasively but they may need to be operatively disconnected.

Shunt occlusion should be considered as a prelude to transplantation, particularly in those with TIPS or surgical shunts, if they are otherwise suitable.

Liver transplantation

The development of hepatic encephalopathy has a significant negative effect on survival in patients with cirrhosis [79]. The Model of End-stage Liver Disease (MELD) system used to prioritize patients on liver transplant lists does not include information on neuropsychiatric status. Thus, at present, no priority is give to patients with severe recurrent or persistent hepatic encephalopathy. The effect of hepatic encephalopathy on survival is independent of MELD so its inclusion in this scoring system might provide additional prognostic information [163]. Selection for transplantation, if based solely on the presence of hepatic encephalopathy, particularly if liver function is well preserved, requires careful exclusion of other neuropsychiatric conditions and clear evidence of an inadequate response to the best possible therapy.

The features of overt hepatic encephalopathy usually resolve following liver transplantation, even in patients with major physical manifestations such as spastic paraparesis [164,165] and parkinsonian features resistant to treatment [166]. In addition, resolution of the EEG [167], cerebral MRI, cerebral MRS [76,168] and cerebral PET abnormalities [169] have also been reported. Cognitive function also improves following transplantation but

not necessarily completely [170–173]. This may reflect: (1) unmasking of other pre-existing but unrecognized abnormalities; (2) the development of neurological complications of the transplant procedure such as intra-operative hypoxia, osmotic and other metabolic stresses [174]; (3) the effects of immunosuppressive therapy and; (4) the effects of of comorbidities such as systemic hypertension and diabetes.

The prevalence of neurological complications following liver transplantation is 10 to 47% [174]. Neuropathological abnormalities have been described in 60 to 70% of transplant recipients who die [175]. Patients with hepatic encephalopathy are more at risk of perioperative neurological insults and to the neurotoxic effects of immunosuppressive agents. Hepatic encephalopathy is an important predictor of neurological dysfunction following transplantation [176].

Artificial liver support systems

Patients with decompensated cirrhosis who develop severe hepatic encephalopathy do not respond well to conventional therapy. Supporting the liver to allow time for correction of any precipitating events might aid recovery or act as a bridge to transplantation.

The Molecular Adsorption Recirculating System (MARS; Teraklin AG, Rostock, Germany) is the most extensively studied of the artificial liver support systems. It purifies the blood by removal of both lipophilic albumin-bound and water-soluble molecules. The system might benefit patients with hepatic encephalopathy by removing circulating ammonia, endotoxin and inflammatory mediators, and by improving cerebral haemodynamics.

In a large controlled trial, patients with cirrhosis and severe hepatic encephalopathy treated with MARS dialysis showed earlier improvement in their mental state than those treated conventionally [177] but no difference in survival.

Colectomy/ colonic exclusion

Surgical approaches to reducing the intestinal production of ammonia, such as colectomy or colonic exclusion, have been used to treat hepatic encephalopathy refractory to other measures [178]. The operative morbidity and mortality rates are high. Today these patients would be considered for liver transplantation.

Potential future therapies

The treatment of hepatic encephalopathy is largely based on strategies aimed at reducing the production and absorption of ammonia from the colon. However, other sites, for example the small intestine, kidney and muscle, are also involved in the metabolism of ammonia and may provide targets for future therapy (Fig. 8.15).

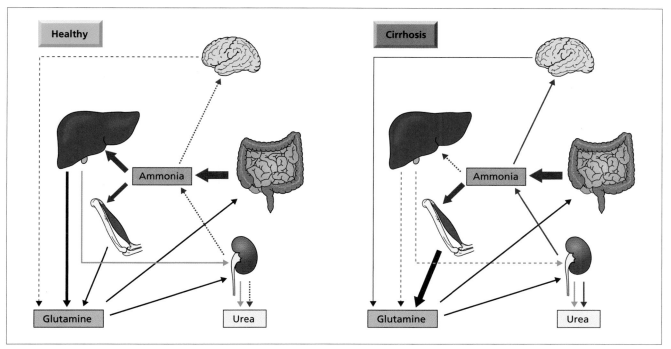

Fig. 8.15. A simple schematic of interorgan trafficking of ammonia both in healthy individuals and in patients with cirrhosis. Red arrows, ammonia; black arrows, glutamine; green arrows, urea. Ammonia is produced in the intestine from dietary protein, deamination of glutamine via glutaminase and bacterial action in the colon. It is also produced in the kidney from glutamine via glutaminase. In healthy individuals, the ammonia generated in the gut and kidney is metabolized in the periportal hepatocytes to form urea, which is then excreted in the urine. A small proportion is detoxified to glutamine via glutamine synthetase (GS) in the perivenous hepatocytes. Ammonia is also detoxified to glutamine in muscle and, to a much lesser extent, in the brain, via GS. A small proportion of the ammonia produced by the kidney is excreted in the urine. The glutamine produced in the liver, skeletal muscle and brain is released back into the circulation and subsequently undergoes degradation by glutaminase in the gut and kidney to form ammonia. In patients with cirrhosis, circulating ammonia levels rise because the liver's capacity for urea synthesis is reduced and portal–systemic shunting allows blood to bypasses the main route of ammonia detoxification. Under these circumstances the synthesis of glutamine via GS becomes the most important, though temporary, pathway for ammonia detoxification. In the presence of hyperammonaemia a greater proportion of the ammonia generated in the kidney is released into urine reducing the amount released into the systemic circulation. Additional ammonia is also detoxified in muscle with the production of glutamine; this is in turn broken down to ammonia by glutaminase in enterocytes or else excreted by the kidney as ammonia. Likewise additional ammonia is metabolized to glutamine in the brain but the capacity is small compared to that of skeletal muscle.

The intestine is an important source of ammonia generation through the uptake and breakdown of glutamine by enterocytes [179]. Non-absorbable disaccharides interfere directly with the uptake of glutamine by the intestinal wall and its subsequent metabolism [120]. Phosphate-activated glutaminase (PAG) is the main glutamine-catabolizing enzyme in the small intestine. Duodenal PAG activity is nearly four times higher in patients with cirrhosis than in healthy controls [180]; the major factors regulating intestinal ammonia production in cirrhotic patients, via PAG, are portal hypertension and systemic inflammation. Inhibiting PAG activity in the small intestine might reduce circulating blood ammonia levels with therapeutic benefit.

The kidneys both produce and excrete ammonia [181]. In patients with cirrhosis plasma expansion leads to an increase in renal ammonia excretion and a reduction in plasma ammonia. Thus, the kidneys can be manipulated to facilitate ammonia excretion [182].

Ammonia can be detoxified in muscle when circulating ammonia levels are high, through conversion to glutamine [183]. Ornithine promotes glutamine synthesis in the muscles; phenylacetate facilitates renal excretion of glutamine as phenylacetylglutamine. Preliminary studies in animal models indicate that the compound ornithine phenylacetate may be of value for treating hepatic encephalopathy [184].

In addition, a number of other potentially important pathogenic mechanisms have been identified, in recent years, which suggest possible alternative treatment approaches in man.

L-*carnitine.* This is used therapeutically to treat hyperammonaemia in children with urea-cycle enzyme deficiencies [185] and valproate-induced hyperammonaemia [186]. The protective effects of L-carnitine are centrally mediated by activation of metabotropic glutamate receptors (mGluR) at the level of brain ammonia uptake and/or mitochondrial energy metabolism. Preliminary studies have been undertaken in patients with hepatic encephalopathy but have not been monitored objectively [187].

Rivastigmine. Acetylcholine levels are considerably reduced in the brains of patients with cirrhosis dying in hepatic coma. Rivastigmine, a reversible cholinesterase inhibitor, improves psychometric performance in patient with hepatic encephalopathy when used together with lactulose [110].

Endocarbinoids. Neural intoxication in hepatic encephalopathy disrupts cerebral energy flux; AMP-activated protein kinase (AMPK) rehabilitates cellular energy stores in response to metabolic injury; its activity can be augmented by cannabinoid compounds. Animal studies have confirmed that pharmacological activation of AMPK by endocarbinoids confers neuroprotection in hepatic encephalopathy [188,189].

Sildenafil. Alterations in the function of the glutamate–nitric oxide–cGMP pathway and the subsequent decrease in extracellular cGMP in brain may be responsible for the impairment in learning ability and intellectual function in patients with hepatic encephalopathy. Pharmacological modulation of extracellular cGMP concentrations using sildenafil, an inhibitor of the phosphodiesterase that crosses the blood–brain barrier, restores learning ability in animal models [190].

mGluR1 antagonists. Alterations in glutamatergic neurotransmission in the substantia nigra pars reticulata may contribute to the psychomotor slowing and hypokinesia observed in patients with hepatic encephalopathy. Blocking mGluR1 at this site normalizes motor activity in a rat model of hepatic encephalopathy [191].

Systemic inflammation. Modulation of the systemic inflammatory response with, for example, anti-inflammatory agents, should be explored with the obvious caveats governing use of these agents in patients with cirrhosis.

Finally, a *symptom-related approach* should be considered for some of the more distinct clinical symptoms associated with hepatic encephalopathy such as daytime sleep disturbances, extrapyramidal symptoms, mood disturbances and cognitive decline.

Prevention

All patients with newly diagnosed cirrhosis should be screened for hepatic encephalopathy. Those with obvious features of the syndrome should be further assessed and treatment instigated. Patients with more advanced disease, those with large spontaneous or created portal–systemic shunts and those who have already experienced an episode(s) of overt hepatic encephalopathy are at high risk. They should be given long-life preventative treatment. Long-term treatment should also be considered in patients with minimal hepatic encephalopathy because of its detrimental effects on their health-related quality of life and their risk of developing overt hepatic encephalopathy. However, issues of compliance and the possible adverse events and costs of long-term treatment need to be considered.

References

1 Weissenborn K. Diagnosis of encephalopathy. *Digestion* 1998; **59** (Suppl. 2): 22–24.
2 Ferenci P, Lockwood A, Mullen K *et al.* Hepatic encephalopathy–definition, nomenclature, diagnosis, and quantification: Final report of the working party at the 11th World Congresses of Gastroenterology, Vienna, 1998. *Hepatology* 2002; **35**: 716–721.
3 Montagnese S, Middleton B, Skene D *et al.* Night-time sleep disturbance does not correlate with neuropsychiatric impairment in patients with cirrhosis. *Liver Int.* 2009; **29**: 1372–1382.
4 Challenger F, Walshe JM. Methyl mercaptan in relation to foetor hepaticus. *Biochem. J.* 1955; **59**: 372–375.
5 Victor M, Adams RD, Cole M. The acquired (non Wilsonian) type of chronic hepatocerebral degeneration. *Medicine* 1965; **44**: 345–396.
6 Krieger S, Jauss M, Jansen O *et al.* Neuropsychiatric profile and hyperintense globus pallidus on T1-weighted magnetic resonance images in liver cirrhosis. *Gastroenterology* 1996; **111**: 147–155.
7 Cadranel JF, Lebiez E, DiMartino V *et al.* Focal neurological signs in hepatic encephalopathy in cirrhotic patients: An underestimated entity? *Am. J. Gastroenterol.* 2001; **96**: 515–518.
8 Joebges EM, Heidemann M, Schimke N *et al.* Bradykinesia in minimal hepatic encephalopathy is due to disturbances in movement initiation. *J. Hepatol.* 2003; **38**: 273–280.
9 Miyata Y, Motomura S, Tsuji Y *et al.* Hepatic encephalopathy and reversible cortical blindness. *Am. J. Gastroenterol.* 1988; **83**: 780–782.
10 Averbuch-Heller L, Meiner Z. Reversible periodic alternating gaze deviation in hepatic encephalopathy. *Neurology* 1995; **45**: 191–192.
11 Gilberstadt SJ, Gilberstadt H, Zieve L *et al.* Psychomotor performance defects in cirrhotic patients without overt encephalopathy. *Arch. Intern. Med.* 1980; **140**: 519–521.
12 Schomerus H, Hamster W. Neuropsychological aspects of portal–systemic encephalopathy. *Metab. Brain. Dis.* 1998; **13**: 361–377.
13 Parsons-Smith BG, Summerskill WHJ, Dawson AM *et al.* The electroencephalograph in liver disease. *Lancet* 1957; **2**: 867–871.

14 Van der Rijt CC, Schalm SW, De Groot GH *et al.* Objective measurement of hepatic encephalopathy by means of automated EEG analysis. *Electroencephalogr. Clin. Neurophysiol.* 1984; **7**: 423–426.

15 Chu NS, Yang SS, Liaw YF. Evoked potentials in liver diseases. *J. Gastroenterol. Hepatol.* 1997; **12**: S288–S293.

16 Amodio P, Del Piccolo F, Pettenò E *et al.* Prevalence and prognostic value of quantified electroencephalogram (EEG) alterations in cirrhotic patients. *J. Hepatol.* 2001; **35**: 37–45.

17 Montagnese S, Jackson C, Morgan MY. Spatio-temporal decomposition of the electroencephalogram in patients with cirrhosis. *J. Hepatol.* 2007; **46**: 447–458.

18 Taylor-Robinson SD, Sargentoni J, Mallalieu RJ *et al.* Cerebral phosphorus-31 magnetic resonance spectroscopy in patients with chronic hepatic encephalopathy. *Hepatology* 1994; **20**: 1173–1178.

19 Taylor-Robinson SD, Sargentoni J, Marcus CD *et al.* Regional variations in cerebral proton spectroscopy in patients with chronic hepatic encephalopathy. *Metab. Brain Dis.* 1994; **9**: 347–359.

20 O'Carroll RE, Hayes PC, Ebmeier KP *et al.* Regional cerebral blood flow and cognitive function in patients with chronic liver disease. *Lancet* 1991; **337**: 1250–1253.

21 Lockwood AH, Murphy BW, Donnelly KZ *et al.* Positron-emission tomographic localization of abnormalities of brain metabolism in patients with minimal hepatic encephalopathy. *Hepatology* 1993; **18**: 1061–1068.

22 Häussinger D, Kircheis G, Fischer R *et al.* Hepatic encephalopathy in chronic liver disease: A clinical manifestation of astrocyte swelling and low-grade cerebral edema? *J. Hepatol.* 2000; **32**: 1035–1038.

23 Batki G, Fisch HU, Karlaganis G *et al.* Mechanism of the selective response of cirrhotics to benzodiazepines. Model experiments with triazolam. *Hepatology* 1987; **7**: 629–638.

24 Bajaj JS, Schubert CM, Heuman DM *et al.* Persistence of cognitive impairment after resolution of overt hepatic encephalopathy. *Gastroenterology* 2010; **138**: 2332–2340.

25 Conn HO, Rössle M, Levy L *et al.* Portosystemic myelopathy: spastic paraparesis after portosystemic shunting. *Scand. J. Gastroenterol.* 2006; **41**: 619–625.

26 Pinarbasi B, Kaymakoglu S, Matur Z *et al.* Are acquired hepatocerebral degeneration and hepatic myelopathy reversible? *J. Clin. Gastroenterol.* 2009; **43**: 176–181.

27 Rikkers L, Jenko P, Rudman D *et al.* Subclinical hepatic encephalopathy: Detection, prevalence, and relationship to nitrogen metabolism. *Gastroenterology* 1978; **75**: 462–469.

28 Groeneweg M, Quero JC, De Bruijn I *et al.* Subclinical hepatic encephalopathy impairs daily functioning. *Hepatology* 1998; **28**: 45–49.

29 Schomerus H, Hamster W. Quality of life in cirrhotics with minimal hepatic encephalopathy. *Metab. Brain Dis.* 2001; **16**: 37–41.

30 Schomerus H, Hamster W, Blunck H *et al.* Latent portasystemic encephalopathy. I. Nature of cerebral functional defects and their effect on fitness to drive. *Dig. Dis. Sci.* 1981; **26**: 622–630.

31 Kircheis G, Knoche A, Hilger N *et al.* Hepatic encephalopathy and fitness to drive. *Gastroenterology* 2009; **137**: 1706–1715.

32 Amodio P, Del Piccolo F, Marchetti P *et al.* Clinical features and survival of cirrhotic patients with subclinical cognitive alterations detected by the number connection test and computerized psychometric tests. *Hepatology* 1999; **29**: 1662–1667.

33 Das A, Dhiman RK, Saraswat VA *et al.* Prevalence and natural history of subclinical hepatic encephalopathy in cirrhosis. *J. Gastroenterol. Hepatol.* 2001; **16**: 531–535.

34 Saxena N, Bhatia M, Joshi YK *et al.* Auditory P300 event-related potentials and number connection test for evaluation of subclinical hepatic encephalopathy in patients with cirrhosis of the liver: A follow-up study. *J. Gastroenterol. Hepatol.* 2001; **16**: 322–327.

35 Montagnese S, Amodio P, Morgan MY. Methods for diagnosing hepatic encephalopathy in patients with cirrhosis: a multidimensional approach. *Metab. Brain Dis.* 2004; **19**: 281–312.

36 Conn HO, Leevy CM, Vlahcevic ZR *et al.* Comparison of lactulose and neomycin in the treatment of chronic portal-systemic encephalopathy. A double blind controlled trial. *Gastroenterology* 1977; **72**: 573–583.

37 Blei AT, Córdoba J. Hepatic encephalopathy. *Am. J. Gastroenterol.* 2001; **96**: 1968–1976.

38 Amodio P, Montagnese S, Gatta A *et al.* Characteristics of minimal hepatic encephalopathy. *Metab. Brain Dis.* 2004; **19**: 253–267.

39 Teasdale G, Jennett B. Assessment of coma and impaired consciousness. A practical scale. *Lancet* 1974; **2**: 81–84.

40 Hodkinson HM. Evaluation of a mental test score for assessment of mental impairment in the elderly. *Age Ageing* 1972; **1**: 233–238.

41 Folstein MF, Folstein SE, McHugh PR. 'Mini-mental state.' A practical method for grading the cognitive state of patients for the clinician. *J. Psychiatr. Res.* 1975; **12**: 189–198.

42 Randolph C, Hilsabeck R, Kato A *et al.* Neuropsychological assessment of hepatic encephalopathy: ISHEN practice guidelines. *Liver Int.* 2009; **29**: 629–635.

43 Tarter RE, Hegedus AM, Van Thiel DH *et al.* Nonalcoholic cirrhosis associated with neuropsychological dysfunction in the absence of overt evidence of hepatic encephalopathy. *Gastroenterology* 1984; **86**: 1421–1427.

44 Weissenborn K, Ennen JC, Schomerus H *et al.* Neuropsychological characterization of hepatic encephalopathy. *J. Hepatol.* 2001; **34**: 768–773.

45 Amodio P, Marchetti P, Del Piccolo F *et al.* Study on the Sternberg paradigm in cirrhotic patients without overt hepatic encephalopathy. *Metab. Brain Dis.* 1998; **13**: 159–172.

46 Guérit J-M, Amantini A, Fischer C *et al.* Neurophysiological investigations of hepatic encephalopathy: ISHEN practice guidelines. *Liver Int.* 2009; **29**: 789–796.

47 Kaplan PW. The EEG in metabolic encephalopathy and coma. *J. Clin. Neurophysiol.* 2004; **21**: 307–318.

48 Amodio P, Marchetti P, Del Piccolo F *et al.* Spectral versus visual EEG analysis in mild hepatic encephalopathy. *Clin. Neurophysiol.* 1999; **110**: 1334–1344.

49 Weissenborn K, Scholz M, Hinrichs H *et al.* Neuropsychological assessment of early hepatic encephalopathy. *Electroencephalogr. Clin. Neurophysiol.* 1990; **75**: 289–295.

50 Pellegrini A, Ubiali E, Orsato R *et al.* Electroencephalographic staging of hepatic encephalopathy by an artificial neural network and an expert system. *Clin. Neurophysiol.* 2005; **35**: 162–167.

51 Kircheis G, Wettstein M, Timmermann L *et al.* Critical flicker frequency for quantification of low-grade hepatic encephalopathy. *Hepatology* 2002; **35**: 357–366.

52 Romero-Gómez M, Córdoba J, Jover R *et al.* Value of the critical flicker frequency in patients with minimal hepatic encephalopathy. *Hepatology* 2007; **45**: 879–885.

53 Sharma P, Sharma BC, Puri V *et al.* Critical flicker frequency: diagnostic tool for minimal hepatic encephalopathy. *J. Hepatol.* 2007; **47**: 67–73.

54 Kircheis G, Bode JG, Hilger N *et al.* Diagnostic and prognostic values of critical flicker frequency determination as new diagnostic tool for objective HE evaluation in patients undergoing TIPS implantation. *Eur J. Gastroenterol. Hepatol.* 2009; **21**: 1383–1394.

55 Sharma P, Sharma BC, Sarin SK. Critical flicker frequency for diagnosis and assessment of recovery from minimal hepatic encephalopathy in patients with cirrhosis. *Hepatobiliary Pancreat. Dis. Int.* 2010; **9**: 27–32.

56 Montagnese S, Gordon HM, Jackson C *et al.* Disruption of smooth pursuit eye movements in cirrhosis: relationship to hepatic encephalopathy and its treatment. *Hepatology* 2005; **42**: 772–781.

57 Mullen KD, Amodio P, Morgan MY. Therapeutic studies in hepatic encephalopathy. *Metab. Brain Dis.* 2007; **22**: 407–423.

58 Berding G, Banati RB, Buchert R *et al.* Radiotracer imaging studies in hepatic encephalopathy: ISHEN practice guidelines. *Liver Int.* 2009; **29**: 621–628.

59 Morgan MY. Cerebral magnetic resonance imaging in patients with chronic liver disease. *Metab. Brain Dis.* 1998; **13**: 273–290.

60 Grover VPB, Dresner MA, Forton DM *et al.* Current and future applications of magnetic resonance imaging and spectroscopy of the brain in hepatic encephalopathy. *World J. Gastroenterol.* 2006; **12**: 2969–2978.

61 Inoue E, Hori S, Narumi Y *et al.* Portal-systemic encephalopathy: presence of basal ganglia lesions with high signal intensity on MR images. *Radiology* 1991; **179**: 551–555.

62 Pujol A, Pujol J, Graus F *et al.* Hyperintense globus pallidus on T1-weighted MRI in cirrhotic patients is associated with severity of liver failure. *Neurology* 1993; **43**: 65–69.

63 Thuluvath PJ, Edwin D, Yue NC *et al.* Increased signals seen in the globus pallidus in T1-weighted magnetic resonance imaging in cirrhotics are not suggestive of chronic hepatic encephalopathy. *Hepatology* 1996; **24**: 282–283.

64 Nolte W, Wiltfang J, Schindler C *et al.* Portosystemic hepatic encephalopathy after transjugular intrahepatic portosystemic shunt in patients with cirrhosis: clinical, laboratory, psychometric and electroencephalographic investigations. *Hepatology* 1998; **28**: 1215–1225.

65 Rose C, Butterworth RF, Zayed J *et al.* Manganese deposition in basal ganglia structures results from both portal-systemic shunting and liver dysfunction. *Gastroenterology* 1999; **117**: 640–644.

66 Jayakumar AR, Rama Rao KV, Kalaiselvi P *et al.* Combined effects of ammonia and manganese on astrocytesin cluture. *Neurochem. Res.* 2004; **29**: 2051–2056.

67 Ahboucha S, Butterworth RF. The neurosteroid system: Implication in the pathogenesis of hepatic encephalopathy. *Neurochem. Int.* 2008; **52**: 575–587.

68 Córdoba J, Sanpedro F, Alonso J, Rovira A. 1H magnetic resonance in the study of hepatic encephalopathy in humans. *Metab. Brain Dis.* 2002; **17**: 415-429.

69 Kramer L, Tribl B, Gendo A *et al.* Partial pressure of ammonia versus ammonia in hepatic encephalopathy. *Hepatology* 2000; **31**: 30–34.

70 Hourani BT, Hamilin EM, Reynolds TB. Cerebrospinal fluid glutamine as a measure of hepatic encephalopathy. *Arch. Intern. Med.* 1971; **127**: 1033–1036.

71 Victor M, Adams RD, Cole M. The acquired (non-Wilsonian) type of chronic hepatocellular degeneration. *Medicine* 1965; **44**: 345–396.

72 Kril JJ, Butterworth RF. Diencephalic and cerebellar pathology in alcoholic and nonalcoholic patients with end-stage liver disease. *Hepatology* 1997; **26**: 837–841.

73 Córdoba J, García-Martinez R, Simón-Talero M. Hyponatremic and hepatic encephalopathies: similarities, differences and coexistence. *Metab. Brain Dis.* 2010; **25**: 73–80.

74 Angeli P, Wong F, Watson H *et al.* Hyponatremia in cirrhosis: results of a patient population survey. *Hepatology* 2006; **44**: 1535–1542.

75 Guevara M, Baccaro ME, Torre A *et al.* Hyponatremia is a risk factor of hepatic encephalopathy in patients with cirrhosis: a prospective study with time-dependent analysis. *Am. J. Gastroenterol.* 2009; **104**: 1382–1389.

76 García Martínez R, Rovira A, Alonso J *et al.* A long-term study of changes in the volume of brain ventricles and white matter lesions after successful liver transplantation. *Transplantation* 2010; **89**: 589–594.

77 Rovira A, Mínguez B, Aymerich FX *et al.* Decreased white matter lesion volume and improved cognitive function after liver transplantation. *Hepatology* 2007; **46**: 1485–1490.

78 Poordad FF. Review article: the burden of hepatic encephalopathy. *Aliment. Pharmacol. Ther.* 2007; **25** (Suppl. 1): 3–9.

79 Bustamante J, Rimola A, Ventura PJ *et al.* Prognostic significance of hepatic encephalopathy in patients with cirrhosis. *J. Hepatol.* 1999; **30**: 890–895.

80 Lustik SJ, Chhibber AK, Kolano JW *et al.* The hyperventilation of cirrhosis: progesterone and estradiol effects. *Hepatology* 1997; **25**: 55–58.

81 Baertt JM, Sancetta SM, Gabuzda GJ. Relation of acute potassium depletion to the renal ammonia metabolism in patients with cirrhosis. *N. Eng. J. Med.* 1964; **271**: 1229–1235.

82 Lockwood AH, Yap EW, Wong WH. Cerebral ammonia metabolism in patients with severe liver disease and minimal hepatic encephalopathy. *J. Cereb. Blood Flow Metab.*1991; **11**: 337–341.

83 Szerb JC, Butterworth RF. Effect of ammonium ions on synaptic transmission in the mammalian central nervous system. *Prog. Neurobiol.* 1992; **39**: 135–153.

84 Lai JC, Cooper AJ. Brain alpha-ketoglutarate dehydrogenase complex; kinetic properties, regional distribution, and effects of inhibitors. *J. Neurochem.* 1986; **47**: 1376–1386.

85 Bruton CJ, Corsellis JA, Russell A. Hereditary hyperammonaemia. *Brain* 1970; **93**: 423–434.

86 Haseler LJ, Sibbitt WL Jr, Mojtahedzadeh HN *et al.* Proton MR spectroscopic measurement of neurometabolites in hepatic encephalopathy during oral lactulose therapy. *Am. J. Neuroradiol.* 1998; **19**: 1681–1686.

87 Riggio O, Mannaioni G, Ridola L *et al.* Peripheral and splanchnic indole and oxindole levels in cirrhotic patients: a study on the pathophysiology of hepatic encephalopathy. *Am. J. Gastroenterol.* 2010; **105**: 1374–1381.

88 Häussinger D, Laubenberger J, vom Dahl S *et al.* Proton magnetic resonance spectroscopy on human brain myo-inositol in hypoosmolarity and hepatic encephalopathy. *Gastroenterology* 1994; **107**: 1475–1480.

89 Córdoba J, Alonso J, Rovira A *et al.* The development of low grade cerebral edema in cirrhosis is supported by the evolution of 1H-magnetic resonance abnormalities after liver transplantation. *J. Hepatol.* 2001; **35**: 598–604.

90 Kale RA, Gupta RK, Saraswat VA *et al.* Demonstration of interstitial cerebral edema with diffusion tensor MR imaging in type C hepatic encephalopathy. *Hepatology* 2006; **43**: 698–706.

91 Shah NJ, Neeb H, Kircheis G *et al.* Quantitative T1 and water content mapping in hepatic encephalopathy. In: Häussinger D, Kircheis G, Schliess F, eds. *Hepatic Encephalopathy and Nitrogen Metabolism.* Doordrecht, The Netherlands: Springer Verlag 2006, pp. 273–283.

92 Laubenberger J, Häussinger D, Bayer S *et al.* Proton magnetic resonance spectroscopy of the brain in symptomatic and asymptomatic patients with liver cirrhosis. *Gastroenterology* 1997; **112**: 610–616.

93 Häussinger D, Schliess F. Pathogenetic mechanisms in hepatic encephalopathy. *Gut* 2008; **57**: 1156–1165.

94 Bemeur C, Desjardins P, Butterworth RF. Evidence for oxidative/ nitrosative stress in the pathogenesis of hepatic encephalopathy. *Metab. Brain Dis.* 2010; **25**: 3–9.

95 Song G, Dhodda VK, Blei AT *et al.* GeneChip analysis shows altered mRNA expression of transcripts of neurotransmitter and signal transduction pathways in the cerebral cortex of portacaval shunted rats. *J. Neurosci. Res.* 2002; **68**: 730–737.

96 Felipo V, Butterworth RF. Neurobiology of ammonia. *Prog. Neurobiol.* 2002; **67**: 259–279.

97 Zhou BG, Norenberg MD. Ammonia downregulates GLAST mRNA glutamate transporter in rat astrocyte cultures. *Neurosci. Lett.* 1999; **276**: 145–148.

98 Chan H, Zwingmann C, Pannunzio M *et al.* Effects of ammonia on high affinity glutamate uptake and glutamate transporter EAAT3 expression in cultured rat cerebellar granule cells. *Neurochem. Int.* 2003; **43**: 137–146.

99 Barbaro G, Di Lorenzo G, Soldini M *et al.* Flumazenil for hepatic encephalopathy grade III and IVa in patients with cirrhosis: an Italian multicentre double-blind, placebo-controlled, cross-over study. *Hepatology* 1998; **28**: 374–378.

100 Mousseau DD, Baker GB, Butterworth RF. Increased density of catalytic sites and expression of brain monoamine oxidase A in humans with hepatic encephalopathy. *J. Neurochem.* 1997; **68**: 1200–1208.

101 Bergeron M, Reader TA, Layrargues GP *et al.* Monoamines and metabolites in autopsied brain tissue from cirrhotic patients with hepatic encephalopathy. *Neurochem. Res.* 1989; **14**: 853–859.

102 Rao VL, Butterworth RF. Alterations of [3H]8-OH-DPAT and [3H]ketanserin binding sites in autopsied brain tissue from cirrhotic patients with hepatic encephalopathy. *Neurosci. Lett.* 1994; **182**: 69–72.

103 Vorobioff J, Garcia-Tsao G, Groszmann R *et al.* Long-term haemodynamic effects of ketanserin, a 5-hydroxytryptamine blocker, in portal hypertensive patients. *Hepatology* 1989; **9**: 88–91.

104 Rao VL, Giguère JF, Layrargues GP *et al.* Increased activities of MAOA and MAOB in autopsied brain tissue from cirrhotic patients with hepatic encephalopathy. *Brain Res.* 1993; **621**: 349–352.

105 Mousseau DD, Perney P, Layrargues GP *et al.* Selective loss of pallidal dopamine D2 receptor density in hepatic encephalopathy. *Neurosci. Lett.* 1993; **162**: 192–196.

106 Butterworth RF, Spahr L, Fontaine S *et al.* Manganese toxicity, dopaminergic dysfunction and hepatic encephalopathy. *Metab. Brain Dis.* 1995; **10**: 259–267.

107 Morgan MY, Jakobovits AW, James IM *et al.* Successful use of bromocriptine in the treatment of chronic hepatic encephalopathy. *Gastroenterology* 1980; **78**: 663–670.

108 García-Ayllón MS, Cauli O, Silveyra MX *et al.* Brain cholinergic impairment in liver failure. *Brain* 2008; **131**: 2946–2956.

109 Palomero-Gallagher N, Bidmon HJ, Cremer M *et al.* Neurotransmitter receptor imbalances in motor cortex and basal ganglia in hepatic encephalopathy. *Cell Physiol. Biochem.* 2009; **24**: 291–306.

110 Basu P, Shah NJ, Krishnaswamy N *et al.* Transdermal rivastigmine for treatment of encephalopathy in liver cirrhosis—a randomized placebo controlled trial (TREC Trial). *J. Hepatol.* 2010; **52** (Suppl. 1): S67, 152 (abstract).

111 Cunha RA. Neuroprotection by adenosine in the brain: from A_1 receptor activation to A_{2A} receptor blockade. *Purinergic Signal* 2005; **1**: 111–134.

112 Shawcross DL, Shabbir SS, Taylor NJ *et al.* Ammonia and neutrophil in the pathogenesis of hepatic encephalopathy in cirrhosis. *Hepatology* 2010; **51**: 1062–1069.

113 Liu Q, Duan ZP, Ha DK *et al.* Synbiotic modulation of gut flora: effect on minimal hepatic encephalopathy in patients with cirrhosis. *Hepatology* 2004; **39**: 1441–1449.

114 Morgan MY, Blei A, Grüngreiff K *et al.* The treatment of hepatic encephalopathy. *Metab. Brain Dis.* 2007; **22**: 389–405.

115 Riggio O, Ridola L. Emerging drugs for hepatic encephalopathy. *Expert Opin. Emerg. Drugs* 2009; **14**: 537–549.

116 Plauth M, Cabré E, Riggio O *et al.* ESPEN Guidelines on Enteral Nutrition: Liver disease. *Clin. Nutr.* 2006; **25**: 285–294.

117 Weber FL Jr, Banwell JG, Fresard KM *et al.* Nitrogen in fecal bacterial fibre, and soluble fractions of patients with cirrhosis: effects of lactulose and lactulose plus neomycin. *J. Lab. Clin. Med.* 1987; **110**: 259–263.

118 Córdoba J, López-Hellín J, Planas M *et al.* Normal protein diet for episodic hepatic encephalopathy: results of a randomized study. *J. Hepatol.* 2004; **41**: 38–43.

119 Uribe M, Campollo O, Vargas F *et al.* Acidifying enemas (lactitol and lactulose) vs. nonacidifying enemas (tapwater) to treat acute portal–systemic encephalopathy: a double-blind, randomised clinical trial. *Hepatology* 1987; **7**: 639–643.

120 van Leeuwen PA, van Berlo CL, Soeters PB. New mode of action for lactulose. *Lancet* 1988; **i**: 55–56.

121 Sharma P, Sharma BC, Sarin SK. Predictors of nonresponse to lactulose in patients with cirrhosis and hepatic encephalopathy. *Eur J. Gastroenterol. Hepatol.* 2010; **22**: 526–531.

122 Bajaj JS, Sanyal AJ, Bell D *et al.* Predictors of the recurrence of hepatic encephalopathy in lactulose-treated patients. *Aliment. Pharmacol. Ther.* 2010; **31**: 1012–1017.

123 Morgan MY, Hawley KM. Lactitol vs. lactulose in the treatment of acute hepatic encephalopathy in cirrhotic patients: a double-blind, randomized trial. *Hepatology* 1987; **7**: 1278–1284.

124 Morgan MY, Alonso M, Stranger LC. Lactitol and lactulose for the treatment of subclinical hepatic encephalopathy in cirrhotic patients. A randomized, cross-over study. *J. Hepatol.* 1989; **8**: 208–217.

125 Blanc P, Daures JP, Rouillon JM *et al.* Lactitol or lactulose in the treatment of chronic hepatic encephalopathy: results of a meta-analysis. *Hepatology* 1992; **15**: 222–228.

126 Als-Nielsen B, Gluud LL, Gluud C. Non-absorbable disaccharides for hepatic encephalopathy (Cochrane review). *Cochrane Database Syst. Rev.* 2004; **2**: CD003044.

127 Córdoba J, Mínguez B, Vergara M. Treatment of hepatic encephalopathy. *Lancet* 2005; **365**: 1384–1385.

128 Prasad S, Dhiman RK, Duseja A *et al.* Lactulose improves cognitive function and health-related quality of life in patients with cirrhosis who have minimal hepatic encephalopathy. *Hepatology* 2007; **45**: 549–559.

129 Strauss E, Tramote R, Silva EP *et al.* Double-blind randomized clinical trial comparing neomycin and placebo in the treatment of exogenous hepatic encephalopathy. *Hepatogastroenterology* 1992; **39**: 542–545.

130 Blanc P, Daures JP, Liautard J *et al.* Lactulose–neomycin combination versus placebo in the treatment of acute hepatic encephalopathy. Results of a randomized controlled trial. *Gastroenterol. Clin. Biol.* 1994; **18**: 1063–1068.

131 Bass NM. The current pharmacological therapies for hepatic encephalopathy. *Aliment. Pharmacol. Ther.* 2006; **25**: 23–31.

132 Bass NM, Mullen KD, Sanyal A *et al.* Rifaximin treatment in hepatic encephalopathy. *N. Engl. J. Med.* 2010; **362**: 1071–1081.

133 Leevy CB, Phillips JA. Hospitalizations during the use of rifaximin versus lactulose for the treatment of hepatic encephalopathy. *Dig. Dis. Sci.* 2007; **52**: 737–741.

134 Lighthouse J, Naito Y, Helmy A *et al.* Endotoxinemia and benzodiazepine-like substances in compensated cirrhotic patients: A randomized study comparing the effect of rifaximine alone and in association with a symbiotic preparation. *Hepatol. Res.* 2004; **28**: 155–160.

135 Weber FL, Jr. Lactulose and combination therapy of hepatic encephalopathy: the role of the intestinal microflora. *Dig. Dis.* 1996; **14** (Suppl. 1): 53–63.

136 Lanthier PL, Morgan MY, Ballantyne J. Bromocriptine-associated ototoxicity. *J. Laryngol. Otol.* 1984; **98**: 399–404.

137 Marshall AW, Jakobovits AW, Morgan MY. Bromocriptine-associated hyponatraemia in cirrhosis. *BMJ* 1982; **285**: 1534–1535.

138 Rose C, Michalak A, Pannunzio P *et al.* L-ornithine-L-aspartate in experimental portal-systemic encephalopathy: therapeutic efficacy and mechanism of action. *Metab. Brain Dis.* 1998; **13**: 147–157.

139 Kircheis G, Nilius R, Held C *et al.* Therapeutic efficacy of L-ornithine-L-aspartate infusions in patients with cirrhosis and hepatic encephalopathy: results of a placebo-controlled, double-blind study. *Hepatology* 1997; **25**: 1351–1360.

140 Ahmad I, Khan AA, Alam A *et al.* L-ornithine-L-aspartate infusion efficacy in hepatic encephalopathy. *J. Coll. Physicians Surg. Pak.* 2008; **18**: 684–687.

141 Stauch S, Kircheis G, Adler G *et al.* Oral L-ornithine-L-aspartate therapy of chronic hepatic encephalopathy: results of a placebo-controlled double-blind study. *J. Hepatol.* 1998; **28**: 856–864.

142 Soárez PC, Oliveira AC, Padovan J *et al.* A critical analysis of studies assessing L-ornithine-L-aspartate (LOLA) in hepatic encephalopathy treatment. *Arq. Gastroenterol.* 2009; **46**: 241–247.

143 Iwasa M, Matsumura K, Watanabe Y *et al.* Improvement of regional cerebral blood flow after treatment with branched-chain amino acid solutions in patients with cirrhosis. *Eur. J. Gastroenterol. Hepatol.* 2003; **15**: 733–737.

144 Yamamoto M, Iwasa M, Matsumura K *et al.* Improvement of regional cerebral blood flow after oral intake of branched-chain amino acids in patients with cirrhosis. *World J. Gastroenterol.* 2005; **11**: 6792–6799.

145 Als-Nielsen B, Koretz RL, Kjaergard LL *et al.* Branched-chain amino acids for hepatic encephalopathy. *Cochrane Database Syst. Rev.* 2003; **2**: CD001939.

146 Marchesini G, Bianchi G, Merli M *et al.* Nutritional supplementation with branched-chain amino acids in advanced cirrhosis: a double-blind, randomized trial. *Gastroenterology* 2003; **124**: 1792–1801.

147 Muto Y, Sato S, Watanabe A *et al.* Effects of oral branched-chain amino acid granules on event-free survival in patients with liver cirrhosis. *Clin. Gastroenterol. Hepatol.* 2005; **3**: 705–713.

148 Tomiya T, Inoue Y, Yanase M *et al.* Leucine stimulates the secretion of hepatocyte growth factor by hepatic stellate cells. *Biochem. Biophys. Res. Commun.* 2002; **297**: 1108–1111.

149 Macbeth WAAG, Kass EH, McDermott WV, Jr. Treatment of hepatic encephalopathy by alteration of intestinal flora and Lactobacillus acidophilus. *Lancet* 1965; **1**: 399–403.

150 Read AE, McCarthy CF, Heaton KW *et al. Lactobacillus acidophilus* (Enpac) in treatment of hepatic encephalopathy. *BMJ* 1966; **1**: 1267–1269.

151 Loguercio C, Abbiati R, Rinaldi M *et al.* Long-term effects of *Enterococcus faecium SF68* versus lactulose in the treatment of patients with cirrhosis and grade 1-2 hepatic encephalopathy. *J. Hepatol.* 1995; **23**: 39–46.

152 Sharma P, Sharma BC, Puri V *et al.* An open-label randomized controlled trial of lactulose and probiotics in the treatment of minimal hepatic encephalopathy. *Eur. J. Gastroenterol. Hepatol.* 2008; **20**: 506–511.

153 Malaguarnera M, Gargante MP, Malaguarnera G *et al.* Bifidobacterium combined with fructo-oligosaccharide versus lactulose in the treatment of patients with hepatic encephalopathy. *Eur. J. Gastroenterol. Hepatol.* 2010; **22**: 199–206.

154 Sushma S, Dasarathy S, Tandon RK *et al.* Sodium benzoate in the treatment of acute hepatic encephalopathy: a double-blind randomized trial. *Hepatology* 1992; **16**: 138–144.

155 Grüngreiff K, Presser HJ, Franke D *et al.* Correlations between zinc, amino acids and ammonia in liver cirrhosis. *Z. Gastroenterol.* 1989; **27**: 731–735.

156 Als-Nielsen B, Gluud LL, Gluud C. Benzodiazepine receptor antagonists for hepatic encephalopathy. *Cochrane Database Syst. Rev.* 2004; **2**: CD002798.

157 Riggio O, Efrati C, Catalano C *et al.* High prevalence of spontaneous portalsystemic shunts in persistent hepatic encephalopathy: a case-control study. *Hepatology* 2005; **42**: 1158–1165.

158 Kuramitsu T, Komatsu M, Matsudaira N *et al.* Portal-systemic encephalopathy from a spontaneous gastrorenal

shunt diagnosed by three-dimensional computed tomography and treated effectively by percutaneous vascular embolization. *Liver* 1998; **18**: 208–212.

159 Boixadera H, Tomasello A, Quiroga S *et al.* Successful embolization of a spontaneous mesocaval shunt using the Amplatzer Vascular Plug II. *Cardiovasc. Intervent. Radiol.* 2010; **33**: 1044–1048.

160 Kawanaka H, Ohta M, Hashizume M *et al.* Portosystemic encephalopathy treated with balloon-occluded retrograde transvenous obliteration. *Am. J. Gastroenterol.* 1995; **90**: 508–510.

161 Yamaguchi S, Kawanaka H, Konishi K *et al.* Laparoscopic disconnection of a huge paraumbilical vein shunt for portosystemic encephalopathy. *Surg. Laparosc. Endosc. Percutan. Tech.* 2007; **17**: 212–214.

162 Fanelli F, Salvatori FM, Rabuffi P *et al.* Management of refractory hepatic encephalopathy after insertion of TIPS: long-term results of shunt reduction with hourglass-shaped balloon-expandable stent-graft. *AJR Am. J. Roentgenol.* 2009; **193**: 1696–1702.

163 Stewart CA, Malinchoc M, Kim WR *et al.* Hepatic encephalopathy as a predictor of survival in patients with end-stage liver disease. *Liver Transpl.* 2007; **13**: 1366–1371.

164 Powell EE, Pender MP, Chalk JB *et al.* Improvement in chronic hepatocerebral degeneration following liver transplantation. *Gastroenterology* 1990; **98**: 1079–1082.

165 Weissenborn K, Tietge UJ, Bokemeyer M *et al.* Liver transplantation improves hepatic myelopathy: evidence by three cases. *Gastroenterology* 2003; **124**: 346–351.

166 Larsen FS, Ranek L, Hansen BA *et al.* Chronic portosystemic hepatic encephalopathy refractory to medical treatment successfully reversed by liver transplantation. *Transpl. Int.* 1995; **8**: 246–247.

167 Parkes JD, Murray-Lyon IM, Williams R. Neuropsychiatric and electroencephalographic changes after transplantation of the liver. *Q. J. Med.* 1970; **39**: 515–527.

168 Long LL, Li XR, Huang ZK *et al.* Relationship between changes in brain MRI and (1) H-MRS, severity of chronic liver damage, and recovery after liver transplantation. *Exp. Biol. Med. (Maywood)* 2009; **234**: 1075–1085.

169 Burra P, Dam M, Chierichetti F *et al.* 18F-fluorodeoxyglucose positron emission tomography study of brain metabolism in cirrhosis: Effect of liver transplantation. *Transpl. Proc.* 1999; **31**: 418–420.

170 Tarter RE, Switala JA, Arria A *et al.* Subclinical hepatic encephalopathy: Comparison before and after orthotopic liver transplantation. *Transplantation* 1990; **50**: 632– 637.

171 O'Carroll RE, Couston M, Cossar J *et al.* Psychological outcome and quality of life following liver transplantation: A prospective, national, single-center study. *Liver Transpl.* 2003; **9**: 712–720.

172 Mattarozzi K, Stracciari A, Vignatelli L *et al.* Minimal hepatic encephalopathy: longitudinal effects of liver transplantation. *Arch. Neurol.* 2004; **61**: 242–247.

173 Mechtcheriakov S, Graziadei IW, Mattedi M *et al.* Incomplete improvement of visuo-motor deficits in patients with minimal hepatic encephalopathy after liver transplantation. *Liver Transpl.* 2004; **10**: 77–83.

174 Campagna F, Biancardi A, Cillo U *et al.* Neurocognitive-neurological complications of liver transplantation: a review. *Metab. Brain Dis.* 2010; **25**: 115–124.

175 Blanco R, De Girolami U, Jenkins RL *et al.* Neuropathology of liver transplantation. *Clin. Neuropathol.* 1995; **14**: 109–117.

176 Sotil EU, Gottstein J, Ayala E *et al.* Impact of preoperative overt hepatic encephalopathy on neurocognitive function after liver transplantation. *Liver Transpl.* 2009; **15**: 184–192.

177 Hassanein TI, Tofteng F, Brown RS, Jr *et al.* Randomized controlled study of extracorporeal albumin dialysis for hepatic encephalopathy in advanced cirrhosis. *Hepatology* 2007; **46**: 1853–1862.

178 Dagenais MH, Bernard D, Marleau D *et al.* Surgical treatment of severe postshunt hepatic encephalopathy. *World J. Surg.* 1991; **15**: 109–113.

179 Olde Damink SW, Deutz N, Redhead D *et al.* Interorgan ammonia and amino acid metabolism in metabolically stable patients with cirrhosis and a TIPSS. *Hepatology* 2002; **36**: 1163–1171.

180 Romero-Gómez M, Ramos-Guerrero R, Grande L *et al.* Intestinal glutaminase activity is increased in liver cirrhosis and correlates with minimal hepatic encephalopathy. *J. Hepatol.* 2004; **41**: 49–54.

181 Olde Damink SW, Jalan R, Deutz NE *et al.* The kidney plays a major role in the hyperammonemia seen after simulated or actual GI bleeding in patients with cirrhosis. *Hepatology* 2003; **37**: 1277–1285.

182 Jalan R, Kapoor D. Reversal of diuretic-induced hepatic encephalopathy with infusion of albumin but not colloid. *Clin. Sci.* 2004; **106**: 467–474.

183 Olde Damink SW, Jalan R, Redhead DN *et al.* Interorgan ammonia and amino acid metabolism in metabolically stable patients with cirrhosis and a TIPSS. *Hepatology* 2002; **36**: 1163–1171.

184 Davies NA, Wright G, Ytrebø LM *et al.* L-ornithine and phenylacetate synergistically produce sustained reduction in ammonia and brain water in cirrhotic rats. *Hepatology* 2009; **50**: 155–164.

185 Matsuda I, Ohtani Y, Ohyanagi K *et al.* Hyperammonemia related to carnitine metabolism with particular emphasis on ornithine transcarbamylase deficiency. *Enzyme* 1987; **38**: 251–255.

186 Raskind JY, El-Chaar GM. The role of carnitine supplementation during valproic acid therapy. *Ann. Pharmacother.* 2000; **34**: 630–638.

187 Malaguarnera M, Pistone G, Elivra R *et al.* Effect of L-carnitine in patients with hepatic encephalopathy. *World J. Gastroenterol.* 2005; **11**: 7197–7202.

188 Dagon Y, Avraham Y, Ilan Y *et al.* Cannabinoids ameliorate cerebral dysfunction following liver failure via AMP-activated protein kinase. *FASEB J.* 2007; **21**: 2431–2441.

189 Magen I, Avraham Y, Ackerman Z *et al.* Cannabidiol ameliorates cognitive and motor impairments in mice with bile duct ligation. *J. Hepatol.* 2009; **51**: 528–534.

190 Erceg S, Monfort P, Hernandez-Viadel M *et al.* Oral administration of sidenafil restore learning ability in rats with hyperammonemia and with portacaval shunts. *Hepatology* 2005; **41**: 299–306.

191 Canales JJ, Elayadi A, Errami M *et al.* Chronic hyperammonemia alters motor and neurochemical responses to activation of group I metabotropic glutamate receptors in the nucleus accumbens in rats in vivo. *Neurobiol. Dis.* 2003; **14**: 380–390.

CHAPTER 9

The Hepatic Artery, Portal Venous System and Portal Hypertension: the Hepatic Veins and Liver in Circulatory Failure

Andrew K. Burroughs

Royal Free Sheila Sherlock Liver Centre, Royal Free Hospital and University College, London, UK

Learning points

- The hepatic artery forms a capillary plexus around the bile ducts. Thrombosis or ischaemia of the hepatic artery leads to bile duct injury, such as due to surgical injury, or after liver transplantation.

- Hepatic arterial flow increases in cirrhosis and is modulated together with portal venous inflow. Hepatic arterial flow is the main blood supply to liver tumours.

- Portal vein thrombosis is frequently associated with prothrombotic conditions; in cirrhosis it is also associated with the severity of the liver disease.

- Portal hypertension develops due to increasing hepatic fibrosis, together with increased splanchnic venous flow. There is a component of reversible intrahepatic resistance. A collateral circulation develops, including varices in the oesophagus and stomach, which can bleed.

- Increased portal pressure and its surrogate the hepatic venous pressure gradient, are associated with the development of complications and mortality in cirrhosis, independently from the severity of liver dysfunction.

- Primary prevention of bleeding from varices or portal hypertensive gastropathy is best undertaken with non-selective beta-blockers, with banding ligation of varices as an alternative. Secondary prevention is best undertaken with combined ligation and non-selective-beta blockers.

- Acute variceal bleeding is best treated with combined vasoactive drugs and endotherapy, together with antibiotics. Failure can be managed with transjugular intrahepatic portosystemic shunt (TIPS), variceal injection of adhesive glue and temporarily with balloon or stent tamponade.

- Hepatic venous outflow obstruction is mainly due to thrombosis of the hepatic veins, frequently associated with thrombophilic conditions. Constrictive pericarditis should always be excluded. Anticoagulation and venoplasty often cure the condition, TIPS is used for failures. Liver transplantation may be needed.

- Hypoxic hepatitis results from severe hypotension, such as shock, and is also seen with heart failure. Treatment is of the primary cause.

The hepatic artery

The hepatic artery is a branch of the coeliac axis. It runs along the upper border of the pancreas to the first part of the duodenum where it turns upwards between the layers of the lesser omentum, lying in front of the portal vein and medial to the common bile duct. Reaching the porta hepatis it divides into right and left branches. Its branches include the right gastric artery and the gas-troduodenal artery. Aberrant branches are common. Surgical anatomy has been defined in donor livers [1]. The common hepatic artery usually rises from the coeliac axis to form the gastroduodenal and proper hepatic artery which divides into right and left branches. A replaced or accessory right hepatic artery may originate from the superior mesenteric artery. A replaced or accessory left hepatic artery may arise from the left gastric artery. Rarely, the entire common hepatic artery

Sherlock's Diseases of the Liver and Biliary System, Twelfth Edition. Edited by
James S. Dooley, Anna S.F. Lok, Andrew K. Burroughs, E. Jenny Heathcote.
© 2011 by Blackwell Publishing Ltd. Published 2011 by Blackwell Publishing Ltd.

arises as a branch of the superior mesenteric or directly from the aorta. Such anomalies are of great importance in liver transplantation.

Anastomoses occur between the right and left branches, with subcapsular vessels of the liver and with the inferior phrenic artery.

Intrahepatic anatomy

The hepatic artery enters sinusoids adjacent to the portal tracts [2]. Direct arterioportal venous anastomoses are not seen in man [2].

The hepatic artery forms a capillary plexus around the bile ducts. Interference with this hepatic arterial supply leads to bile duct injury—surgical and laparoscopic (Fig. 9.1) [3]. Diseases of the hepatic artery, such as polyarteritis nodosa, may present as biliary strictures [4].

The connective tissue in the portal zones is supplied by the hepatic artery.

Hepatic arterial flow

In man, during surgery, the hepatic artery supplies 35% of the hepatic blood flow and 50% of the liver's oxygen supply [5]. The hepatic arterial flow serves to hold total hepatic blood flow constant. It regulates blood levels of nutrients and hormones by maintaining blood flow, and thereby hepatic clearance, as steady as possible [6].

The proportion of hepatic arterial flow increases greatly in cirrhosis, related to the extent of portal–systemic venous shunting. It is the main blood supply to tumours. A drop in systemic blood pressure from haemorrhage, or any other cause, lowers the oxygen content of the portal vein and the liver becomes more and more dependent on the hepatic artery for oxygen. The hepatic artery and the portal vein adjust the volume

of blood and oxygen they supply to the liver according to demand [6].

Hepatic arteriography

Hepatic arteriography can be used for the diagnosis of space-occupying lesions of the liver, but cross-sectional imaging has greatly reduced this indication. Lesions include cysts, abscesses and benign and malignant tumours (Chapter 35), as well as vascular lesions such as aneurysms (Fig. 9.2) or arteriovenous fistulae. Embolization via a catheter is used for treating tumours and hepatic trauma, and in the management of

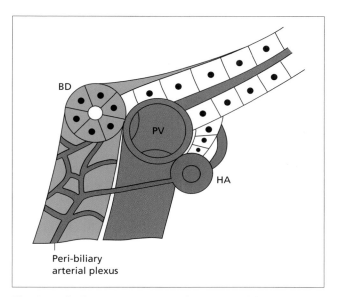

Fig. 9.1. The hepatic artery (HA) forms a peribiliary plexus supplying the bile duct (BD). PV, portal vein.

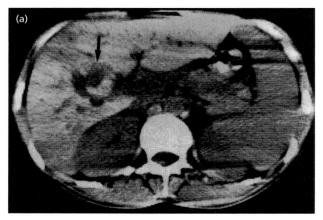

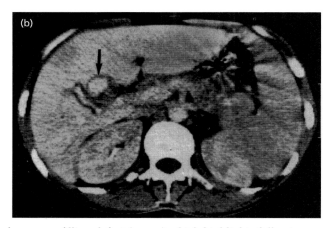

Fig. 9.2. Hepatic artery aneurysm in a patient with subacute bacterial endocarditis. CT scans of the upper abdomen: (a) before and (b) after contrast enhancement. The aneurysm shows as a filling defect (arrow) which highlights following contrast injection.

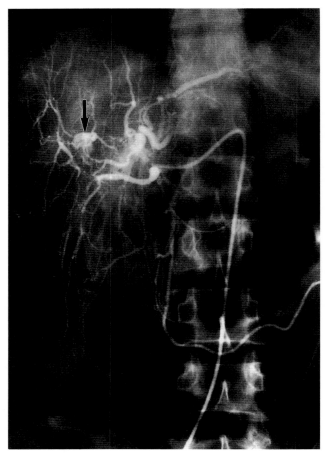

Fig. 9.3. Subacute bacterial endocarditis. Coeliac arteriogram showing a 3-cm false aneurysm (arrow) of one of the intrahepatic branches of the right hepatic artery, 2.5 cm lateral to its major bifurcation.

hepatic arterial aneurysms or arteriovenous fistulae (Figs 9.3, 9.4).

Hepatic arterial catheterization is used to introduce cytotoxic drugs or radioactive beads into hepatocellular neoplasms and for pump perfusion in patients with metastases, particularly from colorectal cancer (Chapter 35).

Spiral CT is of great value in diagnosing hepatic arterial thrombosis after liver transplant [7] and variations in intrahepatic anatomy before liver resection [8].

Hepatic artery occlusion

The effects depend on the site and extent of available collateral circulation. If the division is distal to the origins of the gastric and gastroduodenal arteries the patient may die. Survivors develop a collateral circulation. Slow thrombosis is better than sudden block. Simultaneous occlusion of the portal vein is nearly always fatal.

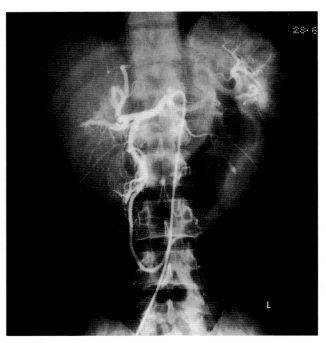

Fig. 9.4. Same patient as in Fig. 9.3. Coeliac angiogram immediately postembolization showing obliteration of the aneurysm and its feeding vessels [8].

The size of the infarct depends on the extent of the collateral arterial circulation. It rarely exceeds 8 cm in diameter and has a pale centre with a surrounding congested haemorrhagic band. Liver cells in the infarcted area are jumbled together in irregular collections of eosinophilic, granular cytoplasm without glycogen or nuclei. Subcapsular areas escape because they have an alternative arterial blood supply.

Hepatic infarction can develop without arterial occlusion in shock, cardiac failure, diabetic ketosis, toxaemia of pregnancy [9], after liver transplant or systemic lupus erythematosus [10]. If sought by scanning, small hepatic infarcts are frequent after percutaneous liver biopsy.

Aetiology

Occlusion of the hepatic artery is very rare. Hitherto it was regarded as a fatal condition. However, hepatic angiography has allowed earlier diagnosis and the prognosis has improved. Some of the causes are polyarteritis nodosa, giant cell arteritis and embolism in patients with acute bacterial endocarditis. A branch of the artery may be tied during cholecystectomy but recovery is usual. Trauma to the right hepatic or cystic artery may complicate laparoscopic cholecystectomy [11]. Hepatic arterial dissection may follow abdominal trauma or hepatic arterial catheterization. Gangrenous cholecystitis can complicate hepatic artery emboliza-tion [12].

Clinical features

The condition is rarely diagnosed ante-mortem. The patient exhibits the features of the cause, such as bacterial endocarditis or polyarteritis nodosa, or has undergone a difficult upper abdominal operation. Sudden pain in the right upper abdomen is followed by collapse and hypotension. Right upper quadrant tenderness develops and the liver edge is tender. Jaundice deepens rapidly. There is usually fever and leucocytosis and liver function tests show hepatocellular damage. The prothrombin time rises precipitously and haemorrhages develop. With major occlusions the patient passes into coma and is dead within 10 days.

Hepatic arteriography. This is essential. The obstruction to the hepatic artery may be shown. Intrahepatic arterial collaterals develop in the portal zones and subcapsular areas. Extrahepatic collaterals form in the suspensory ligaments and with adjacent structures.

Scanning. The infarcts are round, oval or wedge-shaped and are centrally located. Early lesions are hypoechoic on ultrasound. CT shows infarcts as low attenuation, peripheral wedged-shaped lesions. Occluded arterial vessels may be identified. Later lesions are confluent with distinct margins. MRI shows a lesion of low signal intensity on T_1-weighted images and with high signal intensity on T_2-weighted images [10]. Bile lakes follow large infarcts and these may contain gas.

Treatment. The causative lesion must be treated. Antibiotics and antifungals may prevent secondary infection in the anoxic liver. The general management is that of acute hepatocellular failure. Trauma to the artery is treated by percutaneous arterial embolization.

Hepatic arterial lesions following liver transplantation

The term *ischaemic cholangitis* is used to describe bile duct damage due to ischaemia [13]. It follows post-transplant-associated thrombosis or stenosis of the hepatic artery or occlusion of peribiliary arteries [14] and is associated with a poor quality donor liver such as one from a non-heart-beating donor. Later, thrombosis or stenosis of the hepatic artery or occlusion of peribiliary arterials leads to segmental hepatic infarction with abscesses and biloma [14]. The picture may be asymptomatic or present as relapsing bacteraemia.

Early diagnosis is made by duplex ultrasound. Spiral CT is highly accurate [7].

Retransplantation is the only management for lesions of the hepatic artery following transplant.

Ischaemic cholangitis manifesting as segmental strictures and cholangiectases with resultant impaired bile flow can also follow hepatic arterial chemotherapy and systemic vasculitis.

Aneurysms of the hepatic artery

These are rare but make up about one-fifth of all visceral aneurysms. The aneurysm may complicate bacterial endocarditis, polyarteritis nodosa or arteriosclerosis. Trauma is becoming increasingly important, including motor vehicle accidents and iatrogenic causes such as biliary tract surgery, liver biopsy and interventional radiological procedures. Pseudoaneurysms may complicate chronic pancreatitis with pseudocyst formation. Bile leaks are significantly associated with pseudoaneurysm [15]. It may be congenital. The aneurysm may be extra- or intrahepatic and may vary in size from a pin point to a grapefruit: it may be congenital.

Clinical presentation. The classical triad of jaundice [16], abdominal pain and haemobilia is present in only about one-third. Abdominal pain is frequent and may last as long as 5 months before the aneurysm ruptures. Between 60 and 80% of patients present for the first time with rupture into the peritoneum, biliary tree or gastrointestinal tract with resultant haemoperitoneum, haemobilia or haematemesis.

Diagnosis. The diagnosis is suggested by sonography and confirmed by hepatic arteriography and a CT scan after enhancement (Fig. 9.2) [17]. Pulsed Doppler ultrasound may show turbulent flow in the aneurysm [18].

Treatment. Intrahepatic aneurysms are treated by angiographic embolization (Figs 9.3, 9.4). Aneurysms of the common hepatic artery may also be treated surgically by proximal and distal ligation.

Hepatic arteriovenous shunts

These are usually secondary to blunt trauma, liver biopsy or neoplasms, usually primary liver cancer. Multiple shunts may be part of hereditary haemorrhagic telangiectasia, when they can be so extensive that congestive heart failure follows.

Large shunts cause a bruit in the right upper quadrant. The diagnosis is confirmed by hepatic angiography. Embolization with particles and/or placement of occluding devices is the usual treatment.

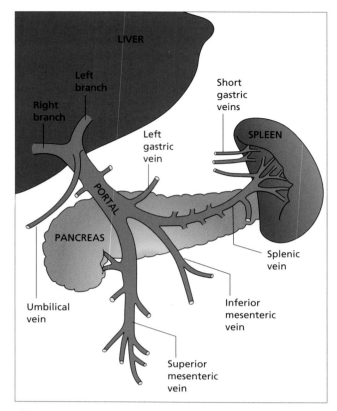

Fig. 9.5. The anatomy of the portal venous system. The portal vein is posterior to the pancreas.

The portal venous system

The portal system includes all veins that carry blood from the abdominal part of the alimentary tract, the spleen, pancreas and gallbladder. The portal vein enters the liver at the porta hepatis in two main branches, one to each lobe; it is without valves in its larger channels (Fig. 9.5) [19].

The *portal vein* is formed by the union of the superior mesenteric vein and the splenic vein just posterior to the head of the pancreas at about the level of the second lumbar vertebra. It extends slightly to the right of the midline for a distance of 5.5–8 cm to the porta hepatis. The portal vein has a segmental intrahepatic distribution, accompanying the hepatic artery.

The *superior mesenteric vein* is formed by tributaries from the small intestine, colon and head of the pancreas, and irregularly from the stomach via the right gastroepiploic vein.

The *splenic veins* (5–15 channels) originate at the splenic hilum and join near the tail of the pancreas with the short gastric vessels to form the main splenic vein. This proceeds in a transverse direction in the body and head of the pancreas, lying below and in front of the artery. It receives numerous tributaries from the head of

the pancreas, and the left gastroepiploic vein enters it near the spleen. The *inferior mesenteric vein*, bringing blood from the left part of the colon and rectum, usually enters its medial third. Occasionally, however, it enters the junction of the superior mesenteric and splenic veins.

Portal blood flow in man is about 1000–1200 mL/min.

The fasting *arterioportal oxygen difference* is only 1.9 volumes per cent (range 0.4–3.3 volumes per cent) and the portal vein contributes 40 mL/min or 72% of the total oxygen supply to the liver. During digestion, the arterioportal venous oxygen difference increases due to increased intestinal utilization.

Stream-lines in the portal vein: there is no consistent pattern of hepatic distribution of portal inflow. Sometimes splenic blood goes to the left and sometimes to the right. Crossing-over of the bloodstream can occur in the portal vein. Flow is probably stream-lined rather than turbulent.

Portal pressure is about 7 mmHg (Fig. 9.6).

Collateral circulation

When the portal circulation is obstructed, whether it be within or outside the liver, a remarkable collateral circulation develops to carry portal blood into the systemic veins (Figs 9.7, 9.8).

Intrahepatic obstruction (cirrhosis)

Normally 100% of the portal venous blood flow can be recovered from the hepatic veins, whereas in cirrhosis only 13% is obtained [20]. The remainder enters collateral channels which form four main groups.

Group I: where protective epithelium adjoins absorptive epithelium:

(a) At the cardia of the stomach, where the left gastric vein, posterior gastric [21] and short gastric veins of the portal system anastomose with the intercostal, diaphragmo-oesophageal and azygos minor veins of the caval system. Deviation of blood into these channels leads to varicosities in the submucous layer of the lower end of the oesophagus and fundus of the stomach.

(b) At the anus, the superior haemorrhoidal vein of the portal system anastomoses with the middle and inferior haemorrhoidal veins of the caval system. Deviation of blood into these channels may lead to rectal varices.

Group II: in the falciform ligament through the paraumbilical veins, relics of the umbilical circulation of the fetus (Fig. 9.9).

Group III: where the abdominal organs are in contact with retroperitoneal tissues or adherent to the abdominal wall. These collaterals run from the liver to

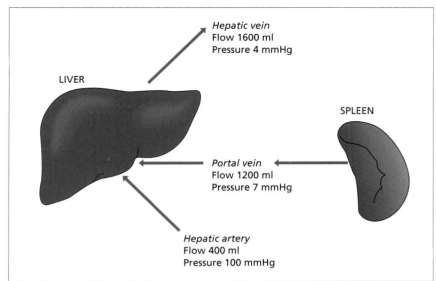

Fig. 9.6. The flow and pressure in the hepatic artery, portal vein and hepatic vein.

Inside figure 9.6:

LIVER

Hepatic vein
Flow 1600 ml
Pressure 4 mmHg

SPLEEN

Portal vein
Flow 1200 ml
Pressure 7 mmHg

Hepatic artery
Flow 400 ml
Pressure 100 mmHg

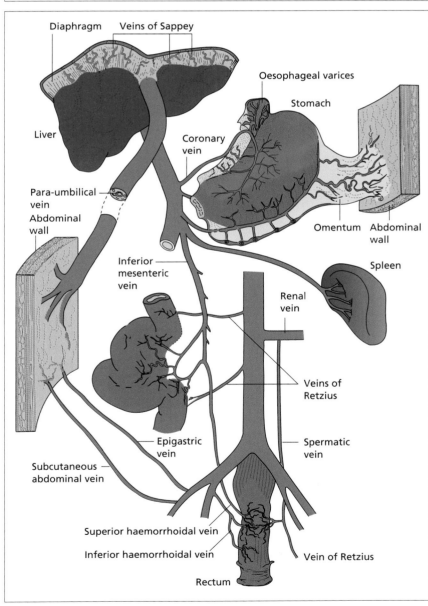

Fig. 9.7. The sites of the portal–systemic collateral circulation in cirrhosis of the liver.

Inside figure 9.7:

Diaphragm
Veins of Sappey
Oesophageal varices
Stomach
Liver
Coronary vein
Para-umbilical vein
Abdominal wall
Omentum
Abdominal wall
Inferior mesenteric vein
Spleen
Renal vein
Veins of Retzius
Epigastric vein
Spermatic vein
Subcutaneous abdominal vein
Superior haemorrhoidal vein
Inferior haemorrhoidal vein
Vein of Retzius
Rectum

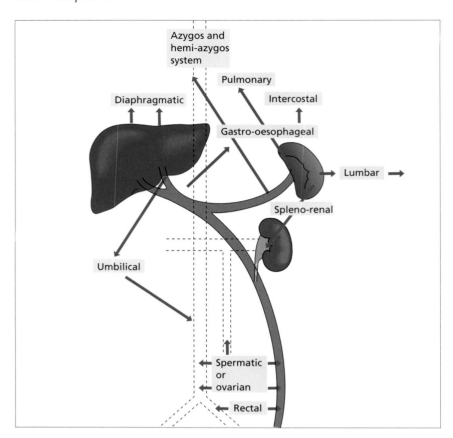

Fig. 9.8. The sites of the collateral circulation in the presence of intrahepatic portal vein obstruction.

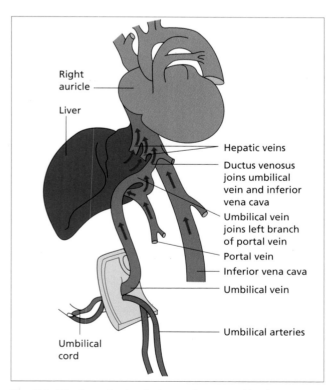

Fig. 9.9. The hepatic circulation at the time of birth.

diaphragm and in the splenorenal ligament and omentum. They include lumbar veins and veins developing in scars of previous operations or in small or large bowel stomas.

Group IV: portal venous blood is carried to the left renal vein. This may be through blood entering directly from the splenic vein or via diaphragmatic, pancreatic, left adrenal or gastric veins.

Blood from gastro-oesophageal and other collaterals ultimately reaches the superior vena cava via the azygos or hemiazygos systems. A small volume enters the inferior vena cava. An intrahepatic shunt may run from the right branch of the portal vein to the inferior vena cava [22]. Collaterals to the pulmonary veins have also been described.

Extrahepatic obstruction

With extrahepatic portal venous obstruction, additional collaterals form, attempting to bypass the block and return blood *towards* the liver. These enter the portal vein in the porta hepatis beyond the block. They include the veins at the hilum, venae comitantes of the portal vein and hepatic arteries, veins in the suspensory ligaments of the liver and diaphragmatic and omental veins. Lumbar collaterals may be very large.

Effects

When the liver is cut off from portal blood by the development of the collateral circulation, it depends more on blood from the hepatic artery. It shrinks and shows impaired capacity to regenerate. This might be due to lack of hepatotrophic factors, including insulin and glucagon, which are of pancreatic origin.

Collaterals usually imply portal hypertension, although occasionally if the collateral circulation is very extensive portal pressure may fall. Conversely, portal hypertension of short duration can exist without a demonstrable collateral circulation.

A large portal–systemic shunt may lead to hepatic encephalopathy, septicaemias due to intestinal organisms, and other circulatory and metabolic effects.

Pathology of portal hypertension

Collateral venous circulation is disappointingly insignificant at autopsy. The oesophageal varices collapse.

The spleen is enlarged with a thickened capsule. The surface oozes dark blood (*fibrocongestive splenomegaly*). Malpighian bodies are inconspicuous. Histologically, sinusoids are dilated and lined by thickened epithelium (Fig. 9.10). Histiocytes proliferate with occasional erythrophagocytosis. Periarterial haemorrhages may progress to siderotic, fibrotic nodules.

The *splenic artery and portal vein* are enlarged and tortuous and may be aneurysmal. The portal and splenic vein may show endothelial haemorrhages, mural thrombi and intimal plaques and may calcify (see Fig. 9.7). Such veins are usually unsuitable for portal surgery.

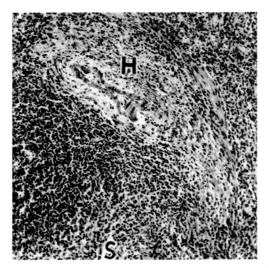

Fig. 9.10. The spleen in portal hypertension. The sinusoids (S) are congested and the sinusoidal wall is thickened. A haemorrhage (H) lies adjacent to an arteriole of a Malpighian corpuscle. (H & E,×70.)

In 50% of patients with cirrhosis small, deeply placed splenic arterial aneurysms are seen [23].

Hepatic changes depend on the cause of the portal hypertension.

The height of the portal venous pressure correlates poorly with the apparent degree of cirrhosis and in particular of fibrosis. There is a much better correlation with the degree of nodularity.

Varices

Oesophageal

The major blood supply to oesophageal varices is the left gastric vein. The posterior branch usually drains into the azygos system, whereas the anterior branch communicates with varices just below the oesophageal junction and forms a bundle of thin parallel veins that run in the junction area and continue in large tortuous veins in the lower oesophagus. There are four layers of veins in the oesophagus (Fig. 9.11) [24]. *Intraepithelial veins* may correlate with the red spots seen on endoscopy and which predict variceal rupture. The *superficial venous plexus* drains into larger, *deep intrinsic veins. Perforating veins* connect the deeper veins with the fourth layer which is the adventitial plexus. Typical large varices arise from the main trunks of the deep intrinsic veins and these communicate with gastric varices.

The connection between portal and systemic circulation at the gastro-oesophageal junction is extremely complex [25]. Its adaptation to the cephalad and increased flow of portal hypertension is ill-understood. A palisade zone is seen between the gastric zone and the perforating zone (Fig. 9.12). In the palisade zone, flow is bidirectional and this area acts as a water shed between the portal and azygos systems. Turbulent flow in perforating veins between the varices and the perioesophageal veins at the lower end of the stomach may explain why rupture is frequent in this region [26]. Recurrence

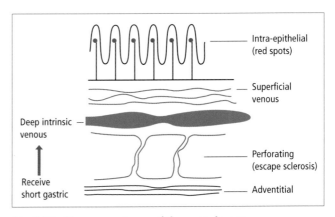

Fig. 9.11. Venous anatomy of the oesophagus.

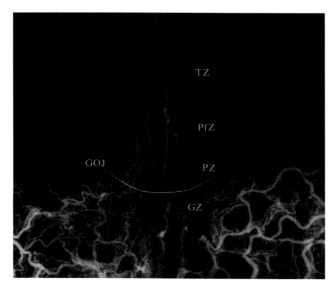

Fig. 9.12. Radiograph of a specimen injected with barium–gelatine, opened along the greater curvature. Four distinct zones of normal venous drainage are identified: the gastric zone (GZ), palisade zone (PZ), perforating zone (PfZ) and truncal zone (TZ). A radio-opaque wire demarcates the transition between the columnar and stratified squamous epithelium. GOJ, gastro-oesophageal junction [25].

of varices after endoscopic sclerotherapy may be related to the communications between various venous channels or perhaps to enlargement of veins in the superficial venous plexus. Failure of sclerotherapy may also be due to failure to thrombose the perforating veins.

Gastric

These are largely supplied by the short gastric veins and drain into the deep intrinsic veins of the oesophagus. They are particularly prominent in patients with extra-hepatic portal obstruction.

Duodenal varices show as filling defects. Bile duct collaterals may be life-threatening at surgery [27].

Colorectal

These develop secondary to inferior mesenteric–internal iliac venous collaterals [28]. They may present with haemorrhage. They are visualized by colonoscopy. Colonic varices are more frequent in association with splanchnic thrombosis.

Collaterals between the superior haemorrhoidal (portal) veins and the middle and inferior haemorrhoidal (systemic) veins lead to anorectal varices [29].

Portal hypertensive intestinal vasculopathy

Chronic portal hypertension may not only be associated with discrete varices but with a spectrum of intestinal mucosal changes due to abnormalities in the microcirculation [30].

Portal hypertensive gastropathy. This is almost always associated with cirrhosis and is seen in the fundus and body of the stomach. Histology shows vascular ectasia in the mucosa. The risk of bleeding is increased, for instance from non-steroidal anti-inflammatory drugs (NSAIDs). These gastric changes may be increased after sclerotherapy. They are relieved only by reducing the portal pressure [31].

Gastric antral vascular ectasia. This is marked by increased arteriovenous communications between the muscularis mucosa and dilated precapillaries and veins [32]. Gastric mucosal perfusion is increased. This must be distinguished from portal hypertensive gastropathy. It is not directly related to portal hypertension, but is influenced by liver dysfunction [33].

Congestive jejunopathy and colonopathy. Similar changes are seen in the duodenum and jejunum. Histology shows an increase in size and number of vessels in jejunal villi [34]. The mucosa is oedematous, erythematous and friable [35]. Congestive colonopathy is shown by dilated mucosal capillaries with thickened basement membranes but with no evidence of mucosal inflammation [30].

Others

Portal–systemic collaterals form in relation to bowel–abdominal wall adhesions secondary to previous surgery or pelvic inflammatory disease. Varices also form at mucocutaneous junctions, for instance, at the site of an ileostomy or colostomy.

Haemodynamics of portal hypertension

This has been considerably clarified by the development of animal models such as the rat with a ligated portal vein or bile duct or with carbon tetrachloride-induced cirrhosis. Portal hypertension is related both to vascular resistance and to portal blood flow (Fig. 9.13). The fundamental haemodynamic abnormality is an increased resistance to portal flow. This is mechanical due to the disturbed architecture and nodularity of cirrhosis or due to an obstructed portal vein and also due to dynamic changes related to dysfunction of the endothelium and reduced bioavailability of nitric oxide (NO) [36]. Other intrahepatic factors such as collagen deposition in the space of Disse [37] leading to loss of fenestrae (capillarization of the sinusoids), hepatocyte swelling [38,39] and the resistance offered by portal–systemic collaterals contribute.

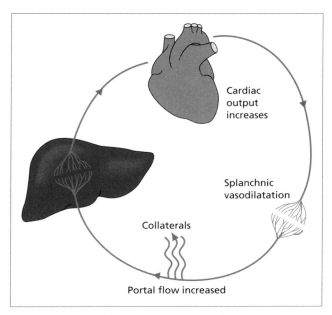

Fig. 9.13. Forward flow theory of portal hypertension.

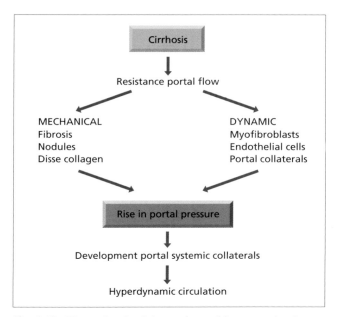

Fig. 9.15. The pathophysiology of portal hypertension in cirrhosis.

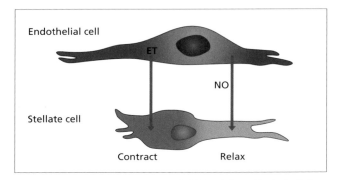

Fig. 9.14. Regulation of sinusoidal blood flow. Endothelial and stellate cells are potential sources of endothelin (ET) which is contractile on stellate cells. Nitric oxide (NO) relaxes stellate cells. NO synthase is the precursor of NO and is produced by endothelial and stellate cells.

There is also a dynamic increase in intrahepatic vascular resistance [36].

Stellate (Ito) cells have contractile properties that can be modulated by vasoactive substances [40]. These include NO which is vasodilatory [41] (Chapter 7) and endothelin which is a vasoconstrictor [42]. These may modulate intrahepatic resistance and blood flow, especially at a sinusoidal level (Fig. 9.14) [43].

Collaterals develop when the pressure gradient between the portal vein and hepatic vein rises above a certain threshold, a process which involves angiogenic factors [44]. At the same time portal flow increases in the splanchnic bed due to splanchnic vasodilatation and increased cardiac output. It is uncertain whether the hyperdynamic circulation is the cause or the consequence of the portal hypertension or both. It is related to the severity of liver failure. Cardiac output increases further and there is generalized systemic vasodilatation (Fig. 9.15). Arterial blood pressure is normal or low (Chapter 7).

Splanchnic vasodilatation is probably the most important factor in maintaining the hyperdynamic circulation. Azygous blood flow is increased. Gastric mucosal blood flow rises. The increased portal flow raises the oesophageal variceal transmural pressure. The increased flow refers to *total* portal flow (hepatic and collaterals). The actual portal flow reaching the liver is reduced. The factors maintaining the hyperdynamic splanchnic circulation are multiple. There seems to be an interplay of vasodilators and vasoconstrictors. These might be formed by the hepatocyte, fail to be inactivated by it or be of gut origin and pass through intrahepatic or extrahepatic venous shunts.

Endotoxins and cytokines, largely formed in the gut, are important triggers [45]. NO and endothelin-1 are synthesized by vascular endothelium in response to endotoxin. *Prostacyclin* is produced by portal vein endothelium and is a potent vasodilator [46]. It may play a major role in the circulatory changes of portal hypertension due to chronic liver disease.

Glucagon is vasodilatory after pharmacological doses but is not vasoactive at physiological doses. It is not a primary factor in the maintenance of the hyperkinetic circulation in established liver disease [47].

Table 9.1. Investigation of a patient with suspected portal hypertension

---

History

  Relevant to cirrhosis or chronic hepatitis (Chapter 7)

  Gastrointestinal bleeding: number, dates, amounts, symptoms, treatment

  Results of previous endoscopies

  Patient history: alcoholism, blood transfusion, hepatitis B, hepatitis C, intra-abdominal, neonatal or other sepsis, oral contraceptives, myeloproliferative disorder

Examination

  Signs of hepatocellular failure

  Abdominal wall veins:

    site

    direction of blood flow

  Splenomegaly

  Liver size and consistency

  Ascites

  Oedema of legs

  Rectal examination

  Endoscopy of oesophagus, stomach and duodenum

Additional investigations

  Liver biopsy

  Hepatic vein catheterization

  Splanchnic arteriography

  Hepatic ultrasound, CT scan or MRI

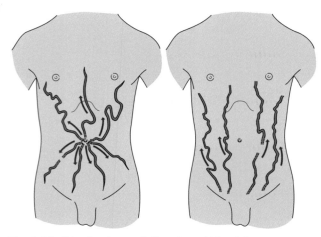

Fig. 9.16. Distribution and direction of blood flow in anterior abdominal wall veins in portal venous obstruction (left) and in inferior vena caval obstruction (right).

Clinical features of portal hypertension

History and general examination (Table 9.1)

Cirrhosis is the commonest cause. Aetiological factors should be looked for. Past abdominal inflammation, especially neonatal, is important in extrahepatic portal vein thrombosis. Prothrombotic factors, inherited or acquired, and drugs, such as sex hormones, predispose to portal and hepatic venous thrombosis.

Haematemesis is the commonest presentation. The number and severity of previous haemorrhages should be noted, together with their immediate effects, whether there was associated confusion or coma and whether blood transfusion was required. Melaena, without haematemesis, may result from bleeding varices. The absence of dyspepsia and epigastric tenderness and a previously normal endoscopy help to exclude haemorrhage from peptic ulcer.

The stigmata of cirrhosis include jaundice, vascular spiders and palmar erythema. Anaemia, ascites and precoma should be noted.

Abdominal wall veins

In intrahepatic portal hypertension, some blood from the left branch of the portal vein may be deviated via paraumbilical veins to the umbilicus, whence it reaches veins of the caval system (Fig. 9.16). In extrahepatic portal obstruction, dilated veins may appear in the left flank.

Distribution and direction. Prominent collateral veins radiating from the umbilicus are termed *caput Medusae*. This is rare and usually only one or two veins, frequently epigastric, are seen (Figs 9.16, 9.17). The blood flow is away from the umbilicus, whereas in inferior vena caval obstruction the collateral venous channels carry blood upwards to reach the superior vena caval system (Fig. 9.16). Tense ascites may lead to functional obstruction of the inferior vena cava and cause difficulty in interpretation.

Murmurs. A venous hum may be heard, usually in the region of the xiphoid process or umbilicus. A thrill, detectable by light pressure, may be felt at the site of maximum intensity and is due to blood rushing through a large umbilical or paraumbilical channel to veins in the abdominal wall. A venous hum may also be heard over other large collaterals such as the inferior mesenteric vein. An arterial systolic murmur usually indicates primary liver cancer or alcoholic hepatitis.

The association of dilated abdominal wall veins and a loud venous murmur at the umbilicus is termed the *Cruveilhier–Baumgarten syndrome* [48,49]. This may be due to congenital patency of the umbilical vein, but more usually to a well-compensated cirrhosis [48–50].

The paraxiphoid umbilical hum and caput Medusae indicate portal obstruction beyond the origin of the umbilical veins from the left branch of the portal vein.

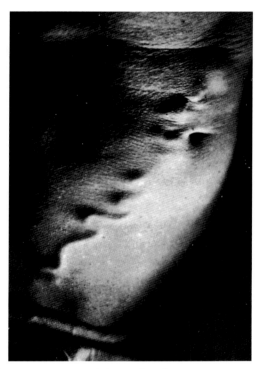

Fig. 9.17. An anterior abdominal wall vein in a patient with cirrhosis of the liver.

They therefore indicate intrahepatic portal hypertension (cirrhosis).

Spleen

The spleen enlarges progressively. The edge is firm. Size bears little relation to the portal pressure. It is larger in young people and in macronodular rather than micronodular cirrhosis.

An enlarged spleen is the single most important diagnostic sign of portal hypertension. If the spleen cannot be felt or is not enlarged on imaging, the diagnosis of portal hypertension is questionable.

The *peripheral blood* shows a pancytopenia associated with an enlarged spleen (*secondary 'hypersplenism'*). This is related more to reticuloendothelial hyperplasia than to the portal hypertension and is unaffected by lowering the pressure by a portacaval shunt.

Liver

A small liver may be as significant as hepatomegaly, and size should be evaluated by careful percussion. It correlates poorly with the height of portal pressure.

Liver consistency, tenderness or nodularity should be recorded. A soft liver suggests extrahepatic portal venous obstruction. A firm liver supports cirrhosis.

Ascites

This is rarely due to portal hypertension alone, although a particularly high pressure may be a major factor. The portal hypertension raises the capillary filtration pressure, and determines fluid localization to the peritoneal cavity. Ascites in cirrhosis always indicates liver cell failure in addition to portal hypertension.

Rectum

Anorectal varices are visualized by sigmoidoscopy and may bleed. They are found in 44% of patients with cirrhosis, increasing in those who have bled from oesophageal varices [51]. They must be distinguished from simple haemorrhoids which are prolapsed vascular cushions and which do not communicate with the portal system.

X-ray of the abdomen and chest

This is useful to delineate liver and spleen. Rarely, a calcified portal vein may be shown (Fig. 9.18) [52].

Branching, linear gas shadows in the portal vein radicles, especially near the periphery of the liver and due to gas-forming organisms, may rarely be seen in adults with intestinal infarction or infants with enterocolitis. Portal gas may be associated with disseminated intravascular coagulation. CT and ultrasound may detect portal gas more often, for instance in suppurative cholangitis when the prognosis is not so grave [53].

Tomography of the azygos vein may show enlargement (Fig. 9.19) as the collateral flow enters the azygos system.

A widened left paravertebral shadow may be due to lateral displacement of the pleural reflection between the aorta and vertebral column by a dilated hemiazygos vein.

Massively dilated paraoesophageal collaterals may be seen on the chest radiograph as a retrocardiac posterior mediastinal mass.

Diagnosis of varices

Barium studies have largely been replaced by endoscopy. Oesophageal varices show as filling defects in the regular contour of the oesophagus (Fig. 9.20). They are most often in the lower third, but may spread upwards so that the entire oesophagus is involved. Widening and finally gross dilatation are helpful signs.

Gastric varices pass through the cardia, line the fundus in a worm-like fashion and may be difficult to distinguish from mucosal folds.

Occasionally gastric varices show as a lobulated mass in the gastric fundus simulating a carcinoma. Portal venography is useful in differentiation.

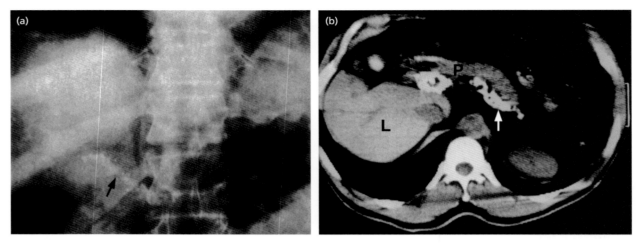

Fig. 9.18. (a) Plain X-ray of the abdomen. Calcification can be seen in the line of the splenic and portal vein (arrow). (b) CT scan confirms the calcified splenic vein (arrow). L, liver; P, pancreas.

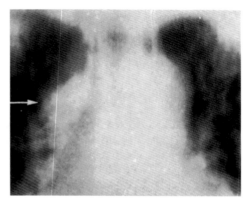

Fig. 9.19. Tomography of the mediastinum of a patient with large portosystemic collaterals, showing enlargement of the azygos vein (arrow).

Endoscopy is the best screening test to detect varices. The size of the varix should be graded (Figs 9.21, 9.22) [54]. Varices are small (≤5 mm diameter) or large (>5 mm diameter) when assessed with full insufflation.

The larger the varix the more likely it is to bleed. Varices usually appear white and opaque (Fig. 9.23). Red colour correlates with blood flow through dilated subepithelial and communicating veins. Dilated subepithelial veins may appear as raised cherry-red spots (Fig. 9.24) and red wheal markings (longitudinal dilated veins resembling whip marks). They lie on top of large subepithelial vessels. The haemocystic spot is approximately 4 mm in diameter (Fig. 9.25). It represents blood coming from the deeper extrinsic veins of the oesophagus straight out towards the lumen through a communicating vein into the more superficial submucosal veins. Red colour is usually associated with larger varices. All these signs are associated with a higher risk of variceal bleeding. Intraobserver error may depend on

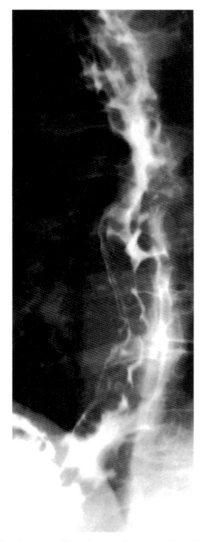

Fig. 9.20. Barium swallow X-ray shows a dilated oesophagus. The margin is irregular. There are multiple filling defects representing oesophageal varices.

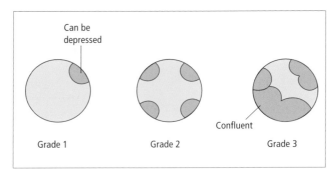

Fig. 9.21. Endoscopic classification of oesophageal varices (adapted from [54]).

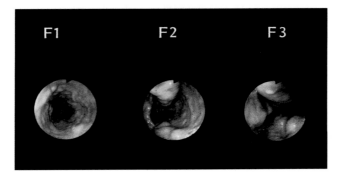

Fig. 9.22. The form (F) of the oesophageal varices (from [54]).

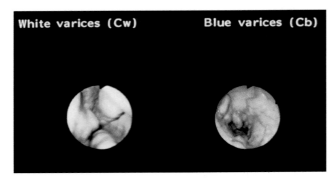

Fig. 9.23. Variceal colour through the endoscope (from [54]).

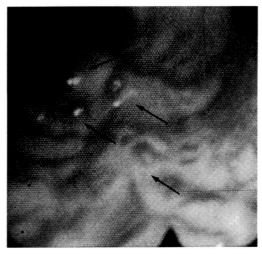

Fig. 9.24. Endoscopic view of cherry-red spots on oesophageal varices (arrows).

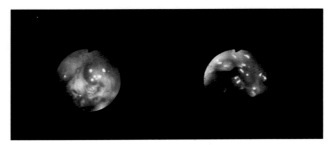

Fig. 9.25. Haemocystic spots on oesophageal varices (from [54]).

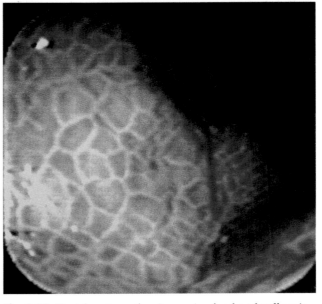

Fig. 9.26. Portal gastropathy. A mosaic of red and yellow is seen together with petechial haemorrhages.

the skill and experience of the endoscopist. Intraobserver agreement is only good for size and presence of red signs [55].

Portal hypertensive gastropathy is seen largely in the fundus and antrum, but can extend throughout the stomach (Fig. 9.26). It is shown as a mosaic-like pattern with small polygonal areas, surrounded by a whitish-yellow depressed border [56]. Red point lesions and cherry-red spots predict a high risk of bleeding. Black–brown spots are due to intramucosal haemorrhage. Sclerotherapy may increase the gastropathy [57]. Capsule endoscopy is an accurate diagnostic tool to detect oesophageal varices and portal hypertensive gastropathy, but not as good as endoscopy [58]. Its use should be confined to patients in whom endoscopy is contraindicated. If neither type of endoscopy is possible the presence of oesophageal varices can be predicted using platelet count/ spleen diameter ratio [59] with a positive likelihood ratio of 2.77 and negative likelihood ratio of 0.13.

Variceal (azygos) blood flow can be assessed during diagnostic endoscopy by a Doppler ultrasound probe passed down the biopsy channel of the standard gastroscope.

Portal hypertensive colopathy is seen in about half the patients with portal hypertension, usually in those with gastropathy. Colonoscopy may be needed to diagnose lower gastrointestinal bleeding in patients with cirrhosis [60].

Imaging the portal venous system

Ultrasound

Longitudinal scans at the subcostal margins and transverse scans at the epigastrium are essential (Fig. 9.27). The portal and superior mesenteric veins can always be seen. The normal splenic vein may be more difficult.

A large portal vein suggests portal hypertension, but this is not diagnostic. If collaterals are seen, this confirms portal hypertension. Portal vein thrombosis is accurately diagnosed and echogenic areas can sometimes be seen within the lumen.

Doppler ultrasound

Doppler ultrasound demonstrates the anatomy of the portal veins and hepatic artery (Table 9.2). Satisfactory results depend on technical expertise. Small cirrhotic livers are difficult to see as are those of the obese. Colour-coded Doppler improves visualization (Fig. 9.28). Portal venous obstruction is demonstrated by Doppler ultrasound as accurately as by angiography provided the Doppler is technically optimal.

Doppler ultrasound shows spontaneous hepatofugal flow in portal, splenic and superior mesenteric veins in 8.3% of patients with cirrhosis [61]. Its presence correlates with severity of cirrhosis and with encephalopathy. Variceal bleeding is more likely if the flow is hepatopetal.

Abnormalities of the intrahepatic portal veins can be shown. These are important if surgery is contemplated.

Colour Doppler is a good way of demonstrating portal–systemic shunts and the direction of flow in them. These include surgical shunts but also transjugu-

Table 9.2. Clinical uses of Doppler ultrasound

Portal vein
  Patency
  Hepatofugal flow
  Anatomical abnormalities
  Portal–systemic shunt patency
  Acute flow changes
Hepatic artery
  Patency (post-transplant)
  Anatomical abnormalities
Hepatic veins
  Screening Budd–Chiari syndrome

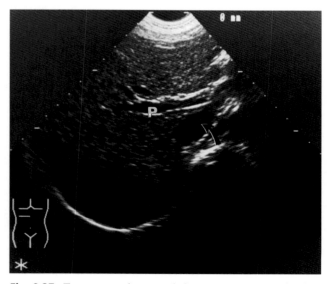

Fig. 9.27. Transverse ultrasound shows a patent portal vein (P); the arrow indicates the inferior vena cava.

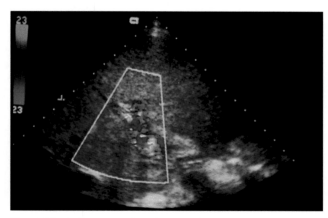

Fig. 9.28. Colour Doppler ultrasound of the porta hepatis shows the hepatic artery in red and portal vein in blue.

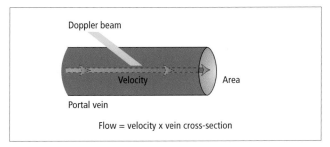

Fig. 9.29. The Doppler real-time ultrasound method of measuring portal venous flow.

lar intrahepatic portosystemic shunts (TIPS). Intrahepatic portal–systemic shunts may be visualized [62].

Colour Doppler screening is useful for patients suspected of the Budd–Chiari syndrome.

The hepatic artery is more difficult than the hepatic veins to locate because of its small size and direction. Nevertheless, duplex Doppler is the primary screening procedure to show a patent hepatic artery after liver transplantation.

Duplex Doppler has been used to measure portal blood flow. The average velocity of blood flowing in the portal vein is multiplied by the cross-sectional area of the vessel (Fig. 9.29). There are observer errors in measurement. The method is most useful in measuring rapid, large, acute changes in flow rather than monitoring chronic changes in portal haemodynamics.

Portal blood flow velocity correlates with the presence and size of oesophageal varices. In cirrhosis, the portal vein velocity tends to fall and when less than 16 cm/s portal hypertension is likely.

Computed Tomography

After contrast, portal vein patency can be established and retroperitoneal, perivisceral and paraoesophageal varices may be visualized (Fig. 9.30). Oesophageal varices may be shown as intraluminal protrusions enhancing after contrast. The umbilical vein can be seen. Gastric varices show as rounded structures, indistinguishable from the gastric wall.

CT arterioportography is done by rapid CT scanning during selective injection of contrast into the superior mesenteric vein via a catheter [63]. It is particularly useful in showing focal lesions, the collateral circulation and arteriovenous shunts [64], but is rarely used due to the improvement of dynamic scanning with CT or MR following intravenous contrast.

Magnetic resonance angiography

Magnetic resonance angiography gives excellent depiction of blood vessels as regions of absent signal (Figs

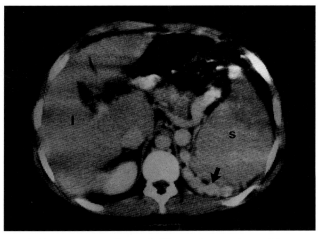

Fig. 9.30. Contrast-enhanced CT scan in a patient with cirrhosis and a large retroperitoneal retrosplenic collateral circulation (arrow). l, liver; s, spleen.

9.31–9.33). Portal patency, morphology and flow of velocity may be demonstrated. Magnetic resonance angiography is more reliable than Doppler [65].

Venography

If the portal vein is patent by scanning, confirmation by venography is not necessary even when portal surgery or hepatic transplantation is being considered.

Patency of the portal vein is important, particularly in the diagnosis of splenomegaly in childhood and in excluding invasion by a hepatocellular carcinoma in a patient with cirrhosis.

Anatomy of the portal venous system must be known before such operations as portal–systemic shunt, or transjugular intrahepatic stent shunt, hepatic resection or hepatic transplantation. The patency of a surgical shunt may be confirmed.

The demonstration of a large portal collateral circulation is essential for the diagnosis of chronic hepatic encephalopathy (Figs 9.8, 9.30).

A filling defect in the portal vein or in the liver due to a space-occupying lesion may be demonstrated. Intrasplenic pulp pressure is an index of portal hypertension [66], but has been replaced by direct intrahepatic puncture of the portal vein.

Venographic appearances

When the portal circulation is normal, the splenic and portal veins are filled but no other vessels are outlined. A filling defect may be seen at the junction of the splenic and superior mesenteric veins due to mixing with non-opacified blood. The size and direction of the splenic and portal veins are very variable. The intrahepatic

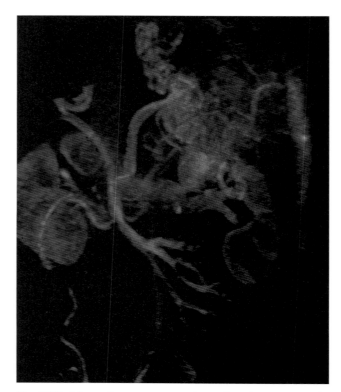

Fig. 9.31. Magnetic resonance angiography of a patient with cirrhosis showing the right kidney (K), superior mesenteric vein (SMV), portal vein (PV), left gastric vein (LGV), left branch of portal vein (LBR), gastro-oesophageal collateral veins (V) and the inferior vena cava (IVC).

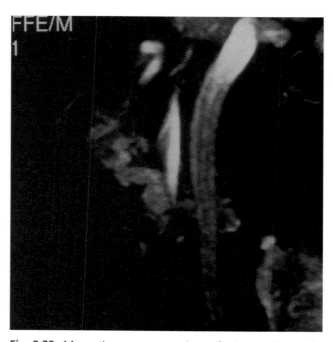

Fig. 9.32. Magnetic resonance angiography in a patient with portal vein thrombosis showing the portal vein replaced by collaterals (PV), the inferior vena cava (IVC) and the aorta (A).

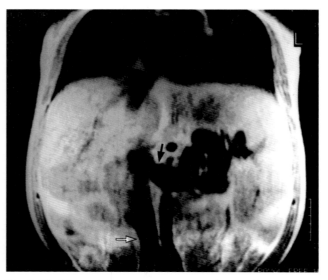

Fig. 9.33. Magnetic resonance angiography showing a spontaneous splenorenal shunt to the inferior vena cava. Black arrow, renal vein; open arrow, vena cava.

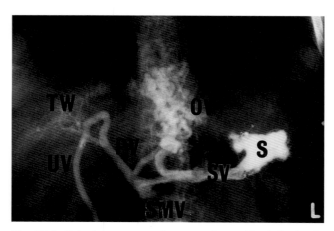

Fig. 9.34. Splenic venogram from a patient with cirrhosis of the liver. The gastro-oesophageal collateral circulation can be seen and the intrahepatic portal vascular tree is distorted ('tree in winter' appearance). OV, oesophageal veins; PV, portal vein; S, splenic pulp; SMV, superior mesenteric vein; SV, splenic vein; TW, 'tree in winter' appearance; UV, umbilical vein.

branches of the portal vein show a gradual branching and reduction in calibre. Later the liver becomes opaque due to sinusoidal filling. The hepatic veins may rarely be seen in later films.

In cirrhosis, the venogram varies widely. It may be completely normal or may show filling of large numbers of collateral vessels with gross distortion of the intrahepatic pattern ('tree in winter' appearance) (Fig. 9.34).

In extrahepatic portal or splenic vein obstruction, large numbers of vessels run from the spleen and splenic

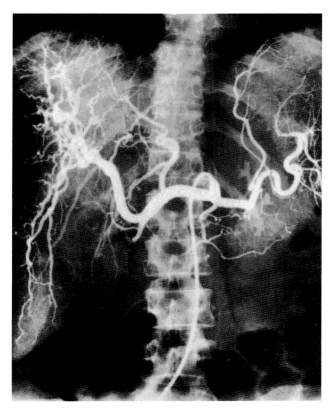

Fig. 9.35. Selective coeliac angiogram showing an intrahepatic arterial pattern. A Riedel's lobe is shown.

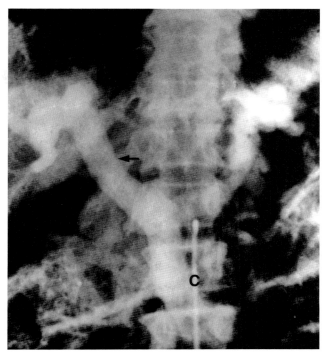

Fig. 9.36. Venous phase of selective coeliac angiogram showing patent portal (arrow) and splenic veins. C, catheter in coeliac axis.

vein to the diaphragm, thoracic cage and abdominal wall. Intrahepatic branches are not usually seen, although, if the portal vein block is localized, paraportal vessels may short circuit the lesion (Fig. 9.32) and produce a delayed but definite filling of the vein beyond.

Visceral angiography

Safety has increased with the use of smaller (French 5) arterial catheters. New contrast materials are less toxic to kidneys and other tissues and hypersensitivity reactions are rare. However, diagnostic angiography is rarely needed except to demonstrate shunting and when evaluating patients with hepatocellular carcinoma for targeted radioactive bead therapy, and for hepatic arterial problems after liver transplantation.

The coeliac axis is catheterized via the femoral artery and contrast is injected. The material that flows into the splenic artery returns through the splenic and portal veins and produces a splenic and portal venogram. Similarly, a bolus of contrast introduced into the superior mesenteric artery returns through the superior mesenteric and portal veins, which can be seen in radiographs exposed at the appropriate intervals (Figs 9.35, 9.36).

Visceral angiography demonstrates the hepatic arterial system, so allowing space-filling lesions in the liver to be identified. A tumour circulation may diagnose hepatocellular cancer or another tumour.

Knowledge of splenic and hepatic arterial anatomy is useful if surgery is contemplated. Haemangiomas, other space-occupying lesions and aneurysms may be identified.

The portal vein may not opacify if flow in it is hepatofugal or if there is 'steal' by the spleen or by large collateral channels. A superior mesenteric angiogram will confirm that the portal vein is in fact patent.

Digital subtraction angiography

The contrast is given by selective arterial injection with immediate subtraction of images. The portal system is very well visualized free of other confusing images (Fig. 9.37). Spatial resolution is poorer than with conventional film-based angiography. The technique is particularly valuable for the parenchymal phase of hepatic angiography and for the diagnosis of vascular lesions such as haemangiomas or arteriovenous malformations.

Splenic venography

Contrast material, injected into the pulp of the spleen, flows into the portal venous system with sufficient

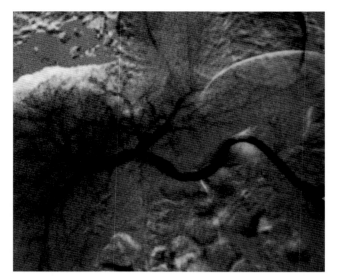

Fig. 9.37. Digital subtraction angiography showing a normal portal venous system.

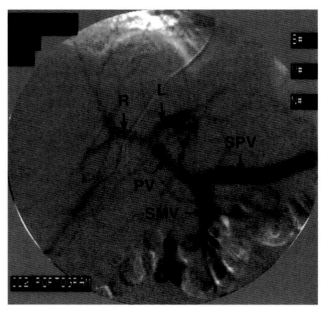

Fig. 9.38. Carbon dioxide portal venography real-time imaging following the injection of carbon dioxide into the wedged hepatic vein. PV, portal vein (L, left branch; R, right branch); SMV, superior mesenteric vein; SPV, splenic vein.

rapidity to outline splenic and portal veins (Fig. 9.34). The collateral circulation is particularly well visualized [67]. Splenic venography has now been replaced by less invasive procedures.

Carbon dioxide occluded venography

Injection of carbon dioxide into a catheter in the wedged hepatic venous position allows an excellent venogram of the hepatic venous and portal venous tree (Fig. 9.38) [68].

Portal pressure measurement

A balloon catheter is introduced into the femoral vein or internal jugular vein and, under fluoroscopic control, into the hepatic vein (Fig. 9.39). Measurements are taken in the wedged hepatic venous pressure (WHVP) and free hepatic venous pressure (FHVP) positions by inflating and deflating the balloon in the tip of the catheter [67,69]. The hepatic venous pressure gradient (HVPG) is the difference between WHVP and FHVP. This is the portal (sinusoidal) venous pressure. When the cause of portal hypertension is mainly sinusoidal (alcohol, viral hepatitis) the WHVP is the same as the portal pressure, but this relationship does not hold when there is a large presinusoidal component [70]. The normal HVPG is 5–6 mmHg and values of 10 mmHg or more represent clinically significant portal hypertension when complications of cirrhosis (decompensation) can occur [71]. Measurements can be performed at the same time as transjugular liver biopsy [72].

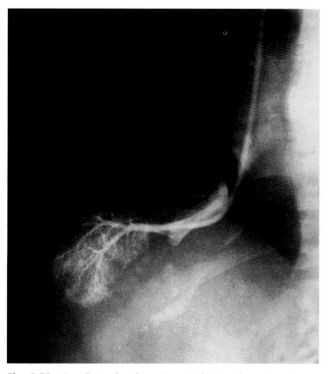

Fig. 9.39. A catheter has been inserted into a hepatic vein via the jugular vein. The wedged position is confirmed by introducing a small amount of contrast, which has entered the sinusoidal bed.

HVPG is related to survival [73] and also to prognosis in patients with bleeding oesophageal varices [74]. The procedure may be used to monitor therapy, for instance the effect of beta-blockers such as propranolol, with optimal target reduction of HVPG by 20% from baseline or to less than 12 mmHg, which results in a reduced risk of bleeding [75].

Variceal pressure

An *endoscopic pressure gauge* may be fixed to the end of the endoscope. The level of venous pressure is a major factor predicting variceal haemorrhage [76].

Pressure may be recorded by *direct puncture* of varices at the time of sclerotherapy [77]. It is about 15.5 mmHg in cirrhotic patients, significantly lower than the main portal pressure of about 18.8 mmHg. An *endoscopic balloon* has been developed to measure variceal pressure and this gives comparable results to direct puncture [78].

Estimation of hepatic blood flow

Constant infusion method

Hepatic blood flow may be measured by a constant infusion of indocyanine green (ICG) and catheterization of the hepatic vein [79,80]. Flow is calculated by the Fick principle.

Plasma disappearance method

Hepatic blood flow can be measured after an intravenous injection of ICG followed by analysis of the disappearance curve in a peripheral artery and hepatic vein. If the extraction of a substance is about 100%, for instance, using ^{131}I heat-denatured albumin colloidal complex, hepatic blood flow can be determined by peripheral clearance without hepatic vein catheterization. However, in patients with cirrhosis, as up to 20% of the blood perfusing the liver may not go through normal channels and hepatic extraction is reduced, hepatic vein catheterization is necessary to estimate extraction and thus hepatic blood flow.

Azygos blood flow

Most of the blood flowing through gastro-oesophageal varices terminates in the azygos system. Azygos blood flow can be measured using a double thermodilution catheter directed under fluoroscopy into the azygos vein [81]. Alcoholic cirrhotic patients who have bled from varices show a flow of about 600 mL/min. Azygos flow is markedly reduced by propranolol.

Experimental portal venous occlusion and hypertension

Survival following acute occlusion depends on the development of an adequate collateral circulation. In the rabbit, cat or dog this does not develop and death supervenes rapidly. In the monkey or man, the collateral circulation is adequate and survival is usual.

Acute occlusion of one branch of the portal vein is not fatal. The liver cells of the ischaemic lobe atrophy, but bile ducts, Kupffer cells and connective tissues survive. The unaffected lobe hypertrophies.

Experimentally, portal hypertension can be produced by occluding the portal vein, injecting silica into the portal vein, infecting mice with schistosomiasis, by any experimental type of cirrhosis or by biliary obstruction. An extensive collateral circulation develops, the spleen enlarges but ascites does not form.

Classification of portal hypertension

Portal hypertension usually follows obstruction to the portal blood flow anywhere along its course. *Portal hypertension* has been classified into two types: (1) *presinusoidal* (extrahepatic or intrahepatic); and (2) a larger group of *hepatic* causes (intrahepatic 'sinusoidal' and postsinusoidal) (Fig. 9.40, Table 9.3). This distinction is a practical one. The presinusoidal forms, which include obstruction to the sinusoids by Kupffer and other cellular proliferations, are associated with relatively normal hepatocellular function. Consequently, if patients with this type suffer a haemorrhage from varices, liver failure is rarely a consequence. In contrast, patients with the hepatic type may develop liver failure after bleeding.

Extrahepatic portal venous obstruction

This causes extrahepatic presinusoidal portal hypertension. The obstruction may be at any point in the course of the portal vein, usually due to thrombosis. The *venae comitantes* enlarge in an attempt to deliver portal blood to the liver, so assuming a leash-like cavernous appearance. The portal vein, represented by a fibrous strand, is recognized with difficulty in the multitude of small vessels. This cavernous change follows any block in the main vein (see Fig. 9.32). Confluent thrombosis may extend to the splenic and/or superior mesenteric vein [82].

Aetiology

Infections

Umbilical infection with or without catheterization of the umbilical vein may be responsible in neonates [83].

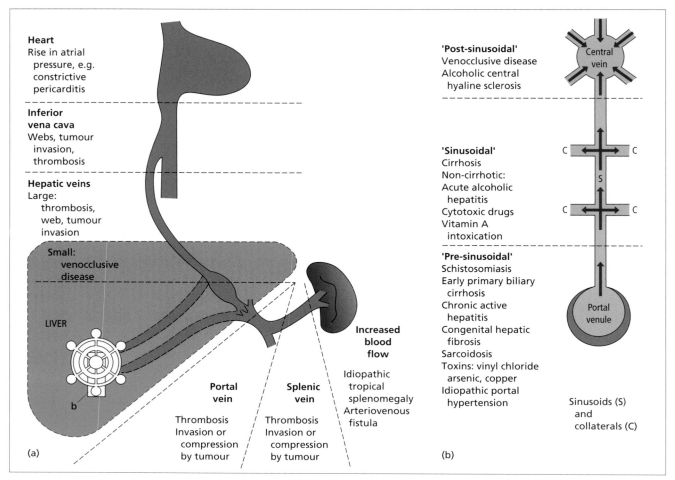

Fig. 9.40. Causes of portal hypertension. (a) Pre- and posthepatic. (b) Intrahepatic (NB an overlap exists; wedge hepatic vein pressure may be high in patients with 'presinusoidal' causes, especially as the disease progresses, indicating sinusoidal and/or collateral involvement. Some 'postsinusoidal' conditions may also have a sinusoidal component).

Table 9.3. Classification of portal hypertension

Presinusoidal	Extrahepatic	Blocked portal vein
		Increased splenic flow
	Intrahepatic	Portal zone infiltrates
		Toxic
		Hepatoportal sclerosis
Hepatic	Intrahepatic (sinusoidal)	Cirrhosis
	Postsinusoidal	Other nodules
		Blocked hepatic vein

The infection spreads along the umbilical vein to the left portal vein and hence to the main portal vein. Acute appendicitis and peritonitis are causative in older children.

Portal vein occlusion is particularly common in India, accounting for 20–30% of all variceal bleeding. Neonatal dehydration and infections may be responsible.

Ulcerative colitis and Crohn's disease can be complicated by portal or hepatic vein thrombosis.

Portal vein obstruction may be secondary to biliary infections due, for instance, to gallstones or primary sclerosing cholangitis.

Postoperative

The portal and splenic veins commonly thrombose after splenectomy, especially when, preoperatively, the patient had a normal platelet count. The thrombosis spreads from the splenic vein into the main portal vein. It is especially likely in patients with myeloid metaplasia. A similar sequence follows occluded surgical portosystemic shunts.

The portal vein may thrombose as a complication of major, difficult hepatobiliary surgery, for instance repair of a stricture or removal of a choledochal cyst.

Trauma

Portal vein injury may rarely follow vehicle accidents or stabbing. Laceration of the portal vein is 50% fatal and ligation may be the only method to control the bleeding.

Hypercoagulable state

This is a frequent cause of portal vein thrombosis in adults and less often in children [84]. It is commonly due to a myeloproliferative disorder which may be latent, or the presence of G20210A prothrombin gene mutation, and/or one or more heterozygous or homozygous deficiency states for protein C, S, antithrombin III or other prothrombotic tendencies [85]. At autopsy, thrombotic lesions are found in macroscopic and microscopic portal veins of patients dying with portal hypertension and myelometaplasia [86]. Ascites and oesophageal varices are associated.

Invasion and compression

The classic example is hepatocellular carcinoma. Carcinoma of the pancreas, usually of the body, and of other adjacent organs may lead to portal vein thrombosis. Chronic pancreatitis is frequently associated with splenic vein obstruction, but involvement of the portal vein is rare (5.6%) [82,87].

Congenital

Congenital obstruction can be produced anywhere along the line of the right and left vitelline veins from which the portal vein develops. The portal vein may be absent with visceral venous return passing to systemic veins, particularly the inferior vena cava [88]. Hilar venous collaterals are absent.

Congenital abnormalities of the portal vein are usually associated with congenital defects elsewhere [88,89].

Cirrhosis

Portal vein thrombosis is not infrequent as a complication of cirrhosis [90]. Invasion by a hepatocellular carcinoma is a frequent cause. Postsplenectomy thrombocytosis is another aetiological factor. Mural thrombi found at autopsy are probably terminal. It is easy to over-diagnose thrombosis by finding a non-filled portal vein on imaging. This usually represents 'steal' into massive collaterals or into a large spleen [90].

Miscellaneous

Portal vein thrombosis has very rarely been associated with pregnancy and with oral contraceptives, especially in older women and with long usage [91] and with thrombophlebitis migrans and other general disease of veins.

In retroperitoneal fibrosis, the portal venous system may be encased by dense fibrous tissue.

Portal vein occlusion with recanalization is a common manifestation of Behçet's disease [92].

Unknown

In about half of patients the aetiology remains obscure. Some of these patients have associated autoimmune disorders such as hypothyroidism, diabetes, pernicious anaemia, dermatomyositis or rheumatoid arthritis [82]. In some instances, the obstruction may have followed undiagnosed intra-abdominal infections such as appendicitis or diverticulitis.

Clinical features

The patient may present with features of the underlying disease, for instance polycythaemia rubra vera [86] or primary liver cancer. Children may have growth retardation [93].

Bleeding from oesophagogastric varices is the most common presentation. In those of neonatal origin, the first haemorrhage is at about the age of 4 years (Fig. 9.41). The frequency increases between 10 and 15 years and decreases after puberty. However, some patients with portal venous thrombosis never bleed and in others haemorrhage may be delayed for as long as 12 years. If blood replacement is adequate, recovery usually ensues in a matter of days. Apart from frank bleeds, intermittent minor blood loss is probably common. This is diagnosed only if the patient is having repeated checks for faecal blood or iron deficiency anaemia.

Especially in children, haemorrhage may be initiated by a minor, intercurrent infection. The mechanism is unclear. Aspirin or a similar drug may be the precipitating factor. Excessive exertion or swallowing a large bolus does not seem to initiate bleeding.

The spleen is always enlarged and symptomless splenomegaly may be a presentation, particularly in children. Periumbilical veins are not seen but there may be dilated abdominal wall veins in the left flank.

The liver is normal in size and consistency. Stigmata of hepatocellular disease, such as jaundice or vascular spiders, are absent. With acute portal venous thrombosis, ascites is early and transient, subsiding as the collateral circulation develops. Ascites is usually related to an additional factor that has depressed hepatocellular

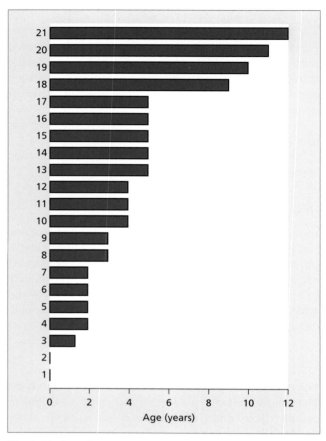

Fig. 9.41. Portal vein occlusion in neonates. Age at time of first haemorrhage in 21 patients in whom the portal vein block occurred in the neonatal period.

function, such as a haemorrhage or a surgical exploration. It may be seen in the elderly where it is related to the deterioration of liver function with ageing [94].

Hepatic encephalopathy is not uncommon in adults, usually following an additional insult such as haemorrhage, infection or anaesthetic. Chronic encephalopathy may be seen in elderly patients with a particularly large portal–systemic circulation. Rarely, compression of the common bile duct can occur, termed 'portal biliopathy' [95], which may cause jaundice.

Imaging

Ultrasound shows echogenic thrombus within the portal vein and colour Doppler shows slow flow velocity in the cavernous collaterals and no portal venous signal [96,97].

CT shows the thrombus as a non-enhancing filling defect within the lumen of the portal vein and dilatation of many small veins at the hilum (Fig. 9.42).

MRI shows an area of abnormal signal within the lumen of the portal vein which appears isointense on a T_1-weighted image with a more intense signal on a T_2-weighted image.

Angiography in the portal venous phase shows a filling defect or non-opacification of the portal vein. However, the portal vein may not be visualized if blood is diverted away from it into extensive collaterals.

Haematology

Haemoglobin is normal unless there has been blood loss. Leucopenia and thrombocytopenia are related to

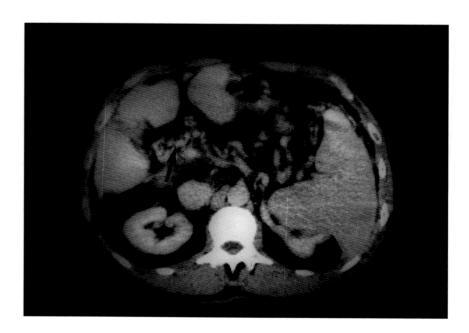

Fig. 9.42. Abdominal CT scan with contrast showing the main portal vein replaced by a leash of small veins (arrow).

the enlarged spleen. Circulating platelets and leucocytes, although in short supply, are adequate and function well.

Hypersplenism is not an indication for splenectomy. Blood coagulation is normal.

Serum biochemistry

All the usual tests of 'liver function' are normal. Elevation of serum globulin may be related to intestinal antigens, bypassing the liver through collaterals. Mild pancreatic hypofunction is related to interruption of the venous drainage of the pancreas [98].

Prognosis

This depends on the underlying disease [82]. The outlook is much better than for cirrhosis as liver function is normal. The prognosis is surprisingly good in the child and, with careful management of recurrent bleeding, survival to adult life is expected. The number of bleeds seems to reduce as time passes. Women may bleed in pregnancy but this is unusual; their babies are normal.

Treatment

Any cause must be identified and treated. This may be more important than the portal hypertension. For instance, hepatocellular carcinoma, invading the portal vein, precludes aggressive therapy for bleeding oesophageal varices. If the variceal bleeding is related to polycythaemia rubra vera, reduction of the platelet count must precede any surgical therapy; anticoagulants may be needed [82].

Prophylactic treatment of varices is not indicated. They may never rupture and as time passes collaterals open up.

With acute portal vein thrombosis, anticoagulant therapy will result in recanalization in one-third of patients [99]. If diagnosed early, anticoagulants may prevent spreading thrombosis and intestinal infarction or severe bleeding. Presence of ascites and splenic vein thrombosis should lead to alternative therapies [99].

Children should survive haemorrhage with proper management, including transfusion. Care must be taken to give compatible blood and to preserve peripheral veins. Aspirin ingestion should be avoided. Upper respiratory any other infections should be treated seriously as they seem to precipitate haemorrhage.

Endoscopic therapy is valuable as an emergency procedure; balloon tamponade may be needed.

Major or recurrent bleeds may be treated by repeated sclerotherapy, particularly in children, or ligation. Unfortunately this does not treat gastric fundal varices and the congestive gastropathy remains.

Definitive surgery to reduce portal pressure maybe impossible as there are no suitable veins for a shunt. Even apparently normal-looking veins seen on venography turn out to be in poor condition, presumably related to extension of the original thrombotic process. In children, veins are very small and difficult to anastomose.

Results for all forms of surgery are unsatisfactory. Splenectomy is the least successful.

A shunt (portacaval, mesocaval or splenocaval) is the most satisfactory treatment. In children a mesentericoportal shunt, anastomosing to a patent left portal vein branch, not only prevents bleeding, but improves growth [100].

When the patient is exsanguinating, despite massive blood transfusion, an oesophageal transection may have to be performed. Here again gastric varices are not treated. Postoperative complications are common.

TIPS may be possible providing the superior mesenteric vein is patent [101].

Splenic vein obstruction

Isolated splenic vein obstruction causes sinistral (left-sided) portal hypertension. It may be due to any of the factors causing portal vein obstruction (Fig. 9.43).

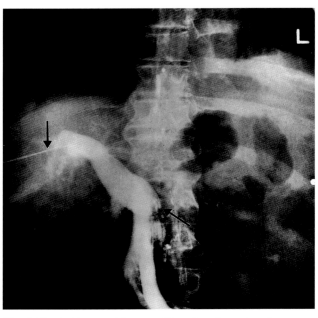

Fig. 9.43. A 64-year-old man with polycythaemia rubra vera. Transhepatic portal venogram (transhepatic needle marked by upper arrow) showing a thrombosed splenic vein (marked by the lower arrow) with patent superior mesenteric and portal veins. This patient, after preliminary reduction of red cell and platelet count by radioactive phosphorus, was successfully treated by splenectomy.

Pancreatic disease such as carcinoma (18%), pancreatitis (65%), pseudocyst and pancreatectomy are particularly important [87].

If the obstruction is distal to the entry of the left gastric vein, a collateral circulation bypasses the obstructed splenic vein through short gastric veins into the gastric fundus and lower oesophagus, so reaching the left gastric vein and portal vein. This leads to very prominent varices in the fundus of the stomach but few in the lower oesophagus.

The selective venous phase of an angiogram, an enhanced CT scan or MRI are diagnostic. Splenectomy, by blocking arterial inflow, is usually curative but unnecessary if the patient has not bled from varices [102].

Hepatic arterioportal venous fistulae

Portal hypertension results from increased portal venous flow. Increase in intrahepatic resistance due to a rise in portal flow may also be important. Portal zones show thickening of small portal radicles with accompanying mild fibrosis and lymphocyte infiltration. The increased intrahepatic resistance may persist after obliteration of the fistula.

These fistulae are usually congenital, traumatic (including after liver biopsy) or related to adjacent malignant neoplasm [103]. Inferior mesenteric arteriovenous fistulae may be associated with acute ischaemic colitis.

With large fistulae, a loud arterial bruit is heard in the right upper abdomen. Pain may be pronounced. Others present with portal hypertension.

Ultrasound and enhanced CT show an enlarged hepatic artery and a dilated intrahepatic portal vein. The diagnosis is confirmed by arteriography.

Selective non-invasive embolization of fistulae has replaced surgery.

Portohepatic venous shunts

These are probably congenital and represent persistence of the omphalomesenteric venous system. They may be between the main portal and hepatic veins or between the right or left portal vein and hepatic veins [104]. They are diagnosed by ultrasound, enhanced CT scan, MRI and colour Doppler imaging and confirmed by arteriography.

Presinusoidal intrahepatic and sinusoidal portal hypertension (Fig. 9.44)

Portal tract lesions

In *schistosomiasis*, the portal hypertension results from the ova causing a reaction in the minute portal venous radicles.

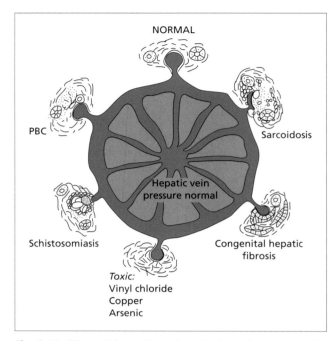

Fig. 9.44. The aetiology of presinusoidal intrahepatic portal hypertension. PBC, primary biliary cirrhosis.

In *congenital hepatic fibrosis*, the portal hypertension is probably due to a deficiency of terminal branches of the portal vein in the fibrotic portal zones.

Portal hypertension has been reported with *myeloproliferative diseases* including myelosclerosis, myeloid leukaemia and Hodgkin's disease [105]. The mechanism is complex. In part it is related to infiltration of the portal zones with haemopoietic tissue, but thrombotic lesions in major and minor portal vein radicles and nodular regenerative hyperplasia contribute [86].

In *systemic mastocytosis*, portal hypertension is related to increased intrahepatic resistance secondary to mast cell infiltration. Increased splenic flow, perhaps with splenic arteriovenous shunting and with histamine release, may contribute.

In *primary biliary cirrhosis*, portal hypertension may be a presenting feature long before the development of the nodular regeneration characteristic of cirrhosis (Chapter 15). The mechanism is uncertain, although portal zone lesions and narrowing of the sinusoids because of cellular infiltration have been incriminated. The portal hypertension of *sarcoidosis* may be similar. Massive fibrosis is usually associated.

Toxic causes

The injurious substance is mainly taken up by hepatic stellate cells in Disse's space; these are fibrogenic. Minute portal vein radicles are obstructed and intrahepatic portal hypertension results.

Inorganic arsenic has caused portal hypertension in patients being treated for psoriasis.

Liver disease in vineyard sprayers in Portugal may be related to exposure to *copper*. Angiosarcoma may be a complication.

Exposure to the vapour of the polymer of *vinyl chloride* leads to sclerosis of portal venules with portal hypertension and angiosarcoma.

Reversible portal hypertension may follow *vitamin A intoxication*—vitamin A being stored in hepatic stellate cells. Prolonged use of *cytotoxic drugs*, such as methotrexate, 6-mercaptopurine and azathioprine, can lead to perisinusoidal fibrosis and portal hypertension.

Hepatoportal sclerosis

This is marked by splenomegaly, hypersplenism and portal hypertension without occlusion of portal and splenic veins and with no obvious pathology in the liver [106]. It has also been termed non-cirrhotic portal fibrosis, non-cirrhotic portal hypertension and idiopathic portal hypertension. *Banti's syndrome*, an obsolete term, probably fell into this group. Injury to intrahepatic portal venous radicles and sinusoidal endothelial cells is the common denominator.

An increase in intrahepatic resistance indicates an obstruction to hepatic blood flow. Increased lymph flow may help to reduce the high portal pressure [107].

The aetiology may be infectious, toxic or, in many instances, unknown (Fig. 9.45). In childhood, intrahepatic thrombosis of small portal veins could be the primary disorder.

In Japan, it affects largely middle-aged women. A very similar condition in India, called *non-cirrhotic portal*

fibrosis, largely affects young males [108]. It has been related to arsenic taken in drinking water and in unorthodox medicines. In both countries, it is probably due to the effects of multiple intestinal infections on the liver. It is therefore decreasing with improved hygiene.

Somewhat similar patients have been reported from the USA [109] and the UK [110].

Liver biopsy shows sclerosis and sometimes obliteration of the intrahepatic venous bed but the changes, and especially the fibrosis, may be minimal. Large portal veins near the hilum may be thickened and narrow, but this is usually seen only at autopsy. Some of the changes seem to be secondary to partial thrombosis of small portal venous channels with recanalization. Perisinusoidal fibrosis is usually present but may be seen only by electron microscopy.

Portal venography shows small portal vein radicles to be narrowed and sparse. The peripheral branches may be irregular with acute-angle division. Some of the large intrahepatic portal branches may be non-opacified with an increase of very fine vasculature around the large intrahepatic portal branches. Hepatic venography confirms the vascular abnormalities and vein-to-vein anastomoses are frequent.

Tropical splenomegaly syndrome

This is marked by residence in a malarial area, splenomegaly, hepatic sinusoidal lymphocytosis and Kupffer cell hyperplasia, raised serum IgM and malarial antibody titres and response to prolonged antimalarial chemotherapy. Portal hypertension is not marked and variceal bleeding is rare [108].

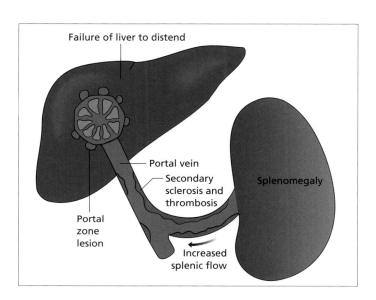

Fig. 9.45. Factors concerned in so-called idiopathic 'primary' portal hypertension.

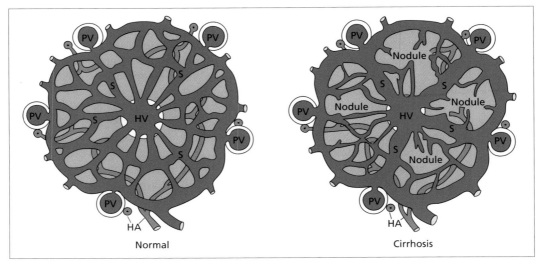

Fig. 9.46. Cirrhosis of the liver showing the formation of portal venous (PV) / hepatic venous (HV) anastomoses or internal Eck fistulae at the site of pre-existing sinusoids (S).

Note that the regeneration nodules are supplied by the hepatic artery (HA).

Intrahepatic sinusoidal portal hypertension

Cirrhosis

All forms of cirrhosis lead to portal hypertension and the primary event is obstruction to portal blood flow [20]. Portal venous blood is diverted into collateral channels and some bypasses the liver cells and is shunted directly into the hepatic venous radicles in the fibrous septa. These portohepatic anastomoses develop from pre-existing sinusoids enclosed in the septa (Fig. 9.46) [111]. The hepatic vein is displaced further and further outwards until it lies in a fibrous septum linked with the portal venous radicle by the original sinusoid. The regenerating nodules become divorced from their portal blood supply and are nourished by the hepatic artery. Even larger portohepatic venous anastomoses are found in the cirrhotic liver. About one-third of the total blood flow perfusing the cirrhotic liver may bypass sinusoids, and hence functioning liver tissue, through these channels [112].

The obstruction to portal flow is partially due to nodules which compress hepatic venous radicles (Fig. 9.47) [113]. This would lead to a postsinusoidal portal hypertension. However, in cirrhosis, the wedged hepatic venous (sinusoidal) and main portal pressures are virtually identical and the stasis must extend to the portal inflow vessels. Sinusoids probably provide the greatest resistance to flow. Changes in the space of Disse, particularly collagenization, result in sinusoidal narrowing and this may be particularly important in the alcoholic. Hepatocyte swelling in the alcoholic may also reduce sinusoidal flow [38]. Obstruction is

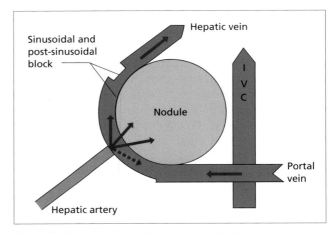

Fig. 9.47. The circulation in hepatic cirrhosis. A nodule obstructs the sinusoids and hepatic veins. The nodule is supplied mainly by the hepatic artery. IVC, inferior vena cava.

therefore believed to be at all levels from portal zones through the sinusoids to the hepatic venous outflow (Fig. 9.48).

The hepatic artery provides the liver with a small volume of blood at a high pressure. The portal vein delivers a large volume at a low pressure (see Fig. 9.6). The two systems are equilibrated in sinusoids. Normally, the hepatic artery probably plays little part in maintaining portal venous pressure. In cirrhosis, more direct arterioportal shunting has been suspected. Hypertrophy of the hepatic artery and relative increase in flow help to maintain sinusoidal perfusion.

Non-cirrhotic nodules

See Chapter 34.

Bleeding oesophageal varices

Predicting rupture

The first appearance and subsequent growth of gastro-esophageal varices following diagnosis of cirrhosis is approximately 7% per year [114,115].

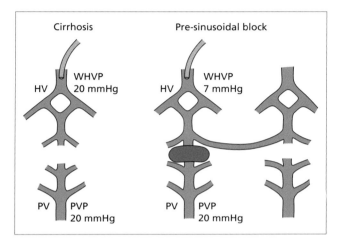

Fig. 9.48. In patients with cirrhosis the wedged hepatic venous pressure (WHVP) (20 mmHg) is equal to the pressure in the main portal vein (PVP) (20 mmHg) (measured via umbilical vein). Resistance to flow extends from the central hepatic vein, through the sinusoids to the portal vein (PV). In presinusoidal portal hypertension normal anastomoses exist between small vascular units and prevent the blocking catheter from producing a large area of stasis. WHVP (7 mmHg) is therefore less than the pressure in the main portal vein (20 mmHg).

The precipitating event is not known, but may be an inflammatory response or infection [116], on a background of raised intravariceal pressure. The first variceal haemorrhage occurs within the first year after diagnosis of varices in approximately 12%, depending on the size of varices, red signs on varices and the degree of liver dysfunction, which are the best predictors of bleeding (Fig. 9.49) [54]. Patients with moderate to severe liver dysfunction, irrespective of the size of varices and presence of red signs, should receive prophylaxis.

Intravariceal pressure is less important than size and appearance of varices, although a portal pressure above 10 mmHg appears necessary for varices to form and 12 mmHg for them to subsequently bleed [117]. Patients with alcoholic cirrhosis may be at most risk [118]. Doppler sonography may predict likelihood of bleeding, based on velocity and diameter of the portal vein, spleen size and the presence of collaterals [119].

Child's grade is used to assess hepatocellular function in cirrhosis (Table 9.4). Every patient should be assigned a grade. It is the most important predictor of the likelihood of bleeding. It correlates with variceal size and with the presence of endoscopic red signs and with the response to emergency treatment.

Prevention of first bleeding [120]

Liver function must be improved, for instance, by abstaining from alcohol. Aspirin and NSAIDs should be avoided. No protection comes from avoiding certain foods such as spices or from taking long-term H_2-blockers.

Propranolol or nadalol are non-selective beta-blockers which reduce portal pressure by splanchnic vasoconstriction and, to a lesser extent, by reducing cardiac output. Hepatic arterial blood flow falls [121,122]. The drug is given in a dose which reduces the resting pulse

Fig. 9.49. Increasing variceal size (small (S), medium (M) and large (L)) combine with red wheals (RW) on varices (absent, moderate, severe) and Child's grade (A, B, C) to define probability of bleeding at 1 year (adapted from [54]).

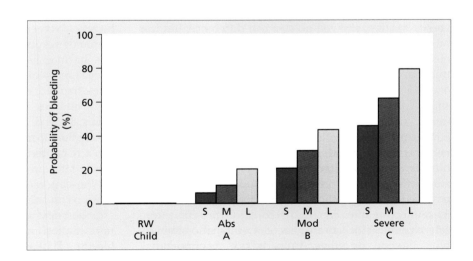

Table 9.4. Child's classification of hepatocellular function in cirrhosis

Group designation	A	B	C
Serum bilirubin* (mg/dL)	Below 2.0	2.0–3.0	Over 3.0
Serum albumin (g/dL)	Over 3.5	3.0–3.5	Under 3.0
Ascites	None	Easily controlled	Poorly controlled
Neurological disorder	None	Minimal	Advanced coma
Nutrition	Excellent	Good	Poor: 'wasting'

*1 mg = 17 μmol/L.

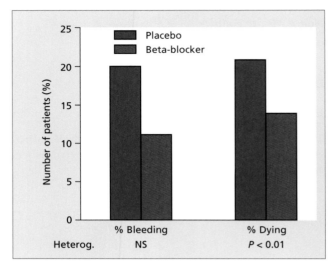

Fig. 9.50. Meta-analysis of six trials of prophylactic propranolol (beta-blocker) therapy. Data on dying cannot be relied upon because of significant heterogeneity (Heterog.) in groups. There is, however, a significant reduction in those bleeding [124].

rate to that best tolerated by the patient, but not below 55/min. There is marked individual variation in the lowering of the portal pressure. Even with large doses, 60–70% of patients do not respond in optimal fashion, especially those with advanced cirrhosis [123]. The optimal HVPG reduction is to or below 12 mmHg and/ or a 20% fall from baseline. However, the low risk of first bleeding with therapy makes HVPG measurement not very applicable outside of research protocols.

Propranolol should not be given to patients with obstructive airways disease. No fatal effects have been reported. If resuscitation is difficult intravenous glucagon can be given. Propranolol causes some mental depression, sometimes impotence and fatigue. Nadolol has similar effects.

Randomized trials of non-selective beta blockers against placebo or no treatment showed a significant reduction in bleeding, but survival was not statistically different [124] (Fig. 9.50). Sclerotherapy is potentially harmful [121]; banding ligation is safer. A meta-analysis of randomized trials of non-selective beta-blockers versus ligation, showed no survival difference, but less bleeding with ligation [125]. However, to avoid one bleeding episode in the ligation group, one needs to treat five to six patients and perform about 33 sessions of endoscopy [126], so that it is not cost effective. Ligation should be used when there are contraindications or intolerance to non-selective beta-blockers. One study has compared carvedilol versus banding ligation [127], resulting in less bleeding with carvedilol. However, the dose used was smaller than in other studies in which side effects of carvedilol precluding continuation occurred, and the efficacy of banding was one of the least effective rates reported [128]. Studies versus non-selective beta-blockers are needed. Combination therapy with ligation or other drugs is not recommended.

Isosorbide mononitrate may worsen fluid retention, particularly in patients over 50 years old [129].

Diagnosis of bleeding

The *clinical features* are those of gastrointestinal bleeding with the added picture of portal hypertension.

Bleeding is most often a sudden haematemesis, but may be a slow ooze with melaena, and sometimes presents with iron deficiency anaemia usually due to portal hypertensive gastropathy or colopathy. The intestines may be full of blood before the haemorrhage is recognized and the bleeding episode is liable to continue for days.

Bleeding varices in cirrhosis have injurious effects on the liver cells. These may be due to anaemia diminishing hepatic oxygen supply, or to increased metabolic demands resulting from the protein catabolism following haemorrhage or to secondary stimulation and release of cytokines. The fall in blood pressure diminishes hepatic arterial flow, on which the regenerating liver nodules depend, and ischaemic hepatitis may ensue as well as renal injury. The increased nitrogen absorption from the intestines often leads to hepatic coma (Chapter 8). Deteriorating liver cell function may precipitate jaundice or ascites, and renal impairment.

Non-variceal bleeding from duodenal ulcers, gastric erosions and the Mallory–Weiss syndrome is frequent.

Endoscopy should always be performed following resuscitation and within 12 h to confirm the source of the bleeding [130] (Fig. 9.51). Bleeding varices may be diag-

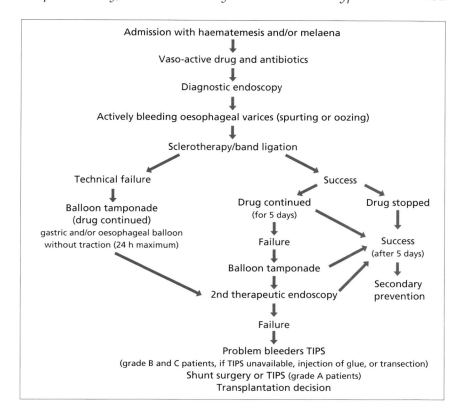

Admission with haematemesis and/or melaena
↓
Vaso-active drug and antibiotics
↓
Diagnostic endoscopy
↓
Actively bleeding oesophageal varices (spurting or oozing)
↓
Sclerotherapy/band ligation

Technical failure   Success

Balloon tamponade
(drug continued)
gastric and/or oesophageal balloon
without traction (24 h maximum)

Drug continued
(for 5 days)   Drug stopped
↓
Failure   Success
↓   (after 5 days)
Balloon tamponade   ↓
↓   Secondary
2nd therapeutic endoscopy   prevention
↓
Failure
↓
Problem bleeders TIPS
(grade B and C patients, if TIPS unavailable, injection of glue, or transection)
Shunt surgery or TIPS (grade A patients)
Transplantation decision

Fig. 9.51. Common practice for the management of oesophageal varices actively bleeding at diagnosis. Acute therapeutic endoscopy should only be performed by an experienced endoscopist [130].

nosed endoscopically when an ooze of blood is seen from an area within 5 cm of the gastroesophageal junction or as a venous spurt (active bleeding). Alternatively a platelet 'plug' (a white raised spot) may indicated a varix that has bled [131]; if no other lesion is seen in the upper gastrointestinal tract, varices are considered to be the source of bleeding.

Prognosis

Sixty-five per cent of varices in patients with cirrhosis will not rupture within 2 years of diagnosis [54].

The prognosis is determined by the severity of the hepatocellular disease, with death within 6 weeks between 0 and 10% for Child A cirrhosis and 20 and 40% for Child C cirrhosis. Survival has improved over the past decades [132]. The 1-year survival in good-risk (Child grade A and B) patients is about 85% and in bad-risk (Child grade C) patients about 30% (Table 9.5). Survival scores [74] can be based on a combination of variables reflecting severity of liver disease and bleeding and the presence of active bleeding [133], encephalopathy, prothrombin time and the number of units transfused in the previous 72 h. Abstention from alcohol considerably improves the prognosis. Patients with continuing chronic hepatitis do poorly. Patients with primary biliary cirrhosis tolerate the haemorrhage reasonably well [134], particularly if not very jaundiced.

Table 9.5. Deaths from upper gastrointestinal bleeding in cirrhosis

Sources of bleeding	Number of patients	Deaths within 6 weeks
All sources	465	92 (20%)
Variceal	336	70 (21%)
Non-variceal	114	17 (15%)
Undefined	15	5 (33%)

The importance of hepatocellular function is emphasized by the relatively good prognosis for bleeding in patients where hepatocellular function is relatively well preserved, as in schistosomiasis, the non-cirrhotic portal hypertension of India and Japan, and portal vein thrombosis.

Management of acute variceal bleeding [74,130] (Fig. 9.51)

Child's grade is recorded (Table 9.4). Bleeding is likely to continue and observations must be close. If possible, the patient should be managed by an experienced intensive care team. Haemodynamic monitoring (central venous pressure) and peripheral drip are instigated. The patient is transfused to a 0.3 haematocrit or haemoglobin to less than or equal to 8 g/L. Over-transfusion is avoided. Systolic blood pressure is maintained at equal or greater than 90 mmHg. Saline infusions are avoided.

Fresh frozen plasma and platelet transfusions may be necessary to prevent further worsening of coagulation by dilution of transfused blood. Vitamin K_1 intravenously is routine. Acid secretion is suppressed although there is little controlled evidence of benefit; H_2 receptor antagonists have less risk of inducing *Clostridium difficile* infections than proton pump inhibitors. However, stress-induced mucosal ulcers are frequent.

Liver function is monitored and electrolyte balance and renal function maintained.

Prophylactic antibiotics, currently third-generation cephalosporins, are given immediately as they prevent infection [135], reduce bleeding and improve survival [136,137]. Pneumonia is prevented by special care during endoscopy, and endotracheal intubation is warranted if the patient has encephalopathy.

Hepatic encephalopathy is prevented by lactulose and phosphate enemas.

Sedatives should be avoided, and, if essential low-dose zopiclone should be used. Oral chlormethiazole or chlordiazepoxide may be required to treat or prevent delirium tremens in alcoholics.

If ascites is very tense, intra-abdominal pressure may be reduced by a cautious paracentesis and intravenous albumin replacement and the use of spironolactone.

Management requires the availability of many therapeutic options and these may need to be combined in the individual patient (Fig. 9.51). They include vasoactive drugs, endoscopic sclerotherapy and variceal banding, the Sengstaken tube, or other tamponade devices, TIPS and very rarely emergency surgery.

Vasoactive drugs

Vasoactive drugs lower portal venous pressure and should be started even before diagnostic and therapeutic endoscopy [130,138]. Treatment can be given even before the patient is admitted to hospital and certainly in the emergency room. Early treatment facilitates the ease with which endoscopic therapy can be done as active bleeding has been reduced.

Vasopressin and terlipressin lower portal venous pressure by constriction of the splanchnic arterioles, so causing an increase in resistance to the inflow of blood to the gut (Fig. 9.52). They control variceal bleeding by lowering the portal venous pressure. Terlipressin has replaced vasopressin in countries where it is available.

Vasopressin and terlipressin can cause coronary vasoconstriction and an electrocardiogram should be taken before they are given. Abdominal colicky discomfort and evacuation of the bowels together with facial pallor are usual during the infusion. Myocardial intestinal

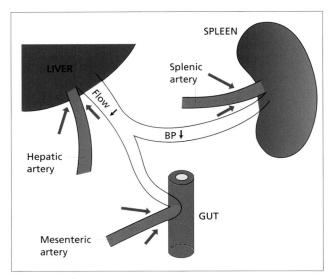

Fig. 9.52. The mode of action of vasopressin on the splanchnic circulation. Hepatic, splenic and mesenteric arteries are shown. Splanchnic blood flow (including hepatic blood flow) and portal venous pressure are reduced by arterial vasoconstriction (blue arrows). BP, blood pressure.

ischaemia and rarely infarction are other possible complications.

Terlipressin is given in a dose of 2 mg intravenously every 6 h for 48 h. It may be continued for a further 3 days at 1 mg every 4–6 h. It is the only vasoactive drug for which there is evidence for improved survival.

Somatostatin reduces the portal pressure by increasing splanchnic arterial resistance. It also inhibits a number of vasodilatory peptides, including glucagon. It has less side effects than vasopressin or terlipressin [139], but does not substantially reduce blood transfusion requirement [140]. An intravenous bolus of 250 μg or 500 μg is given followed by an infusion of 6 mg/24 h for 120 h [130,138].

Octreotide and *vapreotide* are synthetic analogues of somatostatin. They have a much longer half-life (1–2 h). Trials have given conflicting results and data are far less robust than for terlipressin and somatostatin in acute variceal bleeding [140].

Sengstaken–Blakemore tube (Figs 9.53, 9.54) and self-expanding oesophageal stent

The use of oesophageal tamponade has decreased markedly with the use of vasoactive drugs, oesophageal sclerotherapy and TIPS. The four-lumen tube has an oesophageal and a gastric balloon, an aspirating channel for the stomach and a fourth lumen for continuous aspiration above the oesophageal balloon. Ideally, endotracheal intubation should be performed first, but this may not be possible. If so two, but preferably three, assistants

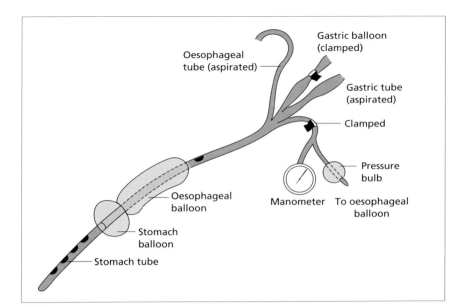

Fig. 9.53. Sengstaken–Blakemore oesophageal compression tube modified by Pitcher. Note the fourth oesophageal tube which aspirates the oesophagus above the oesophageal balloon.

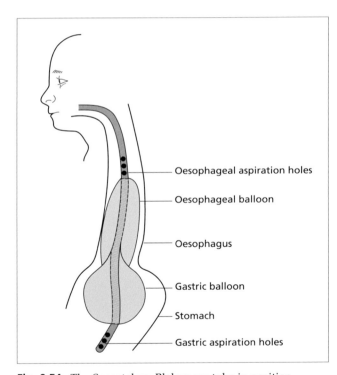

Fig. 9.54. The Sengstaken–Blakemore tube in position.

are required. The tube is easier to insert if it has been allowed to stiffen in the icebox of a refrigerator. The stomach is emptied. A new, tested and lubricated tube is passed through the mouth into the stomach. The gastric balloon is inflated with 250 mL of air and doubly clamped. The gastric tube is aspirated continuously. The whole tube is pulled back until resistance is encountered

and the oesophageal tube is then inflated to a pressure of 40 mmHg, greater than that expected in the portal vein. The tube should be taped securely to the side of the face to provide adequate traction. Too little traction means that the gastric balloon falls back into the stomach. Too much causes discomfort with retching, and also potentiates gastro-oesophageal ulceration. The initial position of the tube is checked by X-ray (Fig. 9.54). The head of the bed is raised.

The oesophageal tube has continuous low-pressure suction and occasional aspiration. Tube traction and oesophageal balloon pressure are checked hourly. After 12 h, traction is released and the oesophageal balloon deflated, leaving the gastric balloon inflated. If bleeding recurs, the traction is reapplied and the oesophageal balloon reinflated until emergency therapeutic endoscopy or TIPS can be performed. A further procedure should always follow tamponade as rebleeding reoccurs in over 50% after withdrawal. If bleeding is not controlled the tube has slipped or the source of bleeding is fundal varices or another lesion.

Complications include obstruction to upper airways. If the gastric balloon bursts or deflates, the oesophageal balloon may migrate into the oropharynx causing asphyxia. The oesophageal balloon must be deflated, and if necessary the tube cut through immediately with scissors.

Ulceration of the lower oesophagus complicates prolonged or repeated use. Aspiration of secretions into the lung is prevented by continuous suction above the oesophageal balloon. Oesophagel rupture can occur, usually when the gastric balloon is wrongly inflated in the oesophagus.

The Sengstaken tube is the most certain method for continued control of oesophageal bleeding over hours. Complications are frequent and are in part related to the experience of the operating team. It is unpleasant for the patient. It is useful when transferring patients from one centre to another, when haemorrhage is torrential and when variceal ligation or injection, TIPS or surgery are not immediately available. The oesophageal tube should not be kept inflated for more than 24 h.

A new self-expanding, covered oesophageal stent device, which can be subsequently removed endoscopically, also results in tamponade, but allows the patient to eat and drink. It can also be used to treat oesophageal tears caused by the Sengstaken tube [141]. It requires expertise to place the tube, but this can also be done solely under radiological screening [141,142].

Endoscopic banding ligation and injection of varices

The combination of immediate use of a vasoactive agent and endoscopic banding ligation or injection is the therapeutic gold standard for the acute treatment of bleeding varices in the oesophagus and for subcardial gastric varices. In over 85% of patients the haemorrhage will be controlled with one or two sessions of endoscopic therapy [74].

Both banding ligation and injection of oesophageal varices are effective in treating bleeding from oesophageal or subcardial gastric varices. Banding ligation is slightly more effective compared to injection sclerotherapy with 5% ethanolamine or 1% sodium tetradecylsulphate, particularly when there is no active bleeding (Fig. 9.55), but survival following either procedure is the same [143]. The endoscopist must use the procedure that he/she is most used to, and judge the risk of lung aspiration if using ligation, as a further endoscopic intubation is required in order to fit the banding device.

If the patient rebleeds, a second emergency ligation or injection may be given. If more sessions are necessary, the salvage rate is poor and alternative therapy, such as injection of glue or TIPS [144] should be considered (Fig. 9.51) [74].

Patients who are likely to fail one session of therapeutic endoscopy are Child C patients with more severe bleeding at presentation. These patients often have higher (≥20 mmHg) HVPG [145]. In this group earlier switch to alternative therapies if available (or their use as first-line therapy) can be considered [74], such as injection of cyanoacrylate glue, oesophageal stenting or TIPS [146]. Double-channel endoscopies are preferred as continued suction is possible to obtain clearer views at the same time as applying bands to varices or injecting them. An assessment must be made regarding protection of the airway. If in doubt, endotracheal intubation rather than sedation must be used. Injection is made just

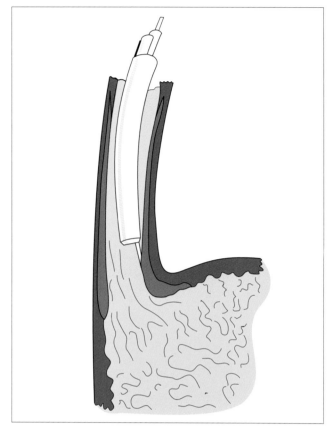

Fig. 9.55. Direct injection of oesophageal varices with an unmodified fibre optic endoscope.

above the gastro-oesophageal junction, and rarely more than 2 mL per varix is needed. More than 4 mL per varix should be avoided. Ligation requires loading of the ligation device at the tip of the endoscope and then ligation is started at the gastro-oesophageal junction and confined to the lower 3–5 cm of the oesophagus. The varices are strangulated by the application of small elastic O rings (Fig. 9.56) pulling a trip wire threaded through the operating channel of the endoscope. At least one band is applied to each varix in a spiral fashion. There is no current evidence that more bands per varix are more effective. Both injection and ligation can result in transient dysphagia, retrosternal chest pain and sometimes fever. Aspiration pneumonia must be avoided. Oesophageal ulcers are almost a universal consequence of therapy and sometimes cause recurrent bleeding. Sucralfate can speed up healing and prevent bleeding. Injection of cyanoacrylate glue is particularly indicated for bleeding gastric varices in the fundus [147] as it is more effective than ligation or sclerotherapy. Bleeding from fundal varices is often severe and has a higher mortality than from bleeding oesophageal varices. TIPS is also a first-line therapy [144,146].

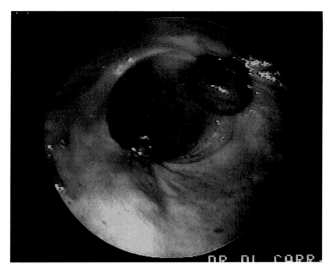

Fig. 9.56. Endoscopic variceal ligation. The varices have been strangulated by an elastic ring introduced via the endoscope.

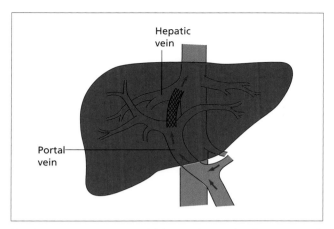

Fig. 9.57. TIPS. An expandable metal stent has been inserted between the portal vein and the hepatic vein producing an intrahepatic portosystemic shunt.

Emergency transjugular intrahepatic stent shunt [144,146]

TIPS is a radiological procedure, which in the emergency situation is best performed under general anaesthetic, but can be done under simple sedation and local anaesthesia. The internal jugular vein is punctured and the hepatic vein (usually middle right) is cannulated. Using ultrasound localization a needle puncture of the portal vein is made, and a track, which is then ballooned, is fashioned between the hepatic and portal veins. Then a self-expanding metal stent, covered in its central area by PTFE, is placed through the track. Care must be taken not to encroach on the inferior vena cava and nor to place the stent too far into the portal vein, as either can render future liver transplantation difficult (Figs 9.57, 9.58). The use of PTFE stents [148] has greatly reduced the rate of occlusion compared to bare metal stents [149], due to reduced pseudointimal hyperplasia as well as thrombosis [150,151].

An adequate portocaval gradient pressure reduction must be achieved by using the correct diameter stent (10–12 mm), usually to 12 mmHg. More than one stent may be required.

Control of bleeding

TIPS controls bleeding resulting from portal hypertension, whether it be oesophageal, gastric, intestinal, colonic or stomal. It is of particular value as salvage therapy in acute variceal bleeding which cannot be controlled by endoscopy and vasoactive drugs [74,144,152]. Embolization of collaterals performed during TIPS may

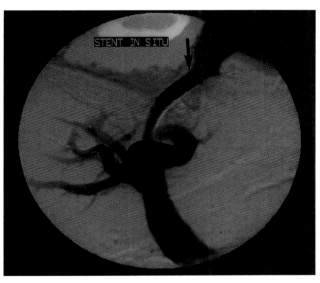

Fig. 9.58. TIPS. A portal venogram showing a portohepatic venous shunt; the stent is *in situ* (arrow).

also be necessary, particularly for bleeding from ectopic varices [153]. This is a difficult technique and a skilled interventional radiologist must be part of the team. The technical failure rate is about 5–10% and control of bleeding achieved in over 90% (Table 9.6).

Complications

Procedural mortality is less than 1%. Complications include haemorrhage, due to liver capsule puncture, or intrahepatic and which may result in intra-abdominal or bleeding into the biliary tract. TIPS can be placed in patients with thrombosis confined to the main portal vein [101].

Table 9.6. Complications of non-covered and covered TIPS in a randomized trial

Complication	Non-covered (%)	Covered (%)
Technical failure	0	0
Shunt thrombosis	7	0
Shunt stenosis	32	5
Severe hepatic encephalopathy	20	15
Shunt dysfunction	44	15
Overall mortality	46	30

Infections are prevented by a careful aseptic technique and early removal of central venous lines.

Intravascular haemolysis may be related to damage to erythrocytes by the steel mesh of the stent [154], which is much less frequent with covered stents. Hyperbilirubinaemia developing postshunt has a poor prognosis [155]. Hypersplenism and, in particular, thrombocytopenia is unaffected [154,156].

Follow-up of shunt patency is essential. This may be done by routine portography or Doppler sonography [157]. Shunt occlusion is treated by revision of the shunt under local anaesthesia. The shunt may be dilated by percutaneous catheterization or a further stent may be inserted [158]. Selected patients with stenosed TIPS, can be treated with distal splenorenal shunt if they have Child's A and B cirrhosis [159].

Emergency surgery

This is hardly ever required, but may be needed if TIPS is not available and other measures have failed. An emergency end-to-side portacaval shunt is effective in stopping bleeding [160]. Mortality is high in grade C patients, and the postsurgical encephalopathy rate is also high. If a shunt must be avoided or if there is portal vein occlusion, emergency oesophageal transection may be done using a staple gun technique [161,162]. Varices recur, enlarge and frequently rebleed [162].

Prevention of rebleeding

Following variceal bleeding, rebleeding occurs without prevention within 1 year in up to 70% of patients, more frequently if Child C grade. All patients should receive preventative therapy before discharge from hospital and replacement of depleted iron stores.

The most effective therapy is a combination of repeated endoscopic band ligation (which is more effective than repeated sclerotherapy) with non-selective beta-blockers [163]. Varices are rebanded at 2 to 3-week intervals allowing ulcers to heal in these intervals, until the varices are rendered too small to band or are eradicated. Follow-up endoscopies should be scheduled as varices can regrow. Non-selective beta-blockers are given in maximal doses as tolerated by the patient providing the pulse rate is above 55/min; they are also effective in prevention of bleeding from portal hypertensive gastropathy [164].

Portal–systemic shunt procedures (Fig. 9.59)

The aim is to reduce portal venous pressure, maintain total hepatic and, particularly, portal blood flow and, above all, not have a high incidence of hepatic encephalopathy. There is no currently available procedure that fulfils all these criteria. Hepatic reserve determines survival. Hepatocellular function deteriorates after shunting. Surgically fashioned shunts are rarely performed if TIPS can be placed.

Portacaval

In 1877, Eck [165] first performed a portacaval shunt in dogs and this remains the most effective way of reducing portal hypertension in man.

The portal vein is joined to the inferior vena cava either end-to-side, with ligation of the portal vein, or side-to-side, maintaining its continuity. The portal blood pressure falls, hepatic venous pressure falls and hepatic arterial flow increases.

Portacaval shunts are rarely performed because of the high incidence of postshunt encephalopathy. Liver function deteriorates due to reduction of portal perfusion. Subsequent hepatic transplantation can be made more difficult. It is still used, after the bleeding episode has been controlled, in patients with good liver reserve, who do not have optimal access to tertiary care including TIPS. It is useful in some patients who have had proven variceal bleeding and a patent portal vein, with early primary biliary cirrhosis, congenital hepatic fibrosis with good hepatocellular function and those with portal vein obstruction at the hilum of the liver. Patients with cirrhosis should preferably be aged less than 50 years. After the age of 40, survival is reduced and encephalopathy is twice as common.

The patient should not have a history of hepatic encephalopathy, and should be Child's grade A or B.

Mesocaval

This shunt is made between the superior mesenteric vein and the inferior vena cava using a Dacron graft (Fig. 9.60) [166]. It is technically easy. Shunt occlusion is usual with time and is followed by rebleeding [166]. It does not interfere with subsequent hepatic transplantation.

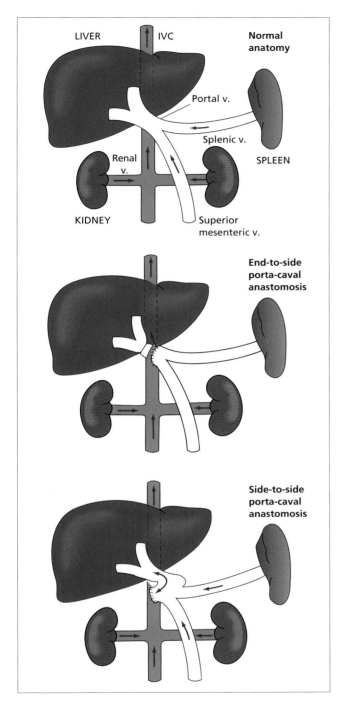

Fig. 9.59. The types of surgical portal–systemic shunt operation performed for the relief of portal hypertension. IVC, inferior vena cava.

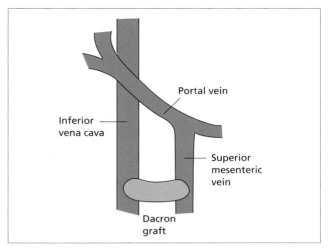

Fig. 9.60. The mesocaval shunt using a Dacron graft.

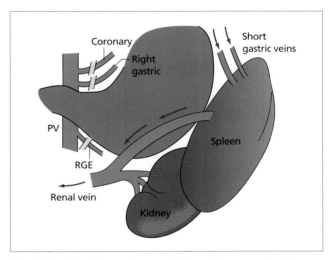

Fig. 9.61. The distal splenorenal shunt. The veins feeding the varices (coronary, right gastric, right gastroepiploic— RGE) are ligated. A splenorenal shunt is made, preserving the spleen; retrograde flow in the short gastric veins is possible. Portal blood flow to the liver is preserved. PV, portal vein.

The mortality and encephalopathy results are similar to those reported for non-selective shunts. Better results are reported in non-alcoholic patients and where gastric varices are the main problem. The operation does not interfere with a subsequent liver transplant.

Selective splenorenal shunt is technically difficult and fewer and fewer surgeons are able or willing to perform it.

General results of portal–systemic shunts

The mortality rate in good-risk patients is about 5%. For poor-risk patients the mortality is 50%.

Selective 'distal' splenorenal (Fig. 9.61)

Veins feeding the oesophagogastric collaterals are divided while allowing drainage of portal blood through short gastric–splenic veins through a splenorenal shunt to the inferior vena cava. Portal perfusion is maintained, but only for between 1 and 2 years [167,168].

Bleeding from gastro-oesophageal varices is prevented or greatly reduced. Variceal size decreases and varices may disappear within 6 months to 1 year.

Blood pressure and hepatic blood flow fall so that hepatic function deteriorates. Postoperative jaundice is related to this and to haemolysis. Ankle oedema is due to a fall in portal venous pressure while serum albumin level remains low. Increased cardiac output with failure may contribute. Shunt patency is confirmed by ultrasound, CT, MRI, Doppler or angiography.

Hepatic encephalopathy may be transient. Chronic changes develop in 20–40% and personality deterioration in about one-third (Chapter 8). The incidence increases with the size of the shunt. Encephalopathy is more common in older patients

Myelopathy with paraplegia and parkinsonian cerebellar syndrome are rare (Chapter 8).

TIPS (transjugular intrahepatic portosystemic shunt)

As for surgical shunts, TIPS should not be used as first-line therapy for prevention of rebleeding as survival is not increased [169].Health-care costs may not be less than with surgical shunts [170]. It is more effective than endoscopic therapy in terms of rebleeding, but there is no difference in survival and there is more encephalopathy [168].

TIPS encephalopathy

This is a side-to-side portal–systemic shunt and is followed by encephalopathy in about the same percentage (25–30%) as that following surgically performed portacaval shunts [171]. Encephalopathy is related to the age of the patient, Child's grade and shunt size [172]. It declines after the first 3 months perhaps due to cerebral adaptation [173] and is reduced if the shunt occludes. It can be treated by placing a smaller stent within the intrahepatic shunt. Resistant encephalopathy may be an indication for liver transplant.

Circulatory changes

The hyperdynamic circulation of cirrhosis persists [174] and systemic vasodilitation is initially increased. Cardiac output and systemic blood volume increase. Patients with underlying cardiac problems may be precipitated into heart failure. In alcoholic cirrhotic patients, a pre-clinical cardiomyopathy may be unmasked [175]. Pulmonary hypertension may develop [176].

Other indications

TIPS effectively controls ascites in Child's grade B patients, and survival can be improved (Chapter 10), as

well as nutritional status. Hepatic hydrothorax may be resolved completely. Budd–Chiari syndrome can be effectively treated (see below).

Renal function may improve in some patients with the hepatorenal syndrome (Chapter 10).

Hepatic transplantation

Patients with cirrhosis and bleeding varices die because their hepatocytes fail, not from blood loss *per se*. The end-point is death or a liver transplant. Previous endoscopic therapy or portal–systemic shunts do not affect post-transplant survival [177]. Liver transplant must be considered for variceal bleeding occurring with end-stage liver disease [178], or if there have been at least two episodes of bleeding from varices despite optimal therapy.

Previous surgical shunts make the transplant technically more difficult, particularly if there has been dissection at the hepatic hilum. Splenorenal and mesocaval shunts and TIPS are not contraindications, but migrated or misplaced TIPS can cause complications [179].

Most of the haemodynamic and humoral changes of cirrhosis are reversed by liver transplant [180].

Pharmacological control of the portal circulation and reduction of HVPG

Portal hypertension is part of a hyperdynamic state with increased cardiac output and reduced peripheral resistance. There are profound changes in autonomic nervous system activity. The various hormonal factors probably involved make pharmacological control possible. Theoretically, portal blood pressure (and flow) could be reduced by lowering cardiac output, by reducing inflow through splanchnic vasoconstriction, by splanchnic venodilatation, by reducing intrahepatic vascular resistance or, of course, by surgical portacaval shunting (Fig. 9.62). It is preferable to reduce pressure by lowering resistance rather than decreasing flow as hepatic blood flow and function will be maintained. New therapies ideally should not worsen systemic haemodynamics, but act specifically on the liver microcirculation without reducing portal inflow. Statin agents fulfil this function, and induce further reduction of HVPG added to non-selective beta-blockers. Monitoring of HVPG reduction and adjustment of therapy to achieve a HVPG less than 12 mmHg or a 20% reduction from baseline is recommended by some [181], but not by others [182]. However, a HVPG guided therapy, although achieving target reductions in more patients, does not result in less rebleeding than in non-monitored patients treated with combined ligation and drug therapy [183].

There is evidence that non-selective beta-blockers may have important therapeutic effects at lesser reduc-

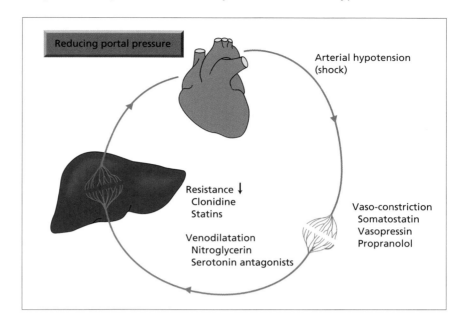

Fig. 9.62. The portal pressure can be reduced by arterial hypotension, splanchnic vasoconstriction, portal venodilatation or reduction in intrahepatic resistance.

tions of HVPG [184], even if rebleeding is not effectively prevented [185]. Bacterial translocation may be reduced as spontaneous bacterial peritonitis is prevented compared to no treatment [186]. Mechanisms may include increased intestinal transit and decreased mucosal congestion [187]. Abstention reduces HVPG and improves liver function [188]. Complications other than bleeding are also reduced by lowering HVPG [189,190]. Simvastatin lowers HVPG with or without beta-blockers; long-term studies may show further reduction in bleeding [191].

Summary

Variceal bleeding still has a high mortality, particularly if patients have more severe liver function or they have developed previous jaundice, ascites or encephalopathy. However, survival has improved steadily over the past decades, through use of prophylactic antibiotics, better use of specific therapies and better general care of the patient. Bleeding as a direct cause of death is rare. Rebleeding has been reduced by about 40–50%, and first bleeding by a similar proportion. Reduction in HVPG reduces complications and improves survival. Practice guidelines are based on many dozens of randomized trials (second only to the number in viral hepatitis) [138].

The hepatic veins

The hepatic veins begin in zone 3. They join the sublobular veins and merge into large hepatic veins, which enter the inferior vena cava while it is still partly embedded in the liver. The number, size and pattern of hepatic veins are very variable. Generally, there are three large veins, one draining segments 2, 3 and 4, and the other two draining segments 5, 6, 7 and 8 (Fig. 9.63). There are variable numbers of small accessory veins, particularly from the *caudate lobe* [192].

In the normal liver there are no direct anastomoses between the portal vein and hepatic vein, which are linked only by the sinusoids (Fig. 9.64). In the cirrhotic liver there are anastomoses between the portal and hepatic veins so that the blood bypasses the regenerating liver cell nodules (see Fig. 9.46). There is no evidence, either in the normal or cirrhotic liver, of anastomoses between the hepatic artery and the hepatic vein.

Functions

The pressure in the free hepatic vein is approximately 6 mmHg.

The hepatic venous blood is only about 67% saturated with oxygen.

Dogs have muscular hepatic veins near their caval orifices which form a sluice mechanism. The hepatic veins in man have little muscle.

The hepatic venous blood is usually sterile since the liver is a bacterial filter.

Visualizing the hepatic vein

Hepatic venography. This is performed by injection of contrast into a hepatic vein radicle with a wedged

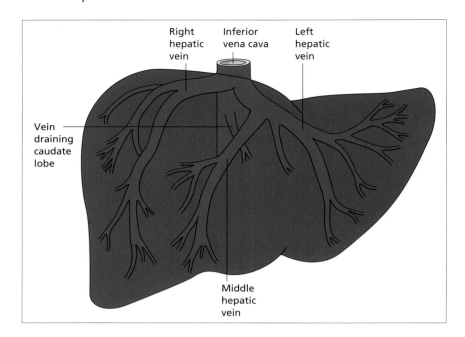

Fig. 9.63. The anatomy of the hepatic venous system. Note the separate vein draining the caudate lobe.

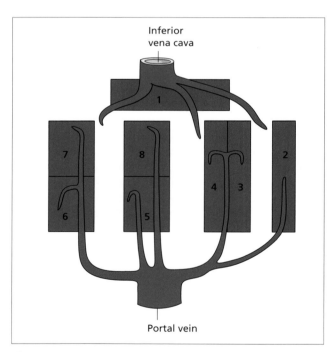

Fig. 9.64. Diagram of the distribution of the four main portal veins to the segments of the liver and the hepatic venous drainage to the inferior vena cava.

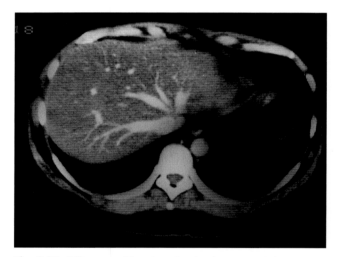

Fig. 9.65. CT scan, without contrast enhancement, in a patient with a fatty liver showing the hepatic venous anatomy well.

catheter or occluded with a balloon catheter and results in filling of the sinusoidal area draining into the catheter and also in retrograde filling of the portal venous system in that area. The portal radicle then carries the contrast medium to other parts of the liver and so other hepatic vein branches become opacified. Cirrhotic nodules and tumour deposits are surrounded by portal vein–hepatic vein anastomoses and may be outlined. In cirrhosis the sinusoidal pattern is coarsened, beady and tortuous, and gnarled hepatic radicles may be seen. The extent of filling of the main portal vein may indicate the extent to which the portal vein has become the outflow tract of the liver.

Scanning. The main hepatic veins may be visualized by ultrasound, colour Doppler imaging, enhanced CT scan and MRI. A CT scan without contrast enhancement in a patient with a fatty liver shows excellent hepatic venous anatomy (Fig. 9.65).

Experimental hepatic venous obstruction

The usual method is to constrict the inferior vena cava by a band placed above the entry of the hepatic veins, and so obstruct the venous return from the liver [193]. Zone 3 haemorrhage and necrosis with fibrosis follow. The hepatic lymphatics dilate and lymph passes through the capsule of the liver forming ascites with a high protein content.

Budd–Chiari (hepatic venous obstruction) syndrome [194]

This condition is usually associated with the names of Budd and Chiari although Budd's description [195] omitted the features, and Chiari's paper [196] was not the first to report the clinical picture. The syndrome comprises hepatomegaly, abdominal pain, ascites and hepatic histology showing zone 3 sinusoidal distension and pooling. It may arise from obstruction to hepatic veins at any site from the efferent vein of the acinus to the entry of the inferior vena cava into the right atrium (Fig. 9.66). It occurs in 1/100 000 of the general population [197]. A similar syndrome may be produced by constrictive pericarditis or right heart failure.

Myeloproliferative diseases, particularly polycythaemia rubra vera, are associated in up to 50% of cases

[198]. These may be covert and diagnosed only by the erythroid bone marrow colony test, although the JAK2 mutation is found in 80% of cases with polycythaemia rubra vera and 50% of idiopathic myelofibrosis patients [199]. The patient is often a young female. Multiple thrombophilic conditions may be present in the same patient [198].

The Budd–Chiari syndrome has been associated with systemic lupus erythematosus [200] and with circulating lupus anticoagulant [200], sometimes with disseminated intravascular coagulation. The antiphospholipid syndrome may be primary or secondary to systemic lupus [201]. Idiopathic granulomatous venulitis is another cause, which is treated successfully with corticosteroids [202].

Paroxysmal nocturnal haemoglobinuria in up to 35% of cases may be associated with Budd–Chiari syndrome, the severity varying from the asymptomatic to a fatal syndrome [203].

The Budd–Chiari syndrome is associated with deficiency of anticoagulant factors and impairment of fibrinolysis [204]. These include antithrombin III deficiency, whether primary or secondary to proteinuria [205], protein S and protein C deficiency [194], which may be difficult to diagnose due to poor hepatic synthesis. A normal factor II concentration together with a 20% or more reduction in protein C or S confirms a true deficiency; factor V Leiden mutation occurs in 20% [194,205,206]. Thromboelastography can detect hypercoagulability even if specific defects are not found [207].

Hepatic vein thrombosis complicating Behçet's disease is a sudden event, usually related to extension of a caval thrombosis to the osteum of hepatic veins [208].

The risk in users of oral contraceptives is about the same as other thrombotic complications [209]. Oral contraceptives may act synergistically in those predisposed to clotting [210].

Hepatic vein thrombosis has been reported in pregnancy (Chapter 27) [211]. Trauma may lead to membranous obstruction to the inferior vena cava in those with a hypercoagulable state [212].

The hepatic veins may be mechanically compressed by severe, polycystic liver disease [213].

Obstruction to the inferior vena cava is secondary to thrombosis in malignant disease, for instance an adrenal or renal carcinoma or invasion by a hepatocellular cancer [214] or angiosarcoma [215]. Rare tumours include leiomyosarcoma of the hepatic veins [216]. Wilms' tumour metastases may involve the inferior vena cava and hepatic veins [217].

Myxoma of the right atrium and metastases to the right atrium can cause hepatic outflow obstruction. Invasion of hepatic veins by masses of aspergillosis and compression by amoebic abscesses has been reported.

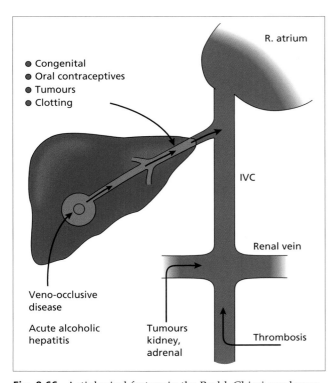

Fig. 9.66. Aetiological factors in the Budd–Chiari syndrome. IVC, inferior vena cava.

The Budd–Chiari picture also follows central hepatic vein involvement in the alcoholic and in veno-occlusive disease (Chapter 24).

Liver transplantation may be followed by small hepatic vein stenosis with some of the features of veno-occlusive disease. It is usually associated with azathioprine and with cellular rejection [218]. Small for size syndrome also has features of venous outflow obstruction [219].

Membranous obstruction of the suprahepatic segment of the inferior vena cava by a web is usually a sequel to thrombosis. It may be associated with infection or with a hypercoagulable state [220]. The web varies from a thin membrane to a thick fibrous band. It is particularly frequent in Japan where it has a strong association with hepatocellular carcinoma [221] and in South Africa and, to a lesser extent, in India and Nepal [222]. It may affect children. Its incidence is falling in India [223]. The clinical picture is milder than for classical Budd–Chiari syndrome. Markedly enlarged subcutaneous veins over the trunk are conspicuous. The picture has been termed *obliterative hepatocavopathy* [224].

The Budd–Chiari syndrome is being diagnosed more frequently and in milder forms, probably due to the routine use of imaging, especially ultrasound [194].

Pathological changes

The hepatic veins show occlusion at points from the ostia to the smaller radicles. Thrombus may have spread from an occluded inferior vena cava. Thrombus may be purulent or may contain malignant cells, depending on the cause. In chronic cases, the vein wall is thickened and there may be some recanalization. In others it is replaced by a fibrous strand; a fibrous web may be seen.

Involvement of large hepatic veins is usually thrombotic. Isolated obstruction to the inferior vena cava or small hepatic veins is usually non-thrombotic [194].

The liver is enlarged, purplish and smooth. Venous congestion is gross and the cut surface shows a 'nutmeg' change. Hepatic veins proximal to the obstruction and, in the acute stage, subcapsular lymphatics, are dilated and prominent.

In the chronic case, the caudate lobe is enlarged and compresses the inferior vena cava as it passes posterior to the liver (Fig. 9.67). Areas less affected by obstruction form nodules. The fibrosis and regenerative nodules continue to evolve after the first hepatic vein thrombosis and often progress to involve the portal venous system. The spleen may enlarge and a portal–systemic circulation develops. Mesenteric vessels may thrombose.

Histology shows zone 3 venous dilatation with haemorrhage and necrosis (Figs 9.68, 9.69). The parenchymal response depends on the distribution of vascular obstruction [224]. Persisting hepatic venous obstruction

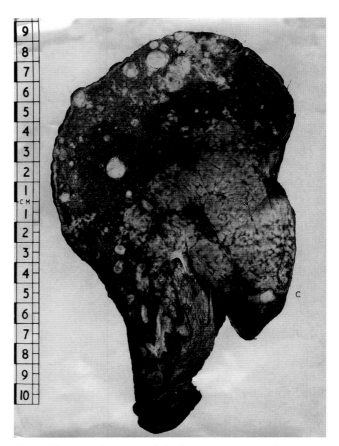

Fig. 9.67. Vertical section of the liver at autopsy in hepatic venous obstruction. The pale areas represent regeneration and the dark areas are congested. Note the marked hypertrophy of the caudate lobe (C).

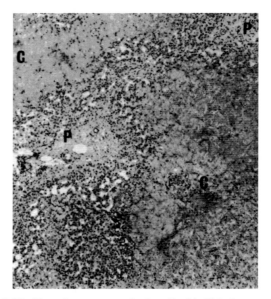

Fig. 9.68. Hepatic venous occlusion (Budd–Chiari syndrome). Hepatic histology showing marked zone 3 haemorrhage (C). The liver cells adjoining the portal zones (P) are spared. (H & E, ×100.)

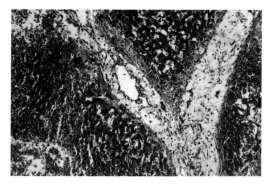

Fig. 9.69. Budd–Chiari syndrome. Longitudinal section of hepatic venules showing fibrosis in the lumen, thickening of the wall and surrounding loss of hepatocytes. (Chromophobe aniline blue.)

results in venocentric cirrhosis, so-called reverse lobulation. Portal vein involvement leads to venoportal cirrhosis and mixed forms exist. Large regenerative nodules are usual and are related to a new arterial supply. Nodular regenerative hyperplasia is frequent with long-standing arterialization [225].

Clinical features

These depend on the speed of occlusion, severity of liver dysfunction, anatomical sites of thrombosis and aetiology [194]. The picture varies from a fulminant course, the patient presenting with encephalopathy (and usually with ascites) and dying within 2–3 weeks, to a presentation as chronic hepatocellular disease, with ascites (often not responding to diuretics), and causing confusion with other forms of cirrhosis. The differing presentations are due to sudden massive thrombosis, or repeated thromboses overtime with variable recannalization [194].

In the most *acute form* the picture is of an ill patient, often suffering from some other condition—for instance renal carcinoma, hepatocellular cancer, thrombophlebitis migrans or polycythaemia. The presentation is with abdominal pain, vomiting, liver enlargement, ascites and mild icterus. Watery diarrhoea, following mesenteric venous obstruction, is a terminal, inconstant feature. If the hepatic venous occlusion is total, delirium and coma with hepatocellular failure and death occurs within a few days.

In the more usual *chronic form* the patient presents with pain over an enlarged tender liver and ascites developing over 1–6 months. Jaundice is mild or absent, unless zone 3 necrosis is marked. Pressure over the liver may fail to fill the jugular vein (negative *hepatojugular reflux*). As portal hypertension increases, the spleen becomes palpable. The enlarged caudate lobe, palpable in the epigastrium, may simulate a tumour.

Asymptomatic patients, who account for up to 15% of cases, may have no ascites, hepatomegaly or abdominal pain [226]. Hepatic outflow is diagnosed fortuitously, either by imaging or by the investigation of abnormal liver function tests. It may be explained by remaining patency of one large hepatic vein or development of a large venous collateral.

If the inferior vena cava is blocked, oedema of the legs is gross and veins distend over the abdomen, flanks and back. Albuminuria is found.

The condition may develop over months as ascites and wasting.

Serum bilirubin rarely exceeds 2 mg/100 mL (34 μmol/L). The serum alkaline phosphatase level is raised and the albumin value reduced. Serum transaminase values increase and, if very high, concomitant blockage of the portal vein is suggested. The prothrombin time is markedly increased, especially in the acute type. Hypoproteinaemia may be due to protein-losing enteropathy.

The protein content of the ascites should, theoretically, be high (total protein >25 g/L) but this is not always so.

Hepatic venous outflow obstruction is classified according to the site of obstruction and the presence or absence of portal vein thrombosis (PVT) [194]: (1) hepatic vein thrombosis or obstruction without obstruction or compression of the inferior vena cava (IVC); (2) hepatic vein thrombosis or obstruction with IVC obstruction (as a result of compensatory hypertrophy of the caudate lobe, or thrombosis); (3) isolated hepatic vein webs; and (4) isolated IVC webs. Diagnosis of portal vein thrombosis and/or IVC thrombosis and measurement of infrahepatic and suprahepatic caval pressures are needed to plan therapeutic options [194].

Ultrasound shows hepatic vein abnormalities, caudate lobe hypertrophy, increased reflectivity and compression of the inferior vena cava. The appearances are hypoechogenic in the early stages of acute thrombosis and hyperechogenic with fibrosis in the later stages. Ascites is confirmed.

Doppler ultrasound shows abnormalities in the direction of flow in the hepatic vein and retrohepatic inferior vena cava. The blood flow in the inferior vena cava and hepatic veins may be absent, reversed, turbulent or continuous. Colour Doppler imaging shows abnormalities in the hepatic veins, portal vein and inferior vena cava and correlates well with venographic appearances [227].

Detection of intrahepatic collateral vessels is important in the distinction from cirrhosis or where hepatic veins are inconspicuous on ultrasound [227].

CT scan (Fig. 9.70) shows enlargement of the liver with diffuse hypodensity before and patchy enhancement after contrast. Heterogeneous hepatic parenchymal patterns are related to regional differences in portal flow.

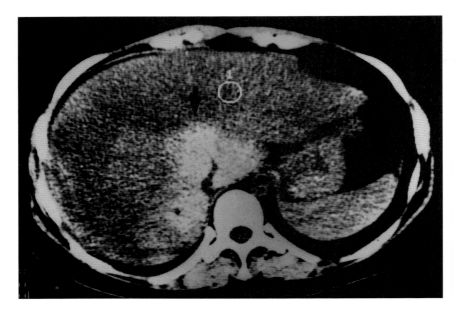

Fig. 9.70. CT scan (unenhanced) showing the caudate lobe (arrow) with surrounding underperfused parenchyma.

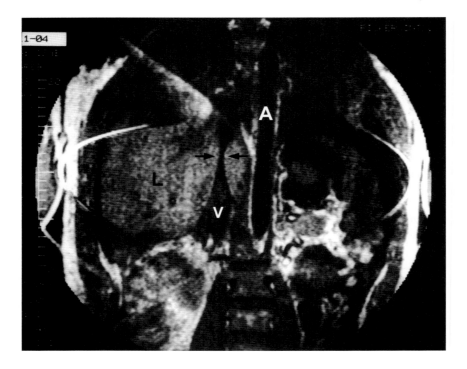

Fig. 9.71. Magnetic resonance scan in a patient with the Budd–Chiari syndrome showing a liver (L) which is dyshomogeneous, the aorta (A) and the inferior vena cava (V). The side-to-side narrowing of the inferior vena cava (arrows) is due to the enlarged caudate lobe.

Areas with complete hepatic vein obstruction remain hypodense after contrast, probably due to portal flow inversion. Subcapsular areas may enhance.

In the unenhanced scan, the caudate lobe appears dense with surrounding underperfused parenchyma (Fig. 9.70).

Thrombi in the inferior vena cava and/or hepatic vein may be seen as intraluminal filling defects that are not changed by contrast [228].

The CT appearances are easily confused with those of hepatic metastases.

MRI shows absence of normal hepatic venous drainage into the inferior vena cava, collateral hepatic veins and signal intensity alterations in the hepatic parenchyma (Fig. 9.71). The caudate lobe can be seen deforming the inferior vena cava.

Early diagnosis depends on Doppler ultrasound and MRI [197,229,230].

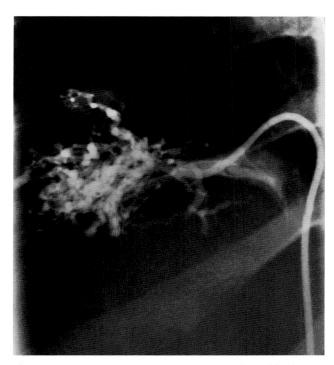

Fig. 9.72. Hepatic venogram in a patient with Budd–Chiari syndrome. Note the lace-like spider-web pattern.

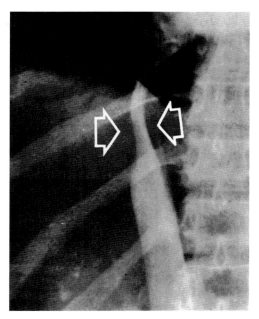

Fig. 9.73. Inferior vena cavogram. Anteroposterior view showing side-to-side narrowing and distortion of the inferior vena cava (arrows). Extrinsic compression from the left is due to an enlarged caudate lobe.

Table 9.7. Hepatic vein occlusion (Budd–Chiari syndrome)

Presentation
Abdominal pain
Hepatomegaly
Ascites
Liver biopsy
Zone 3 congestion
Imaging
MRI (contrast enhanced)
Doppler ultrasound
Aetiology
Myeloproliferative diseases
Anticoagulant deficiency
Paroxysmal nocturnal haemoglobinuria
Malignant disease
Management
Cause
anticoagulants, venesection
cytotoxic drugs
Ascites (Chapter 10)
Surgical
portacaval shunt
TIPS
orthotopic transplant

From *needle liver biopsy* speckled zone 3 areas can be distinguished from the pale portal areas. Histologically, the picture is of zone 3 congestion (Figs 9.68, 9.69). Alcoholic hepatitis or phlebitis of the hepatic veins should be noted.

Hepatic venography may fail or show narrow occluded hepatic veins. Adjacent veins show a tortuous, lace-like spider-web pattern (Fig. 9.72) [197]. This probably represents abnormal venous collaterals. The catheter cannot be advanced the usual distance along the hepatic vein and wedges 2–12 cm from the diaphragm.

Inferior vena cavography establishes the patency of the inferior vena cava. The hepatic segment may show side-to-side narrowing due to distortion from the enlarged caudate lobe (Fig. 9.73). Pressure measurements should be taken in the inferior vena cava along its length to confirm its patency and to quantify the extent of any membranous or caudate lobe obstruction.

From *selective coeliac arteriography* the hepatic artery appears small. Branches appear stretched and displaced, producing the appearance of multiple space-occupying lesions simulating metastases. The venous phase shows delayed emptying of the portal venous bed.

Diagnosis

The condition should be suspected if a patient with a tendency to thrombosis, or with malignant disease in or near the liver, or on oral contraceptives, develops tender hepatomegaly with ascites (Table 9.7). Diagnosis, prognosis and correct treatment are only possible if the disease is staged by imaging [194].

Heart failure and constrictive pericarditis must be excluded. Tense ascites *per se* can elevate the jugular venous pressure and displace the cardiac apex.

Cirrhosis must be distinguished and liver biopsy is helpful. The ascitic protein is usually lower in cirrhosis.

Portal vein thrombosis rarely leads to ascites. Jaundice is absent and the liver is not very large.

Inferior vena caval thrombosis results in distended abdominal wall veins but without ascites. If the renal vein is occluded, albuminuria is gross. Hepatic venous and inferior vena caval thrombosis may, however, coexist.

Hepatic metastases are distinguished clinically and by the liver biopsy.

A thrombophilia screen must be performed on all patients and myeloproliferative disorder requires screening of the V617F mutation in Janus tyrosine kinase-2 gene of granulocytes in blood [231]; if this is negative a bone marrow should be performed. Paroxysmal nocturnal haemoglobinuria requires flow cytometry of peripheral blood cells for detection of CD55 and CD59 deficient clones for diagnosis.

Prognosis

In symptomatic untreated patients, 90% will die by 3 years [232]. With treatment mortality rates have fallen over recent years [226,232], and survival has reached 75% at 5 years. However, specific therapy may have less beneficial effect than previously thought [232]. Severity of liver and renal dysfunction are important as predictors of survival [194]. If liver function is reflected in a low Child–Pugh score and renal function is normal, 5 year survival is over 95% [226,233]. Hepatocellular carcinoma develops in about 10%, during a mean follow-up of 5 years [234].

The fulminant form is usually fatal unless liver transplantation is carried out. Variceal haemorrhage can occur, as well as extension of the thrombus. Histopathological features do not help to determine prognosis [235]; in fact almost 60% of patients with an acute presentation have features of chronic disease [236]. Japan patients with obliterative cavopathy have a 25% mortality rate over 15 years, dying from variceal bleeding and hepatocellular carcinoma [237].

Treatment

Early treatment of an underlying haematological disorder improves long-term survival [238,239]. This can include anticoagulants in those with hypercoagulation or reduction of haemoglobin and platelets by venesection, cytotoxic drugs in those with polycythaemia and thrombocytosis and molecular therapies for such as eculizumab for paroxysmal nocturnal haemoglobinuria. Progressive loss of hepatic veins can be halted as large intrahepatic and portal–systemic collaterals develop

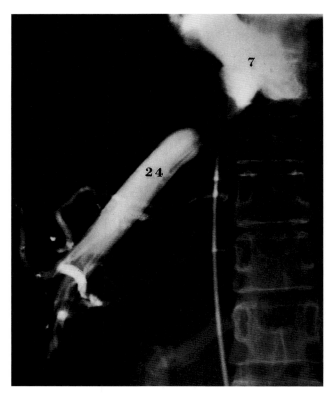

Fig. 9.74. Hepatic venogram in a patient with the Budd–Chiari syndrome due to obstruction of the right main hepatic vein. The right hepatic venous pressure is 24 mmHg distal to the obstruction and 7 mmHg proximal to it. (Courtesy of D.S. Zimmon.)

[226]. Long-term anticoagulation is given for all patients irrespective of whether a thrombophilic condition is diagnosed. It can be sufficient to control disease in about 10% [194].

Ascites is treated with a low sodium diet, diuretics and paracentesis. Severe cases demand ever increasing doses of potent diuretics and eventually the patient is overtaken by inanition and renal failure, unless a TIPS is placed. Some milder cases, however, respond slowly and require less treatment with time.

The timing of radiological or surgical intervention is difficult. On the one hand, some revascularization may continue. On the other hand, the long-term results of medical therapy are so poor that as time passes, radiological or surgical treatment becomes mandatory [194].

Percutaneous transluminal angioplasty

This has been used to dilate webs (Fig. 9.74) and also for hepatic vein obstruction after liver transplant. It is particularly useful if the suprahepatic portion of the inferior vena cava is involved. As for hepatic vein webs, multiple dilatations are usually necessary [240].

Intravascular metallic stents may be introduced after the dilatation [241]. Stents are usually reserved for those in whom angioplasty has failed. Together with anticoagulation this treats Budd–Chiari syndrome in up to 30% of cases in series from Western countries.

Transjugular intrahepatic stent shunt

If anticoagulation and percutaneous angioplasty, if performed, fail, TIPS is the next step [194]. The aim is to decompress the liver and reverse portal venous flow, in effect acting as a side-to-side portal caval shunt. TIPS has greatly improved treatment for Budd–Chiari syndrome. It avoids laparotomy, overcomes caudate lobe compression and occlusion of the IVC, with less mortality than surgical shunting. It does not hinder further surgical management [242] and, in fulminant Budd–Chiari syndrome, if emergency transplantation is not available it may rescue some patients [242].

Survival at 5 years is currently 70% or more [243]. If the hepatic vein cannot be entered a transcaval approach is used, and even if the portal vein is occluded a TIPS placement is possible [244].

Long-term patency (with anticoagulation) should be improved by PTFE-covered stents. An estimate suggests about 60% of patients in Western countries will need to undergo TIPS [194].

Surgical portal–systemic shunts

Surgical shunts are indicated only if TIPS is not available or cannot be fashioned, and liver transplantation is not feasible. It should be avoided in acute Budd–Chiari syndrome as liver failure may be precipitated requiring salvage transplantation [194,245,246]. Results on the whole are unsatisfactory due to thrombosis of the shunt, especially in those with haematological disorders or where stents have been used. If the shunt remains patent, 5-year survival is 87%, falling to 38% if the shunt thromboses [247]. No survival benefit has been clearly shown when taking into account the initial severity of disease [194]. Life-long anticoagulation is essential, but may not be sufficient to maintain patency [191].

Liver function usually deteriorates slowly and the patient becomes a candidate for transplant [246]. Morbidity for transplantation is greater with a previous shunt.

The enlarged caudate lobe increases pressure in the infrahepatic inferior vena cava so that it may exceed the portal venous pressure. If it exceeds 20 mmHg shunting is precluded [194] unless an inferior vena caval stent is placed [248]. The anatomical bulk of the caudate lobe makes a technical approach to the portal vein difficult [194].

If the portal vein is also occluded, shunts will not function.

Clinically, shunts such as side-to-side portacaval or mesocaval are technically difficult. Interposition grafts are often needed, increasing the likelihood of thrombosis [194,246]. A mesocaval interposition shunt has given good results and does not affect the subsequent hepatic transplantation. Mesoatrial shunt is used rarely when the inferior vena cava is obstructed. Posterocranial liver resection can render liver transplantation impossible and is a redundant intervention due to advances in interventional radiology [249].

Liver transplantation

This is indicated when the patient deteriorates despite aggressive medical and radiological therapy. The patient has usually progressed to cirrhosis with hepatocellular failure [246]. The transplant may have been preceded by a TIPS, so allowing more time to procure the donor liver. Surgical shunt may have failed. [191,239,240]. The 1-year survival is 85% and 5 year survival of 80% [250,251]. Post-transplant thrombosis remains a problem and early anticoagulation is essential [252]. In the case of an underlying thrombotic condition, anticoagulation must be life long; despite curing protein C [253], S and antithrombin III deficiency, multiple, including as yet unknown, thrombotic conditions may co-exist, so anticoagulation must still be used [94]. After transplantation, obstruction to hepatic venous drainage can be improved by balloon angioplasty [254].

Veno-occlusive disease

See Chapter 24.

Spread of disease by the hepatic veins

The hepatic veins link the portal and systemic venous systems. Malignant disease of the liver is spread by the hepatic veins to the lungs and hence to other parts. Liver abscesses can burst into the hepatic vein and metastatic abscesses may result. Parasitic disease, including amoebiasis, hydatid disease and schistosomiasis, is spread by this route. The portohepatic venous anastomoses developing in cirrhosis may allow intestinal organisms to cause septicaemia.

Circulatory failure

A rise in pressure in the right atrium is readily transmitted to the hepatic veins. Liver cells are particularly vulnerable to diminished oxygen supply, so that a failing heart, lowered blood pressure or reduced hepatic blood flow are reflected in impaired hepatic function. The left lobe of the liver may suffer more than the right.

Hepatic changes in acute heart failure and shock

Hepatic changes are common in acute heart failure and in shock. Ischaemic changes follow cessation of hepatic blood flow during the course of hepatic transplantation or tumour resection.

Some patients show mild icterus. Cardiac causes accounted for 1% of referrals for jaundice to a special access clinic [255]. Jaundice has been recorded in severely traumatized patients. Serum transaminase levels increase markedly and the prothrombin time rises.

Light microscopy shows a congested zone 3 with local haemorrhage (Fig. 9.75). Focal necrosis with eosinophilic hepatocytes, hydropic change and polymorph infiltration is usual. The reticulin framework is preserved within the necrotic zone. With recovery, particularly after trauma, mitoses may be prominent. Diffuse hepatic calcification can follow shock [256]. This might be related to the disturbance of intracellular Ca^{2+} homeostasis as a result of ischaemia.

Mechanisms of the hepatic changes

The changes can be related to duration. The fall in blood pressure leads to reduction in liver blood flow and hepatic arterial vasoconstriction. The oxygen content of the blood is reduced. The cells in zone 3 receive blood at a lower oxygen tension than zone 1 cells and therefore more readily become anoxic and necrotic. Intense selective splanchnic vasoconstriction follows.

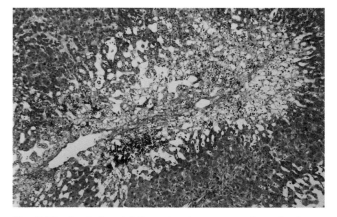

Fig. 9.75. Acute heart failure due to coronary thrombosis with prolonged hypotension. Zone 3 (stained blue) shows disappearance and necrosis of liver cells. The sinusoids are dilated with areas of haemorrhage. (Picro–Mallory stain, × 25.)

The hepatocyte injury is largely hypoxic. Insufficient substrates and accumulation of metabolites contribute. The mechanisms are multiple. The absence of available oxygen results in loss of mitochondrial oxidative phosphorylation. Impaired membrane function and reduced protein synthesis contribute. There are alterations in hepatocellular ion homeostasis [257].

Hypoxia can induce hydrogen peroxide in hepatocytes and this induces apoptosis in sinusoidal endothelial cells [258]. Much of the tissue damage develops during reperfusion, when there is a large flux of oxygen-derived 'free' radicles [259]. These initiate lipid peroxidation with disruption of membrane integrity. Experimentally, superoxide, formed during reperfusion, may combine with nitric oxide (NO) to cause hepatocellular injury [260]. Free radical peroxynitrite may be responsible. Lysosomal membranes may be peroxidized with the release of enzymes into the cytoplasm. Treatment is unsatisfactory. 'Free' radicle trapping agents such as vitamin E, glutathione and ascorbic acid are being evaluated.

Hypoxic or ischaemic hepatitis

This term is defined as marked and rapid elevation of serum transaminases in the setting of an acute fall in cardiac output. *Acute hepatic infarction* is a term sometimes used. The picture simulates acute viral hepatitis.

The patient usually suffers from cardiac disease, often ischaemic or a cardiomyopathy and less often chronic respiratory failure, and toxic septic shock [261]. It is particularly frequent in patients in coronary care units where it affects 22% of those with a low cardiac output, a decreased hepatic blood flow and passive venous congestion [261]. Zone 3 necrosis, without inflammation, results. Clinical evidence of hepatic failure is absent. Congestive cardiac failure is inconspicuous. True circulatory shock may be absent except in cases associated with sepsis. It may be associated with renal impairment and hyperglycaemia [262].

Ischaemic hepatitis may complicate variceal haemorrhage in patients with cirrhosis [263].

Severe arterial hypoxaemia due to obstructive sleep apnoea may be causative [264].

Serum bilirubin and alkaline phosphatase values increase slightly, but serum transaminases and lactic dehydrogenase values rise rapidly and strikingly [265]. Values return speedily towards recovery in less than 1 week. Mortality is high (58.6%) and depends on the underlying cause and not the liver injury [265]. If the liver has been previously damaged by chronic congestive heart failure, acute circulatory failure may lead to the picture of fulminant hepatic failure and the cardiac cause misdiagnosed [266,267].

Postoperative jaundice

Jaundice developing *soon* after surgery may have multiple causes. Increased serum bilirubin follows blood transfusion, particularly of stored blood. Extravasated blood in the tissues gives an additional bilirubin load.

Impaired hepatocellular function follows operation, anaesthetics and shock. Severe jaundice develops in approximately 2% of patients with shock resulting from major trauma [268]. Hepatic perfusion is reduced particularly if the patient is in incipient circulatory failure and the cardiac output is already reduced. Renal blood flow also falls.

Anaesthetics and other drugs used in the operative period must be considered. Sepsis, *per se*, can produce deep jaundice which may be cholestatic.

Rarely, a *cholestatic jaundice* may be noted on the first or second postoperative day. It reaches its height between the fourth and tenth day, and disappears by 14–18 days. Serum biochemical changes are variable. Sometimes, but not always, the alkaline phosphatase and transaminase levels are increased. Serum bilirubin can rise to levels of 23–39 mg/100 mL. The picture simulates extrahepatic biliary obstruction. Patients have all had an episode of shock, and have been transfused. Hepatic histology shows only minor abnormalities. The mechanism of the cholestasis is uncertain. This picture must be recognized and, if necessary, needle biopsy of the liver performed.

Severely ill patients in intensive care following severe trauma or postoperative intra-abdominal sepsis may develop jaundice, which reflects severe multiple organ failure and a poor prognosis [269]. The jaundice is usually of cholestatic type with raised conjugated serum bilirubin and alkaline phosphatase levels and only slightly increased transaminases.

Endotoxaemia and sepsis may activate inflammatory mediators leading to vascular damage, increased permeability and oedema and impaired oxygen transport [270].

Bile flow falls following the reduction in hepatic arterial perfusion (*ischaemic cholangitis*) [271].

Ischaemia in the rat liver is followed by ATP depletion in the cholangiocytes with changes in membrane and membrane–skeletal structures [272].

Jaundice after cardiac surgery

Jaundice develops in 20% of patients having cardiopulmonary bypass surgery [273,274]. It carries a bad prognosis. The jaundice is detected by the second postoperative day. Serum bilirubin is conjugated and the level returns to normal in 2–4 weeks in those who survive. Serum alkaline phosphatase may be normal or only slightly increased and transaminases are raised, often to very high levels. Older patients are particularly at risk. Jaundice is significantly associated with multiple valve replacement, high blood transfusion requirements and a longer bypass time.

Many factors contribute. The liver may have already suffered from prolonged heart failure. Operative hypotension, shock and hypothermia contribute. Infections, drugs (including anticoagulants) and anaesthetics must be considered.

Liver blood flow falls. The serum bilirubin load is increased by blood transfusion. The pump may contribute by decreasing erythrocyte survival and by adding gaseous microemboli and platelet aggregates and debris to the circulation.

Virus B and C hepatitis are rare nowadays. Cytomegalovirus hepatitis may develop.

The liver in congestive heart failure

Pathological changes [275]

Hepatic autolysis is particularly rapid in the patient dying with heart failure [276]. Autopsy material is therefore unreliable for assessment.

Macroscopic changes. The liver is enlarged, and purplish with rounded edges. Nodularity is inconspicuous but nodular masses of hepatocytes (*nodular regenerative hyperplasia*) may be seen. The cut surface (Fig. 9.76)

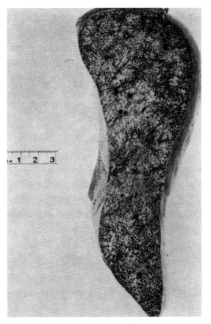

Fig. 9.76. Cut surface of the liver from a patient dying with congestive heart failure. Note the dilated hepatic veins. Light areas corresponding to peripheral fatty zones alternate with dark areas corresponding to zone 3 congestion and haemorrhage.

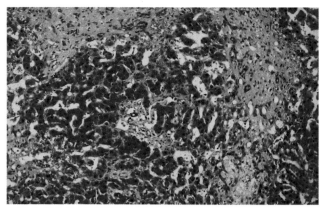

Fig. 9.77. Cardiac cirrhosis. Zone 3 fibrosis is increased and septa extend to link other central veins isolating nodules of liver cells. (H & E.)

shows prominent hepatic veins which may be thickened. The liver drips blood. Zone 3 is prominent with alternation of yellow (fatty change) and red (haemorrhage) areas.

Histological changes. The hepatic venule is dilated, and the sinusoids entering it are engorged for a variable distance towards the periphery. In severe cases, there is frank haemorrhage with focal necrosis of liver cells. The liver cells show a variety of degenerative changes but each zone 1 is surrounded by relatively normal cells to a depth that varies inversely with the extent of the zone 3 atrophy. Biopsy sections show significant fatty change in only about a third of cases. This contrasts with the usual post-mortem picture. Cellular infiltration is inconspicuous.

Zone 3 degenerating cells are often packed with brown lipochrome pigment. As they disintegrate, pigment lies free. Bile thrombi, particularly in zone 1, may be seen in the deeply jaundiced. Zone 3 PAS-positive, diastase-resistant hyaline globules may be seen [277].

Zone 3 reticulin condenses. Collagen increases and the central vein shows phlebosclerosis. Eccentric thickening or occlusion of the walls of zone 3 veins and perivenular scars extends into the lobule [268]. If the heart failure continues or relapses, bridges develop between central veins so that the unaffected portal zone is surrounded by a ring of fibrous tissue (*reversed lobulation*) (Fig. 9.77). Later the portal zones are involved and a complex cirrhosis results. A true cardiac cirrhosis is extremely rare.

Mechanism (Fig. 9.78)

Hypoxia causes degeneration of the zone 3 liver cells, dilatation of sinusoids and slowing of bile secretion.

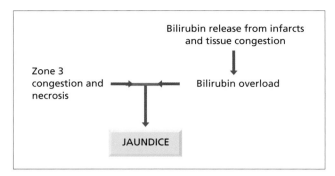

Fig. 9.78. Mechanisms of hepatic jaundice developing in patients with cardiac failure.

Endotoxins diffusing through the intestinal wall into the portal blood may augment this effect [278]. The liver attempts to compensate by increasing the oxygen extracted as the blood flows across the sinusoidal bed. Collagenosis of Disse's space may play a minor role in impairing oxygen diffusion.

Necrosis correlates with a low cardiac output [278]. The hepatic venous pressure increases and this correlates with zone 3 congestion [279].

Thrombosis begins in the sinusoids and may propagate to the hepatic veins with secondary local, portal vein thrombosis, ischaemia, parenchymal loss and fibrosis [280].

Clinical features

Mild jaundice is common but deeper icterus is rare and associated with chronic congestive failure. In hospital in-patients, cardiorespiratory disease is the commonest cause of a raised serum bilirubin level. Oedematous areas escape, for bilirubin is protein-bound and does not enter oedema fluid with a low protein content.

Jaundice is partly hepatic, for the greater the extent of zone 3 necrosis the deeper the icterus (Fig. 9.79) [276].

Bilirubin released from infarcts or simply from pulmonary congestion, provides an overload on the anoxic liver. Patients in cardiac failure who become jaundiced with minimal hepatocellular damage usually have pulmonary infarction [276]. The serum shows unconjugated bilirubinaemia.

The patient may complain of right abdominal pain, probably due to stretching of the capsule of the enlarged liver. The firm, smooth, tender lower edge may reach the umbilicus.

A rise in right atrial pressure is readily transmitted to the hepatic veins. This is particularly so in tricuspid incompetence when the hepatic vein pressure tracing resembles that obtained from the right atrium. Palpable systolic pulsation of the liver can be related to this transmission of pressure. Presystolic hepatic pulsation occurs

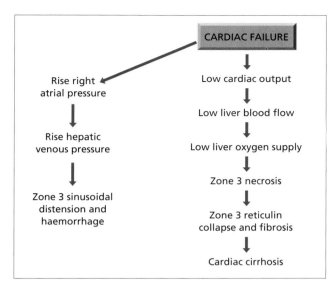

Fig. 9.79. Possible mechanisms of the hepatic histological changes in heart failure.

in tricuspid stenosis. The expansion may be felt bimanually. This expansibility distinguishes it from the palpable epigastric pulsation due to the aorta or a hypertrophied right ventricle. Correct timing of the pulsation is important.

In heart failure, pressure applied over the liver increases the venous return and the jugular venous pressure rises due to the inability of the failing right heart to handle the increased blood flow. The *hepatojugular reflux* is of value for identifying the jugular venous pulse and to establish that venous channels between the hepatic and jugular veins are patent. The reflux is absent if the hepatic veins are occluded or if the main mediastinal or jugular veins are blocked. It is useful for diagnosing tricuspid regurgitation [281].

Atrial pressure is reflected all the way to the portal system. Doppler sonography shows increased pulsatility in the portal vein depending on the severity of the heart failure [282].

Ascites is associated with a particularly high venous pressure, a low cardiac output and severe zone 3 necrosis. In patients with mitral stenosis and tricuspid incompetence or constrictive pericarditis, the ascites may be out of proportion to the oedema and symptoms of congestive heart failure. The ascitic fluid protein content is raised to 2.5 g/dL or more, similar to that observed in the Budd–Chiari syndrome [283].

Confusion, lethargy and coma are related to cerebral anoxia. Occasionally the whole picture of impending hepatic coma may be seen. Splenomegaly is frequent. Other features of portal hypertension are usually absent except in very severe cardiac cirrhosis associated with constrictive pericarditis.

Contrast-enhanced CT shows retrograde hepatic venous opacification on the early scans and a diffusely mottled pattern of hepatic enhancement during the vascular phase [284].

Cardiac cirrhosis should be suspected in patients with prolonged, decompensated mitral valve disease with tricuspid incompetence or in patients with constrictive pericarditis. The prevalence has fallen since both these conditions are relieved surgically.

Biochemical changes

The biochemical changes are small and proportional to the severity of the heart failure.

In congestive failure the serum bilirubin level usually exceeds 1 mg/dL and in about one-third it is more than 2 mg/dL [276]. The jaundice may be deep, exceeding 5 mg/dL and even up to 26.9 mg/dL. Patients with advanced mitral valve disease and a normal serum bilirubin concentration have a normal hepatic bilirubin uptake but diminished capacity to eliminate conjugated bilirubin related to reduced liver blood flow [285]; this contributes to postoperative jaundice.

Serum alkaline phosphatase is usually normal or slightly increased. Serum albumin values may be mildly reduced. Protein loss from the intestine may contribute.

Serum transaminases are higher in acute than chronic failure and are proportional to the degree of shock and the extent of zone 3 necrosis. The association of very high values with jaundice may simulate acute viral hepatitis.

Prognosis

The prognosis is that of the underlying heart disease. Cardiac jaundice, particularly if deep, is always a bad omen.

Cardiac cirrhosis *per se* does not carry a bad prognosis. If the heart failure responds to treatment, the cirrhosis compensates.

The liver in constrictive pericarditis

The clinical picture and hepatic changes are those of the Budd–Chiari syndrome.

Marked thickening of the liver capsule simulates sugar icing (*zuckergussleber*). Microscopically, the picture is of cardiac cirrhosis.

Jaundice is absent. The liver is enlarged and hard and may pulsate [286]. Ascites is gross.

A differential diagnosis must be made from ascites due to cirrhosis or to hepatic venous obstruction [287]. This is done by the paradoxical pulse, the venous pulse, the calcified pericardium, the echocardiogram, the electrocardiogram and by cardiac catheterization.

Treatment is that of the cardiac condition. If pericardectomy is possible, prognosis as regards the liver is good although recovery may be slow. Within 6 months of a successful operation, liver function tests improve and the liver shrinks. The cardiac cirrhosis will not resolve completely, but fibrous bands become narrower and avascular.

References

1 Hiatt JR, Gabbay J, Busuttil RW. Surgical anatomy of the hepatic arteries in 1000 cases. *Ann. Surg.* 1994; **220**: 50–52.

2 Yamamoto K, Sherman I, Phillips MJ *et al.* Three-dimensional observations of the hepatic arterial terminations in rat, hamster and human liver by scanning electron microscopy of micro vascular casts. *Hepatology* 1985; **5**: 452–456.

3 Sherlock S. The syndrome of disappearing intrahepatic bile ducts. *Lancet* 1987; **ii**: 493–496.

4 Barquist ES, Goldstein N, Zinner MJ. Polyarteritis nodosa presenting as a biliary stricture. *Surgery* 1991; **109**: 16–19.

5 Tygstrup N, Winkler K, Mellengaard K *et al.* Determination of the hepatic arterial blood flow and oxygen supply in man by clamping the hepatic artery during surgery. *J. Clin. Invest.* 1962; **41**: 447–454.

6 Lautt WW, Greenaway CV. Conceptual review of the hepatic vascular bed. *Hepatology* 1987; **7**: 952–963.

7 Legmann P, Costes V, Tudoret L. Hepatic artery thrombosis after liver transplantation: diagnosis with spiral CT. *Am. J. Roentgenol.* 1995; **164**: 97–101.

8 Soyer P, Bluemke DA, Choit MA *et al.* Variations in the intrahepatic portions of the hepatic and portal veins: findings on helical CT scans during arterial portography. *Am. J. Roentgenol.* 1995; **164**: 103–108.

9 Kronthal AJ, Fishman EK, Kuhlman JE *et al.* Hepatic infarction in pre-eclampsia. *Radiology* 1990; **177**: 726–728.

10 Khoury G, Tobi M, Oren M *et al.* Massive hepatic infarction in systemic lupus erythematosus. *Dig. Dis. Sci.* 1990; **35**: 1557–1560.

11 Bacha EA, Stieber AC, Galloway JR *et al.* Non-biliary complication of laparoscopic cholecystectomy. *Lancet* 1994; **344**: 896–897.

12 Simons RK, Sinanan MN, Coldwell DM. Gangrenous cholecystitis as a complication of hepatic artery embolization: case report. *Surgery* 1992; **112**: 106–110.

13 Ludwig J, Batts KP, MacCarthy RL. Ischemic cholangitis in hepatic allografts. *Mayo Clin. Proc.* 1992; **67**: 519–526.

14 Gunsar F, Rolando N, Pastacaldi S *et al.* Late hepatic artery thrombosis after orthotopic liver transplantation. *Liver Transpl.* 2003; **9**: 605–11.

15 Croce MA, Fabian TC, Spiers JP *et al.* Traumatic hepatic artery pseudoaneurysm with haemobilia. *Am. J. Surg.* 1994; **168**: 235–238.

16 Zachary K, Geier S, Pellecchia D *et al.* Jaundice secondary to hepatic artery aneurysm: radiological appearance and clinical features. *Am. J. Gastroenterol.* 1986; **81**: 295–298.

17 Kibbler CC, Cohen DL, Cruickshank JK *et al.* Use of CT scanning in the diagnosis and management of hepatic artery aneurysm. *Gut* 1985; **26**: 752–756.

18 Falkoff GE, Taylor KJW, Morse S. Hepatic artery pseudoaneurysm: diagnosis with real-time and pulsed Doppler US. *Radiology* 1986; **158**: 55–56.

19 Douglass BE, Baggenstoss AH, Hollinshead WH. Variations in the portal systems of veins. *Proc. Mayo Clin.* 1950; **25**: 26.

20 McIndoe AH. Vascular lesions of portal cirrhosis. *Arch. Path.* 1928; **5**: 23.

21 Kimura K, Ohto M, Matsutani S *et al.* Relative frequencies of portosystemic pathways and renal shunt formation through the 'posterior' gastric vein: portographic study in 460 patients. *Hepatology* 1990; **12**: 725–728.

22 Park JH, Cha SH, Han JK *et al.* Intrahepatic portosystemic venous shunt. *Am. J. Roentgenol.* 1990; **155**: 527–528.

23 Manenti F, Williams R. Injection of the splenic vasculature in portal hypertension. *Gut* 1966; **7**: 175–180.

24 Kitano S, Terblanche J, Kahn D *et al.* Venous anatomy of the lower oesophagus in portal hypertension: practical implications. *Br. J. Surg.* 1986; **73**: 525–531.

25 Vianna A, Hayes PC, Moscoso G *et al.* Normal venous circulation of the gastroesophageal junction. A route to understanding varices. *Gastroenterology* 1987; **93**: 876–889.

26 McCormack TT, Rose JD, Smith PM *et al.* Perforating veins and blood flow in oesophageal varices. *Lancet* 1983; **ii**: 1442–1444.

27 Dan SJ, Train JS, Cohen BA *et al.* Common bile duct varices: cholangiographic demonstration of a hazardous portosystemic communication. *Am. J. Gastroenterol.* 1983; **78**: 42–3.

28 Gudjonsson H, Zeiler D, Gamelli R *et al.* Colonic varices. Report of an unusual case diagnosed by radionuclide scanning, with review of the literature. *Gastroenterology* 1986; **91**: 1543–1547.

29 Weinshel E, Chen W, Falkenstein DB *et al.* Hemorrhoids or rectal varices: defining the cause of massive rectal hemorrhage in patients with portal hypertension. *Gastroenterology* 1986; **90**: 744–747.

30 Viggiano TR, Gostout CJ. Portal hypertensive intestinal vasculopathy: a review of the clinical, endoscopic, and histopathologic features. *Am. J. Gastroenterol.* 1992; **87**: 944–954.

31 Panés J, Piqué JM, Bordas JM *et al.* Reduction of gastric hyperemia by glypressin and vasopressin administration in cirrhotic patients with portal hypertensive gastropathy. *Hepatology* 1994; **19**: 55–60.

32 Payen J-L, Calès P, Voigt J-J *et al.* Severe portal hypertensive gastropathy and antral vascular ectasia are distinct entities in patients with cirrhosis. *Gastroenterology* 1995; **108**: 138–144.

33 Spahr L, Villeneuve J-P, DuFresne MP *et al.* Gastric antral vascular ectasia in cirrhotic patients: absence of relation with portal hypertension. *Gut* 1999; **44**: 739–742.

34 Nagral AS, Joshi AS, Bhatia SJ *et al.* Congestive jejunopathy in portal hypertension. *Gut* 1993; **34**: 694–697.

35 Scandalis N, Archimandritis A, Kastanas K *et al.* Colonic findings in cirrhotics with portal hypertension. A prospec-

tive colonoscopic and histological study. *J. Clin. Gastroenterol.* 1994; **18**: 325–328.

36 Iwakiri Y, Groszmann RJ. Vascular endothelial dysfunction in cirrhosis. *J. Hepatol.* 2007; **46**: 927–934

37 Bhathal PS, Grossman HJ. Reduction of the increased portal vascular resistance of the isolated perfused cirrhotic rat liver by vasodilators. *J. Hepatol.* 1985; **1**: 325–337.

38 Blendis LM, Orrego H, Crossley IR *et al.* The role of hepatocyte enlargement in hepatic pressure in cirrhotic and non-cirrhotic liver disease. *Hepatology* 1982; **2**: 539–546.

39 Grossman HJ, Gorssman VL, Bhathal PS. The effect of hepatocyte enlargement on the haemodynamic characteristics of the isolated perfused rat liver preparation. *Hepatology* 1998; **27**: 446–451.

40 Rockey D. The cellular pathogenesis of portal hypertension: stellate cell contractility, endothelin and nitric oxide. *Hepatology* 1997; **25**: 2–5.

41 Sogni P, Moreau R, Gadano A *et al.* The role of nitric oxide in the hyperdynamic circulatory syndrome associated with portal hypertension. *J. Hepatol.* 1995; **23**: 218–224.

42 Gerbes AL, Bilzer M, Gulberg V. Role of endothelins. *Digestion* 1998; **59**: 410–412.

43 Wheatley AM, Zhang X-Y. Intrahepatic modulation of portal pressure and its role in portal hypertension. *Digestion* 1998; **59**: 424–428.

44 Fernandez M, Mejias M, Garcia-Pras E *et al.* Reversal of portal hypertension and hyperdynamic splanchnic circulation by combined vascular endothelial growth factor and platelet derived growth factor blockade in rats. *Hepatology* 2007; **46**: 1208–1217.

45 Groszmann RJ. Hyperdynamic circulation of liver disease 40 years later: pathophysiology and clinical consequences. *Hepatology* 1994; **20**: 1359–1363.

46 Oberti F, Sogni P, Cailmail S *et al.* Role of prostacyclin in haemodynamic alterations in conscious rats with extrahepatic or intrahepatic portal hypertension. *Hepatology* 1993; **18**: 621–627.

47 Pak J-M, Lee SS. Glucagon in portal hypertension. *J. Hepatol.* 1994; **20**: 825–832.

48 Cruveilhier J. *Anatomie pathologique du corps humain*, vol. I. XVI livr. pl. vi, Maladies du Veines. Paris: J.B. Baillière, 1829–1835.

49 Baumgarten P von. Über völlstandiges Offenbleiben der Vena umbilicalis: zugleichein Beitrag zur Frage des Morbus Bantii. *Arb. Path. Anat. Inst. Tübingen* 1907; **6**: 93.

50 Bisseru B, Patel JS. Cruveilhier–Baumgarten disease. *Gut* 1989; **30**: 136–137.

51 Hosking SW, Smart HL, Johnson AG *et al.* Anorectal varices, haemorrhoids and portal hypertension. *Lancet* 1989; **i**: 349–352.

52 Ayuso C, Luburich P, Vilana R *et al.* Calcifications in the portal venous system: comparison of plain films, sonography, and CT. *Am. J. Roentgenol.* 1992; **159**: 321–323.

53 Dennis MA, Pretorius D, Manco-Johnson ML *et al.* CT detection of portal venous gas associated with suppurative cholangitis and cholecystitis. *Am. J. Roentgenol.* 1985; **145**: 1017–1018.

54 North Italian Endoscopic Club for Study and Treatment of Esophageal Varices. Prediction of the first variceal haemorrhage in patients with cirrhosis of the liver and esophageal varices. A prospective multicentre study. *N. Engl. J. Med.* 1988; **319**: 983–989.

55 Calès P, Zabotto B, Meskens C *et al.* Gastroesophageal endoscopic features in cirrhosis. Observer variability, interassociations, and relationship to hepatic dysfunction. *Gastroenterology* 1990; **98**: 156–162.

56 Spina GP, Arcidiacono R, Bosch J *et al.* Gastric endoscopic features in portal hypertension: final report of a consensus conference, Milan, Italy, 19 September 1992. *J. Hepatol.* 1994; **21**: 461–467.

57 D'Amico G, Montalbano L, Traina M *et al.* Natural history of congestive gastropathy in cirrhosis. *Gastroenterology* 1990; **99**: 1558–1564.

58 de Franchis R, Risen GM, Laine L *et al.* Esophageal capsule endoscopy for screening and surveillance of esophageal varices in patients with portal hypertension. *Hepatology* 2008; **47**: 1595–1603.

59 Giannini EG, Zaman A, Kreil A *et al.* Platelet count/spleen diameter ratio for the non-invasive diagnosis of oesophageal varices: results of a multicentre prospective validation study. *Am. J. Gastroenterol.* 2006; **101**: 2511–2519.

60 Ganguly S, Sarin SK, Bhatia V *et al.* The prevalence and spectrum of colonic lesions in patients with cirrhotic and noncirrhotic portal hypertension. *Hepatology* 1995; **21**: 1226–1231.

61 Gaiani S, Bolondi L, Li Bassi S *et al.* Prevalence of spontaneous hepatofugal portal flow in liver cirrhosis. *Gastroenterology* 1991; **100**: 160–167.

62 Kudo M, Tomita S, Tochio H *et al.* Intrahepatic portosystemic venous shunt: diagnosis by colour Doppler imaging. *Am. J. Gastroenterol.* 1993; **88**: 723–729.

63 Redvanly RD, Chezmar JL. CT arterial portography: technique, indications and applications. *Clin. Radiol.* 1997; **52**: 256–268.

64 Taylor CR. Computed tomography in the evaluation of the portal venous system. *J. Clin. Gastroenterol.* 1992; **14**: 167–172.

65 Finn JP, Kane RA, Edelman RR *et al.* Imaging of portal venous system in patients with cirrhosis: MR angiography vs. duplex Doppler sonography. *Am. J. Roentgenol.* 1993; **161**: 989–994.

66 Atkinson M, Sherlock S. Intrasplenic pressure as an index of the portal venous pressure. *Lancet* 1954; **i**: 1325–1327.

67 Groszmann RJ, Glickman M, Blei AT *et al.* Wedged and free hepatic venous pressure measured with a balloon catheter. *Gastroenterology* 1979; **76**: 253–258.

68 Vlachogiannakos J, Patch D, Watkinson A *et al.* Carbondioxide portography: an expanding role? *Lancet* 2000; **355**: 987–988.

69 Burroughs AK, Thalheimer U. Hepatic venous pressure gradient in 2010: optimal measurement is key. *Hepatology* 2010; **51**: 1894–1896.

70 Thalheimer U, Leandro G, Samonakis DN *et al.* Assessment of the agreement between wedge hepatic vein pressure and portal vein pressure in cirrhosis patients. *Dig. Liv. Dis.* 2005; **37**: 601–608.

71 Ripoll C, Groszmann RJ, Garcia-Tsao G *et al.* Hepatic venous pressure gradient predicts clinical decompensation in patients with compensated cirrhosis. *Gastroenterology* 2007; **133**: 481–488.

72 Senzolo M, Burra P, Cholongitas E *et al.* The transjugular route: the key hole to the liver world. *Dig. Liver Dis.* 2007; **39**: 105–116.

73 Armonis A, Patch D, Burroughs A. Hepatic venous pressure measurement: an old test as a new prognostic marker in cirrhosis. *Hepatology* 1997; **25**: 245–248.

74 Burroughs AK, Triantos CK. Predicting failure to control bleeding and mortality in acute variceal bleeding. *J. Hepatol.* 2008; **48**: 185–188.

75 Triantos CK, Nikolopoulou V, Burroughs AK. Review article: the therapeutic and prognostic benefit of portal pressure reduction in cirrhosis. *Aliment. Pharmacol. Therap.* 2008; **28**: 943–952.

76 Nevens F, Bustami R, Scheys I *et al*. Variceal pressure is a factor predicting the risk of a first variceal bleeding. A prospective cohort study in cirrhotic patients. *Hepatology* 1998; **27**: 15–19.

77 Hou MC, Lin HC, Kou BIT *et al*. Sequential variceal pressure measurement by endoscopic needle puncture during maintenance sclerotherapy: the correlation between variceal pressure and variceal rebleeding. *J. Hepatol.* 1998; **29**: 772–778.

78 Gertsch P, Fischer G, Kleber G *et al*. Manometry of esophageal varices: comparison of an endoscopic balloon technique with needle puncture. *Gastroenterology* 1993; **105**: 1159–1166.

79 Bradley SE, Ingelfinger FJ, Bradley GP *et al*. Estimation of hepatic blood flow in man. *J. Clin. Invest.* 1945; **24**: 890–897.

80 Caesar J, Shaldon S, Chiandussi L *et al*. The use of indocyanine green in the measurement of hepatic blood flow and as a test of hepatic function. *Clin. Sci.* 1961; **21**: 43–57.

81 Bosch J, Groszmann RJ. Measurement of azygous venous blood flow by a continuous thermal dilution technique: an index of blood flow through gastroesophageal collaterals in cirrhosis. *Hepatology* 1984; **4**: 424–429.

82 Webster GJ, Burroughs AK, Riordan SM. Portal vein thrombosis—new insigts into aetiology and management. *Aliment. Pharmacol. Therap.* 2005; **21**: 1–9.

83 Thompson EN, Sherlock S. The aetiology of portal vein thrombosis with particular reference to the role of infection and exchange transfusion. *Q. J. Med.* 1964; **33**: 465–480.

84 Dubuisson C, Boyer-Neumann C, Wolf M *et al*. Protein C, protein S and antithrombin III in children with portal vein obstruction. *J. Hepatol.* 1997; **27**: 132–135.

85 Valla D, Casadevall N, Huisse MG *et al*. Etiology of portal thrombosis in adults. *Gastroenterology* 1988; **94**: 1063–1069.

86 Wanless IR, Peterson P, Das A *et al*. Hepatic vascular disease and portal hypertension in polycythemia vera and agnogenic myeloid metaplasia: a clinicopathological study of 145 patients examined at autopsy. *Hepatology* 1990; **12**: 1166–1174.

87 Bernades P, Baetz A, Lévy P *et al*. Splenic and portal venous obstruction in chronic pancreatitis. A prospective longitudinal study of a medical-surgical series of 266 patients. *Dig. Dis. Sci.* 1992; **37**: 340–346.

88 Morse SS, Taylor KJW, Strauss EB *et al*. Congenital absence of the portal vein in oculoauriculo-vertebral dysplasia (Goldenhar syndrome). *Pediatr. Radiol.* 1986; **16**: 437–439.

89 Odièvre M, Pigé G, Alagille D. Congenital abnormalities associated with extrahepatic portal hypertension. *Arch. Dis. Child.* 1977; **52**: 383–385.

90 Tsochatzis EA, Senzolo M, Germani G *et al*. Systemic review:portal vein thrombosis in cirrhosis. *Aliment. Pharmacol. Therap.* 2010; **31**: 366–374.

91 Capron JP, LeMay JL, Muir JF *et al*. Portal vein thrombosis and fatal pulmonary thromboembolism associated with oral contraceptive treatment. *J. Clin. Gastroenterol.* 1981; **3**: 295–298.

92 Bayraktar Y, Balkanci F, Kansu E *et al*. Cavernous transformation of the portal vein: a common manifestation of Behçet's disease. *Am. J. Gastroenterol.* 1995; **90**: 1476–1479.

93 Sarin SK, Bansal A, Sasan S, Nigram A. Portal vein obstruction in children leads to growth retardation. *Hepatology* 1992; **15**: 229–233.

94 Thompson EN, Williams R, Sherlock S. Liver function in extra-hepatic portal hypertension. *Lancet* 1964; **ii**: 1352–1356.

95 Senzolo M, Cholongitas E, Tibballs J *et al*. Relief of biliary obstruction due to portal vein cavernoma using a transjugular intrahepatic portosystemic shunt (TIPS) without need for long term stenting. *Endoscopy* 2006; **38**: 760.

96 Konno K, Ishida H, Uno A *et al*. Cavernous transformation of the portal vein (CTPV): role of colour Doppler sonography in the diagnosis. *Eur. J. Ultrasound* 1996; **3**: 231–240.

97 Parvey HR, Raval B, Sandler CM. Portal vein thrombosis: imaging findings. *Am. J. Roentgenol.* 1994; **162**: 77–81.

98 Webb L, Smith-Laing G, Lake-Bakaar G *et al*. Pancreatic hypofunction in extrahepatic portal venous obstruction. *Gut* 1980; **21**: 227–231.

99 Plessier A, Darwish-Murad S, Hernandez-Guerra M *et al*. Acute portal vein thrombosis unrelated to cirrhosis: a prospective multi-centre follow up study. *Hepatology* 2010; **51**: 210–218.

100 De Ville de Goyet J, Alberti D, Clapuyt P *et al*. Direct by passing of extrahepatic portal venous obstruction in children: a new technique for combined hepatic portal revscularisation and treatment of extra hepatic portal hypetension. *J. Surg.* 1998; **33**: 597–601.

101 Senzolo M, Tibballs J, Cholangitas E *et al*. Transjugular intrahepatic portosystemic shunt for portal vein thrombosis with and witout cavernous transformation. *Aliment. Pharmacol. Therap.* 2006; **23**: 767–775.

102 Loftus JP, Nagorney DM, Ilstrup D *et al*. Sinistral portal hypertension. Splenectomy or expectant management. *Ann. Surg.* 1993; **217**: 35–40.

103 Shields SJ, Byse BH, Grace ND. Arterioportal fistula: a role for pre-TIPSS arteriography and hepatic venous pressure measurements. *Am. J. Gastroenterol.* 1992; **87**: 1828–1832.

104 Chagnon SF, Vallee CA, Barge J *et al*. Aneurysmal portal hepatic venous fistula: report of two cases. *Radiology* 1986; **159**: 693–695.

105 Dubois A, Dauzat M, Pignodel C *et al*. Portal hypertension in lymphoproliferative and myeloproliferative disorders: haemodynamic and histological correlations. *Hepatology* 1993; **17**: 246–250.

106 Ludwig J, Hashimoto E, Obata H *et al*. Idiopathic portal hypertension. *Hepatology* 1993; **17**: 1157–1162.

107 Oikawa H, Masuda T, Sato S-I *et al*. Changes in lymph vessels and portal veins in the portal tract of patients with idiopathic portal hypertension; a morphometric study. *Hepatology* 1998; **27**: 1607–1610.

108 Sarin SK. Progress report. Non-cirrhotic portal fibrosis. *Gut* 1989; **30**: 406–415.

109 Mikkelsen WP. Extrahepatic portal hypertension in children. *Am. J. Surg.* 1966; **111**: 333–340.

110 Kingham JG, Levinson DA, Stansfeld AG *et al*. Non-cirrhotic intrahepatic portal hypertension. A long-term follow-up study. *Q. J. Med.* 1981; **50**: 259–268.

111 Popper H, Elias H, Petty DE. Vascular pattern of the cirrhotic liver. *Am. J. Clin. Path.* 1952; **22**: 717–729.

112 Shaldon S, Chiandussi L, Guevara L *et al*. The measurement of hepatic blood flow and intrahepatic shunted blood flow by colloid heat denatured human serum albumin labelled with I131. *J. Clin. Invest.* 1961; **40**: 1346–1354.

113 Kelty RH, Baggenstoss AH, Butt HR. The relation of the regenerated liver nodule to the vascular bed in cirrhosis. *Gastroenterology* 1950; **15**: 285–295.

114 Groszmann RJ, Garcia-Tsao G, Bosch J *et al*. Beta-blockers to prevent gastro-oesophageal varices in patients with cirrhosis. *N. Engl. J. Med.* 2005; **353**: 2254–2261.

115 Merli M, Nicolini G, Angeloni S *et al*. Incidence and natural history of small oesophageal varices in cirrhotic patients. *J. Hepatol.* 2003; **38**: 266–272.

116 Goulis J, Patch D, Burroughs AK. Bacterial infection in the pathogenesis of variceal bleeding. *Lancet* 1999; **353**: 1102.

117 Lebrec D, de Fleury P, Rueff B. Portal hypertension, size of esophageal varices and risk of gastrointestinal bleeding in alcoholic cirrhosis. *Gastroenterology* 1980; **79**: 1139–1144.

118 Kleber G, Sauerbruch T, Ansari H *et al*. Prediction of variceal hemorrhage in cirrhosis: a prospective follow-up study. *Gastroenterology* 1991; **100**: 1332–1337.

119 Schmassmann A, Zuber M, Livers M *et al*. Recurrent bleeding after variceal haemorrhage: predictive value of portal venous duplex sonography. *Am. J. Roentgenol.* 1993; **160**: 41–47.

120 Burroughs AK, Patch D. Primary prevention of bleeding from esophageal varices. *N. Engl. J. Med.* 1999; **340**: 1033–1035.

121 Groszmann RJ, Bosch J, Grace ND *et al*. Hemodynamic events in a prospective randomized trial of propranolol vs placebo in the prevent of a first variceal hemorrhage. *Gastroenterology* 1990; **99**: 1401–1407.

122 Mastai R, Bosch J, Bruix J *et al*. Beta-blockade with propranolol and hepatic artery blood flow in patients with cirrhosis. *Hepatology* 1989; **10**: 269–272.

123 Garcia-Tsao G, Grace ND, Groszmann RJ *et al*. Short-term effects of propranolol on portal venous pressure. *Hepatology* 1986; **6**: 101–106.

124 Pagliaro L, D'Amico G, Sorensen TIA *et al*. Prevention of first bleeding in cirrhosis. A meta-analysis of randomized trials of nonsurgical treatment. *Ann. Intern. Med.* 1992; **117**: 59–70.

125 Gludd LL, Klingenberg S, Nikolova D *et al*. Banding ligation versus beta-blockers as primary prophylaxis in oesophageal varices: a systematic review of randomized trials. *Am. J. Gastroenterol.* 2007; **102**: 2842–2848.

126 Tsochatzis E, Triantos C, Burroughs AK. Non-selective beta-bockers and prevention of first variceal bleeding. *J. Hepatol.* 2010; **52**: 946–948..

127 Tripathi D, Ferguson JW, Kochar N *et al*. Randomized controlled trial of carvedilol versus variceal band ligation for the prevention of first variceal bleed. *Hepatology* 2009; **50**: 825–833.

128 Tsochatzis EA, Christos CK, Burroughs AK. Variceal bleeding: carvedilol the best beta-blocker for primary prophylaxis? *Nat. Rev. Gastroenterol. Hepatol.* 2009; **6**: 992–994.

129 Groszmann RJ. Beta-adrenergic blockers and nitrovasodilators for the treatment of portal hypertension: the good, the bad, the ugly. *Gastroenterology* 1997; **113**: 1794–1797.

130 Burroughs AK, Planas R, Svoboda P. Optimizing care of upper gastrointestinal bleeding in cirrhotic patients. *Scand. J. Gastroenterol.* 1998; **226**: 14–24.

131 Siringo S, McCormick PA, Mistry PA *et al*. Prognostic significance of the white nipple sign in variceal bleeding. *Gastrointest. Endoscopy* 1991; **37**: 51–55.

132 McCormick PA, O'Keefe C. Improving prognosis following a first variceal haemorrhage over 4 decades. *Gut* 2001; **49**: 682–685.

133 Ben-Ari Z, Cardin F, McCormick PA *et al*. A predictive model for failure to control bleeding during acute variceal haemorrahge. *J. Hepatol.* 1999; **31**: 443–450.

134 Vlachogiannakos J, Carpenter J, Goulis J *et al*. Variceal bleeding in primary biliary cirrhosis patients: a subgroup with improved prognosis and a model to predict survival after first bleeding. *Eur. J. Gastroenterol. Hepatol.* 2009; **21**: 701–707.

135 Bernard B, Grange J-D, Khac EN *et al*. Antibiotic prophylaxis for the prevention of bacterial infections in cirrhotic patients with gastrointestinal bleeding; a meta-analysis. *Hepatology* 1999; **29**: 1655–1661.

136 Hou MC, Lin HC, Liu TT *et al*. Antibiotic prophylaxis after endoscopic therapy prevents rebleeding in acute variceal haemorrhage: a randomized trial. *Hepatology* 2004; **39**: 746–753.

137 Jun CH, Park CH, Lee WS *et al*. Antibiotic prophylaxis using third generation cephalosporins can reduce the risk of early rebleeding in the first acute gastroesophageal variceal haemorrhage. A prospective randomized study. *J. Korean Med. Sci.* 2006; **21**: 883–890.

138 de Franchis R, Baveno V Faculty. Revising consensus in portal hypertension:report of the Baveno V consensus workshop on methodology of diagnosis and therapy in portal hypertension. *J. Hepatol.* 2010; **53**: 762–768.

139 Kravetz D, Bosch J, Teres J *et al*. Comparison of intravenous somatostatin and vasopressin infusions in treatment of acute variceal haemorrhage. *Hepatology* 1984; **4**: 442–446.

140 Gotzsche PC, Hrobjartsson A. Somatostatin analogues for acute bleeding oesophageal varices. *Cochrane Database Syst. Rev.* 2008; **3**: CD000193.

141 Wright G, Lewis H, Hogan B *et al*. A self expanding metal stent for complicated variceal haemorrhage: experience at a single centre. *Gastrointest. Endoscopy* 2010; **71**: 71–78.

142 Zehetner J, Shamiyeh A, Wayand W, Hubmann R. Results of a new method to stop acute bleeding from oesophageal varices: implantation of self expanding stent. *Endoscopy* 2008; **22**: 2140–2152.

143 Triantos CK, Goulis J, Patch D *et al*. An evaluation of emergency sclerotherapy of varices in randomized trials: looking at the needle in the eye. *Endoscopy* 2006; **38**: 797–807.

144 Chau TN, Patch D, Chan YW *et al*. 'Salvage' transjugular intrahepatic portosystemic shunts: gastric fundal compared with esophageal variceal bleeding. *Gastroenterology* 1998; **114**: 981–987.

145 Monescillo A, Martinex-Langares F, Ruiz del Arbo L *et al.* Influence of portal hypertension and its early decompression by TIPS placement on the outcome of variceal bleeding. *Hepatology* 2004; **40**: 793–801.

146 Garcia-Pagan JC, Caca K, Bureau C *et al.* Early use of TIPS in patients with cirrhosis and variceal bleeding. *N. Engl. J. Med.* 2010; **362**: 2370–2379.

147 Tan PC, Hou MC, Lin HC *et al.* A randomized trial of endoscopic treatment of acute gastric variceal haemorrhage: N butyl-2 cyanoacrylate injection versus band ligation. *Hepatology* 2006; **43**: 690–7 (erratum 2006; **43**: 1410).

148 Bureau C, Garcia-Pagan JC, Otal P *et al.* Improved clinical outcome using polytetrafluoroethylene coated stents for TIPS: results of a randomized study. *Gastroenterology* 2004; **126**: 469–475.

149 Rössle M, Haag K, Ochs A *et al.* The transjugular intrahepatic portosystemic stent-shunt procedure for variceal bleeding. *N. Engl. J. Med.* 1994; **330**: 165–171.

150 Ducoin H, El-Khoury J, Rousseau H *et al.* Histopathologic analysis of transjugular intrahepatic portosystemic shunts. *Hepatology* 1997; **25**: 1064–1069.

151 Sanyal AJ, Contos MJ, Yager D *et al.* Development of pseudointima and stenosis after transjugular intrahepatic portosystemic shunts; characterization of cell phenotype and function. *Hepatology* 1998; **28**: 22–32.

152 Sanyal A, Freedman AM, Luketic VA *et al.* Transjugular intrahepatic portosystemic shunts for patients with active variceal haemorrhage unresponsive to sclerotherapy. *Gastroenterology* 1996; **111**: 138–146.

153 Vangeli M, Patch D, Terreni N et al. Bleeding ectopic varices—treatment with transjugular intrahepatic portosystemic shunt (TIPS) and embolisation. *J. Hepatol.* 2004; **41**: 560–566.

154 Sanyal AJ, Freedman AM, Purdum PP *et al.* The haematologic consequences of transjugular intrahepatic portosystemic shunts. *Hepatology* 1996; **23**: 32–39.

155 Rouillard SS, Bass NM, Roberts JP *et al.* Severe hyperbilirubinemia after creation of transjugular intrahepatic portosystemic shunts: natural history and predictors of outcome. *Ann. Intern. Med.* 1998; **128**: 374–377.

156 Jabbour N, Zajko A, Orons P *et al.* Does transjugular intrahepatic portosystemic shunt (TIPS) resolve thrombocytopenia associated with cirrhosis? *Dig. Dis. Sci.* 1998; **43**: 2459–2462.

157 Lind CD, Malish TW, Chong WK *et al.* Incidence of shunt occlusion or stenosis following transjugular intrahepatic portosystemic shunt placement. *Gastroenterology* 1994; **106**: 1277–1283.

158 LaBerge JM, Somberg KA, Lake JR *et al.* Two-year outcome following transjugular intrahepatic portosystemic shunt for variceal bleeding: results in 90 patients. *Gastroenterology* 1995; **108**: 1143–1151.

159 Selim N, Fendley MJ, Boyer TD *et al.* Conversion of failed transjugular intrahepatic portosystemic shunt to distal splenorenal shunt in patients with Child's A or B cirrhosis. *Ann. Surg.* 1998; **227**: 600–603.

160 Orloff MJ, Bell RH Jr, Orloff MS *et al.* Prospective randomized trial of emergency portacaval shunt and emergency medical therapy in unselected cirrhotic patients with bleeding varices. *Hepatology* 1994; **20**: 863–872.

161 Burroughs AK, Hamilton G, Philips A *et al.* A comparison of sclerotherapy with staple transaction of the oesophagus for the emergency control of bleeding from oesophageal varices. *N. Engl. J. Med.* 1989; **321**: 857–862.

162 McCormick PA, Kaye GL, Greenslade L *et al.* Esophageal staple transection as a salvage procedure after failure of acute injection sclerotherapy. *Hepatology* 1992; **15**: 403–406.

163 Gonzalez R, Zamora J, Gomez-Camero J *et al.* Combination endoscopic and drug therapy to prevent variceal rebleeding in cirrhosis. *Ann. Intern. Med.* 2008; **149**: 109–122.

164 Perez-Ayuso RM, Pique JP, Bosch J *et al.* Propranolol in prevention of recurrent bleeding from severe portal hypertensive gastropathy in cirrhosis. *Lancet* 1991; **337**: 1431–1434.

165 Eck NV. On the question of ligature of the portal vein (trans. title). *Voyenno Med. J. (St Petersburg)* 1877; **130**: Sect. 2.1.

166 Dowling JB. Ten years' experience with mesocaval grafts. *Surg. Gynecol. Obstet.* 1979; **149**: 518–522.

167 Millikan WJ, Warren WD, Henderson JM et al. The Emory prospective randomized trial selective vs non-selective shunt to control variceal bleeding. Ten year follow up. *Ann. Surg.* 1985; **201**: 712–722.

168 Spina GP, Henderson JM, Rikkers LF *et al.* Distal splenorenal sunt ersus endoscopic sclerotherapy in prevention of variceal rebleeding. A meta analysis of 4 randomized clinical trials. *J. Hepatol.* 1992; **16**: 338–345.

169 Burroughs AK, Vangeli M. Transjugular intrahepatic portosystemic shunt versus endoscopic therapy: randomized trials for secondary prophylaxis of variceal bleeding: an updated meta-analysis. *Scan. J. Gastroenterol.* 2002; **37**: 249–252.

170 Zacks SL, Sandler RS, Biddle AK *et al.* Decision analysis of transjugular intrahepatic portosystemic shunt vs. distal splenorenal shunt for portal hypertension. *Hepatology* 1999; **29**: 1399–1405.

171 Sanyal AJ, Freedman AM, Shiffman ML *et al.* Portosystemic encephalopathy after transjugular intrahepatic portosystemic shunt: results of a prospective controlled study. *Hepatology* 1994; **20**: 46–55.

172 Riggio O, Merli M, Pedretti G *et al.* Hepatic encephalopathy after transjugular intrahepatic portosystemic shunt. Incidence and risk factors. *Dig. Dis. Sci.* 1996; **41**: 578–584.

173 Nolte W, Wiltfang J, Schindler C *et al.* Portosystemic hepatic encephalopathy after transjugular intrahepatic portosystemic shunt in patients with cirrhosis: clinical, laboratory, psychometric and electroencephalographic investigations. *Hepatology* 1998; **28**: 1215–1225.

174 Guevara M, Gines P, Bandi JC *et al.* Transjugular intrahepatic portosystemic shunt in hepatorenal syndrome: effects on renal function and vasoactive systems. *Hepatology* 1998; **28**: 416–422.

175 Huonker M, Schumacher YO, Ochs A *et al.* Cardiac function and haemodynamics in alcoholic cirrhosis and effects of the transjugular intrahepatic portosystemic stent shunt. *Gut* 1999; **44**: 743–748.

176 Van der Linden P, Le Moine O, Ghysels M *et al.* Pulmonary hypertension after transjugular intrahepatic portosystemic shunt: effects on right ventricular function. *Hepatology* 1996; **23**: 982–987.

177 Ho K-S, Lashner BA, Emond JC *et al.* Prior esophageal variceal bleeding does not adversely affect survival after

orthotopic liver transplantation. *Hepatology* 1993; **18**: 66–72.

178 Ewaga H, Keeffe EB, Dort J *et al*. Liver transplantation for uncontrollable variceal bleeding. *Am. J. Gastroenterol.* 1994; **89**: 1823–1826.

179 Guerrini GP, Pleguezuelo M, Maimone S *et al*. Impact of TIPS pre-liver transplantation for the outcome post transplantation. *Am. J. Transplant.* 2009; **9**: 192–200.

180 Navasa M, Feu F, Garcia-Pagán JC *et al*. Hemodynamic and humoral changes after liver transplantation in patients with cirrhosis. *Hepatology* 1993; **17**: 355–360.

181 D'Amico G, Garcia-Pagan JC, Luca A, Bosch J. Hepatic vein pressure gradient reduction and prevention of variceal bleeding in cirrhosis: a systematic review. *Gastroenterology* 2006; **131**: 1611–1624.

182 Thalheimer V, Mela M, Patch D, Burroughs AK. Monitoring target reduction in hepatic venous pressure gradient during pharmacological therapy of portal hypertension: a core look at the evidence. *Gut* 2004; **53**: 143–148.

183 Villaneuva C, Aracil C, Colomo A *et al*. Clinical trial: a randomized controlled study on the prevention of variceal rebleeding comparing nadolol and ligation vs hepatic venous pressure gradient guided pharmacological therapy. *Aliment. Pharmacol. Therap.* 2009; **29**: 397–408.

184 Thalheimer U, Bosch J, Burroughs AK. How to prevent varices from bleeding: shades of grey—the case for nonselective beta blockers. *Gastroenterology* 2007; **133**: 2029–2036.

185 Lo GH, Cheu WC, Lin CK *et al*. Improved survival in patients receiving medical therapy as compared with banding ligation for the prevention of esophageal variceal rebleeding. *Hepatology* 2008; **48**: 580–587.

186 Senzolo M, Cholongitas E, Burra P *et al*. Beta-blockers protect against spontaneous bacterial peritonitis in cirrhotic patients: a meta-analysis. *Liver Int.* 2009; **29**: 1189–1193.

187 Thalheimer U, Triantos CK, Samonakis DN *et al*. Infection, coagulation and variceal bleeding in cirrhosis. *Gut* 2005; **54**: 556–563.

188 Vorobioff J, Groszmann RJ, Picabea E *et al*. Prognostic value of hepatic venous pressure gradient measurements in alcoholic cirrhsis: a 10 year prospective study. *Gastroenterology* 1996; **111**: 701–709.

189 Abraldes JG, Tarantino I, Turnes J *et al*. Haemodynamic response to pharmacological treatment of portal hypertension and influence on complications of cirrhosis. *Hepatology* 2003; **37**: 902–908.

190 Villaneuva C, Lopez-Balaguer JM, Aracil C *et al*. Maintenance of haemodynamic response to treatment for portal hypertension and influence on complications of cirrhosis. *J. Hepatol.* 2004; **40**: 757–765.

191 Abraldes JG, Albillos A, Banares R *et al*. Simvastatin lowers portal pressure in patients with cirrhosis and portal hypertension: a randomized controlled trial. *Gastroenterology* 2009; **136**: 1651–1658.

192 Dodds WJ, Erickson SJ, Taylor AJ *et al*. Caudate lobe of the liver: anatomy, embryology, and pathology. *Am. J. Roentgenol.* 1990; **154**: 87–93.

193 Bolton C, Barnard WG. The pathological occurrences in the liver in experimental venous stagnation. *J. Path. Bact.* 1931; **34**: 701.

194 Senzolo M, Cholongitas E, Patch D, Burroughs AK. Update on the classification, assessment of prognosis and therapy of Budd-Chiari syndrome. *Nat. Clin. Pract. Gastroenterol. Hepatol.* 2005; **2**: 182–190.

195 Budd G. *On Diseases of the Liver*, 3rd edn. Philadelphia: Blanchard & Lea, 1857.

196 Chiari H. Ueber die selbständige Phlebitis obliterans der Hauptstämme der Venae hepaticae als Todesurache. *Beitr. Path. Anat.* 1899; **26**: 1.

197 Valla DC. The diagnosis and management of the Budd-Chiari syndrome: consensus and controversies. *Hepatology* 2003; **38**: 793–803.

198 Denninger MH, Chait Y, Casadevall N *et al*. Cause of portal or hepatic venous thrombosis in adults: the role of multiple concurrent factors. *Hepatology* 2000; **31**: 587–591.

199 Hussein K, Bock O, Kreipe J. Histological and molecular classifications of chronic myeloproliferative disorders in the age of JAK2: persistence of old questions despite new answers. *Pathobiology* 2007; **74**: 72–80.

200 Pomeroy C, Knodell RG, Swaim WR *et al*. Budd–Chiari syndrome in a patient with the lupus anticoagulant. *Gastroenterology* 1984; **86**: 158–161.

201 Pelletier S, Landi B, Piette J-C *et al*. Antiphospholipid syndrome as the second cause of non-tumorous Budd–Chiari syndrome. *J. Hepatol.* 1994; **21**: 76–80.

202 Young ID, Clark RN, Manley PN *et al*. Response to steroids in Budd–Chiari syndrome caused by idiopathic granulomatous venulitis. *Gastroenterology* 1988; **94**: 503–507.

203 Hoekstra J, Leebeek FW, Plessier A *et al*. Paroxysmal nocturnal hemoglobinuria in Budd-Chiari syndrome: findings form a cohort study. *J. Hepatol.* 2009; **51**: 696–706.

204 Hoekstra J, Guimaraes AHC, Leebeek FWG *et al*. Impaired fibrinolysis as a risk factor for Budd-Chiari syndrome. *Blood* 2010; **115**: 388–395.

205 Das M, Carroll SF. Antithrombin III deficiency: an aetiology of Budd–Chiari syndrome. *Surgery* 1985; **97**: 242–246.

206 Janssen HL. Factor V Leiden mutation, prothrombin gene mutation and deficiencies in coagulation inhibitors associated with Budd-Chiari syndrome and portal vein thrombosis: results of a case controlled study. *Blood* 2000; **96**: 2369–2368.

207 Salooja N, Perry D. Thromboelastography. *Blood Coagul. Fibrinolysis* 2001; **12**: 327–337.

208 Bayraktar Y, Balkanci F, Bayraktar M *et al*. Budd–Chiari syndrome: a common complication of Behçet's disease. *Am. J. Gastroenterol.* 1997; **92**: 858–862.

209 Valla D, Le MG, Poynard T *et al*. Risk of hepatic vein thrombosis in relation to recent use of oral contraceptives: a case–control study. *Gastroenterology* 1986; **90**: 807–811.

210 Minnema MC. Budd-Chiari syndrome: combination of genetic defects and the use of oral contraceptives leading to hypercoagulability. *J. Heptol.* 2000; **33**: 509–512.

211 Khuroo MS, Datta V. Budd-Chiari syndrome following pregnancy. Report of 16 cases with roentgenologic haemodynamia and histological studies of the hepatic outflow tract. *Am. J. Med.* 1980; **68**: 113–121.

212 Balian A, Valla D, Naveau S *et al*. Post-traumatic membranous obstruction of the inferior vena cava associated with a hypercoagulable state. *J. Hepatol.* 1998; **28**: 723–726.

213 Uddin W, Ramage JK, Portmann B *et al*. Hepatic venous outflow obstruction in patients with polycystic liver disease: pathogenesis and treatment. *Gut* 1995; **36**: 142–145.

214 Takayasu K, Muramatsu Y, Moriyama N *et al.* Radiological study of idiopathic Budd–Chiari syndrome complicated by hepatocellular carcinoma. A report of four cases. *Am. J. Gastroenterol.* 1994; **88**: 249–253.

215 Schluger LK, Cubukcu O, Klion F *et al.* Unexplained Budd–Chiari syndrome in a young man. *Hepatology* 1995; **21**: 584–588.

216 MacMahon HE, Ball HG III. Leiomyosarcoma of hepatic vein and the Budd–Chiari syndrome. *Gastroenterology* 1971; **61**: 239–243.

217 Schraut WH, Chilcote RR. Metastatic Wilms' tumour causing acute hepatic-vein occlusion (Budd–Chiari syndrome). *Gastroenterology* 1985; **88**: 576–579.

218 Dhillon AP, Burroughs AK, Hudson M *et al.* Hepatic venular stenosis after orthotopic liver transplantation. *Hepatology* 1994; **19**: 106–111.

219 Kiuchi T. Small for size graft in living donor liver transplantation: how far should we go. *Liver Transpl.* 2003; **9**: 529–S35.

220 Blanshard C, Dodge G, Pasi J *et al.* Membranous obstruction of the inferior vena cava in a patient with factor V Leiden: evidence for prothrombotic aetiology. *J. Hepatol.* 1997; **26**: 731–735.

221 Okuda K, Kage M, Shrestha SM. Proposal of a new nomenclature for Budd–Chiari syndrome: hepatic vein thrombosis vs. thrombosis of the inferior vena cava at its hepatic portion. *Hepatology* 1998; **28**: 1191–1198.

222 Shrestha SM. Endemicity and clinical picture of liver disease due to obstruction of the hepatic portion of the inferior vena cava in Nepal. *J. Gastroenterol. Hepatol.* 1996; **11**: 170–179.

223 Amarapurkar DN, Punamiya SJ, Patel ND. Changing spectrum of Budd-Chiari syndrome in India with special reference to non-surgical treatment. *World J. Gastroenterol.* 2008; **14**: 278–285.

224 Tanaka M, Wanless IR, Pathology of the liver in Budd–Chiari syndrome: portal vein thrombosis and the histogenesis of veno-centric cirrhosis, veno-portal cirrhosis, and large regenerative nodules. *Hepatology* 1998; **27**: 488–496.

225 Casals-Hatem D, Vilgrain V, Genin P *et al.* Arterial and portal circulation and parenchymal changes in Budd-Chiari syndrome: a study in 17 explanted lviers. *Hepatology* 2003; **37**: 510–519.

226 Hadengue A, Poliquin M, Vilgrain V *et al.* The changing scene of hepatic vein thrombosis: recognition of asymptomatic cases. *Gastroenterology* 1994; **106**: 1042–1047.

227 Millener P, Grant EG, Rose S *et al.* Color Doppler imaging findings in patients with Budd–Chiari syndrome: correlation with venographic findings. *Am. J. Roentgenol.* 1993; **161**: 307–312.

228 Mori H, Maeda H, Fukuda T *et al.* Acute thrombosis of the inferior vena cava and hepatic veins in patients with Budd–Chiari syndrome: CT demonstration. *Am. J. Roentgenol.* 1989; **153**: 987–991.

229 Kane R, Eustace S. Diagnosis of Budd–Chiari syndrome: comparison between sonography and magnetic resonance angiography. *Radiology* 1995; **195**: 117–121.

230 Miller WJ, Federle MP, Straub EH *et al.* Budd–Chiari syndrome: imaging with pathologic correlation. *Abdom. Imaging* 1993; **18**: 329–335.

231 James C, Ugo V, Le Couedic JP *et al.* A unique clonal JAK2 mutation leading to constitutive signalling causes polycythaemia vera. *Nature* 2005; **434**: 1134–1148.

232 Zeitoun G. Outcome of Budd-Chiari syndrome: a multivariate analysis of factors related to survival including surgical portosystemic shunting. *Hepatology* 1999; **30**: 84–89.

233 Darwish Murad S, Plessier A, Hernandez-Guerra M *et al.* Etiology, management and outcome of the Budd-Chiari syndrome. *Ann. Intern. Med.* 2009; **151**: 167–175.

234 Moucari R, Rautou PE, Cazals-Hatem D *et al.* Hepatocellular carcinoma in Budd-Chiari syndrome: characteristics and risk factors. *Gut* 2008; **57**: 828–835.

235 Tang TJ. The prognostic value of histology in the assessment of patients with Budd-Chiari syndrome. *J. Hepatol.* 2001; **35**: 338–343.

236 Singh V. Budd-Chiari syndrome: our experience of 71 patients. *J. Gastroenterol. Hepatol.* 2000; **15**: 550–554.

237 Okuda H. Epidemiological and clinical features of Budd-Chiari syndrome in Japan. *J. Hepatol.* 1995; **22**: 1–9.

238 Ganguli SC, Ramzan NN, McKusick MA *et al.* Budd–Chiari syndrome in patients with haematological disease: a therapeutic challenge. *Hepatology* 1998; **27**: 1157–1161.

239 Min AD, Atillasoy EO, Schwartz ME *et al.* Reassessing the role of medical therapy in the management of hepatic vein thrombosis. *Liver Transpl. Surg.* 1997; **3**: 423–429.

240 Martin LG, Henderson JM, Millikan WJ Jr *et al.* Angioplasty for long-term treatment of patients with Budd–Chiari syndrome. *Am. J. Roentgenol.* 1990; **154**: 1007–1010.

241 Venbrux AC, Savader SJ, Mitchell SE *et al.* Interventional management of Budd-Chiari syndrome. *Semin. Intervent. Radiol.* 1994; **11**: 312.

242 Mancuso A, Fung K, Mela M *et al.* TIPS for acute and chronic Budd-Chiari syndrome: a single centre experience. *J. Hepatol.* 2003; **38**: 751–754.

243 Garcia-Pagan JC, Heydtmann M, Raffia S *et al.* TIPS for Budd Chiari syndrome: long term results and prognostic factors in 124 patients. *Gastroenterology* 2008; **135**: 808–815.

244 Mancuso A, Watkinson A, Tibbals J *et al.* Budd Chiari syndrome with portal, splenic and superior mesenteric thrombosis treated with TIPS: who dares wins. *Gut* 2003; **52**: 438.

245 Thompson NP, Miller AD, Hamilton G *et al.* Emergency rescue hepatic Transplantation following shunt surgery for Budd-Chiari Syndrome. *Eur. J. Gastroenterol.* 1994; **6**: 836–837.

246 Ringe B, Lang H, Oldhafer K-J *et al.* Which is the best surgery for Budd–Chiari syndrome: venous decompression or liver transplantation? A single-centre experience with 50 patients. *Hepatology* 1995; **21**: 1337–1344.

247 Panis Y, Belghiti J, Valla D *et al.* Portosystemic shunt in Budd–Chiari syndrome: long-term survival and factors affecting shunt patency in 25 patients in Western countries. *Surgery* 1994; **115**: 276–281.

248 Gillams A, Dick R, Platts A *et al.* Dilitation of the inferior vena cava using an expandable metal stent in Budd-Chiari syndrome. *J. Hepatol.* 1991; **13**: 149–151.

249 Senning A. Transcaval posterocranial resection of the liver as treatment for the Budd-Chirari syndrome. *World J. Surg.* 1983; **7**: 632–640.

250 Mentha G, Giostra E, Majno PE *et al*. Liver transplantation for Budd Chiari syndrome: a European study on 248 patients from 51 centres. *J. Hepatol.* 2006; **44**: 529–528.

251 Segev DL, Nguyen GC, Locke JE *et al*. Twenty years of liver transplantation for Budd-Chiari syndrome: a national registry analysis. *Liver Transpl.* 2007; **13**: 1285–1294.

252 Campbell DA Jr, Rolles K, Jamieson N *et al*. Hepatic transplantation with perioperative and long-term anticoagulation as treatment for Budd–Chiari syndrome. *Surg. Gynecol. Obstet.* 1988; **166**: 511–518.

253 Casella JF, Bontempo FA, Markel H *et al*. Successful treatment of homozygous protein C deficiency by hepatic transplantation. *Lancet* 1988; **i**: 435–438.

254 Zajko AB, Claus D, Clapuyt P *et al*. Obstruction to hepatic venous drainage after liver transplantation: treatment with balloon angioplasty. *Radiology* 1989; **170**: 763–765.

255 Van Lingen R, Warshow U, Dalton HR, Hussaini SH. Jaundice as a presentation of heart failure. *J. Soc. Med.* 2005; **98**: 357–359.

256 Shibuya A, Unuma T, Sugimoto M *et al*. Diffuse hepatic calcification as a sequelae to shock liver. *Gastroenterology* 1985; **89**: 196–201.

257 Berger ML, Reynolds RC, Hagler HK *et al*. Anoxic hepatocyte injury: role of reversible changes in elemental content and distribution. *Hepatology* 1989; **9**: 219–228.

258 Motoyama S, Minamiya Y, Saito S *et al*. Hydrogen peroxide derived from hepatocytes induces sinusoidal cell apoptosis in perfused hypoxic rat liver. *Gastroenterology* 1998; **114**: 153–163.

259 Weisiger RA. Oxygen radicals and ischemic tissue injury. *Gastroenterology* 1986; **90**: 494–496.

260 Ma TT, Ischiropoulos H, Brass CA. Endotoxin-stimulated nitric oxide production increases injury and reduces rat liver chemiluminescence during reperfusion. *Gastroenterology* 1995; **108**: 463–469.

261 Henrion J, Schapira M, Luwaert R *et al*. Hypoxic hepatitis. Clinical and haemodynamic study in 142 consecutive cases. *Medicine* 2003; **82**: 392–406.

262 Gitlin N, Serio KM. Ischemic hepatitis: widening horizons. *Am. J. Gastroenterol.* 1992; **87**: 831–836.

263 Kamiyama T, Miyakawa H, Tajiri K. Ischemic hepatitis in cirrhosis. Clinical features and prognostic implications. *J. Clin. Gastroenterol.* 1996; **22**: 126–130.

264 Mathurin P, Durand F, Ganne N *et al*. Ischemic hepatitis due to obstructive sleep apnea. *Gastroenterology* 1995; **109**: 1682–1684.

265 Hickman PE, Potter JM. Mortality associated with ischaemic hepatitis. *Aust. NZ J. Med.* 1990; **20**: 32–34.

266 Denis C, de Kerguennec C, Bernuau J *et al*. Acute hypoxic hepatitis ("liver shock"): still a frequently overlooked cardiological diagnosis. *Eur. J. Heart Failure* 2004; **6**: 561–565.

267 Nouel O, Henrion J, Bernuau J *et al*. Fulminant hepatic failure due to transient circulatory failure in patients with chronic heart disease. *Dig. Dis. Sci.* 1980; **25**: 49–52.

268 Nunes G, Blaisdell FW, Margaretten W. Mechanism of hepatic dysfunction following shock and trauma. *Arch. Surg.* 1970; **100**: 646.

269 te Boekhorst T, Urlus M, Doesburg W *et al*. Etiologic factors of jaundice in severely ill patients: a retrospective study in patients admitted to an intensive care unit with severe trauma or with septic intra-abdominal complications following surgery and without evidence of bile duct obstruction. *J. Hepatol.* 1988; **7**: 111–117.

270 Carrico JC, Meakins JL, Marshall JC *et al*. Multiple-organ failure syndrome. *Arch. Surg.* 1986; **121**: 196.

271 Batts KP. Ischemic cholangitis. *Mayo Clin. Proc.* 1998; **73**: 380–385.

272 Doctor RB, Dahl RH, Salter KD *et al*. Reorganization of cholangiocyte membrane domains represents an early event in rat liver ischaemia. *Hepatology* 1999; **29**: 1364–1374.

273 Chu C-M, Chang C-H, Liaw Y-F *et al*. Jaundice after open heart surgery: a prospective study. *Thorax* 1984; **39**: 52–56.

274 Collins JD, Bassendine MF, Ferner R *et al*. Incidence and prognostic importance of jaundice after cardiopulmonary bypass surgery. *Lancet* 1983; **i**: 1119–1123.

275 Lefkowitch JH, Mendez L. Morphologic features of hepatic injury in cardiac disease and shock. *J. Hepatol.* 1986; **2**: 313–327.

276 Sherlock S. The liver in heart failure; relation of anatomical, functional and circulatory changes. *Br. Heart J.* 1951; **13**: 273–293.

277 Klatt EC, Koss MN, Young TS *et al*. Hepatic hyaline globules associated with passive congestion. *Arch. Pathol. Lab. Med.* 1988; **112**: 510–544.

278 Shibayama Y. The role of hepatic venous congestion and endotoxaemia in the production of fulminant hepatic failure secondary to congestive heart failure. *J. Pathol.* 1987; **151**: 133–138.

279 Arcidi JM Jr, Moore GM, Hutchins GM. Hepatic morphology in cardiac dysfunction. A clinicopathologic study of 1000 subjects at autopsy. *Am. J. Pathol.* 1981; **104**: 159–166.

280 Wanless IR, Liu JJ, Butany J. Role of thrombosis in the pathogenesis of congestive hepatic fibrosis (cardiac cirrhosis). *Hepatology* 1995; **21**: 1232–1237.

281 Maisel AS, Atwood JE, Goldberger AL. Hepatojugular reflux: useful in the bedside diagnosis of tricuspid regurgitation. *Ann. Intern. Med.* 1984; **101**: 781–782.

282 Hosoki T, Arisawa J, Marukawa T *et al*. Portal blood flow in congestive heart failure: pulsed duplex sonographic findings. *Radiology* 1990; **174**: 733–736.

283 Runyon BA. Cardiac ascites: a characterization. *J. Clin. Gastroenterol.* 1988; **10**: 410–412.

284 Moulton JS, Miller BL, Dodd GD III *et al*. Passive hepatic congestion in heart failure: CT abnormalities. *Am. J. Roentgenol.* 1988; **151**: 939–942.

285 Bohmer T, Kjekshus E, Nitter-Hauge S. Studies on the elevation of bilirubin preoperatively in patients with mitral valve disease. *Eur. Heart J.* 1994; **15**: 1016.

286 Coralli RJ, Crawley IS. Hepatic pulsations in constrictive pericarditis. *Am. J. Cardiol.* 1986; **58**: 370–373.

287 Lowe MD, Harcombe AA, Grace AA *et al*. Restrictive-constrictive heart failure masquerading as liver disease. *Br. Med. J.* 1999; **318**: 585.

CHAPTER 10
Ascites

Guadalupe Garcia-Tsao

Yale University School of Medicine, New Haven, and VA-CT Healthcare System, West Haven, CT, USA

Learning points

- Ascites is the most common decompensating event in cirrhosis.

- Its pathophysiology is mostly explained by splanchnic and peripheral vasodilatation that lead to a decrease in effective blood volume.

- The natural history of ascites results from a progressively more deranged circulatory status; with ascites that initially responds to diuretics, then becoming refractory to diuretics, at which time the patient may develop hyponatraemia and, finally, hepatorenal syndrome.

- Most patients respond to diuretics. Patients who no longer respond should be treated with repeated large-volume paracenteses. Transjugular intrahepatic porto-systemic shunt (TIPS) should be considered in those requiring frequent paracenteses. Fluid restriction is recommended in patients with hyponatraemia. Vasoconstrictors may reverse hepatorenal syndrome and are useful as a bridge to liver transplantation.

- Ascites *per se* is not lethal unless it becomes infected (spontaneous bacterial peritonitis). Infection often precipitates the hepatorenal syndrome leading to death. Antibiotic prophylaxis is indicated for secondary prevention of spontaneous bacterial peritonitis and in high-risk patients.

Ascites is free fluid within the peritoneal cavity. It forms because of conditions directly involving the peritoneum (infection, malignancy), or diseases remote from the peritoneum (liver disease, heart failure, hypoproteinaemia). Cirrhosis is the commonest cause of ascites in the Western world (~75%), followed by peritoneal malignancy (12%), cardiac failure (5%) and peritoneal tuberculosis (2%) [1] (Fig. 10.1). In patients with cirrhosis, the development of ascites marks the transition from compensated to decompensated cirrhosis [2,3]; and is the

most frequent first decompensating event, occurring in 48% [4].

The mechanisms of ascites formation in cirrhosis are complex but portal (sinusoidal) hypertension and renal retention of sodium are universal. The natural history of cirrhotic ascites progresses from diuretic-responsive (uncomplicated) ascites to the development of dilutional hyponatraemia, refractory ascites, and finally, hepatorenal syndrome (HRS) (Fig. 10.2). While 1-year survival in patients who develop ascites is 85%, it decreases to 25% once it has progressed to hyponatraemia, refractory ascites or HRS [4].

Treatment of ascites has not resulted in a significant improvement in survival. However, treating ascites is important, not only because it improves quality of life but because spontaneous bacterial peritonitis (SBP), a lethal complication of cirrhosis, does not occur in the absence of ascites. New treatments are being evaluated that modify its pathophysiology, such as the transjugular intrahepatic portosystemic shunt (TIPS) for refractory ascites and vasoconstrictors for HRS. Liver transplantation is the ultimate therapy and should be considered when the patient first presents with ascites.

Mechanisms of ascites formation

In cirrhosis, the source of ascites is mainly the hepatic sinusoids. Therefore sinusoidal hypertension is the initial mechanism that determines leakage of ascites into the peritoneal space [5,6]. Sinusoidal hypertension results from hepatic venous outflow block secondary to regenerative nodules and fibrosis. The other essential factor in the pathogenesis of cirrhotic ascites is sodium and water retention which allows for the replenishment of the intravascular volume and maintenance of ascites formation [7]. Inappropriate sodium retention is either secondary to vascular changes (*underfill and peripheral*

Sherlock's Diseases of the Liver and Biliary System, Twelfth Edition. Edited by James S. Dooley, Anna S.F. Lok, Andrew K. Burroughs, E. Jenny Heathcote.
© 2011 by Blackwell Publishing Ltd. Published 2011 by Blackwell Publishing Ltd.

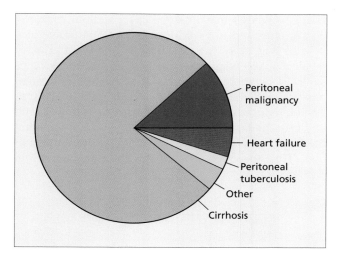

Fig. 10.1. Causes of ascites.

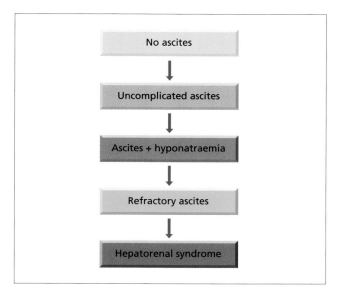

Fig. 10.2. Natural history of cirrhotic ascites.

Table 10.1. Sequence of events for the hypotheses of ascites formation

	Underfill/ peripheral arterial vasodilatation theory	Overfill theory
Primary event	Vascular	Renal
Secondary event	Renal	Vascular

arterial vasodilatation hypotheses) or as a primary event (*overfill theory*) (Table 10.1).

Sinusoidal hypertension

Similar to gastro-oesophageal varices, in which a minimal portal pressure gradient of 12 mmHg is needed

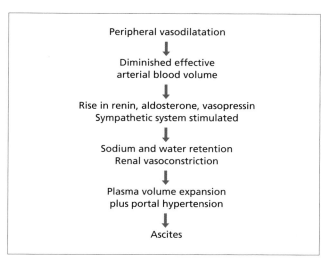

Fig. 10.3. The peripheral arterial vasodilatation hypothesis for ascites formation in cirrhosis [7].

for their presence [8]; the development of ascites also requires a minimal portal pressure gradient of 12 mmHg [5,6]. A threshold portal pressure gradient of 10 mmHg or more has been defined as 'clinically significant portal hypertension' because it best predicts the development of complications of cirrhosis, such as ascites [9,10].

Sodium retention

In patients with cirrhosis and ascites, the normal regulation of sodium balance is lost. Sodium is retained avidly; urinary sodium excretion is often below 5 mmol/day. Inappropriate sodium retention occurs even in the absence of ascites [11].

Vasodilatation theory (Fig. 10.3)

Arterial vasodilatation, a haemodynamic abnormality typical of the patient with cirrhosis, is the most likely mechanism that explains sodium retention [7]. An increased production of the vasodilator nitric oxide (NO) is considered the main cause of vasodilatation [12]. In experimental models of cirrhosis, inhibition of NO synthase increases systemic blood pressure and renal sodium excretion, resulting in a reduced volume of ascites [13,14]. Other vasodilators implicated in the vasodilatation of cirrhosis include adrenomedullin, carbon monoxide, endocannabinoids, prostacyclin, tumour necrosis factor alpha and urotensin [15].

Arterial vasodilatation results in a reduction in 'effective' arterial blood volume and a decrease in systemic arterial pressure, leading to the activation of the renin–angiotensin–aldosterone system (RAAS) and the sympathetic nervous system (through carotid sinus baroreceptors). Renin is produced by the kidney (juxtaglomerular apparatus) in response to low blood volume and β-adrenergic stimulation. Under the influence of renin, angiotensinogen (produced by the liver) is converted to angiotensin I (a decapeptide), which in turn is converted to angiotensin II (an octapeptide) by angiotensin-converting enzyme (ACE). Angiotensin II is the main stimulant to the synthesis and secretion of aldosterone, a mineralocorticoid, from the glomerular cells of the adrenal cortex. Aldosterone acts on cells in the collecting duct(ule) and, through a cytoplasmic interaction, increases both luminal uptake and basolateral passage of sodium (Fig. 10.3). Natriuresis after spironolactone, an aldosterone antagonist, supports hyperaldosteronism as a major contributor to sodium retention in cirrhosis [16].

In addition to sodium (and water) retention, angiotensin II is a potent vasoconstrictor (both venules and arterioles), a potent stimulant for the non-osmotic release of antidiuretic hormone (ADH) from the posterior pituitary and a potent activator of the adrenergic system (Fig. 10.4).

Bacterial translocation to mesenteric lymph nodes with increased endotoxin production and consequent stimulation of cytokine synthesis plays a major role in enhancing vasodilatation in animals with cirrhosis and ascites [17,18]. Further vasodilatation, with further activation of the RAAS, leads to hyponatraemia (through secretion of ADH) [19], and to the HRS (through maximal renal vasoconstriction) [7]. The time course of circulatory, neurohumoral and renal function abnormalities is depicted in Fig. 10.5 [20].

Overfill theory (Fig. 10.6)

The presence of normal or low levels of plasma renin activity in about a third of patients with cirrhosis and ascites, suggests that in some cases sodium retention occurs unrelated to vasodilatation. An alternative proposal is that, early on in the process, there is a primary renal change—responding to hepatic insufficiency or sinusoidal hypertension—that leads to sodium retention (overfill theory). Several signals have been suggested: reduced hepatic synthesis of a natriuretic agent, reduced hepatic clearance of a sodium-retaining hormone, or a 'hepatorenal reflex' of unknown aetiology. This theory is based on findings of sodium

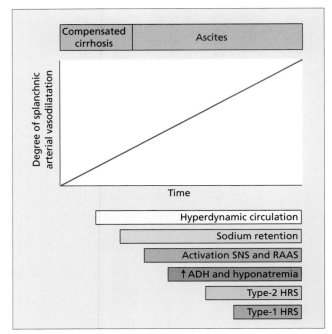

Fig. 10.5. Time course of circulatory, neurohormonal and renal function abnormalities in cirrhosis (in sequence of peripheral arterial vasodilation theory). ADH, antidiuretic hormone; HRS, hepatorenal syndrome; RAAS, renin–angiotensin–aldosterone system; SNS, sympathetic nervous system. (From [20] with permission.)

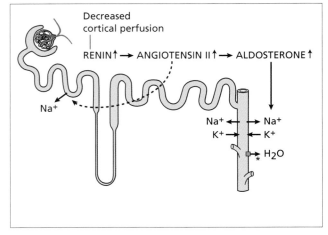

Fig. 10.4. Mechanisms of increased sodium and water reabsorption in cirrhosis. * Increased ADH-stimulated water reabsorption in collecting ducts.

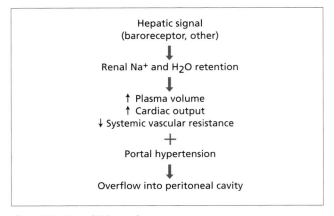

Fig. 10.6. Overfill hypothesis.

handling abnormalities, in the absence of systemic vasodilatation or arterial under-filling, when patients with preascitic cirrhosis are challenged with a sodium load [21]. This hypothesis proposes that primary sodium and water retention lead to expansion of the plasma volume, an increase in cardiac output and a fall in systemic vascular resistance (vasodilatation).

Whether vasodilatation is a primary or secondary event, therapy that counteracts the mechanisms that lead to vasodilatation (e.g. NO inhibition) or vasodilatation itself (e.g. vasoconstrictors), improves renal haemodynamics and increases sodium excretion [13,22].

Other renal factors

Atrial natriuretic peptides (ANP)

The plasma concentration of ANP is markedly increased in patients with cirrhosis and ascites, regardless of plasma levels of renin, aldosterone and noradrenaline (norepinephrine). This is a potent natriuretic peptide released from the cardiac atria, probably in response to intravascular volume expansion. In compensated cirrhosis, ANF may maintain sodium homeostasis despite the presence of mild antinatriuretic factors. In later stages, renal resistance to ANF develops, rendering it ineffective [23]. Therefore, sodium retention in cirrhosis cannot be explained on the basis of a deficient synthesis of natriuretic peptides.

Prostaglandins

Several prostaglandins are synthesized in the kidney and have both vascular and tubular actions. Although they are not primary regulators, they modulate the effects of other factors and hormones locally. Prostaglandin (PG) I$_2$ and E$_2$ are vasodilators, and also increase sodium excretion through vasodilatation and a direct effect on the loop of Henle. They inhibit cyclic adenosine monophosphate (cAMP) synthesis, thereby interfering with the action of vasopressin (ADH). PGI$_2$ is synthesized in the tubules and increases sodium and water excretion. Therefore, prostaglandins have a significant role in sodium and water homeostasis. In conditions where there is a reduced circulating volume, which includes cirrhosis, there is increased prostaglandin synthesis. This counterbalances renal vasoconstriction by antagonizing the local effects of renin, angiotensin II, endothelin 1, vasopressin and catecholamines.

The importance of this role is demonstrated clinically by the renal dysfunction precipitated by the administration non-steroidal anti-inflammatory agents to decompensated [24] and compensated [25] patients with cirrhosis. Without the vasodilatory influence of prostaglandins, renal blood flow and glomerular filtration rate

fall because of unopposed vasoconstriction due to renin and other factors. Such an imbalance may be a trigger for HRS.

Circulation of ascites

Once formed, ascitic fluid can exchange with blood through a large capillary bed under the visceral peritoneum. This plays a vital, dynamic role, sometimes actively facilitating transfer of fluid into ascites and sometimes retarding it. Ascitic fluid is continuously circulating, with about half entering and leaving the peritoneal cavity every hour, there being a rapid transit in both directions. The constituents of the fluid are in dynamic equilibrium with those of the plasma. Rate of ascitic fluid reabsorption is limited to 700–900 mL daily.

Summary (Fig. 10.5)

Ascites in cirrhosis results from sinusoidal hypertension and sodium retention. The most accepted theory for sodium retention is the *peripheral arterial vasodilatation hypothesis,* which proposes that renal sodium (and water retention) is due to reduced effective blood volume secondary to peripheral arterial vasodilatation (Figs 10.3, 10.4, 10.5). The renal changes are mediated by stimulation of the RAAS, an increase in sympathetic function, and other systemic and local peptide and hormone disturbances. The *overfill* view suggests that renal retention of sodium is primary with secondary vascular changes and accumulation of ascites and oedema. Depending on the degree of circulatory changes (Table 10.2), these same mechanisms will lead to hyponatraemia and, at the extreme end of severity of renal and vascular changes, HRS develops (Fig. 10.5).

Clinical features

Symptoms

The most frequent symptoms are *increased abdominal girth* (the patient notices tightness of the belt or garments around the waist) and recent *weight gain* [26]. As

Table 10.2. Circulatory changes in patients with cirrhosis

Increased	Plasma/ total blood volume
	Non-central blood volume
	Cardiac output
	Portal pressure and flow
Reduced	Central blood volume
	Arterial blood pressure
	Splanchnic vascular resistance
	Systemic vascular resistance
	Renal blood flow

fluid continues to accumulate, it leads to elevation of the diaphragm that may cause *shortness of breath*. Fluid accumulation may also be associated with a feeling of *satiety* and *generalized abdominal pain*. The rapid onset of symptoms in a matter of weeks in ascites helps to distinguish it from obesity, which develops over a period of months to years.

Examination

The presence of ascites in patients with cirrhosis denotes a decompensated, more advanced stage of cirrhosis, therefore stigmata of cirrhosis are usually present (spider angiomata, palmar erythema, muscle wasting). There may also be jaundice and signs of portal hypertension, such as splenomegaly and abdominal wall collaterals. Inferior vena caval collaterals result from a secondary, functional block of the inferior vena cava due to pressure of the peritoneal fluid. They commonly run from the groin to the costal margin or flanks and disappear when the ascites is controlled and intra-abdominal pressure is reduced.

Physical examination is relatively insensitive for detecting ascitic fluid, particularly when the amount is small and/or the patient is obese. Patients must have at least 1500 mL of fluid to be detected reliably on physical examination. The clinical diagnosis of ascites will be questionable or incorrect in roughly a third of the cases [27]. When present in small amounts, ascites can be identified by bulging flanks. Flank dullness is very sensitive in detecting ascites [28]. When flank dullness is detected, it is useful to see whether it shifts with rotation of the patient (shifting dullness). This sign is the most sensitive finding (compared to abdominal distension, bulging flanks and fluid wave) [29]. The fluid wave sign has the poorest sensitivity in the diagnosis of peritoneal fluid, even though its specificity is high [26,28,29]. With tense ascites it is difficult to palpate abdominal viscera, but with moderate amounts of fluid the liver or spleen may be ballotted. The presence of a ballotable liver is a good indicator of the presence of ascites [26].

Associated conditions

Umbilical hernias. Increased intra-abdominal pressure favours the development of diastasis recti or hernias in the umbilical, femoral or inguinal regions or through old abdominal incisions. Hernias develop in about 20 % of patients with cirrhosis and ascites (whereas only 3% have hernias without ascites), and may increase to up to 70% in patients with long-standing, recurrent, tense ascites [30]. The main risks of these hernias are rupture [31] and incarceration, the latter complication observed mostly in patients in whom ascites has reduced after paracentesis, peritoneovenous shunt or after transjugular intrahepatic portosystemic shunt [32]. Once ascites is optimally

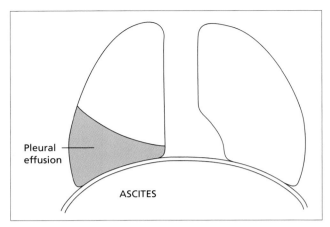

Fig. 10.7. A right-sided pleural effusion may accompany ascites and is related to defects in the diaphragm.

treated, elective hernia repair with permanent mesh is the best treatment for symptomatic hernias, with far less complications than following emergent repair [33].

Hepatic hydrothorax. Pleural effusion develops in about 5–10% of patients with cirrhosis [34] and although it usually develops in patients with ascites, hepatic hydrothorax may develop in patients without detectable ascites [35]. Pleural effusion is right-sided in 85%, left-sided in 13% and bilateral in 2% of the cases [36]. It is due to defects in the diaphragm allowing ascites to pass into the pleural cavity (Fig. 10.7). Examination of pleural and ascitic fluid may not be reliable to differentiate an effusion due to local pleural disease from that due to hepatic hydrothorax [37]. The diagnosis of hepatic hydrothorax can be established by radionuclide scanning of the chest after the intraperitoneal injection of Tc-99m-labelled sulphur colloid or macroaggregated serum albumin [35]. Presence of radiotracer in the pleural space is demonstrated generally within 2 hours following its intraperitoneal injection [38]. Although large amounts of ascites can accumulate in the peritoneal cavity before resulting in significant patient discomfort, the accumulation of smaller amounts of fluid (1–2 litres) in the pleural space results in severe shortness of breath and hypoxaemia. As pleural fluid is in equilibrium with peritoneal fluid, control depends on medical treatment of ascites. Aspiration is followed by rapid filling up of the pleural space by ascitic fluid. TIPS have been successful [39]; pleurodesis following complete drainage is less successful.

Peripheral oedema. This usually follows ascites and is related to hypoproteinaemia. A functional inferior vena caval block due to pressure of the abdominal fluid is an additional factor. The presence of oedema without ascites should therefore lead to investigations of causes of fluid retention other than ascites.

Ascitic fluid

Diagnostic paracentesis (of about 30 mL) should always be performed in a patient with new-onset ascites, however obvious its cause. In patients with known cirrhotic ascites, diagnostic paracentesis should be performed at every hospital admission and whenever SBP is suspected. Diagnostic paracentesis is a safe procedure with a very low incidence of serious complications, mostly transfusion-requiring haematomas that occur at a rate of 0.2 to 0.9% [40,41].

Fluid appearance is clear, green, straw-coloured or bile-stained. The volume is variable and up to 70 litres have been recorded. A blood-stained fluid indicates malignant disease or a recent paracentesis or an invasive investigation, such as liver biopsy or transhepatic cholangiography.

Ascites total protein and *serum-ascites albumin gradient (SAAG)* are two inexpensive tests that, taken together, are most useful in determining the source of ascites (Table 10.3). A high (>2.5 g/dL) ascites total protein occurs with peritoneal involvement (malignancy, tuberculosis) due to leakage of high protein mesenteric lymph from obliterated lymphatics and/or from an inflamed peritoneal surface. A high ascites total protein also occurs in cases of postsinusoidal or posthepatic sinusoidal hypertension when sinusoids are normal and protein-rich lymph leaks into the peritoneal cavity [42]. In cirrhosis, an abnormally low protein content of liver lymph has been demonstrated as a result of deposition of fibrous tissue in the sinusoids ('capillarization of the sinusoid'), which renders the sinusoid less leaky to macromolecules [43]. On the other hand, the SAAG, which involves subtracting ascites fluid albumin concentration from serum albumin, has been shown to correlate with hepatic sinusoidal pressure [44]. A SAAG more than 1.1 g/dL indicates that there is sinusoidal hypertension and that the source of ascites is the hepatic sinusoid as in the case of cirrhosis, heart failure or Budd–Chiari syndrome [45] (Table 10.3).

Ascites polymorphonuclear cells increase with peritoneal infection or with other intra-abdominal inflammatory conditions such as diverticulitis, cholecystitis. The diagnosis of SBP is established with a polymorphonuclear cell count of more than 250/mm^3 [46]. In sterile ascites, ascitic fluid white blood cell count is usually less than 100/mm^3 with a predominance of mononuclear cells and a low number of polymorphonuclear cells.

Ascites bacteriological culture is negative in approximately 40% of patients with clinical manifestations suggestive of SBP and increased ascites polymorphonuclear cells [46]. Nevertheless, aerobic and anaerobic cultures should be performed. The percentage of positive cultures increases when ascitic fluid is inoculated directly into blood culture bottles at the bedside, which is the recommended method of culture [46].

Electrolyte concentrations are those of other extracellular fluids.

The *rate of accumulation of fluid* is variable and depends on the dietary intake of sodium and the ability of the kidneys to excrete it.

Ascitic fluid protein and white cell count, but not polymorph concentration, increase during diuresis.

Radiological features

Plain X-ray of the abdomen shows a diffuse ground-glass appearance. Distended loops of bowel simulate intestinal obstruction. Ultrasound and CT scan show a space around the liver and these can be used to demonstrate quite small amounts of fluid (Fig. 10.8).

Differential diagnosis

Heart failure/ constrictive pericarditis. Diagnostic points include jugular vein distension and, in constrictive pericarditis, the paradoxical pulse and the radiological demonstration of a calcified pericardium [47]. In both cases SAAG will be more than 1.1 mg/dL and ascites protein will be more than 2.5 g/dL [48]. Right and left

Table 10.3. Differential diagnosis among the three most common causes of ascites

	Serum-ascites albumin gradient (cutoff 1.1 g/dL)	Ascites protein (cutoff 2.5 g/dL)	Hepatic vein pressures*		
			WHVP	FHVP	HVPG
Cirrhosis	High	Low	High	Normal	High
Cardiac ascites	High	High	High	High	Normal
Peritoneal malignancy/ peritoneal TB	Low	High	Normal	Normal	Normal

*Only to be performed in equivocal cases. WHVP, wedged hepatic venous pressure; FHVP, free hepatic venous pressure; HVPG, hepatic venous pressure gradient.

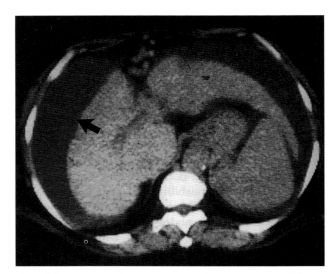

Fig. 10.8. CT scan showing an irregular cirrhotic small liver, splenomegaly and ascites (arrow).

heart catheterization and transjugular liver biopsy with measurements of hepatic venous pressure gradient may be necessary to make the differential between cardiac and cirrhotic ascites [27] (Table 10.3).

Malignant ascites. There may be symptoms and localizing signs due to the primary tumour. After paracentesis, the liver may be enlarged and nodular. Fluid cytological exam should be performed, although normal endothelial cells in the peritoneum can resemble malignant cells. Massive hepatic metastasis can lead to the development of ascites but since the mechanism of ascites formation is sinusoidal hypertension, these cases of 'malignant ascites' will have the characteristics of cirrhotic ascites [49,50].

Tuberculous ascites. This should be suspected particularly in the severely malnourished alcoholic who may be febrile. Rarely, lumps of matted omentum can be palpated after paracentesis. Ascitic fluid has many lymphocytes. When suspected, ascites should be stained for tubercle bacilli, and suitable cultures set up.

Mixed aetiology ascites. In patients with mixed ascites (e.g. cirrhosis with superimposed peritoneal malignancy or tuberculosis), the SAAG is high and the ascites protein is low, that is the findings of ascites due to cirrhosis predominate [48,50].

Chylous ascites. This results from accumulation of fat, predominantly chylomicrons, in the ascitic fluid. Its appearance is milky and diagnosis is confirmed on a triglyceride ascites content more than 200 mg/dL. The most common cause of chylous ascites is postsurgical disruption of lymphatics. The most common cause of

Table 10.4. Spontaneous bacterial peritonitis

Suspect grade B and C cirrhosis with ascites
Clinical features may be absent and peripheral WBC normal
Ascitic protein usually <1 g/dL
Usually monomicrobial and Gram-negative
Start antibiotics if ascites >250 mm polymorphs
Concomitant albumin use if renal dysfunction or jaundice
20% die
69% recur in 1 year

non-surgical chylous ascites is cirrhosis [51,52]. Management is of the underlying cause and a low-fat medium chain triglyceride diet for 3 weeks, or if this fails total parenteral nutrition for 4–6 weeks.

Hepatic venous obstruction (Budd–Chiari syndrome). This must be considered, especially if the protein content of the ascitic fluid is high and the SAAG is high.

Pancreatic ascites. Ascites is rarely gross. It develops as a complication of acute pancreatitis with pseudocyst rupture, or from pancreatic duct disruption. The amylase content of the ascitic fluid is very high.

Ovarian tumour. This is suggested by resonance in the flanks. The maximum bulge is anteroposterior and the maximum girth is below the umbilicus.

Spontaneous bacterial peritonitis (Table 10.4) [46]

The most common infection in cirrhosis is spontaneous bacterial peritonitis (SBP). It is called spontaneous because it occurs in the absence of a contiguous source of infection (e.g. intestinal perforation, intra-abdominal abscess) and in the absence of an intra-abdominal inflammatory focus (e.g. abscess, acute pancreatitis, cholecystitis). SBP occurs in 9% of hospitalized patients with cirrhosis and accounts for 25% of all infections [53]. It is particularly frequent in severely decompensated cirrhosis. Spontaneous bacterial empyema is an entity akin to SBP in which hepatic hydrothorax becomes infected. Its diagnosis and management are the same as for SBP [54].

SBP is blood-borne and in 90% monomicrobial. Bacteria of gut origin are the most commonly isolated causative organisms. Therefore, migration of enteric bacteria across the intestinal mucosa to extraintestinal sites and the systemic circulation (bacterial translocation) has been implicated in its pathogenesis [55]. In cirrhosis, an overactive sympathetic nervous system slows gut motility and facilitates bacterial stasis and overgrowth, thereby facilitating bacterial translocation.

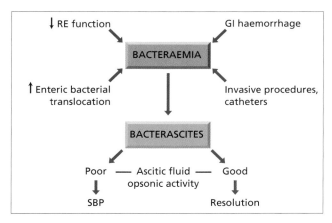

Fig. 10.9. The pathogenesis of spontaneous bacterial peritonitis (SBP) in patients with cirrhosis. GI, gastrointestinal; RE, reticuloendothelial.

Persistence of bacteria in extraintestinal sites is favoured by impaired host defences. In cirrhosis, host defences are abnormal because of portosystemic shunting and impaired reticuloendothelial function. Neutrophils are abnormal in the alcoholic. Decreased synthesis of proteins, such as complement and fibronectin, result in diminished adhesiveness and decreased bacterial phagocytosis [56]. Ascitic fluid favours bacterial growth and deficient ascitic opsonins lead to defective coating of bacteria which are indigestible by polymorphs. The opsonic activity of the ascitic fluid is proportional to protein concentration and SBP is more likely if ascitic fluid protein is less than 1 g/dL [57] (Fig. 10.9). Infection with more than one organism or with fungi is likely to be associated with colonic perforation or dilatation, or any intra-abdominal source of infection (i.e. secondary peritonitis).

SBP should be suspected when a patient with cirrhosis deteriorates, particularly with encephalopathy and/or jaundice. Patients with variceal bleeding or with previous SBP are at particular risk. Pyrexia, local abdominal pain and tenderness, and systemic leukocytosis may be noted. These features, however, may be absent and the diagnosis is made following a high index of suspicion with examination of the ascitic fluid.

The diagnosis of SBP is established with an ascites polymorophonuclear count more than 250/ mm³ [46]. The infecting organisms are commonly *Escherichia coli* or group D streptococci [58]. Anaerobic bacteria are rarely found. Blood cultures are positive in 50%.

Bacterascites (positive culture, polymorphonuclear cells <250/mm³) may resolve without treatment but can progress to SBP [59].

Patients with SBP are particularly at risk of renal complications, probably related to systemic vascular changes secondary to inflammatory response to infection generated by tumour necrosis factor and interleukin 6 [60].

Prognosis

With SBP, 10–20% of patients will die during that hospital admission. The 1-year probability of SBP recurrence is 69% and median survival of a patient who develops SBP is 9 months [61]. Mortality depends on the development of renal dysfunction [62] and the site of acquisition of the infection, with nosocomial infection being an important predictor of death [63–65].

SBP resolution and immediate survival are 100% in community-acquired SBP that is uncomplicated (i.e. no renal dysfunction, no encephalopathy) whether patients receive oral or intravenous antibiotics [66].

Treatment

Antibiotics should be started empirically in all patients with ascites showing more than 250 polymorphonuclear cells/mm³, except in those in whom a local inflammatory reaction is identified (e.g. diverticulitis, cholecystitis, etc.).

Five to seven days of a third-generation cephalosporin such as cefotaxime administered intravenously is usually effective [67,68]. For cefotaxime the optimal cost-effective dosage is 2 g every 12 h. Amoxycillin-clavulanic acid is as effective as cefotaxime [69].

The antibiotic choice should be reviewed once results of ascitic culture and sensitivity of the bacterial isolates are known. Because of renal toxicity, aminoglycosides should be avoided.

In a randomized study the administration of intravenous albumin to patients with SBP treated with cefotaxime significantly reduced the incidence of renal impairment (10 vs. 33%) and hospital mortality (10 vs. 29%) [62]. Patients that benefit most from the use of albumin are those with renal dysfunction at baseline (creatinine >1.0 mg/dL and/or blood urea nitrogen >30 mg/dL) and serum bilirubin more than 4 mg/dL [62,70,71].

Success rates for cefotaxime and amoxicillin-clavulanic may be as low as 44% in nosocomial SBP because of the presence of multidrug-resistant organisms [72,73]. Extended spectrum antibiotics (e.g. carbapenems, piperacillin/ tazobactam) should be used as initial empirical therapy in patients with hospital-acquired SBP, particularly in those who had been on beta-lactams during admission, had been recently hospitalized or on quinolone prophylaxis [72].

Secondary bacterial peritonitis should be suspected when a suspected SBP fails to respond to antibiotic therapy.

Because of reduced survival, SBP is an indication to consider hepatic transplantation, particularly if recurrent.

Prophylaxis

Long-term prophylaxis will lead to the emergence of resistant bacteria [53]. Therefore, only patients at the highest risk of developing SBP should receive antibiotic prophylaxis.

The risk of SBP is particularly high in patients with cirrhosis with upper gastrointestinal haemorrhage. Oral administration of norfloxacin (400 mg/12 h for a minimum of 7 days) is currently recommended for this group [46]. However, intravenous ceftriaxone should be considered in high quinolone resistance settings or in patients with two or more of the following: malnutrition, ascites, encephalopathy or serum bilirubin more than 3 mg/dL [74]. SBP and other infections should be ruled out by bacterial cultures before starting prophylaxis.

In patients with a previous episode of SBP, the risk of recurrence during the subsequent year is 40–70%. Oral administration of norfloxacin (400 mg/day) is recommended in such patients, who should then be evaluated for liver transplantation [46,75].

There is currently insufficient evidence to recommend prophylaxis for patients with a low ascitic fluid protein (<1 g/dL). However, norfloxacin prophylaxis appears justified in patients with advanced liver failure (Child–Pugh score >9 points with serum bilirubin level >3 mg/dL) or impaired renal function (serum creatinine level >1.2 mg/dL, blood urea nitrogen level >25 mg/dL, or serum sodium level <130 mEq/L). In these patients, the 1-year probability of first SBP is 60% and is significantly reduced with norfloxacin [76] .

In patients with a high ascitic fluid protein (>1 g/dL) without a past history of SBP, prophylaxis is not necessary as the 1-year probability of SBP is nil [77].

Treatment of cirrhotic ascites [78,79]

Therapy of ascites, whether by diuretics or paracentesis, reduces clinical symptoms and improves quality of life. However, although the initial clinical response may be excellent, if fluid loss is excessive it may lead to hyponatraemia, hyperkalaemia, renal failure or encephalopathy. Treatment must therefore be appropriate to the clinical state and the response properly monitored. The approach must be tailored to the patient. The spectrum of therapeutic intervention ranges from sodium restriction alone (rarely used), to diuretic use, therapeutic paracentesis (Table 10.5), and, for the most severe groups, TIPS and eventually liver transplantation.

Indications for treatment include the following:
• *Symptomatic ascites* with abdominal distension sufficient to be obvious and produce physical or emotional distress requires treatment with sodium restriction and diuretics. The presence of subclinical ascites (that seen only on ultrasound without clinical symptoms) may not require active treatment, although to prevent deterioration advice on a reduction in sodium intake is wise. Inappropriate introduction of excessive treatment for ascites may lead to symptomatic hypotension, muscle cramps, dehydration, and renal dysfunction.
• *Large ascites*, causing abdominal discomfort or pain and/or dyspnoea most often demands paracentesis.
• *Tense ascites* with pain may lead to eversion and ulceration of an umbilical hernia, which is near to rupture. This complication has a very high mortality, due to shock, renal failure and sepsis, and urgent paracentesis is indicated.

Monitoring during treatment is mandatory. The patient should be weighed daily as it provides a satisfactory guide to progress. Urinary electrolyte (sodium, potassium) determinations are helpful in determining dosage, monitoring the response and assessing compliance. Serum electrolytes and creatinine should be measured two to three times per week while the patient is in hospital. Where liver disease is due to alcohol, the patient should be encouraged to abstain. The mild case is managed as an out-patient by diet and diuretics, but if admitted to hospital, paracentesis is usually a first procedure. In a survey of European hepatologists, 50% used paracentesis initially, followed by diuretics [80]. Fifty per cent regarded complete control of ascites as

Table 10.5. General management of ascites

Diagnostic paracentesis with first presentation or with any symptom/ sign suggestive of SBP
70–90 mmol sodium diet; weigh daily; check serum creatinine and electrolytes
Spironolactone 100 mg daily
If tense ascites consider paracentesis (see Table 10.7)
After 4 days consider adding frusemide (furosemide) 40 mg daily; check serum creatinine and electrolytes
Maximum daily weight loss 0.5 kg/day (1.0 kg/day in those with peripheral oedema)
Stop diuretics if precoma ('flap'), hypokalaemia, azotaemia or alkalosis
Continue to monitor weight; increase diuretics as necessary
Avoid non-steroidal anti-inflammatory drugs

SBP, spontaneous bacterial peritonitis.

desirable, whereas the other half was satisfied with symptomatic relief without removing all the ascites. Thus consensus on standardized treatment regimes is difficult to reach because of the clinical spectrum of ascites, the clinical success of the different regimens and the lack of evidence-based studies comparing individual approaches.

Bed rest used to be a feature of initial therapy. Evidence for benefit is sparse but as part of an overall strategy in combination with diuretics it has been found to be beneficial [81]. This may be related to increased renal perfusion and portal venous blood flow during recumbency.

Sodium restriction/ diet

The patient with cirrhosis who is accumulating ascites on an unrestricted sodium intake excretes less than 10 mmol (approximately 0.2 g) sodium daily in the urine. Extrarenal loss is about 0.5 g. Sodium taken in excess of 0.75 g will result in ascites, with every gram retaining 200 mL of fluid. Historically, such patients were recommended a diet containing 22–40 mmol/day of sodium (approximately 0.5–1.0 g/day). However, such diet is unpalatable and also compromises protein and calorie intake, which in patients with cirrhosis is critical for proper nutrition. Current recommendations are to use a 'no added salt' diet (approximately 70–90 mmol or approximately 1.5–2.0 g/day) combined with diuretics to increase urinary sodium excretion (Table 10.6). In this diet, salt should not be used at the table or when cooking. Also, various foods containing sodium should be restricted or avoided (Table 10.6). Many low-sodium foods are now available.

A few patients with ascites may respond to this regimen alone, but usually the first line of treatment for ascites includes diuretics. Patients prefer the combination of diuretics and a modest restriction of sodium to severe sodium restriction alone. Very occasionally if there is a good response, diuretics may be withdrawn and the patient maintained on dietary sodium restriction alone.

Good responders are liable to be those:
• with ascites and oedema presenting for the first time in an otherwise stable patient;
• with a normal creatinine clearance (glomerular filtration rate);
• with an underlying reversible component of liver disease such as alcoholic hepatitis;
• in whom the ascites has developed acutely in response to a treatable complication such as infection or bleeding, or after a non-hepatic operation;
• with ascites following excessive sodium intake, such as in sodium-containing antacids or purgatives, or mineral waters with a high sodium content.

Diuretics

The major reason for sodium retention in cirrhosis is hyperaldosteronism due to increased activity of the renin–angiotensin system. There is avid reabsorption of sodium from the distal tubule and collecting duct (Fig. 10.4).

Diuretics can be divided into two main groups (Fig. 10.10) according to their site of action. The first group inhibits Na^+–K^+–Cl^- (NKCC2) cotransporter in the ascending limb of the loop of Henle and includes frusemide (furosemide) and bumetamide. It is not appropriate to use these alone since the sodium remaining in the tubule as a result of diuretic action is reabsorbed in the distal tubule and collecting duct because of hyperaldosteronism. A randomized controlled trial has shown frusemide alone to be less effective than spironolactone [16]. Thiazides inhibit sodium in the distal convoluted tubule, have a longer half-life, may cause hypotension, and should not be used in the treatment of ascites.

The second group, spironolactone (an aldosterone antagonist), amiloride and triamterene, (inhibitors of the sodium channel) block sodium reabsorption in the distal tubule and collecting duct. They are the drugs of first choice in the treatment of ascites due to cirrhosis. They are weakly natriuretic but conserve potassium. Potassium supplements are not usually necessary— indeed this type of diuretic sometimes needs to be temporarily stopped because of hyperkalaemia [82].

There are two therapeutic approaches that can be used initially: spironolactone alone, or a combination of spironolactone with frusemide. Both have their advocates and may be chosen depending on the degree of ascites [82,83].

Spironolactone alone. The starting dose is 50–100 mg/day according to the degree of ascites. If there has been insufficient clinical response after 3–4 days (weight loss less than 300 g/day), then the dose is increased by 100 mg/day every 4 days to a maximum of 400 mg/day, unless hyperkalaemia develops. Lack of clinical response indicates the need to check the urinary sodium, because a high value will identify the occasional patient who is exceeding the prescribed low sodium diet.

The disadvantage of starting with spironolactone alone is the delay before its clinical effect and associated hyperkalaemia [82].

If there is insufficient clinical response or no response on spironolactone alone (when taking 200 mg/day) or associated hyperkalaemia, a loop diuretic such as frusemide is added at a dose of 20–40 mg/day.

Combination therapy. Treatment is started with the combination of spironolactone (100 mg) and frusemide (40 mg) daily. The disadvantage of starting with

Table 10.6. Advice for 'no added salt diet' (70–90 mmol/day or 1.5–2.0 g/day)

Omit

Anything containing baking powder or baking soda (contains sodium bicarbonate): pastry, biscuits, crackers, cakes, self-raising flour and ordinary bread (see restriction below)

All commercially prepared foods (unless designated low salt—check packet)

Dry breakfast cereals except Shredded Wheat, Puffed Wheat or Sugar Puffs

Tinned/ bottled savouries: pickles, olives, chutney, salad cream, bottled sauces

Tinned meats/ fish: ham, bacon, corned beef, tongue, oyster, shellfish

Meat and fish pastes; meat and yeast extracts

Tinned/ bottled vegetables, soups, tomato juice

Sausages, kippers

Cheese, ice-cream

Candy, pastilles, milk chocolate

Salted nuts, potato crisps, savoury snacks

Drinks: especially Lucozade, soda water, mineral waters according to sodium content (essential to check sodium content of mineral waters, varies from 5 to 1000 mg/L)

Restrict

Milk (300 mL = half pint/day)

Bread (two slices/day)

Free use

Fresh and home-cooked fruit and vegetables of all kinds

Meat/poultry/fish (100 g/day) and one egg; egg may be used to substitute 50 g meat (2 oz)

Unsalted butter or margarine, cooking oils, double cream

Boiled rice, pasta (without salt), semolina

Seasonings help make restricted salt meal more palatable: include lemon juice, onion, garlic, pepper, sage, parsley, thyme, marjoram, bay leaves

Fresh fruit juice, coffee, tea

Mineral water (check sodium content)

Marmalade, jam

Dark chocolate, boiled sweets, peppermints, chewing gum

Salt substitutes (not potassium chloride)

Salt-free bread, crispbread, crackers or matzos

combination therapy may be the need for closer laboratory monitoring [83].

Monitoring of daily weight is necessary. The rate of ascitic fluid reabsorption is limited to 700–900 mL/day. If a diuresis of 2–3 litres is induced, much of the fluid must come from non-ascitic, extracellular fluids including oedema fluid and the intravascular compartment. This is safe so long as oedema persists. Indeed diuresis may be rapid (greater than 2 kg daily) until oedema disappears [84]. To avoid the risk of renal dysfunction there should be a maximum daily weight loss of 0.5 kg/day, with a maximum of 1.0 kg/day in those with oedema.

Intravascular volume expansion with intravenous albumin increases natriuresis in response to diuretics, but is expensive and not cost-effective [85].

Long-term spironolactone causes painful gynaecomastia in males and should then be replaced by 10–15 mg/day of amiloride. However, this is less effective than spironolactone.

Before diuretic therapy is deemed to have failed (diuretic-refractory ascites) non-compliance with sodium

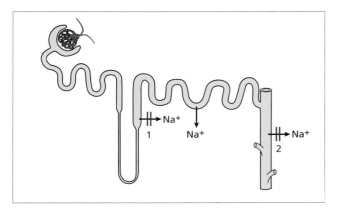

Fig. 10.10. Site of action of diuretics. 1 = loop diuretics: frusemide (furosemide), bumetamide. 2 = distal tubule/collecting duct: spironolactone, amiloride, triamterene.

restriction should be ruled out by measuring 24-h urinary sodium excretion. If this is greater than the 'prescribed dietary' sodium intake the patient is not complying with the restriction. Another cause of a lack of response to diuretics are concomitant use of non-steroidal anti-inflammatory agents, and angiotensin converting enzyme blockers or angiotensin receptor blockers [86].

Failure to respond to diuretics often occurs in those with very poor hepatocellular function who have a poor prognosis without liver transplantation. In such refractory patients, diuretics have eventually to be withdrawn because of intractable uraemia, hypotension or encephalopathy.

Complications

Rising urea and creatinine reflect contraction of the extracellular fluid volume and reduced renal circulation (prerenal azotaemia). Hepatorenal syndrome may be precipitated. It is necessary to interrupt or reduce diuretic therapy and use plasma expansion with albumin in more severe cases.

Encephalopathy may follow any profound diuresis and is usually associated with prerenal azotaemia, hypokalaemia and hypochloraemic acidosis.

Hyperkalaemia reflects the effect of spironolactone, which should be reduced or interrupted according to the level of serum potassium. If the level of potassium is not dangerous, frusemide can be added to therapy at this point.

Painful gynaecomastia may be caused by spironolactone, which should be reduced or discontinued and substituted by amiloride.

Muscle cramps may be a problem. They indicate the need to review the dose of diuretic, but can occur without their use. Quinine sulphate 300 mg given at night is often helpful to prevent cramps [87], otherwise quinine water can be recommended; weekly intravenous albumin is also effective [87].

Follow-up advice

The out-patient should adhere to the low-sodium diet, and abstain from alcohol where this is the cause of liver disease. Bathroom scales should be used to allow a record of daily weight at the same time of day, nude or with similar clothing. This daily record should be kept and brought to the physician at each visit.

The dose of diuretics depends upon the degree of ascites and the severity of the liver disease. A usual regime is 100–200 mg spironolactone (or 10–20 mg amiloride) daily with frusemide 40–80 mg daily for the patient with more marked ascites initially, or with a poor response to spironolactone alone. Serum electrolytes, creatinine, urea and liver function tests are monitored every 4 weeks for the stable out-patient. In the patient who has been treated initially as an in-patient, an earlier check at 1 week after discharge allows an adjustment to the management plan before electrolyte or clinical imbalance has occurred. As liver function improves and the oedema and ascites resolve, it may be possible to stop the frusemide first and then the spironolactone. Symptoms such as postural dizziness and thirst indicate over-enthusiastic treatment. The 'no added salt' (70–90 mmol/day or 1.5–2.0 g/day) is maintained in the majority of patients.

Therapeutic abdominal paracentesis (Table 10.7)

This procedure was abandoned in the 1960s because of the fear of causing acute renal failure. Moreover, the loss of approximately 50 g of protein in a 5-litre paracentesis led to patients becoming severely malnourished. New interest came with the observation that a 5-litre paracentesis was safe in fluid- and salt-restricted patients with ascites and peripheral oedema [88]. This work was extended to daily 4–5-litre paracenteses with 40 g salt-poor albumin infused intravenously over the same period [81]. Finally, a single total paracentesis, about 10 litres in 1 h combined with intravenous albumin (6–8 g/L ascites removed) was shown to be equally effective and safe (Table 10.7) [89,90].

In a controlled trial, serial large-volume paracenteses (LVP) reduced hospital stay compared with standard diuretic treatment [81]. However, readmissions to hospital, survival and causes of death did not differ significantly between the LVP and diuretic groups. Total paracentesis results in hypovolaemia as reflected by a rise in plasma renin levels [88], and can lead to hypotension and renal failure (postparacentesis circulatory syndrome) [88].

Table 10.7. Therapeutic paracentesis

Selection
Large or tense ascites
Routine
No volume limit
i.v. salt-poor albumin: 6–8 g/L removed
No need to perform cell count unless symptoms/ signs suggestive of SBP
Advantages
Comfort
Shortens hospital stay
SBP, spontaneous bacterial peritonitis.

Table 10.8. Hyponatraemia

Serum sodium <130 mEq/L
Present in 22% of patients with ascites
May contribute to encephalopathy and poor quality of life
Water restriction (1–1.5 L/day)
'Vaptans' correct sodium but are still under investigation
Poor prognostic marker

Albumin replacement is more effective in preventing postparacentesis hypovolaemia and hyponatraemia than less costly plasma expanders such as dextran 70, dextran 40 and polygeline [91].

Major complications, mostly bleeding, have been associated with therapeutic but not diagnostic procedures and tend to be more prevalent in patients with low platelet count (<50 000) and Child–Pugh class C [92]. Major bleeding occurs rarely but may be lethal [93] and is mostly related to puncture of collaterals rather than as a result of coagulopathy. In a series of over 1000 LVPs there was no significant bleeding, even in patients with marked thrombocytopenia or prothrombin time prolongation [94]. Therefore clotting abnormalities should not be considered a contraindication to LVP. Leakage of ascitic fluid is rare and occurs when extraction of ascites is incomplete. Therefore, this complication can be solved by completing the LVP, preferably in a site remote from the leaking puncture site. Similarly, another rare complication of paracentesis is the development of sudden scrotal oedema that results from subcutaneous tracking of peritoneal fluid into the scrotum and which should be treated by elevation of the scrotum [95].

Summary

Paracentesis is a safe, cost-effective treatment for cirrhotic ascites. However, approximately 90% of patients with ascites respond to sodium restriction and diuretics, and paracentesis is generally a second-line treatment except for patients with tense and refractory ascites (see below). Despite this, many clinicians opt for early paracentesis rather than waiting for diuretics to be effective [81]. Intravenous salt-poor albumin should be used concomitant to LVP, particularly when more than 5 litres are

removed. The paracentesis must be followed by an optimal salt-restricted diet and diuretic regimen.

Hyponatraemia [96] (Table 10.8)

Hyponatraemia develops in approximately 20–30% of cirrhotic patients with ascites and is defined as a serum sodium concentration less than 130 mEq/L [97,98]. Hyponatraemia in cirrhosis is dilutional. Although hyponatraemia is usually asymptomatic, some patients may complain of anorexia, nausea and vomiting, lethargy and occasionally seizures. Hyponatraemia has been associated with a further reduction in brain organic osmolytes, particularly myoinositol, suggesting that it may play a role in the pathogenesis of hepatic encephalopathy [99].

Serum sodium concentrations of less than 130 mmol/L are treated by fluid restriction, to avoid further reduction in concentrations. Advances in the understanding of the pathogenesis are leading to pharmacological approaches to treatment.

Mechanism

Eighty per cent of the water in the glomerular filtrate is reabsorbed in the proximal tubule and descending limb of Henle. The ascending limb of Henle and distal tubule are impermeable to water. Control of the volume of water passed in urine is dependent on the amount of water reabsorbed in the collecting tubule and collecting duct. This is under the control of vasopressin, which interacts with V2 receptors on the cells of the renal collecting ducts (Fig. 10.4). Vasopressin receptor activation stimulates the translocation of the water channel aquaporin 2 from a cytoplasmic vesicular compartment to the apical membrane. This mechanism may be affected by prostaglandins which inhibit vasopressin-stimulated water reabsorption.

Vasopressin is produced in the hypothalamus. Production is controlled in two ways: by osmoreceptors in the anterior hypothalamus under the influence of plasma osmolarity, and by parasympathetic stimulation as a result of activation of baroreceptors in the atria, ventricles, aortic arch and carotid sinus. Water retention in patients with cirrhosis and ascites is due to excess vasopressin as a result of baroreceptor stimulation. This is thought to be related to the reduced effective circulating volume as a result of splanchnic and systemic vasodilatation—the same circulatory abnormality which leads to activation of the renin–angiotensin–aldosterone axis and the sympathetic nervous system and sodium retention. However, alterations in sodium and water handling are not synchronous, sodium abnormalities occurring first (Fig. 10.5).

Vasopressin concentrations are not grossly elevated in cirrhosis. However, the normal inhibition of vasopressin by a water load is blunted or absent. Although there is reduced hepatic metabolism of vasopressin in patients with cirrhosis, related to the severity of disease, this is not thought to be the primary reason for water retention.

Treatment

Hyponatraemia reflects reduced free water clearance. In the patient with severe hepatocellular dysfunction it may also indicate the passage of sodium into the cells. If the serum sodium falls below 130 mmol/L, fluid intake should be restricted to 1–1.5 litres per day [19]. Intravenous albumin is beneficial but its effect is transient [100].

Several approaches are being studied to increase free water clearance. Drugs such as *kappa-opioid receptor agonists*, which inhibit vasopressin release, and *demeclocycline*, which interferes with generation and action of cAMP in collecting ducts, have been reported to be effective but their use has been abandoned due to important side effects [101,102].

V2 receptor antagonists ('vaptans') have been the most investigated aquaretic agents. The short-term (7–14 days) use of lixivaptan [103,104] or satavaptan [105] was effective in increasing serum sodium. However, their use was associated with severe side-effects, dehydration and Q–T prolongation, respectively, and has led to their withdrawal. In a large multicenter randomized trial, tolvaptan used for 30 days in patients with euvolaemic or hypervolaemic hyponatraemia (of whom 63 had cirrhosis), was associated with a rapid improvement in serum sodium and significant weight loss compared to placebo, without significant side effects [106]. Longer-term trials targeting patients with cirrhosis are awaited.

Summary

Although advances are being made in pharmacological approaches to correct water retention and the associated hyponatraemia, these are not yet clinically applicable. The mainstay of treatment is fluid restriction. Intravenous albumin infusion may be effective in the short term [100]. Whichever approach is used, it should be recog-

nized that hyponatraemia is a predictor of reduced survival in cirrhotic patients with ascites [107,108] and is a risk factor for encephalopathy and the HRS syndrome [96,98]. Liver transplantation should be considered providing serum sodium can be increased to 125 mmol/L or more.

Refractory ascites [109,110] (Table 10.9)

This is defined as ascites that cannot be mobilized or prevented from recurring by medical therapy. It is divided into *diuretic-resistant* (ascites is not mobilized despite maximal diuretic dosage) and *diuretic-intractable* ascites (development of diuretic-induced complications that preclude the use of an effective diuretic dosage) [109]. Dietary history, use of NSAID or angiotension converting enzyme or angiotensin II receptor blockers [86], and patient compliance with the treatment regimen must be reviewed before confirming the diagnosis.

Treatment

The therapeutic options for patients with refractory ascites include repeated LVPs, TIPS, peritoneovenous (Le Veen) shunting and liver transplantation.

Therapeutic paracentesis

This has been discussed above as initial treatment for the patient with tense severe ascites. For refractory ascites repeated LVP plus albumin is the most accepted initial therapy. It is easy to perform and relatively inexpensive compared to other therapies such as the peritoneovenous shunt. In this group of patients recurrence of ascites is the rule because paracentesis is symptomatic therapy that does not act on the mechanisms responsible for ascites formation. Patients generally require paracentesis every 2 to 4 weeks. Reintroduction of diuretic treatment after paracentesis lengthens time to recurrence [111] in patients with a urinary sodium greater

Table 10.9. Refractory ascites

First line:	Serial therapeutic paracenteses
	Relapse is the rule
Second line:	TIPS
	When paracenteses >1–2/month
	MELD <15
	?Survival benefit
Third line:	Peritoneovenous shunt
	Non-LVP, non-TIPS candidates

TIPS, transjugular intrahepatic portosystemic shunt; MELD, Model for End Stage Liver Disease; LVP, large-volume paracenteses.

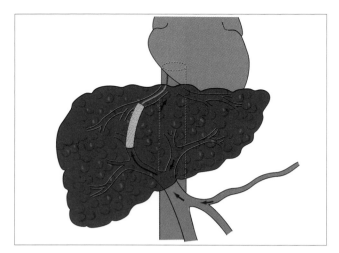

Fig. 10.11. The transjugular intrahepatic portosystemic shunt (TIPS) decompresses hepatic sinusoids.

than 30 mEq/L. In others, diuretics should be discontinued, particularly if associated with complications [110].

Transjugular intrahepatic portosystemic shunt (TIPS)

Side-to-side portacaval shunts, unlike end-to-side shunts, decompress the hepatic sinusoids (Fig. 10.11) and had been shown to be effective in the treatment of ascites. However, they have been abandoned because of the associated morbidity and mortality of major surgery and the advent of TIPS, which is a less invasive procedure that achieves the same decompression of the sinusoid [112].

Early experience with TIPS showed a reduction in diuretic requirements, and a fall in plasma renin and aldosterone activities. However, TIPS may precipitate hepatic encephalopathy and/or liver failure.

Not surprisingly, since TIPS acts on the pathophysiological mechanisms responsible for ascites TIPS is more effective than LVP in preventing recurrence of ascites in randomized comparative trials [113,114], but had a higher risk for severe encephalopathy, without differences in mortality. A meta-analysis of individual patient data in randomized studies showed that mortality was significantly lower in patients treated with TIPS and identified a Model for End Stage Liver Disease (MELD) score above 15 as having a high risk of death [115]. In trials performed to date, uncovered TIPS stents were used. Uncovered stents frequently obstruct (18 to 78%) [116] and have been largely substituted by polytetrafluoroethylene-covered stents which are associated with a significantly lower obstruction rate. [117]. Until results of ongoing trials using covered stents are available, TIPS should be considered second-line treatment for refractory ascites, and reserved for patients who require frequent paracentesis

and have reasonable hepatic reserve with normal or minimal renal dysfunction.

Peritoneovenous (Le Veen) shunt

This consists of a plastic tube with multiple holes that is placed in the peritoneal cavity and is connected to a unidirectional pressure-sensitive valve lying extraperitoneally, from which a silicone rubber tube passes subcutaneously to the neck and thence to the internal jugular vein and superior vena cava (SVC). When the diaphragm descends during inspiration, the intraperitoneal fluid pressure rises while that in the intrathoracic SVC falls. This allows ascitic fluid to pass from the peritoneal cavity into the general circulation. It is generally inserted under general anaesthesia. Flow of ascites along the shunt depends upon this pressure gradient between peritoneal cavity and SVC.

The peritoneovenous shunt may control ascites over many months. It produces sustained expansion of the circulating blood volume and a fall in plasma levels of renin–angiotensin, noradrenaline and antidiuretic hormone. Renal function and nutrition improve.

In uncontrolled studies, peritoneovenous shunts resulted in frequent blockage, severe complications (disseminated intravascular coagulation, pulmonary oedema, variceal haemorrhage) and high perioperative mortality. However, randomized trials comparing peritoneovenous shunt with LVP and albumin replacement resulted in similar efficacy, with similar complication rates and survival [89,118]. Since paracentesis with albumin replacement is simpler and can be done on an out-patient basis, it is the preferred procedure. Additionally, peritoneovenous shunt may hinder future placement of TIPS and may complicate liver transplant surgery due to peritoneal adhesions. Therefore, it is mostly indicated in patients who require LVP frequently and who are not candidates for TIPS [119].

Hepatorenal syndrome [120]

Hepatorenal syndrome (HRS) is the development of renal failure in patients with severe liver disease in the absence of any identifiable renal pathology. It is a functional rather than structural disturbance in renal function. The histology of the kidney is virtually normal. Such kidneys have been successfully transplanted, following which they functioned normally. After liver transplantation, kidney function also usually returns to normal.

The mechanism is not fully understood, but the renal disturbance is thought to represent the severest form of vascular and neurohumoral changes associated with severe liver disease, which in a less severe form results in ascites (Figs 10.5, 10.12) [7].

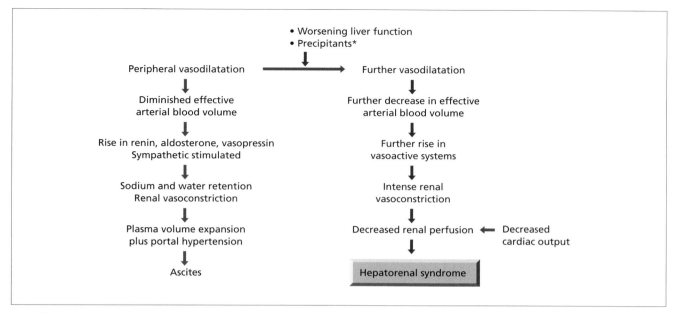

Fig. 10.12. Mechanism for hepatorenal syndrome. *Precipitants include bacterial infections (particularly spontaneous bacterial peritonitis), hypovolaemia (gastrointestinal haemorrhage, over-diuresis, diarrhoea), vasodilators.

Table 10.10. Criteria for diagnosis of hepatorenal syndrome [122]

1   Cirrhosis with ascites
2   Serum creatinine >1.5 mg/dL (>133 µmol/L)
3   No improvement in serum creatinine (decrease to 1.5 mg/dL or less) after at least 2 days of diuretic withdrawal and expansion of plasma volume with albumin (1 g/kg of body weight/day up to a maximum of 100 g/day)
4   Absence of shock
5   No current or recent treatment with nephrotoxic drugs or vasodilators
6   Absence of parenchymal kidney disease as indicated by proteinuria >500 mg/day, microhaematuria (>50 red blood cells per high power field), and/or abnormal renal ultrasonography

HRS is a rare but severe complication in patients with cirrhosis and ascites. From first presentation with ascites, the 5-year probability of developing HRS is 11% [97], with increasing probability in patients who develop hyponatraemia or refractory ascites. Without liver transplantation and prior to the recent studies of treatment using vasocontrictors, recovery of renal function was unusual (<5% of patients) and prognosis was poor with a median survival of 2 weeks [121].

Diagnostic criteria (Table 10.10)

These are based largely on abnormal creatinine, the absence of other causes of renal failure and the absence of sustained improvement in renal function after diuretic withdrawal and plasma volume expansion [122]. The occurrence of shock before deterioration of renal function precludes a diagnosis of HRS and is more indicative of acute tubular necrosis (ATN) [120].

Additional criteria describe the characteristics of urine volume and content, but since these may be present with other types of renal failure, for example ATN, they are not considered essential for the diagnosis of HRS [120].

Classification

HRS syndrome may be classified into two types:
Type 1. Patients have a rapidly progressive (less than 2 weeks) reduction of renal function with doubling of the initial serum creatinine to greater than 2.5 mg/dL (220 µmol/L) [122]. However, as recently proposed [120], a diagnosis of HRS (type 1) should be considered whenever there are criteria for acute kidney injury, namely an abrupt increase in serum creatinine ≥0.3 mg/dL (≥26.4 µmol/L) or an increase ≥150% (1.5-fold) from baseline [123]. This ensures that treatment is not unnecessarily delayed as baseline creatinine is a predictor of HRS reversal with vasoconstrictors [124].
Type 2. Patients satisfy the criteria for the diagnosis of HRS but the renal failure does not progress rapidly [122]. These patients usually have relatively preserved

hepatic function with refractory ascites. Survival is reduced compared with patients with cirrhosis and ascites and normal renal function.

Mechanism

The peripheral arterial vasodilatation theory for the formation of ascites proposes initial splanchnic and systemic arterial dilatation with consequent stimulation of the sympathetic nervous system (raised noradrenaline) and the renin–angiotensin system. This is the result of activation of volume receptors responding to vascular under-filling. Initially, despite changes in vasoconstrictors and vasodilators, renal function is preserved. HRS occurs with extreme vasodilatation, decrease in cardiac output [125] and an imbalance between systemic and intrarenal vasodilator and vasoconstrictor mechanisms, with increases in vasoconstrictors such as thromboxane A2 and endothelin [126] and decreases in vasodilators such as prostaglandin E2 and nitric oxide [127].

Clinical features

Many features are associated with an increased risk for HRS including marked sodium (<5 mmol/L) and water retention (hyponatraemia), low mean arterial blood pressure (<80 mmHg) and marked elevation of the RAAS [121], all indicative of a worsening haemodynamic status. A lower cardiac output (<6 L/min) (in the setting of severe arterial vasodilatation) has also been identified as an independent predictor of HRS [125].

Patients with HRS characteristically have advanced liver disease (median Child–Pugh score 11.2), difficult to control ascites, a low mean arterial pressure and hyponatraemia [120]. Hyperkalaemia is unusual. Death is due to liver failure; survival depends on the reversibility of the liver disease.

Differential diagnosis

Prerenal azotaemia (or volume-responsive acute kidney injury). In a patient with cirrhosis this must be differentiated from HRS as the management and prognosis are different (Table 10.11). Causes include over-diuresis and severe diarrhoea, for example due to lactulose. Bacterial infection, particularly SBP, may present with reversible impairment of renal function. Non-steroidal anti-inflammatory drugs reduce renal prostaglandin production, thereby reducing the glomerular filtration rate and free water clearance.

Intrinsic renal failure. Nephrotoxic drugs should be identified, including aminoglycosides and X-ray contrast media. Glomerular mesangial IgA deposits, accompanied by complement deposition, complicate cirrhosis,

Table 10.11. Iatrogenic causes of acute kidney injury in cirrhosis

Drugs	Treatment
Diuretics	Volume expansion
Lactulose	Volume expansion
NSAID (prostaglandin inhibition)	Stop drug
Aminoglycosides	Diagnose urine β2-microglobulins
Ciclosporin	Haemofiltration

NSAID, non-steroidal anti-inflammatory drug.

usually in the alcoholic. Hepatitis B and C are associated with immune-related glomerulonephritis. These lesions are diagnosed by finding proteinuria with microscopic haematuria and casts. The main differential diagnosis and the most difficult to make is ATN. A history of shock, increased urine sodium and granular casts indicate ATN, however all these findings can also be present in HRS.

Prevention

The risk of HRS syndrome is reduced by careful use and monitoring of diuretic therapy, and the early recognition of any complication such as electrolyte imbalance, haemorrhage or infection. Nephrotoxic drugs should be avoided. The risk of renal deterioration after large volume paracentesis is reduced by the administration of salt-poor albumin. The risk of further worsening renal failure in patients with SBP is prevented by intravenous albumin and concomitant antibiotics [62]. The risk of SBP and HRS in high-risk patients without a prior episode of SBP is reduced by prophylactic antibiotics [76].

Treatment

General measures

Since renal dysfunction may be related to hypovolaemia and since assessment of volume status may be uncertain, diuretics are stopped and intravascular volume is assessed by measuring central venous pressure (CVP). A normal or increased CVP indicates that the cause of renal failure is not volume-related, but this must be interpreted in relation to diaphragmatic pressure secondary to ascites. Intravascular volume should be expanded with intravenous albumin at a dose of 1 g/kg body weight up to a maximum of 100 g [122]. This dose can be repeated in 12 hours if the serum creatinine has not normalized, provided that the CVP is less than 10 mmHg. A reduction in serum creatinine indicates that acute kidney injury is due to prerenal azotaemia.

Intravenous albumin is preferred over saline solution as a volume expander.

Potentially nephrotoxic drugs, diuretics and vasodilators are stopped. A search for sepsis is made. Ascites is tapped for white cell count, Gram stain and culture. Blood, urine and cannula tips are cultured. A broadspectrum antibiotic is started if infection is suspected.

Renal replacement therapy (mainly continuous arteriovenous and venovenous haemofiltration) should be started if there is severe volume overload, acidosis or hyperkalaemia. However, it does not lead to renal recovery, unless liver transplantation occurs. Complications occur, including arterial hypotension, coagulopathy, sepsis and gastrointestinal haemorrhage, and many patients die during this treatment.

Suitability for liver transplantation needs to be rapidly evaluated as this is the only curative therapy for HRS. New therapeutic pharmacological approaches may act as a bridge to liver transplantation by lengthening survival time.

Liver transplantation

Liver transplantation is the only definitive therapy for HRS, and the only therapy that results in improved survival. However, it is important to try to reverse HRS prior to transplantation because lower pretransplantation serum creatinine is associated with improved posttransplantation outcomes [128,129]. Patients with HRS have longer stays in intensive care units (21 vs. 4.5 days) and haemodialysis is required more often post-transplant (35 vs. 5%). Since calcineurin inhibitors may con-

tribute to renal deterioration, it has been suggested that azathioprine and steroids or interleukin 2 receptor blockers, be given until a diuresis has started—usually by 48–72 hours [130]. In patients with type 2 HRS, liver transplantation results in return of acceptable renal function in 90%, and the overall survival rates are similar to those without HRS [130].

Pharmacological treatment [120]

Vasodilators. These have been used in an attempt to reverse renal vasoconstriction. Dopamine at renal support doses has a renal vasodilatory effect, however it has no effect in HRS [131]. Prostaglandin administration is not associated with significant improvement in renal function.

Vasoconstrictors (Table 10.12). The rationale for use of these agents is to reverse the intense splanchnic and systemic vasodilatation. Administration of vasoconstrictors (ornipressin, terlipressin, octreotide with midodrine, noradrenaline) for periods greater than 3 days is associated with significant increases in mean arterial pressure, decreased serum creatinine and plasma renin activity as well as an increase in serum sodium [131–134].

The best evidence supports the use of terlipressin, a synthetic analogue of vasopressin. It has intrinsic vasoconstrictor effects and *in vivo* slow conversion to vasopressin, with a longer biological half-life. It has fewer side effects than ornipressin. Terlipressin is more effective than control therapy in randomized controlled trials

Table 10.12. Vasoconstrictors in HRS: doses used and adverse events

Drug	Dose range	Observed adverse events
Terlipressin	0.5–2.0 mg i.v. every 4–6 h	Cardiac: arrhythmia, angina, myocardial infarction GI: abdominal cramps, diarrhoea, nausea, vomiting, intestinal ischaemia Peripheral: livedo reticularis, finger ischaemia, cutaneous necrosis at the infusion site, scrotal necrosis Others: arterial hypertension, dyspnoea, bronchospasm, respiratory acidosis
Vasopressin	0.01–0.8 U/min (continuous intravenous infusion)	None reported although expectedly same as for terlipressin
Noradrenaline	0.5–3.0 mg/h (continuous i.v. infusion)	Chest pain with or without ventricular hypokinesia
Octreotide + midodrine	100–200 μg subcutaneously three times a day 7.5–12.5 mg orally three times a day 25 μg → 25 μg/h (continuous intravenous infusion) 2.5 mg/day orally	Diarrhoea Tingling Goosebumps

i.v., intravenous; GI, gastrointestinal.

[135–138], the largest being a double-blind, placebo-controlled trial [138]. Meta-analysis of these studies shows that vasoconstrictors are associated with significantly higher HRS-1 reversal rates compared to controls (46% vs. 11%) and a decreased risk of death, although mortality is still very high in patients treated with vasoconstrictors (58 vs. 74% in controls)[139]. Survival is significantly better in terlipressin 'responders'. Terlipressin should be started at a dose 0.5–1 mg i.v. every 4–6 hours. If there is no early response (>25% decrease in creatinine levels) after 2 days of therapy, the dose can be doubled every 2 days up to a maximum of 12 mg/day (i.e. 2 mg i.v. every 4 hours). Treatment can be stopped if serum creatinine does not decrease by at least 50% after 7 days at the highest dose, or if there is no reduction in creatinine after the first 3–4 days. In patients with early response, treatment should be extended until reversal of HRS (decrease in creatinine below 1.5 mg/dL or 130 μmol/L) or for a maximum of 14 days [122]. The dose of vasoconstrictors can be adjusted by monitoring mean arterial blood pressure (an indirect indicator of vasodilatation).

Alternative pharmacological approaches have used intravenous noradrenaline infusion [134] with one small randomized trial showing it to be equivalent to terlipressin [140], vasopressin infusion [141] or long-term midodrine (an α-adrenergic agonist) combined with octreotide (an inhibitor of the release of glucagon) and intravenous albumin [142]. Randomized trials for the latter are lacking.

Transjugular intrahepatic portosystemic shunt (TIPS)

Uncontrolled studies have shown that TIPS may improve renal perfusion and reduce the activity of the RAAS. In a prospective study of 31 non-transplantable patients, approximately 75% had improvement in renal function after TIPS [143]. The 1-year survival was significantly better in type 2 than type 1 patients (70 vs. 20%). This study excluded patients with a Child score above 12, serum bilirubin above 15 mg/dL (250 μmol/L) and severe spontaneous encephalopathy. Sequential treatment with vasoconstrictors and albumin followed by TIPS also resulted long-term success in some patients [144]. TIPS can be considered if HRS recurs after discontinuation of successful vasoconstrictor therapy, with creatinine returning to near normal values, particularly if transplantation is not likely in the near future and the patient has refractory ascites [120].

Extracorporeal albumin dialysis

A small randomized trial of the molecular absorbent recirculating system, has shown benefit for patients with type 1 HRS syndrome [145]. This modified dialysis method uses an albumin-containing dialysate. Studies are ongoing to establish whether it has a role in such patients as a bridge to transplantation.

Summary

New approaches offer hope that HRS syndrome, which previously had a dismal outlook, may be improved or reversed. Once the diagnosis of HRS is suspected, specific treatment with vasoconstrictors and intravenous albumin should be initiated. The best evidence supports the use of terlipressin, which should be started at a dose of 0.5 mg i.v. every 6 hours.

Prognosis

The prognosis is poor when ascites develops in a patient with cirrhosis. While median survival in patients with compensated cirrhosis is around 9 years [146], once decompensation occurs, median survival decreases to 1.6–1.8 years [146,147]; with ascites, mortality is about 20% per year [148,149]. An analysis of over 200 patients with cirrhosis admitted to hospital for the treatment of ascites showed four variables with independent prognostic value. These were renal water excretion (diuresis after water load), mean arterial pressure, Child–Pugh class and serum creatinine [150]. Except for the Child–Pugh score, which is indicative of a poor liver function, all other parameters indicate a worsened haemodynamic status (that is, a more vasodilated state) and are consistent with other studies that have shown that hyponatraemia and renal dysfunction are predictors of a poor survival in cirrhosis [97,151,152].

Because of the poor prognosis, liver transplantation should be considered in all patients with ascites. Early assessment is needed and a decision taken before the clinical decline associated with refractory ascites or hepatorenal syndrome.

References

1 Runyon BA. Ascites. In: Schiff L, Schiff ER, eds. *Diseases of the Liver*. Philadelphia: Lippincott Company, 1993; pp. 990–1015.
2 Gines P, Quintero E, Arroyo V *et al.* Compensated cirrhosis: natural history and prognostic factors. *Hepatology* 1987; **7**: 122–128.
3 D'Amico G, Garcia-Tsao G, Pagliaro L. Natural history and prognostic indicators of survival in cirrhosis. A systematic review of 118 studies. *J. Hepatol.* 2006; **44**: 217–231.
4 Planas R, Balleste B, Alvarez MA *et al.* Natural history of decompensated hepatitis C virus-related cirrhosis. A study of 200 patients. *J. Hepatol.* 2004; **40**: 823–830.
5 Morali GA, Sniderman KW, Deitel KM *et al.* Is sinusoidal portal hypertension a necessary factor for the development of hepatic ascites? *J. Hepatol.* 1992; **16**: 249–250.

6 Casado M, Bosch J, Garcia-Pagan JC *et al.* Clinical events after transjugular intrahepatic portosystemic shunt: correlation with hemodynamic findings. *Gastroenterology* 1998; **114**: 1296–1303.

7 Schrier RW, Arroyo V, Bernardi M *et al.* Peripheral arterial vasodilation hypothesis—A proposal for the initiation of renal sodium and water retention in cirrhosis. *Hepatology* 1988; **8**: 1151–1157.

8 Garcia-Tsao G, Groszmann RJ, Fisher RL *et al.* Portal pressure, presence of gastroesophageal varices and variceal bleeding. *Hepatology* 1985; **5**: 419–424.

9 D'Amico G, Garcia-Tsao G, Cales P *et al.* Diagnosis of portal hypertension: how and when. In: DeFranchis R, ed. *Portal Hypertension III. Proceedings of the Third Baveno International Consensus Workshop on Definitions, Methodology and Therapeutic Strategies.* Oxford: Blackwell Science, 2001, p. 36–64.

10 Ripoll C, Groszmann R, Garcia-Tsao G *et al.* Hepatic venous pressure gradient predicts clinical decompensation in patients with compensated cirrhosis. *Gastroenterology* 2007; **133**: 481–488.

11 Wong F, Liu P, Blendis L. Sodium homeostasis with chronic sodium loading in preascitic cirrhosis. *Gut* 2001; **49**: 847–851.

12 Wiest R, Groszmann RJ. The paradox of nitric oxide in cirrhosis and portal hypertension: Too much, not enough. *Hepatology* 2002; **35**: 478–491.

13 Martin PY, Ohara M, Gines P *et al.* Nitric oxide synthase (NOS) inhibition for one week improves renal sodium and water excretion in cirrhotic rats with ascites. *J. Clin. Invest.* 1998; **101**: 235–242.

14 Lee FY, Colombato LA, Albillos A *et al.* N-ω-nitro-L-arginine administration corrects peripheral vasodilation and systemic capillary hypotension, and ameliorates plasma volume expansion and sodium retention in portal hypertensive rats. *Hepatology* 1993; **17**: 84–90.

15 Iwakiri Y, Groszmann RJ. The hyperdynamic circulation of chronic liver diseases: from the patient to the molecule. *Hepatology* 2006; **43**: S121–S131.

16 Perez-Ayuso RM, Arroyo V, Planas R *et al.* Randomized comparative study of efficacy of furosemide versus spironolactone in nonazotemic cirrhosis with ascites. Relationship between the diuretic response and the activity of the renin-aldosterone system. *Gastroenterology* 1983; **84**: 961–968.

17 Wiest R, Das S, Cadelina G *et al.* Bacterial translocation to lymph nodes of cirrhotic rats stimulates eNOS-derived NO production and impairs mesenteric vascular contractility. *J. Clin. Invest.* 1999; **104**: 1223–1233.

18 Wiest R, Cadelina G, Milstien S *et al.* Bacterial translocation up-regulates GTP-cyclohydrolase I in mesenteric vasculature of cirrhotic rats. *Hepatology* 2003; **38**: 1508–1515.

19 Gines P, Berl T, Bernardi M *et al.* Hyponatremia in cirrhosis: from pathogenesis to treatment. *Hepatology* 1998; **28**: 851–863.

20 Arroyo V, Jimenez W. Complications of cirrhosis. II. Renal and circulatory dysfunction. Lights and shadows in an important clinical problem. *J. Hepatol.* 2000; **32**: 157–170.

21 Girgrah N, Liu P, Collier J *et al.* Haemodynamic, renal sodium handling, and neurohormonal effects of acute administration of low dose losartan, an angiotensin II receptor antagonist, in preascitic cirrhosis. *Gut* 2000; **46**: 114–120.

22 Krag A, Moller S, Henriksen JH *et al.* Terlipressin improves renal function in patients with cirrhosis and ascites without hepatorenal syndrome. *Hepatology* 2007; **46**: 1863–1871.

23 Gerbes AL, Wernze H, Arendt RM *et al.* Atrial natriuretic factor and renin-aldosterone in volume regulation of patients with cirrhosis. *Hepatology* 1989; **9**: 417–422.

24 Boyer TD, Zia P, Reynolds TB. Effect of indomethacin and prostaglandin A1 on renal function and plasma renin activity in alcoholic liver disease. *Gastroenterology* 1979; **77**: 215–222.

25 Wong F, Massie D, Hsu P *et al.* Indomethacin-induced renal dysfunction in patients with well-compensated cirrhosis. *Gastroenterology* 1993; **104**: 869–876.

26 Simel DL, Halvorsen RA Jr, Feussner JR. Quantitating bedside diagnosis: clinical evaluation of ascites. *J. Gen. Intern. Med.* 1988; **3**: 423–428.

27 Khalid SK, Garcia-Tsao G. Ascites: Clinical features, diagnosis and natural history. In: Sanyal AJ, Shah V, ed. *Portal Hypertension. Pathobiology, Evaluation and Treatment.* Totowa: Humana Press, 2005, p. 285–299.

28 Cattau EL Jr, Benjamin SB, Knuff TE *et al.* The accuracy of the physical examination in the diagnosis of suspected ascites. *JAMA* 1982; **247**: 1164–1166.

29 Cummings S, Papadakis M, Melnick J *et al.* The predictive value of physical examinations for ascites. *West. J. Med.* 1985; **142**: 633–636.

30 Belghiti J, Durand F. Abdominal wall hernias in the setting of cirrhosis. *Semin. Liver Dis.* 1997; **17**: 219–226.

31 Kirkpatrick S, Schubert T. Umbilical hernia rupture in cirrhotics with ascites. *Dig. Dis. Sci.* 1988; **33**: 762–765.

32 Trotter JF, Suhocki PV. Incarceration of umbilical hernia following transjugular intrahepatic portosystemic shunt for the treatment of ascites. *Liver Transpl. Surg.* 1999; **5**: 209–210.

33 Trianto CK, Kehagias I, Nikolopoulou V, *et al.* Surgical repair of umbilical hernias. *Am. J. Med. Sci.* 2010 doi 10.1097/MAJ.0b013e3181f31982.

34 Lieberman FL, Hidemura R, Peters RL *et al.* Pathogenesis and treatment of hydrothorax complicating cirrhosis with ascites. *Ann. Intern. Med.* 1966; **64**: 341–351.

35 Rubinstein D, McInnes IE, Dudley FJ. Hepatic hydrothorax in the absence of clinical ascites: diagnosis and management. *Gastroenterology* 1985; **88**: 188–191.

36 Strauss RM, Boyer TD. Hepatic hydrothorax. *Sem. Liver Dis.* 1997; **17**: 227–232.

37 Ackerman Z, Reynolds TB. Evaluation of pleural fluid in patients with cirrhosis. *J. Clin. Gastroenterol.* 1997; **25**: 619–622.

38 Bhattacharya A, Mittal BR, Biswas T *et al.* Radioisotope scintigraphy in the diagnosis of hepatic hydrothorax. *J. Gastroenterol. Hepatol.* 2001; **16**: 317–321.

39 Strauss RM, Martin LG, Kaufman SL *et al.* Transjugular intrahepatic portal systemic shunt for the management of symptomatic cirrhotic hydrothorax. *Am. J. Gastroenterol.* 1994; **89**: 1522.

40 Runyon BA. Management of adult patients with ascites caused by cirrhosis. *Hepatology* 1998; **27**: 264–272.

41 McVay PA, Toy PT. Lack of increased bleeding after paracentesis and thoracentesis in patients with mild coagulation abnormalities. *Transfusion* 1991; **31**: 164–171.

42 Witte CL, Witte MH. The congested liver. In: Lautt WW, ed. *Hepatic Circulation in Health and Disease.* New York: Raven Press, 1981, p. 307–323.

43 Henriksen JH, Horn T, Christoffersen P. The blood-lymph barrier in the liver. A review based on morphological and functional concepts of normal and cirrhotic liver. *Liver* 1984; **4**: 221–232.

44 Hoefs JC. Serum protein concentration and portal pressure determine the ascitic fluid protein concentration in patients with chronic liver disease. *J. Lab. Clin. Med.* 1983; **102**: 260–273.

45 Pare P, Talbot J, Hoefs JC. Serum-ascites albumin concentration gradient: a physiologic approach to the differential diagnosis of ascites. *Gastroenterology* 1983; **85**: 240–244.

46 Rimola A, Garcia-Tsao G, Navasa M *et al.* Diagnosis, treatment and prophylaxis of spontaneous bacterial peritonitis: a consensus document. *J. Hepatol.* 2000; **32**: 142–153.

47 Van der MS, Dens J, Daenen W *et al.* Pericardial disease is often not recognised as a cause of chronic severe ascites. *J. Hepatol.* 2000; **32**: 164–169.

48 Runyon BA, Montano AA, Akriviadis EA *et al.* The serum-ascites albumin gradient is superior to the exudate-transudate concept in the differential diagnosis of ascites. *Ann. Intern. Med.* 1992; **117**: 215–220.

49 Runyon BA, Hoefs JC, Morgan TR. Ascitic fluid analysis in malignancy-related ascites. *Hepatology* 1988; **8**: 1104–1109.

50 Albillos A, Cuervas-Mons V, Millan I *et al.* Ascitic fluid polymorphonuclear cell count and serum to ascites albumin gradient in the diagnosis of bacterial peritonitis. *Gastroenterology* 1990; **98**: 134–140.

51 Runyon BA, Akriviadis EA, Keyser AJ. The opacity of portal hypertension-related ascites correlates with the fluid's triglyceride concentration. *Am. J. Clin. Pathol.* 1991; **96**: 142–143.

52 Rector WG Jr. Spontaneous chylous ascites of cirrhosis. *J. Clin. Gastroenterol.* 1984; **6**: 369–372.

53 Fernandez J, Navasa M, Gomez J *et al.* Bacterial infections in cirrhosis: epidemiological changes with invasive procedures and norfloxacin prophylaxis. *Hepatology* 2002; **35**: 140–148.

54 Xiol X, Castellvi JM, Guardiola J *et al.* Spontaneous bacterial empyema in cirrhotic patients: a prospective study. *Hepatology* 1996; **23**: 719–723.

55 Garcia-Tsao G, Lee FY, Barden GE *et al.* Bacterial translocation to mesenteric lymph nodes is increased in cirrhotic rats with ascites. *Gastroenterology* 1995; **108**: 1835–1841.

56 Homann C, Varming K, Hogasen K *et al.* Acquired C3 deficiency in patients with alcoholic cirrhosis predisposes to infection and increased mortality. *Gut* 1997; **40**: 544–549.

57 Runyon BA. Patients with deficient ascitic fluid opsonic activity are predisposed to spontaneous bacterial peritonitis. *Hepatology* 1988; **8**: 632–635.

58 Garcia-Tsao G. Spontaneous bacterial peritonitis. *Gastro. Clin. North Am.* 1992; **21**: 257–275.

59 Runyon BA. Monomicrobial nonneutrocytic bacterascites: a variant of spontaneous bacterial peritonitis. *Hepatology* 1990; **12**: 710–715.

60 Navasa M, Follo A, Filella X *et al.* Tumor necrosis factor and interleukin-6 in spontaneous bacterial peritonitis in cirrhosis: relationship with the development of renal impairment and mortality. *Hepatology* 1998; **27**: 1227–1232.

61 Tito L, Rimola A, Gines P *et al.* Recurrence of spontaneous bacterial peritonitis in cirrhosis: frequency and predictive factors. *Hepatology* 1988; **8**: 27–31.

62 Sort P, Navasa M, Arroyo V *et al.* Effect of intravenous albumin on renal impairment and mortality in patients with cirrhosis and spontaneous bacterial peritonitis. *N. Engl. J. Med.* 1999; **341**: 403–409.

63 Toledo C, Salmeron JM, Rimola A *et al.* Spontaneous bacterial peritonitis in cirrhosis: predictive factors of infection resolution and survival in patients treated with cefotaxime. *Hepatology* 1993; **17**: 251–257.

64 Bert F, Panhard X, Johnson J *et al.* Genetic background of Escherichia coli isolates from patients with spontaneous bacterial peritonitis: relationship with host factors and prognosis. *Clin. Microbiol. Infect.* 2008; **14**: 1034–1040.

65 Cheong HS, Kang CI, Lee JA *et al.* Clinical significance and outcome of nosocomial acquisition of spontaneous bacterial peritonitis in patients with liver cirrhosis. *Clin. Infect. Dis.* 2009; **48**: 1230–1236.

66 Navasa M, Follo A, Llovet JM *et al.* Randomized, comparative study of oral ofloxacin versus intravenous cefotaxime in spontaneous bacterial peritonitis. *Gastroenterology* 1996; **111**: 1011–1017.

67 Rimola A, Salmeron JM, Clemente G *et al.* Two different dosages of cefotaxime in the treatment of spontaneous bacterial peritonitis in cirrhosis: results of a prospective, randomized, multicenter study. *Hepatology* 1995; **21**: 674–679.

68 Runyon BA, McHutchison JG, Antillon MR *et al.* Short-course versus long-course antibiotic treatment of spontaneous bacterial peritonitis. *Gastroenterology* 1991; **100**: 1737–1742.

69 Ricart E, Soriano G, Novella M *et al.* Amoxicillin-clavulanic acid versus cefotaxime in the therapy of bacterial infections in cirrhotic patients. *J. Hepatol.* 2000; **32**: 596–602.

70 Sigal SH, Stanca CM, Fernandez J *et al.* Restricted use of albumin for spontaneous bacterial peritonitis. *Gut* 2007; **56**: 597–599.

71 Terg R, Gadano A, Cartier M *et al.* Serum creatinine and bilirubin predict renal failure and mortality in patients with spontaneous bacterial peritonitis: a retrospective study. *Liver Int.* 2009; **29**: 415–419.

72 Acevedo J, Fernandez J, Castro M *et al.* Current efficacy of recommended empirical antibiotic therapy in patients with cirrhosis and bacterial infection. *J. Hepatol.* 2009; **50** (Suppl. 1): S5 (abstract).

73 Umgelter A, Reindl W, Miedaner M *et al.* Failure of current antibiotic first-line regimens and mortality in hospitalized patients with spontaneous bacterial peritonitis. *Infection* 2009; **37**: 2–8.

74 Fernandez J, Ruiz DA, Gomez C *et al.* Norfloxacin vs ceftriaxone in the prophylaxis of infections in patients with advanced cirrhosis and hemorrhage. *Gastroenterology* 2006; **131**: 1049–1056.

75 Gines P, Rimola A, Planas R *et al.* Norfloxacin prevents spontaneous bacterial peritonitis recurrence in cirrhosis: results of a double-blind, placebo-controlled trial. *Hepatology* 1990; **12**: 716–724.

76 Fernandez J, Navasa M, Planas R *et al.* Primary prophylaxis of spontaneous bacterial peritonitis delays hepatorenal syndrome and improves survival in cirrhosis. *Gastroenterology* 2007; **133**: 818–824.

77 Llach J, Rimola A, Navasa M *et al.* Incidence and predictive factors of first episode of spontaneous bacterial peritonitis in cirrhosis with ascites: relevance of ascitic fluid protein concentration. *Hepatology* 1992; **16**: 724–727.

78 Runyon BA. Management of adult patients with ascites due to cirrhosis: an update. *Hepatology* 2009; **49**: 2087–2107.

79 Garcia-Tsao G, Lim JK. Management and treatment of patients with cirrhosis and portal hypertension: recommendations from the Department of Veterans Affairs Hepatitis C Resource Center Program and the National Hepatitis C Program. *Am. J. Gastroenterol.* 2009; **104**: 1802–1829.

80 Arroyo V, Gines A, Salo J. A European survey on the treatment of ascites in cirrhosis. *J. Hepatol.* 1994; **21**: 667–672.

81 Gines P, Arroyo V, Quintero E *et al.* Comparison of paracentesis and diuretics in the treatment of cirrhotics with tense ascites: Results of a randomized study. *Gastroenterology* 1987; **93**: 234–241.

82 Angeli P, Fasolato S, Mazza E *et al.* Combined versus sequential diuretic treatment of ascites in nonazotemic patients with cirrhosis: results of an open randomized clinical trial. *Gut* 2010; **59**: 98–104

83 Santos J, Planas R, Pardo A *et al.* Spironolactone alone or in combination with furosemide in the treatment of moderate ascites in nonazotemic cirrhosis. A randomized comparative study of efficacy and safety. *J. Hepatol.* 2003; **39**: 187–192.

84 Pockros PJ, Reynolds TB. Rapid diuresis in patients with ascites from chronic liver disease: the importance of peripheral edema. *Gastroenterology* 1986; **90**: 1827–1833.

85 Gentilini P, Casini-Raggi V, Di Fiore G *et al.* Albumin improves the response to diuretics in patients with cirrhosis and ascites: results of a randomized, controlled trial. *J. Hepatol.* 1999; **30**: 639–645.

86 Vlachogiannakos J, Tang AKW, Patch D *et al.* Angiotensin converting enzyme inhibitors and angiotensin II antagonists as therapy in chronic liver disease. *Gut* 2001; **49**: 303–308

87 Corbani A, Manousou P, Calvaruso V *et al.* Muscle cramps in cirrhosis. The therapeutic value of quinine. Is it underused? *Dig. Liver Dis.* 2008; **40**: 794–799

88 Kao HW, Rakov NE, Savage E *et al.* The effect of large volume paracentesis on plasma volume—a cause of hypovolemia? *Hepatology* 1985; **5**: 403–407.

89 Tito L, Gines P, Arroyo V *et al.* Total paracentesis associated with intravenous albumin management of patients with cirrhosis and ascites. *Gastroenterology* 1990; **98**: 146–151.

90 Gines P, Arroyo V, Vargas V *et al.* Paracentesis with intravenous infusion of albumin as compared with peritoneovenous shunting in cirrhosis with refractory ascites. *N. Engl. J. Med.* 1991; **325**: 829–835.

91 Gines A, Fernandez-Esparrach G, Monescillo A *et al.* Randomized trial comparing albumin, dextran-70 and polygeline in cirrhotic patients with ascites treated by paracentesis. *Gastroenterology* 1996; **111**: 1002–1010.

92 De Gottardi A, Thevenot T, Spahr L *et al.* Risk of complications after abdominal paracentesis in cirrhotic patients: a prospective study. *Clin. Gastroenterol. Hepatol.* 2009; **7**: 906–909.

93 Arnold C, Haag K, Blum HE *et al.* Acute hemoperitoneum after large-volume paracentesis. *Gastroenterology* 1997; **113**: 978–982.

94 Grabau CM, Crago SF, Hoff LK *et al.* Performance standards for therapeutic abdominal paracentesis. *Hepatology* 2004; **40**: 484–488.

95 Conn HO. Sudden scrotal edema in cirrhosis: a postparacentesis syndrome. *Ann. Intern. Med.* 1971; **74**: 943–945.

96 Gines P, Guevara M. Hyponatremia in cirrhosis: pathogenesis, clinical significance, and management. *Hepatology* 2008; **48**: 1002–1010.

97 Angeli P, Wong F, Watson H *et al.* Hyponatremia in cirrhosis: Results of a patient population survey. *Hepatology* 2006; **44**: 1535–1542.

98 Planas R, Montoliu S, Balleste B *et al.* Natural history of patients hospitalized for management of cirrhotic ascites. *Clin. Gastroenterol. Hepatol.* 2006; **4**: 1385–1394.

99 Restuccia T, Gomez-Anson B, Guevara M *et al.* Effects of dilutional hyponatremia on brain organic osmolytes and water content in patients with cirrhosis. *Hepatology* 2004; **39**: 1613–1622.

100 McCormick PA, Mistry P, Kaye G *et al.* Intravenous albumin infusion is an effective therapy for hyponatraemia in cirrhotic patients with ascites. *Gut* 1990; **31**: 204–207.

101 Carrilho F, Bosch J, Arroyo V *et al.* Renal failure associated with demeclocycline in cirrhosis. *Ann. Intern. Med.* 1977; **87**: 195–197.

102 Gadano A, Moreau R, Pessione F *et al.* Aquaretic effects of niravoline, a kappa-opioid agonist, in patients with cirrhosis. *J. Hepatol.* 2000; **32**: 38–42.

103 Wong F, Blei AT, Blendis LM *et al.* A vasopressin receptor antagonist (VPA-985) improves serum sodium concentration in patients with hyponatremia: a multicenter, randomized, placebo-controlled trial. *Hepatology* 2003; **37**: 182–191.

104 Gerbes AL, Gulberg V, Gines P *et al.* Therapy of hyponatremia in cirrhosis with a vasopressin receptor antagonist: a randomized double-blind multicenter trial. *Gastroenterology* 2003; **124**: 933–939.

105 Gines P, Wong F, Watson H *et al.* Effects of satavaptan, a selective vasopressin V(2) receptor antagonist, on ascites and serum sodium in cirrhosis with hyponatremia: a randomized trial. *Hepatology* 2008; **48**: 204–213.

106 Schrier RW, Gross P, Gheorghiade M *et al.* Tolvaptan, a selective oral vasopressin V2-receptor antagonist, for hyponatremia. *N. Engl. J. Med.* 2006; **355**: 2099–2112.

107 Heuman DM, Abou-Assi SG, Habib A *et al.* Persistent ascites and low serum sodium identify patients with cirrhosis and low MELD scores who are at high risk for early death. *Hepatology* 2004; **40**: 802–810.

108 Kim WR, Biggins SW, Kremers WK *et al.* Hyponatremia and mortality among patients on the liver-transplant waiting list. *N. Engl. J. Med.* 2008; **359**: 1018–1026.

109 Arroyo V, Gines P, Gerbes AL *et al.* Definition and diagnostic criteria of refractory ascites and hepatorenal syndrome in cirrhosis. *Hepatology* 1996; **23**: 164–176.

110 Moore KP, Wong F, Gines P *et al.* The management of ascites in cirrhosis: report on the consensus conference of the International Ascites Club. *Hepatology* 2003; **38**: 258–266.

111 Fernandez-Esparrach G, Guevara M, Sort P *et al.* Diuretic requirements after therapeutic paracentesis in nonazotemic patients with cirrhosis. A randomized double-blind trial of spironolactone versus placebo. *J. Hepatol.* 1997; **26**: 614–620.

112 Ferral H, Bjarnason H, Wegryn SA *et al.* Refractory ascites: early experience in treatment with transjugular intrahepatic portosystemic shunt. *Radiology* 1993; **189**: 795–801.

113 D'Amico G, Luca A, Morabito A *et al.* Uncovered transjugular intrahepatic portosystemic shunt for refractory ascites: a meta-analysis. *Gastroenterology* 2005; **129**: 1282–1293.

114 Albillos A, Banares R, Gonzalez M *et al.* A meta-analysis of transjugular intrahepatic portosystemic shunt versus paracentesis for refractory ascites. *J. Hepatol.* 2005; **43**: 990–996.

115 Salerno F, Camma C, Enea M *et al.* Transjugular intrahepatic portosystemic shunt for refractory ascites: a meta-analysis of individual patient data. *Gastroenterology* 2007; **133**: 825–834.

116 Boyer TD, Haskal ZJ. The role of transjugular intrahepatic portosystemic shunt in the management of portal hypertension. *Hepatology* 2005; **41**: 386–400.

117 Bureau C, Garcia-Pagan JC, Otal P *et al.* Improved clinical outcome using polytetrafluoroethylene-coated stents for TIPS: results of a randomized study. *Gastroenterology* 2004; **126**: 469–475.

118 Gines A, Planas R, Angeli P *et al.* Treatment of patients with cirrhosis and refractory ascites by LeVeen shunt with titanium tip. Comparison with therapeutic paracentesis. *Hepatology* 1995; **22**: 124–131.

119 Dumortier J, Pianta E, Le Derf Y *et al.* Peritoneovenous shunt as a bridge to liver transplantation. *Am. J. Transplant.* 2005; **5**: 1886–1892.

120 Garcia-Tsao G, Parikh CR, Viola A. Acute kidney injury in cirrhosis. *Hepatology* 2008; **48**: 2064–2077.

121 Gines A, Escorsell A, Gines P *et al.* Incidence, predictive factors, and prognosis of the hepatorenal syndrome in cirrhosis with ascites. *Gastroenterology* 1993; **105**: 229–236.

122 Salerno F, Gerbes A, Gines P *et al.* Diagnosis, prevention and treatment of the hepatorenal syndrome in cirrhosis. A consensus workshop of the international ascites club. *Gut* 2007; **56**: 1310–1318.

123 Mehta RL, Kellum JA, Shah SV *et al.* Acute Kidney Injury Network: report of an initiative to improve outcomes in acute kidney injury. *Crit. Care* 2007; **11**: R31.

124 Sanyal AJ, Boyer TD, Garcia-Tsao G *et al.* A randomized prospective, double-blind, placebo-controlled trial of terlipressin for type 1 hepatorenal syndrome. *Gastroenterology* 2008; **134**: 1360–68

125 Ruiz-del-Arbol L, Monescillo A, Arocena C *et al.* Circulatory function and hepatorenal syndrome in cirrhosis. *Hepatology* 2005; **42**: 439–447.

126 Moore K, Wendon J, Frazer M *et al.* Plasma endothelin immunoreactivity in liver disease and the hepatorenal syndrome. *N. Engl. J. Med.* 1992; **327**: 1774–1778.

127 Martin PY, Gines P, Schrier RW. Nitric oxide as a mediator of hemodynamic abnormalities and sodium and water retention in cirrhosis. *N. Engl. J. Med.* 1998; **339**: 533–541.

128 Gonwa TA, McBride MA, Anderson K *et al.* Continued influence of preoperative renal function on outcome of orthotopic liver transplant (OLTX) in the US: where will MELD lead us? *Am. J. Transplant.* 2006; **6**: 2651–2659.

129 Weismuller TJ, Prokein J, Becker T *et al.* Prediction of survival after liver transplantation by pre-transplant parameters. *Scand. J. Gastroenterol.* 2008; **43**: 736–746.

130 Gonwa TA, Morris CA, Goldstein RM *et al.* Long-term survival and renal function following liver transplantation in patients with and without hepatorenal syndrome—experience in 300 patients. *Transplantation* 1991; **51**: 428–430.

131 Angeli P, Volpin R, Piovan D *et al.* Acute effects of the oral administration of midodrine, an α-adrenergic agonist, on renal hemodynamics and renal function in cirrhotic patients with ascites. *Hepatology* 1998; **28**: 937–943.

132 Lenz K, Hortnagel H, Druml W *et al.* Ornipressin in the treatment of functional renal failure in decompensated liver cirrhosis. Effects on renal haemodynamics and atrial natriuretic factor. *Gastroenterology* 1991; **101**: 1060–1067.

133 Uriz J, Gines P, Cardenas A *et al.* Terlipressin plus albumin infusion: an effective and safe therapy of hepatorenal syndrome. *J. Hepatol.* 2001; **33**: 43–48.

134 Duvoux C, Zanditenas D, Hezode C *et al.* Effects of noradrenalin and albumin in patients with type I hepatorenal syndrome: A pilot study. *Hepatology* 2002; **36**: 374–380.

135 Solanki P, Chawla A, Garg R *et al.* Beneficial effects of terlipressin in hepatorenal syndrome: a prospective, randomized placebo-controlled clinical trial. *J. Gastroenterol. Hepatol.* 2003; **18**: 152–156.

136 Neri S, Pulvirenti D, Malaguarnera M *et al.* Terlipressin and albumin in patients with cirrhosis and type I hepatorenal syndrome. *Dig. Dis. Sci.* 2008; **53**: 830–835.

137 Martin-Llahi M, Pepin MN, Guevara M *et al.* Terlipressin and albumin vs albumin in patients with cirrhosis and hepatorenal syndrome: a randomized study. *Gastroenterology* 2008; **134**: 1352–1359.

138 Sanyal AJ, Boyer T, Garcia-Tsao G *et al.* A randomized, prospective, double-blind, placebo-controlled trial of terlipressin for type 1 hepatorenal syndrome. *Gastroenterology* 2008; **134**: 1360–1368.

139 Gluud LL, Christensen K, Christensen E *et al.* Systematic review of randomized trials on vasoconstrictor drugs for hepatorenal syndrome. *Hepatology* 2009; **50**: 1–9

140 Sharma P, Kumar A, Shrama BC *et al.* An open label, pilot, randomized controlled trial of noradrenaline versus terlipressin in the treatment of type 1 hepatorenal syndrome and predictors of response. *Am. J. Gastroenterol.* 2008; **103**: 1689–1697

141 Kiser TH, Fish DN, Obritsch MD *et al.* Vasopressin, not octreotide, may be beneficial in the treatment of hepatorenal syndrome: a retrospective study. *Nephrol. Dial. Transplant.* 2005; **20**: 1813–1820.

142 Angeli P, Volpin R, Gerunda G *et al.* Reversal of type 1 hepatorenal syndrome with the administration of midodrine and octreotide. *Hepatology* 1999; **29**: 1690–1697.

143 Brensing KA, Textor J, Perz J *et al.* Long-term outcome after transjugular intrahepatic portosystemic stent-shunt in non-transplant cirrhotics with hepatorenal syndrome: a phase II study. *Gut* 2000; **47**: 288–295.

144 Wong F, Pantea L, Sniderman K. Midodrine, octreotide, albumin, and TIPS in selected patients with cirrhosis and type 1 hepatorenal syndrome. *Hepatology* 2004; **40**: 55–64.

145 Mitzner SR, Stange J, Klammt S *et al.* Improvement of hepatorenal syndrome with extracorporeal albumin dialysis MARS: results of a prospective randomized, controlled clinical trial. *Liver Transpl.* 2000; **6**: 277–286.

146 Gines P, Quintero E, Arroyo V. Compensated cirrhosis: natural history and prognosis. *Hepatology* 1987; **7**: 122–128.

147 D'Amico G, Morabito A, Pagliaro L *et al.* Survival and prognostic indicators in compensated and decompensated cirrhosis. *Dig. Dis. Sci.* 1986; **31**: 468–475.

148 Salerno F, Borroni G, Moser P *et al.* Survival and prognostic factors of cirrhotic patients with ascites: a study of 134 outpatients. *Am. J. Gastroenterol.* 1993; **88**: 514–519.

149 D'Amico G. Natural history of compensated cirrhosis and varices. In: Boyer TD, Groszmann RJ. *Complications of Cirrhosis: Pathogenesis, Consequences and Therapy.* American Association for the Study of Liver Diseases, 2001, p. 118–123.

150 Fernandez-Esparrach G, Sanchez-Fueyo A, Gines P *et al.* A prognostic model for predicting survival in cirrhosis with ascites. *J. Hepatol.* 2001; **34**: 46–52.

151 Arroyo V, Rodes J, Gutierrez Lizarraga MA *et al.* Prognostic value of spontaneous hyponatremia in cirrhosis with ascites. *Am. J. Dig. Dis.* 1976; **21**: 249–256.

152 Llach J, Gines P, Arroyo V *et al.* Prognostic value of arterial pressure, endogenous vasoactive systems, and renal function in cirrhotic patients admitted to the hospital for the treatment of ascites. *Gastroenterology* 1988; **94**: 482–487.

CHAPTER 11
Jaundice and Cholestasis

Elwyn Elias

University of Birmingham, Birmingham, UK

Learning points

- Involvement of the sclera helps distinguish jaundice from other causes of cutaneous pigmentation.

- Bilirubin is an end-product of haem catabolism, the majority (80–85%) of which is derived from haemoglobin.

- Unconjugated bilirubin is non-polar (lipid soluble) and transported in the plasma tightly bound to albumin. Competitive binders in the neonate can cause kernicterus.

- Microsomal bilirubin uridine diphosphate glucuronosyl transferase (UGT) is the enzyme that converts unconjugated bilirubin to conjugated bilirubin mono- and diglucuronide. Its deficiency causes Gilbert's and Crigler–Najjar syndromes.

- Bile formation is dependent on energy-dependent transport processes in the basolateral and canalicular membranes of the hepatocyte and cholangiocytes and largely independent of perfusing blood pressure. Conjugated bilirubin, bile salts, cholesterol, phospholipids, proteins, electrolytes and water are secreted by the liver cell into the canaliculus.

- Biliary excretion of bilirubin glucuronides is mediated by the ATP-dependent multidrug resistance protein-2 (MRP-2) and is the rate-limiting factor in the transport of bilirubin from plasma to bile. Its deficiency causes the Dubin–Johnson syndrome.

- The human liver synthesizes the primary bile acids—cholic acid ($3\alpha,7\alpha,12\alpha$ trihydroxy cholanoic acid), chenodeoxycholic acid ($3\alpha,7\alpha$ dihydroxycholanoic acid) and a little (1%) ursodeoxycholic acid, the 7β isomer of chenodeoxycholic acid. Their dehydroxylation by bacteria in the intestine produces deoxycholic acid ($3\alpha,12\alpha$ dihydroxy) and lithocholic acid (3α monohydroxy), known as secondary bile acids. The liver conjugates both primary and secondary bile acids with either glycine or taurine.

- Cholestasis refers to impaired formation or flow of bile, due to any cause, between the basolateral (sinusoidal) membrane of the hepatocyte and the ampulla of Vater.

- Familial intrahepatic cholestasis may be caused by identifiable, genetically determined defects in specific canalicular transporters such as the bile salt export pump.

- Jaundice is not a constant finding in cholestasis. Prominent features of cholestasis, both acute and chronic, are itching and malabsorption of fat and fat-soluble nutrients.

- Prolonged cholestasis may cause deficiency of vitamin A, D, E or K, and require parenteral replacement therapy for prevention and treatment of complications.

- Investigation of jaundice and cholestasis aims at identification of its cause and treatment, which may be expectant and medicinal or require interventional radiology, therapeutic endoscopy and abdominal surgery.

Introduction

Jaundice is the yellow discoloration of sclera, mucous membranes and skin caused by bilirubin. Involvement of the sclera helps distinguish jaundice from other causes of cutaneous pigmentation such as melanin, hypercarotenaemia and mepacrine therapy. In medicine, icterus, from the Greek *ikteros*, is used synonymously with jaundice although it can also refer to a disease of plants in which the leaves turn yellow, or a certain yellowish-green bird.

Classification of jaundice

Classification is into three types: prehepatic, hepatic and cholestatic (Fig. 11.1). There is much overlap, particularly between the hepatic and cholestatic varieties.

Prehepatic. This may be due to an increased load of bilirubin arriving at the liver, as in haemolysis, or diminished hepatic capacity for conjugation of bilirubin, as in Gilbert's and Crigler–Najjar syndrome. The circulating

---

Sherlock's Diseases of the Liver and Biliary System, Twelfth Edition. Edited by James S. Dooley, Anna S.F. Lok, Andrew K. Burroughs, E. Jenny Heathcote.
© 2011 by Blackwell Publishing Ltd. Published 2011 by Blackwell Publishing Ltd.

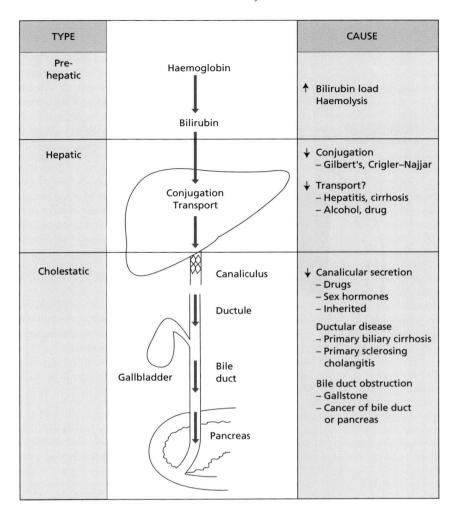

TYPE		CAUSE
Pre-hepatic	Haemoglobin ↓ Bilirubin	↑ Bilirubin load Haemolysis
Hepatic	Conjugation Transport	↓ Conjugation – Gilbert's, Crigler–Najjar ↓ Transport? – Hepatitis, cirrhosis – Alcohol, drug
Cholestatic	Canaliculus Ductule Gallbladder Bile duct Pancreas	↓ Canalicular secretion – Drugs – Sex hormones – Inherited Ductular disease – Primary biliary cirrhosis – Primary sclerosing cholangitis Bile duct obstruction – Gallstone – Cancer of bile duct or pancreas

Fig. 11.1. Classification and causes of jaundice.

serum bilirubin is largely unconjugated and the serum transaminase and alkaline phosphatase are normal. Bilirubin cannot be detected in urine.

Hepatic. Hepatocyte damage results in reduced efficiency of bilirubin excretion into bile. Conjugated bilirubin refluxes into the circulation and is found in urine. Serum biochemistry shows an increase in hepatic enzymes according to the underlying cause.

Cholestatic. This is due to failure of adequate amounts of bile to reach the duodenum, either through a specific failure of canalicular secretion or physical obstruction to bile flow at any level. The serum shows increases in conjugated bilirubin, biliary alkaline phosphatase, γ-glutamyl transpeptidase (γ-GT), total cholesterol and conjugated bile acids. Lack of bile acids to form micelles may cause steatorrhoea and malabsorption of calcium and the fat-soluble vitamins A, D, E and K.

Physiology and pathophysiology

Bilirubin metabolism and transport

Bilirubin is an end-product of haem catabolism, the majority (80–85%) of which is derived from haemoglobin and only a small fraction from other haem-containing proteins such as cytochrome P450 (Fig. 11.2), myoglobin and immature bone marrow cells. Approximately 300 mg bilirubin is formed daily.

The enzyme that converts haem to bilirubin is microsomal haem oxygenase (Fig. 11.3). Cleavage of the porphyrin ring occurs selectively at the α-methane bridge. The α-bridge carbon atom is converted to carbon monoxide and the original bridge function is replaced by two oxygen atoms which are derived from molecular oxygen. The resulting linear tetrapyrrole has the structure of IX α-biliverdin, which is converted to IX α-bilirubin by biliverdin reductase, a cytosolic enzyme.

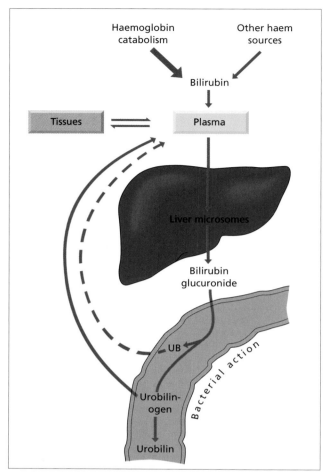

Fig. 11.2. The metabolism of bilirubin. UB, unconjugated bilirubin.

Such a linear tetrapyrrole should be water soluble, but realignment of the pyrrole ring allows internal hydrogen bonding to mask the propionic acid side chains and thus make bilirubin poorly soluble in aqueous solvents. The bonding is broken by alcohol in the diazo (van den Bergh) reaction converting unconjugated, indirect bilirubin to direct reacting bilirubin. *In vivo* hepatic esterification of bilirubin's propionic groups by glucuronic acid makes it water soluble. Unconjugated bilirubin is non-polar (lipid soluble) and transported in the plasma tightly bound to albumin. Only a very small amount is dialysable, but this can be increased by substances such as fatty acids, organic anions and drugs, which compete with bilirubin for albumin-binding sites. Avoidance of such competitive binders is vitally important in the neonate when diffusion of unbound bilirubin into the brain can cause kernicterus [1].

Bilirubin is efficiently removed from albumin and internalized by the liver where it is bound initially to cytosolic carrier proteins such as glutathione-*S*-transferase (ligandin), then glucuronidated and excreted into bile.

Microsomal bilirubin uridine diphosphate glucuronosyl transferase (UGT) is the enzyme that converts unconjugated bilirubin to conjugated bilirubin mono- and diglucuronide. The gene expressing bilirubin UGT is on chromosome 2. The structure of the gene is complex (Fig. 11.4) [2]. Exons 2–5 at the 3′ end are constant components of all isoforms of UGT but, to complete their expression, one of several first exons can be employed. Each exon 1 sequence has different substrate specificity and enzyme characteristics. Exon 1*1 encodes the variable region for bilirubin UGT1*1, responsible for virtually all conjugation of bilirubin to both its monoglucuronide and diglucuronide. The major conjugate in human bile is the diglucuronide, though sulphate, xylose and glucose conjugation also occur to a small extent and may be increased in cholestasis. Biliary excretion of the glucuronide is mediated by the ATP-dependent multidrug resistance protein-2 (MRP-2) [3,4] and is the rate-limiting factor in the transport of bilirubin from plasma to bile.

Bilirubin diglucuronide is not reabsorbed from the small intestine but in the colon may be hydrolysed by bacterial β-glucuronidases, producing urobilinogens and urobilin which are excreted in the stool or urine. In cholangitis, bacterial hydrolysis of bilirubin glucuronide in the biliary tree produces unconjugated bilirubin which may result in production of pigment gallstones.

Secretion of bile

Bile is produced by hepatocytes and modified by cholangiocytes lining the bile ducts. Bile formation is dependent on energy-dependent transport processes in the basolateral and canalicular membranes of the hepatocyte and cholangiocytes and largely independent of perfusing blood pressure. Conjugated bilirubin, bile salts, cholesterol, phospholipids, proteins, electrolytes and water are secreted by the liver cell into the canaliculus. The bile secretory apparatus comprises the *canalicular membrane* with its carrier proteins, the *intracellular organelles* and the *cytoskeleton* of the hepatocyte. *Tight junctions* between hepatocytes seal the biliary space from the blood compartment (Fig. 11.5).

The canalicular membrane contains carrier proteins which transport bile acids, bilirubin, cations and anions (Fig. 11.6). Canalicular secretion is modified by water and electrolytes passing between hepatocytes across the tight junction (*paracellular flow*) in response to osmotic gradients between canalicular bile and the intercellular fluid which is in continuity with the space of Disse [5]. Canaliculi empty their bile into ductules, sometimes called cholangioles or canals of Hering, which connect with interlobular bile ducts, the first bile channels to be

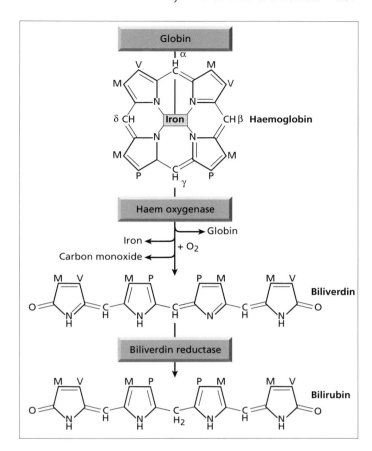

Fig. 11.3. The metabolism of haemoglobin to bilirubin. M, methyl; P, proprionate; V, vinyl.

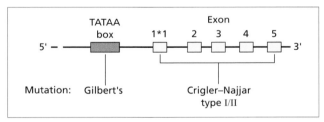

Fig. 11.4. Structure of the gene for bilirubin UGT1*1 with five exons and the promoter region (TATAA box). There are several other possible first exons (not shown) that can be spliced to exons 2–5, and have other substrate specificities.

accompanied by a branch of the hepatic artery and portal vein to form the triad which is characteristically found in portal tracts. Cholangiocytes, whose properties differ between small and large ducts, contribute a further 150 mL/day [6,7].

The passage of conjugated bile salts into the biliary canaliculus is the most important factor promoting bile formation. Water follows the osmotically active bile salts and there is a tight relationship between bile flow and bile salt secretion. Total bile flow in man is about 600 mL/day. The hepatocyte provides two components: bile salt dependent (approximately 225 mL/day) and bile salt independent (approximately 225 mL/day).

When bile flow is plotted against bile salt secretion, bile salt independent flow is the value obtained when bile salt excretion is extrapolated to zero. In this case other osmotically active solutes, such as glutathione and bicarbonate, generate water flow.

Cellular mechanisms

Sinusoidal uptake

Bile formation requires the uptake of bile acids and other organic and inorganic ions from plasma across the basolateral (sinusoidal) membrane, transport through the hepatocyte and excretion across the canalicular membrane (Fig. 11.6). Na^+/K^+–ATPase, which is found only on the basolateral membrane, exchanges three intracellular sodium ions for two extracellular potassium ions, thus maintaining the sodium (high outside:low inside) and potassium (low outside:high inside) gradients. In addition, because of the imbalance of electrical exchange, the cell interior is negatively charged ($-35\,mV$) compared with the exterior, favouring uptake of positively charged ions and excretion of those with a negative charge.

The sodium gradient drives the Na^+-dependent taurocholate cotransporter protein which internalizes

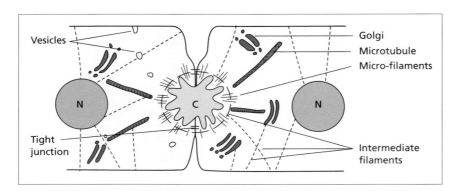

Fig. 11.5. The biliary secretory apparatus. Diagram of the ultrastructure of the bile canaliculus (C), cytoskeleton, and organelles (N, nucleus).

plasma bile acids conjugated with taurine or glycine. The organic anion transporter protein is sodium independent and carries several molecules, including bile acids, bromsulphthalein and other organic anions. There is also an organic cation transporter. Less well-defined carriers are thought to transport bilirubin into the hepatocyte [8].

Other ion transporters on the basolateral surface are the Na$^+$–H$^+$ exchanger involved in control of intracellular pH. A Na$^+$–HCO$_3$ cotransporter also serves this function. The basolateral membrane also contains uptake processes for sulphate, non-esterified fatty acids and organic cations.

Canalicular secretion (Figs 11.6, 11.7, 11.8)

The canalicular membrane, which accounts for only 1% of the hepatocyte's surface area, contains transporters [10] which secrete molecules into bile against steep concentration gradients as well as enzymes such as alkaline phosphatase and γ-GT. The transporters mainly belong to the family of ATP-binding cassette (ABC-) proteins, of which several hundred have been identified across many organisms. Canalicular MRP-2 (a member of the multidrug resistance protein family) excretes glucuronide and glutathione-*S*-conjugates, for example bilirubin diglucuronide [8]. The canalicular bile salt export pump [11] carries bile acids and is in part driven by the negative intracellular electric potential.

Two members of the P-glycoprotein family are important in canalicular transport; both are ATP dependent. MDR1 (multiple drug resistance 1) is a transporter of hydrophobic organic cations, and derives its name from being responsible for transporting cytotoxic drugs out of cancer cells, rendering them resistant to these drugs. The endogenous substrate is not known. MDR3 is a phospholipid flippase, which selectively enriches the canalicular (outer) surface of the membrane bilayer with phosphatidyl choline (lecithin) from where it is leeched by bile acids to become the major phospholipid in bile [12]. Hepatocytic active transport of the various

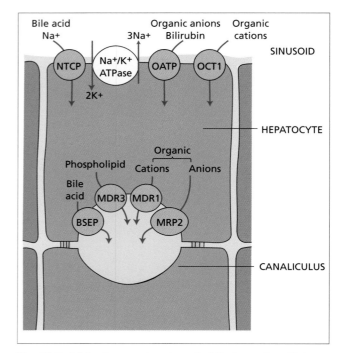

Fig. 11.6. Major transport systems in bile formation. Note the Na$^+$/K$^+$ ATPase or sodium pump (centre top), the sinusoidal Na$^+$ taurocholate co-transporting protein (NTCP), the sinusoidal multispecific organic anion transporter (OATP) and the organic cation transport 1 (OCT1). The canalicular membrane transporters are: BSEP, the bile salt export pump; MRP2, the multispecific organic anion transporter; MDR1, the ATP-dependent transporter of organic cations; and MDR3, an ATP-dependent phospholipid transporter (flippase). Other transport systems include a sinusoidal Na$^+$–H$^+$ exchanger, and canalicular bicarbonate transporter.

biliary solutes into the canaliculus creates the osmotic and electrochemical gradients which result in diffusion of water and inorganic ions (in particular sodium) into the canaliculus. The rate of bile secretion is influenced by many hormones and second messengers including

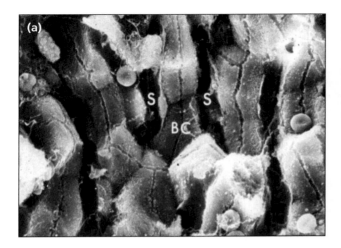

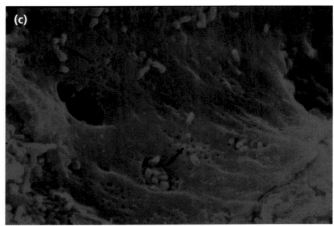

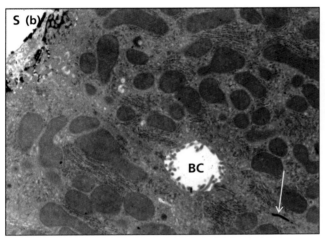

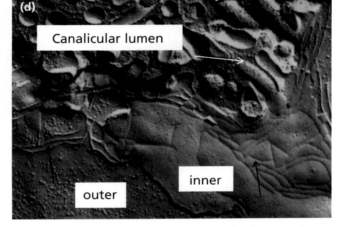

Fig. 11.7. Specialized domains of the hepatocyte membrane are illustrated by freeze fracture (a,c,d). On transmission electron microscopy (b) the basolateral intercellular space is marked with an electron dense marker (white arrow). In (a) the bile canaliculus (BC) can be seen running along the surface of a trabeculum of hepatocytes whose basolateral surfaces are in contact with blood within the sinusoids (S) on each side. (c) The sinusoidal endothelial cell is fenestrated, allowing the microvilli of hepatocytes (arrows) to come into direct contact with blood. (d) The canalicular and basolateral membrane domains are separated by tight junctions (zonula occludens, black arrows). Canalicular microvilli are indicated by white arrows. The inner and outer surfaces of the basolateral membrane of adjacent hepatocytes are marked.

cyclic AMP and protein kinase C. Passage of bile along the canaliculus involves the action of contractile microfilaments.

Ductular modification of bile

Cholangiocytes lining the larger bile ducts participate in hormone-regulated ductal secretion of a bicarbonate-rich solution, so-called *ductular bile flow*. They express secretin receptors, the cystic fibrosis transmembrane conductance regulator (CFTR), the chloride–bicarbonate exchanger and somatostatin receptors. Interaction of secretin with its receptor increases intracellular cyclic AMP synthesis and activates protein kinase A (PKA) which activates the chloride channel (CFTR). Function of the chloride– bicarbonate exchanger depends upon the transport of chloride ions by CFTR into the bile duct. Chloride within the bile duct lumen is reabsorbed into cholangiocytes in exchange for bicarbonate [13]. Interaction of somatostatin with its receptor (SSTR2) on the basolateral surface of large cholangiocytes depresses cyclic AMP synthesis, a reversal of the above [7]. Bombesin and vasoactive intestinal peptide (VIP) increase bile flow through stimulation of the chloride–bicarbonate exchanger. Gastrin, insulin and endothelin inhibit secretin-induced bicarbonate-rich choleresis. Acetyl choline increases basal- and secretin-stimulated bicarbonate secretion. Secretin triggers the insertion of aquaporin 1 into the apical membrane of the cholangi-ocyte and this facilitates transport of water into bile. Aquaporin 4, in the basolateral membrane, subserves entry of water into the cell [14].

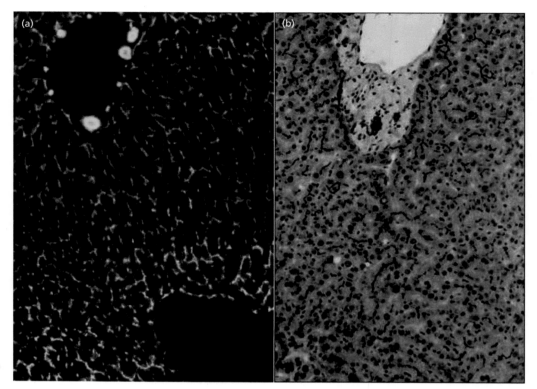

Fig. 11.8. (a) Bile flow is made visible within the canaliculi by the presence of the fluoroscein-conjugated bile acid, cholyl lysyl fluoroscein [9]. (b) Immunostaining (dark brown) by antibodies to the bile acid transporter (BSEP) show its expression to be confined to the canalicular membrane.

Ursodeoxycholic acid and other bile acids with a p*Ka* which is sufficiently high that it enables them to exist within bile in their non-ionized (protonated) state, may be reabsorbed across the biliary epithelium by non-ionic diffusion. Such bile acid 'short circuits' from bile duct to liver ('cholehepatic shunting') explain the choleretic effect and high biliary bicarbonate secretion associated with ursodeoxycholic acid and nor-bile acids [15].

Bile acid metabolism and transport

The human liver synthesizes the primary bile acids—cholic acid (3α,7α,12α trihydroxy cholanoic acid), chenodeoxycholic acid (3α,7α dihydroxycholanoic acid) and a little (1%) ursodeoxycholic acid, the 7β isomer of chenodeoxycholic acid (see Chapter 2). Their dehydroxylation by bacteria in the intestine produces deoxycholic acid (3α,12α dihydroxy) and lithocholic acid (3α monohydroxy), known as secondary bile acids. The liver conjugates both primary and secondary bile acids with either glycine or taurine. The bile acids circulate from liver to intestine and back about 6–10 times per day, about 5% being replaced by *de novo* hepatic synthesis to compensate for their loss in faeces. Provided bile acid loss in faeces does not exceed 20%, a constant bile acid pool size is sustained. This is through feedback regulation of *de novo* bile acid synthesis by the farnesoid X receptor as well as by cytokines and by a peptide (FGF-19) liberated by bile acids from the ileal enterocyte [15,16]. Protection against the potentially severe toxicity of lithocholic acid is coordinated by the pregnane X receptor which has the potential to switch on all the genes required for its safe metabolism and elimination, including hydroxylation by cytochrome P450 3A, sulphation by sulphotransferase (SULT2A1) and transporter promoted excretion in faeces [17,18] (Fig. 11.9).

Syndrome of cholestasis

Definition

Cholestasis is impaired formation or flow of bile. This can occur at any level between the basolateral (sinusoidal) membrane of the hepatocyte and the ampulla of Vater.

Morphologically, cholestasis is recognized from accumulation of biliary constituents in liver cells and biliary passages.

Clinically, cholestasis results in retention in blood of substances normally excreted in bile typically with elevated levels of serum alkaline phosphatase (biliary isoenzyme), γ-GT and cholesterol. Itching (pruritus) is

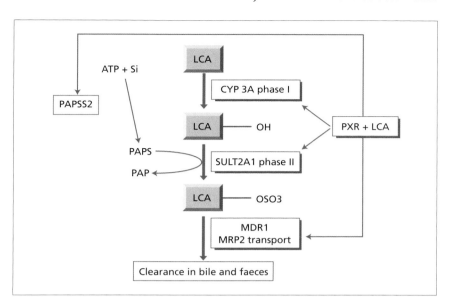

Fig. 11.9. The pregnane X receptor (PXR) is the hepatocyte's ligand for the potentially toxic secondary bile acid, lithocholic acid (LCA) as well as a vast array of other toxic substances. The nuclear receptor coordinates enhanced synthesis of the substrate donor (3'-phosphoadenosine 5'-phosphosulfate synthetase, PAPS) for sulphation, expression of the enzymes required in hydroxylation and sulphation of LCA, (phase I and II biotransformation) as well as expression of the active transport pumps which eliminate the metabolites in bile. CYP 3A, cytochrome P450 3A; SULT 2A1, sulphotransferase 2A1; MDR, multidrug resistance protein.

the most typical symptom but not always present. Bilirubin darkens the urine. Lack of sufficient bile acids for micellar solubilization of the products of intestinal fat digestion causes steatorrhoea and may result in deficiencies of the fat-soluble vitamins A, D, E and K which can not be absorbed in the absence of bile acids.

Classification

Cholestasis may be classified as intra- or extrahepatic, and acute or chronic.

Clinical features

Jaundice is not a constant finding in cholestasis. Patients have been treated for a decade or more on the basis of a mistaken diagnosis of dermatological disease when pruritus was not accompanied by jaundice. The sclerae are yellowed in jaundice but not by other causes of yellowing of the skin. The basal ganglia may be stained yellow in the newborn (kernicterus) due to the high concentration of circulating unconjugated bilirubin having an affinity for neural tissue. Circulating protein-bound bilirubin does not easily enter protein-low tissue fluids; thus exudates tend to be more icteric than transudates. The extremely rare symptom of xanthopsia (seeing yellow) is typically due to deficiency of vitamin A caused by the cholestasis and resolves within a few hours of parenteral administration of vitamin A.

Typically, the cholestatic patient feels well. The *liver* is usually enlarged with a firm smooth non-tender edge. *Splenomegaly* is unusual except in biliary cirrhosis where portal hypertension has developed. Stools become pale, their colour giving a good indication of whether

cholestasis is total, intermittent or decreasing. Prominent features of cholestasis, both acute and chronic, are itching and malabsorption of fat and fat-soluble nutrients. Hence, chronic cholestasis is associated with bone disease (hepatic osteodystrophy), cutaneous deposition of cholesterol (xanthoma, xanthelasma) and darkening of the skin by melanin. In steatorrhoea stools are loose, pale, bulky and offensive, mandating a reduction of dietary fat intake to prevent associated weight loss; caloric substitution can be achieved with medium-chain triglycerides as they are absorbed directly into the portal vein, by-passing the requirement for lipolysis, micelle formation and lymphatic chylomicron transportation which are essential components of long-chain triglyceride assimilation (Table 11.1).

Itching (Fig. 11.10). Itching is typically mild before breakfast and at its worst in the evenings, hindering sleep. Night-time fasting permits catch-up concentration of biliary elements in the gallbladder, but during the day they re-accumulate in the systemic circulation due to impaired hepatic clearance of each meal-stimulated enterohepatic cycle of bile. The anion-binding resin cholestyramine is therefore most efficacious if present in the duodenum during vigorous gallbladder emptying stimulated by a good breakfast. The association of pruritus with cholestasis suggests that it is caused by a substance normally excreted in bile, and the efficacy of cholestyramine in providing relief from pruritus strongly suggests that the pruritogenic factor has an enterohepatic circulation. Nevertheless, the severity of pruritus does not correlate with the concentration of any naturally occurring bile acid in serum or skin [19]. Disappearance of itching when end-stage liver failure

Table 11.1. Dietary management of the cholestatic patient

Nutrient	Deficiency state	Diagnosis	Management
Fat	Steatorrhoea	History Inspection and/ or analysis of stool	Dietary neutral fat should be restricted if steatorrhoea is associated with weight loss Calorie intake can be maintained with MCT*
Protein	Muscle wasting, growth failure	Monitor mid arm circumference	High protein diet; nutritional supplements.
Vitamin A	Night blindness, xerophthalmia	Visual evoked responses	Oral or parenteral replacement
Vitamin D	Osteomalacia, tetany, proximal myopathy	*Fasting* plasma phosphate and calcium levels should be monitored	Oral or parenteral replacement
Vitamin E	Spinocerebellar degeneration, haemolysis	Areflexia, ataxia, decreased proprioception and vibration sense, abnormal eye movements; plasma vitamin E levels	Oral or parenteral replacement
Vitamin K	Excessive bleeding and bruising	Prothrombin time	Oral or parenteral replacement †

*MCT: medium-chain triglycerides are absorbed into the portal vein, thus by-passing the need for digestion, micelle formation and lymphatic transport which are essential for long-chain triglyceride assimilation. MCT can be given as Liquigen (Scientific Hospital Supplies Ltd, UK) or as MCT (coconut) oil for cooking or in salads.
†Parenteral vitamin K (10 mg) should correct prothrombin time within a day if prolongation due to deficiency alone.

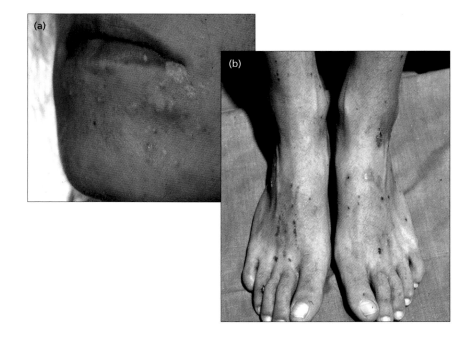

Fig. 11.10. A patient with cholestatic jaundice who demonstrates the classical features of (a) cutaneous cholesterol deposits and (b) scratch marks in response to pruritus.

ensues suggests that the agent responsible is manufactured by the liver. Despite these clues as to its identity the exact cause of pruritus remains unknown. Attention has turned towards agents that may produce itching by a central neurotransmitter mechanism [20]. Opiate agonists induce opioid receptor mediated scratching activity of central origin. Cholestatic animals have evidence of increased opioidergic tone, reversible by naloxone. Opiate antagonists reduce scratching in cholestatic patients [21] and may produce opioid withdrawal-like reactions.

Fatigue. This is troublesome in 70–80% of patients with chronic cholestatic liver disease. Experimental data show behavioural changes in cholestasis and suggest a central mechanism involving serotoninergic neurotransmission and/or neuroendocrine defects in the corticotrophin-releasing hormone axis [22].

Fat-soluble vitamins [23] (Table 11.1). Before any invasive techniques are embarked upon for investigation and treatment of cholestasis, it may be necessary to administer *vitamin K* parenterally to correct the prolonged prothrombin time. In prolonged cholestasis, plasma *vitamin A* levels fall due to poor absorption, and hepatic reserves may become exhausted, resulting in failure of dark adaption (night blindness). *Vitamin D deficiency* may lead to osteomalacia. Spinocerebellar degeneration has been reported in adolescents with cholestasis and cystic fibrosis-induced *vitamin E deficiency* [24]. The picture is of cerebellar ataxia, posterior column dysfunction, peripheral neuropathy and retinal degeneration. If the serum bilirubin level exceeds $100\,\mu mol/L$ ($6\,mg/dL$) almost all adult patients with cholestasis will have subnormal vitamin E levels.

Xanthomas. Flat or slightly raised yellow skin deposits are usually noted around the eyes (xanthelasma) (Fig. 11.10) but may also appear in palmar creases, below the breast and on the neck, chest or back. Tuberous (nodular) lesions are found on extensor surfaces, on pressure points and in scars. Cholesterol deposits may regress and disappear during treatment with statins, following resolution of cholestasis or with advancing hepatocellular failure.

Hepatic osteodystrophy [23] (Table 11.2)

Bone disease is a complication of chronic liver disease, particularly chronic cholestasis. Untreated, it can lead to bone pain and fractures. Studies show that *osteoporosis* is responsible for the bone changes in the majority of patients with primary biliary cirrhosis and primary sclerosing cholangitis, although the potential for *osteomalacia* also exists. In osteoporosis there is loss of bone,

Table 11.2. Factors increasing risk of bone disease in chronic cholestasis

General	Reduced physical activity
	Low body mass index
	Increasing age
	Female sex
	Reduced sunlight exposure
Cholestasis	Vitamin D and K deficiency
	Reduced calcium availability
	Increased serum bilirubin
Genetic	Vitamin D receptor genotype
Hormonal	Menopause/ hypogonadism
	Steroid therapy

both matrix and mineral. In osteomalacia there is defective mineralization of osteoid. Risk factors for osteoporosis include low body mass index, steroid treatment, increasing age and female sex [25]. One-third of patients with primary biliary cirrhosis and approximately 10% of those with primary sclerosing cholangitis had a bone density value below the fracture threshold, osteoporosis generally being associated with advanced disease [26]. In a more recent study, no increase was found in the incidence of metabolic bone disease in primary biliary cirrhosis patients who had been treated with regular calcium and vitamin D supplements [27].

Bone disease manifests as loss of height, back pain (usually midthoracic or lumbar), collapsed vertebrae and fractures with minimal trauma, particularly of ribs. Spinal X-rays may show vertebrae of low density, as well as compression. *Bone mineral density* may be measured by dual photon absorptiometry. The cause of osteoporosis in chronic cholestatic liver disease is multifactorial. Factors that may play a role include vitamin D, calcitonin, parathyroid hormone, growth hormone and sex steroids. External influences in cholestatic patients include immobility, poor nutrition and reduced muscle mass. Vitamin D levels may be reduced due to malabsorption, inadequate diet and reduced exposure to the sun. Activation of vitamin D, by 25-hydroxylation in liver and 1-hydroxylation in the kidney, is normal. In patients with primary biliary cirrhosis, polymorphisms of the vitamin D receptor (VDR) gene correlate with the degree of osteoporosis and vertebral fracture [28].

Early experience with liver transplantation showed that improved bone density was delayed until 1–5 years after transplant. Before recovery, spontaneous bone fractures were common, occurring in 35% of patients with primary biliary cirrhosis in the first year. Heavy exposure to corticosteroids for immunosuppression probably played a part in this increased fracture rate. Vitamin D levels may not return to normal for several months after transplantation and supplementation has been recommended [29].

It is important to consider vitamin D deficiency in patients with chronic cholestasis. Cholestatic patients may fail to go out in the sun or take an adequate diet. Absorption is poor due to steatorrhoea. As chelation by cholestyramine may exacerbate the deficiency, vitamin D supplements, ursodeoxycholic acid and lipid-soluble medications such as digoxin should be taken in the evening to distance them from possible chelation by cholestyramine taken with breakfast. Vitamin D deficiency may be masked by secondary hyperparathyroidism, which will result in a compensatory mobilization of calcium from bones to normalize serum levels. Therefore blood testing for osteomalacia needs to be after an overnight fast when hypophosphataemia due to secondary hyperparathyroidism is most easily detected. Confirmation that vitamin D deficiency is the cause can be obtained by measurement of plasma vitamin D levels.

A rarer manifestation of bone disease is painful *osteoarthropathy* in the wrists and ankles [30], a non-specific complication of chronic liver disease.

Changes in copper metabolism

Approximately 80% of absorbed copper is normally excreted in bile and lost in faeces. In chronic cholestasis (as in primary biliary cirrhosis, biliary atresia or sclerosing cholangitis), hepatic copper levels may equal or exceed those found in Wilson's disease. However, in cholestasis the retained copper is sequestered and not hepatotoxic. Kayser–Fleischer rings may be seen. Finding copper-associated protein on orcein staining of liver tissue supports a diagnosis of cholestasis.

Development of hepatocellular failure

Initially, liver cells appear to function well despite the presence of cholestasis. However, if unrelieved for several years cholestasis will ultimately lead to liver cell failure as indicated by rapidly deepening jaundice, ascites, oedema and a lowered serum albumin level. Pruritus declines and the bleeding tendency is not controlled by parenteral vitamin K. Hepatic encephalopathy is terminal.

Extrahepatic effects

Deep cholestatic jaundice may result in serious complications when the patient is stressed by dehydration, blood loss or investigative and therapeutic procedures of a surgical or non-surgical nature. It confers a high susceptibility to sepsis, acute renal failure, haemorrhage and wound dehiscence. Cardiovascular responses are abnormal and peripheral vasoconstriction in response to hypotension is impaired. The kidneys have an increased susceptibility to hypotension and hypoxic damage [31]. Processes involved in responding to sepsis and in wound healing are impaired. The prolonged prothrombin time is correctable with vitamin K but coagulation may still be abnormal due to platelet dysfunction. The gastric mucosa is more susceptible to ulceration.

Haematology

Iron deficiency anaemia in a patient presenting with obstructive jaundice may indicate bleeding from carcinoma of the papilla of Vater. A polymorphonuclear leucocytosis suggests cholangitis or underlying neoplastic disease.

Biochemistry

In cholestatic jaundice the *serum conjugated bilirubin level* is raised. When the cholestasis is relieved, serum bilirubin values fall slowly to normal. This is in part due to bilirubin which has become covalently bound to albumin. The *serum alkaline phosphatase level* is raised, usually to more than three times the upper limit of normal. *Serum γ-GT levels* are raised. In chronic cholestasis plasma cholesterol and phospholipid levels are greatly increased, probably reflecting increased hepatic synthesis, regurgitation from bile and reduced lecithin cholesterol acyl transferase activity. Atheroma is not a complication of prolonged cholestasis and florid hypercholesterolaemia does not produce atherosclerosis in primary biliary cirrhosis [32]. Serum cholesterol values fall terminally.

The lipoproteins of cholestasis differ from those found in atherosclerosis. The abnormal lipoproteins appear by electron microscopy as disc-shaped particles. *Lipoprotein-X* is a spherical particle, 70 nm in diameter, increased in both intra- and extrahepatic cholestasis.

In cholestasis, conjugated bilirubin is present in urine. Urinary urobilinogen is excreted in proportion to the amount of bile reaching the duodenum. Bile salts accumulate in the blood. Measurement of serum bile acids (normal less than 15 μmol/L) is particularly useful in diagnosis of cholestasis of pregnancy when pruritus may be deemed insignificant on the basis of normal values of alkaline phosphatase and γ-GT.

Bacteriology

In the febrile patient with bile duct obstruction or primary sclerosing cholangitis, blood cultures should be performed. Septicaemia, especially due to Gram-negative organisms, complicates ductal gallstones, and occurs following invasive cholangiography if complete resolution of obstruction was not achieved at the end of the procedure.

Investigation of the jaundiced patient

A careful history and physical examination with routine biochemical and haematological tests are essential. Stool should be inspected and occult blood examination performed. Urine is tested for bilirubin and urobilinogen excess. The place of special tests such as ultrasound, liver biopsy and cholangiography will depend on the category of jaundice. Clinical features from an accurate history and physical examination often suggest the cause of the cholestasis. *Pain* can be related to duct stones, tumour or gallbladder disease. *Fever* and *rigors* may indicate cholangitis due to duct stone or biliary stricture (*Charcot's intermittent biliary fever*). The patient may have taken *drug treatment* that coincides with the development of cholestasis. *Ulcerative colitis* raises the possibility of primary sclerosing cholangitis. On examination, hepatic nodularity may indicate metastatic *malignancy*. A palpable gallbladder suggests non-calculous biliary obstruction. Other abdominal masses may indicate a primary lesion such as carcinoma of the stomach or colon. Endoscopy, rectal examination and sigmoidoscopy may indicate carcinoma.

Clinical history

The onset is extremely important.

Cholestatic jaundice may develop slowly with an antecedent history of pruritus for months or years. Biliary colic typically involves an episode, persisting for several hours, of severe epigastric or right upper quadrant abdominal pain with radiation to the tip of the right scapula which antedates the onset of jaundice by a day or two. Associated dyspepsia and intolerance of dietary fat support a diagnosis of choledocholithiasis. Pyrexia with rigors strongly suggests cholangitis associated with gallstones or biliary stricture. Jaundice after biliary tract surgery suggests residual calculus, injury to the bile duct at the time of surgery or drug-induced hepatitis. Persistent central back pain which causes the patient to lean forward usually indicates pancreatic carcinoma. Progressive weight loss favours an underlying carcinoma or a marked chronic pancreatitis, for example autoimmune [33]. Jaundice in a patient with prior history of malignancy may be due to hepatic metastases. Jaundice occurring in seriously ill hospitalized patients is often caused by sepsis and/or shock, or drug [34].

The patient is asked about previous *drug treatment*. Treatment with co-amoxiclavulanic acid may precede onset of jaundice by several weeks. Cholestatic jaundice may persist for many months following adverse reactions to certain drugs, including erythromycin, flucloxacillin and chlorpromazine (see Chapter 24).

Nausea, anorexia and an aversion to smoking (in smokers) which have preceded the onset of jaundice by a few days suggest viral hepatitis or drug jaundice. *Contact* with jaundiced persons, particularly in nurseries, camps, hospitals and schools, is noted. Close contact with patients on renal units or with drug abusers is recorded, as is any *injection* in the preceding 6 months. 'Injections' include blood tests, drug abuse, tuberculin testing, dental treatment and tattooing, and any parenterally administered therapy including blood or plasma transfusions. Consumption of *shellfish* and previous *travel* to areas where hepatitis is endemic should be noted.

Occupation should be noted, particularly employment involving alcohol or contact with water carrying risk of Weil's disease.

Place of origin (Mediterranean, African or Far East) may suggest carriage of hepatitis B or C.

Family history is important with respect to jaundice, hepatitis and anaemia. Positive histories are helpful in diagnosing haemolytic jaundice, congenital hyperbilirubinemia and hepatitis.

Examination (Fig. 11.11)

Age and sex. A parous, middle-aged, obese female is likely to develop gallstones. The probability of malignant biliary obstruction increases with age. Drug jaundice is very rare in childhood. The incidence of type A hepatitis decreases as age advances but no age is exempt from type B, D and C.

General examination. Anaemia may indicate haemolysis, cancer or cirrhosis. Gross weight loss suggests cancer or severe malabsorption. The patient with haemolytic jaundice is a mild yellow colour, with hepatocellular jaundice is orange and with prolonged biliary obstruction has a deep greenish hue. A hunched-up position suggests pancreatic carcinoma. In alcoholics, the skin signs of cirrhosis should be noted. Sites to be examined for a primary tumour include breasts, thyroid, stomach, colon, rectum and lung. Lymphadenopathy is noted, and Virchow's node sought.

Mental state. Slight intellectual deterioration with minimal personality change suggests hepatocellular jaundice. Fetor hepaticus and 'flapping' tremor indicate impending hepatic coma.

Skin changes. In chronic cholestasis, scratch marks, melanin pigmentation, finger clubbing, xanthoma on the eyelids (xanthelasma), extensor surfaces and palmar creases, and hyperkeratosis may be found.

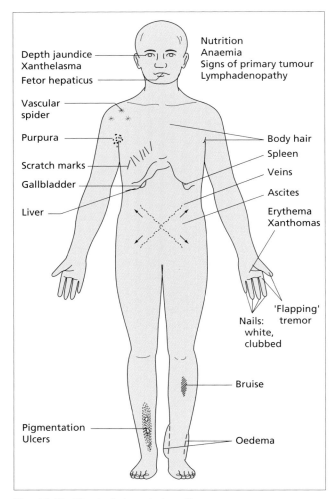

Fig. 11.11. Physical signs in jaundice.

Bruising may indicate a clotting defect. Purpuric spots, most often noticed on forearms, axillae or shins, may be related to the thrombocytopenia of cirrhosis. Other cutaneous manifestations of cirrhosis include vascular spiders, palmar erythema, white nails and loss of secondary sexual hair.

Pigmentation of the shins and ulcers may be seen in some forms of congenital haemolytic anaemia.

Multiple venous thromboses suggest carcinoma of the body of the pancreas. Ankle oedema may indicate cirrhosis, or obstruction of the inferior vena cava due to thrombosis, hepatic or pancreatic malignancy.

Abdominal examination. A very large nodular liver suggests cancer. A small liver may indicate severe hepatitis or cirrhosis, and excludes extrahepatic cholestasis in which the liver is enlarged and smooth. The edge may be tender in hepatitis, congestive heart failure, alcohol-

ism and bacterial cholangitis. In choledocholithiasis the gallbladder area may be tender and Murphy's sign positive. A palpable, and sometimes visibly enlarged, gallbladder suggests pancreatic cancer (Courvoisier's sign).

Splenomegaly occurs with haemolytic states, infiltrative disorders such as Hodgkin's disease and portal hypertension. Ascites may be due to cirrhosis or to malignant disease within the abdomen.

Laboratory investigation

Serum biochemical tests

Serum bilirubin confirms jaundice, indicates depth and is used to follow progress. Serum alkaline phosphatase values more than three times normal strongly suggest cholestasis if bone disease is absent and γ-GT is elevated.

Serum albumin and globulin levels are little changed in jaundice of short duration. In more chronic hepatocellular jaundice the albumin is depressed and globulin increased.

Serum transaminases are more highly elevated in hepatitis with variable but lower levels in cholestatic jaundice. Higher values may sometimes be found transiently with acute bile duct obstruction due to a stone.

Haematology

Increased leucocyte counts are found with acute cholangitis, underlying malignant disease and alcoholic hepatitis. If the prothrombin time is prolonged due to cholestasis vitamin K_1 10 mg parenterally leads to its correction within a few hours, whereas patients with hepatocellular jaundice show little response.

If haemolysis is suspected, investigations should include a reticulocyte count and examination of the blood film. Brisk intravascular haemolysis reflected by haemoglobinuria and fragmented red cells on blood film is classically seen in Wilson's disease, and may be caused by hepatitis A in individuals affected by glucose-6-phosphate dehydrogenase deficiency or by parvovirus infection in hereditary spherocytosis.

Diagnostic routine

Clinical evaluation allows the clinical picture to be categorized into hepatocellular, infiltrative, possible extrahepatic biliary obstruction and likely extrahepatic biliary obstruction. Various algorithms are possible. The sequence employed depends on the clinical evaluation, the facilities available and the risk of each investigation. Cost plays a part.

Radiology

A chest film is taken to show primary and secondary tumours and any irregularity and elevation of the right diaphragm due to an enlarged or nodular liver.

Visualization of the bile ducts (see Chapter 12)

The first procedure should be real-time ultrasound, which allows the distinction between cholestasis with dilated bile ducts and cholestasis without duct dilatation. If ultrasound does not show dilated ducts the next step depends upon the clinical data.

If ultrasound shows dilated ducts, cholangiography is necessary with magnetic resonance cholangiopancreatography (MRCP) being the procedure of choice. Endoscopic retrograde cholangiopancreatography (ERCP) has more risks and is reserved for additional diagnostic modalities such as biliary cytology or therapy to relieve obstruction caused by stones and strictures. For direct cholangiography ERCP is generally the first choice. However, if access to the duodenal papilla is impossible because of duodenal stenosis or a previous hepaticojejunostomy or when ERCP has failed to drain an obstructed and potentially infected biliary system then percutaneous cholangiography (PTC) should be undertaken.

Liver biopsy

If intrahepatic cholestasis due to a drug or infiltration is likely from clinical data and scanning then liver biopsy may be appropriate following correction of the prothrombin time with vitamin K.

Differential diagnosis

Extrahepatic cholestasis

Extrahepatic cholestasis encompasses conditions where there is physical obstruction to the bile ducts. The commoner causes include: a stone in the common duct (Chapter 12); carcinoma of the pancreas or ampulla of Vater (Chapter 13); benign bile duct strictures (Chapter 12); primary or secondary sclerosing cholangitis, for example autoimmune cholangitis (with or without autoimmune pancreatitis) (Chapter 16); and cholangiocarcinoma (Chapter 13).

Intrahepatic cholestasis

The cause of intrahepatic cholestasis lies within the hepatic lobules. The general clinical and biochemical picture is the same as for extrahepatic cholestasis. Febrile cholangitis is absent. The liver is not necessarily enlarged and is not tender. The five main types are discussed here.

Hepatocellular

Cholestasis is complex. Hepatic injury has as one of its major effects impaired bile formation and secretion.

Viral hepatitis (Chapter 17) is sometimes purely cholestatic, more commonly in those on oral contraceptives. The history of exposure to risk factors and the nature of the prodromal symptoms may be helpful. The liver biopsy appearances are those of acute viral hepatitis.

Acute alcoholic hepatitis (Chapter 25) can be cholestatic. The history of alcohol abuse, the large tender liver and cutaneous spider naevi are helpful points. Chronic pancreatitis may be associated.

Cholestasis develops with *prolonged parenteral nutrition* especially in neonates (Chapter 29) but also in adults [35]. The cholestasis of *intrahepatic atresia* (infantile cholangiopathy) (Chapter 29) may be related to viral injury to intrahepatic bile ducts.

Zellweger's syndrome [36]. This is very rare and presents before 6 months of age with progressive cholestasis and hepatomegaly. There is associated mental retardation, a characteristic facies, hypotonia and renal cysts. It is caused by a defect in hepatic peroxisomes and bile acid oxidation is abnormal with the appearance of C27 bile acids in serum and bile. Affected individuals have a short survival of only a few years. Oral bile acid therapy should be considered [37].

In some patients with *cryptogenic macronodular cirrhosis* cholestasis may be prominent.

Canalicular membrane changes

Sometimes cholestasis occurs in a 'pure' form with absence of any cellular infiltrate or other evidence of liver injury. Cholestatic reactions to oral contraceptives (Chapter 24) and pregnancy (Chapter 30) fall into this group.

Drugs include the promazine group, long-acting sulphonamides, antibiotics and antithyroid drugs (Chapter 24). The history is important and liver biopsy aids diagnosis.

Genetic defects in transporters [38]

The syndromes of benign recurrent intrahepatic cholestasis (BRIC) and progressive familial intrahepatic cholestasis (PFIC) comprise subgroups for which genetic defects have been found or mapped.

Benign recurrent intrahepatic cholestasis (BRIC)

This rare condition presents as recurrent episodes of cholestatic jaundice. Main bile duct obstruction must be excluded by ultrasonography and magnetic resonance imaging (MRCP). Other causes known to produce cholestasis, such as drugs, should be ruled out. There should be symptom-free intervals of several months or years. The first patient described survived 22 episodes and three laparotomies [39]. Another patient had 27 attacks over 38 years.

The onset is with itching, occasionally with influenza-type illness and vomiting. Twenty-five to 50% of patients suffer abdominal pain. There is often fatigue, anorexia and weight loss. Serum alkaline phosphatase levels increase but transaminases are virtually normal. Jaundice appears and typically persists for 3–4 months.

Hepatic histology shows cholestasis with bile plugs, portal zone expansion, mononuclear cells and some liver cell degeneration, mainly in zone 1. Hepatic histology and liver function are normal in remission.

Aetiology. The disease is autosomal recessive and the gene locus involved has been mapped to the *FIC1* locus as for *PFIC1* [40]. Environmental factors are suggested by the allergic diathesis; some patients have rashes. The condition may recur at particular times of the year.

Treatment. The attacks are self-limiting and vary in duration. Corticosteroid treatment is probably of little benefit. *S*-adenosylmethionine is ineffective. Results with ursodeoxycholic acid are conflicting. Rifampicin has been highly effective in some [41].

Progressive familial intrahepatic cholestasis (PFIC) [42]

This is a group of rare, autosomal recessive diseases characterized by cholestasis in infancy (see also Chapter 29, Table 29.5). Three types are recognized.

PFIC type 1 (Byler's disease) is an autosomal recessive disease described in the Amish population (descendants of Jacob and Nancy Byler). Recurrent episodes of intrahepatic cholestasis lead to permanent cholestasis, fibrosis, cirrhosis and liver failure. Liver transplantation may be necessary in the first decade of life. Characteristically serum γ-GT is not or only slightly increased. Genetic studies have mapped the *PFIC1* locus in Amish descendants to chromosome 18q21–q22. This region contains the gene *FIC1* which encodes a P-type ATPase and in Amish patients with FIC a single specific mutation is found [40]. The pathogenetic mechanism causing this condition is not clear.

FIC2 is due to mutations in the bile salt export pump [43]. In contrast to FIC1, FIC2 often begins as a non-specific giant cell hepatitis which may not be distinguishable from intrahepatic neonatal giant cell hepatitis. Mutation of gene and absence of canalicular bile salt export pump have been shown in patients with FIC2. Affected individuals may or may not be jaundiced.

There may be progressive cholestasis requiring liver transplantation.

FIC3 is due to mutations in the *MDR3* gene (phosphoflippase). Serum γ-GT is usually markedly elevated. Lack of the biliary phospholipid required for assimilation of bile acids into mixed micelles results in abnormally high concentrations of non-micellar biliary bile acids which are toxic to cholangiocytes and hepatocytes. There is extensive bile duct proliferation on biopsy. In this group symptoms appear later in life than in FIC types 1 and 2 and presentation in adult life is reported [44]. Liver transplantation is often necessary. Cholestasis in pregnancy has been reported in a family with FIC type 3 but can also be seen in other FIC subtypes.

Obstruction to the lumen of canaliculi and ductules

Following massive haemolytic episodes such as sickle cell crisis, the lumen of bile canaliculi may be expanded and occluded by solid biliary precipitate. A similar picture occurs in hereditary protoporphyria when the biliary concretions show typical Maltese cross signs on imaging with polarized light (Fig. 11.12).

Canalicular concretions and inspissated casts in ductules were also seen due to benoxaprofen, an antirheumatoid drug withdrawn from the market because of fatalities due to its hepatotoxicity [45]. Bile plugs in dilated periportal cholangioles are highly characteristic of cholestasis in *severe bacterial infections*, particularly in childhood or postoperatively. Inspissated bile is also seen in cholestasis associated with *cystic fibrosis*.

Ductopenia

Inspection of portal tracts in some patients with cholestasis reveals the triad is incomplete and that in more than 50%, the portal vein and hepatic artery have no accompanying interlobular bile duct. This ductopenia is termed either *paucity of intrahepatic bile ducts* or the *vanishing bile duct syndrome*.

Adults and adolescents with *paucity of intrahepatic bile ducts* are being increasingly described. The condition may be familial [46] or drug-induced [47], or a late-onset form of the non-syndromic type seen in children [48].

Extreme irreversible ductopenia may occur as part of chronic allograft rejection following liver transplantation, in drug jaundice (flucloxacillin, coamoxyclavulanic acid) [49] and Hodgkin's disease [50]. In severe cases all trace of interlobular bile ducts is lost and bile has the appearance of clear water. Lesser degrees of ductopenia are seen in sarcoid, primary sclerosing cholangitis (Chapter 16) and primary biliary cirrhosis (Chapter 15).

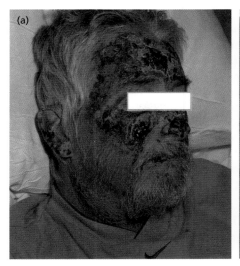
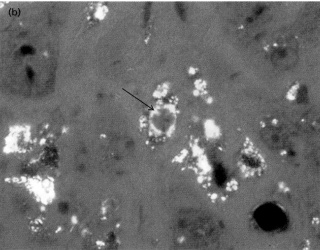

Fig. 11.12. (a) Severe sunburn is seen as a result of photosensitivity due to protoporphyria. (b) Biliary canaliculi and ductules are occluded by protoporphyrin pigment which demonstrates the classical Maltese cross sign on exposure to polarized light (arrow).

Treatment

Biliary decompression: resection

The choice between non-surgical and surgical treatment will depend upon the cause of obstruction and the clinical state of the patient. Common duct stones are treated by endoscopic sphincterotomy and removal (Chapter 12). In malignant obstruction the resectability of the tumour is assessed. If judged inoperable or irresectable, a stent is inserted to drain the bile duct by endoscopy or, if that fails, by the percutaneous route in patients with severe pruritus. A laparotomy for by-pass with hepaticojejunostomy and Roux-en-Y is the alternative. The approach employed depends upon the patient, the facilities and the expertise available.

Preparation of the patient for any of these procedures is critical in order to avoid complications that include renal failure, which may occur in 5–10% of patients [31] and sepsis. *Coagulation* is corrected with parenteral vitamin K. *Dehydration* and *hypotension*, which can lead to acute tubular necrosis, are prevented by intravenous hydration, usually with 0.9% NaCl, and close monitoring of fluid balance. *Mannitol* is given to protect renal function but patients must be well hydrated before its use. A trial has questioned its benefit [51]. Postoperative renal dysfunction may in part be caused by circulating endotoxin derived from increased intestinal absorption. To reduce absorption of endotoxin, oral deoxycholate or lactulose have been given and appear to protect against renal impairment after surgery [52]. For all these reasons surgery may not be appropriate if no prolongation of life is expected. To reduce the risk of septic complications after both non-surgical and surgical intervention,

antibiotic is given beforehand. The duration of continued antibiotic treatment after the procedure will depend upon whether or not there is evidence of sepsis, and how successful biliary decompression has been.

The important factors associated with increased postoperative morbidity and mortality are an initial haematocrit of 30% or less, a serum bilirubin value exceeding 200 µmol/L (12 mg/dL) and malignancy. Deep jaundice can be relieved preoperatively by percutaneous external drainage or endoscopic stenting but randomized controlled studies have not shown benefit [53].

Medical

Pruritus [54] (Table 11.3)

Pruritus is relieved in patients with biliary obstruction by external or internal *biliary drainage*. Itching disappears or is much improved after 24–48 h.

Cholestyramine [55] should always be taken to mix with breakfast in the stomach. Pruritus is least at this time of day and the pruritic factor has probably been concentrated in the gallbladder during overnight fasting. In most patients with chronic cholestasis and partial biliary obstruction this will provide relief after a week or so. If not, another sachet (4 g) may be given after breakfast. Further doses can be taken with meals later in the day but with greatly diminished efficacy. This, together with the need to avoid mixing cholestyramine with other medications, makes it wise to avoid the resin in the evening when other prescribed medications can be ingested. The maintenance dose is usually 4 g/day but occasionally patients may tolerate as much as 12 g/day. Relief from pruritus is delayed for several days and

Table 11.3. Drug treatment of pruritus

Routine	Cholestyramine
Careful use	Rifampicin (often highly effective)
Experimental	Naloxone, nalmefene; ondansetron; S-adenosyl methionine; propofol
Variable effect	Antihistamine; ursodeoxycholic acid; phenobarbitone (little role)

patients may need encouragement to persevere with it as the drug causes nausea and increases faecal fat. It is particularly valuable for itching associated with primary biliary cirrhosis, primary sclerosing cholangitis, biliary atresia and biliary stricture. The dose should be the smallest one that controls pruritus. Supplements of fat-soluble vitamins may be necessary if it is used long term.

Ursodeoxycholic acid (13–15 mg/kg per day) can reduce itching in patients with primary biliary cirrhosis, perhaps by a choleretic effect or by reducing toxic bile salts. Although its use has been associated with biochemical resolution of drug-induced cholestasis, it is unproven as an antipruritic agent in this and other cholestatic syndromes.

Antihistamines are of value only for their sedative action.

Phenobarbitone may relieve itching in patients resistant to other therapy.

Naloxone, an opiate antagonist given as an intravenous infusion, reduced itching in a randomized controlled trial, but is not appropriate for long-term use. An oral opiate antagonist, nalmefene, is also effective and clinical trials of another orally active opiate antagonist, naltrexone, have also shown benefit [21]. Both oral agents are experimental and not yet in clinical use.

S-adenosyl-L-methionine, which among many effects improves membrane fluidity and acts as an antioxidant, has been used to treat cholestatic syndromes but results are inconsistent.

Rifampicin (300–450 mg daily) relieves pruritus within 7 days [56,57]. It acts via the pregnane X receptor as a powerful inducer of anticholestatic genes involved in biotransformation by the liver coordinated with their active transport into bile and intestine for excretion [17] (Fig. 11.9). Potential side effects include increased risk of gallstone formation, reduction in 25-OH-cholecalciferol levels, drug interactions, hepatotoxicity and emergence of resistant organisms, although successful longer-term use (mean 18 months) is reported in children without clinical or biochemical toxicity [58]. Patients treated with this agent should be carefully selected and frequently monitored.

Bright light therapy (10 000 lux) has been studied and found beneficial in a pilot study [59]. Its use is based on the circadian pattern of cholestatic pruritus.

Interruption of the enterohapatic circulation by *surgical by-pass of the terminal 15% of ileum* decreases pruritus and improves quality of life in children with cholestasis and intractable itching [60].

Plasmapheresis has been used to treat intractable pruritus as well as hypercholesterolaemia associated with xanthomatous neuropathy. The procedure is temporarily effective but costly and labour intensive.

The wide range of partially effective and experimental therapies underlines the difficulty in treating some patients with long-standing cholestasis. Intractable itching may be an indication for *liver transplantation*.

Familial non-haemolytic hyperbilirubinaemias (Table 11.4)

Gilbert's syndrome

This is named after Augustin Gilbert (1858–1927), a Parisian physician. It is defined as benign, familial, mild, unconjugated hyperbilirubinaemia (serum bilirubin 17–85 μmol/L (1–5 mg/dL)) not due to haemolysis and with normal routine tests of liver function and hepatic histology. It affects some 2–5% of the population.

It may be diagnosed by chance at a routine medical examination or when the blood is being examined for another reason. It has an excellent prognosis. Jaundice is mild and intermittent. Deepening follows an intercurrent infection or fasting and may be associated with malaise, nausea and often discomfort over the liver. These symptoms are probably no greater than in normal controls. There are no other abnormal physical signs; the spleen is not palpable.

Patients with Gilbert's syndrome have a deficiency in hepatic bilirubin glucuronidation—about 30% of normal. The bile contains an excess of bilirubin monoglucuronide over the diglucuronide. The genetic basis for Gilbert's syndrome has been clarified by the finding that the promoter region (A(TA)$_6$TAA) of the gene encoding UGT1*1 (Fig. 11.4) has an additional TA dinucleotide, resulting in a change to (A(TA)$_7$TAA) [61]. There is a close relationship between the promoter region genotype and the expression of hepatic bilirubin UGT enzyme activity [62]. Individuals with the 7/7 genotype have the lowest enzyme activity. Heterozygotes (6/7 genotype) have an enzyme activity intermediate between 7/7 and normal wild-type 6/6. Patients with other variations of the A(TA)$_n$TAA allele have also shown elevated serum total bilirubin levels, including the genotypes 5/6, 5/7 and 7/8.

Although a reduced enzyme level is necessary for Gilbert's syndrome, it is not sufficient alone to cause overt jaundice, and other factors such as reduced hepatic uptake of bilirubin (or occult haemolysis) may play a role in the development of hyperbilirubinaemia. Thus

Table 11.4. Isolated rise in serum bilirubin

Type	Diagnostic points
Unconjugated	
Haemolysis	Splenomegaly, blood film, reticulocytosis, Coombs' test, etc.
Gilbert's syndrome	Clinical: jaundice spotted during fasting (e.g. with intercurrent illness); normal serum transaminases; familial
	No bilirubin in urine; no haemolysis (normal reticulocyte count)
	Research: liver biopsy normal but conjugating enzyme reduced; DNA analysis
Crigler–Najjar syndrome	
type I	No conjugating enzyme in liver; no response to phenobarbitone; risk of kernicterus; liver transplantation effective
type II	Severely deficient conjugating enzyme in liver; response to phenobarbitone
Conjugated	
Dubin–Johnson syndrome	Bilirubinuria; black-liver biopsy; no concentration of cholecystographic media; secondary rise in BSP test
Rotor type	Normal liver biopsy; cholecystography normal; BSP test no uptake

BSP, bromsulphalein.

there may be a mild impairment of bromsulphalein (BSP) and tolbutamide clearance (a drug that does not need conjugation) [63].

The variant of the TATAA box found in Gilbert's syndrome is a major factor determining the unconjugated hyperbilirubinaemia in ABO-incompatible neonates and also neonates with prolonged unconjugated hyperbilirubinaemia, persistent unconjugated hyperbilirubinaemia after liver transplantation [64], inherited haemolytic diseases and β thalassaemia where there is also an association with gallstone formation [65].

Specialist diagnostic tests include the increase in serum bilirubin on fasting (Fig. 11.13a) [66], the fall on taking phenobarbitone which induces the hepatic conjugating enzyme (Fig. 11.13b), and the increase following intravenous nicotinic acid which raises the osmotic fragility of red blood cells—but these tests are rarely necessary.

Demonstration of a raised bilirubin level that is predominantly unconjugated, with normal liver enzymes and no evidence of haemolysis, is usually sufficient to reassure the patient who is otherwise asymptomatic and has no abnormal physical signs.

Patients with Gilbert's syndrome have a normal life expectancy and reassurance is the only necessary treatment. Hyperbilirubinaemia is life long, is not associated with increased morbidity but increases with fasting. Thus 'sufferers' should be warned that jaundice can follow an intercurrent infection, repeated vomiting or missed meals. The 'sufferer' is a normal risk for life insurance.

Crigler–Najjar syndrome

This extreme form of familial non-haemolytic jaundice is associated with very high serum unconjugated bilirubin values. Inheritance is autosomal recessive. Deficiency of conjugating enzyme can be demonstrated in the liver. Total pigment in the bile is minimal.

Type I

In untreated patients the serum bilirubin is in excess of 350 μmol/L. No bilirubin conjugating enzyme can be detected in the liver. Bile contains only traces of bilirubin conjugates. Since the serum bilirubin levels eventually stabilize, the patient must have some alternative pathway of bilirubin metabolism.

The molecular defect is in one of the five exons (1*1–5) of the bilirubin UGT1*1 gene (Fig. 11.4). Analysis of the Crigler–Najjar type I mutations by expression in COS cells or fibroblasts shows no bilirubin conjugating activity [68].

By 1999, around 170 cases of Crigler–Najjar type I had been reported in the world literature [2]. Before phototherapy was used, patients died at between 1 and 2 years of age from kernicterus. Phototherapy gives only temporary benefit. Phototherapy degrades unconjugated bilirubin into products including lumibilirubin, which is water soluble and can be secreted into the bile. Some of the photodegradation products may spontaneously revert to natural isomers of unconjugated bilirubin and the oral administration of calcium salts prevents

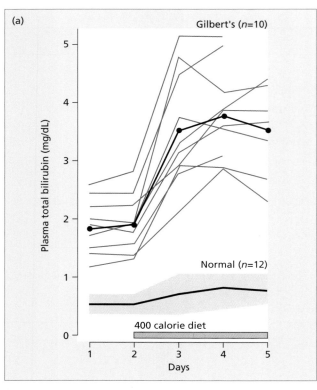

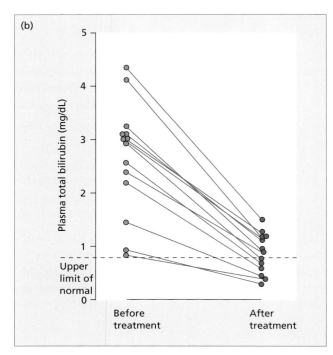

Fig. 11.13. Gilbert's syndrome. (a) The serum unconjugated bilirubin level increases during a 400 calorie diet [66]. (b) The effect of phenobarbitone (60 mg, three times a day) on the serum bilirubin level [67].

their reabsorption. Oral calcium phosphate makes phototherapy more effective [69]. An alternative approach is to inhibit the enzyme haem oxygenase, responsible for formation of bilirubin from haem (Fig. 11.3). Tin protoporphyrin, a haem oxygenase inhibitor, has been demonstrated to give a temporary (5–7 weeks) decrease in plasma unconjugated bilirubin of around 30% [70]. Unconjugated bilirubin *in vitro* damages neurones and astrocytes through increased apoptosis; bilirubin encephalopathy may lead to central deafness, oculomotor palsy, ataxia, choreoathetosis, mental retardation, seizures, spasticity and death. This complication of the Crigler–Najjar syndrome is usually seen in the very young patient but may occur later particularly if patient has a prolonged period of fasting, for example postoperatively.

Orthotopic or orthotopic-auxiliary liver transplantation is the only definitive therapy for Crigler–Najjar type I. It has been recommended that this should be performed at a young age, particularly where reliable phototherapy cannot be guaranteed. Phototherapy, although initially successful, becomes less efficient after puberty. There is always a risk of kernicterus because of lack of compliance and/or events that precipitate hyperbilirubinaemia, including infection, drug interactions, trauma and surgical procedures.

In a survey of 57 patients with Crigler–Najjar type I, 37% had received a liver transplant [71]. Twenty-six per cent had suffered brain damage and in half of these damage was mild.

Experimental treatment using percutaneous, transhepatic intraportal administration of normal hepatocytes successfully reduced the serum bilirubin and the duration of phototherapy in a case report [72].

In Gunn rats, a mutant strain of the Wistar rat in which bilirubin UGT is absent, gene therapy has been attempted [73] with varying success. The metabolic defect has been corrected experimentally by site-specific repair using a chimeric oligonucleotide [74].

Type II

Bilirubin conjugating enzyme in the liver is reduced to less than 10% of normal. The serum bilirubin usually does not exceed 350 μmol/L. Jaundice is present in about half of patients within the first year of life, but can occur as late as 30 years of age. Acute exacerbations of hyperbilirubinaemia may occur during fasting or intercurrent illnesses and bilirubin encephalopathy can develop. The jaundice responds to phenobarbitone and patients survive into adulthood.

DNA analysis of the bilirubin UGT1*1 gene (Fig. 11.4) has shown mutations in exons 1*1–5 [2]. However, expression analysis of these mutants has shown residual enzyme activity, explaining the lower serum bilirubin concentration than those found in Crigler–Najjar type I, the presence of glucuronides in bile and the beneficial effect of phenobarbitone.

Some relatives of patients with Crigler–Najjar syndrome have an elevated serum bilirubin concentration, below that of true Crigler–Najjar but higher than that of Gilbert's syndrome. Analysis of the UGT1*1 gene has suggested that these patients are compound heterozygotes, one allele having the Gilbert's TATAA box mutation, and the other having a Crigler–Najjar mutation [61].

Type II is not always benign and phototherapy and phenobarbitone should be given to keep the serum bilirubin level less than 340 μmol/L (26 mg/dL).

The distinction between type I and type II Crigler–Najjar syndrome is made by observing the response to phenobarbitone treatment. There is no response in patients with type I and type II is confirmed if serum bilirubin level falls by more than 25%. An alternative approach is to analyse duodenal bile after phenobarbitone. In type II there is an increase in biliary mono- and diconjugates. In type I only minimal traces of monoconjugate bilirubin are found.

Dubin–Johnson syndrome

This is a chronic, benign, intermittent jaundice with conjugated hyperbilirubinaemia and bilirubinuria. It is autosomal recessive, and is most frequent in the Middle East among Iranian Jews. The mutation responsible is in the gene encoding MRP-2 which transports bilirubin glucuronides across the canalicular membrane [3]. The defect in this transporter explains the diagnostic pattern seen in the prolonged BSP test [75]. After intravenous injection of BSP there is an initial fall in serum level but the value at 120 min exceeds that seen at 45 min (Fig. 11.14) due to regurgitation into the circulation of its glutathione conjugate, which is normally excreted into bile via MRP-2. The defect in this transporter also explains the increased urinary excretion of coproporphyrin I. Studies in the TR⁻ rat, which has a mutation in the homologous canalicular transporter cMOAT, has allowed characterization of these and other biochemical defects.

The liver, macroscopically, is greenish-black (black-liver jaundice) (Fig. 11.15b). In sections the liver cells show a brown pigment which is neither iron nor bile (Fig. 11.15a). There is no correlation between liver pigment and serum bilirubin levels. The chemical nature of the pigment is not certain. Previously thought due to

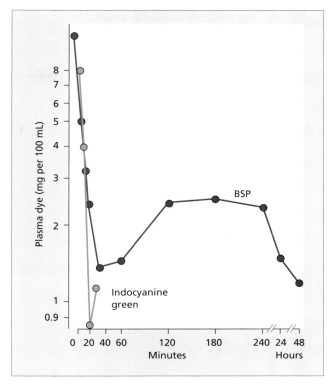

Fig. 11.14. Bromsulphalein (BSP) tolerance test (5 mg/kg i.v.) in a patient with Dubin–Johnson syndrome. At 40 min, the BSP level has almost returned to normal. An increase is then seen at 120, 180 and 240 min. Dye can still be detected in the blood at 48 h. The indocyanine green test is also shown and is normal at 20 min, but also has a tendency to increase at 30 min.

melanin, recent data support the proposal that impaired secretion of anionic metabolites of tyrosine, phenylalanine and tryptophan is responsible. Electron microscopy shows the pigment in dense bodies related to lysosomes (Fig. 11.15c).

Pruritus is absent and the serum alkaline phosphatase and bile acid levels are normal.

In Dubin–Johnson syndrome the contrast media used in intravenous cholangiography are not transported into bile; nevertheless transport of ⁹⁹ᵐTc-HIDA for biliary visualization by scintigraphy is normal.

Rotor type

Rotor syndrome resembles the Dubin–Johnson syndrome in being a form of chronic familial conjugated hyperbilirubinaemia, the main difference being absence of brown pigment in hepatocytes in Rotor type. Electron microscopy may show abnormalities of mitochondria and peroxisomes [76].

The condition also differs from the Dubin–Johnson type in that the gallbladder opacifies on cholecystography and there is no secondary rise in the BSP test. The

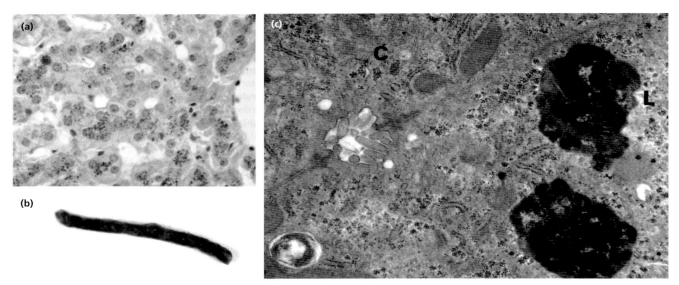

Fig. 11.15. (a) Dubin–Johnson hyperbilirubinaemia. The liver cells and Kupffer cells are packed with a dark pigment which gives the staining reactions of lipofuscin. (H & E, ×275.) (b) This needle liver biopsy from a patient with Dubin–Johnson syndrome is blackish-brown. (c) Lysosomes (L) are enlarged, irregularly shaped and contain granular material and often membrane-bound lipid droplets (normal bile canaliculus, C).

abnormality causing BSP retention appears to be related to a defect in hepatic uptake rather than of biliary excretion as in the Dubin–Johnson syndrome. ^{99m}Tc-HIDA excretion gives no visualization of the liver, gallbladder or biliary tree.

Total urinary coproporphyrins are raised, as in cholestasis.

Family studies make an autosomal inheritance probable. The Rotor type has an excellent prognosis.

References

1 Watchko JF. Kernicterus and the molecular mechanisms of bilirubin-induced CNS injury in newborns. *Neuromolecular Med.* 2006; **8**: 513–529.

2 Jansen PLM. Diagnosis and management of Crigler–Najjar syndrome. *Eur. J. Paediatr.* 1999; **158** (Suppl. 2): S89–94.

3 Paulusma CC, Kool M, Bosma PJ *et al.* A mutation in the human canalicular multispecific organic anion transporter gene causes the Dublin–Johnson syndrome. *Hepatology* 1997; **25**: 1539–1542.

4 Payen L, Sparfel L, Courtois A *et al.* The drug efflux pump MRP2: regulation of expression in physiopathological situations and by endogenous and exogenous compounds. *Cell Biol. Toxicol.* 2002; **18**: 221–233.

5 Layden TJ, Elias E, Boyer JL. Bile formation in the rat: the role of the paracellular shunt pathway. *J. Clin. Invest.* 1978; **62**: 1375–1385.

6 Baiocchi L, LeSage G, Glaser S *et al.* Regulation of cholangiocyte bile secretion. *J. Hepatol.* 1999; **31**: 179–191.

7 Kanno N, LeSage G, Glaser S *et al.* Functional heterogeneity of the intrahepatic biliary epithelium. *Hepatology* 2000; **31**: 555–561.

8 Kamisako T, Kobayashi Y, Takeuchi K *et al.* Recent advances in bilirubin metabolism research: the molecular mechanism of hepatocyte bilirubin transport and its clinical relevance. *J. Gastroenterol.* 2000; **35**: 659–664.

9 Mills CO, Rahman K, Coleman R *et al.* Cholyl-lysylfluorescein: synthesis, biliary excretion in vivo and during single-pass perfusion of isolated perfused rat liver. *Biochim. Biophys. Acta* 1991; **1115**: 151–156.

10 Kosters A, Karpen SJ. Bile acid transporters in health and disease. *Xenobiotica* 2008; **38**: 1043–1071.

11 Stieger B, Meier Y, Meier PJ. The bile salt export pump. *Pflugers Arch.* 2007; **453**: 611–620.

12 Oude Elferink RP, Paulusma CC. Function and pathophysiological importance of ABCB4 (MDR3 P-glycoprotein). *Pflugers Arch.* 2007; **453**: 601–610.

13 Banales JM, Prieto J, Medina JF. Cholangiocyte anion exchange and biliary bicarbonate excretion. *World J. Gastroenterol.* 2006; **12**: 3496–511.

14 Jessner W, Zsembery A, Graf J. Transcellular water transport in hepatobiliary secretion and role of aquaporins in liver. *Wien. Med. Wochenschr.* 2008; **158**: 565–569.

15 Hofmann AF. Biliary secretion and excretion in health and disease: current concepts. *Ann. Hepatol.* 2007; **6**: 15–27.

16 Zollner G, Marschall HU, Wagner M *et al.* Role of nuclear receptors in the adaptive response to bile acids and cholestasis: pathogenetic and therapeutic considerations. *Mol. Pharm.* 2006; **3**: 231–251.

17 Elias E, Mills CO. Coordinated defence and the liver. *Clin. Med.* 2007; **7**: 180–184.

18 Stahl S, Davies MR, Cook DI *et al.* Nuclear hormone receptor-dependent regulation of hepatic transporters and their role in the adaptive response in cholestasis. *Xenobiotica* 2008; **38**: 725–777.

19 Freedman MR, Holzbach RT, Ferguson DR. Pruritus in cholestasis: no direct causative role for bile acid retention. *Am. J. Med.* 1981; **70**: 1011–1016.

20 Jones EA, Bergasa NV. The pruritis of cholestasis. *Hepatology* 1999; **29**: 1003–1006.

21 Wolfhagen FJH, Sternieri E, Hop WCJ *et al.* Oral naltrexone treatment for cholestatic pruritus: a double-blind, placebo-controlled study. *Gastroenterology* 1997; **113**: 1264–1269.

22 Bergasa NV, Mehlman JK, Jones EA. Pruritus and fatigue in primary biliary cirrhosis. *Baillieres Best Pract. Clin. Gastroenterol.* 2000; **14**: 643–655.

23 EASL (European Association for the Study of the Liver). Clinical Practice Guidelines: management of cholestatic liver diseases. *J. Hepatol.* 2009; **51**: 237–267.

24 Elias E, Muller DPR, Scott J. Association of spinocerebellar disorders with cystic fibrosis or chronic childhood cholestasis and very low serum vitamin E. *Lancet* 1981; **2**: 1219–1221.

25 Ormarsdottir S, Ljunggren O, Mallmin H *et al.* Low body mass and use of corticosteroids, but not cholestasis, are risk factors in patients with chronic liver disease. *J. Hepatol.* 1999; **31**: 84–90.

26 Angulo P, Therneau TM, Jorgensen RA *et al.* Bone disease in patients with primary sclerosing cholangitis: prevalence, severity and prediction of progression. *J. Hepatol.* 1998; **29**: 729–735.

27 Bennetti A, Crosignani A, Varenna M *et al.* Primary biliary cirrhosis is not an additional risk factor for bone loss in women receiving regular calcium and vitamin D supplementation: a controlled longitudinal study. *J. Clin. Gastroenterol.* 2008; **42**: 306–311.

28 Springer JE, Cole DEC, Rubin LA *et al.* Vitamin D-receptor genotypes as independent genetic predictors of decreased bone mineral density in primary biliary cirrhosis. *Gastroenterology* 2000; **118**: 145–151.

29 Mells G, Neuberger J. Long-term care of the liver allograft recipient. *Semin. Liver Dis.* 2009; **29**: 102–120.

30 Epstein O, Dick R, Sherlock S. Prospective study of periostitis and finger clubbing in primary biliary cirrhosis and other forms of chronic liver disease. *Gut* 1981; **22**: 203–206.

31 Fogarty BJ, Parks RW, Rowlands BJ *et al.* Renal dysfunction in obstructive jaundice. *Br. J. Surg.* 1995; **82**: 877–884.

32 Sorokin A, Brown JL, Thompson PD. Primary biliary cirrhosis, hyperlipidemia, and atherosclerotic risk: a systematic review. *Atherosclerosis* 2007; **194**: 293–299.

33 Finkelberg DL, Sahani D, Deshpande V *et al.* Autoimmune pancreatitis. *N. Engl. J. Med.* 2006; **355**: 2670–2676.

34 Whitehead MW, Hainsworth I, Kingham JGC. The causes of obvious jaundice in South West Wales: perceptions versus reality. *Gut* 2001; **48**: 409–413.

35 Quigley EM, Marsh MN, Shaffer JL *et al.* Hepatobiliary complications of total parenteral nutrition. *Gastroenterology* 1993; **104**: 286–301.

36 FitzPatrick DR. Zellweger syndrome and associated phenotypes. *J. Med. Genet.* 1996; **33**: 863–868.

37 Setchell KD, Bragetti P, Zimmer-Nechemias L *et al.* Oral bile acid treatment and the patient with Zellweger syndrome. *Hepatology* 1992; **15**: 198–207.

38 Oude Elferink RP, Paulusma CC, Groen AK. Hepatocanicular transport defects: pathophysiologic mechanisms of rare diseases. *Gastroenterology* 2006; **130**: 908–925.

39 Williams R, Cartter MA, Sherlock S *et al.* Idiopathic recurrent cholestasis: a study of the functional and pathological lesions in four cases. *Q. J. Med.* 1964; **33**: 387–399.

40 Bull LN, Juijn JA, Liao M *et al.* Fine-resolution mapping by haplotype evaluation: the examples of PFIC1 and BRIC. *Human Genet.* 1999; **104**: 241–248.

41 Trauner M, Wagner M, Fickert P *et al.* Molecular regulation of hepatobiliary transport systems: clinical implications for understanding and treating cholestasis. *J. Clin. Gastroenterol.* 2005; **39** (Suppl. 2): S111–124.

42 Carlton VE, Pawlikowska L, Bull LN. Molecular basis of intrahepatic cholestasis. *Ann. Med.* 2004; **36**: 606–617.

43 Plass JR, Mol O, Heegsma J *et al.* A progressive familial intrahepatic cholestasis type 2 mutation causes an unstable, temperature-sensitive bile salt export pump. *J. Hepatol.* 2004; **40**: 24–30.

44 Jacquemin E, De Vree JML, Cresteil D *et al.* The wide spectrum of multidrug resistance 3 deficiency: from neonatal cholestasis to cirrhosis of adulthood. *Gastroenterology* 2001; **120**: 1448–1458.

45 Zimmerman HJ, Lewis JH. Drug-induced cholestasis. *Med. Toxicol.* 1987; **2**: 112–160.

46 Burak KW, Pearson DC, Swain MG *et al.* Familial idiopathic adulthood ductopenia: a report of five cases in three generations. *J. Hepatol.* 2000; **32**: 159–163.

47 Degott C, Feldmann G, Larrey D *et al.* Drug-induced prolonged cholestasis in adults: a histological semiquantitative study demonstrating progressive ductopenia. *Hepatology* 1992; **15**: 244–251.

48 Bruguera M, Llach J, Rodes J. Non-syndromic paucity of intrahepatic bile ducts in infancy and idiopathic ductopenia in adulthood: the same syndrome? *Hepatology* 1992; **15**: 830–834.

49 Davies MH, Harrison RF, Elias E *et al.* Antibiotic-associated acute vanishing bile duct syndrome: a pattern associated with severe, prolonged, intrahepatic cholestasis. *J. Hepatol.* 1994; **20**: 112–116.

50 Hubscher SG, Lumley MA, Elias E. Vanishing bile duct syndrome: a possible mechanism for intrahepatic cholestasis in Hodgkin's lymphoma. *Hepatology* 1993; **17**: 70–77.

51 Gubern JM, Sancho JJ, Simo J *et al.* A randomised trial on the effect of mannitol on postoperative renal function in patients with obstructive jaundice. *Surgery* 1988; **103**: 39–44.

52 Pain JA, Cahill CJ, Gilbert JM *et al.* Prevention of postoperative renal dysfunction in patients with obstructive jaundice: a multicentre study of bile salts and lactulose. *Br. J. Surg.* 1991; **78**: 467–469.

53 Lai ECS, Mok FPT, Fan ST *et al.* Preoperative endoscopic drainage for malignant obstructive jaundice. *Br. J. Surg.* 1994; **81**: 1195–1198.

54 Kremer AE, Beuers U, Oude-Elferink RP *et al.* Pathogenesis and treatment of pruritus in cholestasis. *Drugs* 2008; **68**: 2163–2182.

55 Datta DV, Sherlock S. Treatment of pruritus of obstructive jaundice with cholestyramine. *BMJ* 1963; **5325**: 216–219.

56 Cynamon HA, Andres JM, Iafrate RP. Rifampin relieves pruritus in children with cholestatic liver disease. *Gastroenterology* 1990; **98**: 1013–1016.

57 Ghent CN, Carruthers SG. Treatment of pruritis in primary biliary cirrhosis with rifampin. Results of a double-blind, crossover, randomized trial. *Gastroenterology* 1988; **94**: 488–493.

58 Yerushalmi B, Sokol RJ, Narkewicz MR *et al.* Use of rifampin for severe pruritus in children with chronic cholestasis. *J. Pediatr. Gastroenterol. Nutr.* 1999; **29**: 442–447.

59 Bergasa NV, Link MJ, Keogh M *et al.* Pilot study of bright-light therapy reflected towards the eyes for pruritus of chronic liver disease. *Am. J. Gastroenterol.* 2001; **96**: 1563–1570.

60 Modi BP, Suh MY, Jonas MM *et al.* Ileal exclusion for refractory symptomatic cholestasis in Alagille syndrome. *J. Pediatr. Surg.* 2007; **42**: 800–805.

61 Bosma PJ, Chowdhury JR, Bakker C *et al.* The genetic basis of the reduced expression of bilirubin UDP-glucuronosyltransferase 1 in Gilbert's syndrome. *N. Engl. J. Med.* 1995; **333**: 1171–1175.

62 Raijmakers MTM, Jansen PLM, Steegers EAP *et al.* Association of human liver bilirubin UDP-glucuronyltransferase activity with a polymorphism in the promoter region of the UGT1A1 gene. *J. Hepatol.* 2000; **33**: 348–351.

63 Persico M, Persico, E, Bakker CTM *et al.* Hepatic uptake of organic anions affects the plasma bilirubin level in subjects with Gilbert's syndrome mutations in UGT1A1. *Hepatology* 2001; **33**: 627–632.

64 Jansen PL, Bosma PJ, Bakker C *et al.* Persistent unconjugated hyperbilirubinemia after liver transplantation due to an abnormal bilirubin UDP-glucuronosyltransferase gene promotor sequence in the donor. *J. Hepatol.* 1997; **27**: 1–5.

65 Premawardhena A, Fisher CA, Fathiu F *et al.* Genetic determinants of jaundice and gallstones in haemoglobin E α thalassaemia. *Lancet* 2001; **357**: 1945–1946.

66 Owens D, Sherlock S. The diagnosis of Gilbert's syndrome: role of the reduced caloric intake test. *Br. Med. J.* 1973; **iii**: 559–563.

67 Black M, Sherlock S. Treatment of Gilbert's syndrome with phenobarbitone. *Lancet* 1970; **i**: 1359–1361.

68 Seppen J, Bosma PJ, Goldhoorn BG *et al.* Discrimination between Crigler–Najjar type I and II by expression of mutant bilirubin uridine diphosphate glucuronosyl transferase. *J. Clin. Invest.* 1994; **94**: 2385–2391.

69 van der Veere CN, Jansen PLM, Sinaasappel M *et al.* Oral calcium phosphate: a new therapy for Crigler–Najjar disease? *Gastroenterology* 1997; **112**: 455–462.

70 Rubaltelli FF, Guerrini P, Reddie E *et al.* Tin-protoporphyrin in the management of children with Crigler–Najjar disease. *Pediatrics* 1989; **84**: 728–731.

71 van der Veere CN, Sinaasappel M, McDonagh AF *et al.* Current therapy of Crigler–Najjar syndrome type I: report of a world registry. *Hepatology* 1996; **24**: 311–315.

72 Fox IJ, Chowdhury JR, Kaufman SS *et al.* Treatment of the Crigler–Najjar syndrome type I with hepatocyte transplantation. *N. Engl. J. Med.* 1998; **338**: 1422–1426.

73 Tiribelli C, Ostrow JD. New concepts in bilirubin and jaundice: report of the Third International Bilirubin Workshop, April 6–8, 1995, Trieste, Italy. *Hepatology* 1996; **24**:1296–1311.

74 Kren BT, Parashar B, Bandyopadhyay P *et al.* Correction of the UDP-glucuronosyltransferase gene defect in the Gunn rat model of Crigler–Najjar syndrome type I with a chimeric oligonucleotide. *Proc. Natl. Acad. Sci. USA* 1999; **96**: 10349–10354.

75 Mandema E, De Fraiture WH, Nieweg HO *et al.* Familial chronic idiopathic jaundice (Dubin–Sprinz disease) with a note on bromsulphalein metabolism in this disease. *Am. J. Med.* 1960; **28**: 42–50.

76 Evans J, Lefkowitch J, Lim CK *et al.* Fecal porphyrin abnormalities in a patient with features of Rotor's syndrome. *Gastroenterology* 1981; **81**: 1125–1130.

CHAPTER 12

Gallstones and Benign Biliary Diseases

James S. Dooley

University College London Medical School and the Royal Free Hampstead NHS Trust, London, UK

Learning points

- Presentation of benign biliary disease is often non-specific; imaging is central in management, ultrasonography being the first approach used.

- Gallstone formation is multifactorial, though lifestyle has an important influence. Genetic markers of increased risk are now recognized in humans.

- Laparoscopic cholecystectomy is the standard surgical approach for patients with cholecystitis. Open cholecystectomy is still needed in some cases, and because of the comorbidities in this selected patient group has a higher complication rate and mortality.

- Bile duct damage at cholecystectomy occurs in around 1 in 200 patients; management requires a multidisciplinary team approach (radiologist, endoscopist, surgeon).

- Biliary tract intervention has a greater risks in patients with cirrhosis.

The spectrum of benign biliary disease is wide (Table 12.1), although the majority of clinical events are due to gallstones, either in gallbladder or bile duct. Symptoms and laboratory tests are likely to be suggestive but non-specific, but this does not obviate the careful assessment of history, examination findings and blood tests. An orderly work-up usually starts with ultrasonography. For the hepatologist, there will be the added complication of benign biliary disease coexisting or developing in a patient with primary hepatic disease, which may complicate normal approaches to management. Less difficult to recognize are the biliary complications of cholecystectomy and liver transplantation, although their management may be complex.

Gallbladder disease is in the differential diagnosis of right upper quadrant pain, some features of which particular suggest this origin. However, there are many other sources of similar pain or discomfort, emphasizing the need for collateral evidence from scanning.

Cholestatic liver function tests with or without jaundice, itching, pain or fever focus attention on possible bile duct disease, although again these features are not specific for bile duct obstruction.

Examination may be useful in showing characteristic pain or tenderness in the right upper quadrant, or a large nodular liver suspicious of malignancy. Jaundice and scratch marks suggest cholestasis. Splenomegaly raises the question of chronic liver disease, although haematological and other causes need to be remembered.

Liver function tests (bilirubin, transaminases, alkaline phosphatase, γ-glutamyl transpeptidase) will generally be normal in gallbladder disease, although there may be mild abnormalities with sepsis. However, abnormalities have to raise the possibility of bile duct disease. Characteristically, serum alkaline phosphatase and γ-glutamyl transpeptidase, with or without bilirubin, are high when bile drainage is impaired. However a sudden rise (and usually fall) of transaminases may be seen when acute obstruction occurs due to a stone, leading to an initial search for a hepatitis. Polymorph leucocytosis will relate to underlying infection.

In these situations, as in most liver-related algorithms, ultrasonography is the first imaging approach of choice. It is effective in showing gallbladder disease, and bile duct dilatation. It may show all that is required; if not, other modalities are used. A single flow chart for all clinical scenarios is not appropriate. Direct cholangiography (percutaneous cholangiography (PTC), endoscopic retrograde cholangiopancreatography (ERCP)) are now done with a specific purpose, therapeutic or to obtain tissue, such is the effectiveness of modern scanning. These techniques compliment management approaches where surgery is an alternative, and this emphasizes the need for a multidisciplinary team.

Cholestatic jaundice without or with pain may be due to malignant disease of the biliary system, described in Chapter 13.

Sherlock's Diseases of the Liver and Biliary System, Twelfth Edition. Edited by
James S. Dooley, Anna S.F. Lok, Andrew K. Burroughs, E. Jenny Heathcote.
© 2011 by Blackwell Publishing Ltd. Published 2011 by Blackwell Publishing Ltd.

Table 12.1. Benign biliary diseases

Gallbladder		
	Stones	
	Cholecystitis	
		calculous
		—acute
		—chronic
		acalculous
		—acute
		—chronic
		—gallbladder dyskinesia
		empyema
	Polyps	
		inflammatory
		neoplastic
	Miscellaneous	
		adenomyomatosis
		cholesterolosis
		porcelain
		xanthogranulomatous
		congenital anomalies
		associated with infections (e.g. HIV related, Salmonella)
Bile duct		
	Stones	
		Common duct
		—asymptomatic
		—without cholangitis
		—with cholangitis
		Intrahepatic
	Strictures	
		Postoperative
		—cholecystectomy
		—transplantation (Chapter 36)
		—anastomotic
		Primary sclerosing cholangitis (Chapter 16)
		Chronic pancreatitis
	Others	
		Sphincter of Oddi dysfunction
		Autoimmune pancreatitis
		Haemobilia
		Mirizzi syndrome
		Parasites

Imaging

Gallbladder

Ultrasonography (US) after fasting is the most effective investigation. It is quick, does not involve radiation and is 95% accurate in the demonstration of gallbladder stones [1] (Fig. 12.1). US will also show whether the gallbladder is tender, whether the gallbladder wall is thickened and whether there is pericholecystic fluid, all features of acute cholecystitis (Fig. 12.2). Failure to show a gallbladder may also be an important finding.

Scintigraphy with technetium-labelled iminodiacetic acid derivatives (which track bile flow) also has an accu-

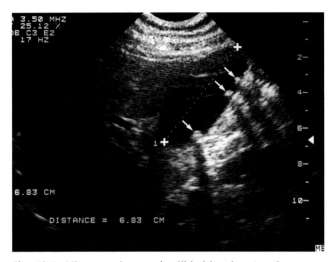

Fig. 12.1. Ultrasound scan of gallbladder showing three stones (arrowed) which cast acoustic shadows.

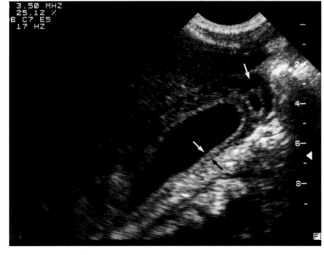

Fig. 12.2. Ultrasound scan in acute cholecystitis. Note the thickened wall of the gallbladder (between black and white arrows) with some pericholecystic fluid (single arrow).

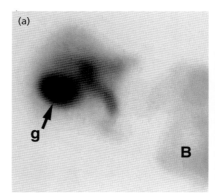
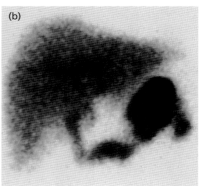

Fig. 12.3. Cholescintigraphy (^{99m}Tc Iodida). (a) Normal scan. At 30 min the gallbladder (g) has filled. Isotope has already entered the bowel (B). (b) Acute cholecystitis. Gallbladder has not filled by 60 min.

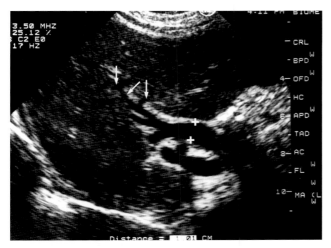

Fig. 12.4. Ultrasound scan showing dilated intrahepatic ducts (arrowed) and common bile duct (marked + +).

racy of 95% for acute cholecystitis (non-filling of gall-bladder) (Fig. 12.3), but is may be more difficult to arrange quickly, takes longer and involves radioisotope. US takes precedence as the diagnostic approach.

CT and MRI scanning can show stones, but are most complementary in showing gallbladder size, wall thickness and evidence of inflammation as in acute cholecystitis [1]. They are second-line approaches after US.

Bile duct

US is also the method of choice in patients with cholestatic features where the primary question is whether there is evidence of bile duct dilatation or disease. The major intrahepatic bile ducts are normally 2 mm in diameter, the common hepatic duct less than 4 mm and the common bile duct less than 5–7 mm. Dilated bile ducts usually (but not always) characterize large bile duct obstruction (Fig. 12.4). US is 95% accurate in diag-

nosis of bile duct obstruction if the serum bilirubin level exceeds 170 µmol/L (10 mg/dL). False negatives occur if obstruction is of short duration or intermittent. US diagnoses the correct level and cause of obstruction in about 60% and less than 50% of cases, respectively, largely due to failure to visualize the complete biliary tree, particularly the periampullary region. Thus the sensitivity of US for showing common bile duct stones has been reported at 63% [2].

CT scanning may follow US, particularly if there is suspicion of malignant disease (see Chapter 13). It is more likely than US to show the level and cause of disease, and conventional CT has been reported to be around 70% sensitive in showing duct stones [2]. Helical CT-cholangiography is more sensitive but involves intravenous contrast and has no advantage over MRCP.

Magnetic resonance cholangiopancreatography (MRCP) allows excellent non-invasive cholangiography. Overall, it has an accuracy of greater than 90% in showing common bile duct stones [3] (Fig. 12.5). The sensitivity is lower for stones less than 6 mm in diameter. MRCP also has a high accuracy in showing bile duct strictures and is as sensitive as ERCP in detecting pancreatic carcinoma. It also shows changes of primary sclerosing cholangitis (Fig. 12.6) (see Chapter 16). MRCP is particularly useful in patients who are poor candidates for ERCP such as the elderly with comorbidity.

Endoscopic ultrasound (EUS) has a sensitivity and accuracy for choledocholithiasis of 96% and 99%, respectively, and is more accurate than transabdominal US [2]. However, the performance of EUS is not statistically better than MRCP [3]. Thus although EUS has been found to be valuable in specific situations, for example the patient with recent acute pancreatitis in whom a stone cannot be seen with non-invasive imaging [4], other techniques come first for most patients. EUS has, however, a role in the evaluation for malignant biliary tract disease (Chapter 13), and in difficult diagnostic situations to help to differentiate between benign and

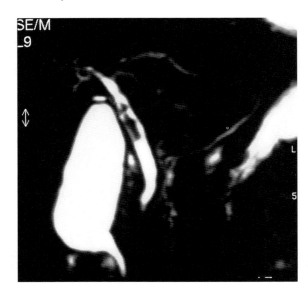

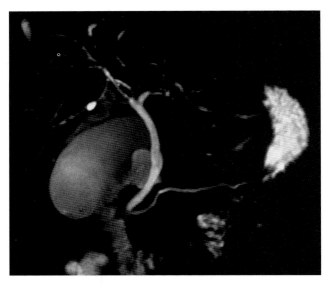

Fig. 12.5. Magnetic resonance cholangiopancreatography in a 39-year-old woman with right upper quadrant discomfort. Ultrasound showed a bile duct of 1 cm but no stones were seen. Gallbladder was normal. Liver function tests were normal apart from marginally abnormal γ-glutamyl transpeptidase. The MRCP shows filling defects in the mid bile duct and stones were removed after endoscopic sphincterotomy.

Fig. 12.6. Magnetic resonance cholangiopancreatography in a 40-year-old woman with chronic cholestasis of unknown aetiology. There are dilatations and strictures of the intrahepatic and perihilar bile ducts. Diagnosis: sclerosing cholangitis.

malignant periampullary stricture—with the option of fine needle aspiration cytology or biopsy.

Oral cholecystography (OCG) and intravenous cholangiography have been superseded by other techniques for showing gallbladder stones and bile duct disease. On the rare occasion when it is necessary to show whether patients are appropriate for non-surgical treatment of gallbladder stones, however, OCG is valuable (see below).

Scintigraphy has a limited role for bile duct diseases, but can be valuable to demonstrate a biliary leak, as after cholecystectomy (Fig. 12.7), or non-invasively to document the degree of functional obstruction to intra- or extrahepatic bile ducts.

Endoscopic retrograde cholangiopancreatography (ERCP) is now widely available (Fig. 12.8). It may be performed in out-patients with only selected patients being admitted afterwards for observation [5].The development of CT, MRI and MRCP, and EUS has led to the majority of ERCPs being planned therapeutic procedures. Sphincterotomy, stone removal, stent insertion, cytological sampling, balloon dilatation and manometry are all feasible. However, ERCP is an invasive procedure and carries the risk of complications. These include pancreatitis (generally ranging between 1 and 7%), cholangitis, bleeding and perforation (after sphincterotomy), as well as the risks of sedation and cardiovascular events in susceptible patients.

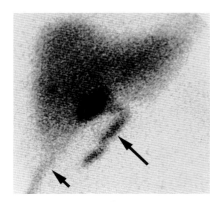

Fig. 12.7. Cholescintigraphy (^{99m}Tc Iodida). Postcholecystectomy bile leak. Isotope tracks laterally from gallbladder bed (short arrow) and T-tube track (long arrow).

The overall complication rate is around 4–7% with a mortality of 0.1–0.4% [6–8]. Complications are related to several factors including the underlying pathology, the difficulty of the procedure and the skill and experience of the operator. One particular focus of discussion currently is around approaches to reduce the risk of post-ERCP pancreatitis, particularly with consideration of placement of a temporary pancreatic duct stent in selected high-risk patients [9–11]. A selective rather than global prophylactic antibiotic policy is reported as being equally effective in preventing septic complications [12]. Despite the associated risks, ERCP rather than PTC is usually the first choice for direct cholangiography.

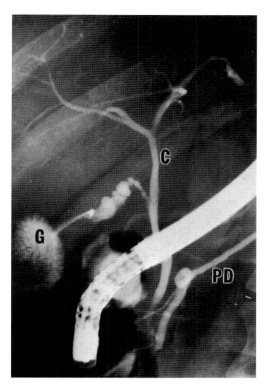

Fig. 12.8. Endoscopic retrograde cholangiopancreatography, normal appearances. C, common bile duct; G, gallbladder; PD, pancreatic duct.

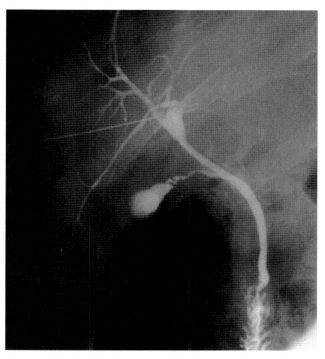

Fig. 12.9. Percutaneous transhepatic cholangiogram showing normal right and left intrahepatic ducts and common bile duct, and free flow of contrast into duodenum. The gallbladder is beginning to fill.

Percutaneous transhepatic cholangiography (PTC) is done by passing a fine-gauge needle through the liver under fluoroscopic control and injecting contrast to identify and fill the biliary system (Fig. 12.9). Most PTC procedures are interventional and the biliary system is then entered with a catheter (PT drainage, PTD). Usually this is prior to insertion of an internal/external biliary drain, or an internal endoprosthesis for malignant disease. However, PTC/D may be used for a combined procedure after failed ERCP access. A wire is passed down the bile duct, through the ampulla and retrieved by the endoscopist. Also, PTD can be done for acute cholangitis when ERCP and drainage has failed.

PTC, however, carries a potentially greater risk than ERCP since catheters are passed through the vascular liver. Haemorrhage, bile leakage with peritonitis and cholangitis may follow. It is rarely used in patients with benign bile duct disease, unless ERCP has failed or previous surgery (e.g. hepaticojejunostomy) has made the ampulla inaccessible.

The nature of biliary tract disease is such that it presents to general physicians and surgeons as well as hepatologists and hepatobiliary surgeons. Cases are often straightforward, but a multidisciplinary approach with physician, radiologist, pathologist and surgeon is optimal to avoid inappropriate diagnostic and therapeutic approaches.

Composition of gallstones

There are three major types of gallstone: cholesterol, black pigment and brown pigment (Fig. 12.10, Table 12.2). In the Western world most are cholesterol stones. Although these consist predominantly of cholesterol (51–99%) they, along with all types, have a complex content and contain a variable proportion of other components including calcium carbonate, phosphate, bilirubinate and palmitate, phospholipids, glycoproteins and mucopolysaccharides. The nature of the nucleus of the stone is uncertain—pigment, glycoprotein and amorphous material have all been suggested.

Formation of cholesterol stones

Three major factors determine the formation of cholesterol gallstones. These are: altered composition of hepatic bile, nucleation of cholesterol crystals and impaired gallbladder function (Fig. 12.11).

The complexity is demonstrated by the finding that although cholesterol supersaturation is a prerequisite for gallstone formation, it does not alone explain the pathogenesis. Other factors must be important since bile supersaturated with cholesterol is frequently found in individuals *without* cholesterol gallstones [13].

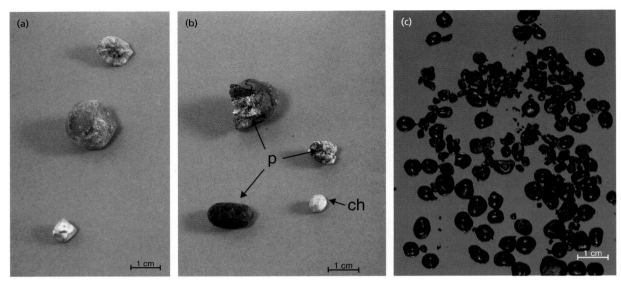

Fig. 12.10. (a) Two faceted cholesterol gallstones. The fragment above shows the concentric structure formed as layer upon layer of cholesterol crystals aggregate.

(b) Stones removed from the common bile duct (ch, cholesterol gallstone; p, brown pigment stone). (c) Black pigment gallstones.

Table 12.2. Classification of gallstones

	Cholesterol	Black pigment	Brown pigment
Location	Gallbladder, ducts	Gallbladder, ducts	Ducts
Major constituents	Cholesterol	Bilirubin pigment polymer	Calcium bilirubinate
Consistency	Crystalline with nucleus	Hard	Soft, friable
% Radio-opaque	15%	60%	0%
Associations			
Infection	Rare	Rare	Usual
Other diseases	See Fig. 12.11	Haemolysis, cirrhosis	Chronic partial biliary obstruction

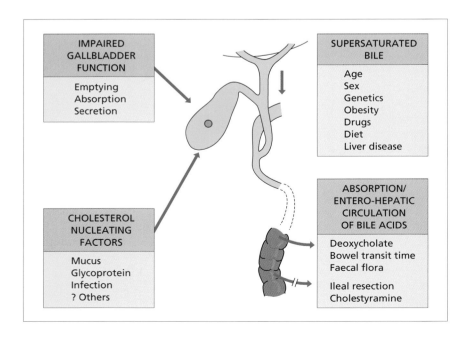

Fig. 12.11. Major factors in cholesterol gallstone formation are supersaturation of the bile with cholesterol, increased deoxycholate formation and absorption, cholesterol crystal nucleation and impaired gallbladder function.

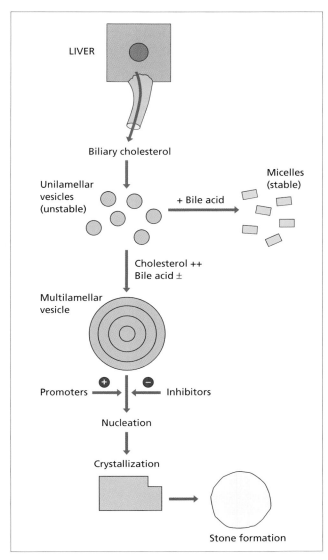

Fig. 12.12. Pathway for cholesterol crystallization in bile.

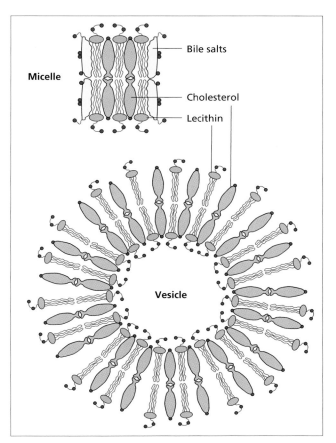

Fig. 12.13. Structure of mixed micelles and cholesterol/phospholipid vesicles.

Altered hepatic bile composition

Bile is 85–95% water. Other components are cholesterol, phospholipids, bile acids, bilirubin, electrolytes and a range of proteins and mucoproteins.

Cholesterol is insoluble in water. It is secreted from the canalicular membrane in unilamellar phospholipid vesicles (Fig. 12.12). Solubilization of cholesterol in bile depends upon whether there is sufficient bile salt and phospholipid (predominantly phosphatidylcholine (lecithin)) to house the cholesterol in mixed micelles (Fig. 12.13). If there is excess cholesterol or reduced phospholipids and/or bile acid, multilamellar vesicles form and it is from these that there is nucleation of cholesterol crystals and ultimately sludge and stone formation (Fig. 12.12).

Biliary cholesterol concentration is unrelated to serum cholesterol level and depends only to a limited extent on the bile acid pool size and bile acid secretory rate.

Changes in bile acid type also reduce the capacity for cholesterol solubilization. A higher proportion of deoxycholate (a secondary bile acid produced in the intestine and absorbed) is found in gallstone patients. This is a more hydrophobic bile salt and when secreted into bile extracts more cholesterol from the canalicular membrane, increasing cholesterol saturation. It also accelerates cholesterol crystallization.

Cholesterol nucleation

Nucleation of cholesterol monohydrate crystals from multilamellar vesicles is a crucial step in gallstone formation (Fig. 12.12).

One distinguishing feature between those who form gallstones and those who do not is the ability of the bile to promote or inhibit nucleation of cholesterol. The time taken for this process ('nucleation time') is significantly shorter in those with gallstones than in those without and in those with multiple as opposed to solitary stones

[14]. Biliary protein concentration is increased in lithogenic bile. Proteins that accelerate nucleation (pronucleators) include gallbladder mucin and immunoglobulin G. Cholesterol gallstones have bilirubin at their centre, and a protein pigment complex might provide the surface for nucleation of cholesterol crystals from gallbladder bile.

Factors that slow nucleation (inhibitors) include apolipoprotein A1 and A2 [15] and a 120-kDa glycoprotein [16]. Ursodeoxycholic acid, as well as decreasing cholesterol saturation, also prolongs the nucleating time [17]. Aspirin reduces mucus biosynthesis by gallbladder mucosa which explains why this drug and other nonsteroidal anti-inflammatory drugs inhibit gallstone formation [18].

Gallbladder function

The gallbladder fills with hepatic bile during fasting, concentrates the bile and contracts in response to a meal, resulting in the passage of bile into the duodenum. The gallbladder must be capable of emptying so as to clear itself of microcrystals, sludge and debris that might initiate stone formation.

The concentration of bile salts, bilirubin and cholesterol, for which the gallbladder wall is essentially impermeable, may rise 10-fold or more as water and electrolytes are absorbed. The concentration of these constituents does not, however, rise in parallel and the cholesterol saturation index may decrease with concentration of bile because of the absorption of some cholesterol.

Gallbladder contraction is under cholinergic and hormonal control. *Cholecystokinin* (CCK), derived from the intestine, contracts and empties the gallbladder and increases mucosal fluid secretion with dilution of gallbladder contents. *Atropine* reduces the contractile response of the gallbladder to CCK [19]. Other hormones found to have an influence on the gallbladder include *motilin* (stimulatory) and *somatostatin* (inhibitory).

Immune processes and inflammation in the gallbladder also appear to effect contraction and promote the production of pronucleators [20].

That gallbladder stasis has a role clinically in the formation of gallstones is suggested by the relationship between impaired gallbladder emptying and the increased incidence of gallstones in patients on long-term parenteral nutrition, and in pregnant women [21].

Biliary sludge

Biliary sludge is a viscous suspension of a precipitate which includes cholesterol monohydrate crystals, calcium bilirubinate granules and other calcium salts/sludge. It usually forms as a result of reduced gallbladder motility related to decreased food intake or parenteral nutrition. After formation, sludge disappears in 70% of patients [22]. Twenty per cent of patients develop complications of gallstones or acute cholecystitis. Whether treatment of sludge would reduce the incidence of complications is not known.

Epidemiology [23]

The prevalence of gallstones varies considerably between and within populations studied. However there are broad differences which are consistent. The highest known prevalence is among American Indians with up to 60–70% of females having cholelithiasis or gallbladder disease in some studies. The prevalence in Chilean Indians is also high. The lowest frequencies are in Black Africans (<5%). In the Western world the prevalence of gallbladder stones is about 5–15%, for example in White Americans and in the UK and Italy, around twofold greater in women than in men. Studies suggest a slightly greater prevalence in Norway and Sweden, but lower in China and Japan. The prevalence is likely to rise as lifestyles change.

Factors in cholesterol stone formation

Genetics

Studies have shown genetic risk and have implicated genes, with a clear link to physicochemical changes in cholesterol and phospholipids.

Analysis of mono- and dizygotic twins suggests that genetic factors account for 25% of the difference in the prevalence of gallstones [24]. In an American family study, around 29% of the chance of having symptomatic gallstones was inherited [25].

Candidate gallstone genes have been identified in mouse models, and recent human studies in sib pairs and cohorts identified a common variant (p.D19H) of the hepatocanalicular cholesterol transporter *ABCG5/ABG8* to be a risk factor for gallstone formation (sevenfold in homozygotes). This variant appears to contribute up to 11% of the total gallstone risk [26].

In a group of individuals with indicators of a risk of cholesterol stones (and also cholestasis), point mutations in *ABCB4* (the transporter for phosphatidyl choline) were found in over 50% of patients [27]. Since ursodeoxycholic acid may reduce the risk in such patients, it has been suggested that checking for mutations in this gene in high-risk patients may be appropriate [28].

Variants in a nuclear receptor (farnesoid X, FXR or NR1H4), which induces *ABCB11* and *ABCB4*, also relate to gallstone formation [29].

Lifestyle

Lack of physical activity [30] is also an association. There also is an association with the metabolic syndrome, and related conditions of obesity, type 2 diabetes and dyslipidaemia [31]. At the molecular level this appears to relate to insulin resistance leading to biliary cholesterol hypersecretion and impaired synthesis of bile acids [32].

Obesity

This seems to be more common among gallstone sufferers than in the general population [33] and is a particular risk factor in women less than 50 years old. Obesity is associated with increased cholesterol synthesis. There are no consistent changes in postprandial gallbladder volume. Fifty per cent of markedly obese patients have gallstones at surgery.

Dieting (2100 kJ/day) can result in biliary sludge and the formation of symptomatic gallstones in obese individuals [34].

Gallstone formation during weight loss following gastric bypass surgery for obesity is prevented by giving ursodeoxycholic acid [35].

Dietary factors

Epidemiological studies show that chronic over-nutrition with refined carbohydrates and triglycerides increases the risk [36].

Increasing dietary cholesterol increases biliary cholesterol but there is no epidemiological or dietary data to link cholesterol intake with gallstones.

In Western countries, gallstones have been linked to dietary fibre deficiency and a longer intestinal transit time [37]. This increases deoxycholic acid in bile, and renders bile more lithogenic. Deoxycholate is derived from dehydroxylation of cholic acid in the colon by faecal bacteria. There is an enterohepatic circulation. Gallstone patients have significantly prolonged small bowel transit times [38] and increased bacterial dehydroxylating activity in faeces [39].

A diet low in carbohydrate and a shorter overnight fasting period protects against gallstones, as does a moderate alcohol intake in males [40]. Vegetarians get fewer gallstones irrespective of their tendency to be slim [41].

Age

There is a steady increase in gallstone prevalence with advancing years, probably due to the increased cholesterol content in bile. By age 75, around 20% of men and 35% of women in some Western countries have gallstones. Clinical problems present most frequently between the ages of 50 and 70.

Sex and oestrogens

Gallstones are twice as common in women as in men, and this is particularly so before the age of 50.

The incidence is higher in multiparous than in nulliparous women. Incomplete emptying of the gallbladder in late pregnancy leaves a large residual volume and thus retention of cholesterol crystals. Biliary sludge occurs frequently but is generally asymptomatic and disappears spontaneously after delivery in two-thirds [42]. In the postpartum period gallstones are present in 8–12% of women (nine times that in a matched group) [43]. One-third of those with a functional gallbladder are symptomatic. Small stones disappear spontaneously in 30%.

The bile becomes more lithogenic when women are placed on birth control pills. Women on long-term oral contraceptives have a twofold increased incidence of gallbladder disease over controls [44]. Postmenopausal women taking oestrogen-containing drugs have a significant increase frequency (around 1.8 times) of gallbladder disease [45]. In men given oestrogen for prostatic carcinoma the bile becomes saturated with cholesterol and gallstones may form [46].

Serum factors

The highest risk of gallstones (both cholesterol and pigment) is associated with low HDL levels and high triglyceride levels, which may be more important than body mass [47]. High serum cholesterol is not a determinant of gallstone risk.

Cirrhosis

About 30% of patients with cirrhosis have gallstones. The risk of developing stones is most strongly associated with Child's grade C and alcoholic cirrhosis with a yearly incidence of about 5% [48]. The mechanisms are uncertain. All patients with hepatocellular disease show a variable degree of haemolysis. Although bile acid secretion is reduced, the stones are usually of the black pigment type. Phospholipid and cholesterol secretion are also lowered so that the bile is not supersaturated.

Cholecystectomy in patients with cirrhosis carries an increased morbidity and mortality [49,50]. In Child's group A and B the laparoscopic approach is preferred to open cholecystectomy because of lower morbidity and mortality. In Child C patients and those with a higher MELD score the risk of cholecystectomy is particularly high, making management decisions more difficult [49,50]. In such patients with symptomatic gallbladder and bile duct stones, non-surgical techniques have to be considered as alternatives to surgery.

Infection

Although infection is thought to be of little importance in cholesterol stone formation, bacterial DNA is found in these stones [51]. Conceivably, bacteria might deconjugate bile salts, allowing their absorption and reducing cholesterol solubility.

Diabetes mellitus

Diabetics have a higher prevalence of gallstones (or a history of cholecystectomy) than non-diabetics, particularly females (42 versus 23%) [52]. The older diabetic tends to be obese, and this may be the important factor in gallstone formation.

Patients with diabetes may have large, poorly contracting and poorly filling gallbladders [53]. A 'diabetic neurogenic gallbladder' syndrome has been postulated.

Patients with diabetes mellitus undergoing cholecystectomy, whether emergency or elective, have an increased risk of complications. These are probably related to associated cardiovascular or renal disease and to more advanced age.

Other factors

Hepatitis C is associated with a higher incidence of gallbladder stones than patients with hepatitis B, or those without hepatitis B or C (11.7 vs. 5.4 vs. 6.0% respectively [54]), but the reason for the link is not known.

Ileal resection breaks the enterohepatic circulation of bile salts, reduces the total bile salt pool and is followed by gallstone formation. The same is found in subtotal or total colectomy [55].

Gastrectomy increases the incidence of gallstones [56].

Long-term cholestyramine therapy increases bile salt loss with a reduced bile acid pool size and gallstone formation.

Parenteral nutrition leads to a dilated, sluggish gallbladder containing stones.

Endoscopic sphincterotomy improves gallbladder emptying and decreases the lithogenicity of bile in patients with gallstone disease [57]. Patients with gallbladder stones have significantly higher sphincter of Oddi tone [58].

Pigment gallstones

This term is used for stones containing less than 30% cholesterol. There are two types: black and brown (see Table 12.2).

Black pigment stones are largely composed of an insoluble bilirubin pigment polymer mixed with calcium phosphate and carbonate. There is no cholesterol. The mechanism of formation is not well understood, but supersaturation of bile with unconjugated bilirubin, changes in pH and calcium, and overproduction of an organic matrix (glycoprotein) play a role [59]. Overall, 20–30% of gallbladder stones are black. The incidence rises with age. They may pass into the bile duct. Black stones accompany chronic haemolysis, usually hereditary spherocytosis or sickle cell disease, and mechanical prostheses, for example heart valves, in the circulation. They show an increased prevalence with all forms of cirrhosis, particularly alcoholic [48]. Patients with ileal Crohn's disease may form pigment stones because of increased colonic absorption of bilirubin due to failure of ileal absorption of bile acid [60].

Brown pigment stones contain calcium bilirubinate, calcium palmitate, and stearate, as well as cholesterol. The bilirubinate is polymerized to a lesser extent than in black stones.

Brown stones are rare in the gallbladder. They form in the bile duct and are related to bile stasis and infected bile. They are usually radiolucent. Bacteria are present in more than 90%. Stone formation is related to the deconjugation of bilirubin diglucuronide by bacterial β-glucuronidase [59]. Insoluble unconjugated bilirubinate precipitates.

Brown pigment stones form above biliary strictures in sclerosing cholangitis and in the dilated segments of Caroli's disease. There is an association with juxtapapillary duodenal diverticula [61]. In Oriental countries, these stones are associated with parasitic infestations of the biliary tract such as *Clonorchis sinensis* and *Ascaris lumbricoides*. These stones are frequently intrahepatic.

Natural history of gallbladder stones
(Fig. 12.14)

Gallstones can be dated from the atmospheric radiocarbon produced by nuclear bomb explosions. This suggests a time lag of about 12 years between initial stone formation and symptoms culminating in cholecystectomy [62].

However, gallbladder stones are usually asymptomatic and diagnosed by chance by imaging or during investigation for some other condition. A small proportion develop symptoms. Around 8–10% of patients with asymptomatic gallstones developed symptoms within 5 years and only 5% required surgery [63,64]. Only about half the patients with symptomatic gallstones come to cholecystectomy within 6 years of diagnosis. Patients with gallstones seem to tolerate their symptoms for long periods of time, preferring this to cholecystectomy. If

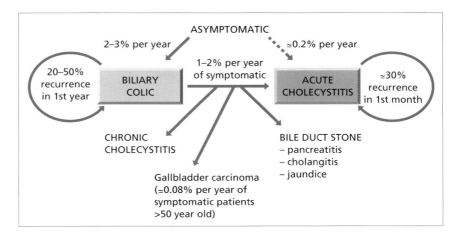

Fig. 12.14. The natural history of gallstones.

symptoms develop, they are unlikely to present as an emergency.

Data suggest that elective cholecystectomy is an appropriate choice for patients with biliary colic [65].

Prophylactic cholecystectomy should not be performed for asymptomatic gallbladder stones [66]. It should not be done to prevent gallbladder cancer since the risk is small and less than that of cholecystectomy [67].

Migration of a stone to the neck of the gallbladder causes *obstruction of the cystic duct* and a rise in gallbladder pressure. There is chemical irritation of the gallbladder mucosa by the retained bile, followed by bacterial invasion. According to the severity of the changes, *acute* or *chronic cholecystitis* results. Empyema may follow; perforation, fistula formation and emphysematous cholecystitis are rare.

Migration of a stone into the bile duct may present with pain, jaundice, cholangitis or pancreatitis.

Possible association of stones with gallbladder and bile duct cancer

Population surveys have investigated the link between stones and malignancy of the gallbladder and extrahepatic bile ducts.

The relative risk of gallbladder carcinoma is 2.4 if gallbladder stones are 2.0–2.9 cm in diameter, and greater with larger stones [68]. The issue is whether this is causative or an association, meaning that there is a common factor(s) that predisposes to both stones and carcinoma. This remains a possibility [69] and difficult to rule in or out.

There appears to be a lower risk of extrahepatic bile duct carcinoma during follow up of patients who had cholecystectomy, raising the question of a link between gallbladder stones or gallbladders containing stones with extrahepatic bile duct malignant changes [70].

Acute calculous cholecystitis

Aetiology

In 95% of patients the cystic duct is obstructed by a gallstone. The imprisoned bile salts have a toxic action on the gallbladder wall. Lipids may penetrate the Rokitansky–Aschoff sinuses and exert an irritant reaction. The rise in pressure compresses blood vessels in the gallbladder wall; infarction and gangrene may follow.

Pancreatic enzymes may also cause acute cholecystitis, presumably by regurgitation into the biliary system when there is a common biliary and pancreatic channel.

Bacterial inflammation is an integral part of acute cholecystitis. Bacterial deconjugation of bile salts may produce toxic bile acids which can injure the mucosa.

Pathology

The gallbladder is usually distended, but after previous inflammation the wall becomes thickened and contracted. There may be vascular adhesions to adjacent structures.

Histology shows haemorrhage and moderate oedema reaching a peak by about the fourth day and diminishing by the seventh day. As the acute reaction subsides it is replaced by fibrosis.

Bacteriology. Cultures of both gallbladder wall and bile usually show organisms of intestinal type, including anaerobes. Common infecting organisms are *Escherichia coli*, *Streptococcus faecalis* and *Klebsiella*, often in combination. Anaerobes are present, if sought, and are usually found with aerobes. They include *Bacteroides* and *Clostridium sp.*

Clinical features

These vary according to whether there is only mild inflammation or more severe disease such as fulminating gangrene of the gallbladder wall. The acute attack is often an exacerbation of underlying chronic cholecystitis.

The sufferers are often obese, female and over 40, but no type, age or sex is immune.

Pain often occurs late at night or in the early morning, usually in the right upper abdomen or epigastrium and is referred to the angle of the right scapula, to the right shoulder [71], or rarely to the left side. It may simulate angina pectoris.

The pain usually rises to a plateau and can last 30–60 min without relief, unlike the short spasm of biliary colic. Attacks may be precipitated by late-night, heavy meals or fatty food.

Distension pain coming in waves is due to the gallbladder contracting to overcome the blocked cystic duct.

Peritoneal pain is superficial with skin tenderness, hyperaesthesia and muscular rigidity. The fundus of the gallbladder is in apposition to the diaphragmatic peritoneum, which is supplied by the phrenic and last six intercostal nerves. Stimulation of the anterior branches produces right upper quadrant pain and of the posterior cutaneous branch leads to the characteristic right infrascapular pain.

Examination

The patient appears ill. The temperature rises with bacterial invasion. Jaundice usually indicates associated stones in the common bile duct.

The gallbladder is usually impalpable; occasionally a tender mass of gallbladder and adherent omentum may be felt. *Murphy's sign* is positive.

The *leucocyte count* may be raised with a moderate increase in polymorphs. In the febrile patient blood cultures may be positive.

For the patient with acute abdominal pain of uncertain cause, a plain X-ray will be taken during the work-up, but if acute cholecystitis is suspected scanning is indicated. Only about 10% of gallstones are radio-opaque, compared with 90% of renal calculi.

Imaging

The diagnosis of gallbladder disease depends upon scanning because of the overall lack of power of any specific symptom [72]. As described earlier, ultrasound is the test of choice. Scintigraphy is also accurate but second line.

Gallstones cast intense echoes with obvious posterior acoustic shadows (see Fig. 12.1). They change in position with turning of the patient. Stones 3 mm or more in size are usually seen. Diagnostic accuracy is 96% but less experienced operators may not achieve this success.

Acute calculous cholecystitis is suggested by the finding of stones with:
- a thickened gallbladder wall (>5 mm) (see Fig. 12.2);
- a positive sonographic Murphy sign—the presence of maximum tenderness, elicited by direct pressure of the transducer, over a sonographically localized gallbladder;
- gallbladder distension;
- pericholecystic fluid;
- subserosal oedema (without ascites);
- intramural gas;
- a sloughed mucosal membrane.

Cholescintigraphy. Technetium-labelled iminodiacetic acid derivatives (IDA) are cleared from the plasma by hepatocellular organic anion transport and excreted in the bile (see Fig. 12.3a).

Hepatic IDA scanning may be used to determine patency of the cystic duct in suspected acute cholecystitis. If the gallbladder fails to visualize, despite common bile duct patency and intestinal visualization (Fig. 12.3b), the probability of acute cholecystitis is 80–90%. False-negative results are more common the later the gallbladder fills [73].

CT and MRI scanning are not indicated as the initial assessment of a patient with suspected acute cholecystitis.

Differential diagnosis

Acute cholecystitis is liable to be confused with other causes of sudden pain and tenderness in the right hypochondrium. Below the diaphragm, acute retrocaecal appendicitis, intestinal obstruction, a perforated peptic ulcer or acute pancreatitis may produce similar clinical features.

Myocardial infarction should always be considered.

Referred pain from muscular and spinal root lesions may cause similar pain.

Prognosis

Spontaneous recovery follows disimpaction of the stone in 85% of patients. Recurrent acute cholecystitis may follow—approximately a 30% chance over the next 3 months [74].

Rarely, acute cholecystitis proceeds rapidly to gangrene or empyema of the gallbladder, fistula formation, hepatic abscesses or even generalized peritonitis. The acute fulminating disease is becoming less common because of earlier antibiotic therapy and more frequent cholecystectomy for recurrent gallbladder symptoms.

Treatment

Medical. This depends upon the clinical severity for which a grading has been described [75,76]. This is based on the white cell count, clinical findings, duration and features of systemic/ multisystem signs or complications. General measures during the acute phase include intravenous fluids, nothing given orally, analgesia and antibiotics. Tokyo guidelines recommend management depending upon the severity [75,76].

Antibiotic(s) are given if there is clinical evidence of sepsis, and should have a spectrum to cover the likely micro-organisms. Choice is according to hospital policy, but a second or third-generation cephalosporin or combination of a quinolone with metronidazole are usually adequate for the stable patient with pain and mild fever. Patients with features of severe sepsis require broader-spectrum antibiotics such as piperacillin/ tazobactam, combined if necessary with an aminoglycoside. The elderly, and those with diabetes or immunodeficiency, are at particular risk of severe sepsis.

Cholecystectomy (see below). For those with mild acute cholecystitis, early cholecystectomy is recommended [75,76]. Meta-analysis of randomized controlled trials shows that this approach (within 1 week) is superior to delayed cholecystectomy (2 to 3 months later) because of avoidance of gallstone-related complications during the waiting period [65,77]. These could lead to emergency surgery which is known to carry a higher risk than elective operation, particularly in elderly patients over 75 years old and in the diabetic patient where early elective cholecystectomy is preferred once symptoms have developed [78].

For moderate acute cholecystitis there may be early or delayed cholecystectomy, but if early laparoscopic surgery is done, it should be by a highly experienced surgeon so that decisions to alter the approach can be made and carried out if the operation becomes complicated [75,76].

For severe acute cholecystitis, based on the Tokyo guidelines, initial intensive medical treatment with antibiotics is recommended with, if needed, percutaneous cholecystostomy [75,76]; surgical decisions are then customized for individual patients according to the clinical course and degree of surgical risk.

Empyema of the gallbladder

If the cystic duct remains blocked by a stone and infection sets in, empyema may develop. Symptoms may be of an intra-abdominal abscess (fever, rigors, pain), although the elderly patient may appear relatively well.

Treatment is with antibiotics and surgery. There is a high postoperative rate of septic complications [79]. Percutaneous cholecystostomy is considered if the patient is unfit for surgery.

Emphysematous cholecystitis

The term is used to denote infection of the gallbladder with gas-producing organisms (*Escherichia coli, Clostridium welchii*) or anaerobic streptococci. The primary lesion is occlusion of the cystic duct or cystic artery. Infection is secondary [80]. The condition classically affects male diabetics who develop features of severe, toxic, acute cholecystitis. An abdominal mass may be palpable.

On a plain abdominal Xray the gallbladder may be seen as a sharply outlined pear-shaped gas shadow. Occasionally air may be seen infiltrating the wall and surrounding tissue. Gas is not apparent in the cystic duct, which is blocked by a gallstone. In the erect position, a fluid level is seen in the gallbladder. However, plain abdominal X-ray may not show the characteristic changes. Ultrasound is diagnostic in around 50% of cases. CT may also show characteristic features.

Standard treatment is with antibiotics and emergency cholecystectomy. In the severely ill patient percutaneous cholecystostomy is an alternative [81].

Chronic calculous cholecystitis

This is the commonest type of clinical gallbladder disease. The association of chronic cholecystitis with stones is almost constant. Aetiological factors therefore include all those related to gallstones. The chronic inflammation may follow acute cholecystitis, but usually develops insidiously.

Pathology

The gallbladder is usually contracted with a thickened, sometimes calcified, wall. Stones are seen lying loosely embedded in the wall or in meshes of an organizing fibrotic network. One stone is usually lodged in the neck. Histologically, the wall is thickened and congested with lymphocytic infiltration and occasionally complete destruction of the mucosa.

Clinical features

Chronic cholecystitis is difficult to diagnose because of the ill-defined symptoms. Episodes of acute cholecystitis punctuate the course.

Abdominal distension or epigastric discomfort, especially after a fatty meal, may be temporarily relieved by belching. Nausea is common, but vomiting is unusual unless there are stones in the common bile duct. Apart from a constant dull ache in the right hypochondrium and epigastrium, pain may be experienced in the right scapular region, substernally or at the right shoulder. Postprandial pain may be relieved by alkalis.

Local tenderness over the gallbladder and a positive Murphy sign are very suggestive.

Investigations

The temperature, leucocyte count, haemoglobin and erythrocyte sedimentation rate are within normal limits. A plain abdominal X-ray may show calcified gallstones. However, the imaging technique of first choice is ultrasound, which may show gallstones within a fibrosed gallbladder with a thickened wall. Non-visualization of the gallbladder is also a significant finding. CT scan may show gallstones but this technique is not usually appropriate in the diagnostic work-up. Endoscopy may be necessary to rule out gastric or duodenal inflammation or ulceration.

Differential diagnosis

Fat intolerance, flatulence and postprandial discomfort are common symptoms. Even if associated with imaging evidence of gallstones, the calculi are not necessarily responsible since stones are frequently present in the symptom-free.

Other disorders producing a similar clinical picture must be excluded before cholecystectomy is advised, otherwise symptoms persist postoperatively. These include peptic ulceration or inflammation, hiatus hernia, irritable bowel syndrome and functional dyspepsias.

Since approximately 10% of young to middle-aged adults have gallstones, symptomatic gallbladder disease may be over-diagnosed. Conversely, ultrasound is only about 95% accurate and symptomatic gallbladder disease may therefore sometimes be unrecognized.

Prognosis

This chronic disease is compatible with good life expectancy. However, once symptoms, particularly biliary colic, are experienced, the patients tend to remain symptomatic with about a 40% chance of recurrence within 2 years [82]. Gallbladder cancer is a rare, later development (see above).

Treatment

Medical measures may be tried if the diagnosis is uncertain and a period of observation is desirable. This is especially so when indefinite symptoms are associated with a well-functioning gallbladder. The general condition of the patient may contraindicate surgery. The infrequent place of medical dissolution and shock-wave lithotripsy of radiolucent stones is discussed later.

Obesity should be addressed. A low-fat diet is advisable.

If the patient is symptomatic, particularly with repeated episodes of pain, cholecystectomy (see below) is indicated.

Acalculous cholecystitis

Acute

About 5–10% of acute cholecystitis in adults and about 30% in children occurs in the absence of stones. The most frequent predisposing cause is an associated critical condition such as after major non-biliary surgery, multiple injuries, major burns, recent childbirth, severe sepsis, mechanical ventilation and parenteral nutrition.

The pathogenesis is unclear and probably multifactorial, but bile stasis (lack of gallbladder contraction), increased bile viscosity and lithogenicity, and gallbladder ischaemia are thought to play a role. Administration of opiates, which increase sphincter of Oddi tone, may also reduce gallbladder emptying.

Clinical features should be those of acute calculous cholecystitis with fever, leucocytosis and right upper quadrant pain but diagnosis is often difficult because of the overall clinical state of the patient who may be intubated, ventilated and receiving narcotic analgesics.

There may be laboratory features of cholestasis with a raised bilirubin and alkaline phosphatase. Ultrasound and CT are complementary and useful in showing a thickened gallbladder wall (>5mm), pericholecystic fluid or subserosal oedema (without ascites), intramural gas or a sloughed mucosal membrane. The sensitivity of ultrasound varies widely between studies (30–100%), but prospective studies have suggested that this is a useful technique [83,84].Cholescintigraphy is reported to have a sensitivity of 60–90% for acalculous cholecystitis [85,86], but moving patients to the imaging unit for the time required for scanning may not be practical.

Because of the difficulties of diagnosis a high index of suspicion is needed, particularly in patients at risk. Gangrene and perforation of the gallbladder are common. The mortality is high, 41% in one series [85], often due to delayed diagnosis.

Treatment is emergency cholecystectomy. In the critically ill patient percutaneous cholecystostomy under ultrasound guidance may be life saving (see below).

Chronic (including gallbladder dyskinesia)

This is a difficult diagnosis as the clinical condition resembles others, particularly irritable bowel syndrome and functional dyspepsias. A description of biliary-like pain has been endorsed by the Rome committee on functional biliary and pancreatic disorders [87]: an episodic, severe, constant pain, in epigastrium or right upper quadrant, lasting at least 30 min, severe enough to interrupt daily activities or lead to consultation with a physician. Laboratory investigations (liver enzymes, conjugated bilirubin, amylase, lipase) are normal; routine transabdominal ultrasound scan shows a normal gallbladder.

Cholescintigraphy with measurement of the gallbladder ejection fraction 15 min after CCK infusion has been used to try and identify patients who have putative gallbladder pathology and would benefit from cholecystectomy. Normal individuals have an ejection fraction of around 70%. In those with a low ejection fraction (usually regarded as less than 35–40%) or who develop pain during the infusion, symptom relief after cholecystectomy is reported in between 70 and 90% of patients [88–90]. However, decisions on management based on the results of a single isotope scan alone may not appear appropriate. There are many issues regarding the actual technique used (e.g. dose and rate of CCK infusion) and that a low ejection fraction is not specific for functional gallbladder disease [91]. Results of scanning should be taken in the context of the other clinical features of the patient. Of note is that EUS may detect small gallbladder stones missed by transabdominal US and in these patients cholecystectomy resulted in loss of pain [92].

In patients with acalculous gallbladder disease undergoing cholecystectomy, chronic cholecystitis, cholesterolosis, muscle hypertrophy and/or a narrowed cystic duct have been shown in patients in whom symptoms were relieved [89,90].

Cholecystectomy

Laparoscopic cholecystectomy, introduced in the late 1980s, is the current standard treatment for symptomatic gallbladder stones, and mild and moderate acute cholecystitis, based on superior outcomes compared with open cholecystectomy [93–95]. *Open cholecystectomy* is still required where the laparoscopic approach fails, or is not possible. Thus expertise is still needed for the open operation.

Operative approach for laparoscopic cholecystectomy

Under general anaesthesia the abdominal cavity is insufflated with CO_2 and the laparoscope and operating channels inserted. Cystic duct and vessels to the gall-bladder are carefully identified and clipped. Haemostasis is achieved by electrocautery or laser. The gallbladder is dissected from the gallbladder bed on the liver and removed whole. When necessary large stones are fragmented while they are still within the gallbladder to allow its delivery through the anterior abdominal wall.

Results

Systemic reviews and meta-analyses show that there is no overall difference in outcome measures of mortality and complications between open, small-incision and laparoscopic cholecystectomy [93,96]. However, the minimally invasive methods (laparoscopic and small incision) were associated with a significantly shorter postoperative hospital stay (around 3 days) compared with open cholecystectomy, and convalescence was shortened (around 22 days). The results from laparoscopic and small incision cholecystectomy were similar. The smaller incision approach interestingly had a shorter operative time and possible lower cost than laparoscopic cholecystectomy.

The Cochrane review raises the question of why laparoscopic rather than mini-incision cholecystectomy has become the standard approach for patients with symptomatic disease, and suggests that to address this other outcomes need more concerted analysis, such as symptom relief and complications. One study involving minilaparotomy and laparoscopic cholecystectomy evaluated pain scores, physical function and psychological health 1 week after operation and found that the laparoscopic approach gave a significantly better outcome [97] (Fig. 12.15). The wide use of laparoscopic cholecystectomy also appears to reflect patient preference and the overall pattern of practice available. Thus practitioners of mini-incision surgery are in the minority, because of its technical difficulty and the fewer opportunities for training.

Laparoscopic cholecystectomy is successful in about 95% of patients. In the remainder, the operation has to be converted to open cholecystectomy. This is more likely if there is acute cholecystitis, particularly with empyema [98]. In these cases, initial laparoscopic assessment is appropriate and conversion to open operation made if indicated. In experienced hands laparoscopic cholecystectomy for acute and gangrenous cholecystitis is as safe and effective as open cholecystectomy although there is a moderately high conversion rate (16%) to the open procedure [99].

Complications

The perioperative mortality lies between 0 and 0.3% [65,96]. The complication rate is around 5% [96], and includes bile duct injury, biliary leak, postoperative

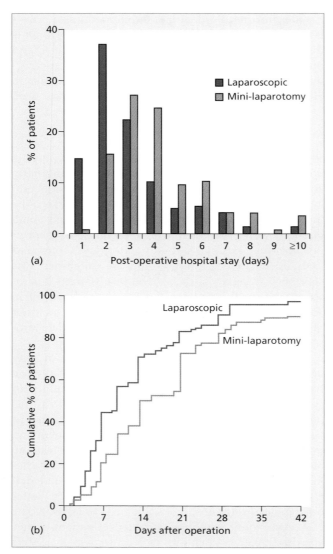

Fig. 12.15. Laparoscopic versus minicholecystectomy. (a) Postoperative hospital stay. (b) Return to work in the home. (From [97] with permission.)

bleeding and wound infection. Complication rates have been reported to be associated with patient characteristics (age, comorbidities) rather than surgeon or hospital operative volume [100]. Bile duct injury occurs in around 0.4–0.6% of patients [101,102], and this is considered as being higher than in the era of open cholecystectomy (0.2–0.3%)[101]. This emphasizes the need for caution at surgery and for rigorous training. Duct injury may occur even with an experienced surgeon.

The reported risks of open cholecystectomy (collected recently) are now greater than laparoscopic, but this predominantly reflects the patient characteristics of those chosen for open operation preoperatively, and those converted from laparoscopic to open at the time of surgery. Thus differences in 30-day morbidity (18.7 % vs. 4.8%; open versus laparoscopic respectively) and

30-day mortality (2.4% vs. 0.4%) reflect these patient factors, including ASA (American Society of Anesthesiologists) class, patient comorbidities, functional status, age, previous abdominal surgery, emergency status and albumin [103].

Cholangiography

Of patients having cholecystectomy, 10–15% have common duct stones. Preoperative ERCP is appropriate for patients with criteria suggestive of a duct stone—recent jaundice, cholangitis, pancreatitis, abnormal liver function tests or duct dilatation on ultrasound. If the data raise the question of a duct stone but are not considered enough for ERCP, MRCP is indicated. If there is a duct stone it is removed after sphincterotomy.

Intraoperative cholangiography at laparoscopic cholecystectomy needs experience. Some advocate its routine use to define bile duct anatomy, anomalies and stones, but this prevents only the minority of bile duct injuries [104].

Laparoscopic common bile duct exploration

In experienced hands duct stones can be removed in 90% of patients [105]. However, this technique is not routine because of lack of expertise and the need for special equipment. Laparoscopic removal of common duct stones is as effective and safe as endoscopic sphincterotomy [106]. Management should be customized according to local expertise, resources and patient considerations.

Percutaneous cholecystostomy

This has a particular place in the elderly patient with acute complicated cholecystitis with comorbid disease [107]. The method can either be done under ultrasound control or fluoroscopy after initial opacification using a skinny needle. A drainage catheter can be left to drain the gallbladder, or aspiration of the fluid and pus can be done without continued drainage [108]. Both methods are combined with intensive antibiotic therapy. Bile/pus is sent for culture. There is usually rapid relief of clinical symptoms.

In the severely ill patient, percutaneous transhepatic cholecystostomy is effective. Resolution of sepsis has been recently reported in 87% of 23 patients, with a 30-day mortality of 8.7%, and one procedure-related death (4.3%) [109].

This technique may allow the patient to be brought to elective surgery in a better clinical condition. In the inoperable patient, after recovery, if a percutaneous catheter has been left in place, it can be removed and the patient treated conservatively, often without recurrence [107].

In the situation of the patient not being a surgical candidate, and/or having a coagulopathy or ascites that precludes cholecystostomy, ERCP with selective cannulation of the cystic duct and nasobiliary tube or stent placement in the gallbladder is possible [110], although technically difficult. A systematic review reported over 90% technical and 80–90% clinical success, with complications in 1–4% [111].

Postcholecystectomy bile duct damage

Bile duct damage occurs in around 0.4–0.6% of patients [101,102]. Injuries include bile leak from cystic duct or gallbladder bed, complete transection of the duct and complete or partial stricture due to clips or damage during dissection.

Several factors contribute to duct injury. There may be mistaken interpretation of the anatomy due to oedema or haemorrhage around an inflamed gallbladder, anomalies of the cystic duct or right hepatic duct (Fig. 12.16), or lack of operator experience.

Risk factors for *laparoscopic bile duct injury* include obesity, bleeding, acute cholecystitis and scarring in Calot's triangle (the area between the cystic duct and common hepatic duct). Uncertain anatomy, inexperi-

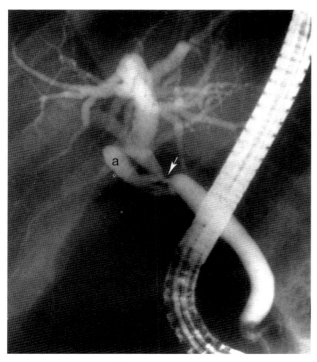

Fig. 12.16. Benign bile duct stricture following laparoscopic cholecystectomy (arrow). Note anomalous right-sided bile duct (a).

ence and a long procedure are also associated with damage [112,113]. The threshold at which the decision is made to convert from laparoscopic to open surgery is also important.

Clinical features

Complete ligation, clipping or transection will become clear clinically in the immediate perioperative period. With partial injury, the occlusion develops slowly. About 60% of patients with bile duct injury present within 3 months of operation, and 80% within 1 year [114].

If unrecognized at the time of cholecystectomy, presentation depends upon the degree of damage. Postoperative anorexia, nausea, vomiting, pain, abdominal distension, ileus and delayed recovery should raise the possibility of damage [112], although the presentation is usually more obvious.

The appearance of bile-stained fluid in the surgical drain raises the possibility of duct damage. Complete transection of the main bile duct usually gives pain (bile peritonitis), fever and cholestatic jaundice 3–7 days postoperatively. Alternatively, an external biliary fistula develops. The fistula may drain intermittently with episodes of jaundice when it is closed. Subhepatic abscesses may develop.

Ligation or clipping the main duct, or a later stricture, gives escalating cholestatic jaundice with or without cholangitis.

With current awareness of the complications of laparoscopic cholecystectomy, and the availability of ERCP and other imaging techniques, patients should not develop the chronic complications of biliary obstruction. Biliary cirrhosis with portal hypertension and splenomegaly will develop with time if the obstruction is not recognized and relieved effectively.

Patients unfortunate enough to suffer bile duct damage at cholecystectomy may become increasingly introspective as the months pass. Some keep the most detailed notes of their symptoms and, understandably, become querulous and suspicious of their medical advisors. They need considerable support.

Investigations

The history of recent cholecystectomy, the postoperative features and the biochemical and imaging data should lead to cholangiography and the correct diagnosis.

Liver function tests may show cholestasis, but may be normal.

Radiology. The first step is scanning with ultrasound or CT. Where duct damage has led to a bile leak, ultrasound or CT will show an intra-abdominal collection which may be drained under scanning control. Bile

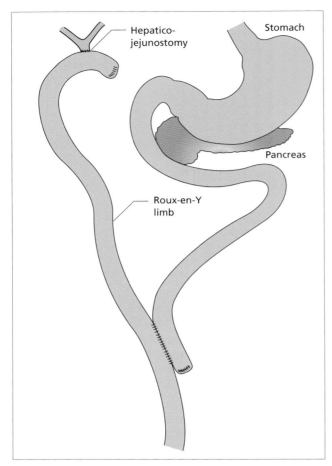

Fig. 12.17. Repair of a high biliary stricture by Roux-en-Y hepaticojejunostomy.

ducts may not be dilated. Biliary scintigraphy detects around 50% of leaks (see Fig. 12.7) [115]. When there is a stricture without a leak, dilated intrahepatic bile ducts are seen.

The route of cholangiography depends upon the clinical data. If bile leakage from a cystic duct or a partial low duct stricture are suspected then ERCP is the first choice (see Fig. 12.16). MRCP may be valuable depending upon the type of injury. For duct transection and discontinuity or a high stricture, percutaneous cholangiography and drainage are appropriate as part of the preoperative work-up and management. *CT or MR angiography* is indicated if vascular injury is suspected, and may be done as a road map for patients with high duct damage.

Classifications

There are many classifications of types of injury, in an attempt to define different patterns and facilitate management decisions [116]. Bergman *et al.* [117] separate

injuries into four major categories and this more often used by biliary endoscopists:
• Type A: cystic duct leak, or leakage from aberrant or peripheral hepatic radicals;
• Type B: major bile duct leak with or without a concomitant bile duct stricture;
• Type C: bile duct stricture without bile leakage;
• Type D: complete transection of the duct, with or without excision of some portion of the biliary tree.

Other classifications are more detailed, such as that by Strasberg *et al.* [118], and are used for planning of surgical repair.

Treatment

Prevention. The majority of strictures would be prevented if: (1) cholecystectomy was only performed by experienced surgeons; (2) the top–down approach was used with thorough dissection at the junction of the gallbladder infundibulum and cystic duct; and (3) there was an appropriate threshold for conversion from laparoscopic to open surgery. This is particularly so in the presence of acute cholecystitis.

Medical. Fluid and electrolyte balance must be maintained, particularly in the jaundiced septic patient and those with a biliary fistula. Antibiotic therapy, based if possible on blood and bile culture, will improve septicaemia but, if there is bile duct obstruction or a leak, bile duct catheterization and drainage by the endoscopic or percutaneous route is essential to treat sepsis. Bile collections may need percutaneous drainage under scanning control.

The overriding principle is the importance of early referral to a specialist hepatobiliary centre where there will be a multidisciplinary approach by surgeon, radiologist and endoscopist [119].

Interventional endoscopy and radiology; surgical repair. Bile leakage from a cystic duct stump or tiny ducts in the gallbladder bed can usually be managed endoscopically by stent insertion [116]. This is the first-choice procedure.

For the incomplete stricture, endoscopic balloon dilatation and stenting, using repeat procedures with graded increase in balloon diameter and number of stents, over a year gives a successful outcome in 80–90% of postcholecystectomy strictures [120–122]. Success with strictures at the hilar confluence is lower.

An analysis of mesh metal stents in this scenario suggests that they should not be used unless life expectancy is less than 2 years, because of occlusion [123]. Whether removable covered mesh metal stents have any role awaits outcome analysis.

For the completely obstructed or transected bile duct, surgery is necessary after investigation and preparatory percutaneous bile drainage, as appropriate to the individual patient. The endoscopic route is likely to be of no value. These are complex patients requiring a specialist multidisciplinary team.

Preoperative percutaneous transhepatic biliary drainage is performed. Intra-abdominal collections are drained. Other preoperative investigations are done, including angiography to detect vascular damage. Surgery may then be performed electively in the subsequent weeks under optimal conditions.

The operation chosen will depend mainly on two factors—the site and length of the stricture and the amount of duct available for repair. Any operation must provide excision of the stricture with mucosal apposition between the duct lining and the intestinal mucosa. The anastomosis must be as large as possible and not under tension.

Even if sufficient duct is available proximally, excision of the stricture and end-to-end anastomosis of the duct is rarely performed. Differences between the calibre of the duct above and below the stricture are too great for a satisfactory anastomosis. Recurrent stricture occurs in 60% of cases.

The usual operation is between the bile duct and a Roux-en-Y segment of jejunum (*choledochojejunostomy*). In the case of high stricture, the hepatic duct is used (*hepaticojejunostomy*) (Fig. 12.17).

Successful long-term results of hepaticojejunostomy (mean 5 years) have been reported in 50 of 54 patients in one series [124]. Predictors of poor outcome were peritonitis at the time of reconstruction, combined vascular and bile duct injuries and injury at or above the level of the biliary bifurcation. Another series also analysed associations with a poor outcome which included three or more attempts at operative repair before referral, hypoalbuminaemia, high serum bilirubin, the presence of liver disease and portal hypertension [125].

Stenosis of a hepaticojejunostomy done either as the primary repair, or after failed other approaches, may be managed by interventional radiological approaches, or by surgical revision (see below).

Postcholecystectomy syndromes

About 90–95% of those *with gallstones* are freed of symptoms or improved postoperatively. The absence of stones questions the original diagnosis. These patients may have been suffering from a psychosomatic or some other disorder including non-visceral pain [126]. Results of surgery are poor when done for vague symptoms such as abdominal bloating or dyspepsia, or in patients using psychiatric medication [127,128]. A biliary cause is likely

if stones are found at cholecystectomy and if a period of relief follows the operation. The colon and pancreas are common alternative culprits.

Postoperative symptoms may be related to technical difficulties at the time of surgery. These include traumatic *biliary stricture* and *residual calculi* (see below).

Amputation neuromas can be demonstrated in some patients but removal offers no relief and this seems unlikely to be the cause of the symptoms.

Chronic pancreatitis, a common association of *choledocholithiasis*, may persist postoperatively.

US is the first test to image the bile duct. Depending on the result and the clinical features MRCP may be indicated. Despite all these, ERCP is usually necessary. Residual calculi, stricture, ampullary stenosis or normal appearances are significant findings.

Sphincter of Oddi dysfunction [129,130]

This has been an area of controversy but now appears to be a cause of postcholecystectomy pain in some patients. Two forms exist.

Papillary stenosis is defined as narrowing of all or part of the sphincter of Oddi. There is fibrosis. It may follow injury due to stones [131], operative instrumentation, biliary infection or pancreatitis. There may be episodes of pain associated with abnormal liver function tests. On ERCP the bile duct is dilated and drains slowly. The basal sphincter tone is raised on manometry and is not reduced by smooth muscle relaxants. Endoscopic sphincterotomy is helpful [132].

Sphincter of Oddi (biliary) dyskinesia is a more difficult area. Biliary manometry shows a range of abnormalities including sphincter spasm, increased phasic contraction frequency (tachyoddia), paradoxical contraction response to CCK and abnormal propagation of phasic waves.

Clinical features (Table 12.3) are valuable in management decisions. Group I benefit from sphincterotomy in around 90% of cases. In group II manometry is important. Patients with an elevated basal sphincter pressure have had greater benefit from sphincterotomy than those with a normal pressure (91 vs. 42%) [133], although a recent expert review suggests a lower success rate (50–70% vs. 30%) based on manometry result [130]. Studies continue in group III. Duodenal distension reproduces the symptoms in most patients [134]. Sphincterotomy in those with abnormal manometry may be beneficial in only 20–30% of patients [130]. This is a difficult group of patients, and it has been suggested that such patients should first have a trial of medical therapy (including proton pump inhibitors and/or calcium channel blockers (nifedipine)) before considering ERCP and manometry, with the attendant risks, in those without a response [135].

Table 12.3. Sphincter of Oddi dysfunction: classification (modified according to [130])

Group I (definite)	
Biliary-type pain	
Abnormal liver function tests (serum transaminases or alkaline phosphatase > 1.5 × normal) documented on two or more occasions, with normalization between attacks	
Dilated common bile duct > 8mm	Manometry unnecessary
Group II (presumptive)	
Biliary-type pain and one of other group I criteria	Manometry essential
Group III (possible)	
Biliary-type pain only. No other abnormalities	Manometry essential if intervention contemplated

Non-surgical treatment of gallstones in the gallbladder

The widespread availability and acceptance of laparoscopic cholecystectomy has markedly reduced the use of non-surgical treatments for gallbladder stones. However, a small group of patients remain where these approaches need to be considered, including those unfit for or refusing surgery.

Dissolution therapy with ursodeoxycholic acid [136]

Ursodeoxycholic acid decreases biliary cholesterol secretion as well as cholesterol absorption and increases solubility of cholesterol by the formation of liquid crystals [28]. Ursodeoxycholic acid also prolongs nucleation time.

Indications

The patient must be compliant and prepared for at least 2 years of treatment. Symptoms must be mild to moderate and silent stones should not be treated. On oral cholecystography the cystic duct must be patent ('functioning gallbladder') and stones radiolucent, preferably floating. They should be less than 15mm in diameter. Best results are for stones less than 5mm diameter.

Unfortunately, no imaging technique accurately determines the composition of gallstones and therefore solubility. Ultrasound is of little value. CT can be useful and, because of the expense of bile acid therapy, cost-effective in assessing stones. Stones with an attenuation value of less than 100 Hounsfield units (reflecting low calcium content) are more likely to dissolve [137].

Results

The dose of ursodeoxycholic acid is at least 10mg/kg per day with more being needed if the patient is mark-

edly obese. The overall success rate for oral bile acid therapy is approximately 40%, rising to 60% with careful patient selection [138]. Stones of 5mm or less in diameter that float dissolve more quickly (80–90% complete dissolution by 12 months). Larger non-floating stones take longer or never disappear.

The effect of bile acid therapy on symptoms is variable. Biliary pain is less frequent in those patients on long-term ursodeoxycholic acid therapy [139]. Stone recurrence develops in 25–50% of patients at a rate of 10% per year. They are most likely in the first 2 years and unlikely after the first 3 years. Recurrence is higher in those with multiple rather than solitary stones.

Side effects are absent. During treatment the stones may undergo surface calcification [140], but this is probably of little significance.

Extracorporeal shock-wave therapy [141]

Gallbladder stones can be fragmented by shock waves generated extracorporeally using the same principle as that developed for kidney stones. Ultrasound is usually used to target stones. Oral bile acid therapy is given to dissolve those fragments remaining in the gallbladder, although when pulverization is achieved bile acid therapy is not necessary [141]. The gallbladder shows bruising and oedema after the shock waves but these are reversible.

Results

These vary from one machine, centre and protocol to another. Only 20–25% of patients referred satisfy the treatment criteria which included: three or fewer radiolucent gallbladder stones with a total diameter of less than 30mm, in a functioning gallbladder (on cholecystography), in a symptomatic patient who is otherwise healthy.

Studies have shown overall complete clearance rates at 12 months of 70–90%. However, long-term results are disappointing with recurrence rates of more than 40% after 5 year [142]. Because of this and the development of laparoscopic cholecystectomy, this method is now used rarely.

Other gallbladder pathology [143]

Gallbladder polyps

Polypoid lesions of the gallbladder are seen in around 5% of patients scanned by ultrasound (Fig. 12.18). The majority of these are pseudopolyps—that is cholesterol polyps, inflammatory polyps and adenomyomas, but some (15 of 130 in one series) are neoplastic polyps [144]. Of these most are adenomatous, but dysplasia and malignant change are seen, so that carcinoma of the gallbladder is a risk. Most patients with polyps do not have symptoms. Ultrasound does not differentiate the potentially malignant polyp.

Most studies have recommended cholecystectomy for symptomatic patients, and/or for solitary sessile polypoid lesions greater than 10 mm. Surveillance by ultrasound at set (but not well defined) intervals has been recommended for 'polyps' less than 10 mm, with cholecystectomy done when enlargement is detected, or the threshold of 10 mm reached. These recommendations have been recently questioned, mainly because neoplasia, with in some cases a risk of malignancy, has been found in 'polyps' less than 10 mm diameter [144,145]. The rationale is that the threshold for removal may have to be lowered, because development of malignancy (carcinoma of the gallbladder) in general has a poor prognosis. The data from a recent study found that reducing the threshold diameter to 6 mm gave an 18.5% positive and 100% negative predictive value for neoplastic change, and dropped the false negative rate to 0% [144].

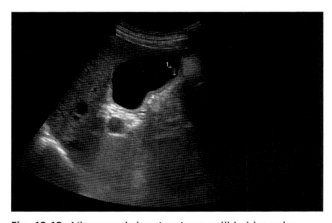

Fig. 12.18. Ultrasound showing 4 mm gallbladder polyp, which does not move on repositioning and does not caste an acoustic shadow.

On the other hand, a study showing no change during follow up (5 years) in 91% of polypoid lesions advised a 'wait and see policy'. Histology, however, was not done in this study (no patient had cholecystectomy) [146]. These recent papers do raise re-examination of the previous recommendation based on a threshold of 10 mm diameter for intervention. However, the use of a lower threshold recognizes that in some patients no lesion is found in a proportion of patients, 27% in the series quoted [144].

Cholecystectomy in polyps is recommended in lesions that show growth, vascularity, invasion, as well as those that are symptomatic, and in those where surveillance is not possible. Age (>50) and the presence of gallstones are also factors to take in account in the decision [147]. To what extent EUS would be able to separate those with and without a malignant potential is unclear.

The risk of malignancy in polyps is considered greater in patients with primary sclerosing cholangitis, and thus cholecystectomy has been recommended in all such patients [148].

Thus, for asymptomatic patients with lesions seen on US less than 6 mm diameter, surveillance is the agreed approach. For polypoid lesions larger than this, there is agreement that those enlarging or greater than 10 mm diameter be removed by cholecystectomy. Whether the threshold for removal is better reduced below 10 mm is conjectural. The presence of other risk factors may favour removal.

Adenomyomatosis

This may affect the gallbladder wall profusely or locally. There is epithelial proliferation with muscular hypertrophy and mural diverticulae (Rokitansky–Aschoff sinuses), which may be seen as spots of contrast medium outside the lumen of the gallbladder on oral cholecystography after a fatty meal. The changes may also be shown by US, CT and MRI. Demonstration of Rokitansky–Aschoff sinuses is important so as to make the diagnosis—and differentiate the thickened gallbladder wall from other causes. Adenomyomatosis may cause chronic symptoms, which are relieved by cholecystectomy.

Cholesterolosis

There is accumulation of cholesterol and triglyceride in the gallbladder wall. It is present in 50% of patients with gallstones, and 35% of symptomatic patients without stones having cholecystectomy for polyp or adenomyomatosis [149].

Cholesterol esters and other lipids are deposited in the submucosal and epithelial cells as small, yellow, lipid specks. As more lipid is deposited, it projects into the lumen as polyps which may become pedunculated.

The change is confined to the gallbladder and never extends to the ducts.

The cholesterolosis is related to the biliary, not blood, cholesterol concentration.

The aetiology is uncertain. The gallbladder mucosa may simply be taking up excess cholesterol from bile. Other possibilities are a defect in submucosal macrophages, impaired transport of cholesterol out of the mucosa [149] or increased cholesterol ester synthesis by the gallbladder mucosa [150].

There is controversy concerning the relation of cholesterolosis to symptoms. However, cholesterolosis may sometimes cause right upper quadrant pain and features causing confusion with the irritable bowel syndrome. Diagnosis is from histology since the changes are generally not shown radiologically.

Xanthogranulomatous cholecystitis

This is an uncommon inflammatory disease of the gallbladder characterized by a focal or diffuse destructive inflammatory process with lipid-laden macrophages. Macroscopically, areas of xanthogranulomatous cholecystitis appear as yellow masses within the wall of the gallbladder. The gallbladder wall is invariably thickened and cholesterol or mixed gallstones are usually present.

The pathogenesis is uncertain, but an inflammatory response to extravasated bile, possibly from ruptured Rokitansky–Aschoff sinuses, is likely.

Symptoms often begin with an episode of acute cholecystitis which persist. There is extension of yellow tissue into adjacent organs. US and/or CT may show hypoechoic or low attenuation areas or bands in the gallbladder wall [143]. Because of the difficulty in pre- and perioperative differentiation from carcinoma of the gallbladder in some cases, extended resection as for malignant disease has been reported [151].

Porcelain gallbladder

This rare condition (0.4–0.8% at cholecystectomy) is due to extensive calcification of the gallbladder wall. Circumferential calcification is seen on abdominal X-ray or CT [143]. Ultrasound is helpful in showing the extent of involvement of the gallbladder wall. It was thought that porcelain gallbladder has a relationship to gallbladder carcinoma, although this is conjectural. Particular patterns of calcification may be relate to risk (see Chapter 13).

Typhoid cholecystitis

Circulating typhoid bacilli are filtered by the liver and excreted in the bile. The biliary tract, however, is infected in only about 0.2% of patients with typhoid fever. Colonization may be facilitated by biofilm formation on cholesterol gallstones [152].

Acute typhoid cholecystitis is becoming very rare. Signs of acute cholecystitis appear at the end of the second week or even during convalescence, and are sometimes followed by perforation of the gallbladder.

Chronic typhoid fever cholecystitis and the typhoid carrier state. The typhoid carrier passes organisms in the faeces derived from a focus of infection in the gallbladder or biliary tract. Chronic typhoid cholecystitis is symptomless. The carrier state is not cured by antibiotic therapy. Cholecystectomy is successful if there is no associated infection of the biliary ducts. Chronic typhoid cholecystitis is not an important cause of gallstones, but carries an increased risk of gallbladder carcinoma [153].

Biliary carriers of other salmonellae have been reported and treated with ampicillin and cholecystectomy.

Acute cholecystitis in AIDS

This is thought to occur because of gallbladder stasis and increased bile lithogenicity in the critically ill patient, opportunistic pathogens such as cytomegalovirus (CMV) and cryptosporidium, or vascular insufficiency due to oedema or infection. Calculous and acalculous cholecystitis are seen.

Patients present with fever, right upper quadrant pain and tenderness. The white cell count is often normal but with a left shift of neutrophils. Ultrasound shows features of acute cholecystitis.

Treatment is by cholecystectomy. In the late1980s, this carried a mortality of around 30% due to sepsis [154]. However, a mortality of 2% was reported in a series of 53 patients with acute cholecystitis in 1999 from the same group, thought due to improvement in medical treatment [155]. Highly active antiretroviral therapy (HAART) is associated with a reduction in postoperative complications after cholecystectomy [156].

Acute cholecystitis is one part of the spectrum of hepatobiliary disease seen in patients with HIV. There may be parenchymal liver disease (see Chapter 22). Pancreatitis may be seen from HIV-related medications or less often opportunistic infections. AIDS-related diseases include not only acalculous cholecystitis, but also Kaposi's sarcoma, gallstones and AIDS cholangiopathy [157,158].

AIDS cholangiopathy has several patterns: papillary stenosis with bile duct dilatation above; a sclerosing cholangitis-like appearance of intra- and extrahepatic ducts; a combination of the two; or segmental extrahepatic strictures. Patients may be asymptomatic, or present with malaise, fever or right upper quadrant pain. US and CT may be useful, but the combination of

MRI and MRCP is valuable [159]. ERCP allows biopsies and bile to be taken, and if appropriate sphincterotomy to be done. Since the introduction of HAART, the incidence of AIDS cholangiography has declined (as with other AIDS-related diseases), and survival with this entity has improved significantly [157]. A worse outcome is associated with opportunistic infections (especially *Cryptosporidia*) and an alkaline phosphatase of greater than eight times normal.

Other associations including infection

Diseases involving the *cystic artery*, such as polyarteritis nodosa, may lead to cholecystitis [160].

The gallbladder may be involved in *Crohn's disease*.

Actinomycosis can very rarely involve the gallbladder, as may *Vibrio cholerae* [161] and *Leptospirosis* [162], which have been associated with acalculous cholecystitis. The pathological significance of *Helicobacter* spp. in the biliary tree still seems uncertain.

Congenital gallbladder anomalies (see Chapter 14)

Possible gallbladder anomalies include absence, double, left-sided, intrahepatic and folded. Accessory bile ducts and anomalous cystic duct are seen. All are rare, as is floating gallbladder with torsion [163] which may present with pain.

Altrhough these congenital defects seem rarely related to symptoms the range of case reports show that awareness of them is of importance to the radiologist and to the biliary and hepatic transplant surgeon.

Perforation of the gallbladder

Acute calculous cholecystitis may lead to complete necrosis of the gallbladder wall and perforation. The gallstone may erode the necrotic wall; alternatively, dilated infected Rokitansky–Aschoff sinuses may provide a weak point for rupture.

Rupture usually takes place at the fundus which is the least well-vascularized part of the gallbladder. Discharge into the free peritoneal cavity is rare and, more usually, adhesions form between adjacent organs with local abscess formation. Rupture into adjacent viscera leads to internal biliary fistula.

The patient presents with nausea, right upper quadrant pain and vomiting. A right upper quadrant mass is palpable in 50%, and a similar number are febrile. The diagnosis is often overlooked. CT and ultrasound are of value in showing peritoneal fluid, abscess and gallstones.

There are three clinical types:

1 *Acute with bile peritonitis.* A history of gallbladder disease is rare. Associated systemic conditions include vascular insufficiency or immunodeficiency such as atherosclerosis, diabetes mellitus, collagen diseases, corticosteroid use or decompensated cirrhosis. The diagnosis should be suspected in any immunocompromised patient, such as a patient with AIDS with an acute abdomen. Prognosis is poor with a mortality of about 30%. Treatment is by massive antibiotics and restoration of the fluid balance. The gangrenous gallbladder wall is removed or drained percutaneously or surgically. Any abscess must also be drained.

2 *Subacute with pericholecystic abscess.* These patients have chronic gallstone disease and the picture is intermediate between the acute and chronic types.

3 *Chronic* with cholecystenteric fistula formation, such as between the gallbladder and colon (see below and Fig. 12.19).

Biliary fistulae

External

These follow procedures such as cholecystotomy, transhepatic biliary drainage or T-tube choledochotomy, after the tube or catheter has been removed.

Because of the sodium and bicarbonate content of bile, patients with large leaks run a risk of hyponatraemic acidosis and impaired renal function.

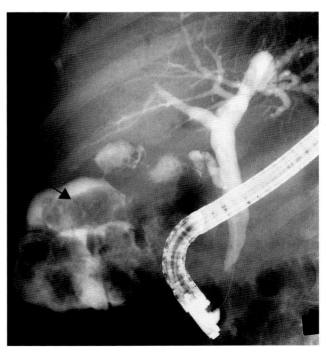

Fig. 12.19. Endoscopic retrograde cholangiopancreatography showing a fistula between the gallbladder and colon (large arrow).

Distal bile duct obstruction may contribute to the failure of a fistula to heal and the placement of an endoscopic stent is likely to be beneficial.

Internal

In 80% these are due to long-standing calculous cholecystitis. The inflamed gallbladder, containing stones, adheres and ruptures into a segment of the intestine, usually the duodenum and less often the colon (Fig. 12.19). The ejected gallstones may be passed or cause intestinal obstruction (*gallstone ileus*), usually in the terminal ileum.

Biliary fistulae may also follow rupture of a chronic duodenal ulcer into the gallbladder or common bile duct. Fistulae may also develop between the colon and biliary tract in ulcerative colitis or Crohn's disease.

Clinical features

The fistula may be symptomless and, when the gallstones have discharged into the intestine successfully, the fistula closes. Such instances are often diagnosed only at the time of a later cholecystectomy.

About one-third give a history of jaundice or are jaundiced on admission. Pain may be absent or as severe as biliary colic. The features of cholangitis may be present. In cholecystocolic fistula the common bile duct may be filled with calculi, putrefying matter and faeces, which cause the severe cholangitis. Bile salts entering the colon produce severe diarrhoea.

Radiological features

These include gas in the biliary tract and the presence of a gallstone in an unusual position. The biliary tree may be filled from barium meal in the case of a cholecystoduodenal fistula, or at barium enema, in the case of a cholecystocolic fistula. ERCP should be diagnostic (Fig. 12.19).

Treatment

Fistulae due to gallbladder disease are treated surgically.

Endoscopic treatment of common duct stones can result in closure of cholecystocolic and bronchobiliary fistulae [164].

Gallstone ileus

A gallstone over 2.5 cm in diameter entering the intestine causes obstruction, usually of the ileum, less often of the duodenojejunal junction, duodenal bulb, pylorus

or colon [165]. The impacted gallstone may excite an inflammatory reaction in the intestinal wall, or cause intussusception. Gallstone ileus is very rare but is a cause of non-strangulated intestinal obstruction.

The patient is usually an elderly, afebrile female, possibly with a preceding history suggestive of chronic cholecystitis. The onset is insidious, with nausea, occasional vomiting, colicky abdominal pain and a somewhat distended but flaccid abdomen. There is obstruction to the bowel, and 'ileus' is a misnomer.

A plain X-ray of the abdomen may show loops of distended bowel with fluid levels and possibly the obstructing stone. Gas may be seen in the biliary tract and gallbladder, indicating a biliary fistula.

The plain film on admission is diagnostic in about 50% of patients. Ultrasound, barium studies and CT provide diagnostic information in a further 25%.

Preoperative diagnosis is made in about 70% of cases [165].

Treatment

The intestinal obstruction should be relieved surgically. Whether fistula repair and cholecystectomy are done at the time of the first operation to relieve intestinal obstruction is debated [166]. The decision may be based on the clinical state of the patient and the operative feasibility [165]. If not done at the initial operation, subsequent cholecystectomy is not mandatory. Recurrent gallstone ileus has been reported at 17% with such treatment [165]. Surgical mortality in series is reported from 10 to 30%.

Bile peritonitis

Aetiology

Postcholecystectomy. Bile may leak from small bile channels between the gallbladder and liver or from an imperfectly ligated cystic duct (see also pg 274). If the biliary pressure is raised, perhaps by a residual common duct stone or papillary stenosis, leakage is facilitated and the subsequent paraductal bile accumulation favours the development of biliary stricture.

Post-transplantation. Leakage of bile from the bile duct anastomosis is a recognized complication of liver transplantation (see Chapter 36).

Rupture of the gallbladder. Empyema or gangrene of the gallbladder may lead to rupture and the formation of an abscess; this is localized by previous inflammatory adhesions.

Trauma. Crushing or gunshot wounds may involve the biliary tree. Needle biopsy of the liver or percutaneous cholangiography may rarely be complicated by puncture of the gallbladder or of a dilated intrahepatic bile duct in a patient with deep cholestasis. Oozing of bile rarely follows operative liver biopsy.

Spontaneous. Biliary peritonitis may develop in patients with prolonged, deep obstructive jaundice without demonstrable breach of the biliary tree. This is presumably due to bursting of minute superficial intrahepatic bile ducts.

Common bile duct perforation is exceedingly rare. The factors concerned are similar to those for perforated gallbladder. They include increases of intraductal pressure, calculous erosion and necrosis of the duct wall secondary to thrombosis [167].

Spontaneous perforation of the extrahepatic bile ducts is a rare cause of jaundice in infancy, the most common site being at the confluence of the cystic and common hepatic duct. The pathogenesis is unknown (see Chapter 14).

Clinical picture

This depends on whether the bile is localized or free in the peritoneal cavity, sterile or infected. Free rupture of bile into the peritoneal cavity causes severe shock. Due to the irritant effect of bile salts, large quantities of plasma are poured into the ascitic fluid. The onset is with excruciating, generalized, abdominal pain. Examination shows a shocked patient, with low blood pressure and persistent tachycardia. There is board-like rigidity of the diffusely tender abdomen. Paralytic ileus is a frequent complication. Bile peritonitis should always be considered in any patient with unexplained intestinal obstruction. In a matter of hours secondary infection follows and the temperature rises while abdominal pain and tenderness persist.

Laboratory findings are non-contributory. Abdominal paracentesis reveals bile, usually infected. Serum bilirubin rises and this is followed by an increase in alkaline phosphatase levels. Cholescintigraphy or cholangiography will show the leakage of bile.

Treatment

Rupture of the gallbladder is treated by cholecystectomy. Biliary leakage from the common bile duct can be treated by endoscopic stenting (with or without sphincterotomy) or nasobiliary drainage. If the leak does not seal over in 7–10 days, surgery may be necessary. Scanning-guided drainage of collections may be necessary.

Association between cholecystectomy and colorectal cancer

Both cohort studies and meta-analyses have suggested a possible increase in carcinoma of the proximal colon after cholecystectomy [168–170]. This is not seen in all populations studied, and some have suggested that some bias may be present in the studies. The data relating cholecystectomy (and cholelithiasis) to colonic adenoma are even less secure and prospective data in larger populations have been suggested. The putative mechanism for any risk relates to possible changes in faecal bile acids and cholesterol metabolites, which may promote colorectal oncogenesis. Cholecystectomy may allow greater exposure of conjugated primary bile acids to anaerobic intestinal bacteria and so increase production of carcinogens. Since cholecystectomy is done for clinical reasons this possible association is of questionable clinical relevance—particularly with the development of surveillance programmes for colonic tumour.

Common duct stones

The majority of stones in the common bile duct have passed from the gallbladder. Migration is related to the size of the stone relative to the cystic and common bile duct. Stones may pass uneventfully into the duodenum, cause acute pancreatitis, acute cholangitis, isolated abdominal pain or remain clinically silent in the duct. They may result in partial *obstruction to the common bile duct* with intermittent obstructive jaundice. Infection behind the obstruction, *cholangitis*, is common and is one cause of liver abscess.

After cholecystectomy stones may be left unintentionally in the common bile duct, or slip there from the cystic duct stump. These present in a similar way.

Stones not of gallbladder origin but forming in the duct usually follow partial biliary obstruction due to other residual calculi, traumatic stricture, sclerosing cholangitis or congenital biliary abnormalities. Infection may be the initial event. Stones are brown (see Fig. 12.10b), single or multiple, often oval and conforming to the long axis of the duct.

Effects of common bile duct stones

Bile duct obstruction is usually partial and intermittent since the calculus exerts a ball-valve effect at the lower end of the common bile duct.

Asymptomatic. Duct stones are sometimes discovered incidentally on scanning after investigation of mildly cholestatic liver function tests, or when another system is being scanned (e.g. virtual colonoscopy). It is often surprising that the patient has had no symptoms. In the elderly, they may present simply as general malaise, or mental and physical debility [171].

Pain with abnormal liver tests. Pain occurs in about three-quarters of patients, is usually severe, colicky and intermittent and needs analgesics for its relief. Sometimes it is a constant, sharp, severe pain. The site may be right upper quadrant or epigastric. It radiates to the back and to the right scapula. It is associated with vomiting. Palpation of the epigastrium is painful. The serum has the changes of cholestasis with one or more of raised alkaline phosphatase, γ-glutamyl transpeptidase and conjugated bilirubin. In acute obstruction the transaminase levels may be briefly very high. Full blood count may show neutrophilia.

Cholangitis. The classical picture is of jaundice, abdominal pain, chills and fever (Charcot's triad). This triad also is not specific to duct stones, and can be seen occasionally in viral hepatitis.

It is important to make a judgement on the severity of cholangitis, since this has a major influence on management. Most patients have mild or moderate cholangitis, based on clinical and laboratory data and the response to antibiotic therapy [172]. In those who do not respond to antibiotic therapy, or have features of septic shock, resuscitation and urgent biliary decompression is necessary. Confusion and hypotension added to Charcot's triad has been termed Reynold's pentad, which was associated with *acute obstructive suppurative cholangitis*, and the need to perform urgent bile duct drainage [173]. Grades of severity of cholangitis have been defined recently in the Tokyo Guidelines [174] with the severe type being that with associated organ dysfunction (one only of hypotension, confusion, respiratory or renal dysfunction (creatinine >170μmol/L), or raised INR >1.5 or platelets <100×10^9/L). Mild and moderate cholangitis (by definition without organ dysfunction) separate according to the response to antibiotics. The message is clear – severe cholangitis must be recognized and managed urgently.

The bile is infected, probably from the duodenum. However the presence of bacteria alone is insufficient to give signs of systemic infection. The biliary pressure must rise due to bile duct blockage. Sepsis may be intermittent or constant. *Blood culture* should be performed during the febrile episode. *Escherichia coli* is the commonest infecting organism. Others include *Klebsiella*, *Streptococcus*, *Pseudomonas*, *Bacteroides* and *Clostridium sp.*.

Acute pancreatitis is due to a stone wedging at, or passing through, the ampulla. The patient presents with an acute abdomen with or without vomiting, and systemic collapse if severe. Serum amylase is raised.

Imaging

As already discussed, where there is suspect biliary tract disease, ultrasonography is the investigation of choice. Dilated ducts and the stone may be seen, but the absence of these should not be regarded as definitive. If the symptoms are strongly suggestive of bile duct stone and there are gallbladder stones, then investigation should be taken further. MRCP is valuable (see Fig. 12.5). Alternatives are EUS or CT. The aim is to detect the duct stone before ERCP is done, usually with sphincterotomy.

Management of duct stones

This depends on the clinical situation—emergency or elective—on the age and general condition of the patient and on the facilities and clinical expertise available. Antibiotics will be given for their systemic effect to treat or prevent septicaemia, and this is probably more relevant than their entry into bile. They are only temporarily effective in controlling the septicaemia if the bile duct is completely obstructed. Decompression is needed. Other measures include control of fluid and electrolyte balance and intravenous vitamin K, if the prothrombin time is prolonged.

Common duct stones without cholangitis

These are usually treated by elective ERCP, sphincterotomy and stone removal. Antibiotics are given to cover the procedure. Stone removal without sphincterotomy is possible, in most cases after balloon dilatation of the sphincter [175]. However the risk of pancreatitis appears to higher using this technique than sphincterotomy [176].

Patients with gallbladder *in situ*

Endoscopic sphincterotomy is definitive for residual postcholecystectomy stones with only 10% having further biliary problems [177]—a similar outcome to surgical treatment.

If the gallbladder is still *in situ* and contains stones, subsequent management depends upon the age and clinical state of the patient. In the elderly, several studies have shown that, after endoscopic sphincterotomy, 5–10% need cholecystectomy for gallbladder disease during 1–9 years' follow-up [178]. However, a randomized trial of sphincterotomy alone versus open cholecystectomy with surgical removal of duct stones found that 15% of patients treated by sphincterotomy alone subsequently required cholecystectomy during a mean follow-up of 17 months [179]. This compared with 4%

of the surgical group needing sphincterotomy after the cholecystectomy for a retained duct stone.

In an otherwise fit patient with duct and gallbladder stones, endoscopic sphincterotomy with subsequent cholecystectomy is the favoured approach unless there are medical or other factors rendering the patient unfit for surgery [172].

Acute cholangitis

The strategy is treatment with antibiotics, with appropriate fluid management followed by ERCP and sphincterotomy. The urgency of endoscopic interventional is governed by the clinical state of the patient, the response to antibiotic and the availability of ERCP with an appropriate team.

The choice of antibiotic depends upon the state of the patient and local policy. A cephalosporin usually suffices. Quinolones (e.g. ciprofloxacin) are an alternative. Cholangiography is timed according to the state of the patient and the response to antibiotics. Stones are removed after endoscopic sphincterotomy. If the stones cannot be extracted, bile drainage is provided by insertion of an endoprosthesis or nasobiliary tube.

This management is necessary independent of whether the gallbladder is *in situ* or not. Subsequent decisions on cholecystectomy have been discussed above.

Acute cholangitis is also the frequent presentation of patients with a blocking or blocked stent placed for a biliary stricture. Management is stent replacement, with antibiotics beforehand. Antibiotic choice may be more complicated if patients have received several different agents previously, and have resistant biliary microorganisms. Previous bile culture should be checked to direct the choice.

Multivariate analysis has identified seven features associated with a poor outcome in a mixed group of patients with cholangitis treated surgically and by nonsurgical techniques. These were acute renal failure, cholangitis associated with liver abscess or liver cirrhosis, cholangitis secondary to high malignant biliary strictures or after percutaneous transhepatic cholangiography, female gender and age over 50 years [180].

Acute obstructive suppurative cholangitis

As described above, clinical features that identify this syndrome are fever, jaundice, pain, and, more importantly, features of single or multiple organ dysfunction. Confusion and hypotension may be followed by renal failure and thrombocytopenia, as part of a disseminated intravascular coagulopathy. This situation indicates the need for biliary decompression by the least invasive approach, as soon as the patient's state allows.

Antibiotics should cover Gram-negative colonic bacteria, and/or any organism cultured. There are several alternatives but piperacillin/ tazobactam is a good choice, with an aminoglycoside (e.g. gentamicin) and metronidazole if the clinical picture is life threatening. Aminoglycoside should only be used for as short a period as possible because of the risk of nephro- and ototoxicity. Most cases are caused by common duct stones. ERCP is done with sphincterotomy and stone removal, if coagulation and anatomy permit. If not, then a stent or nasobiliary tube is inserted.

The aim of any procedure is to *guarantee decompression of the biliary system*. The endoscopic approach is now accepted as the first choice, although there is still a mortality of around 5–10% [181,182]. If this method fails, percutaneous transhepatic external bile drainage is the second choice. Every attempt should be made not to raise the biliary pressure more than necessary by contrast injection, simply to place a drain (either by endoscopic or percutaneous approach), to avoid worsening septicaemia. A full diagnostic cholangiogram is not usually necessary. Surgical operation carries a greater mortality than non-surgical techniques, being between 16 and 40% [182].

After biliary decompression there is usually rapid resolution of septicaemia and toxaemia. If not, drainage of the biliary system should be checked, or another source of sepsis sought, such as empyema of the gallbladder or liver abscess.

Acute gallstone pancreatitis

Gallstones travelling down the bile duct may produce acute pancreatitis as they pass through the ampulla. The stones are usually small and pass into the faeces. The inflammation then subsides. Sometimes the stone does not pass out of the ampulla and pancreatitis persists and may be severe. Abnormal liver function tests, particularly transaminases, and ultrasound are the most useful tests to identify the patient with pancreatitis due to gallstones [183]. Early (within 72 h) ERCP and sphincterotomy to remove the stone(s) has been shown to reduce complications and cholangitis in patients with severe, but not mild, biliary pancreatitis, and in those with coincident jaundice or cholangitis [184,185]. The optimal timing and selection of patients awaits further study.

Biliary sludge may also cause attacks of acute pancreatitis [186]. Biliary microscopy or EUS may be useful to define this.

Large common duct stones

Stones greater than 15 mm in diameter are sometimes difficult or impossible to remove with a standard basket

Table 12.4. Non-surgical treatment options for large common duct stones

Mechanical lithotripsy ('crushing basket')
Endoprosthesis
Extracorporeal shock-wave lithotripsy
Electrohydraulic lithotripsy
Laser lithotripsy

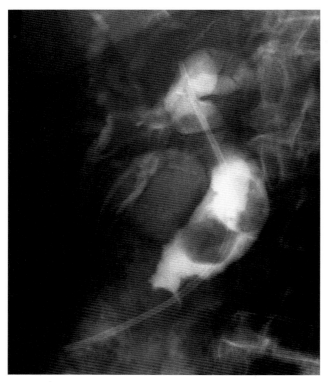

Fig. 12.20. Endoscopic retrograde cholangiopancreatography in a patient with acute cholangitis. The common bile duct contains a large stone which could not be removed. A stent was inserted to provide drainage.

or balloon after sphincterotomy. There are several options (Table 12.4), which will depend upon local expertise.

Mechanical lithotripsy may crush the stone but is limited by basket design and stone shape and size. However 90% success is possible [187].

Extracorporeal shock-wave lithotripsy can fragment 70–90% of large common duct stones with subsequent clearance of fragments through the sphincterotomy in the majority of patients, with less than a 1% 30-day mortality [188,189].

Endoscopic electrohydraulic and *laser lithotripsy*, if available, may be used for difficult stones [190].

The easiest method, particularly in the poor-risk patient, is the insertion of an *endoprosthesis* (Fig. 12.20),

which may be long term, or temporary before surgical or endoscopic duct clearance. Early complications are seen in 12%, with a mortality of 4% [191]. Biliary colic, cholangitis and cholecystitis are late complications [192]. Stones may become smaller after stenting and may then be easier to remove at later ERCP [193].

Trans T-tube tract removal of stones

Retained stones can be removed percutaneously along the T-tube tract in 77–96% of patients [194] with a complication rate of 2–4% (cholangitis, pancreatitis, tract perforation). The T-tube should have been in place for 4–5 weeks before stone removal to allow a fibrous tract to form. Because of the availability of endoscopic techniques including sphincterotomy, percutaneous removal is now infrequently used. With a T-tube in place the endoscopic approach is successful in about 75% [194].

Mirizzi syndrome

Impaction of a gallstone in the cystic duct or neck of the gallbladder can cause partial common hepatic duct obstruction [195]. Jaundice and/or recurrent cholangitis follows and the stone may erode into the common hepatic duct creating a single cavity [196].

Ultrasound shows dilated intrahepatic and common hepatic ducts, but the cause may not been seen or correctly interpreted. Cholangiography shows mid-duct obstruction (Fig. 12.21). There may be the appearances of a stone, and from the outset it may be obvious that this is in cystic rather than bile duct. However, the appearances may initially suggest a common duct stone and only when attempts have failed to remove it does it become clear that the situation is more complicated. The operator must be alert to the possibility of a cystic duct stone and Mirizzi syndrome. Endoscopic therapy is possible (stent insertion) to decompress the biliary system before surgery. Endoscopic stone retrieval is occasionally possible [197]. Surgery consists of removing the diseased gallbladder and the impacted stone.

A higher frequency of gallbladder carcinoma has been reported in Mirizzi syndrome than with long-standing gallstone disease alone [198].

Intrahepatic gallstones

Stones in the intrahepatic ducts are particularly common in certain parts of the world such as the Far East and Brazil, where they are associated with recurrent pyogenic cholangitis and parasitic infestation (see Chapter 32). Gallstones form in chronically obstructed bile ducts due to such conditions as anastomotic biliary–enteric stricture, primary sclerosing cholangitis or Caroli's disease. They are usually of brown pigment type.

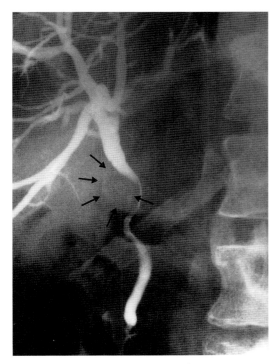

Fig. 12.21. Percutaneous cholangiography in Mirizzi syndrome shows a large gallstone impacted in the cystic duct (arrowed) which has caused obstruction to the common hepatic duct.

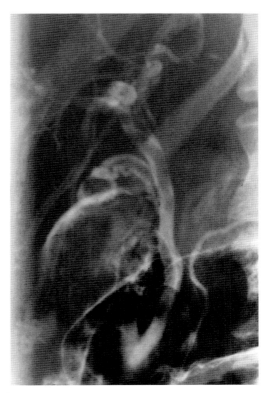

Fig. 12.22. Endoscopic retrograde cholangiopancreatography in haemobilia shows filling defects, representing blood clot in the bile ducts.

Secondary hepatic infection may result in multiple abscesses.

Percutaneous techniques using large-bore transhepatic catheters, combined with surgery if necessary, can clear stones in over 90% of patients, leaving the majority symptom free [199]. The percutaneous transhepatic cholangioscopic approach alone can clear intrahepatic stones in over 70%, with a major complication rate of 7.5% [200]. Removal of stones on the right side is more difficult. There is stone recurrence in 40% of patients who have duct strictures, within 5 years. Surgical resection may need to be considered.

Haemobilia [201]

Haemorrhage into the biliary tract may follow trauma including surgical and needle liver biopsy, aneurysms of the hepatic artery or one of its branches, extra- or intrahepatic tumours of the biliary tract, hepatocellular carcinoma, gallstone disease, inflammation of the liver especially helminthic or pyogenic, and rarely varicose veins related to portal hypertension. Iatrogenic disease such as liver biopsy and percutaneous transhepatic cholangiography and bile drainage now accounts for 40%.

Clinical features are pain related to the passage of clots, jaundice and haematemesis and melaena. Minor episodes may be shown only by positive occult blood tests in faeces.

Diagnosis is suspected whenever upper gastrointestinal bleeding is associated with biliary colic, jaundice or a right upper quadrant mass or tenderness.

MRCP, ERCP or percutaneous cholangiography may show the clot in the ducts (Fig. 12.22).

Treatment

Many resolve spontaneously. If bleeding continues angiography with embolization of a bleeding vessel if seen is indicated [202]. If clot obstructs the bile duct or gives colic, ERCP and drainage or sphincterotomy may be necessary [203].

Bile duct–bowel anastomotic stricture

Choledochojejunostomies and hepaticojejunostomies may stricture. Between 10 and 30% of patients with such anastomoses will need a further procedure—surgical or radiological [124,204]. Of the recurrent strictures, two-thirds occur within 2 years and 90% by 5 years [205]. If the patient remains symptom-free for 4 years postoperatively, there is a 90% chance of complete cure. This happy result reduces with the number of operations, but *can* follow many attempts at repair.

Clinical features

Restricturing presents as fever, rigors and jaundice. There may be pain. Previous episodes of mild flu-like symptoms may precede the major attack. Cholangitis does not necessarily indicate restenosis, but can be due to intrahepatic strictures or stones, or improperly constructed enteric loops up to the anastomosis with reflux and increased pressure [206].

Investigations

Investigations in the acute phase show leucocytosis and abnormal liver function tests, often with a transient rise in transaminase (due to short-term acute obstruction) with later elevation of alkaline phosphatase and γ-glutamyl transpeptidase.

Radiology

A plain film of the abdomen may show air in the biliary tree and the site of the stricture. Air in the ducts does not necessarily imply a fully patent anastomosis; the alternative is intermittent obstruction. Ultrasound may show dilated ducts but often does not because of the intermittent nature of the obstruction.

Cholangiography by the percutaneous transhepatic route shows whether the anastomosis is strictured (Fig. 12.23); careful fluoroscopic observation of the rate of flow of contrast across the anastomosis is of equal importance to the fixed images examined later. If there has been prolonged partial obstruction with recurrent cholangitis, the changes of secondary sclerosing cholangitis may be seen.

Investigation of the patient with cholangitis but an apparently patent anastomosis is a challenge, since no one imaging technique can be relied upon to demonstrate the cause [206]. Scintigraphy may be useful. There may be poor drainage through the afferent loop of a Roux-en-Y anastomosis.

Treatment

Usually access to the biliary system is only possible percutaneously. A percutaneous transhepatic balloon catheter is passed across the stricture and the balloon inflated. After dilatation, an internal–external catheter with numerous side holes sitting above and below the dilated stricture is left in place. Dilatation can be repeated. Balloon dilatation is usually used without endoprosthesis insertion.

Success rates of percutaneous approaches vary considerably; balloon dilatation is effective in three-quarters

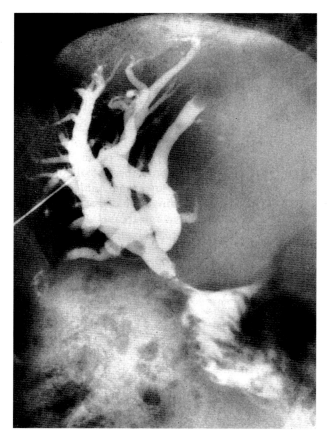

Fig. 12.23. Percutaneous transhepatic cholangiogram in a patient with hepaticojejunostomy following postcholecystectomy stricture. There is restenosis at the anastomosis with dilatation of the ducts in the right lobe.

of patients with a 30-month follow-up [207]. However, the multidisciplinary approach is essential to tailor treatment according to the individual patient in order to reduce the risk of secondary biliary cirrhosis. A retrospective comparison has shown better results with surgical repair than with percutaneous balloon dilatation at around 30 months (90 vs. 65%) [208]. However, the multidisciplinary approach (using both options as necessary) gave a successful outcome in all patients.

Chronic pancreatitis

Pancreatitis, usually of alcoholic aetiology, can cause narrowing of the intrapancreatic portion of the common bile duct. The resultant cholestasis may be transient during exacerbations of acute pancreatitis. This is presumably due to oedema of the pancreas. More persistent cholestasis follows encasement of the low bile duct in a progressively fibrotic pancreatitis. Pseudocysts of the pancreatic head can also cause biliary obstruction.

Bile duct stenosis affects about 8% of patients with chronic alcoholic pancreatitis. It should be suspected if

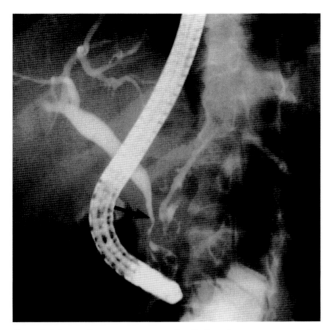

Fig. 12.24. Endoscopic retrograde cholangiopancreatography in a patient with alcoholic chronic pancreatitis. Note the 'rat tail' narrowing of the distal common bile duct (arrow).

the serum alkaline phosphatase is more than twice elevated for longer than 1 month. ERCP shows a smooth narrowing of the lower end of the bile duct, sometimes adopting a rat tail configuration (Fig. 12.24). The main pancreatic duct may be tortuous, irregular and dilated. Pancreatic calcification may be present.

Liver biopsy shows portal fibrosis, features of biliary obstruction and sometimes biliary cirrhosis. Features of alcoholic liver disease are unusual. Hepatic fibrosis regresses after biliary decompression [209].

Management

Early diagnosis is essential as biliary cirrhosis and acute cholangitis can develop in the absence of clinical jaundice.

If alcohol is responsible for the pancreatitis the patient must abstain completely.

The place of surgery is controversial. Clinical, laboratory and imaging data do not necessarily distinguish those patients with significant bile duct obstruction from those with alcoholic liver disease or normal liver histology. Liver biopsy is valuable in deciding whether surgical decompression of the bile duct is necessary.

Plastic stents successfully relieve bile duct obstruction due to chronic pancreatitis. Placement of multiple plastic stents, to preserve wider dilatation of the stricture, for 12 months has led to an effective outcome after 4 years' follow up, though patients with calcific do worse than those with non-calcific pancreatitis [210] Covered meta-

llic stents may have a place but are under study [211]. Acute cholangitis, biliary cirrhosis and protracted jaundice are strong indicators for surgery [212]. Choledochoenterostomy is the usual procedure.

Primary sclerosing cholangitis and autoimmune pancreatitis (see Chapter 16)

Extra- and intrahepatic bile ducts are diffusely involved in approximately 80% of patients with primary sclerosing cholangitis. If the patient develops persistent jaundice or recurrent sepsis, investigations are necessary to show whether there is a dominant stricture, that is one which appears to be causing significant obstruction compared with the diffuse changes elsewhere. Ultrasound may show duct dilatation; MRCP or ERCP will show a dominant stricture if present. Brush cytology is necessary. Differentiation of benign stricturing from cholangiocarcinoma is difficult and often impossible.

In autoimmune pancreatitis the biliary tree may be involved with sclerosing cholangitis-like changes, with or without the characteristic pancreatic changes. Steroids typically reverse the bile duct changes, differentiating this syndrome from classic PSC [213].

Bile duct pathology following liver transplantation

See Chapter 36.

References

1 Gore RM, Thakrar KH, Newmark GM *et al.* Gallbladder imaging. *Gastroenterol. Clin. N. Am.* 2010; **39**: 265–287.
2 Sugiyama M, Atomi Y. Endoscopic ultrasonography for diagnosing choledocholithiasis; a prospective comparative study with ultrasonography and computed tomography. *Gastrointest. Endosc.* 1997; **45**: 143–146.
3 Verma D, Kapadia A, Eisen GM *et al.* EUS v MRCP for detection of choledocholithiasis. *Gastrointest. Endosc.* 2006; **64**: 248–254.
4 Liu CL, Lo CM, Chan JK *et al.* EUS for detection of occult cholelithiasis in patients with idiopathic pancreatitis. *Gastrointest. Endosc.* 2000; **51**: 28–32.
5 Jeurnick SM, Poley JW, Steyerberg EW *et al.* ERCP as an outpatient treatment: a review. *Gastrointest. Endosc.* 2008; **68**: 118–123.
6 Andriulli A, Loperfido S, Napolitano G *et al.* Incidence rates of post-ERCP complications: a systematic survey of prospective studies. *Am. J. Gastroenterol.* 2007; **102**: 1781–1788.
7 Williams EJ, Taylor S, Fairclough P *et al.* Are we meeting the standards set for endoscopy? Results of a large-scale prospective survey of Endoscopic retrograde cholangiopancreatograph practice. *Gut* 2007; **56**: 821–829.
8 Cotton PB, Garrow DA, Gallagher J *et al.* Risk factors for complications after ERCP: a multivariate analysis of 11,497

procedures over 12 years. *Gastrointest. Endosc.* 2009; **70**: 80–88.

9 Freeman ML. Pancreatic stents for prevention of post-ERCP pancreatitis: for everyday practice or for experts only? *Gastrointest. Endosc.* 2010; **71**: 940–944.

10 Dumonceau J-M, Andriulli A, Deviere J *et al.* European Society of Gastrointestinal Endoscopy (ESGE) Guideline: Prophylaxis of post-ERCP pancreatitis. *Endoscopy* 2010; **42**: 503–515.

11 Kennedy PTF, Russo E, Kumar N *et al.* The safety and utility of prophylactic pancreatic duct stents in the prevention of post-ERCP pancreatitis: an analysis of practice in a single UK tertiary referral center. *Surg. Endosc.* 2010; **24**: 1923–1928.

12 Cotton PB, Connor P, Rawls E *et al.* Infection after ERCP and antibiotic prophylaxis: a sequential quality-improvement approach over 11 years. *Gastrointest. Endosc.* 2008; **67**: 471–475.

13 Holzbach RT, Marsh M, Olszewski M *et al.* Cholesterol solubility in bile: evidence that supersaturated bile is frequent in healthy man. *J. Clin. Invest.* 1973; **52**: 1467–1479.

14 Jüngst D, Lang T, von Ritter C *et al.* Cholesterol nucleation time in gallbladder bile of patients with solitary or multiple cholesterol gallstones. *Hepatology* 1992; **15**: 804–808.

15 Kibe A, Holzbach RT, LaRusso NF *et al.* Inhibition of cholesterol crystal formation by apolipoproteins in supersaturated model bile. *Science* 1984; **225**: 514–516.

16 Ohya T, Schwarzendrube J, Busch N *et al.* Isolation of a human biliary glycoprotein inhibitor of cholesterol crystallization. *Gastroenterology* 1993; **104**: 527–538.

17 Portincasa P, van Erpecum KJ, Vanberge-Henegouwen GP. Cholesterol crystallization in bile. *Gut* 1997; **41**: 138–141.

18 Hood K, Gleeson D, Ruppin DC *et al.* Prevention of gallstone recurrence by nonsteroidal anti-inflammatory drugs. *Lancet* 1988; **ii**: 1223–1225.

19 Hopman WP, Jansen JB, Rosenbusch G *et al.* Role of cholecystokinin and the cholinergic system in intestinal stimulation of gallbladder contraction in man. *J. Hepatol.* 1990; **11**: 261–265.

20 Maurer KJ, Carey MC, Fox JG. Roles of infection, inflammation, and the immune system in cholesterol gallstone formation. *Gastroenterology* 2009; **136**: 425–440.

21 Van Bodegraven AA, Böhmer CJM, Manoliu RA *et al.* Gallbladder contents and fasting gallbladder volumes during and after pregnancy. *Scand. J. Gastroenterol.* 1998; **33**: 993–997.

22 Janowitz J, Kratzer W, Zemmler T *et al.* Gallbladder sludge: spontaneous course and incidence of complications in patients without stones. *Hepatology* 1994; **20**: 291–294.

23 Shaffer EA. Epidemiology of gallbladder stone disease. *Best Pract. Res. Clin. Gastroenterol.* 2006; **20**: 981–996.

24 Katsika D, Grjibovski A, Einarsson C *et al.* Genetic and environmental influences on symptomatic gallstone disease: a Swedish study of 43,141 twin pairs. *Hepatology* 2005; **41**: 1138–1143.

25 Nakeeb A, Comuzzie AG, Martin L *et al.* Gallstones: genetics versus environment. *Ann. Surg.* 2002; **235**: 842–849.

26 Grünhage F, Acalovschi M, Tirziu S *et al.* Increased gallstone risk in humans conferred by common variant of hepatic ATP-binding cassette transporter for cholesterol. *Hepatology* 2007; **46**: 793–801.

27 Rosmorduc O, Hermelin B, Boelle PY *et al.* ABCB4 gene mutation-associated cholelithiasis in adults. *Gastroenterology* 2003; **125**: 452–459.

28 Lammert F, Miquel J-F. Gallstone disease: from genes to evidence-based therapy. *J. Hepatol.* 2008; **48**: S124–135.

29 Kovacs P, Kress R, Rocha J *et al.* Variation of the gene encoding the nuclear bile salt receptor FXR and gallstone susceptibility in mice and humans. *J. Hepatol.* 2008; **48**: 116–124.

30 Leitzmann MF, Rimm EB, Willett WC *et al.* Recreational physical activity and the risk of cholecystectomy in women. *N. Engl. J. Med.* 1999; **341**: 777–784.

31 Portincasa P, Moschetta A, Palasciano G. Cholesterol gallstone disease. *Lancet* 2006; **368**: 230–239.

32 Biddinger SB, Haas JT, Yu BB *et al.* Hepatic insulin resistance directly promotes formation of cholesterol gallstones. *Nat. Med.* 2008; **14**: 778–782.

33 Maclure KM, Hayes KC, Colditz GA *et al.* Weight, diet and the risk of symptomatic gallstones in middle-aged women. *N. Engl. J. Med.* 1989; **321**: 563–9.

34 Liddle RA, Goldstein RB, Saxton J. Gallstone formation during weight-reduction dieting. *Arch. Intern. Med.* 1989; **149**: 1750–1753.

35 Sugerman HJ, Brewer WH, Schiffman ML *et al.* A multi-center, placebo-controlled, randomised, double-blind, prospective trial of prophylactic ursodiol for the prevention of gallstone formation following gastric-bypass-induced rapid weight loss. *Am. J. Surg.* 1995; **169**: 91–96.

36 Tsai CJ, Leitzmann MF, Willett WC *et al.* Dietary carbohydrates and glycaemic load and the incidence of symptomatic gall stone disease in men. *Gut* 2005; **54**: 823–828.

37 Heaton KW, Emmett PM, Symes CL *et al.* An explanation for gallstones in normal-weight women: slow intestinal transit. *Lancet* 1993; **341**: 8–10.

38 Azzaroli F, Mazzella G, Mazelo P *et al.* Sluggish small bowel motility is involved in determining increased biliary deoxycholic acid in cholesterol gallstone patients. *Am. J. Gastroenterol.* 1999; **94**: 2453–2459.

39 Wells JE, Berr F, Thomas LA *et al.* Isolation and characterization of cholic acid 7 alpha-dehydroxylating fecal bacteria from cholesterol gallstone patients. *J. Hepatol.* 2000; **32**: 4–10.

40 Attili AF, Scafato E, Marchiolo R *et al.* Diet and gallstones in Italy: the cross-sectional MICOL results. *Hepatology* 1998; **27**: 1492–1498.

41 Pixley F, Wilson D, McPherson K *et al.* Effect of vegetarianism on development of gallstones in women. *Br. Med. J.* 1985; **291**: 11–12.

42 Maringhini A, Ciambra M, Baccelliere P *et al.* Biliary sludge and gallstones in pregnancy: incidence, risk factors, and natural history. *Ann. Intern. Med.* 1993; **119**: 116–120.

43 Valdivieso V, Covarrubias C, Siegel F *et al.* Pregnancy and cholelithiasis: pathogenesis and natural course of gallstones diagnosed in early puerperium. *Hepatology* 1993; **17**: 1–4.

44 Boston Collaborative Drug Surveillance Program. Oral contraceptives and venous thromboembolic disease: surgically confirmed gall-bladder disease and breast tumours. *Lancet* 1973; **i**: 1399–1404.

45 Cirillo DJ, Wallace RB, Rodabough RJ *et al*. Effect of estrogen therapy on gallbladder disease. *JAMA* 2005; **293**: 330–339.

46 Henriksson P, Einarsson K, Eriksson A *et al*. Estrogen-induced gallstone formation in males. *J. Clin. Invest.* 1989; **84**: 811–816.

47 Thijs C, Knipschild P, Brombacher P. Serum lipids and gallstones: a case–control study. *Gastroenterology* 1990; **99**: 843–849.

48 Fornari F, Imberti D, Squillante MM *et al*. Incidence of gallstones in a population of patients with cirrhosis. *J. Hepatol.* 1994; **20**: 797–801.

49 Lucidi V, Buggenhout A, Donckier V. Cholecystectomy in cirrhotic patients: pitfalls and reasonable recommendations. *Acta Chir. Belg.* 2009; **109**: 477–480.

50 Frey JW, Peri RE. Perioperative risk assessment for patients with cirrhosis and liver disease. *Expert Rev. Gastroenterol. Hepatol.* 2009; **3**: 65–75.

51 Swidsinski A, Khilkin M, Pahlig H *et al*. Time dependent changes in the concentration and type of bacterial sequences found in cholesterol gallstones. *Hepatology* 1998; **27**: 662–665.

52 Chapman BA, Wilson IR, Frampton CM *et al*. Prevalence of gallbladder disease in diabetes mellitus. *Dig. Dis. Sci.* 1996; **41**: 2222–2228.

53 Keshavarzian A, Dunne M, Iber FL. Gallbladder volume and emptying in insulin requiring male diabetics. *Dig. Dis. Sci.* 1987; **32**: 824–828.

54 Chang TE-S, Lo SK, Shyr H-Y *et al*. Hepatitis C virus infection facilitates gallstone formation. *J. Gastroenterol. Hepatol.* 2005; **20**: 1416–1421.

55 Makino I, Chijiiwa K, Higashijima H *et al*. Rapid cholesterol nucleation time and cholesterol gall stone formation after subtotal or total colectomy in humans. *Gut* 1994; **35**: 1760–1764.

56 Inoue K, Fuchigami A, Higashide S *et al*. Gallbladder sludge and stone formation in relation to contractile function after gastrectomy. *Ann. Surg.* 1992; **215**: 19–26.

57 Dhiman RK, Phanish MK, Chawla YK *et al*. Gallbladder motility and lithogenicity of bile in patients with choledocholithiasis after endoscopic sphincterotomy. *J. Hepatol.* 1997; **26**: 1300–1305.

58 Cicala M, Habib FI, Fiocca F *et al*. Increased sphincter of Oddi basal pressure in patients affected by gall stone disease: a role for biliary stasis and colicy pain? *Gut* 2001; **48**: 414–417.

59 Leuschner U, Güldütuna S, Hellstern A. Pathogenesis of pigment stones and medical treatment. *J. Gastroenterol. Hepatol.* 1994; **9**: 87–98.

60 Brink MA, Slors JFM, Keulemans YCA *et al*. Enterohepatic cycling of bilirubin: a putative mechanism for pigment gallstone formation in ileal Crohn's disease. *Gastroenterology* 1999; **116**: 1420–1427.

61 Sandstad O, Osnes T, Skar V *et al*. Common bile duct stones are mainly brown and associated with duodenal diverticula. *Gut* 1994; **35**: 1464–1467.

62 Mok HYI, Druffel ERM, Rampone WH. Chronology of cholelithiasis. Dating gallstones from atmospheric radiocarbon produced by nuclear bomb explosions. *N. Engl. J. Med.* 1986; **344**: 1075–1077.

63 McSherry CK, Ferstenberg H, Calhoun WF *et al*. The natural history of diagnosed gallstone disease in symptomatic and asymptomatic patients. *Ann. Surg.* 1985; **202**: 59–63.

64 Halldestam I, Enell E-L, Kullman E *et al*. Development of symptoms and complications in individuals with asymptomatic gallstones. *Br. J. Surg.* 2004; **91**: 734–738.

65 Gurusamy KS, Davidson BR. Surgical treatment of gallstones. *Gastroenterol. Clin. N. Am.* 2010; **39**: 229–244.

66 Ransohoff DF, Gracie WA, Wolfenson LB *et al*. Prophylactic cholecystectomy or expectant management for silent gallstones. *Ann. Intern. Med.* 1983; **99**: 199–204.

67 Diehl AK, Beral V. Cholecystectomy and changing mortality from gallbladder cancer. *Lancet* 1981; **i**: 187–189.

68 Diehl AK. Gallstone size and the risk of gallbladder cancer. *JAMA* 1983; **250**: 2323–6.

69 Misra S, Chaturvedi A, Misra NC *et al*. Carcinoma of the gallbladder. *Lancet Oncol.* 2003; **4**: 167–176.

70 Ekbom A, Hsieh CC, Yuen J *et al*. Risk of extrahepatic bile duct cancer after cholecystectomy. *Lancet* 1993; **342**: 1262–1265.

71 Festi D, Sottili S, Colecchia A *et al*. Clinical manifestations of gallstone disease: evidence from the multicentre Italian study on cholelithiasis (MICOL). *Hepatology* 1999; **30**: 839–846.

72 Berger MY, van der Velden JJIM, Lijmer JG *et al*. Abdominal symptoms: do they predict gallstones? *Scand. J. Gastroenterol.* 2000; **35**: 70–76.

73 Hicks RJ, Kelly MJ, Kalff V. Association between false negative hepatobiliary scans and initial gallbladder visualization after 30 min. *Eur. J. Nucl. Med.* 1990; **16**: 747–753.

74 Ransohoff DF, Gracie WA. Treatment of gallstones. *Ann. Intern. Med.* 1993; **119**: 606–619.

75 Hirota M, Takada T, Kawarada Y *et al*. Diagnostic criteria and severity assessment of acute cholecystitis: Tokyo guidelines. *J. Hepatobiliary. Pancreat. Surg.* 2007; **14**: 78–82.

76 Strasberg SM. Acute calculous cholecystitis. *N. Engl. J. Med.* 2008; **358**: 2804–2811.

77 Papi C, Catarci M, D'Ambrosio L *et al*. Timing of cholecystectomy for acute calculous cholecystitis: a meta-analysis. *Am. J. Gastroenterol.* 2004; **99**: 147–155.

78 Hickman MS, Schwesinger WH, Page CP. Acute cholecystitis in the diabetic. A case control study of outcome. *Arch. Surg.* 1988; **123**: 409–411.

79 Chow WC, Ong CL, Png JC *et al*. Gall bladder empyema—another good reason for early cholecystectomy. *J. R. Coll. Surg. Edin.* 1993; **38**: 213–215.

80 Garcia-SanchoTellez L, Rodriquez-Montes JA, Fernandez de Lis S *et al*. Acute emphysematous cholecystitis. Report of twenty cases. *Hepatogastroenterology* 1999; **46**: 2144–2148.

81 Zeebregts CJ, Wijffels RT, de Jong KP *et al*. Percutaneous drainage of emphysematous cholecystitis associated with pneumoperitoneum. *Hepatogastroenterology* 1999; **46**: 771–774.

82 Thistle JL, Cleary PA, Lachin JM *et al*. The natural history of cholelithiasis: the National Cooperative Gallstone Study. *Ann. Intern. Med.* 1984; **101**: 171–175.

83 Owen CC, Jain R. Acute acalculous cholecystitis. *Curr. Treat. Options Gastroenterol.* 2005; **8**: 99–104.

84 Huffman JL, Schenker S. Acute acalculous cholecystitis: a review. *Clin. Gastroenterol. Hepatol.* 2010; **8**: 15–22.

85 Kalliafas S, Ziegler DW, Flancbaum L *et al.* Acute acalculous cholecystitis: incidence, risk factors, diagnosis, and outcome. *Am. Surg.* 1998; **64**: 471–475.

86 Mariat G, Mahul P, Prév TN *et al.* Contribution of ultrasonography and cholescintigraphy to the diagnosis of acute acalculous cholecystitis in intensive care unit patients. *Intensive Care Med.* 2000; **26**: 1658–1663.

87 Drossman DA, Dumitrascu DL. Rome III: new standard for functional gastrointestinal disorders. *J. Gastrointest. Liver Dis.* 2006; **15**: 307–312.

88 Skipper K, Sligh S, Dunn E *et al.* Laparoscopic cholecystectomy for abnormal hepato-iminodiacetic acid scan: a worthwhile procedure. *Am. Surg.* 2000; **66**: 30–32.

89 Yap L, Wycherley AG, Morphett AD *et al.* Acalculous biliary pain: cholecystectomy alleviates symptoms in patients with abnormal cholescintigraphy. *Gastroenterology* 1991; **101**: 786–793.

90 Sabbaghian MS, Rich BS, Rothberger GD *et al.* Evaluation of surgical outcomes and gallbladder characteristics in patients with biliary dyskinesia. *J. Gastrointest. Surg.* 2008; **12**: 1324–1330.

91 Hansel SL, DiBaise JK. Functional gallbladder disorder: gallbladder dyskinesia. *Gastroenterol. Clin. N. Am.* 2010; **39**: 369–379.

92 Thorboli J, Vilmann P, Hassan H. Endoscopic ultrasonography in detection of cholelithiasis in patients with biliary pain and negative transabdominal ultrasonogrpahy. *Scand. J. Gastroenterol.* 2004; **39**: 267–269.

93 Keus F, Gooszen HG, van Laarhoven CJHM. Open, small-incision, or laparoscopic cholecystectomy for patients with symptomatic cholecystolithiasis. An overview of Cochrane Hepato-Biliary Group reviews. *Cochrane Database Syst. Rev.* 2006; CD008318.

94 Gurusamy KS, Samraj K. Early versus delayed laparoscopic cholecystectomy for acute cholecystitis. *Cochrane Database Syst. Rev.* 2010; CD005440.

95 Yamashita Y, Takada T, Kawarada Y *et al.* Surgical treatment of patients with acute cholecystitis. Tokyo guidelines. *J. Hepatobiliary Pancreat. Surg.* 2007; **14**: 91–97.

96 Keus F, Gooszen HG, Van Laarhoven CJHM. Systematic review: open, small-incision or laparoscopic cholecystectomy for symptomatic cholecystolithiasis. *Aliment Pharmacol. Ther.* 2009; **29**: 359–378.

97 McMahon AJ, Russell IT, Baxter JN *et al.* Laparoscopic vs. minilaparotomy cholecystectomy: a randomised trial. *Lancet* 1994; **343**: 135–138.

98 Cox MR, Wilson TG, Luck AJ *et al.* Laparoscopic cholecystectomy for acute inflammation of the gall bladder. *Ann. Surg.* 1993; **218**: 630–634.

99 Kiviluoto T, Sirén J, Luukkonen P *et al.* Randomised trial of laparoscopic vs. open cholecystectomy for acute and gangrenous cholecystitis. *Lancet* 1998; **351**: 321–325.

100 Murphy MM, Ng SC, Simons JP *et al.* Predictors of major complications after laparoscopic cholecystectomy: surgeon, hospital or patient? *J. Am. Coll. Surg.* 2010; **211**: 73–80.

101 Lillemoe KD, Melton GB, Cameron JL *et al.* Postoperative bile duct strictures: management and outcome in the 1990s. *Ann. Surg.* 2000; **232**: 430–441.

102 Flum DR, Cheadle A, Prela C *et al.* Bile duct injury during cholecystectomy and survival in Medicare beneficiaries. *JAMA* 2003; **290**: 2168–2173.

103 Kaafarani HMA, Smith TS, Neumayer L *et al.* Trends, outcomes, and predictors of open and conversion to open cholecystectomy in Veterans Health Administration hospitals. *Am. J. Surg.* 2010; **200**: 32–40.

104 Barkun JS, Fried GM, Barkun AN *et al.* Cholecystectomy without operative cholangiography: implications for common bile duct injury and retained common bile duct stones. *Ann. Surg.* 1993; **218**: 371–377.

105 Millat B, Fingerhut A, Deleuze A *et al.* Prospective evaluation in 121 consecutive unselected patients undergoing laparoscopic treatment of choledocholithiasis. *Br. J. Surg.* 1995; **82**: 1266–1269.

106 Clayton ES, Connor S, Alexakis N *et al.* Meta-analysis of endoscopy and surgery versus surgery alone for common bile duct stones with the gallbladder in situ. *Br. J. Surg.* 2006; **93**: 1185–1191

107 Van Steenbergen W, Ponette E, Marchal G *et al.* Percutaneous transhepatic cholecystostomy for acute complicated cholecystitis in elderly patients. *Am. J. Gastroenterol.*1990; **85**: 1363–1369.

108 Verbanck JJ, Demol JW, Ghillebert GL *et al.* Ultrasound-guided puncture of the gallbladder for acute cholecystitis. *Lancet* 1993; **341**: 1132–1133.

109 Chok KSH, Chu FSK, Cheung TT *et al.* Results of percutaneous transhepatic cholecystostomy for high surgical risk patients with acute cholecystitis. *ANZ J. Surg.* 2010; **80**: 280–283.

110 Johlin FC, Neil GA. Drainage of the gallbladder in patients with acute acalculous cholecystitis by transpapillary endoscopic cholecystotomy. *Gastrointest. Endosc.* 1993; **39**: 645–651.

111 Itoi T, Coehlo-Prabhu N, Baron TH. Endoscopic gallbladder drainage for management of acute cholecystitis. *Gastrointest. Endosc.* 2010; **71**: 1038–1045.

112 Rossi RL, Schirmer WJ, Braasch JW *et al.* Laparoscopic bile duct injuries: risk factors, recognition, and repair. *Arch. Surg.* 1992; **127**: 596–601.

113 Schol FPG, Go PM, Gouma DJ. Risk factors for bile duct injury in laparoscopic cholecystectomy: analysis of 49 cases. *Br. J. Surg.* 1994; **81**: 1786–1788.

114 Lillemoe KD. Benign postoperative bile duct strictures. *Baillière's Clin. Gastroenterol.* 1997; **11**: 749–79.

115 Kurzawinski TR, Selves L, Farouk M *et al.* Prospective study of hepatobiliary scintigraphy and endoscopic cholangiography for the detection of early biliary complications after orthotopic liver transplantation. *Br. J. Surg.* 1997; **84**: 620–623.

116 Lau WY, Lai ECH, Lau SHY. Management of bile duct injury after laparoscopic cholecystectomy: a review. *ANZ J. Surg.* 2010; **80**: 75–81.

117 Bergman JJGHM, van der Brink GR, Rauws EAJ *et al.* Treatment of bile duct lesions after laparoscopic cholecystectomy. *Gut* 1996; **38**: 141–147.

118 Strasberg SM, Herd M, Soper NJ. An analysis of the problem of bile duct injury during laparoscopic cholecystectomy. *J. Am. Coll. Surg.* 1995; **180**: 101–125.

119 Nuzzo G, Giuliante F, Giovannini I *et al.* Advantages of multidisciplinary management of bile duct injuries occurring during cholecystectomy. *Am. J. Surg.* 2008; **195**: 763–769.

120 Vitale GC, Tran TC, Davis BR *et al.* Endoscopic management of post cholecystectomy bile duct strictures. *J. Am. Coll. Surg.* 2008; **206**: 918–923.

121 Costamagna G, Pandolfi M, Mutignani M *et al.* Long term results of endoscopic management of postoperative bile

duct strictures with increasing number of stents. *Gastrointest. Endosc.* 2001; **54**: 162–168.

122 Kuzela L, Oltman M, Sutka J *et al.* Prospective follow up of patients with bile duct strictures due to laparoscopic cholecystectomy, treated endoscopically with multiple stents. *Hepatogastroenterology* 2005; **52**: 1357–1361.

123 Siriwardana HP, Siriwardana AK. Systemic appraisal of the role of metallic endobiliary stents in the treatment of benign biliary stricture. *Ann. Surg.* 2005; **242**: 10–19.

124 Schmidt SC, Langrehr JM, Hintze RE *et al.* Long-term results and risk factors influencing outcomes of major bile duct injuries following cholecystectomy. *Br. J. Surg.* 2005; **92**: 76–82.

125 Chapman WC, Halevy A, Blumgart LH *et al.* Postcholecystectomy bile duct strictures: management and outcomes in 130 patients. *Arch. Surg.* 1995; **130**: 597–602.

126 Sharpstone D, Colin-Jones DG. Chronic, non-visceral abdominal pain. *Gut* 1994; **35**: 833–836.

127 Luman W, Adams WH, Nixon SN *et al.* Incidence of persistent symptoms after laparoscopic cholecystectomy: a prospective study. *Gut* 1996; **39**: 863–866.

128 Vander Velpen GC, Shimi SM, Cuschieri A. Outcome after cholecystectomy for symptomatic gall stone disease and effect of surgical access: laparoscopic vs. open approach. *Gut* 1993; **34**: 1448–1451.

129 Menees S, Elta GH. Sphincter of Oddi dysfunction. *Curr. Treat. Options Gastrenterol.* 2005; **8**: 109–115.

130 Baillie J. Sphincter of Oddi dysfunction. *Curr. Gastroenterol. Rep.* 2010; **12**: 130–134.

131 Hernandez CA, Lerch MM. Sphincter stenosis and gallstone migration through the biliary tract. *Lancet* 1993; **341**: 1371–1373.

132 Toouli J, Roberts-Thomson IC, Kellow J *et al.* Manometry based randomised trial of endoscopic sphincterotomy for sphincter of Oddi dysfunction. *Gut* 2000; **46**: 98–102.

133 Geenen JE, Hogan WJ, Dodds WJ *et al.* The efficacy of endoscopic sphincterotomy after cholecystectomy in patients with sphincter of Oddi dysfunction. *N. Engl. J. Med.* 1989; **320**: 82–87.

134 Desautels SG, Slivka A, Hutson WR *et al.* Postcholecystectomy pain syndrome: pathophysiology of abdominal pain in sphincter of Oddi type III. *Gastroenterology* 1999; **116**: 900–905.

135 Behar J, Corazziari E, Guelrud M *et al.* Functional gallbladder and sphincter of Oddi disorders. *Gastroenterology* 2006; **130**: 1498–1509.

136 Howard DE, Fromm H. Nonsurgical management of gallstone disease. *Gastroenterol. Clin. North Am.* 1999; **28**: 133–144.

137 Walters JRF, Hood KA, Gleeson D *et al.* Combination therapy with oral ursodeoxycholic and chenodeoxycholic acids: pretreatment computed tomography of the gall bladder improves gall stone dissolution efficacy. *Gut* 1992; **33**: 375–380.

138 Gleeson D, Ruppin DC, Saunders A *et al.* Final outcome of ursodeoxycholic acid treatment in 126 patients with radiolucent gallstones. *Q. J. Med.* 1990; **279**: 711–729.

139 Tomida S, Abei M, Yamaguchi T *et al.* Long-term ursodeoxycholic acid therapy is associated with reduced risk of biliary pain and acute cholecystitis in patients with gallbladder stones: a cohort analysis. *Hepatology* 1999; **30**: 6–13.

140 Bateson MC, Bouchier IAD, Trash DB *et al.* Calcification of radiolucent gallstones during treatment with ursodeoxycholic acid. *Br. Med. J.* 1981; **283**: 645–646.

141 Mulagha E, Fromm H. Extracorporeal shock wave lithotripsy of gallstones revisited: current status and future promises. *J. Gastroenterol. Hepatol.* 2000; **15**; 239–243.

142 Rabenstein T, Radespiel-Tröger M, Höpfner L *et al.* Ten year experience with piezoelectric extracorporeal shockwave lithotripsy of gallbladder stones. *Eur. J. Gastroenterol. Hepatol.* 2005; **17**: 629–639.

143 Ash-Miles J, Roach H, Virjee J *et al.* More than just stones: a pictorial review of common and less common gallbladder pathologies. *Curr. Probl. Diagn. Radiol.* 2008; **37**: 189–202.

144 Zielinski MD, Atwell TD, Davis PW *et al.* Comparison of surgically resected polypoid lesions of the gallbladder to their pre-operative ultrasound characteristics. *J. Gastroenterol. Surg.* 2009; **13**: 19–25.

145 Park JY, Hong SP, Kim YJ *et al.* Long-term follow up of gall bladder polyps. *J. Gastroenterol. Hepatol.* 2009; **24**: 219–222.

146 Colecchia A, Larocca A, Scaioli E *et al.* Natural history of small gallbladder polyps is benign: evidence from a clinical and pathogenetic study. *Am. J. Gastroentrol.* 2009; **104**: 624–629.

147 Gallahan WC, Conway JD. Diagnosis and management of gallbladder polyps. *Gastroenterol. Clin. N. Am.* 2010; **39**: 359–367.

148 Leung UC, Wong PY, Roberts RH *et al.* Gall bladder polyps in sclerosing cholangitis: does the 1-cm rule apply? *ANZ J. Surg.* 2007; **77**: 355–357

149 Sahlin S, Ståhlberg D, Einarsson K. Cholesterol metabolism in liver and gallbladder mucosa of patients with cholesterolosis. *Hepatology* 1995; **21**: 1269–1275.

150 Watanabe F, Hanai H, Kaneko E. Increased acylCoAcholesterol ester acyltransferase activity in gallbladder mucosa in patients with gallbladder cholesterolosis. *Am. J. Gastroenterol.* 1998; **93**: 1518–1523.

151 Spinelli A, Schumacher G, Pascher A *et al.* Extended surgical resection for xanthogranulomatous cholecystitis mimicking advanced gallbladder carcinoma: a case report and review of literature. *World J. Gastroenterol.* 2006; **12**: 2293–2296.

152 Crawford RW, Rosales-Reyes R, Ramirez-Aguilar M de la L *et al.* Gallstones play a significant role in Salmonella spp. gallbladder colonization and carriage. *PNAS* 2010; **107**: 4353–4358.

153 Caygill CPJ, Hill MJ, Braddick M *et al.* Cancer mortality in chronic typhoid and paratyphoid carriers. *Lancet* 1994; **343**: 83–84.

154 LaRaja RD, Rothenberg RE, Odom JW *et al.* The incidence of intra-abdominal surgery in acquired immunodeficiency syndrome: a statistical review of 904 patients. *Surgery* 1989; **105**: 175–179.

155 Ricci M, Puente AO, Rothenberg RE *et al.* Open and laparoscopic cholecystectomy in acquired immunodeficiency syndrome: indications and results in fifty-three patients. *Surgery* 1999; **125**: 172–177.

156 Foschi D, Cellerino P, Corsi F *et al.* Impact of highly active antiretroviral therapy on outcome of cholecystectomy in patients with human immunodeficiency virus infection. *Br. J. Surg.* 2006; **93**: 1383–1389.

157 Ko WF, Cello JP, Rogers SJ *et al*. Prognostic factors for the survival of patients with AIDS cholangiopathy. *Am. J. Gastroenterol.* 2003; **98**: 2176–2181.

158 Liong SY, Sukumar SA. An African woman presenting with acalculous cholecystis and sclerosing cholangiopathy. *Br. J. Radiol.* 2009; **82**: 699–703.

159 Bilgin M, Balci NC, Erdogan A *et al*. Hepatobiliary and pancreatic MRI and MRCP findings in patients with HIV infection. *AJR Am. J. Roentgenol.* 2008; **191**: 228–232.

160 Parangi S, Oz MC, Blume RS *et al*. Hepatobiliary complications of polyarteritis nodosa. *Arch. Surg.* 1991; **126**: 909–912.

161 Gomez NA, Gutierrez J, Leon CJ. Acute acalculous cholecystitis due to *Vibrio cholerae*. *Lancet* 1994; **343**: 1156–1157.

162 Vilaichone RK, Mahachai V, Wilde H. Acute acalculous cholecystitis in leptospirosis. *J. Clin. Gastroenterol.* 1999; **29**: 280–283.

163 Faure JP, Doucet C, Scepi M *et al*. Abnormalities of the gallbladder, clinical effects. *Surg. Radiol. Anat.* 2008; **30**: 285–290.

164 Brem H, Gibbons GD, Cobb G *et al*. The use of endoscopy to treat bronchobiliary fistula caused by choledocholithiasis. *Gastroenterology* 1990; **98**: 490–492.

165 Clavien P-A, Richon J, Burgan S *et al*. Gallstone ileus. *Br. J. Surg.* 1990; **77**: 737–742.

166 Ravikumar R, Williams JG. The operative management of gallstone ileus. *Ann. R. Coll. Surg. Engl.* 2010; **92**: 279–281.

167 Kerstein MD, McSwain NE. Spontaneous rupture of the common bile duct. *Am. J. Gastroenterol.*1985; **80**: 469–471.

168 Schemhammer ES, Leitzmann MF, Michaud DS *et al*. Cholecystectomy and the risk for developing colorectal cancer and distal colorectal adenomas. *Br. J. Cancer* 2003; **88**: 79–83.

169 Lagergren J, Ye W, Ekbom A. Intestinal cancer after cholecystectomy: is bile involved in carcinogenesis? *Gastroenterology* 2001; **121**: 542–547.

170 Reid FD, Mercer PM, Harrison M *et al*. Cholecystecomy as a risk factor for colorectal cancer: a meta-analysis. *Scand. J. Gastroenterol.* 1996; **31**: 160–169.

171 Cobden I, Lendrum R, Venables CW *et al*. Gallstones presenting as mental and physical debility in the elderly. *Lancet* 1984; **i**: 1062–1064.

172 Williams EJ, Green J, Beckingham I *et al*. British Society of Gastroenterology. Guidelines on the management of common bile duct stones (CBDS). *Gut* 2008; **57**: 1004–1021.

173 Reynolds BM, Dargan FL. Acute obstructive cholangitis: a distinct clinical syndrome. *Ann. Surg.* 1959; **150**: 299–303.

174 Wada K, Takada T, Kawarada Y *et al*. Diagnostic criteria and severity assessment of acute cholangitis: Tokyo guidelines. *J. Hepatobiliary Pancreat. Surg.* 2007; **14**: 52–58.

175 Bergman JJ, Rauws EA, Fockens P *et al*. Randomised trial of endoscopic balloon dilation vs. endoscopic sphincterotomy for removal of bileduct stones. *Lancet* 1997; **349**: 1124–1129.

176 Baron TH, Harewood GC. Endoscopic balloon dilatation of the biliary sphincter compared to endoscpic biliary sphincterotomy for removal of common bile duct stones during ERCP: a meta-analysis of randomized, controlled trials. *Am. J. Gastroenterol.*2004; **99**: 1455–1460.

177 Hawes RH, Cotton PB, Vallon AG. Follow-up 6–11 years after duodenoscopic sphincterotomy for stones in patients with prior cholecystectomy. *Gastroenterology* 1990; **98**: 1008–1012.

178 Ingoldby CJH, el-Saadi J, Hall RI *et al*. Late results of endoscopic sphincterotomy for bile duct stones in elderly patients with gallbladder *in situ*. *Gut* 1989; **30**: 1129–1131.

179 Targarona EM, Ayuso RM, Bordas JM *et al*. Randomised trial of endoscopic sphincterotomy with gallbladder left in situ vs. open surgery for common bileduct calculi in high-risk patients. *Lancet* 1996; **347**: 926–929.

180 Gigot JF, Leese T, Dereme T *et al*. Acute cholangitis: multivariate analysis of risk factors. *Ann. Surg.* 1989; **209**: 435–438.

181 Lai EC, Mok FP, Tan ES *et al*. Endoscopic biliary drainage for severe acute cholangitis. *N. Engl. J. Med.* 1992; **326**: 1582–1586.

182 Leung JWC, Sung JY, Chung SCS *et al*. Urgent endoscopic drainage for acute suppurative cholangitis. *Lancet* 1989; **i**: 1307–1309.

183 Davidson BR, Neoptolemos JP, Leese T *et al*. Biochemical prediction of gallstones in acute pancreatitis: a prospective study of three systems. *Br. J. Surg.* 1988; **75**: 213–215.

184 Enns R, Baillie J. The treatment of acute biliary pancreatitis. *Aliment Pharmacol. Ther.* 1999; **11**: 1379–1389.

185 Sharma VK, Howden CW. Metaanalysis of randomized controlled trials of endoscopic retrograde cholangiography and endoscopic sphincterotomy for the treatment of acute biliary pancreatitis. *Am. J. Gastroenterol.* 1999; **94**: 3211–3214.

186 Lee SP, Nicholls JF, Park HZ. Biliary sludge as a cause of acute pancreatitis. *N. Engl. J. Med.* 1992; **326**: 589–593.

187 Shaw MJ, Mackie RD, Moore JP *et al*. Result of a multicentre trial using a mechanical lithotripter for the treatment of large bile duct stones. *Am. J. Gastroenterol.* 1993; **88**: 730–733.

188 Ellis RD, Jenkins AP, Thompson RP *et al*. Clearance of refractory bile duct stones with extracorporeal shockwave lithotripsy. *Gut* 2000; **47**: 728–731.

189 Sackmann M, Holl J, Sauter GH *et al*. Extracorporeal shock wave lithotripsy for clearance of bile duct stones resistant to endoscopic extraction. *Gastrointest. Endosc.* 2001; **53**: 27–32.

190 Swahn F, Edlund G, Enochsson L *et al*. Ten years of Swedish experience with intraductal electrohydraulic lithotripsy and laser lithotripsy for the treatment of difficult bile duct stones: an effective and safe option for octogenarians. *Surg. Endosc.* 2010; **24**: 1011–1016.

191 Navicharen P, Rhodes M, Flook D *et al*. Endoscopic retrograde cholangiopancreatography (ERCP) and stent placement in the management of large common bile duct stones. *Aust. NZ J. Surg.* 1994; **64**: 840–842.

192 Peters R, Macmathuna P, Lombard M *et al*. Management of common bile duct stones with a biliary endoprosthesis. Report on 40 cases. *Gut* 1992; **33**: 1412–1415.

193 Chan AC, Ng EK, Chung SC *et al*. Common bile duct stones become smaller after endoscopic biliary stenting. *Endoscopy* 1998; **30**: 356–359.

194 Nussinson E, Cairns SR, Vaira D *et al*. A 10-year single centre experience of percutaneous and endoscopic extraction of bile duct stones with T tube in situ. *Gut* 1991; **32**: 1040–1043.

195 Freeman ME, Rose JL, Forsmark CE *et al*. Mirizzi syndrome: a rare cause of obstructive jaundice. *Dig. Dis.* 1999; **17**: 44–48.

196 Csendes A, Carlos Diaz J, Burdiles P *et al*. Mirizzi syndrome and cholecystobiliary fistula: a unifying classification. *Br. J. Surg.* 1989; **76**: 1139–1143.

197 England RE, Martin DF. Endoscopic management of Mirizzi's syndrome. *Gut* 1997; **40**: 272–276.

198 Redaelli CA, Büchler MW, Schilling MK *et al*. High coincidence of Mirizzi syndrome and gallbladder carcinoma. *Surgery* 1997; **121**: 58–63.

199 Pitt HA, Venbrux AC, Coleman J *et al*. Intrahepatic stones. The transhepatic team approach. *Ann. Surg.* 1994; **219**: 527–535.

200 Cheung M-T, Wai S-H, Kwok PC-H. Percutaneous transhepatic choledochoscopic removal of intrahepatic stones. *Br. J. Surg.* 2003; **90**: 1409–1415.

201 Bloechle C, Izbicki JR, Rashed MY *et al*. Hemobilia: presentation, diagnosis and management. *Am. J. Gastroenterol.* 1994; **89**: 1537–1540.

202 Czerniak A, Thompson JN, Hemingway AP *et al*. Hemobilia: a disease in evolution. *Arch. Surg.* 1988; **123**: 718–721.

203 Kroser J, Rothstein RD, Kochman ML. Endoscopic management of obstructive jaundice caused by haemobilia. *Gastrointest. Endosc.* 1996; **44**: 618–619.

204 Murr MM, Gigot JF, Nagorney DM *et al*. Long-term results of biliary reconstruction after laparoscopic bile duct injury. *Arch. Surg.* 1999; **134**: 604–609.

205 Pellegrini CA, Thomas MJ, Way LW. Recurrent biliary stricture. Patterns of recurrence and outcome of surgical therapy. *Am. J. Surg.* 1984; **147**: 175–180.

206 Matthews JB, Baer HU, Schweizer WP *et al*. Recurrent cholangitis with and without anastomotic stricture after biliary-enteric bypass. *Arch. Surg.* 1993; **128**: 269–272.

207 Vos PM, van Beek EJR, Smits NJ *et al*. Percutaneous balloon dilatation for benign hepaticojejunostomy strictures. *Abdom. Imaging* 2000; **25**: 134–138.

208 Lillemoe KD, Martin SA, Cameron JA *et al*. Major bile duct injuries during laparoscopic cholecystectomy. Follow-up after combined surgical and radiological management. *Ann. Surg.* 1997; **225**: 459–468.

209 Hammel P, Couvelard A, O'Toole D *et al*. Regression of liver fibrosis after biliary drainage in patients with chronic pancreatitis and stenosis of the common bile duct. *N. Engl. J. Med.* 2001; **333**: 418–423.

210 Dragonov P, Hoffmann B, Marsh W *et al*. Long-term outcome in patients with benign biliary strictures treated endoscopically with multiple stents. *Gastrointest. Endosc.* 2002; **55**: 680–686.

211 Isayama H, Nakai Y, Togawa O *et al*. Covered metallic stents in the management of malignant and benign pancreatobiliary strictures. *J. Hepatobiliary Pancreat Surg.* 2009; **16**: 624–627.

212 Stahl TJ, Allen MO'C, Ansel HJ *et al*. Partial biliary obstruction caused by chronic pancreatitis: an appraisal of indications for surgical biliary drainage. *Ann. Surg.* 1988; **207**: 26–32.

213 Webster GJM, Pereira SP, Chapman RW. Autoimmune pancreatitis/IgG4-associated cholangitis and primary sclerosing cholangitis – overlapping or separate diseases. *J. Hepatol.* 2009; **51**: 398–402.

CHAPTER 13
Malignant Biliary Diseases

Rahul S. Koti & Brian R. Davidson
Royal Free and University College London, London, UK

Learning points

- Biliary and pancreatic malignancies present major challenges in diagnosis and treatment.

- Advances in CT and MRI technology have increased the accuracy of determining the stage of tumour and resectability.

- Laparoscopy is an important component of the staging process. Its potential benefit is in detecting peritoneal disease and occult liver metastases. It is widely accepted that staging laparoscopy should be performed prior to proceeding with definitive surgery.

- Biliary and pancreatic surgery is complex. Early referral to specialist units is recommended. The centralization of biliary and pancreatic surgery in high volume specialist centres has improved outcomes.

- Adjuvant and neoadjuvant treatments have not improved survival for patients with bile duct carcinoma. Adjuvant treatment may have an impact on survival after resection of pancreatic carcinoma but there is no consensus on optimal treatment.

Carcinoma of the gallbladder

This is an uncommon tumour with a poor prognosis. It has a wide geographical variation and is particularly common in Chile, north and central India, and areas of Japan. It is relatively rare in the western world.

Gallstones coexist in about 75% of cases and chronic cholecystitis is a frequent association. There is an association with multiple, large gallbladder stones, but a causal relationship is unproven.

Controversy exists regarding the association of the calcified (*porcelain*) gallbladder with carcinoma, but most authors advise prophylactic cholecystectomy for such patients [1].

An anomalous pancreaticobiliary ductal union, greater than 15 mm from the papilla of Vater, is associated with congenital cystic dilatation of the common bile duct and with gallbladder carcinoma [2]. Regurgitation of pancreatic juice may be tumourigenic [2].

There is indirect evidence for malignant transformation in gallbladder polyps and cholecystectomy is advised for polyps greater than 10 mm in diameter. The common gallbladder cholesterol polyps are not precancerous.

Chronic typhoid infection (*Salmonella typhi* and *Salmonella paratyphi*) of the gallbladder increases the risk of gallbladder carcinoma significantly, emphasizing the need for antibiotic treatment to eradicate the chronic typhoid and paratyphoid carrier state, or for elective cholecystectomy. There may also be an association with infection with *Helicobacter bilis* and *Helicobacter pylori*.

There is a strong association of gallbladder cancer with overweight and obesity.

Pathology

Papillary adenocarcinoma of the gallbladder starts as a wart-like excrescence. It grows slowly into, rather than through, the wall until a fungating mass fills the gallbladder. Mucoid change is associated with more rapid growth, early metastasis and gelatinous peritoneal carcinomatosis. *Squamous cell carcinoma, scirrhous* forms and *anaplastic* (undifferentiated) *type* are recognized. The most common tumour is an adenocarcinoma which may be papillary.

The tumour usually arises in the fundus or neck, but rapid spread may make the original site difficult to locate. The rich lymphatic and venous drainage of the gallbladder leads to early spread to related lymph nodes. Direct invasion of the biliary tree or nodal metastases can produce obstructive jaundice. The liver bed is invaded and there may also be local spread to the duodenum, stomach and colon, resulting in fistulae or external compression.

Sherlock's Diseases of the Liver and Biliary System, Twelfth Edition. Edited by
James S. Dooley, Anna S.F. Lok, Andrew K. Burroughs, E. Jenny Heathcote.
© 2011 by Blackwell Publishing Ltd. Published 2011 by Blackwell Publishing Ltd.

Clinical features

The patient is usually an elderly, white female, complaining of pain in the right upper quadrant, nausea, vomiting, weight loss and possibly jaundice. Sometimes a cholecystectomy is performed for symptomatic gallstones and the cancer is only found at histology. These early stage cancers are often not suspected at the time of operation [3].

Examination may reveal a hard and sometimes tender mass in the gallbladder area.

Serum, *urine* and *faeces* show the changes of cholestatic jaundice if the bile duct is obstructed.

Serum tumour markers (CA 19-9, Ca 125, CA 242 and CA 15-3) may be increased but are not specific to this tumour.

A national French audit of gallbladder carcinoma suggested that in only 50% of patients is the diagnosis made preoperatively

Imaging

Ultrasound scanning shows a mass in the gallbladder lumen or totally replacing the gallbladder. With early lesions the differentiation between gallbladder carcinoma and a thickened gallbladder wall due to acute or chronic cholecystitis is difficult. In advanced disease, ultrasound has a diagnostic sensitivity of 85% [4].

CT scan of the chest and abdomen with contrast enhancement can show a mass in the area of the gallbladder, infiltration of the liver parenchyma and adjacent organs, local vascular involvement and evidence of local (nodal) or distant (liver, lung, bone) metastases. Modern CT technology has increased the accuracy in determining the stage of the gallbladder carcinoma [5]. In a study of 118 patients, multidetector CT had an accuracy of 84% in diagnosing the local extent (T staging) of gallbladder carcinoma [6].

Magnetic resonance cholangiopancreatography (MRCP) and *MR angiography* (MRA) may help in evaluating the extent of biliary and vascular invasion prior to surgery [5]. One study [7] suggested an 'all-in-one' MR protocol, comprising MRI, MRCP and MRA, where the sensitivity and specificity of MR examination were, respectively, 100 and 89% for bile duct invasion, 100 and 87% for vascular invasion, 67 and 89% for hepatic invasion, and 56 and 89% for lymph node metastasis.

Endoscopic ultrasound (EUS) may be useful in staging [8] but there is no current evidence base for its routine use.

Endoscopic retrograde cholangiopancreatography (ERCP) shows external compression of the bile duct in the jaundiced patient and may be used for stent insertion and bile or brush cytology or endobiliary biopsy.

Angiography shows displacement or encasement of the portal blood vessels but has been largely replaced by arterial phase CT or MRA.

PET (positron emission tomography, FDG-PET) for staging of gallbladder carcinoma may be useful in a selected group of patients [9–11].

Staging laparoscopy is useful for patients with potentially resectable gallbladder carcinoma, since CT and MRI rarely detect peritoneal disease. In one study it avoided unnecessary laparotomy in 48% of cases [12].

Treatment

Patients with symptomatic gallstones should undergo cholecystectomy but there is no evidence to support this for patients with asymptomatic gallstones to prevent development of gallbladder carcinoma.

When gallbladder carcinoma is detected incidentally in a cholecystectomy specimen no further surgery is required for carcinoma *in situ* and for tumours invading only as far as the lamina propria. Further surgery should be considered for tumours invading muscularis and beyond. Surgery usually involves gallbladder fossa resection (segmental resection) and lymphadenectomy. There is no role for routine excision of the bile duct unless the cystic duct stump is involved with tumour. If there is involvement of the right hepatic artery or portal vein, then right hepatectomy is required.

When invasive gallbladder cancer is diagnosed preoperatively, resection involves partial hepatectomy and lymphadenectomy.

The impact of surgery on the overall survival of gallbladder cancer is limited since the surgery is complex and high risk, and few patients undergo potentially curative resection. There is no current evidence that adjuvant radiotherapy or chemotherapy are of benefit.

Palliative treatment of gallbladder carcinoma is by endoscopic or percutaneous stent insertion. Chemotherapy has shown modest survival advantage in the few trials that have been performed, and can be considered.

Prognosis

This is generally poor because most patients have advanced and unresectable disease at presentation or have distant metastases. Long-term survivors are mainly those in whom the tumour was found incidentally at cholecystectomy for gallstones (carcinoma *in situ*).

Patients with papillary and well-differentiated adenocarcinomas have longer survival than those with tubular and undifferentiated types. Tumour stage (T stage) and complete cancer clearance at surgery are important prognostic factors. Five-year survival rates after surgery are more than 85% when tumour invasion is limited to

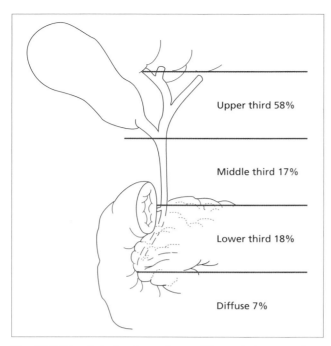

Fig. 13.1. Site of cholangiocarcinoma. The majority occur in the upper third of the bile duct.

lamina propria or muscularis. For tumours perforating the serosa of the gallbladder, 5-year survival after surgery is around 30%. Tumours invading extrahepatic organs are generally unresectable.

Other gallbladder tumours

Rarely other tumours develop in the gallbladder including leiomyosarcoma, rhabdomyosarcoma, oat cell carcinoma and carcinoid tumours.

Carcinoma of the bile duct (cholangiocarcinoma)

Cholangiocarcinoma may arise at any point in the biliary tree from the small intrahepatic bile ducts to the distal bile duct within the pancreas (Fig. 13.1).

The incidence of intrahepatic cholangiocarcinoma is increasing. Studies from England and Wales [13,14] and the USA [15] show a 10-fold increase in incidence and mortality between the early 1970s and the mid-1990s. The explanation is unclear. Although improved diagnostic techniques for cholangiocarcinoma and primary sclerosing cholangitis (PSC) may have played a part, they do not alone explain the marked increase. Mortality from extrahepatic cholangiocarcinoma fell over the same period.

Suspicion of cholangiocarcinoma, for example after ultrasound scan, should lead to direct referral to a specialist unit. This is to co-ordinate the work-up to evalu-ate resectability of the tumour. Modern CT techniques and MRI with MR cholangiography allow a high degree of non-invasive evaluation [16] and the accuracy of tumour staging is reduced by prior biliary stent insertion.

The necessity and timing of ERCP and percutaneous drainage depends on clinical circumstances. They should not be done inappropriately since they may introduce sepsis into the biliary tract which may compromise later treatment [17,18].

These aspects emphasize the importance of a multidisciplinary approach. Staging and formulation of a surgical treatment plan should be the first step. Those patients who have unresectable tumour undergo a planned non-surgical biliary drainage procedure [19].

Associations

PSC predisposes to cholangiocarcinoma with a incidence of up to 40% [20]. The majority of patients with PSC who develop cholangiocarcinoma also have ulcerative colitis [21]. Colonic neoplasia on the background of ulcerative colitis and PSC increases the risk [21]. In a group of 70 patients with PSC followed prospectively for a mean of 30 months, 15 patients died of liver failure. Five of 12 patients having an autopsy had cholangiocarcinoma—7% of the total group [22].

Biliary malignancy is not necessarily a late complication of PSC. In one series, 30% of patients with PSC had a diagnosis of cholangiocarcinoma made within 1 year of the first evidence of underlying liver disease [23]. Clinical features associated with malignancy were epigastric pain, weight loss and raised CA 19-9 and carcinoembryonic antigen (CEA) [23].

Patients with congenital fibrocystic liver disease are predisposed to cholangiocarcinoma. These include congenital hepatic fibrosis, cystic dilatation (Caroli's syndrome), choledochal cyst and von Meyenburg complexes.

Cholangiocarcinoma may be associated with biliary cirrhosis secondary to biliary atresia.

Liver fluke infestations of the Orient may be complicated by intrahepatic cholangiocarcinoma. In the Far East (China, Hong Kong, Korea, Japan), where *Clonorchis sinensis* is prevalent, cholangiocarcinoma accounts for 20% of primary liver tumours. These arise in the heavily parasitized bile ducts near the hilum. *Opisthorchis viverrini* infestation, prevalent in Thailand, Laos and western Malaysia, has a strong association with cholangiocarcinoma [20].

Intrahepatic bile duct stones (hepatolithiasis) is also a risk factor for cholangiocarcinoma [20].

The risk of extrahepatic bile duct carcinoma is significantly lower 10 years or more after cholecystectomy, suggesting a link with gallstones [24] or concentrated gallbladder bile.

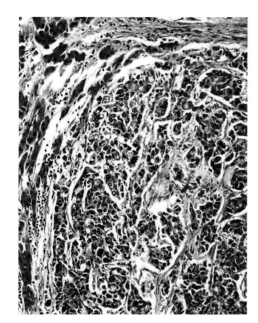

Fig. 13.2. Bile duct carcinoma: with irregular fibrous stroma. (H & E.)

Pathology

The common sites of origin are the confluence of the cystic duct with the main hepatic duct and the junction of the main right and left hepatic ducts at the porta hepatis (Fig. 13.1). Tumours of the hepatic duct confluence extend into the liver. They cause complete biliary obstruction with intrahepatic duct dilatation and enlargement of the liver. The gallbladder is collapsed. If the tumour is restricted to one hepatic duct, biliary obstruction is incomplete and jaundice absent. The lobe of the liver drained by this duct atrophies and the other hypertrophies.

In the common bile duct the tumour presents as a firm nodule or plaque which causes an annular stricture which may ulcerate. It spreads along the bile duct and through its wall.

In autopsy studies local and distant metastases are found in about 50% of patients. They involve peritoneum, abdominal lymph nodes, diaphragm, liver or gallbladder. Blood vessel invasion is rare and extra-abdominal spread is unusual.

Histologically the tumour is usually a mucin-secreting adenocarcinoma with cuboidal or columnar epithelium (Fig. 13.2). Spread along neural sheaths may be noted. Tumours around the hilum are sclerosing with an abundant fibrous stroma. Distal biliary tract cholangiocarcinoma are often nodular or papillary.

Molecular changes

Point mutations in codon 12 of the K-*ras* oncogene are found in cholangiocarcinoma [25]. p53 protein is synthesized particularly in distal duct cholangiocarcinomas

[26]. Aneuploidy (divergence from the normal chromosome content) is found in hilar cholangiocarcinoma [26] and is associated with shorter survival. Many other tumour suppressor genes and oncogenes are altered. Cholangiocarcinoma cells contain somatostatin receptor RNA and cell lines have specific receptors. Cell growth is inhibited both *in vitro* and *in vivo* by somatostatin analogues [27].

Clinical features

This tumour tends to occur in the older age group, patients being about 60 years old. Slightly more males than females are affected. Jaundice is the usual presenting feature, followed by pruritus—a point of distinction from primary biliary cirrhosis where itching usually precedes jaundice.

Jaundice is not usually present in those with intrahepatic cholangiocarcinoma or unilateral main duct involvement.

In those presenting with jaundice, the bilirubin rise is progressive but periods of temporary improvement occur in up to 50% [28].

Pain, usually epigastric and mild, is present in about one-third of patients. Diarrhoea may be related to steatorrhoea or underlying ulcerative colitis. Weakness and weight loss are marked.

Examination. Jaundice is deep. Cholangitis is unusual unless there has been prior cannulation of the biliary tree by ERCP or PTC.

The liver is large and smooth, extending 5–12 cm below the costal margin. The spleen is not felt. Ascites is unusual.

Investigations

Serum biochemical findings are those of cholestatic jaundice. The serum bilirubin, alkaline phosphatase and γ-glutamyl transpeptidase levels may be very high. Fluctuations may reflect incomplete obstruction.

The serum antimitochondrial antibody test is negative and α-fetoprotein is not increased.

The *faeces* are pale and fatty. *Glycosuria* is absent.

Anaemia may be greater than that seen with ampullary carcinoma; the explanation is unknown—it is not due to blood loss. The leucocyte count is high normal with increased polymorphs.

Liver biopsy shows features of large duct obstruction. However, it must be emphasized that liver biopsy on the background of biliary obstruction has a risk of serious complications such as biliary peritonitis, and should be performed only when there is doubt about the diagnosis. In PSC, biliary dysplasia raises the possibility of coexistent cholangiocarcinoma [29].

Cytology taken at the time of ERCP or percutaneous drainage is worthwhile, but requires cytological expertise for interpretation. Brush cytology has a higher sensitivity than analysis of aspirated bile [30].

Percutaneous biopsy is contraindicated in patients with resectable disease due to the risk of needle tract seeding [31]. A tissue diagnosis is required in those with unresectable or metastatic disease prior to palliative therapy. Approaches include biopsy or fine-needle aspiration cytology from the suspected tumour guided by fluoroscopy, transabdominal or endoscopic ultrasound, or cholangioscopy with endobiliary biopsy.

In PSC, brush cytology of dominant strictures at ERCP has a sensitivity of 60% for diagnosis of cholangiocarcinoma [32]. *p53* and K-*ras* mutation analysis does not increase sensitivity but K-*ras* mutations may be found ahead of the diagnosis of cholangiocarcinoma in patients with PSC [33].

The serum concentration of the tumour marker CA 19-9 is often increased in patients with biliary tract malignancy. Extremely high levels are also reported with benign biliary obstruction [34]. The sensitivity for detecting cholangiocarcinoma in PSC is 50–60% [35,36].

Imaging [16]

Ultrasound is usually the initial imaging modality done for patients with cholestasis (see Chapter 12). With a typical hilar cholangiocarcinoma ultrasound shows dilated intrahepatic ducts with a normal extrahepatic biliary tree. A tumour mass may be shown in up to 80% of cases [37]. Ultrasound (real-time together with Doppler) accurately detects neoplastic involvement of the portal vein, both occlusion and wall infiltration, but is less good in showing hepatic arterial involvement [38]. Intraduct ultrasound is still experimental but can provide information on tumour extension in and around the bile duct [39].

Modern helical CT (chest and abdomen) can detect cholangiocarcinoma in more than 90% of patients (as small as 15 mm diameter). It also provides information on parenchymal infiltration and bile duct, portal vein and hepatic artery involvement [40]. Local and distant metastases can also be detected.

However, CT underestimates the extent of bile duct involvement, hepatic arterial invasion, lymph node spread and rarely detects peritoneal disease.

MRI is currently the best imaging modality when ultrasound suggests hilar cholangiocarcinoma [13]. MRCP detects over 90% of biliary strictures [40]. In cholangiocarcinoma (Fig. 13.3) MRI and MRCP correctly delineate duct obstruction and the extent of hilar tumour extension in more than 80% of patients [41]. The accuracy of MRCP in evaluating the level and extent of bile duct involvement is comparable to direct cholangiography by ERCP or PTC [42]. MRI with MRCP is an impor-tant technique for planning the treatment of malignant hilar strictures but does not replace invasive cholangi-ography which also allows brushings to be taken for cytology and bile drainage if indicated. MRA provides information on vascular involvement.

Thus CT and MRI usually demonstrate bile duct obstruction and often a mass but cannot reliably differ-entiate between inflammatory and malignant biliary strictures. If surgical resection is not possible then inva-sive techniques are used to obtain cytology or biopsy.

Detecting cholangiocarcinoma in patients with PSC is difficult. PET scanning using [^{18}F] fluoro-2-deoxy-D-glucose (FDG) can detect cholangiocarcinomas in patients with and without PSC with a sensitivity of 90% [43,44]. However, false-positive scans have been seen in normal individuals [44]. Most biliary cancers are FDG avid and PET or integrated PET-CT may have a role in the detection of unsuspected metastases or lymph node spread which can be underestimated by CT. In a pro-spective study [45] of 123 patients, PET-CT showed sig-nificantly higher accuracy over CT in the diagnosis of regional lymph node metastases and distant metastases. However, PET-CT demonstrated no significant advan-tage over CT and MRI/MRCP in the diagnosis of the primary tumour [45].

Direct cholangiography

Endoscopic or percutaneous cholangiography (Fig. 13.3) prior to staging is only indicated in the septic patient or where there is renal failure associated with severe cholestasis. It is prudent to investigate the patient non-invasively with CT and MRI/MRCP to judge the nature and extent of the hilar lesion, and then consider direct cholangiography, cytology and drainage when the management plan is clear. MRCP is useful to select the duct system for endoscopic or percutaneous drainage.

In hilar cholangiocarcinoma, ERCP shows a normal common bile duct and gallbladder with obstruction at the hilum (Fig. 13.3c). Contrast usually passes through the stricture(s) into dilated bile ducts above. The strict-ure is passed with a guide-wire, brushings taken for cytology and a stent placed.

Percutaneous cholangiography shows the dilated int-rahepatic ducts down to the stricture (Fig. 13.3d). A drain is inserted. When right and left hepatic ducts are individually obstructed, puncture of both systems may be necessary for planning surgical intervention but drainage of one lobe or sector is usually sufficient to relieve jaundice.

Percutaneous cholangiography usually provides more information on tumour extension within the liver and biliary tree compared with endoscopic cholangiography.

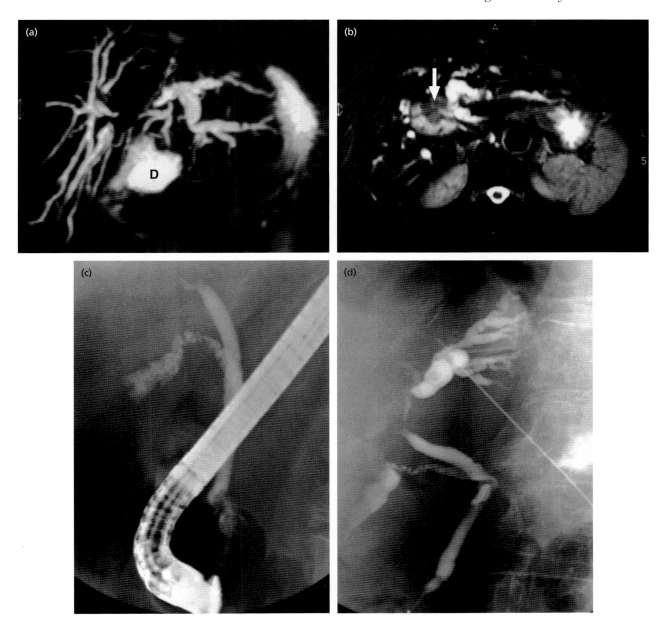

Fig. 13.3. A 75-year-old woman presenting with cholestatic jaundice. Ultrasound showed dilated intrahepatic ducts, a hilar mass and a normal common bile duct. (a) MRCP shows dilated intrahepatic ducts with at least three segments obstructed in the right lobe and the left hepatic system obstructed at the hilum. If non-surgical drainage is to be done, these appearances favour drainage of the left- rather than the right-sided system (D, duodenum). (b) MRI scan shows a mass in the liver (arrow) above the hilum. (c) Non-operative drainage was chosen since the patient was considered inoperable due to inadequate future remnant liver volume. ERCP shows a normal common duct with a hilar stricture. A stent could not be placed. (d) Following on the MRCP appearances, the left-sided duct system was chosen for percutaneous cholangiography and a stent inserted.

Angiography

Hepatic artery and portal vein involvement by tumour often dictates whether resection is feasible. MRA and CT angiography are useful in the assessment of vascular involvement and their diagnostic accuracy is comparable to conventional angiography which is invasive.

New techniques

These include endoscopic ultrasound, intraductal ultrasound and direct cholangioscopy [13,16]. Their use is evolving but as yet their precise role for cholangiocarcinoma is not defined. They are best used within the context of clinical trials [13].

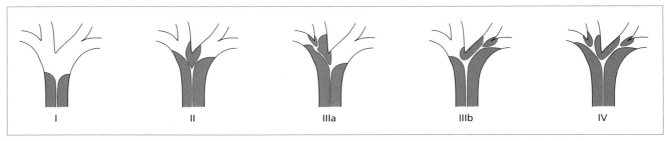

Fig. 13.4. Classification of hilar cholangiocarcinoma according to the involvement of bile ducts. Resectability of type I to III depends on angiographic findings. Type IV (bilateral involvement of secondary hepatic ducts) indicates incurable disease. In inoperable patients median survival after stent insertion depends upon the extent of tumour.

EUS provides good views of the extrahepatic biliary tree and regional lymph nodes. The sensitivity and specificity of EUS in the diagnosis of malignancy is comparable to ERCP [46]. In addition, EUS can facilitate fine-needle aspiration of lesions and lymph nodes. However, the availability and expertise of EUS is limited and poor views are often obtained for hilar strictures.

Cholangioscopy directly views bile duct mucosa and allows endobiliary biopsy. It can be performed perorally via an endoscope or percutaneously. However, this technique is expensive and invasive.

Intraductal ultrasound may have a role in differentiating benign and malignant biliary strictures.

Staging and preparation for surgery

If the clinical state of the patient does not rule out surgery the resectability and stage of tumour must first be assessed as outlined above. If cholangiography shows involvement of the secondary hepatic ducts in both hepatic lobes (Fig. 13.4, type IV) then hilar cholangiocarcinoma would be considered unresectable. Bilateral involvement of hepatic arterial or portal vein branches or both is also considered unresectable disease. Encasement of the main portal vein or common hepatic artery is a relative contraindication to surgery. If the tumour is limited to the hepatic duct bifurcation with or without unilobar portal vein or hepatic artery involvement then the lesion is usually resectable with an extended right or left hepatectomy.

Portal vein embolization

Extended right or left hepatectomy may result in postoperative hepatic insufficiency if the volume of the remnant liver is not adequate. The volume of the future liver remnant can be reliably quantified by MRI or CT. Preoperative portal vein embolization is a safe and effective method of increasing the volume of the future liver remnant and should be considered when the future liver remnant is less than 20% in patients with normal liver function, or less than 40% in patients with compromised liver function [47].

Preoperative biliary drainage

The role of preoperative biliary drainage prior to resection for hilar cholangiocarcinoma is controversial, and there are no prospective randomized trials. The primary concern with preoperative biliary drainage is the associated risk of sepsis. However, malignant obstructive jaundice is associated with liver and kidney failure, and coagulopathy, and many patients will benefit from preoperative biliary drainage. It should be considered in association with preoperative portal vein embolization when the future liver remnant is small.

Laparoscopy

The sensitivity of all the imaging modalities outlined above in detecting peritoneal disease is poor. Laparoscopy is invasive, but can reliably detect peritoneal disease. There are no randomized trials reporting the role of laparoscopy in the staging of cholangiocarcinoma. However, it is widely accepted that staging laparoscopy should be performed before proceeding with definitive surgery as this will prevent unnecessary laparotomy in up to 30% of patients [48].

Treatment

Surgery

Surgical resection is the primary treatment for cholangiocarcinomas. Distal cholangiocarcinomas are resected with pancreatoduodenectomy, with a 5-year survival of about 30%. In patients with spread along the common bile duct, hepatic resection and pancreatoduodenectomy can be performed.

Mid-bile duct cancers are resected with excision of the biliary tree and hilar lymphadenectomy.

Typical hilar (Klatskin) tumours are resected by an extended right or left hepatectomy depending on the extent of involvement of the right or left duct system. The biliary tree is excised and the proximal bile duct(s) drained into a Roux-en-Y loop of intestine. Radical hilar lymphadenectomy is done because of the possibility of lymphatic dissemination. With Klatskin tumours a caudate lobectomy is usually performed since segment 1 ducts drain to the confluence of the hepatic ducts and are likely to be involved by tumour.

The proportion of cholangiocarcinomas being resected has increased from 5–20% of patients in the 1970 and 1980s to 30% or more in specialist centres currently. This is because of improved staging and resection techniques within specialist surgical units.

The challenge is to achieve resection with tumour-negative margins and aggressive, major hepatic resections may increase the likelihood of achieving this. Extended resection including the portal vein to achieve tumour clearance can be performed but at present the role of routine portal vein resection is not clear.

Median survival after aggressive resection of hilar cholangiocarcinoma is 18–40 months with good palliation for most of this time [49].

Local resection can be considered for Bismuth type I and II tumours (Fig. 13.4) with low perioperative mortality.

At present, there is no role for adjuvant chemotherapy or radiotherapy for patients with tumour-negative resection margins. Cancer Research UK is conducting a randomized phase III trial comparing surgery and capecitabine with surgery alone for cancer of the bile duct or gallbladder (BILCAP trial).

Liver transplantation

In general cholangiocarcinoma is a contraindication for liver transplantation. The early experience for unresectable cholangiocarcinoma was disappointing because of early recurrence. In the last decade, however, the University of Nebraska and the Mayo Clinic have published reports where, in highly selected patients with early stage unresectable cholangiocarcinoma, liver transplantation in combination with preoperative chemoradiation was associated with prolonged disease-free and overall survival. These are single institution studies and it is not certain such results could be reproduced uniformly by other transplant centres. Overall, the role of liver transplantation for *de novo* cholangiocarcinoma is not clearly defined and this treatment should be carried out within a prospective trial.

Surgical palliation

These include anastomosis of jejunum to the segment III duct in the left lobe, which is usually accessible above

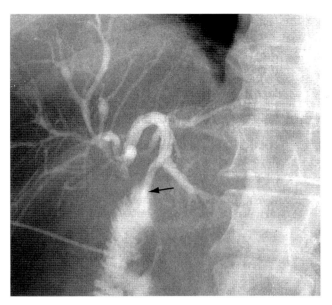

Fig. 13.5. Check cholangiogram after surgical bypass for hilar cholangiocarcinoma. The anastomosis is between the jejunum and the third segment duct of the left lobe (arrow).

the hilar tumour (Fig. 13.5). Jaundice is relieved for at least 3 months in 75% of patients. If segment III bypass is not possible (atrophy, metastases), a right-sided intrahepatic anastomosis to the segment V duct can be done. Surgical approaches for palliation are rarely indicated in centres with specialists in ERCP and percutaneous biliary intervention.

Non-surgical palliation

In those patients unfit for surgery or with irresectable tumours, jaundice and itching may be relieved by placing an endoprosthesis across the stricture either by the endoscopic or percutaneous route.

By the endoscopic route, stents can be inserted successfully in about 90% of patients. The major, early complication is cholangitis (7%). Thirty-day mortality is between 10 and 28% depending upon the extent of the tumour at the hilum and the mean survival is 20 weeks [50]. It is only necessary (initially) to stent one lobe [51]. Scoring systems to predict outcome in patients having palliative stenting are available and can aid decision making in patients with advanced disease [52].

Percutaneous transhepatic endoprosthesis insertion is also effective but carries a higher risk of complications such as bleeding and bile leakage. Metal mesh endoprostheses, which expand to 10 mm diameter in the stricture after insertion on a 5 or 7 French catheter, are more expensive than plastic types, but have longer patency [53,54].

There are no trials comparing surgical versus non-surgical palliation. Generally, non-operative techniques are appropriate for high-risk patients expected to have a shorter survival. If recurrent stent blockage occurs, a surgical bypass can be considered [55].

There is no conclusive evidence to support the role of chemotherapy or radiotherapy in patients with advanced or metastatic disease. The role of external radiotherapy or radiotherapy combined with biliary drainage is unproven. Cytotoxic drugs are ineffective. A UK phase II trial (the UK ABC-01 study) compared gemcitabine alone or in combination with cisplatin in patients with advanced biliary tract cancers [56]. The primary end-point, 6 month progression-free survival, was 57.1% for the combination arm and 47.7% for the single agent arm [56]. This study has been extended into a phase III study (ABC-02) to determine the effect on overall survival and quality of life.

Intraduct photodynamic therapy combined with stenting in patients with unresectable cholangiocarcinoma has shown survival benefit in randomized, controlled trials [57,58]. The treatment is costly but appears to offer good palliation. However, further studies are required to confirm the benefits of photodynamic therapy.

Prognosis

Prognosis depends on the site, stage and treatment of the tumour. Distal cholangiocarcinomas are more likely to be resectable than those at the hilum. Polypoid cancers have the best prognosis.

If unresected, the 1-year survival for cholangiocarcinoma is 50%, with 20% surviving 2 years and 10% at 3 years [59]. This reflects the observation that some tumours are slow growing and metastasize late.

Intrahepatic cholangiocarcinoma [60]

This intrahepatic bile duct-derived tumour is classified as a primary hepatic carcinoma (see Chapter 35). It becomes symptomatic as it enlarges, producing abdominal pain rather than jaundice. It grows rapidly with early metastasis and a particularly poor prognosis. Scanning shows an intrahepatic mass. Distinction from hepatocellular carcinoma may be difficult. Hepatic venous and portal vein involvement is rare. Surgery is the only chance for effective treatment. Resection is possible in 30–60% of cases [61]. One-year survival after resection is 50–60%. Five-year survival rates range from 4.1% [62] to 35% [63]. The results of liver transplantation for intrahepatic cholangiocarcinoma have been poor and at present there is no role for liver transplantation outside of a clinical trial [60].

Other biliary malignancies

Biliary cystadenocarcinoma and mixed hepatocellular and cholangiocarcinoma have been reported but are rare.

Metastases at the hilum

Cholestatic jaundice developing following the diagnosis of carcinoma elsewhere (in particular the breast and colon) may be due to diffuse metastases within the liver or duct obstruction by nodes at the hilum. Differentiation between the two is by ultrasound. If dilated bile ducts are shown and the patient is symptomatic with itching, biliary obstruction can be relieved by insertion of an endoprosthesis by the endoscopic or percutaneous approach [64].

Periampullary carcinoma

The region of the head of the pancreas is a common site for carcinoma. Most arise in the head of the pancreas from ductular epithelium, but may also develop from pancreatic acinar cells, the lining of the low bile duct, the ampulla of Vater (papilla) or rarely the duodenum.

Tumours at these sites usually present with obstructive jaundice. Although they may be grouped as 'cancers of the head of the pancreas' they have a different biological behaviour and prognosis. Resection is possible in 80% of patients with carcinoma of the ampulla compared with 20% for cancer of the head of the pancreas. Five-year survival following resection is 40–70% for ampullary and only 10–20% for pancreatic carcinoma.

Periampullary and pancreatic neuroendocrine tumours are rare but important to recognize. The biological behaviour of these tumours is very different from adenocarcinomas with a better prognosis. More than 70% of pancreatic neuroendocrine tumours present with metastatic disease (except insulinomas which are benign in 90% of cases) but overall 5-year survival is 80% [65]. Surgery for localized pancreatic neuroendocrine tumours is often curative with 5-year survival rates of 60–100% [65].

Genetic and environmental predisposition

In the majority of patients there is no clear aetiological factor.

In some, however, there is a genetic influence either through a strong family history or through hereditary pancreatitis. Individuals with three or more first-degree relatives with pancreatic cancer have a 32-fold increased risk of developing pancreatic cancer. The risk in those with two affected first-degree relatives is 6.4-fold and in those with a single affected first degree relative 4.5-fold [66].

An underlying germline disorder can be found in 5–10% of patients [67]. Those with hereditary pancreatitis (*PRSS1* gene mutation) have a cumulative lifetime risk of pancreatic carcinoma of 40% [68]. Such patients have a 54-fold greater risk than the general population and in those patients who smoke cigarettes this risk rises to 154-fold [69]. Germ line mutations in *BRCA2* (familial breast cancer), *STK11* (Peutz–Jeghers syndrome) and *vHL* (von Hippel–Lindau) genes also have an increased risk of pancreatic cancer [70].

There is no formal recommendation for screening such patients with an increased risk, but EUS, EUS with fine-needle aspiration, CT and ERCP are the most common, current methods [71].

There is a 50% increased relative risk of pancreatic cancer in patients with type 2 diabetes of more than 5 years' duration, suggesting a modest causal relationship [72].

Patients with chronic pancreatitis are reported to have a cumulative risk of 2% per decade [73].

Smoking, alcohol and obesity are also risk factors. There is no strong link between diet and pancreatic cancer.

Some benign pancreatic tumours have the potential for malignant change, including mucinous cystic neoplasms, intraductal papillary mucinous neoplasms and pancreatic intraepithelial neoplasia [74].

Molecular changes [75]

There is uncertainty regarding the cellular origin of pancreatic cancer and the molecular events which lead to invasive carcinoma. K-*ras* gene mutation, particularly at codon 12, is found in the majority of pancreatic carcinomas. Mutations can be detected by polymerase chain reaction on formalin-fixed paraffin-embedded tissue. Abnormally high *p53* gene expression is found in 60% of pancreatic carcinomas, predominantly in ductal tumours. Clinically, K-*ras* mutation analysis remains a research rather than a clinical tool.

K-*ras* mutations may be detected in pancreatic duct brushings in patients with carcinoma [76]. However they are also found in the pancreatic juice of patients with chronic pancreatitis. This may relate to K-*ras* mutations in areas of duct hyperplasia [77]. Over a 2-year follow-up only a minority of K-*ras*-positive patients develop a pancreatic carcinoma [78].

Pathology

Histologically, the tumour is an adenocarcinoma, whether arising from pancreatic duct, acinus or bile duct. Ampullary tumours have a papillary arrangement and are often of low-grade malignancy. They tend to be polypoid and soft, whereas the acinar tumours are usually infiltrative and firm.

Obstruction of common bile duct

This results from direct invasion of the distal bile duct or extrinsic compression.

The bile ducts dilate and the gallbladder enlarges. Ascending cholangitis in the obstructed duct is rare. The liver shows changes of cholestasis.

Pancreatic changes

The main pancreatic duct may be obstructed by tumour. As a result, the ducts and acini distal to the obstruction dilate and later rupture, causing focal areas of pancreatitis, fat necrosis and subsequently fibrosis.

Diabetes mellitus or impaired glucose tolerance is found in 60–80% of patients. This may be due to direct tumour invasion, ductal obstruction with fibrosis or production of islet amyloid polypeptide by islet cells adjacent to the tumour [79].

Spread of the tumour

Local tumour spread results in obstruction to the distal bile duct and obstructive jaundice, the most common presenting feature. The second part of the duodenum may also be invaded resulting in ulceration of the mucosa and secondary haemorrhage. The splenic and portal veins may be invaded and may thrombose with resultant splenomegaly.

Involvement of regional nodes is found in approximately a third of operated cases. Perineural lymphatic spread is common. Blood-borne metastases, with secondaries in liver and lungs, follows invasion of the splenic or portal veins. Transcoelomic spread results in peritoneal and omental metastases.

Clinical features

Both sexes are affected, but males more frequently than females in a ratio of 2:1. The peak incidence is in the sixth and seventh decades. The clinical picture is a composite one of cholestasis with pancreatic insufficiency, and the general and local effects of a malignant tumour (Fig. 13.6).

Jaundice is of gradual onset, usually progressive, but ampullary neoplasms can cause mild and intermittent jaundice. *Itching* is a common but not invariable feature, and when present comes after jaundice. Cholangitis at presentation is unusual.

Cancer of the head of the pancreas is not always painless. Pain may be experienced in the back, the epigas-

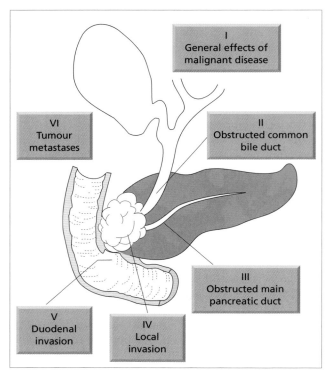

Fig. 13.6. The effects of carcinoma in the ampullary region.
I, General effects of malignant disease—weakness, weight loss.
II, Obstructed common bile duct; dilated gallbladder and bile ducts—jaundice, pruritus.
III, Obstructed pancreatic duct—steatorrhoea, diabetes.
IV, Local invasion: blood vessels (portal, superior mesenteric)—encasement, thrombosis; nerves—back and epigastric pain.
V, Duodenal invasion—occasional duodenal obstruction, positive occult blood.
VI, Tumour metastases—regional glands, liver, lungs, peritoneum.

trium and right upper quadrant, usually a continuous discomfort worse at night and sometimes ameliorated by crouching or leaning forward. It may be aggravated by eating.

Weakness and weight loss are progressive and have usually continued for at least 3 months before jaundice develops.

Although frank steatorrhoea is rare, the patient often complains of a change in bowel habit, usually diarrhoea.

Vomiting and intestinal obstruction follows invasion of the second part of the duodenum and occurs overall in 15–20% of patients. Ulceration of the duodenum can result in haematemesis or, more commonly, occult blood loss.

Often the diagnosis of periampullary cancer is delayed as the symptoms in the early stages are non-specific.

Examination. The patient is jaundiced and shows evidence of recent weight loss. The gallbladder may be enlarged and palpable (*Courvoisier's law*). In practice, the gallbladder is only clinically apparent in about half the patients, although at subsequent laparotomy a dilated gallbladder is found in three-quarters. The liver is enlarged with a sharp, smooth, firm edge. The pancreatic tumour is usually impalpable.

The spleen may be palpable if involvement of the splenic vein has caused thrombosis. Peritoneal invasion may result in ascites. Locoregional lymphatic metastases are common with cancer of the pancreas [80] Occasionally distal nodal metastases are present in the axilla, neck or groin.

Virchow's gland in the left supraclavicular fossa may be palpable.

Pancreatic cancers produce a prothrombotic tendency and may present with an episode of venous thrombosis.

Investigations

Glycosuria occurs in 60–80% and with it there is an impaired oral glucose tolerance test.

Blood biochemistry. The serum bilirubin and alkaline phosphatase level is raised. The serum amylase and lipase concentrations are sometimes persistently elevated in carcinoma of the ampullary region. Hypoproteinaemia with peripheral oedema may be present.

There is no reliable serum tumour marker with sufficient specificity or sensitivity. In a systematic review, the carbohydrate antigen CA 19-9 had a median sensitivity of 79% and median specificity of 82% [81]. However, it can be elevated in benign biliary obstruction and its specificity decreases in the presence of jaundice or cholangitis. Tumour M2-pyruvate kinase has similar efficacy to CA 19-9 [82].

Haematology. Anaemia is mild or absent. The leucocyte count may be normal or raised with a relative increase in neutrophils. The erythrocyte sedimentation rate is usually raised. Prothrombin time may be prolonged due to malabsorption of vitamin K in severely jaundiced patients. Elevated C-reactive protein in patients with pancreatic adenocarcinoma is associated with poor prognosis [83,84] independent of biliary tract obstruction [85].

Differential diagnosis

The diagnosis must be considered in any patient over 40 years with progressive or intermittent jaundice. The suspicion is strengthened by persistent or unexplained abdominal pain, weakness and weight loss, diarrhoea, glycosuria, positive faecal occult blood, hepatomegaly, a palpable spleen or thrombophlebitis migrans.

Diagnosis and staging

Conventional imaging modalities used in the diagnosis and staging of pancreatic cancer include CT, MRI, EUS and ERCP. It is important to exclude extrapancreatic spread of tumour and to determine potential resectability for planning treatment. There are no universally accepted criteria for defining resectability in pancreatic adenocarcinoma but most centres consider local vascular invasion as locally advanced disease.

Dual phase contrast enhanced CT with images obtained during pancreatic phase and hepatic phase (pancreas protocol CT) is currently the most widely used and best validated imaging modality [86]. This has a sensitivity of 89 to 97% for diagnosis of pancreatic carcinoma.

Pancreatic protocol CT is superior to most other imaging techniques in predicting resectability and staging of pancreatic cancer [87]. In a recent meta-analysis, the sensitivity and specificity of CT for determining resectability was 81% and 82% respectively [88].

Three-dimensional CT (3D-CT) is a recent innovation in CT technology. In a single-centre study, preoperative 3D-CT accurately predicted periampullary cancer resectability and a margin-negative resection in 98 and 86% of patients, respectively [89].

MRI has not been shown to perform better than CT in the diagnosis and staging of pancreatic cancer but is useful in characterization of small hepatic lesions [86].

EUS is valuable in the imaging of small pancreatic lesions or when CT findings of locally advanced disease are equivocal [86]. EUS-guided fine-needle aspiration (EUS-FNA) for cytological examination or Trucut biopsies for histological examination, are safe and reliable [90]. For solid pancreatic masses, the diagnostic yield of EUS-FNA is in the range of 86 to 98% and for EUS-biopsy 69 to 89% [90].

Biopsy of a suspected pancreatic tumour is indicated for tissue diagnosis before palliative treatment in patients with unresectable disease, or when neoadjuvant therapy is to be considered in patients with resectable disease. Also, unusual tumours such as lymphoma need to be identified since they may respond to specific therapy. Both CT-guided percutaneous core biopsy and EUS-FNA have high sensitivity for diagnosing pancreatic neoplasms. Biliary brush cytology has a relatively low sensitivity for diagnosing malignancy.

ERCP can demonstrate the pancreatic and bile ducts, allow biopsy of any ampullary lesion (Fig. 13.7), and provide bile or pancreatic juice or brushings from the stricture for cytological examination (Fig. 13.8). An adjacent narrowing of the bile and pancreatic duct (double duct sign) is usually associated with a malignant stric-

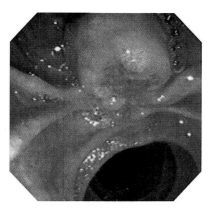

Fig. 13.7. Abnormal ampulla at ERCP. Note irregular surface with nodularity. Biopsy showed adenocarcinoma.

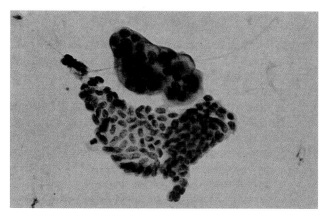

Fig. 13.8. Brush cytology taken from a low common bile duct stricture. There is a sheet of benign biliary epithelial cells and above this a small group of large polymorphic cells characteristic of adenocarcinoma.

ture (Fig. 13.9) but occasionally appearances are deceptive and tissue diagnosis should be sought. Biliary brush cytology has a sensitivity of around 60% for pancreatic carcinoma [91,92].

With advances in imaging technology, the role of ERCP in the diagnosis of pancreatic carcinoma has been challenged. MRCP is as sensitive as ERCP in detecting pancreatic carcinomas and avoids the risks of ERCP, including pancreatitis and cholangitis. The role of routine preoperative biliary drainage by means of ERCP in resectable pancreatic carcinoma is controversial. However, a randomized trial in patients undergoing surgery for cancer of the head of the pancreas has shown that routine preoperative biliary drainage increased postoperative complications [93].

Laparoscopy is an important component of the staging process for pancreatic cancer. The potential benefit is in detecting CT occult metastases and hence avoiding an

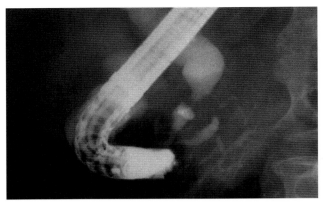

Fig. 13.9. ERCP showing dilated bile duct above a stricture. The pancreatic duct comes to an abrupt halt in the head of the pancreas ('double duct' sign). Appearances are characteristic of carcinoma of the pancreas.

unnecessary laparotomy. The procedure is cost effective [94] and a positive peritoneal cytology correlates with a poor survival [95]. The yield of staging laparoscopy has been debated. Some recommended it for all patients with pancreatic adenocarcinoma [96] whereas others advise selective use in subset of patients with high risk of metastatic disease [97], such as those with considerable weight loss, ascites, markedly elevated CA 19-9 and a large primary tumour.

In the patient with vomiting, oral contrast CT and/or endoscopy will show the extent of duodenal invasion and obstruction.

Treatment

Resection

Pancreatic adenocarcinoma has an aggressive biological behaviour with late onset of symptoms. Most patients (85 to 90%) have locally advanced disease at the time of diagnosis [98]. Overall 5-year survival rate in patients who undergo potentially curative surgical resection is 10 to 20%. Nevertheless, surgery remains the only potentially curative treatment. In experienced centres the perioperative mortality is less than 5%.

Patients with ampullary carcinoma who undergo potentially curative resection have a 5-year survival between 40 and 70% [99]. For distal cholangiocarcinoma, 5-year survival after surgery is 25 to 40% [100].

The classical procedure for a periampullary carcinoma is *pancreaticoduodenectomy (Whipple's operation)* which is performed in one stage with *en masse* removal of the head of the pancreas with distal common bile duct, the entire duodenum, the distal third of the stomach and related lymph nodes. This operation was modified in 1978 to preserve antral and pyloric function (pylorus-preserving pancreaticoduodenectomy). Following resection, reconstruction involves anastomosis of the remaining pancreas, distal bile duct and stomach to the small intestine.

Several technical aspects of the pancreaticoduodenectomy operation have been studied. Both standard Whipple's operation and pylorus-preserving pancreaticoduodenectomy are equally effective and have comparable overall long-term survival, disease-free survival and quality of life [101,102]. The pylorus-preserving procedure offers some minor advantages in the early postoperative period but not in the long term [102].

The pancreatic remnant can be joined to the jejunum or stomach. When pancreaticojejunostomy and pancreaticogastrostomy were compared, there was no advantage of either technique [103]. Both methods have comparable incidence of pancreatic fistula, the most feared complication after pancreaticoduodenectomy, and have a similar overall postoperative complication rate [104].

The extent of lymph node dissection has also been a subject of discussion. It was hoped that extensive retroperitoneal lymphadenectomy and clearance of soft tissue around the pancreas (extended pancreaticoduodenectomy) may improve survival. However, available data does not demonstrate a benefit in long-term survival with extended pancreaticoduodenectomy [105].

Vascular resection with pancreaticoduodenectomy is another area of debate. Invasion of the superior mesenteric vein or portal vein in the presence of pancreatic cancer is considered locally advanced disease and was accepted as a contraindication to resection. In the last decade, some specialists have done *en bloc* resection of the involved segment of the vein. Despite the complexity of the procedure, it can be carried out safely by experienced surgeons and does not adversely impact survival [106,107]. However this approach remains controversial.

Frozen section examination of the pancreatic resection margin is commonly done during surgery to ensure a negative margin [108]. Some studies report that a negative resection margin is a powerful independent predictor of long-term survival [109] whereas others do not show this [110]. Although there is a lack of good data on the value of examining frozen sections during pancreaticoduodenectomy, it is common practice for most surgeons.

Pancreaticoduodenectomy for pancreatic carcinoma is a complex operation. Surgeons should maintain an adequate case load to maintain skill levels, although the threshold number of procedures is not established. After controlling for patient demographics and other factors, pancreatic resection by a 'high-volume' surgeon is independently associated with a 51% reduction in in-hospital mortality [111]. This supports the argument for centralization of pancreatic surgery in high-volume specialist units.

Adjuvant therapy

This may have an impact on survival after resection of pancreatic cancer. However, there is no consensus on the optimal treatment.

Several trials have studied the role of adjuvant chemoradiation and adjuvant chemotherapy in resected pancreatic cancers [112]. Despite some criticisms, the European Study Group for Pancreatic Cancer trial (ESPAC-1 trial) was the first trial to show significant survival benefit with adjuvant 5-fluorouracil (5-FU) and folinic acid based chemotherapy. Some trials, performed prior to the ESPAC-1 trial, suggested benefit with adjuvant chemoradiation, but later trials have not demonstrated a survival benefit.

Overall, there may be benefit with adjuvant chemotherapy and the role of chemoradiation is not clear. At present no definite standard has been established in the adjuvant treatment of resected pancreatic cancers and this is a subject of ongoing trials.

Adjuvant therapy for adenocarcinoma of the ampulla of Vater is controversial. These tumours are relatively uncommon and prospective data for effective treatment options is sparse. At present, adjuvant and neoadjuvant treatments for ampullary adenocarcinoma are not considered standard therapy.

Currently, there is no good evidence to support the use of adjuvant or neoadjuvant treatments for distal cholangiocarcinoma.

Palliative procedures

The choice lies between surgical bypass and endoscopic or percutaneous transhepatic insertion of an endoprosthesis (stent). The two have not as yet been compared in a controlled trial.

Surgical biliary bypass is an option in unresectable patients with a predicted longer survival [113]. For the patient with bile duct obstruction alone, some argue for prophylactic gastric bypass surgery at the time of biliary bypass as about 25% of patients will subsequently develop duodenal obstruction.

Others would try and predict the risk of obstruction based on the size and position of the tumour. For the jaundiced patient with vomiting due to duodenal obstruction, surgery involves gastroenterostomy as well as choledochojejunostomy.

Bile duct and duodenal stenting. Gastric outlet and duodenal stenosis can be treated by endoscopically or radiologically placed self-expandable mesh metal stents [114].

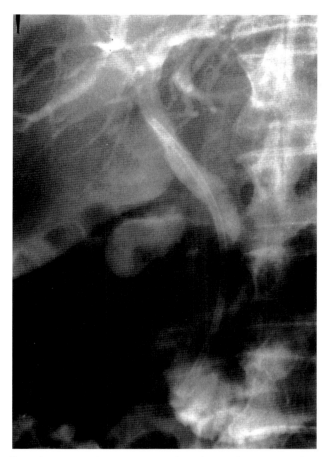

Fig. 13.10. Polyethylene 10 French endoprosthesis inserted across low common bile duct stricture by the endoscopic route. Note good flow of contrast into duodenum and decompressed biliary system.

Endoscopic biliary stent insertion (Fig. 13.10) has a success rate of more than 90% in experienced centres [114] but 5–25% of patients require re-intervention for stent occlusion during the course of the disease [115].When the endoscopic approach fails, a percutaneous or combined percutaneous/endoscopic approach can be used.

Plastic stents are inexpensive and effective but have a short patency rate of approximately 3 to 5 months [114]. Self-expandable metal stents have a higher patency rate [116]. Later metal stent occlusion occurs in 20–30% of patients. When this happens an additional metal or plastic stent can be inserted through the occluded stent [114].

Patients can have intractable pain with advanced periampullary cancers. Coeliac plexus neurolysis can provide good pain relief. Chemical neurolysis can be performed either percutaneously, under fluoroscopic guidance, or with EUS guidance [117,118].

Palliative chemotherapy

Locally unresectable or metastatic pancreatic carcinoma is incurable. Chemotherapy when compared to best supportive care prolongs survival and improves quality of life [119]. Gemcitabine as a single agent therapy is an acceptable palliative treatment for advanced pancreatic carcinoma [119]. 5-FU has poor response rates and 6-month survival. The role of chemoradiation for advanced pancreatic cancer is controversial.

Molecular therapy

Several trials have investigated the role of molecular targeted therapy in advanced pancreatic cancer. Addition of erlotinib, an epidermal growth factor receptor inhibitor to gemcitabine was associated with greater progression-free survival and 1-year survival [120]. However, addition of the following to gemcitabine based regimens has as yet shown no benefit: monoclonal antibody against EGFR receptor (cetuximab), monoclonal antibody to vascular endothelial growth factor (bevacizumab), matrix metalloproteinase inhibitor (marimastat). Similarly the tyrosine kinase inhibitor imatinib was not beneficial. The same is true for several other molecular targets.

Prognosis

Most patients present with locally advanced or metastatic disease. Only 10 to 20% are suitable for surgical resection [121]. Even for patients with surgically resectable disease, the long-term survival is poor. The estimated 5-year survival after pancreaticoduodenectomy is 10 to 20%. The actual 5-year survival rate for these patients has been reported as 4 to 10% [122].

Survival is better for carcinoma of the ampulla of Vater. Pancreaticoduodenectomy for invasive adenocarcinoma of the ampulla has a 5-year survival of 30 to 70% [99].

Resectability rates for distal cholangiocarcinoma range from 22 to 89% [123]. Overall 5-year survival is 24 to 39% [100].

Primary duodenal carcinoma is rare and most studies in the literature have included only a small number of patients. In a recent report median survival after surgery was 34 months [124].

Conclusions

Surgical outcomes of cholangiocarcinoma and periampullary carcinoma have improved in the last two decades. The ability to carry out these major operations successfully is largely based on state of the art advances in diagnosis and staging, and improved surgical techniques. The procedures are complex and require discussions in the context of a multidisciplinary team. The procedures should be carried in specialist units.

References

1 Sakorafas GH, Milingos D, Peros G. Asymptomatic cholelithiasis: is cholecystectomy really needed? A critical reappraisal 15 years after the introduction of laparoscopic cholecystectomy. *Dig. Dis. Sci.* 2007; **52**: 1313–1325.
2 Benjamin IS. Biliary cystic disease: the risk of cancer. *J. Hepatobiliary Pancreat. Surg.* 2003; **10**: 335–339.
3 de Aretxabala X, Roa I, Burgos L *et al.* Gallbladder cancer in Chile. A report on 54 potentially resectable tumors. *Cancer* 1992 ; **69**: 60–65.
4 Hawkins WG, Dematteo RP, Jarnagin WR *et al.* Jaundice predicts advanced disease and early mortality in patients with gallbladder cancer. *Ann. Surg. Oncol.* 2004; **11**: 310–315.
5 Furlan A, Ferris JV, Hosseinzadeh K *et al.* Gallbladder carcinoma update: multimodality imaging evaluation, staging, and treatment options. *AJR Am. J. Roentgenol.* 2008; **191**: 1440–1447.
6 Kim SJ, Lee JM, Lee JY *et al.* Accuracy of preoperative T-staging of gallbladder carcinoma using MDCT. *AJR Am. J. Roentgenol.* 2008; **190**: 74–80.
7 Kim JH, Kim TK, Eun HW *et al.* Preoperative evaluation of gallbladder carcinoma: efficacy of combined use of MR imaging, MR cholangiography, and contrast-enhanced dual-phase three-dimensional MR angiography. *J. Magn. Reson. Imaging* 2002; **16**: 676–684.
8 Sadamoto Y, Kubo H, Harada N *et al.* Preoperative diagnosis and staging of gallbladder carcinoma by EUS. *Gastrointest. Endosc.* 2003; **58**: 536–541.
9 Reddy SK, Clary BM. Surgical management of gallbladder cancer. *Surg. Oncol. Clin. North Am.* 2009; **18**: 307–324, ix.
10 Miller G, Jarnagin WR. Gallbladder carcinoma. *Eur. J. Surg. Oncol.* 2008; **34**: 306–312.
11 Hueman MT, Vollmer CM Jr, Pawlik TM. Evolving treatment strategies for gallbladder cancer. *Ann. Surg. Oncol.* 2009; **16**: 2101–2115.
12 Weber SM, Dematteo RP, Fong Y *et al.* Staging laparoscopy in patients with extrahepatic biliary carcinoma. Analysis of 100 patients. *Ann. Surg.* 2002; **235**: 392–399.
13 Khan SA, Davidson BR, Goldin R *et al.* Guidelines for the diagnosis and treatment of cholangiocarcinoma: consensus document. *Gut* 2002; **51** (Suppl. 6): VI1–VI9.
14 Taylor-Robinson SD, Toledano MB, Arora S *et al.* Increase in mortality rates from intrahepatic cholangiocarcinoma in England and Wales 1968–1998. *Gut* 2001; **48**: 816–820.
15 Patel T. Increasing incidence and mortality of primary intrahepatic cholangiocarcinoma in the United States. *Hepatology* 2001; **33**: 1353–1357.
16 Gakhal MS, Gheyi VK, Brock RE *et al.* Multimodality imaging of biliary malignancies. *Surg. Oncol. Clin. North Am.* 2009; **18**: 225–239, vii–viii.
17 Hochwald SN, Burke EC, Jarnagin WR *et al.* Association of preoperative biliary stenting with increased postoperative infectious complications in proximal cholangiocarcinoma. *Arch. Surg.* 1999; **134**: 261–266.
18 Nakeeb A, Pitt HA. The role of preoperative biliary decompression in obstructive jaundice. *Hepatogastroenterology* 1995; **42**: 332–337.
19 Khan SA, Thomas HC, Davidson BR *et al.* Cholangiocarcinoma. *Lancet* 2005; **366**: 1303–1314.
20 Shaib Y, El-Serag HB. The epidemiology of cholangiocarcinoma. *Semin. Liver Dis.* 2004; **24**: 115–125.

21 Broome U, Lofberg R, Veress B *et al.* Primary sclerosing cholangitis and ulcerative colitis: evidence for increased neoplastic potential. *Hepatology* 1995; **22**: 1404–1408.

22 Rosen CB, Nagorney DM, Wiesner RH *et al.* Cholangiocarcinoma complicating primary sclerosing cholangitis. *Ann. Surg.* 1991; **213**: 21–25.

23 Leidenius M, Hockersted K, Broome U *et al.* Hepatobiliary carcinoma in primary sclerosing cholangitis: a case control study. *J. Hepatol.* 2001; **34**: 792–798.

24 Ekbom A, Hsieh CC, Yuen J *et al.* Risk of extrahepatic bileduct cancer after cholecystectomy. *Lancet* 1993; **342**: 1262–1265.

25 Nehls O, Gregor M, Klump B. Serum and bile markers for cholangiocarcinoma. *Semin. Liver Dis.* 2004; **24**: 139–154.

26 Briggs CD, Neal CP, Mann CD *et al.* Prognostic molecular markers in cholangiocarcinoma: a systematic review. *Eur. J. Cancer* 2009; **45**: 33–47.

27 Tan CK, Podila PV, Taylor JE *et al.* Human cholangiocarcinomas express somatostatin receptors and respond to somatostatin with growth inhibition. *Gastroenterology* 1995; **108**: 1908–1916.

28 Klatskin G. Adenocarcinoma of the hepatic duct at its bifurcation within the porta hepatis. an unusual tumor with distinctive clinical and pathological features. *Am. J. Med.* 1965; **38**: 241–256.

29 Fleming KA, Boberg KM, Glaumann H *et al.* Biliary dysplasia as a marker of cholangiocarcinoma in primary sclerosing cholangitis. *J. Hepatol.* 2001; **34**: 360–365.

30 Selvaggi SM. Biliary brushing cytology. *Cytopathology* 2004; **15**: 74–79.

31 Silva MA, Hegab B, Hyde C *et al.* Needle track seeding following biopsy of liver lesions in the diagnosis of hepatocellular cancer: a systematic review and meta-analysis. *Gut* 2008; **57**: 1592–1596.

32 Ponsioen CY, Vrouenraets SM, van Milligen de Wit AW *et al.* Value of brush cytology for dominant strictures in primary sclerosing cholangitis. *Endoscopy* 1999; **31**: 305–309.

33 Kubicka S, Kuhnel F, Flemming P *et al.* K-ras mutations in the bile of patients with primary sclerosing cholangitis. *Gut* 2001; **48**: 403–408.

34 Robertson AG, Davidson BR. Mirizzi syndrome complicating an anomalous biliary tract: a novel cause of a hugely elevated CA19-9. *Eur. J. Gastroenterol. Hepatol.* 2007; **19**: 167–169.

35 Bjornsson E, Kilander A, Olsson R. CA 19-9 and CEA are unreliable markers for cholangiocarcinoma in patients with primary sclerosing cholangitis. *Liver* 1999; **19**: 501–508.

36 Patel AH, Harnois DM, Klee GG *et al.* The utility of CA 19-9 in the diagnoses of cholangiocarcinoma in patients without primary sclerosing cholangitis. *Am. J. Gastroenterol.* 2000; **95**: 204–207.

37 Hann LE, Greatrex KV, Bach AM *et al.* Cholangiocarcinoma at the hepatic hilus: sonographic findings. *AJR Am. J. Roentgenol.* 1997; **168**: 985–989.

38 Neumaier CE, Bertolotto M, Perrone R *et al.* Staging of hilar cholangiocarcinoma with ultrasound. *J. Clin. Ultrasound* 1995; **23**: 173–178.

39 Tamada K, Ido K, Ueno N *et al.* Preoperative staging of extrahepatic bile duct cancer with intraductal ultrasonography. *Am. J. Gastroenterol.* 1995; **90**: 239–246.

40 Vilgrain V. Staging cholangiocarcinoma by imaging studies. *HPB (Oxford)* 2008; **10**: 106–109.

41 Zidi SH, Prat F, Le GO *et al.* Performance characteristics of magnetic resonance cholangiography in the staging of malignant hilar strictures. *Gut* 2000; **46**: 103–106.

42 Zech CJ, Schoenberg SO, Reiser M *et al.* Cross-sectional imaging of biliary tumors: current clinical status and future developments. *Eur. Radiol.* 2004; **14**: 1174–1187.

43 Keiding S, Hansen SB, Rasmussen HH *et al.* Detection of cholangiocarcinoma in primary sclerosing cholangitis by positron emission tomography. *Hepatology* 1998; **28**: 700–706.

44 Kluge R, Schmidt F, Caca K *et al.* Positron emission tomography with [(18)F]fluoro-2-deoxy-D-glucose for diagnosis and staging of bile duct cancer. *Hepatology* 2001; **33**: 1029–1035.

45 Kim JY, Kim MH, Lee TY *et al.* Clinical role of 18F-FDG PET-CT in suspected and potentially operable cholangiocarcinoma: a prospective study compared with conventional imaging. *Am. J. Gastroenterol.* 2008; **103**: 1145–1151.

46 Rosch T, Meining A, Fruhmorgen S *et al.* A prospective comparison of the diagnostic accuracy of ERCP, MRCP, CT, and EUS in biliary strictures. *Gastrointest. Endosc.* 2002; **55**: 870–876.

47 Palavecino M, Abdalla EK, Madoff DC *et al.* Portal vein embolization in hilar cholangiocarcinoma. *Surg. Oncol. Clin. North Am.* 2009; **18**: 257–267, viii.

48 Joseph S, Connor S, Garden OJ. Staging laparoscopy for cholangiocarcinoma. *HPB (Oxford)* 2008; **10**: 116–119.

49 Lillemoe KD, Cameron JL. Surgery for hilar cholangiocarcinoma: the Johns Hopkins approach. *J. Hepatobiliary Pancreat. Surg.* 2000; **7**: 115–121.

50 Polydorou AA, Cairns SR, Dowsett JF *et al.* Palliation of proximal malignant biliary obstruction by endoscopic endoprosthesis insertion. *Gut* 1991; **32**: 685–689.

51 De Palma GD, Galloro G, Siciliano S. Unilateral vs. bilateral endoscopic hepatic drainage in patients with malignant hilar biliary obstruction: results of a prospective, randomized and controlled study. *Gastrointest. Endosc.* 2001; **53**: 547.

52 Rai R, Dick R, Doctor N *et al.* Predicting early mortality following percutaneous stent insertion for malignant biliary obstruction: a multivariate risk factor analysis. *Eur. J. Gastroenterol. Hepatol.* 2000; **12**: 1095–1100.

53 Lammer J, Hausegger KA, Fluckiger F *et al.* Common bile duct obstruction due to malignancy: treatment with plastic versus metal stents. *Radiology* 1996; **201**: 167–172.

54 Wagner HJ, Knyrim K, Vakil N *et al.* Plastic endoprostheses versus metal stents in the palliative treatment of malignant hilar biliary obstruction. A prospective and randomized trial. *Endoscopy* 1993; **25**: 213–218.

55 Gerhards MF, den Hartog D, Rauws EA *et al.* Palliative treatment in patients with unresectable hilar cholangiocarcinoma: results of endoscopic drainage in patients with type III and IV hilar cholangiocarcinoma. *Eur. J. Surg.* 2001; **167**: 274–280.

56 Valle JW, Wasan H, Johnson P *et al.* Gemcitabine alone or in combination with cisplatin in patients with advanced or metastatic cholangiocarcinomas or other biliary tract tumours: a multicentre randomised phase II study—The UK ABC-01 Study. *Br. J. Cancer* 2009; **101**: 621–627.

57 Ortner ME, Caca K, Berr F *et al.* Successful photodynamic therapy for nonresectable cholangiocarcinoma: a rand-

omized prospective study. *Gastroenterology* 2003; **125**: 1355–1363.

58 Zoepf T, Jakobs R, Arnold JC *et al.* Palliation of nonresectable bile duct cancer: improved survival after photodynamic therapy. *Am. J. Gastroenterol.* 2005; **100**: 2426–2430.

59 Farley DR, Weaver AL, Nagorney DM. 'Natural history' of unresected cholangiocarcinoma: patient outcome after noncurative intervention. *Mayo Clin. Proc.* 1995; **70**: 425–429.

60 Carpizo DR, D'Angelica M. Management and extent of resection for intrahepatic cholangiocarcinoma. *Surg. Oncol. Clin. North Am.* 2009; **18**: 289–305, viii–ix.

61 Chen MF. Peripheral cholangiocarcinoma (cholangiocellular carcinoma): clinical features, diagnosis and treatment. *J. Gastroenterol. Hepatol.* 1999; **14**: 1144–1149.

62 Jan YY, Yeh CN, Yeh TS *et al.* Prognostic analysis of surgical treatment of peripheral cholangiocarcinoma: two decades of experience at Chang Gung Memorial Hospital. *World J. Gastroenterol.* 2005; **11**: 1779–1784.

63 Madariaga JR, Iwatsuki S, Todo S *et al.* Liver resection for hilar and peripheral cholangiocarcinomas: a study of 62 cases. *Ann. Surg.* 1998; **227**: 70–79.

64 Valiozis I, Zekry A, Williams SJ *et al.* Palliation of hilar biliary obstruction from colorectal metastases by endoscopic stent insertion. *Gastrointest. Endosc.* 2000; **51**: 412–417.

65 Oberg K, Jelic S. Neuroendocrine gastroenteropancreatic tumors: ESMO clinical recommendation for diagnosis, treatment and follow-up. *Ann. Oncol.* 2009; **20** (Suppl. 4): 150–153.

66 Klein AP, Brune KA, Petersen GM *et al.* Prospective risk of pancreatic cancer in familial pancreatic cancer kindreds. *Cancer Res.* 2004 1; **64**: 2634–2638.

67 Raimondi S, Maisonneuve P, Lowenfels AB. Epidemiology of pancreatic cancer: an overview. *Nat. Rev. Gastroenterol. Hepatol.* 2009; **6**: 699–708.

68 Lowenfels AB, Maisonneuve P, Dimagno EP *et al.* Hereditary pancreatitis and the risk of pancreatic cancer. International Hereditary Pancreatitis Study Group. *J. Natl. Cancer Inst.* 1997; **89**: 442–446.

69 Lowenfels AB, Maisonneuve P, Whitcomb DC *et al.* Cigarette smoking as a risk factor for pancreatic cancer in patients with hereditary pancreatitis. *JAMA* 2001; **286**: 169–170.

70 Klein AP, Hruban RH, Brune KA *et al.* Familial pancreatic cancer. *Cancer J.* 2001; **7**: 266–273.

71 Greer JB, Lynch HT, Brand RE. Hereditary pancreatic cancer: a clinical perspective. *Best Pract. Res. Clin. Gastroenterol.* 2009; **23**: 159–170.

72 Huxley R, Nsary-Moghaddam A, Berrington de GA *et al.* Type-II diabetes and pancreatic cancer: a meta-analysis of 36 studies. *Br. J. Cancer* 2005; **92**: 2076–2083.

73 Lowenfels AB, Maisonneuve P, Cavallini G *et al.* Pancreatitis and the risk of pancreatic cancer. International Pancreatitis Study Group. *N. Engl. J. Med.* 1993; **328**: 1433–1437.

74 Hruban RH, Maitra A, Kern SE *et al.* Precursors to pancreatic cancer. *Gastroenterol. Clin. North Am.* 2007; **36**: 831–849, vi.

75 Buchholz M, Gress TM. Molecular changes in pancreatic cancer. *Expert Rev. Anticancer Ther.* 2009; **9**: 1487–1497.

76 van Laethem JL, Vertongen P, Deviere J *et al.* Detection of c-Ki-ras gene codon 12 mutations from pancreatic duct brushings in the diagnosis of pancreatic tumours. *Gut* 1995; **36**: 781–787.

77 Rivera JA, Rall CJ, Graeme-Cook F *et al.* Analysis of K-ras oncogene mutations in chronic pancreatitis with ductal hyperplasia. *Surgery* 1997; **121**: 42–49.

78 Queneau PE, Adessi GL, Thibault P *et al.* Early detection of pancreatic cancer in patients with chronic pancreatitis: diagnostic utility of a K-ras point mutation in the pancreatic juice. *Am. J. Gastroenterol.* 2001; **96**: 700–704.

79 Basso D, Greco E, Fogar P *et al.* Pancreatic cancer-associated diabetes mellitus: an open field for proteomic applications. *Clin. Chim. Acta* 2005; **357**: 184–189.

80 Artinyan A, Soriano PA, Prendergast C *et al.* The anatomic location of pancreatic cancer is a prognostic factor for survival. *HPB (Oxford)* 2008; **10**: 371–376.

81 Goonetilleke KS, Siriwardena AK. Systematic review of carbohydrate antigen (CA 19-9) as a biochemical marker in the diagnosis of pancreatic cancer. *Eur. J. Surg. Oncol.* 2007; **33**: 266–270.

82 Kumar Y, Gurusamy K, Pamecha V *et al.* Tumor M2-pyruvate kinase as tumor marker in exocrine pancreatic cancer: a meta-analysis. *Pancreas* 2007; **35**: 114–119.

83 Jamieson NB, Glen P, McMillan DC *et al.* Systemic inflammatory response predicts outcome in patients undergoing resection for ductal adenocarcinoma head of pancreas. *Br. J. Cancer* 2005; **92**: 21–23.

84 Tingstedt B, Johansson P, Andersson B *et al.* Predictive factors in pancreatic ductal adenocarcinoma: role of the inflammatory response. *Scand. J. Gastroenterol.* 2007; **42**: 754–759.

85 Pine JK, Fusai KG, Young R *et al.* Serum C-reactive protein concentration and the prognosis of ductal adenocarcinoma of the head of pancreas. *Eur. J. Surg. Oncol.* 2009; **35**: 605–610.

86 Wong JC, Lu DS. Staging of pancreatic adenocarcinoma by imaging studies. *Clin. Gastroenterol. Hepatol.* 2008; **6**: 1301–1308.

87 Horton KM, Fishman EK. Adenocarcinoma of the pancreas: CT imaging. *Radiol. Clin. North Am.* 2002; **40**: 1263–1272.

88 Bipat S, Phoa SS, van Delden OM *et al.* Ultrasonography, computed tomography and magnetic resonance imaging for diagnosis and determining resectability of pancreatic adenocarcinoma: a meta-analysis. *J. Comput. Assist. Tomogr.* 2005; **29**: 438–445.

89 House MG, Yeo CJ, Cameron JL *et al.* Predicting resectability of periampullary cancer with three-dimensional computed tomography. *J. Gastrointest. Surg.* 2004; **8**: 280–288.

90 Jenssen C, Dietrich CF. Endoscopic ultrasound-guided fine-needle aspiration biopsy and trucut biopsy in gastroenterology—An overview. *Best Pract. Res. Clin. Gastroenterol.* 2009; **23**: 743–759.

91 Kurzawinski TR, Deery A, Dooley JS *et al.* A prospective study of biliary cytology in 100 patients with bile duct strictures. *Hepatology* 1993; **18**: 1399–1403.

92 Stewart CJ, Mills PR, Carter R *et al.* Brush cytology in the assessment of pancreatico-biliary strictures: a review of 406 cases. *J. Clin. Pathol.* 2001; **54**: 449–455.

93 van der Gaag NA, Rauws EA, van Eijck CH *et al.* Preoperative biliary drainage for cancer of the head of the pancreas. *N. Engl. J. Med.* 2010; **362**: 129–137.

94 Enestvedt CK, Mayo SC, Diggs BS *et al.* Diagnostic laparoscopy for patients with potentially resectable pancreatic

adenocarcinoma: is it cost-effective in the current era? *J. Gastrointest. Surg.* 2008; **12**: 1177–1184.

95 Ferrone CR, Haas B, Tang L *et al.* The influence of positive peritoneal cytology on survival in patients with pancreatic adenocarcinoma. *J. Gastrointest. Surg.* 2006; **10**: 1347–1353.

96 Contreras CM, Stanelle EJ, Mansour J *et al.* Staging laparoscopy enhances the detection of occult metastases in patients with pancreatic adenocarcinoma. *J. Surg. Oncol.* 2009; **100**: 663–669.

97 Mayo SC, Austin DF, Sheppard BC *et al.* Evolving preoperative evaluation of patients with pancreatic cancer: does laparoscopy have a role in the current era? *J. Am. Coll. Surg.* 2009; **208**: 87–95.

98 Yokoyama Y, Nimura Y, Nagino M. Advances in the treatment of pancreatic cancer: limitations of surgery and evaluation of new therapeutic strategies. *Surg. Today* 2009; **39**: 466–475.

99 O'Connell JB, Maggard MA, Manunga J Jr *et al.* Survival after resection of ampullary carcinoma: a national population-based study. *Ann. Surg. Oncol.* 2008; **15**: 1820–1827.

100 Seyama Y, Makuuchi M. Current surgical treatment for bile duct cancer. *World J. Gastroenterol.* 2007; **13**: 1505–1515.

101 Tran KT, Smeenk HG, van Eijck CH *et al.* Pylorus preserving pancreaticoduodenectomy versus standard Whipple procedure: a prospective, randomized, multicenter analysis of 170 patients with pancreatic and periampullary tumors. *Ann. Surg.* 2004; **240**: 738–745.

102 Seiler CA, Wagner M, Bachmann T *et al.* Randomized clinical trial of pylorus-preserving duodenopancreatectomy versus classical Whipple resection-long term results. *Br. J. Surg.* 2005; **92**: 547–556.

103 Wente MN, Shrikhande SV, Muller MW *et al.* Pancreaticojejunostomy versus pancreaticogastrostomy: systematic review and meta-analysis. *Am. J. Surg.* 2007; **193**: 171–183.

104 Bassi C, Falconi M, Molinari E *et al.* Reconstruction by pancreaticojejunostomy versus pancreaticogastrostomy following pancreatectomy: results of a comparative study. *Ann. Surg.* 2005; **242**: 767–771.

105 Farnell MB, Aranha GV, Nimura Y *et al.* The role of extended lymphadenectomy for adenocarcinoma of the head of the pancreas: strength of the evidence. *J. Gastrointest. Surg.* 2008; **12**: 651–656.

106 Yekebas EF, Bogoevski D, Cataldegirmen G *et al.* En bloc vascular resection for locally advanced pancreatic malignancies infiltrating major blood vessels: perioperative outcome and long-term survival in 136 patients. *Ann. Surg.* 2008; **247**: 300–309.

107 Tseng JF, Raut CP, Lee JE *et al.* Pancreaticoduodenectomy with vascular resection: margin status and survival duration. *J. Gastrointest. Surg.* 2004; **8**: 935–949.

108 Dillhoff M, Yates R, Wall K *et al.* Intraoperative assessment of pancreatic neck margin at the time of pancreaticoduodenectomy increases likelihood of margin-negative resec-tion in patients with pancreatic cancer. *J. Gastrointest. Surg.* 2009; **13**: 825–830.

109 Wagner M, Redaelli C, Lietz M *et al.* Curative resection is the single most important factor determining outcome in patients with pancreatic adenocarcinoma. *Br. J. Surg.* 2004; **91**: 586–594.

110 Raut CP, Tseng JF, Sun CC *et al.* Impact of resection status on pattern of failure and survival after pancreaticoduodenectomy for pancreatic adenocarcinoma. *Ann. Surg.* 2007; **246**: 52–60.

111 Eppsteiner RW, Csikesz NG, McPhee JT *et al.* Surgeon volume impacts hospital mortality for pancreatic resection. *Ann. Surg.* 2009; **249**: 635–640.

112 Rudloff U, Maker AV, Brennan MF *et al.* Randomized clinical trials in pancreatic adenocarcinoma. *Surg. Oncol. Clin. North Am.* 2010; **19**: 115–150.

113 Taylor MC, McLeod RS, Langer B. Biliary stenting versus bypass surgery for the palliation of malignant distal bile duct obstruction: a meta-analysis. *Liver Transpl.* 2000; **6**: 302–308.

114 Sanders M, Papachristou GI, McGrath KM *et al.* Endoscopic palliation of pancreatic cancer. *Gastroenterol. Clin. North Am.* 2007; **36**: 455–476, xi.

115 van Delden OM, Lameris JS. Percutaneous drainage and stenting for palliation of malignant bile duct obstruction. *Eur. Radiol.* 2008; **18**: 448–456.

116 Moss AC, Morris E, Leyden J *et al.* Malignant distal biliary obstruction: a systematic review and meta-analysis of endoscopic and surgical bypass results. *Cancer Treat. Rev.* 2007; **33**: 213–221.

117 Wong GY, Schroeder DR, Carns PE *et al.* Effect of neurolytic celiac plexus block on pain relief, quality of life, and survival in patients with unresectable pancreatic cancer: a randomized controlled trial. *JAMA* 2004; **291**: 1092–1099.

118 Levy MJ, Wiersema MJ. EUS-guided celiac plexus neurolysis and celiac plexus block. *Gastrointest. Endosc.* 2003; **57**: 923–930.

119 Yip D, Karapetis C, Strickland A *et al.* Chemotherapy and radiotherapy for inoperable advanced pancreatic cancer. *Cochrane Database Syst. Rev.* 2006; **3**: CD002093.

120 Moore MJ, Goldstein D, Hamm J *et al.* Erlotinib plus gemcitabine compared with gemcitabine alone in patients with advanced pancreatic cancer: a phase III trial of the National Cancer Institute of Canada Clinical Trials Group. *J. Clin. Oncol.* 2007; **25**: 1960–1966.

121 Poon RT, Fan ST. Opinions and commentary on treating pancreatic cancer. *Surg. Clin. North Am.* 2001; **81**: 625–636.

122 House MG, Gonen M, Jarnagin WR *et al.* Prognostic significance of pathologic nodal status in patients with resected pancreatic cancer. *J. Gastrointest. Surg.* 2007; **11**: 1549–1555.

123 Veillette G, Castillo CF. Distal biliary malignancy. *Surg. Clin. North Am.* 2008; **88**: 1429–1447, xi.

124 Hurtuk MG, Devata S, Brown KM *et al.* Should all patients with duodenal adenocarcinoma be considered for aggressive surgical resection? *Am. J. Surg.* 2007; **193**: 319–324.

CHAPTER 14
Cysts and Congenital Biliary Abnormalities

Giorgina Mieli-Vergani & Nedim Hadžić
King's College London School of Medicine, King's College Hospital, London, UK

Learning points

- Fibropolycystic liver diseases are heterogeneous, overlapping conditions in which liver cystic lesions are often associated with renal abnormalities.

- There is a wide spectrum of polycystic disease (differing in age of presentation, predominantly renal or liver pathology) based on whether inheritance is autosomal recessive or dominant.

- Congenital hepatic fibrosis (CHF) is mainly diagnosed in childhood or adolescence, with features of portal hypertension or with the incidental finding of isolated firm hepatomegaly. Often there is associated renal pathology.

- Caroli's disease is characterized by congenital, segmental, saccular dilatations of the intrahepatic bile ducts without other hepatic abnormalities. When associated with CHF, it is called Caroli's syndrome.

- Recurrent cholangitis is a serious complication of autosomal recessive polycystic kidney disease, Caroli's disease and CHF, leading to deteriorating liver damage and liver failure.

Cystic lesions of the liver and bile ducts are increasingly being diagnosed because of improved imaging techniques. They comprise several different conditions, some hereditary, some sporadic, some presenting mainly in childhood, others typically in adult life. Liver and bile duct cystic lesions may overlap (Fig. 14.1). According to the underlying pathology, clinical symptoms are variable and encompass those of recurrent jaundice, of a space-occupying lesion, of portal hypertension and of cholangitis (Fig. 14.2).

Fibropolycystic diseases

Fibropolycystic diseases of the liver comprise a heterogeneous group of genetic disorders in which segmental dilatations of the intrahepatic bile ducts are associated with fibrosis. Although classified into specific conditions, there is much overlap with a varied contribution of microscopic and/or macroscopic cystic lesions often associated with fibrocystic anomalies in the kidneys. The severity of the renal lesions may overshadow the liver disease, as in the early presentation of autosomal recessive polycystic kidney disease. Conversely, portal hypertension with preserved liver function may dominate a delayed clinical presentation, as in congenital hepatic fibrosis. Cholangitis may develop, especially when the cysts communicate with the biliary system. Malignant change may be a complication.

Embryologically, the hepatobiliary abnormalities are thought to stem from ductal plate maldevelopment in different parts of the biliary tree [1,2].

The ductal plate is a sleeve of epithelium, one and then two cells thick, which forms in the mesenchyme surrounding portal vein branches from bipotential liver progenitor cells—that is cells that may form either hepatocytes or bile duct epithelium. During the development of the liver and biliary system, ductal plates are remodelled into mature tubular ducts which eventually form (in descending size interhepatically from the hilum) hepatic ducts, segmental ducts, area ducts, interlobular ducts and the smallest bile duct branches. Since the various segments of the intrahepatic duct system develop successively throughout fetal life, it is likely that the timing of the inherited malfunction will determine the type and extent of ductal injury [3].

Ductal plate malformation during embryogenesis may also account for a subgroup of biliary atresia, though in most cases this condition is due to necroinflammatory destruction and fibrous obliteration of normally formed extrahepatic bile ducts.

The various types of fibrocystic disease will be described under separate headings (Table 14.1). This classification is based on the dominant clinicopathological features at presentation. However, the different entities are part of a spectrum and may coexist in various

Sherlock's Diseases of the Liver and Biliary System, Twelfth Edition. Edited by James S. Dooley, Anna S.F. Lok, Andrew K. Burroughs, E. Jenny Heathcote.
© 2011 by Blackwell Publishing Ltd. Published 2011 by Blackwell Publishing Ltd.

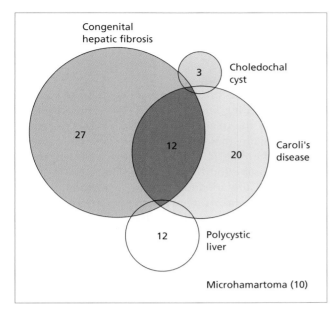

Fig. 14.1. Venn diagram showing one series of 51 patients in which many had more than one fibropolycystic disease. The combination of congenital hepatic fibrosis and Caroli's disease was most striking. Microhamartomas, although reported in only 10 patients in this series, are common [53].

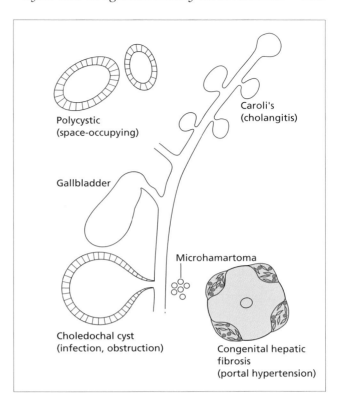

Fig. 14.2. Fibropolycystic disease: spectrum of pathology.

Table 14.1. Hereditary fibrocystic diseases of the liver: clinical presentation and associated renal disorders

Liver disease/ lesion	Age at presentation	Mode of presentation	Associated renal disorder
DPM (CHF) (histological change)	Neonates/ infants	Abdominal distension Renal failure, hypertension Respiratory distress	ARPKD
CHF	Adolescents > children > adults	Portal hypertension ± recurrent cholangitis Late-onset renal failure	ARPKD nephronophthisis medullary sponge kidney
Caroli's syndrome	Adults > adolescents	Recurrent cholangitis Portal hypertension	ARPKD tubular ectasia
Caroli's disease	Any age	Recurrent cholangitis	ARPKD
von Meyenburg complexes	Any age (incidental)	Incidental finding	Unknown
Polycystic liver disease	Adults	Abdominal mass Chronic renal failure	? None ADPKD

DPM, ductal plate malformation; CHF, congenital hepatic fibrosis; ARPKD, autosomal recessive polycystic kidney disease; ADPKD, autosomal dominant polycystic kidney disease.

combinations [3]. In addition to the influence of the genetic mutations identified so far, environmental factors, in particular superimposed infection, may modulate the disease process. Moreover, the natural history of these disorders has been modified by improved treatment such as renal transplantation and successful management of portal hypertension. These enable patients to live longer but with liver complications or late renal failure.

Autosomal recessive polycystic kidney disease

Autosomal recessive polycystic kidney disease (ARPKD) has an estimated incidence of 1/10000 live births and comprises a spectrum of clinical and histopathological manifestations, the constant features being ductal plate malformation of the intrahepatic bile ducts and fusiform dilatation of renal tubules.

The gene for ARPKD, called polycystic kidney and hepatic disease-1 (*PKHD1*), has been mapped to chromosome 6 (6p21.1) [4]. It is a large gene (67 exons) encoding the protein fibrocystin [5,6]. This is expressed in renal collecting ducts and bile ducts, but its biological function is unknown [5,6]. More than 100 mutations are known. Most renal patients are compound heterozygotes. There is no clear genotype/phenotype relationship for predominant renal or hepatic involvement. Mutations leading to truncated transcripts have been described with a severe renal, often lethal, phenotype [7].

Clinical features

The severity of the renal lesion determines the mode of presentation. In the perinatal or infantile period, rapidly progressive renal failure is associated with large symmetrical renal masses due to radially orientated and fusiform corticomedullary cysts. Infants may be stillborn or die in early infancy from renal failure, fluid retention or bronchopneumonia. The liver lesion is usually clinically silent. The affected children may have cardiac anomalies (ventricular septal defect, pulmonary valve stenosis) and dysmorphic features ('Potter face'—squashed nose, micrognathia, large low-set ears, epicanthal folds), possibly secondary to severe hydramnios. Cases with a lesser degree of renal involvement present later in life—late childhood or juvenile forms—with progressive renal failure and/or portal hypertension. The condition then merges with congenital hepatic fibrosis (CHF). Often patients are referred to the hepatologist while on chronic renal dialysis because of complications of portal hypertension, such as splenomegaly with hypersplenism and bleeding varices, and/or cholangitis [8,9].

Pathology

Histologically, the liver lesion in ARPKD ranges from a persistent hyperplastic ductal plate with scanty portal fibrosis to marked excess of ductular structures at the periphery of the fibrotic portal tracts. At an early stage, portal fibrosis resembles primitive mesenchyme; later the collagen is more mature and the lesion is indistinguishable from CHF. There are no visible cysts in the liver, which may be enlarged and firm, showing a fine reticular pattern of fibrosis [10].

Imaging

Plain abdomen X-ray, ultrasound and intravenous pyelogram are the most useful investigations in infancy.

Bile duct abnormalities can be diagnosed by magnetic resonance cholangiopancreatography (MRCP) [11].

Treatment

For those patients presenting in childhood with gastrointestinal bleeding, endoscopic sclerotherapy or banding of varices is the treatment of choice. Failure to control bleeding with these techniques necessitates portosystemic shunting [12]. Combined liver–kidney transplant is advisable for children with established end-stage renal failure and advanced chronic liver disease, since immunosuppression after isolated renal transplant may increase the frequency cholangitis with worsening liver function.

Adult polycystic disease

In adult polycystic disease, liver cysts are probably developmental and are frequently associated with autosomal dominant polycystic kidney disease (PKD). The latter is better understood than the liver disease. At least three different genes appear to be involved.

PKD-1 on chromosome 16p13.3 expresses polycystin 1 which is thought to have a role in epithelial cell differentiation and maturation, and in cell–cell interactions [13,14]. Loss of function of this protein may be one prerequisite for cyst formation but a further somatic event is thought necessary.

PKD-2 on chromosome 4q21–23 expresses polycystin 2. Polycystin 1 and 2 interact through their C-terminal cytoplasmic tails suggesting that they function together through a common signalling pathway. Polycystic kidney disease type 2 is clinically milder than type 1.

Polycystic liver disease is most often associated with autosomal dominant polycystic kidney disease. However, polycystic liver may be an isolated finding and is genetically linked to chromosome 19p13.2–13.1 [15].

The molecular mechanism responsible for cyst formation is not clear. They may arise from failure of supernumerary intrahepatic bile ducts within the hepatic embryonic anlage to involute when the biliary system forms. When the original segment of blind bile ducts is replaced by a second generation of highly active proliferating ducts, redundant ducts may become distorted and form cysts. The second-generation bile ducts are normal so there is no biliary dysfunction.

Pathology

Depending on the number and size of cysts, the liver may be normal or greatly enlarged. Cysts may be scattered diffusely or restricted to one lobe, usually the left. The outer surface may be considerably deformed. A cyst may vary in size from a pin's head to a child's head, the

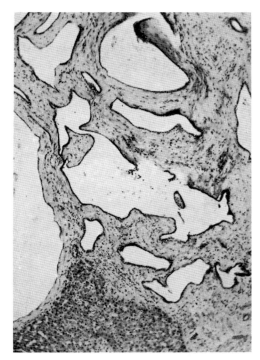

Fig. 14.3. Polycystic disease of the liver. The cysts vary in size and are lined by flattened epithelium. (H & E, ×63.)

largest having a capacity of over 1 litre. They are rarely greater than 10 cm in diameter. The larger ones are probably formed by rupture of septa between adjacent cysts, and the cut liver may display a honeycomb appearance. The cavities are thin walled and contain clear or brown fluid due to altered blood. They never contain bile because they are not in continuity with the biliary tract. They may be complicated by haemorrhage or infection.

Histologically the lobular architecture is unchanged and liver cells are normal. The cystic areas are related to the bile ducts and to biliary microhamartomas in the portal areas. They are surrounded by a fibrous tissue capsule and lined by columnar or cuboidal epithelium (Fig. 14.3).

Frequently, there is cystic disease of other organs, including kidneys, spleen, pancreas, ovary and lungs. About half the patients with polycystic disease of the liver have polycystic kidneys. The majority (50–88%) of patients with polycystic kidneys have a polycystic liver [16]. The prevalence of hepatic cysts increases with age, being approximately 20% in the third decade rising to 75% in the seventh decade.

Cyst fluid

Fluid has been obtained using needle aspiration under ultrasound guidance [17]. The constituents and response to secretin support the concept that cyst fluid is formed by functioning bile duct epithelium lining the cysts.

Clinical features

In many patients the liver lesion is diagnosed incidentally during scanning or at autopsy. Sometimes the patient presents with some other disease or with polycystic kidneys.

Patients with symptoms and signs are usually in the fourth or fifth decade. The patient complains of abdominal distension and dull abdominal pain. Pressure on the stomach and duodenum causes epigastric discomfort, nausea, flatulence and occasional vomiting. Acute pain may be due to rupture of, or haemorrhage into, a cyst.

Cysts tend to be larger in women who have been pregnant [18]. Hormone replacement therapy is associated with an approximate 5% enlargement of the liver over a year [19]. There is no increase in symptoms. On the basis of these data hormone replacement therapy is not withheld when clinically indicated [19].

Ascites, obstructive jaundice and hepatic venous outflow obstruction [20] are rare.

On examination the liver may be impalpable or so large that it seems to fill the whole abdomen. The edge is firm and nodules can be palpated. There may be difficulty in distinguishing cysts from other types of liver nodule. The spleen is not enlarged.

Bilaterally enlarged irregular kidneys may suggest associated renal cysts which may be symptomatic.

Hepatic fumction is excellent because the liver cells are preserved. Serum alkaline phosphatase and γ-glutamyl transpeptidase may be increased but bilirubin is normal.

The serum carbohydrate antigen CA 19-9 may be elevated, and levels correlate with high levels found in cyst fluid and polycystic liver volume [21]. Serum levels increase with liver cyst infection in kidney transplant recipients [22].

Portal venous obstruction rarely may result in oesophageal varices which bleed [23].

Imaging

Ultrasound is the most satisfactory method of diagnosis (Fig. 14.4). CT scanning (Fig. 14.5) is also useful in symptomatic patients with multiple cysts to show how much normal liver remains. This helps with planning surgical options.

Differential diagnosis

Polycystic liver should be suspected in an apparently well person, often over 30 years of age, with nodular hepatomegaly, but no evidence of hepatic dysfunction, associated with polycystic kidney or a positive family history.

Polycystic liver may be confused with *hydatid disease* (Chapter 32).

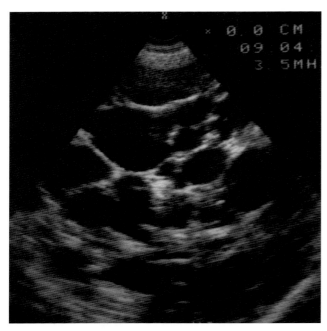

Fig. 14.4. Adult polycystic liver: ultrasound shows numerous echo-free space-occupying lesions.

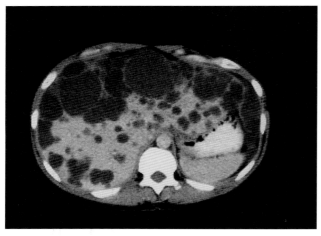

Fig. 14.5. CT scan (contrast enhanced) showing a polycystic liver.

Metastases are accompanied by malaise, weight loss, rapid increase in size of the liver, and, possibly, evidence of a primary neoplasm.

Cirrhosis may be accompanied by signs of hepatocellular disease and the spleen is usually enlarged.

Prognosis and treatment

Polycystic disease of the liver is compatible with long life.

The prognosis is determined by the extent of associated renal cystic disease. Carcinoma is very rare. Surgery is rarely necessary and aspiration under ultrasound

control is easy and effective in controlling acute symptoms. However, the fluid returns.

In clinical trials somatostatin analogues do reduce liver size (by 3–6%) [24,25] and may reduce perception of pain. This approach holds promise for selected patients but is not yet in clinical practice outside trials.

There are several surgical techniques, the choice depending upon the extent of disease [26]. Patients with a limited number of large cysts may be treated by fenestration which can be performed laparoscopically [27]. Where there is localized involvement of liver parenchyma by multiple medium-sized cysts but with adjacent large areas of normal parenchyma shown by CT, operative fenestration with or without hepatic resection produces symptomatic improvement in most cases [28,29]. In patients with massive diffuse involvement of the majority of liver parenchyma by all sizes of liver cysts with only a small amount of normal parenchyma between them, fenestration may be useful but carries a high morbidity and mortality. In patients with severe limitation of daily activity and failed previous treatment, liver transplantation can be done (combined with kidney transplantation if necessary) and has a 1-year survival of 89% [30].

Successful liver transplantation has been reported using a donor liver with polycystic change [31].

Congenital hepatic fibrosis

CHF consists histologically of broad, densely collagenous fibrous bands surrounding otherwise normal hepatic lobules (Fig. 14.6). The bands contain large numbers of microscopic, well-formed bile ducts (Fig. 14.7), some containing bile. Arterial branches are normal or hypoplastic, while the veins appear reduced in size. Inflammatory changes are not seen. It may be associated with congenital dilatation of the intrahepatic bile ducts (Caroli's syndrome).

The disease appears both sporadically and in a familial form. In the latter, the mode of inheritance is autosomal recessive. A ductal plate malformation of interlobular bile ducts has been suggested as the pathogenetic mechanism [1].

Portal hypertension is common. Occasionally, this may be due to defects in the main portal veins. More often it is caused by hypoplasia or fibrous compression of portal vein radicles in the fibrous bands surrounding the nodules.

Associated renal conditions include renal dysplasia, adult-type polycystic kidneys [32] and nephronophthisis (medullary cystic disease).

Clinical features

CHF is diagnosed predominantly in children and adolescents, rarely as an isolated entity, more often in asso-

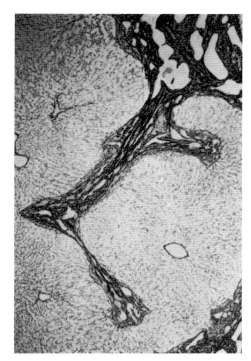

Fig. 14.6. Congenital hepatic fibrosis. Broad bands of fibrous tissue containing bile ducts separate and surround liver lobules. (Silver impregnation, ×36.)

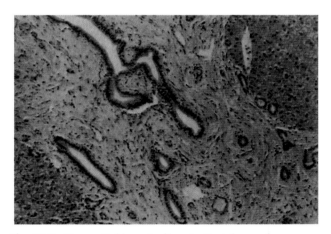

Fig. 14.7. Congenital hepatic fibrosis. Portal area shows dense mature fibrous tissue with a number of abnormal bile ducts. (H & E, ×40.)

ciation with ARPKD, or less frequently with renal medullary cystic lesions, in particular nephronophthisis and medullary sponge kidneys. The clinical presentation is with signs of portal hypertension (splenomegaly with hypersplenism or variceal haemorrhage) or incidental finding of isolated firm hepatomegaly (Fig. 14.8).

The age at presentation is typically between 5 and 13 years [33]. Sexes are equally affected.

CHF is often misdiagnosed as cirrhosis. An important clue is that hepatocellular function remains essentially

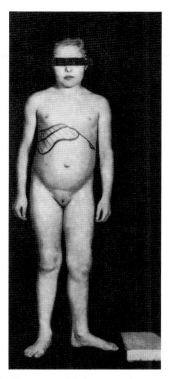

Fig. 14.8. Girl of 8 years with hepatosplenomegaly discovered at routine examination. Liver biopsy showed congenital hepatic fibrosis. Note normal development.

normal. A cholangitic form is recognized with subclinical or symptomatic episodes of recurrent cholangitis requiring exclusion of an associated Caroli's disease. Rarely, recurrent cholangitis may progress to a true biliary cirrhosis with progressive impairment of the liver function. In a few cases the disease manifests in adulthood (latent form) [3].

CHF has been reported in association with familial congenital heart disease [34], pulmonary arteriovenous fistulae [35] and multiple gastric ulcers [36]. A number of malformation syndromes are characterized by hepatic histological changes resembling those of CHF (Table 14.2).

Carcinoma, both hepatocellular and cholangiocarcinoma, may be a complication [45,46] as may adenomatous hyperplasia [47].

CHF is a feature of the rare disorder carbohydrate-deficient glycoprotein syndrome type Ib (CDGS 1b) [48], other features including cyclical vomiting, protein-losing enteropathy and prothrombotic tendency. Abnormal glycosylation is caused by phosphomannose isomerase deficiency, which can be demonstrated by transferrin isoelectric focusing (IEF). Regular mannose supplements bypass the enzymatic pathway, correct the biochemical abnormality and improve the clinical symptoms [49]. Despite difficulties in interpreting a link between the biochemical defect in CDGS 1b and the histological

Table 14.2. Malformation syndromes reported with liver histological changes resembling those of congenital hepatic fibrosis

Meckel's syndrome: encephalocoele, polydactyly and cystic kidneys [37]
Ivemark's syndrome: dysplasia of the pancreas, liver and kidneys, together with cysts in the pancreas and liver in some cases [38,39]
Ellis van Creveld syndrome or chondroectodermal dysplasia [40]
Nephronophthisis–congenital hepatic fibrosis syndrome with retinal lesions, mental retardation, cerebellar hypoplasia and osseous abnormalities [41]
Jeune syndrome: skeletal dysplasia, pulmonary hypoplasia and retinal lesions [42,43]
Laurence–Moon–Biedl syndrome [44]

features of CHF, screening all patients with CHF for glycosylation defect by transferrin IEF appears justified.

Investigations

Serum protein, bilirubin and transaminase levels are usually normal, while serum alkaline phosphatase values are occasionally increased.

Liver biopsy is essential for diagnosis, but because of the tough consistency of the liver it may be difficult. Liver histology shows bridging fibrous septa, which sharply delineate areas of parenchyma with a normal architecture. The fibrous bands contain numerous ductular structures similar to those seen in infants with ARPKD and it is arguable whether CHF is simply a variant of ARPKD. Some are dilated and may contain bile. The portal vein branches are inconspicuous or reduced to numerous thin radicles. Focal cholangiolitis and copper-associated protein deposition may lead to a misleading diagnosis of cirrhosis.

Ultrasound shows very bright areas of echogenicity due to the dense bands of fibrous tissue. Direct cholangiography in patients with congenital hepatic fibrosis alone shows tapered intrahepatic radicals suggesting fibrosis. MR cholangiography may show duct abnormalities including biliary cysts in some patients. The association of these with CHF has been termed Caroli's syndrome. Choledochal cysts may also occasionally be seen [50].

Portal venography reveals the collateral circulation and a normal or distorted intrahepatic portal tree.

Ultrasound, CT, MRI and *intravenous pyelography* may show cystic renal changes or medullary sponge kidney.

Treatment and prognosis

The prognosis of CHF is considerably better than that of cirrhosis.

The treatment is that of portal hypertension. Following variceal haemorrhage these patients should be treated by sclerotherapy or banding, but if these modalities fail to control bleeding, they should undergo portosystemic shunting. However, patients with CHF may eventually require renal and/or liver transplantation and the choice of the type of shunting procedure should take this into account. A lienorenal shunt avoids compromising either the vena cava or the portal vein and is therefore recommended. As the patients are non-cirrhotic, encephalopathy does not develop after shunt surgery [33]. In the cholangitic form, prolonged rotating antibiotic therapy my be successful, but the prognosis remains guarded.

Caroli's disease [51]

Caroli's disease is a rare disorder characterized by congenital, segmental, saccular dilatations of the intrahepatic bile ducts without other hepatic histological abnormalities. The dilated ducts connect with the main duct system and are liable to become infected and contain stones (Fig. 14.9). The cystic dilatation of the intrahepatic bile ducts can affect the entire liver or be segmental or lobar [52]. When the disease is associated with CHF it is referred to as Caroli's syndrome [53].

The inheritance of Caroli's disease is uncertain [54]. In contrast, Caroli's syndrome, characterized by an association between Caroli's cysts and CHF, often with fibrocystic renal changes, probably falls within the autosomal recessive polycystic disorder spectrum.

In Caroli's disease, kidney lesions are usually absent, but renal tubular ectasia and larger cysts have been described.

Clinical features

The condition presents at any age, but usually in childhood or early adult life, as abdominal pain, hepatomegaly and fever with Gram-negative septicaemia [55]. Neonatal presentation has also been reported [56]. About 75% of affected individuals are male.

Jaundice is mild or absent but may increase during the episodes of cholangitis. Portal hypertension is absent, unless CHF is associated (Caroli's syndrome). Complications include abscess formation, septicaemia and intrahepatic lithiasis. Development of cholan-

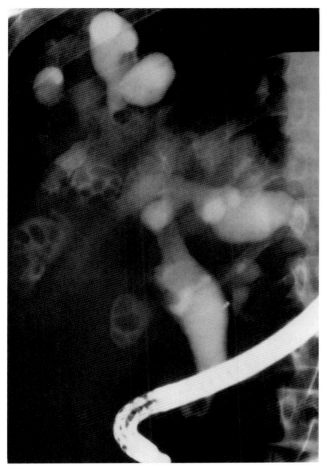

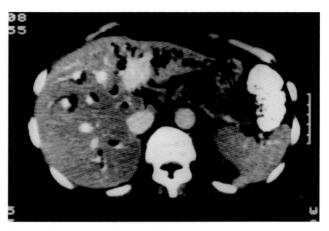

Fig. 14.10. Caroli's disease. CT scan after intravenous contrast shows dilated intrahepatic bile ducts with adjacent enhanced radicles of the portal vein.

Fig. 14.9. Caroli's disease. Endoscopic cholangiography shows bulbous dilatations of the intrahepatic bile ducts, some of which contain multiple gallstones.

giocarcinoma has been reported in about 7% of patients [57]. ARPKD or other forms of renal tubular ectasia are often associated with Caroli's syndrome.

If the biliary system is drained, bile volumes may be high, and flow increased by an infusion of secretin which stimulates ductular secretion. It is likely that the high resting flow arises from the cysts [58].

Imaging

Ultrasound may be helpful as may CT scanning (Fig. 14.10) where portal vein radicles can be seen after enhancement within dilated intrahepatic bile ducts (the 'central dot' sign) [59]. MR cholangiography is diagnostic [60] as is the more invasive endoscopic or percutaneous cholangiography (Fig. 14.9). However, the latter two techniques may introduce sepsis and should be avoided unless therapeutic benefit is clear.

The common bile duct is normal, but the intrahepatic ducts are marked by bulbous dilatations with normal ducts in between. The abnormality may be unilateral

[52]. The appearances contrast with those of primary sclerosing cholangitis where the common bile duct is irregular with strictures and the intrahepatic ducts show irregularities with dilatations.

Treatment and prognosis

Akin to the cholangitic form of CHF, Caroli's disease is managed with aggressive antibiotic therapy. Non-surgical approaches such as percutaneous biliary drainage, extracorporeal shock-wave lythotripsy and transhepatic or endoscopic decompression have been attempted with unconvincing results. Drainage or resection surgery (partial hepatectomy) for recurrent cholangitis have been disappointing except in the rare patients with disease localized to one side of the liver [52,61]. Intrahepatic stones have been successfully treated with ursodeoxycholic acid [62].

The prognosis is generally poor, varying between a mean survival of 9 months [54] to a mortality over 5 years of 20% [55]. Death is related to septicaemia, liver abscess, liver failure and portal hypertension. Episodes of cholangitis, however, can extend over many years.

Liver transplantation may be offered for the diffuse form of the disease affected by uncontrolled, severe, recurrent cholangitis or for uncontrollable portal hypertension secondary to hepatic fibrosis in Caroli's syndrome, though the procedure is risky because of chronic infection.

Death from renal failure is very unusual.

Microhamartoma (von Meyenberg complexes)

These are usually asymptomatic, diagnosed incidentally or found at autopsy. Rarely, they may be associated with

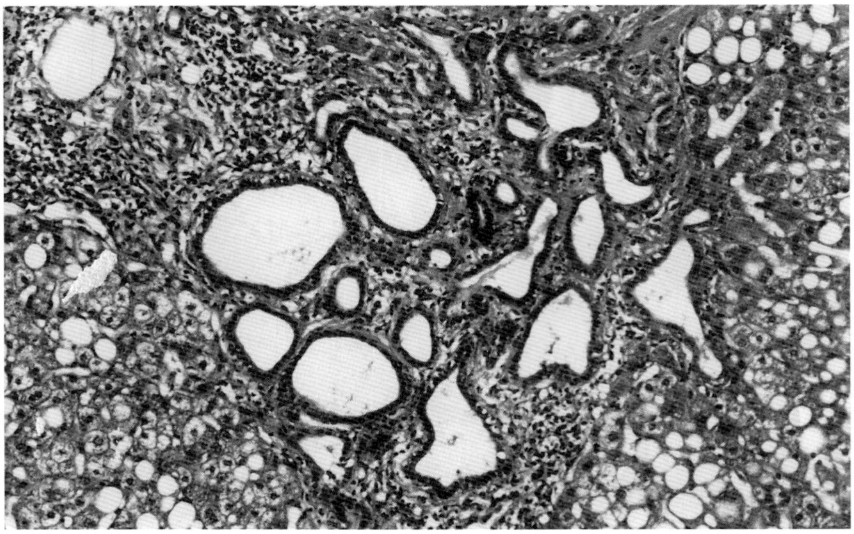

Fig. 14.11. Microhamartoma of the liver. Groups of biliary channels are lined by cuboidal epithelium and are embedded in mature fibrous tissue [53]. (H & E, ×180.)

portal hypertension. Kidneys may show medullary sponge change. Microhamartomas can be associated with polycystic disease.

Histologically, microhamartomas consist of groups of rounded biliary channels, lined by cuboidal epithelium and often containing inspissated bile (Fig. 14.11). These biliary structures are embedded in mature collagenous stroma. They are usually located in, or near, portal tracts. The appearances suggest congenital hepatic fibrosis, but in a localized form.

In a hepatic arteriogram, multiple microhamartomas lead to stretching of the arteries and blushing in the venous phase.

Choledochal cysts

Choledochal cysts are congenital anomalies characterized by cystic dilatations of one or more segments of the biliary tree. When the common duct itself is involved, the gallbladder, cystic duct and proximal hepatic ducts are not dilated, in contrast to the pattern of dilatation of the whole biliary tree above an obstructing lesion. Histologically, the cyst wall consists of dense fibrous tissue with little elastic or muscle tissue and often has no epithelial lining.

No unifying pathological process explains all cysts. Some are associated with a long common channel between the pancreatic duct and the bile duct which predisposes to the reflux of pancreatic enzymes [63]. Many patients, however, do not have this anomaly. There may be infective and molecular genetic factors. Reovirus RNA was detected in tissue taken from eight out of nine infants and children with choledochal cysts [64]. Immunohistochemical studies in patients with choledochal cysts have shown a high expression of inducible nitric oxide synthase, which has been suggested to participate in mucosal hyperplasia and carcinogenesis in choledochal cysts secondary to regurgitation of pancreatic enzymes [65]. Other postulated mechanisms include a congenital weakness of the muscle wall, congenital inflammation or valvular obstruction within the ampulla of Vater, or excessive proliferation of the epithelial cells of the primitive choledochus leading to biliary dilatation when canalization occurs [66].

Classification

Choledochal cysts are classified as follows (Fig. 14.12) [67,68].

Type I: cystic (Ia), segmental (Ib) or fusiform (Ic) dilatation of the extrahepatic bile duct. A further group (Id) has been suggested with multiple extrahepatic cysts. Differentiation between the fusiform type and dilatation of the bile duct secondary to obstruction is based on the absence of a previous history of gallstones or biliary surgery, a common bile duct diameter greater than 30 mm, and the presence of an anomalous bile duct junction shown on cholangiography [67].

Type II: the cyst forms a diverticulum from the extrahepatic bile duct.

Type III: there is cystic dilatation (choledochocele) of the distal common bile duct lying mostly within the duodenal wall.

Type IV: this comprises type I anatomy together with intrahepatic bile duct cysts. It has been proposed that IVa, IVb and IVc describe this picture (type I) with cystic, segmental or fusiform change of the extrahepatic biliary tree [67].

When used, type V denotes Caroli's disease.

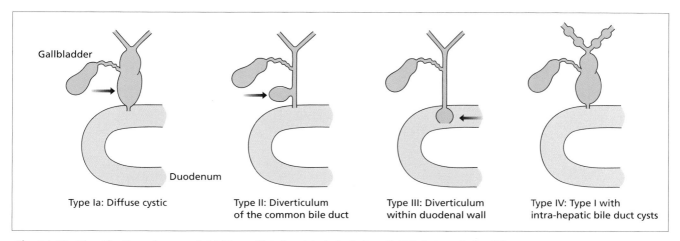

Fig. 14.12. Classification of congenital biliary dilatation (choledochal cyst) (IVb is type I plus III).

The commonest types are I and IV [67,68]. Whether choledochocele (type III) should be classified as a choledochal cyst has been questioned [69].

Rarely, a solitary cystic dilatation of an intrahepatic bile duct is seen [70].

The type I lesion presents as a partially retroperitoneal, cystic tumour varying from 2 to 3 cm in size, to a capacity of 8 litre. The cyst contains thin, dark brown fluid. It is sterile but may become secondarily infected. The cyst can burst.

Biliary cirrhosis is a late complication. Choledochal cysts may obstruct the portal vein leading to portal hypertension. Malignant tumours in the cyst or bile ducts may develop [68].

Clinical features

The infantile form presents as prolonged cholestasis and is the most common surgically correctable cause of jaundice in the neonatal period after biliary atresia. If not diagnosed appropriately, it can lead to biliary cirrhosis and portal hypertension. The distended cyst can directly occlude the portal vein, causing portal hypertension. Spontaneous perforation of the choledochal cyst is common and can result in biliary peritonitis. The cause of the perforation is thought to be biliary epithelial irritation as a result of reflux of pancreatic juice through the common channel rather than increase in ductal pressure [71]. Prenatal diagnosis of choledocal cyst warrants referral to a specialized paediatric hepatology centre, since it could be related to biliary atresia [72].

Later in life, classical symptoms are jaundice, pain and an abdominal tumour. The jaundice is intermittent, of cholestatic type and associated with fever. The pain is colicky and mainly experienced in the right upper abdomen. The tumour is cystic and in the right upper quadrant of the abdomen. It characteristically varies in size and in tenseness. Care must be taken during palpation to avoid rupturing the cyst. Children are more likely to have two or more of this 'classical' triad than adults (82 vs. 25%) [68]. Although formerly regarded as a childhood disease, the diagnosis is now more often made in adult life. One-quarter of individuals affected present with symptoms and signs of pancreatitis [68].

The frequency of choledochal cysts is about 1 in 15000 live births in Western countries and is as high as 1 in 1000 live births in Japan [71]. There is a marked female predominance (4:1), regardless of racial origin.

Choledochal cysts may rarely be associated with congenital hepatic fibrosis or Caroli's disease. Anomalous pancreaticobiliary drainage is important, particularly if the duct junction is right-angular or acute.

Complications include recurrent ascending cholangitis, portal vein thrombosis, hepatic abscess, carcinoma of the cyst wall and gallstones.

Imaging

Plain X-ray of the abdomen may show a soft-tissue mass. The diagnosis of choledochal cyst is characteristically first made on ultrasound. HIDA scanning and CT can show the cystic lesion but MRCP has become the first choice imaging technique for defining these cysts (Fig. 14.13) [73,74]. It does not, however, remove the need for other approaches including endoscopic retrograde or percutaneous cholangiopancreatography in selected patients [73].

Treatment

Because of the risk of subsequent adenocarcinoma or squamous cell carcinoma, radical excision is the method

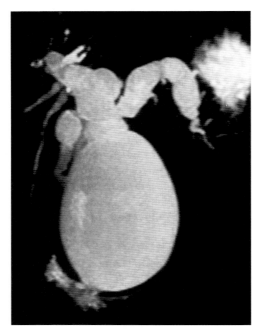

Fig. 14.13. MR cholangiogram in a 40-year-old woman with a type Ia choledochal cyst. The patient presented with acute pancreatitis.

of choice [68,75]. Biliary tract continuity is maintained by hepaticojejunostomy with Roux-en-Y anastomosis.

Anastomosis of the cyst to the intestinal tract without excision is simpler but postoperative cholangitis and subsequent biliary stricturing and stone formation are frequent. The risk of carcinoma remains, perhaps related to dysplasia and metaplasia of the epithelium [76].

For type III cysts, endoscopic sphincterotomy or unroofing of the cyst can give adequate drainage. Occasionally in type IVa and V cysts the intrahepatic involvement is so extensive that hepatectomy and liver transplantation become necessary.

Solitary non-parasitic liver cyst

This is being diagnosed more often due to the increased use of liver scanning. It is probably a variant of polycystic disease.

The lining wall has partitions, which suggest an origin from conglomerate polycystic disease. The fibrous capsule contains aberrant bile ducts and blood vessels. The contents vary from colourless to brown altered blood. The tension is low in contrast to the high pressure of hydatid cysts.

Symptoms are rare and related to abdominal distension, or pressure effects on adjacent organs including the bile ducts, causing intermittent jaundice. The patient should be reassured.

Symptoms follow rupture or haemorrhage into the cyst. These events are extremely rare. Surgical excision is indicated only for complications.

Other cysts

These are all very rare, small and superficial. Their contents vary with the cause. Bile cysts may follow prolonged extrahepatic biliary obstruction of all types.

Blood cysts follow haemorrhage into a simple cyst. They can also follow trauma to the liver. Small cystic spaces containing blood may follow needle biopsy.

Lymphatic cysts are due to obstruction or congenital dilatation of liver lymphatics. They are usually on the surface of the liver.

Biliary cystadenoma and cystadenocarcinoma are rare (see Chapter 34). Malignant pseudocysts from degeneration and softening of secondary malignant growths also occur.

Carcinoma secondary to cystic disease

Tumours may arise in association with microhamartomas, congenital hepatic fibrosis, Caroli's disease [57] and choledochal cyst [68]. Carcinoma is rare in association with non-parasitic cysts [77] or polycystic liver disease. Malignant change is more likely where epithelium is exposed to bile.

Congenital anomalies of the biliary tract

The liver and biliary tract develop from a bud-like outpouching of the ventral wall of the primitive foregut just cranial to the yolk sac. Two solid buds of cells form the right and left lobes of the liver while the original elongated diverticulum forms the hepatic and common bile duct. The gallbladder arises as a smaller bud of cells from this same diverticulum. The biliary tract is patent in early intrauterine life but becomes solid later by epithelial proliferation within the lumen. Eventually, revacuolization takes place, starting simultaneously in different parts of the solid gallbladder bud and spreading until the whole system is recanalized. At 5 weeks the ductal communications of gallbladder, cystic duct and hepatic ducts are completed and at 3 months the fetal liver begins to secrete bile.

The majority of the congenital anomalies can be related to alterations in the original budding from the foregut or to failure of vacuolization of the solid gallbladder and bile duct diverticulum (Table 14.3).

These congenital defects are usually of no importance and cannot be related to symptoms. Occasionally bile duct anomalies lead to bile stasis, inflammation and

Table 14.3. Classification of congenital anomalies of the biliary tract

> ***Anomalies of the primitive foregut bud***
> Failure of bud
>   absent bile ducts
>   absent gallbladder
> Accessory buds or splitting of bud
>   accessory gallbladder
>   bilobed gallbladder
>   accessory bile ducts
> Bud migrates to left instead of right
>   left-sided gallbladder
>
> ***Anomalies of vacuolization of the solid biliary bud***
> Defective bile duct vacuolization
> Congenital obliteration of bile ducts
> Congenital obliteration of cystic duct
> Choledochal cyst
> Defective gallbladder vacuolization
>   rudimentary gallbladder
> Fundal diverticulum
> Serosal type of Phrygian cap
> Hour-glass gallbladder
>
> ***Persistent cystohepatic duct***
> Diverticulum of body or neck of gallbladder
>
> ***Persistence of intrahepatic gallbladder***
>
> ***Aberrant folding of gallbladder anlage***
> Retroserosal type of Phrygian cap
>
> ***Accessory peritoneal folds***
> Congenital adhesions
> Floating gallbladder
>
> ***Anomalies of hepatic and cystic arteries***
> Accessory arteries
> Abnormal relation of hepatic artery to cystic duct

gallstones [78]. They are of importance to the radiologist and to the biliary and hepatic transplant surgeon.

Anomalies of the biliary tree and liver may be associated with congenital lesions elsewhere, including cardiac defects, polydactyly and polycystic kidneys. They can also be related to maternal virus infections, such as rubella.

Absence of the gallbladder [79]

This is a rare congenital anomaly. Two types can be recognized.

Type I is the failure of the gallbladder and cystic duct to develop as an outgrowth from the hepatic diverticulum of the foregut. This type is often found with other anomalies of the biliary passages.

Type II is the failure of the gallbladder to vacuolize from its solid state. This is usually associated with atresia of the extrahepatic ducts. The gallbladder is not absent but

rudimentary. This type is therefore found in infants who present the picture of congenital biliary atresia.

Most cases occur in infants with other major congenital anomalies. Adults are usually healthy and without other anomalies. Some have right upper quadrant pain or jaundice. The inability to show the gallbladder on ultrasound may be interpreted as gallbladder disease and lead to surgery. The possibility of agenesis or an ectopic location must be considered. Cholangiography should be diagnostic. Failure to identify the gallbladder at operation is not proof of its absence. The gallbladder may be intrahepatic, buried in extensive adhesions or atrophied following previous cholecystitis.

An intraoperative cholangiogram should be done.

Double gallbladder

Double gallbladder is very rare. In embryonic life, little pockets often arise from the hepatic or common bile ducts. Occasionally these persist and form a second gallbladder having its own cystic duct (Fig. 14.14). This may enter the hepatic substance directly. If the pouch forms from the cystic duct the two gallbladders share a Y-shaped cystic duct.

Double gallbladder can be recognized by imaging. The accessory organ is frequently diseased.

Bilobed gallbladder is an extremely rare congenital anomaly. Embryologically, the single bud forming the gallbladder becomes paired but the primary connection is maintained, thus forming two separate and distinct fundi with a single cystic duct.

The anomaly is of no clinical significance.

Accessory bile ducts

These are rare. The extra duct is usually a subdivision of the right hepatic system and joins the common hepatic duct somewhere between the junction of the main right and left hepatic ducts and the entry of the cystic duct. It may, however, join the cystic duct, the gallbladder or the common bile duct.

Cholecystohepatic ducts are due to persistence of fetal connections between the gallbladder and the liver parenchyma with failure of recanalization of the right and left hepatic ducts. Continuity is maintained by the cystic duct entering a remaining hepatic duct or common hepatic duct or the duodenum directly.

Accessory ducts are of importance to the biliary and transplant surgeon as they may be inadvertently ligated or cut with resultant biliary stricture or fistula.

Left-sided gallbladder

In this rare anomaly the gallbladder lies under the left lobe of the liver, to the left of the falciform ligament.

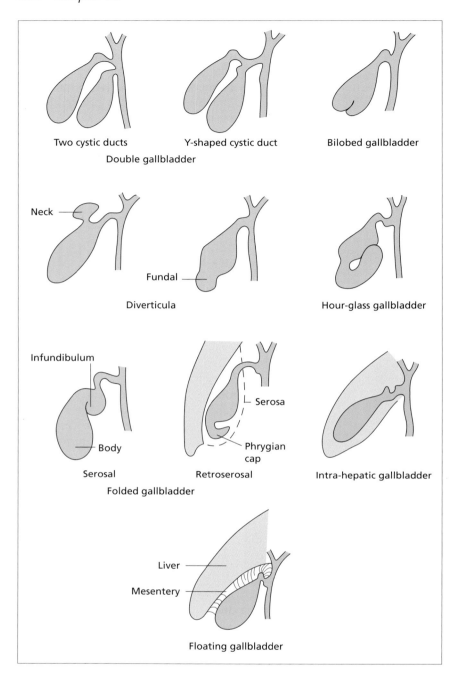

Two cystic ducts   Y-shaped cystic duct   Bilobed gallbladder

Double gallbladder

Neck

Fundal

Diverticula

Hour-glass gallbladder

Infundibulum

Serosa

Body

Phrygian cap

Serosal   Retroserosal   Intra-hepatic gallbladder

Folded gallbladder

Liver

Mesentery

Floating gallbladder

Fig. 14.14. Congenital anomalies of the gallbladder.

This may be caused by the gallbladder migrating to a position under the left lobe of the liver (to the left of the round ligament). The path of the cystic duct is normal. Alternatively, a second gallbladder may develop directly from the left hepatic duct with failure of development or regression of the normal structure on the right side. A left-sided gallbladder formed in this way is of little clinical significance.

In some cases, however, a left-sided gallbladder may be described as such because of its relationship to the round ligament ('a right-sided round ligament'). In these cases the gallbladder is in its normal site. The right-sided round ligament anomaly is important because it is associated with abnormal intrahepatic portal venous branching. This is important to recognize when performing hepatectomy [80].

Rokitansky–Aschoff sinuses of the gallbladder

These consist of hernia-like protrusions of the gallbladder mucosa through the muscular layer (intramural diverticulosis). Although potentially congenital, they are particularly prominent with chronic cholecystitis when intraluminal pressure rises. They may be seen in an oral cholecystogram as a halo-like stippling surrounding the gallbladder.

Folded gallbladder

The gallbladder is deformed so that the fundus appears folded 'bent down to the breaking point after the manner of a *Phrygian cap*'. A Phrygian cap is a conical cap or bonnet, with the peak bent or turned over in front, worn by the ancient Phrygians, and identified with the Cap of Liberty (*Oxford English Dictionary*).

Two varieties are recognized:
1 *Kinking between body and fundus* (*retroserosal Phrygian cap*) (Fig. 14.14). This is due to aberrant folding of the gallbladder within the embryonic fossa.
2 *Kinking between body and infundibulum* (*serosal Phrygian cap*) (Fig. 14.14). This is due to aberrant folding of the fossa itself in the early stages of development. The bend in the gallbladder is fixed by development of fetal ligaments, vestigial septa or constrictions of the lumen following delayed vacuolization of the solid epithelial anlage.

These kinked gallbladders empty at a normal rate and are of no clinical significance. The importance lies in the correct interpretation of the gallbladder imaging.

Hour-glass gallbladder (Fig. 14.14). This probably represents an exaggerated form of Phrygian cap, presumably of the serosal type. The constancy of position of the fundus during contraction and the small size of the opening between the two parts indicate that this is probably a fixed, congenital malformation.

Diverticula of the gallbladder and ducts

Diverticula of the gallbladder body and neck may arise from persistent cystohepatic ducts which run in embryonic life between the gallbladder and the liver.

The fundal variety arises from incomplete vacuolization of the solid gallbladder of embryonic life. An incomplete septum pinches off a small cavity at the tip of the gallbladder (Fig. 14.14).

These diverticula are rare and of no clinical significance. The congenital variety should be distinguished from *pseudodiverticula* developing in the diseased gallbladder as a result of partial perforation. The pseudodiverticulum in these cases usually contains a large gallstone.

Intrahepatic gallbladder

The gallbladder is included and buried in hepatic tissue up to the second month of intrauterine life, thereafter assuming an extrahepatic position. In some instances the intrahepatic condition may persist (Fig. 14.14). The gallbladder is higher than normal and more or less buried but never entirely covered by liver tissue. It is frequently diseased, for the embedded organ has difficulty in contracting and so becomes infected, with subsequent gallstone formation.

Congenital adhesions to the gallbladder

These are very frequent. Developmentally these peritoneal sheets are due to an extension of the anterior mesentery, which forms the lesser omentum. The sheet may run from the common bile duct laterally over the gallbladder down to the duodenum, to the hepatic flexure of the colon and even to the right lobe of the liver, perhaps closing the foramen of Winslow. In a milder form, a band of tissue runs from the lesser omentum across to the cystic duct and anterior to the gallbladder; or a loose veil forms a mesentery to the gallbladder ('floating gallbladder') (Fig. 14.14).

These adhesions are of no clinical importance. Surgically, their presence should be remembered, so that they are not mistaken for inflammatory adhesions.

Floating gallbladder and torsion of the gallbladder

The gallbladder possesses a supporting membrane in 4–5% of specimens. The peritoneal coat surrounding the gallbladder continues as two approximated leaves to form a fold or mesentery to support the gallbladder from under the surface of the liver. This fold may allow the gallbladder to hang as much as 2–3 cm below the inferior hepatic surface.

The mobile gallbladder is apt to twist, and *torsion* results [81]. The blood supply is impaired in the small pedicle and infarction follows.

The condition usually occurs in thin, elderly women. With ageing, omental fat lessens and there is a great caudal displacement of abdominal viscera due to loss of tone in the abdominal and pelvic muscles. The gallbladder with mesentery becomes more pendulous and can twist. It can affect all ages, including children.

Torsion is followed by sudden, severe, constant epigastric and right costal margin pain passing through to the back with vomiting and collapse. Characteristically, a palpable tumour appears, having the features of an enlarged gallbladder. Within a few hours it may disappear. The treatment is cholecystectomy.

Recurrent partial torsion leads to acute episodes. Ultrasound or CT shows a gallbladder situated low in the abdomen and even in the pelvis. It is suspended by a very long, down-curved cystic duct. Early cholecystectomy is indicated.

Anomalies of the cystic duct and cystic artery

In 20% of subjects the *cystic duct* does not join the common hepatic duct directly but first runs parallel to it, lying in the same sheath of connective tissue. Occasionally it makes a spiral turn around the duct.

These variations are extremely important to the surgeon. Unless the cystic duct is carefully dissected and its union with the common hepatic duct identified, the common hepatic duct may be ligated, with disastrous consequences.

The *cystic artery* can arise not, as normally, from the right hepatic artery but from the left hepatic artery or even from the gastroduodenal artery. Accessory cystic arteries usually arise from the right hepatic artery. Again, the surgeon must be careful to identify the cystic artery precisely.

References

1 Desmet VJ. Ludwig symposium on biliary disorders—part 1. Pathogenesis of dutal plate abnormalities. *Mayo Clin. Proc.* 1998; **73**: 80–89.

2 Desmet VJ. Embryology of the liver and intrahepatic biliary tract, and an overview of the malformations of the bile ducts. In: McIntyre N, Benhamou J-P, Bircher J *et al*, eds. *Oxford Textbook of Clinical Hepatology*. Vol 1. Oxford: Oxford University Press; 1991: 497–519.

3 D'Agata IDA, Jonas MM, Perez-Atayde AR *et al*. Combined cystic disease of the liver and kidney. *Semin. Liver Dis.* 1994; **14**: 215–228.

4 Mucher G, Wirth B, Zerres K. Refining the map and defining flanking markers of the gene for autosomal recessive polycystic kidney disease on chromosome 6p21.1 p12. *Am. J. Hum. Genet.* 1994; **55**: 1281–1284.

5 Ward CJ, Hogan MC, Rossetti S *et al*. The gene mutated in autosomal recessive polycystic kidney disease encodes a large, receptor-like protein. *Nat. Genet.* 2002; **30**: 259–269.

6 Onuchic LF, Furu L, Nagasawa Y *et al*. PKHD1, the polycystic kidney and hepatic disease 1 gene, encodes a novel large protein containing multiple immunoglobulin-like plexin-transcription-factor domains and parallel beta-helix 1 repeats. *Am. J. Hum. Genet.* 2002; **70**: 1305–1317.

7 Bergmann C, Senderek J, Küpper F *et al*. PKHD1 mutations in autosomal recessive polycystic kidney disease (ARPKD). *Hum. Mutat.* 2004; **23**: 453–463.

8 Perisic VN. Long term studies on congenital hepatic fibrosis in children. *Acta Pediatr.* 1995; **84**: 695–696.

9 Samyn M, Hadzic N, Portmann B *et al*. Fibropolycystic disease of the liver and kidneys in children. *Hepatology* 1999; **30**: 328A.

10 Ishak KG, Sharp HL. Developmental abnormalities and liver disease in childhood. In: MacSween RNM, Anthony PP, Scheuer PJ *et al*., eds. *Pathology of the Liver*, 3rd ed. 1994 Edinburgh: Churchill Livingstone.

11 Asselah T, Ernst O, Sergent G *et al*. Caroli's disease: a magnetic resonance cholangiopancreatography diagnosis. *Am. J. Gastroenterol.* 1998; **93**: 109–110.

12 McGonigle RJS, Mowat AP, Bewick M *et al*. Congenital hepatic fibrosis and polycystic kidney disease; role of portacaval shunting and transplantation in three cases. *Q. J. Med.* 1981; **50**: 269–278.

13 Hateboer N, van Dijk MA, Bogdanova N *et al*. Comparison of phenotypes of polycystic kidney disease types 1 and 2. *Lancet* 1999; **353**: 103–107.

14 Ibraghimov-Beskrovnaya O, Dackowski WR, Foggensteiner L *et al*. Polycystin: *in vitro* synthesis, *in vivo* tissue expression and subcellular localization identifies a large membrane-associated protein. *Proc. Natl. Acad. Sci. USA* 1997; **94**: 6397–6402.

15 Reynolds DM, Falk CT, Li A *et al*. Identification of a locus for autosomal dominant polycystic liver disease, on chromosome 19p13.2–13.1. *Am. J. Hum. Genet.* 2000; **67**: 1598–1604.

16 Gabow PA. Autosomal dominant polycystic kidney disease. *N. Engl. J. Med.* 1993; **329**: 332–342.

17 Everson GT, Emmett M, Brown WR *et al*. Functional similarities of hepatic cystic and biliary epithelium: studies of fluid constituents and *in vivo* secretion in response to secretin. *Hepatology* 1990; **11**: 557–565.

18 Gabow PA, Johnson AM, Kaehny WD *et al*. Risk factors for the development of hepatic cysts in autosomal dominant polycystic kidney disease. *Hepatology* 1990; **11**: 1033–1037.

19 Sherstha R, McKinley C, Russ P *et al*. Postmenopausal oestrogen therapy selectively stimulates hepatic enlargement in women with autosomal dominant polycystic kidney disease. *Hepatology* 1997; **26**: 1282–1286.

20 Uddin W, Ramage JK, Portmann B *et al*. Hepatic venous outflow obstruction in patients with polycystic liver disease: pathogenesis and treatment. *Gut* 1995; **36**: 142–145.

21 Waanders E, van Keimpema L, Brouwer JT *et al*. Carbohydrate antigen 19-9 is extremely elevated in polycystic liver disease. *Liver Int.* 2009; **29**: 1389–1395.

22 Kanaan N, Goffin E, Pirson Y *et al*. Carbonhydrate antigen 19-9 as a diagnostic marker for hepatic cyst infection in autosomal dominant polycystic kidney disease. *Am. J. Kidney Dis.* 2010; **55**: 916–922.

23 Srinivasan R. Polycystic liver disease: an unusual cause of bleeding varices. *Dig. Dis. Sci.* 1999; **44**: 389–392.

24 Hogan MC, Masyuk TV, Page LJ *et al*. Randomized clinical trial of long-acting somatostatin for autosomal dominant polycystic kidney and liver disease. *J. Am. Soc. Nephrol.* 2010; **21**: 1052–1061.

25 van Keimpema I, Nevens F, Vanslembrouck R *et al*. Lanreotide reduces the volume of polycystic liver: a randomized, double-blind, placebo-controlled trial. *Gastroenterology* 2009; **137**: 1661–1668.

26 Gigot J-F, Jadoul P, Que F *et al*. Adult polycystic liver disease: is fenestration the most adequate operation for long-term management? *Ann. Surg.* 1997; **225**: 286–294.

27 Kabbej M, Sauvanet A, Chauveau D *et al*. Laparoscopic fenestration in polycystic liver disease. *Br. J. Surg.* 1996; **83**: 1697–1701.

28 Farges O, Bismuth H. Fenestration in the management of polycystic liver disease. *World J. Surg.* 1995; **19**: 25–30.

29 Que F, Nagorney DM, Gross JB *et al*. Liver resection and cyst fenestration in the treatment of severe polycystic liver disease. *Gastroenterology* 1995; **108**: 487–494.

30 Swenson K, Seu P, Kinkhabwala M *et al*. Liver transplantation for adult polycystic liver disease. *Hepatology* 1998; **28**: 412–415.

31 Caballero F, Domingo P, Lopéz-Navidad A. Successful liver transplant using a polycystic donor liver. *J. Hepatol.* 1997; **26**: 1428.

32 Cobben JM, Breuning H, Schoots C *et al.* Congenital hepatic fibrosis in autosomal-dominant polycystic kidney disease. *Kidney Int.* 1990; **38**: 880–885.

33 Alvarez F, Bernard O, Brunelle F *et al.* Congenital fibrosis in children. *J. Pediatr.* 1981; **99**: 370–375.

34 Naveh Y, Roguin N, Ludatscher R *et al.* Congenital hepatic fibrosis with congenital heart disease. *Gut* 1980; **21**: 799–807.

35 Maggiore G, Borgana-Pignatti C, Marni E *et al.* Pulmonary arteriovenous fistulas: an unusual complication of congenital hepatic fibrosis. *J. Pediatr. Gastroenterol.* 1983; **2**: 183–186.

36 Bogomoletz WV, Lefaucher CC. Congenital hepatic fibrosis (asymptomatic and latent forms) and multiple gastric ulcers. *Dig. Dis. Sci.* 1979; **24**: 887–890.

37 Miller WA, Gang DL. Case records of the Massachusetts General Hospital: Case 11-1983. *N. Engl. J. Med.* 1983; **308**: 642–648.

38 Strayer DS, Kissane JM. Dysplasia of the kidneys, liver, and pancreas: report of a variant of Ivemark's syndrome. *Hum. Pathol.* 1979; **10**: 228–234.

39 Bernstein J, Chandra M, Creswell J *et al.* Renal-hepatic-pancreatic dysplasia: a syndrome reconsidered. *Am. J. Med. Genet.* 1987; **26**: 391–403.

40 Bohm N, Fukuda M, Staudt R *et al.* Chondroectodermal dysplasia (Ellis van Creveld syndrome) with dysplasia of the renal medulla and bile ducts. *Histopathology* 1978; **2**: 267–281.

41 Witzleben CL, Sharp AR. 'Nephronophthisis congenital hepatic fibrosis': an additional hepatorenal disorder. *Hum. Pathol.* 1982; **13**: 728–733.

42 Langer LO. Thoracic-pelvic-phalangeal dystrophy. *Radiology* 1968; **91**: 447–456.

43 Hudgins L, Rosengren S, Treem W *et al.* Early cirrhosis in survivors with Jeune thoracic dystrophy. *J. Pediatr.* 1992; **120**: 754–756.

44 Nakamura F, Sasaki H, Kajihara H *et al.* Laurence-Moon-Biedl syndrome accompanied by congenital hepatic fibrosis. *J. Gastroenterol. Hepatol.* 1990; **5**: 206–210.

45 Bauman ME, Pound DC, Ulbright TM. Hepatocellular carcinoma arising in congenital hepatic fibrosis. *Am. J. Gastroenterol.* 1994; **89**: 450–451.

46 Yamato T, Sasaki M, Hoso M *et al.* Intrahepatic cholangiocarcinoma arising in congenital hepatic fibrosis: report of an autopsy case. *J. Hepatol.* 1998; **28**: 717–722.

47 Bertheau P, Degott C, Belghiti J *et al.* Adenomatous hyperplasia of the liver in a patient with congenital hepatic fibrosis. *J. Hepatol.* 1994; **20**: 213–217.

48 Jaeken J, Matthijs G, Saudubray J-M *et al.* Phosphomannose isomerase deficiency: A carbohydrate-deficient glycoprotein syndrome with hepatic-intestinal presentation. *Am. J. Hum. Genet.* 1998; **62**: 1535–1539.

49 Nichues R, Hasilik M, Alton G *et al.* Carbohydrate-deficient glycoprotein syndrome type 1b: Phosphomannose isomerase deficiency and mannose therapy. *J. Clin. Invest.* 1998; **191**: 1414–1420.

50 Ernst O, Gottrand F, Calvo M *et al.* Congenital hepatic fibrosis: findings at MR cholangiopancreatopraphy. *Am. J. Roentgenol.* 1998; **170**: 409–412.

51 Taylor ACF, Palmer KR. Caroli's disease. *Eur. J. Gastroenterol. Hepatol.* 1998; **10**: 105–108.

52 Boyle MJ, Doyle GD, McNulty JG. Monolobar Caroli's disease. *Am. J. Gastroenterol.* 1989; **84**: 1437–1444.

53 Summerfield JA, Nagafuchi Y, Sherlock S *et al.* Hepatobiliary fibropolycystic disease: a clinical and histological review of 51 patients. *J. Hepatol.* 1986; **2**: 141–156.

54 Tsuchida Y, Sato T, Sanjo K *et al.* Evaluation of long-term results of Caroli's disease: 21 years' observation of a family with autosomal 'dominant' inheritance, and review of the literature. *Hepatogastroenterology* 1995; **42**: 175–181.

55 Dagli Ü, Atalay F, Sasmaz N *et al.* Caroli's disease: 1977–95 experiences. *Eur. J. Gastroenterol. Hepatol.* 1998; **10**: 105–108.

56 Keane F, Hadzic N, Wilkinson ML *et al.* Neonatal presentation of Caroli's disease. *Arch. Dis. Child* 1997; **77**: F145–146.

57 Dayton MT, Longmire WP Jr, Tompkins PK. Caroli's disease: a premalignant condition? *Am. J. Surg.* 1983; **145**: 41–48.

58 Turnberg LA, Jones EA, Sherlock S. Biliary secretion in a patient with cystic dilation of the intrahepatic biliary tree. *Gastroenterology* 1968; **54**: 1155–1161.

59 Choi BI, Yeon KM, Kim SH *et al.* Caroli disease: central dot sign in CT. *Radiology* 1990; **174**: 161–163.

60 Asselah T, Ernst O, Sergent G *et al.* Caroli's disease: a magnetic resonance cholangiopancreatography diagnosis. *Am. J. Gastroenterol.* 1998; **93**: 109–110.

61 Nagasue N. Successful treatment of Caroli's disease by hepatic resection: report of six patients. *Ann. Surg.* 1984; **200**: 718–723.

62 Ros E, Navarro S, Bru C *et al.* Ursodeoxycholic acid treatment of primary hepatolithiasis in Caroli's syndrome. *Lancet* 1993; **342**: 404–406.

63 Komi N, Takehara H, Kunitomo K. Choledochal cyst: anomalous arrangement of the pancreatico-biliary ductal system and biliary malignancy. *J. Gastroenterol. Hepatol.* 1989; **4**: 63–74.

64 Tyler KL, Sokol RJ, Oberhaus SM *et al.* Detection of reovirus RNA in hepatobiliary tissues from patients with extrahepatic biliary atresia and choledochal cysts. *Hepatology* 1998; **27**: 1475–1482.

65 Zhan JH, Hu XL, Dai CJ *et al.* Expressions of p53 and inducible nitric oxide synthase in congenital choledochal cysts. *Hepatobiliary Pancreat. Dis. Int.* 2004; **3**: 120–123.

66 Kerkar N, Norton K, Suchy FJ. The hepatic fibrocystic diseases. *Clin. Liver Dis.* 2006; **10**: 55–57.

67 Lenriot JP, Gigot JF, Ségol P *et al.* Bile duct cysts in adults: a multi-institutional retrospective study. *Ann. Surg.* 1998; **228**: 159–166.

68 Lipsett PA, Pitt HA, Colombani PM *et al.* Choledochal cyst disease: a changing pattern of presentation. *Ann. Surg.* 1994; **220**: 644–652.

69 Spier LN, Crystal K, Kase DJ *et al.* Choledochocele: newer concepts of origin and diagnosis. *Surgery* 1995; **117**: 476–478.

70 Terada T, Nakanuma Y. Solitary cystic dilation of the intrahepatic bile duct: morphology of two autopsy cases and a review of the literature. *Am. J. Gastroenterol.* 1987; **82**: 1301–1305.

71 Miyano T, Yamataka A. Choledochal cysts. *Curr. Opin. Pediatr.* 1997; **9**: 283–288

72 Hinds R, Davenport M, Mieli-Vergani G *et al.* Antenatal diagnosis of biliary atresia. *J. Pediatr.* 2004; **144**: 43–46.

73 Irie H, Honda H, Jimi M *et al.* Value of MR cholangiopancreatography in evaluating choledochal cysts. *AJR Am. J. Roentgenol.* 1998; **171**: 1381–1385.

74 Lam WWM, Lam TPW, Saing H *et al.* MR cholangiography and CT cholangiography of paediatric patients with choledochal cysts. *Am. J. Roentgenol.* 1999; **173**: 401–405.

75 Ishibashi T, Kasahara K, Yasuda Y *et al.* Malignant change in the biliary tract after excision of choledochal cyst. *Br. J. Surg.* 1997; **84**: 1687–1691.

76 Todani T, Watanabe Y, Toki A *et al.* Carcinoma related to choledochal cysts with internal drainage operations. *Surg. Gynecol. Obstet.* 1987; **164**: 61–64.

77 Nieweg O, Sloof MJH, Grond J. A case of primary squamous cell carcinoma of the liver arizing in a solitary cyst. *HPB Surg.* 1992; **5**: 203–208.

78 Cullingford G, Davidson B, Dooley J *et al.* Case report: hepatolithiasis associated with anomalous biliary anatomy and a vascular compression. *HPB Surg.* 1991; **3**: 129–134.

79 Richards RJ, Raubin H, Wasson D. Agenesis of the gallbladder in symptomatic adults: a case and review of the literature. *J. Clin. Gastroenterol.* 1993; **16**: 231–233.

80 Nagai M, Kubota K, Kawasaki S *et al.* Are left-sided gallbladders really located on the left side? *Ann. Surg.* 1997; **225**: 274–280.

81 Faure JP, Doucet C, Scepi M *et al.* Abnormalities of the gallbladder, clinical effects. *Surg. Radiol. Anat.* 2008; **30**: 285–290.

CHAPTER 15
Primary Biliary Cirrhosis

Margaret F. Bassendine

Medical School, Newcastle University, Newcastle upon Tyne

Learning points

- More than 90% of primary biliary cirrhosis patients are female and test positive for antimitochondrial antibodies in serum.
- Liver biochemistry is cholestatic and liver histology show granulomatous destruction of interlobular bile ducts.
- Ursodeoxycholic acid (UDCA) is the only currently known treatment that can slow disease progression.
- Primary biliary cirrhosis patients who start UDCA treatment at early-stage disease and/or show a biochemical response have a good prognosis.
- Liver transplantation is the only effective treatment for those with end-stage disease.

Primary biliary cirrhosis (PBC) is a disease of unknown cause in which intrahepatic bile ducts are progressively destroyed. It was first described in 1851 by Addison and Gull [1] and later by Hanot [2]. The association with high serum cholesterol levels and skin xanthomas led to the term 'xanthomatous biliary cirrhosis'. Ahrens *et al.* [3] termed the condition 'primary biliary cirrhosis'. The disease is now usually diagnosed in the early stages when cirrhosis is not present.

Clinical features

Presentation (Table 15.1) *[4]*

Ninety per cent of patients with PBC are female. The cause for disease prevalence among women is unknown. The patient is usually 40–60 years of age, but can be as old as 80 or as young as 15. Ten per cent are male, in whom the disease runs a similar course. The disease starts insidiously, most frequently as pruritus without jaundice [5]. Patients may be referred initially to dermatologists. Jaundice may never develop, but in the major-ity appears within 6 months to 2 years of the onset of pruritus. In about a quarter, jaundice and pruritus start simultaneously. The pruritus can start during pregnancy and be confused with cholestatic jaundice of pregnancy but it may not regress following delivery. Chronic right upper quadrant pain is frequent (17%). This may persist or resolve [6]. Magnetic resonance cholangiopancrea-tography (MRCP) may be necessary to exclude a diag-nosis of primary sclerosing cholangitis in patients without detectable antimitochondrial antibody (AMA).

Fatigue is frequent [7] but is not a specific symptom of PBC. Examination shows a well-nourished, some-times pigmented woman. Jaundice is rarely seen at pres-entation. The liver is usually enlarged and firm and the spleen palpable when the patient presents with jaundice.

The asymptomatic patient

Widespread use of biochemical screening has resulted in over 60% of patients being diagnosed when asymp-tomatic, usually by a raised serum alkaline phosphatase level [8]. Antimitochondrial antibody is present. Serum bilirubin may be normal or only minimally increased. Serum cholesterol and transaminases may or may not be elevated. In those with high transaminases, overlap with autoimmune hepatitis should be considered and is characterized by a positive International Autoimmune Hepatitis Group (IAIHG) score [9].

Abnormal physical signs may be absent.

The diagnosis may be made in patients under inves-tigation for a condition known to be associated with PBC, such as thyroid or collagen disease, or in the course of family surveys.

Associated diseases

PBC is associated with almost any autoimmune disease. Sjögren's syndrome with or without CREST (calcinosis,

Sherlock's Diseases of the Liver and Biliary System, Twelfth Edition. Edited by
James S. Dooley, Anna S.F. Lok, Andrew K. Burroughs, E. Jenny Heathcote.
© 2011 by Blackwell Publishing Ltd. Published 2011 by Blackwell Publishing Ltd.

Table 15.1. Diagnosis of primary biliary cirrhosis at presentation [4]

Symptomatic

Middle-aged woman with pruritus followed by slowly progressive jaundice

Liver palpable

Serum bilirubin about twice normal; serum alkaline phosphatase about 4 times normal; serum alanine transaminase about twice normal; serum albumin normal

Serum AMA >1:40

Liver biopsy appearances compatible

MRCP (if diagnosis in doubt, e.g. negative AMA): normal intrahepatic bile ducts

Asymptomatic

Routine laboratory screen or during investigation of other disease, especially collagen or thyroid

Physical signs often absent

Increased serum alkaline phosphatase, normal serum bilirubin

Positive serum AMA

Liver biopsy appearances compatible

AMA, antimitochondrial antibody; MRCP, magnetic resonance cholangiopancreatography.

Raynaud's, oesophageal dysfunction, sclerodatyly and telangectasia) syndrome and Raynaud's disease are particularly frequent [10]. The collagenoses, especially rheumatoid arthritis, dermatomyositis, mixed connective tissue disease and systemic lupus erythematosus are also seen.

Autoimmune thyroiditis affects about 20%. Graves' disease has also been reported.

There is an increased incidence of coeliac disease in PBC. Patients with PBC in whom there is a clinical suspicion of coeliac disease should be screened by tissue transglutaminase antibodies and, if present, confirmed by duodenal biopsy.

PBC has been associated with autoimmune thrombocytopenia and autoimmune haemolytic anaemia.

Renal complications include distal tubular acidosis and IgM-associated membranous glomerular nephritis. Hypouricaemia and hyperuricosuria are further expressions of renal tubular damage. Asymptomatic bacteriuria is not unusual.

There is a small increase in overall cancer incidence and mortality in patients with PBC probably in part due to the higher reported rates of smoking. The risk for lymphoma in patients with PBC is less than 1%.

Pulmonary abnormalities include lymphocyte interstitial pneumonitis leading to pulmonary fibrosis and consequent pulmonary hypertension. Moderate to severe pulmonary hypertension is also associated with portal hypertension and indicates a poor prognosis.

It is not unusual to see enlarged nodes in the gastrohepatic ligament and porta hepatis and even enlarged paracardiac and mesenteric nodes on CT scan.

Natural history (Fig. 15.1)

Most data on natural history relate to patients diagnosed in the pre or early *ursodeoxycholic acid* (UDCA) era. Asymptomatic patients usually survive at least 9 to 10 years (Fig. 15.2) [4,11,12]. In those with symptomatic disease and jaundice the survival is about 7 to 8 years [12,13].

The course of asymptomatic patients is variable but the majority (80%) become symptomatic within 10 years (Table 15.2) and the estimates for developing symptoms in 5 and 20 years are 50 and 95%, respectively [12]. No reliable way has been identified to predict which patients will remain asymptomatic. Some will never become symptomatic and others will run a progressive downhill course (Fig. 15.3).

The natural history of histological changes in PBC (without UDCA) has documented that the majority of patients will progress histologically within 2 years. Liver stiffness measurement (transient elastography), a non-invasive test for assessment of liver fibrosis, may be useful to monitor its progression over time [14].

Fatigue is very common, affecting 60% of sufferers [7]. It is the primary predictor of impaired quality of life,

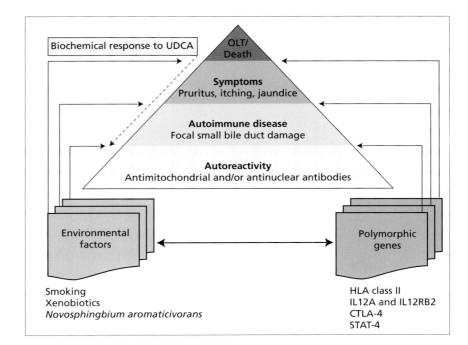

Fig. 15.1. Schematic representation of the stages of PBC from pre-disease (autoreactivity) to asymptomatic, symptomatic and end-stage liver disease. Environmental factors act on a genetically predisposed host to initiate and/or perpetuate disease. Biochemical responders to UDCA have a better prognosis.

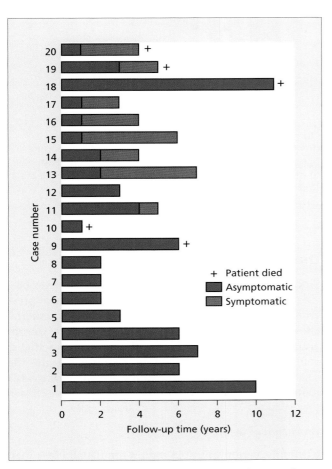

Fig. 15.2. The course of 20 patients with PBC diagnosed when asymptomatic. Note that one patient continued asymptomatic for 10 years [11].

Table 15.2. The progression of untreated primary biliary cirrhosis [35]

Stage			
AMA	Biochemistry	Symptoms	Progression time (years)
+	0	0	80% will progress
+	+	0	40% in 6 years
+	+	+	70% in 10 years (50% in 5 years)

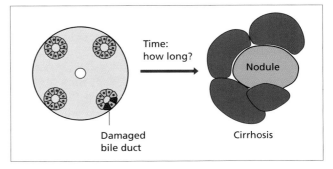

Fig. 15.3. Natural history of PBC: the time taken from acute bile duct damage to end-stage biliary cirrhosis is uncertain [84].

which may be assessed by a PBC-specific score [15]. The pathogenesis of fatigue in PBC is unclear but it cannot be explained by depression. Fatigue does not correlate with the liver disease severity and liver transplantation does not improve fatigue. The fatigue phenotype appears to be highly stable in PBC and it's presence may indicate a poorer prognosis [16,17].

The course is afebrile and abdominal pain is unusual but may persist.

When jaundice is obvious this is complicated by steatorrhoea and consequent weight loss. Skin xanthomas may develop, sometimes acutely, but many patients remain without xanthoma throughout their course. If xanthoma are plentiful, pain in the fingers, especially on opening doors, and in the toes may be due to xanthomatous peripheral neuropathy. There may be a butterfly area over the back which is inaccessible and escapes scratching. These late manifestations of disease are now rarely seen in western countries as liver transplant is performed in most patients before their development.

Osteoporosis in PBC is related to advancing age and disease severity with a possible genetic component and there is a twofold increase in both the absolute and relative fracture risk in people with PBC compared with the general population [18].

Bleeding oesophageal varices may be a presenting feature and rarely before nodules have developed when portal hypertension is related to nodular regenerative hyperplasia. A subgroup of patients with cirrhosis but near normal bilirubin values has a better prognosis than other patients with obvious jaundice. Within a median of 5.6 years, varices have developed in 31% of patients and 48% of these will have bled unless primary prevention manoeuvres have been instituted. Varices are more likely to develop in those with a high serum bilirubin and with an advanced histological stage of the disease. A platelet count of less than 140 000 identifies those patients more likely to benefit from a screening endoscopy [19]. The portohepatic gradient may stabilize or improve with response to ursodeoxycholic acid treatment. Once varices have developed, 83% survive 1 year and 59% 3 years. Survival after the initial bleed is 65% at 1 year and 46% at 3 years.

There is a risk of hepatocellular carcinoma, especially in older males with cirrhosis. Surveillance for hepatocellular carcinoma is recommended is those known to have cirrhosis [20].

Liver-related mortality has been reported as 60% in symptomatic patients but this will vary according to age at initial diagnosis [8]. If liver transplantation is not an option, the terminal stages last about 1 year and are marked by a rapid deepening of jaundice (Fig. 15.4) with the disappearance of both xanthomas and pruritus. Serum albumin and total cholesterol levels fall. Oedema and ascites develop. The final events include episodes of hepatic encephalopathy with uncontrollable bleeding, usually from the oesophageal varices. An intercurrent infection, sometimes a Gram-negative septicaemia, may be terminal.

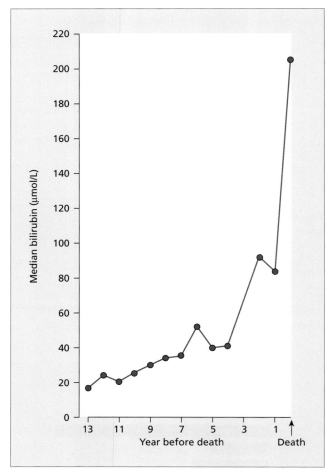

Fig. 15.4. The evolution of liver failure in PBC. This nomogram is derived from the medians of pooled serum bilirubin results in patients followed serially from diagnosis to death. Expected survival can be calculated using the Mayo Risk Score which is available online at http://www.mayoclinic.org/gi-rst/mayomodel1.html (accessed 15 Oct. 2010).

Diagnosis

Since the introduction of routine screening of liver biochemical tests many patients are asymptomatic at presentation. Diagnosis is currently based on three criteria: cholestatic liver biochemical tests, presence of serum antimitochondrial antibodies and liver histology that is compatible with PBC. A definite diagnosis requires the presence of all three criteria and a probable diagnosis requires two of these three.

Biochemical tests

Currently, serum bilirubin values are usually less than 35 μmol/L (2 mg/100 mL) at the time of diagnosis of PBC. Serum alkaline phosphatase and γ-glutamyl transpeptidase (γ-GT) are raised. The total serum cho-

Fig. 15.5. Schematic representation of the four major mitochondrial autoantigens showing similar domain structure. The essential cofactor, lipoic acid, is covalently attached to a lysine residue in each lipoyl domain. [PDC, pyruvate dehydrogenase complex. E3BP, E3 binding protein. BCOADC, branched chain 2-oxo-acid dehydrogenase complex, OGDC, oxoglutarate dehydrogenase complex]. Note xenobiotic incorporation into the inner lipoyl domain of PDC-E2 in place of the cofactor, lipoic acid forming a 'neoantigen' [40].

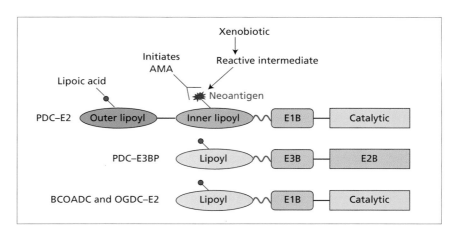

lesterol is increased but not constantly. The serum albumin level is usually normal at presentation and the serum IgM is usually raised. This is not reliable for diagnosis, although an increase may add some diagnostic weight.

Autoantibodies

Over 90% of patients have AMA[21]. The antigens to which the antibodies are directed are localized on the inner mitochondrial membrane. The dominant autoantibody response is directed against two components (dihydrolipoamide acetyltransferase (E2) and E3-binding protein) of the pyruvate dehydrogenase complex (PDC) [22,23]. The E2 components of the other 2-oxo-acid dehydrogenase complexes also react with AMA [24]. These four mitochondrial autoantigens share a highly conserved structure containing a lipoic acid cofactor (Fig. 15.5). Immunodominant B- and T-cell epitopes have been localized to the inner lipoyl domain of PDC-E2 around the lipoic acid attachment site [25,26].

Antinuclear antibodies are found in a minority of patients with primary biliary cirrhosis. Antinuclear antibodies display unique immunofluorescence patterns such as nuclear dots or a nuclear ring-like pattern. PBC-specific nuclear antigens include a 210-kDa glycoprotein of the nuclear-pore membrane (gp 210), nucleoporin p62 and Sp100, an interferon-inducible nucleoprotein.

Patients who lack AMA need careful evaluation (Table 15.3).

They may have AMA-negative PBC, which has been mistakenly termed 'autoimmune cholangitis'. Clinical presentation, biochemistry, liver histology and response to UDCA are no different from those with typical AMA-positive PBC. Nearly all these patients have PBC-specific antinuclear antibodies. IgM levels are lower.

Visualization of the bile ducts, preferably by MR, is necessary in atypical patients particularly males, those with inconclusive liver biopsy findings or with marked abdominal pain and those who lack AMA. In primary sclerosing cholangitis, cholangiography demonstrates the typical bile duct irregularities.

Idiopathic adult ductopenia is marked by absence of interlobular bile ducts but with minimal portal tract inflammation. The aetiology of 'vanishing bile syndromes' are multiple and are sometimes uncertain.

Widespread tissue granulomas may suggest cholestatic sarcoidosis [27]. Liver biopsy shows less bile duct damage than seen in PBC.

Cholestatic drugs reactions are excluded by the history and by the acute onset, with rapidly deepening jaundice developing within weeks of starting the drug.

A small minority of PBC patients may have features of autoimmune hepatitis. This 'overlap' syndrome has higher alanine transaminase and IgG levels than are seen in typical PBC and liver biopsy needs to show moderate or severe periportal or periseptal inflammation. Patients with overlap features demonstrate an increased liver-related mortality [28]. Transition between PBC and autoimmune hepatitis may occur [29] associated with biochemical and serological changes and liver biopsy is needed to confirm the new diagnosis.

Liver biopsy [30]

Many consider liver biopsy to be unnecessary unless the patient tests AMA negative, is at risk of another superimposed liver disease, for example non-alcoholic fatty liver disease, or is a non-responder to treatment with UDCA.

Histologically the only diagnostic lesion is the injured septal or interlobular bile duct. Such ducts may be missed on needle biopsy specimens if the sample contains an inadequate number of portal tracts (≥10 required). They are represented in surgical biopsies (Fig. 15.6).

The disease begins with damage to the epithelium of the small bile ducts. Histometric examinations show

Table 15.3. Differential diagnosis of primary biliary cirrhosis

Disease	Features	AMA	Liver biopsy
Primary biliary cirrhosis	Female	Positive	Bile duct damage
	Pruritus		Lymphoid aggregates
	High serum alkaline phosphatase		Slight PMN
			Intact lobules
			Periseptal cholestasis
AMA negative PBC	Females	Negative	Bile duct damage
	High serum alkaline phosphatase		Lymphoid aggregates
	Serum ANA positive in high titre		Slight PMN
	High IgG		
Primary sclerosing cholangitis	Males predominate	Negative or low titre	Ductular proliferation fibrosis
	Associated ulcerative colitis		
	MRC is diagnostic		Onion-skin duct fibrosis
Cholestatic sarcoidosis	Equal sexes	Negative	Many granulomas throughout liver
	Black patients		Modest bile duct changes
	Pruritus		
	High serum alkaline phosphatase		
	Chest X-ray changes		
Cholestatic drug reactions	History	Negative	Mononuclear portal. reaction , sometimes with eosinophils, granulomas and fatty change
	Usually within 6 weeks of starting drug		
	Acute onset		
	Often jaundiced		

ANA, antinuclear antibodies; AMA, antimitochondrial antibodies; PMN, piecemeal necrosis.

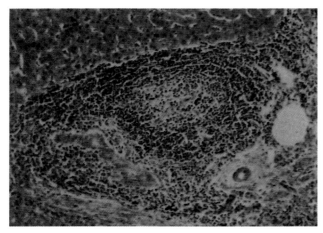

Fig. 15.6. The portal zone contains a well-formed granuloma. An adjacent bile duct shows damage.

that bile ducts less than 70–80 μm in diameter are destroyed, particularly in the early stages. Epithelial cells are swollen, irregular and more eosinophilic. The bile duct lumen is irregular and the basement membrane is disrupted. The bile duct occasionally ruptures. Surrounding the damaged duct is a cellular reaction which includes lymphocytes, plasma cells, eosinophils and histiocytes. Apoptosis of biliary epithelial cells is increased in the presence of inflammation. Granulomas confined to the portal tracts commonly form, usually in zone 1 (Fig. 15.6).

Bile ducts eventually become destroyed. Their sites are marked by aggregates of lymphoid cells, and bile ductules begin to proliferate (Fig. 15.7). Hepatic arterial branches can be identified in zone 1, but without accompanying bile ducts. Fibrosis extends from zone 1 and

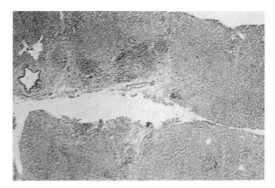

Fig. 15.7. Stage 2 lesion, marked by aggregates of lymphoid cells. Bile ducts begin to proliferate. (H & E, ×10.)

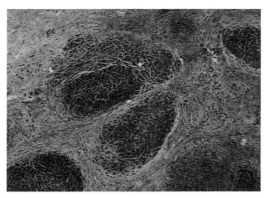

Fig. 15.9. Stage 4: biliary cirrhosis has developed [32].

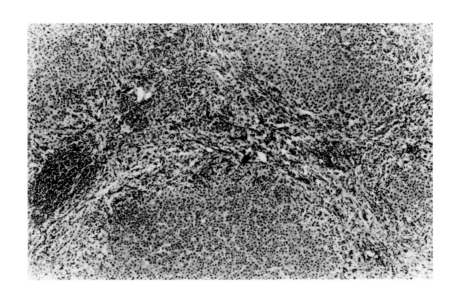

Fig. 15.8. There is scarring and septa contain lymphoid aggregates. Bile ducts are inconspicuous. Hyperplastic 'regeneration' nodules are beginning to develop [4]. (H & E, ×48.)

there is a variable degree of piecemeal necrosis. Piecemeal necrosis is the only histological lesion which significantly enhances the risk of disease progression [31]. Substantial amounts of copper and copper-associated protein can be demonstrated histochemically, due to retention of bile. The fibrous septa gradually distort the architecture of the liver and regeneration nodules form (Figs 15.8, 15.9). These are often irregular in distribution and cirrhosis may be seen in one part of a biopsy but not in another. In the early stages, cholestasis is in zone 1 (portal) but they may be little else seen in terms of diagnostic lesions.

Hepatocellular hyaline deposits, similar to those of alcoholic disease, are found in hepatocytes in about 25% of cases.

The histological appearances have been divided into four stages [32]: stage I, florid bile duct lesions; stage II, ductular proliferation; stage III, scarring (septal fibrosis and bridging); and stage IV, cirrhosis. Such staging is of limited value as the changes in the liver are focal and evolve at different speeds in different parts, hence the stages may overlap. In addition, as PBC is now diagnosed much earlier these stages may not be represented.

Aetiology

The precise aetiology of PBC remains uncertain [33]. The balance of evidence supports an autoimmune process in which autoreactive effector mechanisms are directed at self-epitopes expressed on small-duct biliary epithelial cells [34]. This autoimmune process is thought to be triggered in 'susceptible' individuals by exposure to one or more environmental triggers which initiate and/or perpetuate the disease process.

Autoimmune process

The loss of tolerance to mitochondrial autoantigens is an early event in this progressive disease. AMA are detectable in serum before abnormalities in liver function and long before the onset of symptoms [35]. One hypothesis is that the development of these AMA marks the exposure of a genetically susceptible individual to an initiating environmental factor.

Data exist on effector mechanisms of bile duct destruction. PBC is characterized histologically by autoreactive CD4$^+$ and CD8$^+$T cells surrounding damaged bile ducts. There is a 100-fold increase in autoreactive CD4$^+$ PDC-E2-specific T cells and a 10-fold increase in autoreactive CD8$^+$ T cells in liver infiltrates. CD4$^+$ T cells mature into Th1, Th2, Th17 or T regulatory cell (Treg) phenotypes. Mature Tregs can be reprogrammed and gain the ability to produce interferon-γ (IFN-γ), interleukin-17 (IL-17) and tumour necrosis factor-α (TNF-α). The relative proportions of T-cell subpopulations is probably relevant in autoimmunity. It is reported that patients with PBC have fewer circulating Tregs and an increase in the frequency of IL-17$^+$ lymphocytic infiltration in liver tissue [36].

Targeting of the autoimmune response to biliary epithelium may be explained by abnormal expression of mitochondrial autoantigens on the surface of these cells. Apoptosis of biliary epithelial cells, which occurs in PBC [37], results in the display of immunoreactive PDC-E2 within apoptotic blebs [38,39]. This could lead to recognition of the mitochondrial autoantigen(s) by the immune system.

Environmental factors

The aetiological factors triggering the production of autoantibodies remain enigmatic. Environmental factors such as xenobiotics and micro-organisms have been implicated. They may initiate and/or perpetuate the autoimmune response via molecular (epitope) mimicry.

Xenobiotics are foreign compounds that may complex to self-proteins, inducing a change in the molecular structure of the native protein sufficient to induce an immune response. It has been shown that a xenobiotic can be incorporated into the major mitochondrial autoantigen (PDC-E2) in place of the cofactor, lipoic acid [40] (Fig. 15.5). Certain chemicals found in food flavorings and cosmetics can induce AMA [41]. T-cell clones reactive to mitochondrial antigens can also be activated by peptides derived from xenobiotics [42].

Another source of antigenic mimicry is infectious agents. The mitochondrial autoantigens (E2 components of 2-oxo acid dehydrogenase complexes [24]) are highly conserved in evolution. AMA have been found to cross-react with homologous E2s in a number of micro-organisms including *E. coli*, but at a lower titre [43]. T-cell clones specific for *E. coli* OGDC-E2 react pro-

miscuously with the human mitochondrial equivalents [44]. Clinical [45] and epidemiological studies [41] have found association with urinary tract infections. Another candidate for the induction of AMA is *Novosphingobium aromaticivorans* [46]. This ubiquitous micro-organism metabolizes xenobiotics and activates environmental oestrogens. *Novosphingobium* E2s show high amino acid homology in their lipoyl domains with human PDC-E2.

Epidemiology and genetics

All races are affected but there is a variable frequency worldwide. Annual incidence is estimated between 0.7 and 49 cases per million population. Changing prevalence may depend on increasing physician awareness, better diagnosis and recognition of more asymptomatic patients.

A role for environmental factors in the triggering of PBC is suggested by disease 'hot spots' [47,48]. Cigarette smoking has been associated with an increased risk of PBC. More epidemiological studies are needed.

There is family clustering; mothers and daughters have the highest prevalence [49] with presentation earlier in the second generation. The rate of concordance among monozygotic twins is 60% [50]. Prevalence of circulating antimitochondrial antibodies is increased in first-degree relatives of patients. They have a 50- to 100-fold higher relative risk of PBC compared to the general population, consistent with a genetic influence. Among the genes studied as susceptibility candidates, only major histocompatibility complex (MHC) class II alleles have consistently been associated with primary biliary cirrhosis. There is no association of the disorder with MHC class I antigens.

Polymorphism in cytotoxic T-lymphocyte-associated antigen 4 (CTLA-4) has also been associated with increased susceptibility to PBC.

An immunogenetic predisposition has been confirmed by genome-wide association studies identifying human leucocyte antigens (HLA) class II, IL12A, and IL12RB2 as susceptibility loci [51,52]. There are associations shown between PBC and variants in the four HLA class II genes (DQB1, DPB1, DRB1 and DRA). These studies suggest that the IL-12 immunoregulatory signalling axis is relevant to the pathogenesis of PBC. They confirmed a modest association between PBC and variants in the CTLA-4 locus and found that variants in 11 other loci play a role in susceptibility to PBC.

Genetic factors may also impact on the severity of PBC. Variants of the multidrug resistance protein 3 (*MDR3/ABCB4*) and anion exchanger (*SLC4A2/AE2*) genes may predict progression [53].

Treatment [54,55]

This consists of therapy aimed at modifying the disease process and progression to cirrhosis, and treatment of symptoms and late complications.

Numerous trials of specific immunosuppressive or antifibrotic therapy have been undertaken in the last 40 years. Drugs tested included chlorambucil, D-penicillamine [56], azathioprine, methotrexate, ciclosporin A, corticosteroids and colchicine. Results in terms of survival, biochemical tests and hepatic histology tended to show no benefit or be inconclusive, but few studies have been of adequate size.

Ursodeoxycholic acid (UDCA)

This is a non-hepatotoxic, hydrophilic bile acid. It is the only FDA drug licensed to treat patients with PBC. It is recommended (in a dose of 13–15 mg/kg body weight per day) by the practice guidelines of both the European and the American Associations for the Study of Liver Diseases for patients with abnormal liver biochemical values [54,55]. UDCA may be more effective when initiated at the earlier stages I–II of the disease [57], but moderate or late stage is unlikely to respond.

A meta-analysis [58] that considered dose of UDCA, did not show that this affected outcomes, but most patients had moderate to advanced disease. Another meta-analysis that did not show benefit of UDCA [59] included studies of short duration and/or an inadequate dose of UDCA.

UDCA should be continued indefinitely. Monitoring is done using liver biochemical values. Biochemical response is is related to baseline pretreatment serum bilirubin or histological stage [31]. In asymptomatic patients the development of liver-related symptoms is higher in UDCA non-responders than in those with a biochemical response to UDCA [60].

The mechanism of action of UDCA is uncertain and is probably multifactorial. It protects cell membranes against the detergent effect of hydrophobic bile acids. It stimulates the excretion of toxic bile acids. It increases anion exchange in the liver. It reduces total and IgM-AMA production by down-regulating B-cell activation and nuclear factor-κB (NF-κB) signalling [61]. It induces the expression of a major antimicrobial peptide, cathelicidin, in biliary epithelial cells and may contribute to epithelial cell innate immunity [62].

Absence of a biochemical response to UDCA has prognostic implications [31]. It is a useful tool in identifying patients requiring further therapeutic intervention to retard disease progression. More trials are needed in these UDCA non-responders.

Combination therapy may be beneficial. Budesonide combined with UDCA improves liver histology [63]. It can worsen osteopenia in patients with more advanced disease and monitoring of bone mass density is recommended. Combination therapy using fenofibrate and UDCA is encouraging and needs further evaluation. Bezafibrate is effective in approximately two-thirds of non-icteric patients who have not shown a complete response to UDCA [64,65].

Management of symptoms

Ursodeoxycholic acid is not a panacea for the treatment of PBC. In symptomatic patients it does not improve fatigue or pruritus.

Fatigue in PBC may be associated with the presence of day-time somnolence and modafinil in a dose of 100–200 mg daily has been used with good effect in pilot studies [66], but its use may be associated with untoward side effects [67].

Pruritus is usually controlled by cholestyramine within a few days from starting treatment. The starting dose is 4 g daily which should be increased, in case of therapeutic failure, until a maximum of 16 g. It may interfere with absorption of UDCA and other medications and should be taken 2–4 h before or after UDCA. It is ineffective in about 10 to 20% of the patients. Many patients find cholestyramine unpleasant to take and develop dyspeptic symptoms or diarrhoea or, alternatively, constipation, leading to poor compliance with treatment.

Rifampicin, given at an initial dose of 150 mg/day and increased to up to 600 mg/day, can relief pruritus. Long-term use is associated with occasional hepatotoxicity and monitoring of liver enzymes is essential. There is evidence to suggest that the pruritus of cholestasis is mediated, at least in part, by endogenous opioids. Opioid antagonists are also effective but their use is difficult to institute [68]. This is because an opioid withdrawal-like reaction can occur; this can be avoided by an intravenous induction stage with naloxone increased from a dose of 0.002 μg/kg per min to 0.2 μg/kg per min over 3 days with translation across to 50 mg/day of naltraxone when the highest dose of naloxone is reached [69]. Long-term use of opioid antagonists may induce a chronic pain syndrome.

General measures apply to all patients with cholestasis. They include maintenance of nutrition and fat-soluble vitamin replacement.

Prevention and treatment of *haemorrhage* from oesophageal varices in PBC is as for any other aetiology of cirrhosis: platelet count may be useful to monitor.

Vitamin A and D deficiencies should be screened for and treated by supplementation (Vit D_3 100,000 IU and Vit A 50,000 intramuscularly 3 monthly), or oral supplements, with calcium. Osteomalacia is rare. In patients with osteoporosis alendronate is helpful [70]. Oestrogens stimulate bone formation and hormone replacement therapy is not contraindicated in postmenopausal women with PBC.

Prognosis

Diagnosis of PBC carries important prognostic implications [8]. People with PBC have a threefold mortality increase when compared with the general population. This is somewhat reduced by regular treatment with UDCA [71]. In a population-based study the estimated 10-year probabilities of survival, liver transplantation and transplant-free survival were 73, 6 and 68%, respectively [72].

The biochemical response to UDCA treatment can be used to predict outcome. Patients with a decrease in serum alkaline phosphatase of at least 40% or a decrease to the normal range at 1 year have a prognosis similar to that of an age-matched healthy population [73]. Survival for those with advanced PBC and a biochemical response to UDCA is better than for non-responders [57]. Absence of a biochemical response to UDCA is an important predictive factor for death or liver transplantation [31].

Age, albumin and Log10(bilirubin) may help to predict the advent of ascites and other complications in PBC [74].

The Mayo Clinic prognostic model predicts survival and has the advantage of being independent of liver biopsy. However, the Mayo risk score was calculated based on a population of patients with PBC, 73% of whom had advanced fibrosis and hence its validity is those diagnosed with PBC 20 years after the score was calculated is uncertain. It depends on age, serum bilirubin, albumin and prothrombin time, and the presence or absence of oedema (http://www.mayoclinic.org/gi-rst/mayomodel1.html) [75]. An optimal timing for liver transplantation, as determined by patient survival and resource utilization, appears to be at a Mayo risk score around 8.0. The use of the Mayo model to predict survival remains valid in patients treated with UDCA.

No model can yield a precise estimate of survival for the individual patient. They cannot predict a life-threatening episode such as bleeding varices. A Mayo risk score of more than 4.0 is an independent predictor of oesophageal varices [19].

The patient with end-stage PBC should be considered for possible liver transplantation. Prognosis is particularly important in determining the best time for transplantation. The model for end-stage liver disease (MELD) formula [76] can be used to predict short-term survival. A MELD score more than 16 indicates a survival benefit from transplantation in PBC. Patients should be considered by a transplant centre when the serum bilirubin level approaches 100 µmol/L (6 mg/100 mL) [77] as the patient is unlikely to survive for more than 2 years. The MELD score does not perform better than the Child–Turcotte–Pugh score for patients with cirrhosis on the waiting list and cannot predict post-liver transplantation mortality [78].

Hepatic transplantation

Liver transplantation remains the only effective treatment for those with end-stage disease [79]. Indications are intractable pruritus, hepatic encephalopathy and end-stage liver disease with, for example, an episode of spontaneous bacterial peritonitis. The requirement for liver transplantation for end-stage PBC is falling in both Europe and North America [80]. Survival after transplant is more than 90% at 1 year and more than 80% at 5 years. Graft survival is lower.

Pruritus resolves rapidly after hepatic transplantation but fatigue persists.

Disease recurs in the transplanted liver in 17% of patients at a mean of 3.7 years. It is diagnosed by characteristic histology. Antimitochondrial antibodies are not lost following liver transplant. Ursodeoxycholic acid can be used and some patients have a biochemical response [81], but there is no evidence it alters disease progression. The type of immunosuppression used may be a factor in disease recurrence [82,83]. The consequences of recurrent disease are usually small; very few patients are retransplanted for recurrent PBC.

References

1 Addison T, Gull W. On a certain affection of the skin—vitiligoidea—alpha plana, beta tuberosa. *Guy's Hosp. Rep.* 1851; **7**: 265.

2 Hanot V. *Etude sur une Forme de Cirrhose Hypertrophique de Foie (Cirrhose Hypertrophique avec Ictère Chronique)*. Paris: Baillière, 1876.

3 Ahrens EH Jr, Payne MA, Kunkel HG *et al.* Primary biliary cirrhosis. *Medicine* 1950; **29**: 299–364.

4 Sherlock S, Scheuer PJ. The presentation and diagnosis of 100 patients with primary biliary cirrhosis. *N. Engl. J. Med.* 1973; **289**: 674–678.

5 Sakauchi F, Mori M, Zeniya M *et al.* A cross-sectional study of primary biliary cirrhosis in Japan: utilization of clinical data when patients applied to receive public financial aid. *J. Epidemiol.* 2005; **15**: 24–28.

6 Laurin JM, DeSotel CK, Jorgensen RA *et al.* The natural history of abdominal pain associated with primary biliary cirrhosis. *Am. J. Gastroenterol.* 1994; **89**: 1840–1843.

7 Cauch-Dudek K, Abbey S, Stewart DE *et al.* Fatigue in primary biliary cirrhosis. *Gut* 1998; **43**: 705–710.

8 Prince M, Chetwynd A, Newman W *et al.* Survival and symptom progression in a geographically based cohort of patients with primary biliary cirrhosis; follow up for up to 28 years. *Gastroenterology* 2002; **123**: 1392–1394.

9 Hennes EM, Zeniya M, Czaja AJ *et al.* Simplified criteria for the diagnosis of autoimmune hepatitis. *Hepatology* 2008; **48**: 169–176.

10 Sakauchi F, Oura A, Ohnishi H *et al.* Comparison of the clinical features of Japanese patients with primary biliary cirrhosis in 1999 and 2004: utilization of clinical data when patients applied to receive public financial aid. *J. Epidemiol.* 2007; **17**: 210–214.

11 Long RG, Scheuer PJ, Sherlock S. Presentation and course of asymptomatic primary biliary cirrhosis. *Gastroenterology* 1977; **72**: 1204–1207.

12 Prince MI, Chetwynd A, Craig WL *et al.* Asymptomatic primary biliary cirrhosis: clinical features, prognosis, and symptom progression in a large population based cohort. *Gut* 2004; **53**: 865–870.

13 Sherlock S. Primary biliary cirrhosis (chronic intrahepatic obstructive jaundice). *Gastroenterology* 1959; **31**: 574.

14 Gomez-Dominguez E, Mendoza J, Garcia-Buey L *et al.* Transient elastography to assess hepatic fibrosis in primary biliary cirrhosis. *Aliment. Pharmacol. Ther.* 2008; **27**: 441–447.

15 Jacoby A, Rannard A, Buck D *et al.* Development, validation, and evaluation of the PBC-40, a disease specific health related quality of life measure for primary biliary cirrhosis. *Gut* 2005; **54**: 1622–1629.

16 Jones DE, Bhala N, Burt J *et al.* Four year follow up of fatigue in a geographically defined primary biliary cirrhosis patient cohort. *Gut* 2006; **55**: 536–541.

17 Bjornsson E, Kalaitzakis E, Neuhauser M *et al.* Fatigue measurements in patients with primary biliary cirrhosis and the risk of mortality during follow-up. *Liver Int.* 2010; **30**: 251–258.

18 Solaymani-Dodaran M, Card TR, Aithal GP *et al.* Fracture risk in people with primary biliary cirrhosis: a population-based cohort study. *Gastroenterology* 2006; **131**: 1752–1757.

19 Levy C, Zein CO, Gomez J *et al.* Prevalence and predictors of esophageal varices in patients with primary biliary cirrhosis. *Clin. Gastroenterol. Hepatol.* 2007; **5**: 803–808.

20 Silveira MG, Suzuki A, Lindor KD. Surveillance for hepatocellular carcinoma in patients with primary biliary cirrhosis. *Hepatology* 2008; **48**: 1149–1156.

21 Walker JG, Doniach D, Roitt IM *et al.* Serological tests in the diagnosis of primary biliary cirrhosis. *Lancet* 1965; **i**: 827–831.

22 Gershwin ME, Mackay IR, Sturgess A *et al.* Identification and specificity of a cDNA encoding the 70 kD mitochondrial antigen recognized in primary biliary cirrhosis. *J. Immunol.* 1987; **138**: 3525–3531.

23 Yeaman SJ, Fussey SP, Danner DJ *et al.* Primary biliary cirrhosis: identification of two major M2 mitochondrial autoantigens. *Lancet* 1988; **i**: 1067–1070.

24 Fussey SPM, Guest JR, James OFW *et al.* Identification and analysis of the major M2 autoantigens in primary biliary cirrhosis. *Proc. Natl. Acad. Sci. USA* 1988; **85**: 8654–8658.

25 Quinn J, Diamond AG, Palmer JM *et al.* Lipoylated and unlipoylated domains of human PDC-E2 as autoantigens in primary biliary cirrhosis: significance of lipoate attachment. *Hepatology* 1993; **18**: 1384–1391.

26 Bruggraber SF, Leung PS, Amano K *et al.* Autoreactivity to lipoate and a conjugated form of lipoate in primary biliary cirrhosis. *Gastroenterology* 2003; **125**: 1705–1713.

27 Murphy JR, Sjogren MH, Kikendall JW *et al.* Small bile duct abnormalities in sarcoidosis. *J. Clin. Gastroenterol.* 1990; **12**: 555–561.

28 Neuhauser M, Bjornsson E, Treeprasertsuk S *et al.* Autoimmune hepatitis-PBC overlap syndrome: a simplified scoring system may assist in the diagnosis. *Am. J. Gastroenterol.* 2010; **105**: 345–353.

29 Gossard AA, Lindor KD. Development of autoimmune hepatitis in primary biliary cirrhosis. *Liver Int.* 2007; **27**: 1086–1090.

30 Rubin E, Schaffner F, Popper H. Primary biliary cirrhosis: chronic nonsuppurative destructive cholangitis. *Am. J. Pathol.* 1965; **46**: 387–407.

31 Corpechot C, Abenavoli L, Rabahi N *et al.* Biochemical response to ursodeoxycholic acid and long-term prognosis in primary biliary cirrhosis. *Hepatology* 2008; **48**: 871–877.

32 Scheuer PJ. Primary biliary cirrhosis. *Proc. Roy. Soc. Med.* 1967; **60**: 1257–1260.

33 Hohenester S, Oude-Elferink RP, Beuers U. Primary biliary cirrhosis. *Sem. Immunopathol.* 2009; **31**: 283–307.

34 Jones DE. Pathogenesis of primary biliary cirrhosis. *Gut* 2007; **56**: 1615–24.

35 Metcalf JV, Mitchison HC, Palmer JM *et al.* Natural history of early primary biliary cirrhosis. *Lancet* 1996; **348**: 1399–1402.

36 Lan RY, Salunga TL, Tsuneyama K *et al.* Hepatic IL-17 responses in human and murine primary biliary cirrhosis. *J. Autoimmunity* 2009; **32**: 43–51.

37 Tinmouth J, Lee M, Wanless IR *et al.* Apoptosis of biliary epithelial cells in primary biliary cirrhosis and primary sclerosing cholangitis. *Liver* 2002; **22**: 228–234.

38 Macdonald P, Palmer J, Kirby JA *et al.* Apoptosis as a mechanism for cell surface expression of the autoantigen pyruvate dehydrogenase complex. *Clin. Exp. Immunol.* 2004; **136**: 559–567.

39 Lleo A, Selmi C, Invernizzi P *et al.* Apotopes and the biliary specificity of primary biliary cirrhosis. *Hepatology* 2009; **49**: 871–879.

40 Walden HR, Kirby JA, Yeaman SJ *et al.* Xenobiotic incorporation into pyruvate dehydrogenase complex can occur via the exogenous lipoylation pathway. *Hepatology* 2008; **48**: 1874–1884.

41 Gershwin ME, Selmi C, Worman HJ *et al.* Risk factors and comorbidities in primary biliary cirrhosis: a controlled interview-based study of 1032 patients. *Hepatology* 2005; **42**: 1194–2002.

42 Amano K, Leung PS, Rieger R *et al.* Chemical xenobiotics and mitochondrial autoantigens in primary biliary cirrhosis: identification of antibodies against a common environmental, cosmetic, and food additive, 2-octynoic acid. *J. Immunol.* 2005; **174**: 5874–583.

43 Fussey SP, Ali ST, Guest JR *et al.* Reactivity of primary biliary cirrhosis sera with *Escherichia coli* dihydrolipoamide acetyltransferase (E2p): characterisation of the main immunogenic region. *Proc. Natl. Acad. Sci. USA* 1990; **87**: 3987–3991.

44 Tanimoto H, Shimoda S, Makanura M *et al.* Promiscuous T cells selected by *Escherichia coli*: OGDC-E2 in primary biliary cirrhosis. *J. Autoimmunity* 2003; **20**: 255–263.

45 Burroughs AK, Rosenstein I, Epstein O *et al.* Bacteriuria and Primary Biliary Cirrhosis. *GUT* 1984; **25**: 133–137.

46 Selmi C, Balkwill DL, Invernizzi P *et al.* Patients with primary biliary cirrhosis react against a ubiquitous xenobiotic-metabolizing bacterium. *Hepatology* 2003; **38**: 1250–1257.

47 Prince MI, Chetwynd A, Diggle P *et al.* The geographical distribution of primary biliary cirrhosis is a well-defined cohort. *Hepatology* 2001; **34**: 1083–1088.

48 McNally RJ, Ducker S, James OF. Are transient environmental agents involved in the cause of primary biliary cirrhosis? Evidence from space-time clustering analysis. *Hepatology* 2009; **50**: 1169–1174.

49 Jones DEJ, Watt FE, Metcalf JV *et al.* Familial primary biliary cirrhosis reassessed: a geographically-based population study. *J. Hepatol.* 1999; **30**: 402–407.

50 Selmi C, Mayo MJ, Bach N *et al.* Primary biliary cirrhosis in monozygotic and dizygotic twins: genetics, epigenetics and environment. *Gastroenterology* 2004; **127**: 485–492.

51 Hirschfield GM, Liu X, Xu C *et al.* Primary biliary cirrhosis associated with HLA, IL12A, and IL12RB2 variants. *N. Engl. J. Med.* 2009; **360**: 2544–2555.

52 Liu X, Invernizzi P, Lu Y *et al.* Genome-wide meta-analyses identify three loci associated with primary biliary cirrhosis. *Nature Genetics* 2010; **42**: 658–60.

53 Poupon R, Ping C, Chretien Y *et al.* Genetic factors of susceptibility and of severity in primary biliary cirrhosis. *J. Hepatol.* 2008; **49**: 1038–1045.

54 Lindor KD, Gershwin ME, Poupon RK *et al.* Primary biliary cirrhosis. *Hepatology* 2009; **50**: 291–308.

55 EASL Clinical Practice Guidelines: management of cholestatic liver diseases. *J. Hepatol.* 2009; **51**: 237–267.

56 Gong Y, Klingenberg SL, Gluud C. Systematic review and meta-analysis: D-Penicillamine vs. placebo/no intervention in patients with primary biliary cirrhosis–Cochrane Hepato-Biliary Group. *Aliment. Pharmacol. Ther.* 2006; **24**: 1535–1544.

57 Kuiper EM, Hansen BE, de Vries RA *et al.* Improved prognosis of patients with primary biliary cirrhosis that have a biochemical response to ursodeoxycholic acid. *Gastroenterology* 2009; **136**: 1281–1287.

58 Goulis J, Leandro G, Burroughs AK. Randomized trials of ursodeoxycholic acid in Primary Biliary Cirrhosis. *Lancet* 1999; **354**: 1053–1060.

59 Gong Y, Huang ZB, Christensen E *et al.* Ursodeoxycholic acid for primary biliary cirrhosis. *Cochrane Database of Sys. Rev.* 2008; **3**: CD000551.

60 Azemoto N, Abe M, Murata Y *et al.* Early biochemical response to ursodeoxycholic acid predicts symptom development in patients with asymptomatic primary biliary cirrhosis. *J. Gastroenterol.* 2009; **44**: 630–634.

61 Kikuchi K, Hsu W, Hosoya N *et al.* Ursodeoxycholic acid reduces CpG-induced IgM production in patients with primary biliary cirrhosis. *Hepatol. Res.* 2009; **39**: 448–454.

62 D'Aldebert E, Biyeyeme Bi Mve MJ, Mergey M *et al.* Bile salts control the antimicrobial peptide cathelicidin through nuclear receptors in the human biliary epithelium. *Gastroenterology* 2009; **136**: 1435–1443.

63 Rautiainen H, Karkkainen P, Karvonen AL *et al.* Budesonide combined with UDCA to improve liver histology in primary biliary cirrhosis: a three-year randomized trial. *Hepatology* 2005; **41**: 747–752.

64 Iwasaki S, Ohira H, Nishiguchi S *et al.* The efficacy of ursodeoxycholic acid and bezafibrate combination therapy for primary biliary cirrhosis: A prospective, multicenter study. *Hepatol. Res.* 2008; **38**: 557–564.

65 Hazzan R, Tur-Kaspa R. Bezafibrate treatment of primary biliary cirrhosis following incomplete response to ursodeoxycholic acid. *J. Clin. Gastroenterol.* 2010; **44**: 371–373.

66 Jones DE, Newton JL. An open study of modafinil for the treatment of daytime somnolence and fatigue in primary biliary cirrhosis. *Aliment. Pharmacol. Ther.* 2007; **25**: 471–476.

67 Ian Gan S, de Jongh M, Kaplan MM. Modafinil in the treatment of debilitating fatigue in primary biliary cirrhosis: a clinical experience. *Dig. Dis. Sci.* 2009; **54**: 2242–22246.

68 Tandon P, Rowe BH, Vandermeer B *et al.* The efficacy and safety of bile Acid binding agents, opioid antagonists, or rifampin in the treatment of cholestasis-associated pruritus. *Am. J. Gastroenterol.* 2007; **102**: 1528–1536.

69 McRae CA, Prince MI, Hudson M *et al.* Pain as a complication of use of opiate antagonists for symptom control in cholestasis. *Gastroenterology* 2003; **125**: 591–596.

70 Zein CO, Jorgensen RA, Clarke B *et al.* Alendronate improves bone mineral density in primary biliary cirrhosis: a randomized placebo-controlled trial. *Hepatology* 2005; **42**: 762–771.

71 Jackson H, Solaymani-Dodaran M, Card TR *et al.* Influence of ursodeoxycholic acid on the mortality and malignancy associated with primary biliary cirrhosis: a population-based cohort study. *Hepatology* 2007; **46**: 1131–1137.

72 Myers RP, Shaheen AA, Fong A *et al.* Epidemiology and natural history of primary biliary cirrhosis in a Canadian health region: a population-based study. *Hepatology* 2009; **50**: 1884–1892.

73 Pares A, Caballeria L, Rodes J. Excellent long-term survival in patients with primary biliary cirrhosis and biochemical response to ursodeoxycholic Acid. *Gastroenterology* 2006; **130**: 715–720.

74 Chan CW, Tsochatzis EA, Carpenter JR *et al.* Predicting the advent of ascites and other complications in primary biliary cirrhosis: a multi-staged model approach. *Aliment. Pharmacol. Ther.* 2010; **31**: 573–582.

75 Dickson ER, Grambsch PM, Fleming TR *et al.* Prognosis in primary biliary cirrhosis: model for decision making. *Hepatology* 1989; **10**: 1–7.

76 Kamath PS, Wiesner RH, Malinchoc M *et al.* A model to predict survival in patients with end-stage liver disease. *Hepatology* 2001; **33**: 464–470.

77 Devlin J, O'Grady J. Indications for referral and assessment in adult liver transplantation: a clinical guideline. British Society of Gastroenterology. *Gut* 1999; **45** (Suppl. 6): VI1–VI22.

78 Cholongitas E, Marelli L, Shusang V *et al.* A systematic review of the performance of the model for end-stage liver disease (MELD) in the setting of liver transplantation. *Liver Transpl.* 2006; **12**: 1049–1061.

79 MacQuillan GC, Neuberger J. Liver transplantation for primary biliary cirrhosis. *Clin. Liver Dis.* 2003; **7**: 941–956, ix.

80 Lee J, Belanger A, Doucette JT *et al.* Transplantation trends in primary biliary cirrhosis. *Clin. Gastroenterol. Hepatol.* 2007; **5**: 1313–1315.

81 Charatcharoenwitthaya P, Pimentel S, Talwalkar JA *et al.* Long-term survival and impact of ursodeoxycholic acid treatment for recurrent primary biliary cirrhosis after liver transplantation. *Liver Transpl.* 2007; **13**: 1236–1245.

82 Neuberger J, Gunson B, Hubscher S *et al.* Immunosuppression affects the rate of recurrent primary biliary cirrhosis after liver transplantation. *Liver Transpl.* 2004; **10**: 488–491.

83 Manousou P, Arvaniti V, Tsochatzis E *et al.* Primary biliary cirrhosis after liver transplantation: Influence of immuno-suppression and human leukocyte antigen locus disparity. *Liver Transpl.* 2009; **16**: 64–73.

84 Sherlock S. Therapeutic trials in primary biliary cirrhosis. *Q. J. Med.* 1994; **87**: 701–703.

CHAPTER 16
Sclerosing Cholangitis

Simon Rushbrook[1] & Roger W. Chapman[2]

[1] Department of Gastroenterology, Norfolk and Norwich Hospital, Norwich, UK
[2] Department of Hepatology, John Radcliffe Hospital, Oxford, UK

Learning points

- There has been greater recognition of primary sclerosing cholangitis (PSC) with the advent of magnetic resonance cholangiopancreatography.

- Small-duct PSC has a more favourable prognosis.

- PSC is the major cause of liver disease in patients with inflammatory bowel disease.

- Symptomatic PSC has a poor prognosis in a predominantly young population.

- Preventive strategies are available for sepsis, colon cancer and osteopenia, but there is no curative therapy for PSC.

- The only option is liver transplantation but rarely for those patients with cholangiocarcinoma.

- Management of secondary sclerosing cholangitis depends on its cause.

Introduction

Primary sclerosing cholangitis (PSC) is a chronic disease of the intra- and/or extrahepatic bile ducts. It is characterized by a concentric, obliterative fibrosis that leads to bile duct strictures (Fig. 16.1). In many patients, this in turn progresses to biliary cirrhosis and hepatic failure. Approximately one-third of patients will develop cholangiocarcinoma [1]. PSC is frequently associated with inflammatory bowel disease (IBD), usually ulcerative colitis and those with Crohn's disease predominantly affecting the colon. Approximately three-quarters of Northern Europeans with PSC have concomitant IBD [2]. Patients, usually with IBD, who have normal cholangiography but typical histological features on liver biopsy are diagnosed as small-duct PSC.

The term 'secondary sclerosing cholangitis' is used for a disease where there are similar radiological and histologic features to PSC, but where another cause for the biliary disease can be identified (Table 16.1).

Primary sclerosing cholangitis

Epidemiology

Little is known about the incidence and prevalence of PSC, as good epidemiological studies are extremely difficult to perform.

The true prevalence of PSC associated with IBD is unknown; the estimated prevalence of PSC in patients with ulcerative colitis is 2.5–7.5%. In the USA, based on a prevalence of ulcerative colitis of 40-225 cases per 100000, the prevalence of PSC has been estimated by extrapolation to be two to seven cases per 100000 population. These figures, however, probably underestimate the actual prevalence of PSC, as the disease can occur in patients with normal serum levels of alkaline phosphatase, and 20–30% of patients with PSC have no associated IBD.

Population studies from the Northern Hemisphere have shown an annual incidence of PSC of 0.9–1.3/100000 person-years and point prevalence of 8.5–13.6/100000. This figure appears to be increasing [1–3]. The study from a population in Olmstead County, Minnesota, USA, estimated a prevalence of 20.9 per 100000 men and 6.3 per 100000 women. In a similar report from South Wales, UK, the point prevalence was 12.7 cases per 100000 persons and the annual incidence was calculated at 0.91 cases per 100000, both very similar to the US data [2].

The higher prevalence of PSC found in more recent studies might be attributed to a more complete capture of incident and prevalent cases, and to a higher rate of liver transplantation among prevalent cases (ascertainment bias). It may not reflect a true increase in prevalence. Also easier access to cholangiography provided by magnetic resonance cholangiopancreatography (MRCP) scanning may be playing a part.

Small-duct PSC occurs in about 10% of a PSC population (see below). A study in Canada has shown an incidence of small-duct PSC as 0.15/100000 [4].

Sherlock's Diseases of the Liver and Biliary System, Twelfth Edition. Edited by James S. Dooley, Anna S.F. Lok, Andrew K. Burroughs, E. Jenny Heathcote.
© 2011 by Blackwell Publishing Ltd. Published 2011 by Blackwell Publishing Ltd.

Smoking

Cigarette smoking has been recognized as a protective factor against the development of ulcerative colitis. It may also protect against the development of PSC, unlike primary biliary cirrhosis [1]. This protective effect was more marked in patients with PSC than ulcerative colitis, and interestingly was observed in patients with and without IBD. The mechanism of protection in both disorders remains unknown.

Prevalence of IBD in PSC, and PSC in IBD

In Scandinavia, UK and the USA, 70–80% of those with PSC also have coexisting IBD. In reports from Spain,

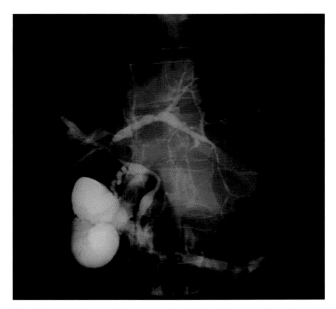

Fig. 16.1. Endoscopic retrograde cholangiogram showing dilatation and stricturing of the extra and intrahepatic biliary tree—the typical changes of primary sclerosing cholangitis.

Italy, India and Japan the prevalence of IBD in PSC is 37–50% although very few underwent total colonoscopy and colonic biopsy [5–8].

Conversely, only 2–7.5% of those with IBD have PSC [9]. However, this is very likely to be an underestimate. As pointed out above, patients with PSC proven on radiological imaging may have normal liver biochemical tests.

Both the development of PSC and its outcome are independent of the activity of colitis. PSC may even occur after proctocolectomy. Similarly IBD may present many years after liver transplant for PSC. The natural history of IBD in patients with PSC, although usually involving the whole colon, has a more benign course than in those patients with IBD alone [10].

Colitis associated with PSC may be a separate disease entity as there is a higher prevalence of rectal sparing in those with PSC (52%) than in those with ulcerative colitis alone (6%). Moreover backwash ileitis occurs in 51% of patients with colitis and PSC, versus only 7% for those with colitis alone [11,12].

It is not known why patients with PSC who have undergone pouch surgery for their ulcerative colitis have a higher rate of pouchitis than those without PSC (63 versus 32%) [13]. Likewise, why colonic resection prior to liver transplant eliminates the risk of recurrent PSC is unknown.

Aetiology and pathogenesis

Immunogenic factors

It has been suggested that PSC results from a maladaptive immune/autoimmune response. This hypothesis is supported by the association with specific human leucocyte antigen (HLA) haplotypes; polymorphisms of other genes involved in the immune response; autoantibodies in serum; and the link with IBD and the consequent 'leaking gut' syndrome [14].

Table 16.1. Causes and mimics of secondary sclerosing cholangitis

Causes
Surgical trauma to bile ducts (with associated cholangitis)
Ischaemic injury, e.g. hepatic artery thrombosis after transplantation, or trans arterial chemotherapy, HHT, PVT
Bile duct gallstones (may be due to *MDR3* mutation)
Viral or bacterial infection, e.g. CMV or cryptosporidiosis, severe sepsis
Caustic injury, e.g. formalin treatment of hydatid cyst
IgG4 associated autoimmune pancreatitis
Mimics on cholangiography
Malignancy, e.g. metastatic carcinoma
Hypereosinophilic syndrome
Polycystic liver disease
Cystic fibrosis
Cirrhosis

HHT, hereditary haemorrhagic telangiectasia; PVT, portal vein thrombosis.

Table 16.2. Key HLA haplotypes associated with primary sclerosing cholangitis (PSC) [1,17]

Haplotype	Association with disease
B8-TNF*2-DRB3*0101-DRB1*0301-DQA1*0501-DQB1*0201	Strong with susceptibility
DRB3*0101-DRB1*1301-DQA1*0103-DQB1*0603	Strong with susceptibility
DRB5*0101-DRB1*1501-DQA1*0102-DQB1*0602	Weak with susceptibility
DRB4*0103-DRB1*0401-DQA1*03-DQB1*0302	Strong with protection against disease
MICA*008	Strong with susceptibility

Table 16.3. Serum autoantibodies in primary sclerosing cholangitis

Antibody*	Prevalence (%)
Antineutrophil cytoplasmic antibodies	33–88
Antinuclear antibody	7–77
Antismooth muscle antibody	13–20
Antiendothelial cell antibody	35
Anticardiolipin antibody	4–66
Thyroperoxidase	7–16
Thyroglobulin	4
Rheumatoid factor	15

*Antimitochondrial antibody is only rarely detected in PSC (<1%). This is useful in differentiating primary sclerosing cholangitis from primary biliary cirrhosis.

There is an increased frequency of the HLA A1 B8 DR3 DRW 52A haplotype in PSC compared with healthy controls. HLA DR2 and HLA DR6 are also associated with PSC. HLA DR4 appears to be less common in PSC populations and may be protective (Table 16.2).

There are other genes outside the HLA region that may play a role in the pathogenesis of PSC. Genome-wide association studies are in progress to identify possible susceptibility genes.

No specific autoantigens have been identified in relation to PSC, although smooth muscle antibodies, antinuclear antibodies and antineutrophil cytoplasmic antibodies (pANCA) are often detected in serum (Table 16.3). A high prevalence of pANCA (33–88%) has been found in patients with PSC, but this autoantibody is not specific to PSC [14]. pANCA is found in ulcerative colitis alone (60–87%), in patients with type I autoimmune hepatitis (50–96%) [15,16] and in primary biliary cirrhosis. Thus it is unlikely that this antibody is involved in the pathogenesis of PSC, and it is not a useful screening test.

PSC is associated, in 25% of patients, with other autoimmune conditions such as diabetes mellitus, celiac and autoimmune thyroid disease (Graves' disease). Rheumatoid arthritis has also been described in association with PSC and may be a clinical marker for those at high risk of rapid progression to cirrhosis [17].

One hypothesis to explain the association between colonic and liver disease is that PSC is mediated by long-lived memory T cells derived from the inflamed gut, which enter the portal circulation and thence reach the liver [14,18]. Aberrant expression of chemokines and adhesion molecules on hepatic endothelial cells may recruit these T cells to the liver. This, in turn, may lead to biliary inflammation, fibrosis and bile duct stricturing.

Infections

Potentially, infectious agents could lead to the development of PSC but to date there is no secure evidence for any of the putative infectious agent studied, including viruses and parasites.

The association of PSC with IBD led to the hypothesis that colonic bacteria plus activated lymphocytes enter the portal circulation through a leaky diseased mucosa [14,18]. Chemokines and cytokines released from within the liver attract macrophages/monocytes, lymphocytes, activated neutrophils and fibroblasts to the site of inflammation. In genetically susceptible individuals, bacterial antigens may act as molecular mimics and cause an immune reaction responsible for initiating PSC.

Clinical features

Nowadays, most individuals with PSC are asymptomatic. Symptoms, when present, are non-specific and relate to cholestasis, for example pruritus, right upper abdominal quadrant pain, fatigue and weight loss. In a few, episodes of fever and chills are predominant. A minority present for the first time with decompensated cirrhosis and portal hypertension, that is ascites and variceal haemorrhage. Nevertheless, hepatomegaly and splenomegaly are the most frequent abnormal physical findings on clinical examination at the time of diagnosis.

Osteopenic bone disease is both a complication of advanced PSC and IBD. Steatorrhoea and malabsorption of fat-soluble vitamins occur only with prolonged cholestasis with jaundice. Presentation with jaundice is uncommon and it is often associated with the presence of underlying cholangiocarcinoma. IgG4-associated sclerosing cholangitis often presents with jaundice, and should be actively excluded by serology and/or histological assessment.

Diagnosis

Laboratory investigations

The finding of cholestatic liver biochemistries, an elevated alkaline phosphatase and γ-glutamyl transpeptidase, in an asymptomatic individual with IBD is suggestive of PSC. Blood tests typically fluctuate over time and some may even return completely to normal.

Autoantibody tests (see above) are of little diagnostic significance. IgM concentrations are increased in about 50% of patients with advanced PSC. The IgG4 level should be measured in all patients with suspected PSC; raised levels are detected in about 10% and associated with a worse outcome if left unrecognized and thus untreated [19].

Radiological features

The diagnosis of PSC depends on typical abnormalities shown on cholangiography. These are diffuse stricturing of intrahepatic and extrahepatic bile ducts with dilatation of the areas between strictures, causing a 'beaded' appearance of the biliary tree. MRCP is the investigation of choice over endoscopic retrograde cholangiopancreatography (ERCP) (Fig. 16.2). MRCP is non-invasive, does not involve radiation and is comparable to ERCP for diagnosis of PSC with good interobserver agreement [20–22]. ERCP should be reserved for either therapeutic purposes or to facilitate diagnosis of cholangiocarcinoma in those with 'suspicious' lesions on MRCP. ERCP

may still have a place in patients where the diagnosis remains uncertain after MRCP. Note that the cholangiographic characteristics can be identical in secondary sclerosing cholangitis, and the clinician should be alert to this possibility, even though unusual.

Histology

Histological examination of the liver is not required to make a diagnosis of primary or secondary cholangitis if the radiological findings show the typical changes described above.

The characteristic early pathological findings of PSC are periductal 'onion-skin' fibrosis and inflammation, with portal oedema and bile ductular proliferation resulting in expansion of portal tracts (Fig. 16.3). The early changes of any cause of sclerosing cholangitis may be focal and non-specific. Later, the fibrotic process progresses, leading to the end-stage of biliary cirrhosis. The severity of fibrosis, however, varies throughout the liver and thus 'staging' degree of fibrosis with liver biopsy is very unreliable [23]. In advanced cases, loss of bile ducts can lead to a 'vanishing bile duct syndrome'. Histology is diagnostic in only one–third, although in another third there may be findings suggestive of biliary disease. Patients with small-duct sclerosing cholangitis have normal cholangiograms with characteristic liver histology of PSC.

Colonoscopy

Since coexisting IBD may be asymptomatic, all patients given a diagnosis of PSC and not already known to have IBD should undergo colonoscopy with multiple biopsies.

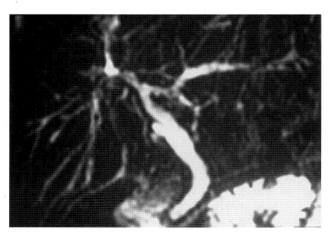

Fig. 16.2. Magnetic resonance cholangiogram showing multiple stricturing and dilatation, the typical changes of sclerosing cholangitis.

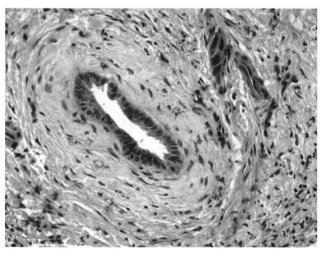

Fig. 16.3. Histology: liver biopsy showing 'onion skin' periductal fibrosis, typical of sclerosing cholangitis.

Special populations

Small-duct PSC

Patients who have cholestatic liver biochemistries and features consistent with a diagnosis of sclerosing cholangitis on liver biopsy, but who have a normal cholangiogram, are described as having small-duct PSC. Of the PSC population 6–16% have small-duct disease [24–26]. For the most part, the course of their disease is milder than for large-duct disease. There is a more favourable prognosis with regard to patient survival, need for transplantation and the development of cholangiocarcinoma. To date, no cases of cholangiocarcinoma have been reported in association with small-duct disease. Over a 10-year follow-up, a quarter of these patients develop typical changes of large-duct PSC on cholangiography [27–31].

Autoimmune hepatitis and sclerosing cholangitis

Patients with simultaneous or sequential PSC and autoimmune hepatitis have been described [32,33]. This has been reported more often in children than adults. Overlap should be considered if the transaminases are greater than twice the upper limit of normal and the serum IgG is elevated. Liver histology will show the diagnostic feature of prominent interface hepatitis. Immunosuppression, particularly in children, appears to be helpful [19,34,35].

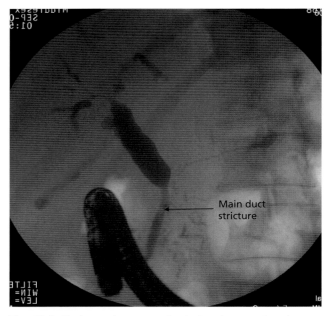

Fig. 16.4. Endoscopic retrograde cholangiogram showing long distal biliary stricture (arrow) with intrahepatic stricturing and dilatation, the typical appearance of IgG4 associated cholangitis.

IgG4-associated cholangitis

IgG4 associated disease is a multisystem disorder which may involve the pancreas, kidneys, lungs, thyroid, retroperitoneal lymph nodes, salivary glands and aorta. Some patients with IgG4 associated autoimmune pancreatitis have biliary strictures. These are often distal but may involve the entire biliary tree similar to PSC (IgG4-associated cholangiography) (Fig. 16.4) [36]. In this male-predominant disease, serum IgG4 levels are variably increased. Importantly, the disease is responsive to steroids. A retrospective study has shown elevated IgG4 levels in a small (9%) proportion of patients with PSC. This untreated subgroup appear to have a more severe disease course with higher bilirubin and alkaline phosphatase, and shorter time to transplant, than PSC patients with a normal IgG4 level. It is possible that these patients really have IgG4-associated systemic disease and therefore may respond to corticosteroid therapy, but this needs further study [19].

Management of complications

The management of the non-hepatic complications of cholestasis that may occur in PSC (pruritus, fatigue and osteoporosis) are discussed elsewhere (see Chapter 11).

Dysplasia and cancer

Patients with ulcerative colitis have an increased risk of colorectal cancer, associated with longevity of disease and the extent of colitis. The risk of colonic dysplasia and colorectal cancer is enhanced in those with coexistent PSC [37–39]. Thus patients with ulcerative colitis and PSC should undergo regular, annual surveillance colonoscopy once the diagnosis of PSC is made. This risk continues after liver transplantation and increases with time [40–42].

Ursodeoxycholic acid (UDCA) treatment in patients with PSC and ulcerative colitis may decrease the risk of colorectal dysplasia and colorectal cancer [43,44].

Cholangiocarcinoma will complicate the clinical course in 8–30% of adult patients with PSC, and can develop in either the intra- or extrahepatic bile ducts [45]. A third of patients with PSC who develop cholangiocarcinoma are diagnosed within 1 year of the diagnosis of their PSC. The incidence of cholangiocarcinoma is approximately 0.5–1.5% per year in those with large-duct PSC.

Symptoms of cholangiocarcinoma are non-specific and include jaundice, weight loss, abdominal pain and, rarely, recurrent cholangitis. Early detection of cholangiocarcinoma is difficult. Unfortunately, computed tomography (CT), ultrasonography and MRCP have poor sensitivity for detecting such tumours [46]. An elevated

CA19-9 (>200 U/L), weight loss as well as presence of a dominant bile duct stricture are suggestive of malignancy. However, CA19-9 has no role in cancer surveillance in PSC since it can be elevated in benign biliary disease as well as other malignancies, including pancreas, colon, stomach and gynaecological cancers [47–49].

Cholangiocarcinoma may be indistinguishable on cholangiography from a benign dominant stricture. Diagnosis is difficult and brush cytology and endoscopic biopsy may need to be performed [50,51]. Survival is poor with a median time to death of 7 months from diagnosis [52]. Most patients are treated palliatively, which may include biliary stenting and photodynamic therapy.

Other hepatobiliary malignancies, particularly gallbladder and hepatocellular carcinoma [53,54], are frequently seen in PSC (Table 16.4). Gallbladder polyps are a risk factor for gallbladder cancer in PSC. HCC are treated conventionally within the accepted criteria. The risk of pancreatic carcinomas (which may be misdiagnosed in patients with autoimmune pancreatitis and cholangitis) may also be increased in PSC [55].

Hepatobiliary malignancy is only detected in a proportion of those in whom it is suspected [56]. This needs to be taken into account when performing and interpreting cholangiograms. Additional risk factors for hepatobiliary cancer include smoking, long duration of IBD and male sex [57].

Other biliary complications

Biliary strictures. Dominant strictures of major bile ducts may develop in patients with PSC and with time. They may cause biliary obstruction and severe cholestasis, but the exact prevalence is unknown there being no population-based studies [58]. Endoscopic balloon dilatation, with or without stent placement may provide relief of symptoms and may improve survival without transplant [59,60]. Dominant strictures are associated with recurrent bacterial cholangitis as well as biliary

Table 16.4. Relative risk for first cancer after diagnosis of primary sclerosing cholangitis (excluding first year after PSC diagnosis)

Site of cancer	Relative risk	95% Confidence ratio
Oesophagus	0.0	0–34.2
Stomach	2.5	0.1–14.1
Small intestine	0.0	0–56.8
Colorectal	6.8	2.7–14
Hepatobiliary	106.9	72.6–151.7
Pancreas	9.7	2–28.4

Modified from Bergquist A *et al.* 2002 [55].

sludge and stones. Before biliary procedures patients should be given antibiotics, such as the quinolone, ciprofloxacin 750 mg, orally approximately 2 h before hand. Thus injecting contrast into an obstructed duct with poor drainage can precipitate acute cholangitis. Other risks of ERCP include pancreatitis, haemorrhage or bile duct perforation.

Recurrent bacterial cholangitis. This is rare in PSC in the absence of previous biliary interventional procedures. It should be treated with broad-spectrum antibiotics such as ciprofloxacin. Prophylaxis using oral quinolones may decrease the frequency of episodes in those with recurrent attacks. All patients should know to rapidly report to Casualty (Emergency Room) should they develop fever and/or chills.

Biliary stones. Choledocholithiasis probably occurs secondary to chronic bacterial contamination of bile. Characteristically the stones are small, and of the mixed brown pigment type. Stones and sludge may be removed by therapeutic ERCP.

Medical treatment

In general, medical therapies, including immunosuppressive agents and antifibrotic therapy, have proved to be disappointing in the treatment of PSC.

UDCA is a naturally occurring bile acid that improves liver biochemistries in PSC. Its effect, however, on survival remains controversial. A recent randomized control study employing high doses, 25–30 mg/kg, of UDCA in patients with advanced PSC was halted before completion because of the greater need for liver transplant and higher death rate in the UDCA group [61,62]. UDCA may, however, decrease the risk of developing colorectal dysplasia in patients with PSC and ulcerative colitis [43,44]. UDCA may also reduce the incidence of biliary tract cancers but this needs further study [53,62].

There is little evidence that steroids are beneficial in patients with PSC, except for those patients with features of both PSC and autoimmune hepatitis, which is more commonly observed in children [33–35]. Steroids are beneficial in those with IgG4-associated autoimmune pancreatitis/autoimmune cholangitis—hence the need to screen for this in all with presumed PSC.

Prognosis

Taking all patients with PSC the estimated median survival from diagnosis to death or liver transplant is 9.6–12 years [63–66]. Patients who are asymptomatic at diagnosis (the majority of whom will develop progressive disease) have a mean survival rate of 88% at 5 years and greater than 70% at 16 years after diagnosis [67,68].

Those who are symptomatic at diagnosis have shorter survival. A persistently raised serum bilirubin for more than 3 months duration from diagnosis is an independent risk factor correlating with poor outcome and high risk of cholangiocarcinoma.

Survival models have been used to evaluate therapy, to stratify patients in clinical trials and to define the time for liver transplantation. The Mayo Clinic model is based on a cohort of 406 patients and uses serum bilirubin, histological stage and the presence of splenomegaly. It may be particularly useful in early cases [67]. The Swedish prognostic model is based on 305 patients and uses age, serum bilirubin and histological stage as bad prognostic features [64]. Cholangiocarcinoma was found at surgery in 8%, and 44% were asymptomatic at the time of its diagnosis.

The Child–Pugh classification was found to be a satisfactory alternative to disease-specific models in both research studies and clinical decision making [68]. Because of the great variability of the disease, models are of less use in individual cases than in primary biliary cirrhosis. These models do not identify the patient with cholangiocarcinoma [64].

Hepatic transplantation

Liver transplantation is still the only treatment option for PSC in those who develop advanced disease. The indications for transplantation and the timing may be difficult as the disease course is unpredictable. Traditionally, the presence of cholangiocarcinoma is a contraindication to transplant; it is usually diagnosed late and patients often have advanced liver disease. One study showed a 5-year survival post-transplant of around 35% for those in whom cholangiocarcinoma was discovered incidentally at operation [53,69]. The prior diagnosis of cholangiocarcinoma is considered an absolute contradiction to liver transplantation, unless the tumour is small and brachytherapy has been given.

Recurrent PSC following liver transplantation is well recognized and seen within 5 years in 10–20% of patients. It is more common in males with an intact colon, and in those who require high-dose prednisone therapy early post-transplant [70]. However, adequate immunosuppression should be maintained after orthotopic liver transplant as rejection is a risk factor for recurrent disease. There are no known therapies to delay the onset or slow the progression of recurrent PSC. However this is rarely responsible for failure of the transplanted organ [70,71].

The results of liver transplantation are good, with a 5-year survival post transplant of 75–80% [72,73]. Gastrointestinal symptoms present post-transplantation—they rarely improve and in most they worsen or stay stable. Ulcerative colitis may even develop *de novo*

[74,75]. Prior IBD may become more severe post-transplant, prompting proctocolectomy, and 5–10% of those with IBD develop colorectal cancer after liver transplantation [76,77]. Thus, annual surveillance colonoscopy is recommended in this particularly high-risk group.

Secondary sclerosing cholangitis

There are several causes of secondary sclerosing cholangitis (Table 16.1) [78], the more common of which are described here.

Vascular cholangitis

The bile ducts are richly supplied by the hepatic artery which forms a peribiliary vascular plexus. Interference with blood flow in these very small vessels leads to ischaemic necrosis of the bile ducts, both extra- and intrahepatic, and to their ultimate disappearance. Injury to hepatic arterial branches, for instance during cholecystectomy or hepatic artery thrombosis or ischaemic reperfusion injury post-transplant, leads to ischaemia of the duct wall, damage to the ductal mucosa and entry of bile into the duct wall so causing fibrosis and stricture [79].

Biliary ischaemia secondary to intimal thickening of hepatic arterioles is a rare feature of chronic allograft rejection in man.

Diffuse small-vessel arteritis, part of a systemic vasculitis, can be followed by bile duct loss. Other causes of reduced blood flow in the hepatobiliary plexus include portal vein thrombosis, hereditary haemorrhagic telangiectasia and patients with severe sepsis in the intensive care unit [80].

Floxuridine (5-FUDR) can be infused by pump into the hepatic artery for the treatment of colorectal hepatic metastases. Biliary strictures can follow [81,82]. The picture resembles PSC.

Bacterial cholangitis

Bacterial cholangitis is rare in the absence of mechanical, usually partial, biliary obstruction. The damaged ducts show infiltration of their walls with neutrophils and destruction of the epithelium. Ultimately, the bile duct is replaced by a fibrous cord. Causes include choledocholithiasis, biliary strictures and stenosis of biliary–enteric anastomoses. The bile duct loss is irreversible and a point comes when, even if the cause of the biliary obstruction can be removed, for instance common duct stones, the bile duct destruction with biliary cirrhosis persists.

If the common bile or hepatic duct is surgically anastomosed to a poorly emptying loop of bowel, continued access of gut organisms to the biliary system can result in bacterial cholangitis without biliary obstruction (sump syndrome). A similar sequence may follow sphincteroplasty.

The sclerosing cholangitis associated with infection by the Chinese liver fluke (*Clonorchis sinensis*) is related to secondary infection, usually with *E. coli*, following biliary obstruction due to the fluke. Multiple pyogenic abscesses, particularly problematic in those with recurrent bacterial cholangitis, may lead to cholangiographic similarities with sclerosing cholangitis (Fig. 16.5) [83].

Immunodeficiency-related opportunistic cholangitis

Opportunistic organisms can invade the bile ducts causing the picture of sclerosing cholangitis. There is usually a background of immunodeficiency which may be congenital or acquired [78].

In the neonate, cytomegalovirus and reovirus type III have a tropism for bile epithelium and an obliterative cholangitis results.

Immunodeficiency syndromes associated with sclerosing cholangitis include familial combined immunodeficiency, hyperimmunoglobulin M immunodeficiency [84], X-linked immunodeficiency [85] and immunodeficiency with transient T-cell abnormalities [86,87]. The usual causative organism is cytomegalovirus or cryptosporidia alone or in combination (Fig. 16.6). *Cryptococcus*,

Candida albicans and *Klebsiella pneumoniae* may be associated [86].

Abnormalities of the biliary system are associated with AIDS [87,88]. In one series, 20 of 26 patients with AIDS and biliary problems had markedly abnormal cholangiograms. In 14 of these, the pattern was that of intrahepatic sclerosing cholangitis with or without papillary stenosis. The combination of intrahepatic duct disease with papillary stenosis is unique to AIDS cholangiography and has not been reported in PSC [78].

PSC and AIDS cholangiopathy differ according to the inflammatory infiltrate surrounding the diseased bile ducts. In PSC, it is rich in T_4 lymphocytes, the subpopulation specifically depleted in patients with AIDS [89].

Drug-related cholangitis

Caustic cholangitis is caused by the injection of a scolicidal solution into a hydatid cyst. Only a part of the biliary tree is usually affected [90]. Within months the strictures can result in jaundice, biliary cirrhosis and portal hypertension.

Histiocytosis X

A cholangiographic picture identical with that of sclerosing cholangitis may complicate histiocytosis X [91]. The biliary lesions progress from a hyperplastic to a granulomatous, xanthomatous and, finally, a fibrotic stage. Clinically, the picture resembles PSC.

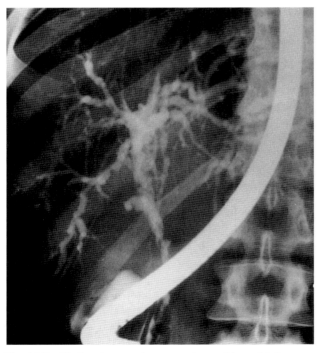

Fig. 16.5. Cholangiogram from a patient with multiple pyogenic liver abscesses showing strictured appearance similar to primary sclerosing cholangitis.

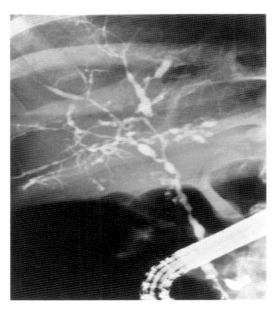

Fig. 16.6. Endoscopic retrograde cholangiogram from an immunodeficient patient infected with *Cryptosporidium*, showing the changes of secondary sclerosing cholangitis indistinguishable from primary sclerosing cholangitis.

References

1 Maggs JR, Chapman RW. An update on primary sclerosing cholangitis. *Curr. Opin. Gastroenterol.* 2008; **24**: 377–383.

2 Kingham JG, Kochar N, Gravenor MB. Incidence, clinical patterns, and outcomes of primary sclerosing cholangitis in South Wales, United Kingdom. *Gastroenterology* 2004; **126**: 1929–1930.

3 Bambha K, Kim WR, Talwalkar J *et al.* Incidence, clinical spectrum, and outcomes of primary sclerosing cholangitis in a United States community. *Gastroenterology* 2003; **125**: 1364–1369.

4 Kaplan GG, Laupland KB, Butzner D *et al.* The burden of large and small duct primary sclerosing cholangitis in adults and children: a population-based analysis. *Am. J. Gastroenterol.* 2007; **102**: 1042–1049.

5 Kochhar R, Goenka MK, Das K *et al.* Primary sclerosing cholangitis: an experience from India. *J. Gastroenterol. Hepatol.* 1996; **11**: 429–433.

6 Okolicsanyi L, Fabris L, Viaggi S *et al.* Primary sclerosing cholangitis: clinical presentation, natural history and prognostic variables: an Italian multicentre study. The Italian PSC Study Group. *Eur. J. Gastroenterol. Hepatol.* 1996; **8**: 685–691.

7 Escorsell A, Parés A, Rodés J *et al.* Epidemiology of primary sclerosing cholangitis in Spain. Spanish Association for the Study of the Liver. *J. Hepatol.* 1994; **21**: 787–791.

8 Takikawa H, Takamori Y, Tanaka A *et al.* Analysis of 388 cases of primary sclerosing cholangitis in Japan; Presence of a subgroup without pancreatic involvement in older patients. *Hepatol. Res.* 2004; **29**: 153–159.

9 Olsson R, Danielsson A, Järnerot G *et al.* Prevalence of primary sclerosing cholangitis in patients with ulcerative colitis. *Gastroenterology* 1991; **100**: 1319–1323.

10 Lundqvist K, Broome U. Differences in colonic disease activity in patients with ulcerative colitis with and without primary sclerosing cholangitis: a case control study. *Dis. Colon. Rectum.* 1997; **40**: 451–456.

11 Oshitani N, Jinno Y, Sawa Y *et al.* Does colitis associated with primary sclerosing cholangitis represent an actual subset of ulcerative colitis? *Hepatogastroenterology* 2003; **50**: 1830–1835.

12 Loftus EV Jr, Harewood GC, Loftus CG *et al.* PSC-IBD: a unique form of inflammatory bowel disease associated with primary sclerosing cholangitis. *Gut* 2005; **54**: 91–96.

13 Penna C, Dozois R, Tremaine W *et al.* Pouchitis after ileal pouch-anal anastomosis for ulcerative colitis occurs with increased frequency in patients with associated primary sclerosing cholangitis. *Gut* 1996; **38**: 234–239.

14 Adams DH, Eksteen B, Curbishley SM. Immunology of gut and liver: a love/hate relationship. *Gut* 2008; **57**: 838–847.

15 Terjung B, Worman HJ. Anti-neutrophil antibodies in primary sclerosing cholangitis. *Best. Pract. Res. Clin. Gastroenterol.* 2001; **15**: 629–642.

16 Lo SK, Fleming KA, Chapman RW. Prevalence of anti-neutrophil antibody in primary sclerosing cholangitis and ulcerative colitis using an alkaline phosphatase technique. *Gut* 1992; **33**: 1370–1375.

17 Gow PJ, Fleming KA, Chapman RW. Primary sclerosing cholangitis associated with rheumatoid arthritis and HLA DR4: is the association a marker of patients with progressive liver disease? *J. Hepatol.* 2001; **34**: 631–635.

18 Grant AJ, Lalor PF, Salmi M *et al.* Homing of mucosal lymphocytes to the liver in the pathogenesis of hepatic complications of inflammatory bowel disease. *Lancet* 2002; **359**: 150–157.

19 Mendes FD, Jorgensen R, Keach J *et al.* Elevated serum IgG4 concentration in patients with primary sclerosing cholangitis. *Am. J. Gastroenterol.* 2006; **101**: 2070–2075.

20 Moff SL, Kamel IR, Eustace J *et al.* Diagnosis of primary sclerosing cholangitis: a blinded comparative study using magnetic resonance cholangiography and endoscopic retrograde cholangiography. *Gastrointest. Endosc.* 2006; **64**: 219–223.

21 Berstad AE, Aabakken L, Smith HJ *et al.* Diagnostic accuracy of magnetic resonance and endoscopic retrograde cholangiography in primary sclerosing cholangitis. *Clin. Gastroenterol. Hepatol.* 2006; **4**: 514–520.

22 Fulcher AS, Turner MA, Franklin KJ *et al.* Primary sclerosing cholangitis: evaluation with MR cholangiography-a case-control study. *Radiology* 2000; **215**: 71–80.

23 Ludwig J. Surgical pathology of the syndrome of primary sclerosing cholangitis. *Am. J. Surg. Pathol.* 1989; **13** (Suppl. 1): 43–49.

24 Bhathal PS, Powell LW. Primary intrahepatic obliterating cholangitis: a possible variant of 'sclerosing cholangitis'. *Gut* 1969; **10**: 886–893.

25 Ludwig J, Barham SS, LaRusso NF *et al.* Morphologic features of chronic hepatitis associated with primary sclerosing cholangitis and chronic ulcerative colitis. *Hepatology* 1981; **1**: 632–640.

26 Wee A, Ludwig J. Pericholangitis in chronic ulcerative colitis: primary sclerosing cholangitis of the small bile ducts? *Ann. Intern. Med.* 1985; **102**: 581–587.

27 Boberg KM, Schrumpf E, Fausa O *et al.* Hepatobiliary disease in ulcerative colitis. An analysis of 18 patients with hepatobiliary lesions classified as small-duct primary sclerosing cholangitis. *Scand. J. Gastroenterol.* 1994; **29**: 744–752.

28 Angulo P, Maor-Kendler Y, Lindor KD. Small-duct primary sclerosing cholangitis: a long-term follow-up study. *Hepatology* 2002; **35**: 1494–1500.

29 Bjornsson E, Boberg KM, Cullen S *et al.* Patients with small duct primary sclerosing cholangitis have a favourable long term prognosis. *Gut* 2002; **51**: 731–735.

30 Broome U, Glaumann H, Lindstöm E *et al.* Natural history and outcome in 32 Swedish patients with small duct primary sclerosing cholangitis (PSC). *J. Hepatol.* 2002; **36**: 586–589.

31 Nikolaidis NL, Giouleme OI, Tziomalos KA *et al.* Small-duct primary sclerosing cholangitis. A single-center seven-year experience. *Dig. Dis. Sci.* 2005; **50**: 324–326.

32 Gohlke F, Lohse AW, Dienes HP *et al.* Evidence for an overlap syndrome of autoimmune hepatitis and primary sclerosing cholangitis. *J. Hepatol.* 1996; **24**: 699–705.

33 Wilschanski M, Chait P, Wade JA *et al.* Primary sclerosing cholangitis in 32 children: clinical, laboratory, and radiographic features, with survival analysis. *Hepatology* 1995; **22**: 1415–1422.

34 Abdalian R, Dhar P, Jhaveri K *et al.* Prevalence of sclerosing cholangitis in adults with autoimmune hepatitis; Evaluating the role of routine magnetic resonance imaging. *Hepatology* 2008; **47**: 949–957.

35 Gregorio GV, Portmann B, Karani J *et al.* Autoimmune hepatitis/sclerosing cholangitis overlap syndrome in childhood: a 16-year prospective study. *Hepatology* 2001; **33**: 544–553.

36 Webster G, Pereira S, Chapman RW. IgG4-associated cholangiography and primary sclerosing cholangitis: overlapping or separate diseases? *J. Hepatol.* 2009; **51**: 398–402.

37 Broome U, Lindberg G, Lofberg R. Primary sclerosing cholangitis in ulcerative colitis—a risk factor for the development of dysplasia and DNA aneuploidy? *Gastroenterology* 1992; **102**: 1877–1880.

38 Kornfeld D, Ekbom A, Ihre T. Is there an excess risk for colorectal cancer in patients with ulcerative colitis and concomitant primary sclerosing cholangitis? A population based study. *Gut* 1997; **41**: 522–525.

39 Brentnall TA, Haggitt RC, Rabinovitch PS *et al.* Risk and natural history of colonic neoplasia in patients with primary sclerosing cholangitis and ulcerative colitis. *Gastroenterology* 1996; **110**: 331–338.

40 Bleday R, Lee E, Jessurun J *et al.* Increased risk of early colorectal neoplasms after hepatic transplant in patients with inflammatory bowel disease. *Dis. Colon. Rectum* 1993; **36**: 908–912.

41 Higashi H, Yanaga K, Marsh JW *et al.* Development of colon cancer after liver transplantation for primary sclerosing cholangitis associated with ulcerative colitis. *Hepatology* 1990; **11**: 477–480.

42 Vera A, Gunson BK, Ussatoff V *et al.* Colorectal cancer in patients with inflammatory bowel disease after liver transplantation for primary sclerosing cholangitis. *Transplantation* 2003; **75**: 1983–1988.

43 Pardi DS, Loftus EV Jr, Kremers WK *et al.* Ursodeoxycholic acid as a chemopreventive agent in patients with ulcerative colitis and primary sclerosing cholangitis. *Gastroenterology* 2003; **124**: 889–893.

44 Tung BY, Emond MJ, Haggitt RC *et al.* Ursodiol use is associated with lower prevalence of colonic neoplasia in patients with ulcerative colitis and primary sclerosing cholangitis. *Ann. Intern. Med.* 2001; **134**: 89–95.

45 Prytz H, Keiding S, Björnsson E *et al.* Dynamic FDG-PET is useful for detection of cholangiocarcinoma in patients with PSC listed for liver transplantation. *Hepatology* 2006; **44**: 1572–1580.

46 Bergquist A, Glaumann H, Persson B *et al.* Risk factors and clinical presentation of hepatobiliary carcinoma in patients with primary sclerosing cholangitis: a case-control study. *Hepatology* 1998; **27**: 311–316.

47 Bjornsson E, Kilander A, Olsson R. CA 19-9 and CEA are unreliable markers for cholangiocarcinoma in patients with primary sclerosing cholangitis. *Liver* 1999; **19**: 501–508.

48 Lindberg B, Arnelo U, Bergquist A *et al.* Diagnosis of biliary strictures in conjunction with endoscopic retrograde cholangiopancreaticography, with special reference to patients with primary sclerosing cholangitis. *Endoscopy* 2002; **34**: 909–916.

49 Murray MD, Burton FR, Di Bisceglie AM. Markedly elevated serum CA 19-9 levels in association with a benign biliary stricture due to primary sclerosing cholangitis. *J. Clin. Gastroenterol.* 2007; **41**: 115–117.

50 Boberg KM, Jebsen P, Clausen OP *et al.* Diagnostic benefit of biliary brush cytology in cholangiocarcinoma in primary sclerosing cholangitis. *J. Hepatol.* 2006; **45**: 568–574.

51 Ponsioen CY, Vrouenraets SM, van Milligen de Wit AW *et al.* Value of brush cytology for dominant strictures in primary sclerosing cholangitis. *Endoscopy* 1999; **31**: 305–309.

52 Burak K, Angulo P, Pasha TM *et al.* Incidence and risk factors for cholangiocarcinoma in primary sclerosing cholangitis. *Am. J. Gastroenterol.* 2004; **99**: 523–526.

53 Leidenius M, Höckersted K, Broomé U *et al.* Hepatobiliary carcinoma in primary sclerosing cholangitis: a case control study. *J. Hepatol.* 2001; **34**: 792–798.

54 Buckles DC, Lindor KD, Larusso NF *et al.* In primary sclerosing cholangitis, gallbladder polyps are frequently malignant. *Am. J. Gastroenterol.* 2002; **97**: 1138–1142.

55 Bergquist A, Ekbom A, Olsson R *et al.* Hepatic and extrahepatic malignancies in primary sclerosing cholangitis. *J. Hepatol.* 2002; **36**: 321–327.

56 Brandsaeter B, Isoniemi H, Broomé U *et al.* Liver transplantation for primary sclerosing cholangitis; predictors and consequences of hepatobiliary malignancy. *J. Hepatol.* 2004; **40**: 815–822.

57 Tischendorf JJ, Meier PN, Strassburg CP *et al.* Characterization and clinical course of hepatobiliary carcinoma in patients with primary sclerosing cholangitis. *Scand. J. Gastroenterol.* 2006; **41**: 1227–1234.

58 Stiehl A, Rudolph G, Klöters-Plachky P *et al.* Development of dominant bile duct stenoses in patients with primary sclerosing cholangitis treated with ursodeoxycholic acid: outcome after endoscopic treatment. *J. Hepatol.* 2002; **36**: 151–156.

59 Bjornsson E, Olsson R. Dominant strictures in patients with primary sclerosing cholangitis-revisited. *Am. J. Gastroenterol.* 2004; **99**: 2281.

60 Baluyut AR, Sherman S, Lehman GA *et al.* Impact of endoscopic therapy on the survival of patients with primary sclerosing cholangitis. *Gastrointest. Endosc.* 2001; **53**: 308–312.

61 Lindor KD, Kowdley KV, Luketic VA *et al.* High dose ursodeoxycholic acid for the treatment of primary sclerosing cholangitis. *Hepatology* 2009; **50**: 808–814.

62 Chapman RW. High dose ursodeoxycholic acid in the reatment of primary sclerosing cholangitis. Throwing the urso out with the bathwater? *Hepatology* 2009; **50**: 671–673.

63 Tischendorf JJ, Hecker H, Krüger M *et al.* Characterization, outcome, and prognosis in 273 patients with primary sclerosing cholangitis: A single center study. *Am. J. Gastroenterol.* 2007; **102**: 107–114.

64 Broome U, Olsson R, Lööf L *et al.* Natural history and prognostic factors in 305 Swedish patients with primary sclerosing cholangitis. *Gut* 1996; **38**: 610–615.

65 Wiesner RH, Grambsch PM, Dickson ER *et al.* Primary sclerosing cholangitis: natural history, prognostic factors and survival analysis. *Hepatology* 1989; **10**: 430–436.

66 Farrant JM, Hayllar KM, Wilkinson ML *et al.* Natural history and prognostic variables in primary sclerosing cholangitis. *Gastroenterology* 1991; **100**: 1710–1717.

67 Dickson ER, Murtaugh PA, Wiesner RH *et al.* Primary sclerosing cholangitis: refinement and validation of survival models. *Gastroenterology* 1992; **103**: 1893–1901.

68 Shetty K, Rybicki L, Carey WD. The Child–Pugh classification as a prognostic indicator for survival in primary sclerosing cholangitis. *Hepatology* 1997; **25**: 1049–1053.

69 Goss JA, Shackleton CR, Farmer DG *et al.* Orthotopic liver transplantation for primary sclerosing cholangitis. A 12-year single center experience. *Ann. Surg.* 1997; **225**: 472–81; discussion 481–483.

70 Charatcharoenwitthaya P, Lindor KD. Recurrence of primary sclerosing cholangits. What do we learn from several transplant centres? *Liver Transpl.* 2008; **14**: 130–132.

71 Cholongitas E, Shusang V, Papatheodoridis GV *et al.* Risk factors for recurrence of primary sclerosing cholangitis after liver transplantation. *Liver Transpl.* 2008; **14**: 138–142.

72 Brandsaeter B, Friman S, Broomé U *et al.* Outcome following liver transplantation for primary sclerosing cholangitis in the Nordic countries. *Scand. J. Gastroenterol.* 2003; **38**: 1176–1183.

73 Roberts MS, Angus DC, Bryce CL *et al.* Survival after liver transplantation in the United States: a disease-specific analysis of the UNOS database. *Liver Transpl.* 2004; **10**: 886–897.

74 MacLean AR, Lilly L, Cohen Z *et al.* Outcome of patients undergoing liver transplantation for primary sclerosing cholangitis. *Dis. Colon Rectum* 2003; **46**: 1124–1128.

75 Riley TR, Schoen RE, Lee RG *et al.* A case series of transplant recipients who despite immunosuppression developed inflammatory bowel disease. *Am. J. Gastroenterol.* 1997; **92**: 279–282.

76 MacFaul GR, Chapman RW. Sclerosing cholangitis. *Curr. Opin. Gastroenterol.* 2004; **20**: 275–280.

77 Dvorchik I, Subotin M, Demetris AJ *et al.* Effect of liver transplantation on inflammatory bowel disease in patients with primary sclerosing cholangitis. *Hepatology* 2002; **35**: 380–384.

78 Abdalian R, Heathcote J. Sclerosing cholangitis: A focus on secondary causes. *Hepatology* 2006; **44**: 1063–1075.

79 Terblanche J, Allison HE, Northover JMA. An ischemic basis for biliary strictures. *Surgery* 1983; **94**: 52–57.

80 Zajko AB, Campbell WL, Logsdon GA *et al.* Cholangiographic findings in hepatic artery occlusion after liver transplantation. *AJR Am. J. Roentgenol.* 1987; **149**: 485–489.

81 Kemeny MM, Battifora H, Blayney DW *et al.* Sclerosing cholangitis after continuous hepatic artery infusion of FUDR. *Ann. Surg.* 1985; **202**: 176–181.

82 Ludwig J, Kim CH, Wiesner RH *et al.* Floxuridine-induced sclerosing cholangitis: an ischemic cholangiopathy? *Hepatology* 1989; **9**: 215–218.

83 Steinhart AH, Simons M, Stone R *et al.* Multiple hepatic abscesses: cholangiographic changes simulating sclerosing cholangitis and resolution after percutaneous drainage. *Am. J. Gastroenterol.* 1990; **85**: 306–308.

84 DiPalma JA, Strobel CT, Farrow JG. Primary sclerosing cholangitis associated with hyperimmunoglobulin M immunodeficiency (dysgammaglobulinemia). *Gastroenterology* 1986; **91**: 464–468.

85 Naveh Y, Mendelsohn H, Spira G *et al.* Primary sclerosing cholangitis associated with immunodeficiency. *Am. J. Dis. Child.* 1983; **137**: 114–117.

86 Davis JJ, Heyman MB, Ferrell L *et al.* Sclerosing cholangitis associated with chronic cryptosporidiosis in a child with a congenital immunodeficiency disorder. *Am. J. Gastroenterol.* 1987; **82**: 1196–1202.

87 Gremse DA, Bucuvalas JC, Bongiovanni GL. Papillary stenosis and sclerosing cholangitis in an immunodeficient child. *Gastroenterology* 1989; **96**: 1600–1603.

88 Cockerill FR, Hurley DV, Malagelada JR *et al.* Polymicrobial cholangitis and Kaposi's sarcoma in blood product transfusion-related acquired immune deficiency syndrome. *Am. J. Med.* 1986; **80**: 1237–1241.

89 Roulot D, Valla D, Brun-Vezinet F *et al.* Cholangitis in the acquired immuno-deficiency syndrome: report of two cases and review of the literature. *Gut* 1987; **28**: 1653–1660.

90 Belghiti J, Benhamou J-P, Heuly S *et al.* Caustic sclerosing cholangitis. A complication of the surgical treatment of hydatid disease of the liver. *Arch. Surg.* 1986; **121**: 1162–1165.

91 Thompson HH, Pitt HA, Lewin KJ *et al.* Sclerosing cholangitis and histocytosis X. *Gut* 1984; **25**: 526–530.

CHAPTER 17
Enterically Transmitted Viral Hepatitis: Hepatitis A and Hepatitis E

Peter Karayiannis & Howard C. Thomas

Department of Hepatology and Gastroenterology, Imperial College, London, UK

Learning points

- Hepatitis A and E viruses are transmitted by the faecal–oral route.

- Hepatitis A and E cause self-limiting acute infections. Hepatitis E may in rare instances, mainly in transplant recipients, result in chronic infection.

- Acute liver failure is uncommon except in pregnant women infected with hepatitis E.

- Vaccines have been developed to prevent hepatitis A and E. Hepatitis A vaccine is safe and highly immunogenic, and has been approved for use in children and adults.

General features of enterically transmitted viral hepatitis

The first reference to epidemic jaundice has been ascribed to Hippocrates. The earliest record in Western Europe is in a letter written in 751 AD by Pope Zacharias to St Boniface, Archbishop of Mainz. Since then there have been numerous accounts of epidemics, particularly during wars. Hepatitis was a problem in the Franco–Prussian War, the American Civil War and World War I. In World War II huge epidemics occurred, particularly in the Middle East and Italy [1].

There are two enterically transmitted viruses: hepatitis A (HAV) and E (HEV). Hepatitis B, C and D are parenterally transmitted (Table 17.1). Hepatitis A is always a self-limited, faecally spread disease. Hepatitis E is also enterically spread, usually via faecally contaminated water, and causes a self-limited hepatitis in developing countries. Cases in developed countries usually occur in individuals returning from visits to high endemic areas such as South East Asia, Indian subcontinent and Mexico. More recently, sporadic hepatitis E has been reported in residents of developed countries

who have not travelled abroad; in these cases the mechanism of spread is unknown but the strain of the virus is similar to that found in the pig populations of these countries. It is of considerable interest that hepatitis E has recently been described as a persistent infection in liver transplant recipients.

Pathology

Changes in the liver

All forms of viral hepatitis have some common histological features. The essential lesion is an acute inflammation of the entire liver [2]. Hepatic cell necrosis is associated with leucocytic infiltration and histiocytic reaction and infiltration. Zone 3 shows the necrosis most markedly and the portal tracts the greatest cellularity (Figs 17.1, 17.2, 17.3). The sinusoids show mononuclear cellular infiltration, polymorphs and eosinophils. Fatty change is rare. Zone 3 liver cells may show eosinophilic change (*acidophil bodies*), ballooning and giant multinucleated cells may be present. Mitoses are sometimes prominent. Zone 3 cholestasis may be found. Focal 'spotty' necrosis may be seen. Bile duct proliferation is usual and damage is an occasional feature [3].

The reticulin network is usually well preserved. Inflammatory cells disappear gradually, and some new zone 1 portal connective tissue can often be found for many months (Fig. 17.4). During recovery reticuloendothelial activity increases throughout. The Kupffer cells contain lipofuscin pigment and iron.

Occasionally, the necrosis may be *confluent* (*submassive*), affecting substantial groups of adjacent liver cells, usually in zone 3.

In *massive fulminant necrosis* the whole acinus is involved. The liver is reduced in size, being smallest in those who

Sherlock's Diseases of the Liver and Biliary System, Twelfth Edition. Edited by James S. Dooley, Anna S.F. Lok, Andrew K. Burroughs, E. Jenny Heathcote.
© 2011 by Blackwell Publishing Ltd. Published 2011 by Blackwell Publishing Ltd.

Table 17.1. Viral hepatitis A, B, C, D and E contrasted

	HAV	HBV	HCV	HDV	HEV
Genome	RNA	DNA	RNA	RNA	RNA
Family	Picornaviridae	Hepadnaviridae	Flaviviridae	Deltavirus	Hepeviridae
Incubation (days)	15–45	30–180	15–150	30–180	15–60
Transmission	Faecal	Blood	Blood	Blood	Faecal
	Oral	Neonatal	Neonatal	–	Oral
		Saliva	Saliva		
		Percutaneous	Percutaneous	Percutaneous	
		Sexual	Sexual	Sexual	
Acute attack	Depends on age	Mild or severe	Usually mild	Mild or severe	Usually mild
Rash	Yes	Yes	Yes	Yes	Yes
Serum diagnosis	IgM anti-HAV	IgM anti-HBc	Anti-HCV	IgM anti-HDV	IgM anti-HEV
		HBsAg	HCV RNA	HDV RNA	
		HBV DNA			
Peak ALT	800–1000	1000–1500	300–800	1000–1500	800–1000
Prevention	Vaccine	Vaccine	None	HBV Vaccine	*Vaccine
Chronicity	No	Yes	Yes	Yes	Rare, in immunocompromised persons
Treatment	Symptomatic	Symptomatic	Symptomatic	Symptomatic	Symptomatic
		Antivirals in severe cases	Antivirals	Antivirals	

ALT, alanine aminotransferase.
*Not licensed yet.

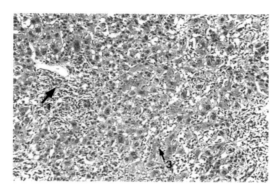

Fig. 17.1. Viral hepatitis: zone 3 (central) (thin arrow) shows marked loss of liver cells. Zone 1 (portal) (thick arrow) shows expansion with cellular infiltration and bile duct proliferation. (H & E, ×40.)

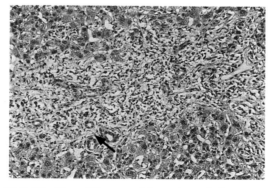

Fig. 17.3. Viral hepatitis: zone 1 (portal tract) shows an acute inflammatory reaction with ductular proliferation (arrow). (H & E, ×50.)

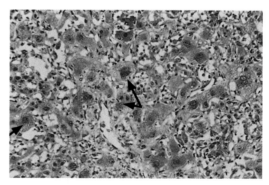

Fig. 17.2. Viral hepatitis: zone 3 shows swollen cells (arrow), mitoses (double arrow) and acidophilic bodies. (H & E, ×80.)

die the soonest. Nodular regeneration is seen in those surviving for more than 2 weeks (Fig. 17.5). The cut surface shows a 'nutmeg' appearance, red areas of haemorrhage alternating with yellow patches of necrosis.

If the necrosis extends from zone 3 to zone 1 the reticulum collapses leaving connective tissue septa. This is termed *bridging* (Fig. 17.6). This may be followed by the development of active fibrous septa, nodules and cirrhosis in the case of hepatitis B and C. More usually it is followed by scar formation (*postnecrotic scarring*) (Fig. 17.7).

Changes in other organs

Regional lymph nodes enlarge. Splenomegaly is related to cellular proliferation and venous congestion secondary to increased portal venous pressure as a result of necroinflammatory changes in the liver. The bone marrow is moderately hypoplastic, but maturation is usually normal.

The brain shows an acute non-specific degeneration of ganglion cells. Occasionally, acute pancreatitis and myocarditis have been noted. These changes are rare and only seen in very severe/fulminant cases.

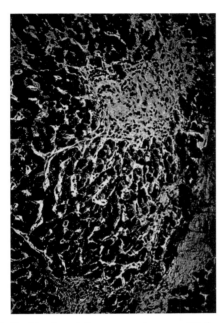

Fig. 17.4. Residual portal zone scarring seen 33 days after the onset of jaundice. (Best's carmine, ×100). From Sherlock S, Walshe VM [10].

Clinical types

Acute hepatitis

Important diagnostic clues can be found in the clinical history. Note is taken of ethnic origin, contacts, recent travel, injections, tattooing, dental treatment, transfusions, sexual preference and ingestion of shellfish. All drugs taken in the previous 2 months are listed.

In general, type A and E hepatitis run the same clinical course often exhibiting a cholestatic phase. Hepatitis B and C may be associated with a serum sickness-like syndrome.

The mildest attack is without symptoms and marked only by a rise in serum transaminase levels. Alternatively, the patient may be anicteric but suffer gastrointestinal and influenza-like symptoms. Such patients are likely to remain undiagnosed unless there is a clear history of

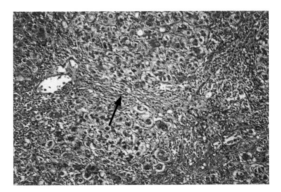

Fig. 17.6. Acute viral hepatitis. A septum (bridge) has formed between zones 1 and 2 (arrow). (H & E, ×40.)

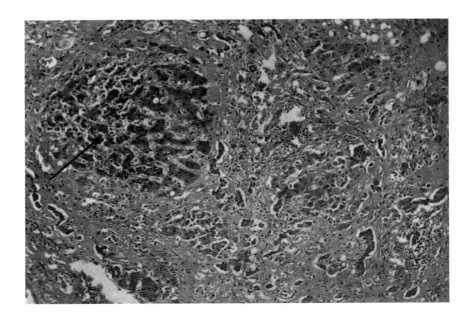

Fig. 17.5. Acute viral hepatitis. Subacute massive necrosis with nodular regeneration (arrow). (H & E, ×120.)

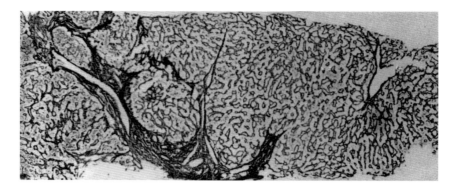

Fig. 17.7. Postnecrotic scarring. The liver biopsy specimen shows scarring, involving and extending from portal tracts. (Reticulin, ×34.)

exposure. Increasing grades of severity are then encountered, ranging from the icteric, from which recovery is usual, through to fulminant, fatal viral hepatitis.

The usual icteric attack in the adult is marked by a prodromal period, usually about 3 or 4 days, even up to several weeks, during which the patient feels generally unwell, suffers digestive symptoms, particularly anorexia and nausea, and may, in the later stages, have mild pyrexia. An ache or feeling of fullness develops in the right upper abdomen. There is loss of desire to smoke or to drink alcohol. Malaise is profound.

Occasionally, fever and headache may be severe and, in children, its association with neck rigidity may suggest meningitis. Protein and lymphocytes in the cerebrospinal fluid may be raised.

The prodromal period is followed by darkening of the urine and lightening of the faeces. This heralds the development of jaundice and symptoms decrease in severity. Pruritus, indicating a cholestatic phase, may appear transiently for a few days. Persistent vomiting and/or drowsiness or confusion indicate urgent hospital referral because they may reflect worsening liver function and incipient liver failure.

The liver is palpable with a smooth, tender edge in 70% of patients. The spleen is palpable in about 20% of patients. A few vascular spiders may appear transiently.

After an icteric period of about 1–4 weeks the adult patient usually makes an uninterrupted recovery. In children, improvement is particularly rapid and jaundice mild or absent. After apparent recovery, lassitude and fatigue persist for some weeks. Clinical and biochemical recovery is usual within 6 months of onset.

Neurological complications, including the Guillain–Barré syndrome, can complicate all forms of viral hepatitis [4].

Prolonged cholestasis

Jaundice appears and deepens, and within 3 weeks the patient starts to itch. After the first few weeks the patient feels well and there are no physical signs apart from icterus and slight hepatomegaly. Jaundice persists for 8–29 weeks and recovery is then complete. It is particularly associated with hepatitis A [5] (7.6% in elderly patients) and E (up to 50% of cases). Liver biopsy shows conspicuous cholestasis which tends to mask the definite, usually mild, hepatitis.

This type must be differentiated from surgical obstructive jaundice [5]. Cholestatic drug jaundice is excluded by the history. If doubt remains, ultrasound and liver biopsy are helpful. The need for liver biopsy should be rare.

The prognosis is usually excellent with complete clinical recovery and restitution of a normal liver [6].

Relapses

These occur in 1.8–15% of cases, particularly with hepatitis A infection. In some the original attack is duplicated, usually in a milder form. More often, the relapse is simply shown by an increase in serum transaminases and sometimes bilirubin. Arthritis, vasculitis and cryoglobulinaemia may be present. Multiple episodes may occur, but recovery is usually complete.

Acute liver failure (fulminant hepatitis)
(see Chapter 5)

This rare form of the disease usually overwhelms the patient within 10 days. It may develop so rapidly that jaundice is inconspicuous. More often, the patient, after a typical acute onset, becomes deeply jaundiced. Ominous signs are repeated vomiting, fetor hepaticus, confusion and drowsiness. The 'flapping' tremor may be only transient. Coma supervenes rapidly. Temperature rises, jaundice deepens and the liver shrinks. Widespread haemorrhages may develop.

Leucocytosis may be found in contrast to the usual leucopenia of viral hepatitis. The biochemical changes are those of acute liver failure (Chapter 5). The height of the serum bilirubin and transaminase are poor indicators of prognosis. Transaminase levels may actually fall as the patient's clinical condition worsens. Blood coagulation is grossly deranged and prothrombin and factor V are the best indicators of prognosis.

The time course depends on whether the cause is A, B, C, D, E or non-A-E hepatitis [7]. Fulminant hepatitis is most often associated with viruses A, B/D and E and rarely hepatitis C. In the USA and Europe, fulminant hepatitis may be due to another cause, presumably viral but not yet identified [8].

When hepatitis E occurs in pregnant women a fulminant course is not infrequent.

There are clinical differences in the fulminant course of the three main types [7]. Pyrexia is most frequent with hepatitis A. The duration of illness before encephalopathy is longer with hepatitis non-A-E. The prothrombin time is greatest with hepatitis B. The bad prognosis in those with a longer duration from onset of illness to encephalopathy is probably related to the greater number of non-A-E hepatitis patients in that group. Acute hepatitis A is more likely to run a fulminant course in persons with underlying chronic hepatitis C than B (41 vs. 0%) [9], including those who are not cirrhotic patients.

Posthepatitis syndrome

Adult patients feel below par for variable periods after acute hepatitis. Usually, this is a matter of weeks but it may extend to months [10]. Features are anxiety, fatigue, failure to regain weight, anorexia and alcohol intolerance, and right upper abdominal discomfort. The liver edge may be palpable and tender.

Treatment consists of reassurance after full investigation. If the acute attack has been type A, chronicity is excluded; if type E, recovery is the normal outcome unless occurring in the context of liver transplantation when viral persistence has been described.

If liver function test abnormalities persist after hepatitis A or E, another cause must be sought. An isolated elevation of unconjugated bilirubin after clinical recovery is usual in patients with coexistence of Gilbert's syndrome. Persistent transaminase elevation may be due to non-alcohol or alcohol-related steatosis or steatohepatitis, or underlying chronic hepatitis B or C.

Investigations

Urine and faeces

Conjugated bilirubin appears in the urine before jaundice, giving a brown coloration. Later it disappears although serum levels remain elevated. Urobilinogenuria is found in the late preicteric phase. At the height of the jaundice, very little bilirubin reaches the intestine, so urobilinogen disappears. Its reappearance indicates commencing recovery. The onset of jaundice is marked by lightening of the faeces due to very little bilirubin entering the intestine, resulting in reduced formation of stercobilinogen in the stool. Reappearance of stool colour denotes impending recovery.

Biochemical changes

Total serum bilirubin levels range widely. Deep jaundice generally implies a prolonged clinical course. An increase in conjugated bilirubin is early, even when the total bilirubin level is still normal.

Serum alkaline phosphatase level is usually less than three times the upper limit of normal and indicates a cholestatic component to the hepatitis, which is fairly common in hepatitis A and E. Serum albumin and globulin are quantitatively unchanged. The serum iron and ferritin levels are raised.

Serum transaminase estimations are useful in early diagnosis, in detecting the anicteric case and for detection of inapparent cases in epidemics. The peak level is found 1 or 2 days before or after onset of jaundice. Later in the course the level falls, even if the clinical condition is worsening. The estimation cannot be used prognostically. Values may remain elevated for 3 to 6 months in those recovering completely.

Haematological changes

The preicteric stage is marked by leucopenia. These revert towards normal as jaundice appears. Some 5–28% of patients show atypical lymphocytes, resembling those seen in infectious mononucleosis. Acute Coombs' test-positive haemolytic anaemia is a rare complication. Haemolysis may develop [11], especially in those with glucose-6-phosphate dehydrogenase deficiency [12].

Aplastic anaemia is very rare. It appears weeks or months after the acute episode and is particularly severe and irreversible. It is not usually associated with A, B/D, C or E infection and may be due to a hitherto unidentified non-A-E hepatitis.

The *prothrombin time* is lengthened in the more severe cases and does not return completely to normal with vitamin K therapy.

The *erythrocyte sedimentation rate* (ESR) is high in the preicteric phase, falls to normal with jaundice and rises again when the jaundice subsides. It returns to normal with complete recovery.

Needle liver biopsy

This is rarely indicated in the acute stage. It may be used to diagnose co-existent second pathology, such as steatosis, causing persistent abnormality of liver function tests continuing for more than 6 months after resolution of the clinical hepatitis A or E.

Differential diagnosis

In the *preicteric stage*, hepatitis can be confused with other acute infectious diseases, with acute surgical abdomen, especially acute appendicitis, and with acute gastroenteritis. Bile in the urine, tender enlargement of the liver and a rise in serum transaminase values are the most helpful points. Viral markers are essential.

In the *icteric stage*, the diagnosis must be made from obstructive jaundice. This is outlined in Chapter 11.

The diagnosis of acute viral hepatitis from drug reactions depends largely on the history and then on the serology. There is real advantage in rapid availability of diagnostic tests for HAV and HEV infections which obviates the need for further testing, particularly ultrasound imaging to exclude biliary obstruction and liver biopsy.

Needle liver biopsy is valuable in the problem case. Attempts at a surgical diagnosis are disastrous.

In the *posticteric stage*, the continuation of transaminase abnormalities necessitates investigations for the diagnosis of chronic hepatitis.

Prognosis

In a survey of 1675 cases of fulminant hepatitis in a group of Boston hospitals, one in eight sufferers from transfusion hepatitis (B and C) succumbed whereas only one in 200 died with type A disease. Since many non-icteric cases are not included in the statistics, the overall mortality rate is undoubtedly very much lower. In the UK, non-A-E hepatitis has the poorest survival [7].

Those who are elderly or in poor general health have a poor prognosis. Fulminant hepatitis is rare in those less than 15 years old. The survival rate is the same for males as for females. The incidence of icteric disease is higher and the prognosis worse in older patients and those with underlying, chronic liver disease.

Treatment

Prevention

Compulsory notification leads to earlier detection and identification of modes of transmission and source of outbreaks, for instance food or water contamination, sexual spread or carriage by blood donors. Vaccination is discussed below.

Treatment of the acute attack

Treatment has little effect in altering the course. At the outset this is unpredictable and it is wise to treat all attacks as potentially serious and to recommend adequate rest.

The traditional low-fat, high-carbohydrate diet is popular because it has proved the most palatable to the anorexic patient. Apart from this, no benefit accrues from a rigid insistence upon a low-fat diet. Supplementary vitamins, amino acids and lipotropic agents are not necessary.

Corticosteroids do not accelerate the rate of healing in viral hepatitis: the usual course of hepatitis A and E is towards spontaneous recovery and any benefit of steroids is not sufficient to justify their use, except occasionally in protracted cholestatic hepatitis A. The steroid whitewash improves the morale of both patient and physician but probably has little effect on the healing process.

Patients with severe nausea or vomiting must be hydrated if necessary with intravenous fluids. Those showing signs of acute hepatocellular failure with coagulopathy or encephalopathy require more active measures and the regimen described in Chapter 5 must be instituted.

Follow-up

The patient should be monitored until symptoms are resolved and liver function tests return to normal. Special attention should be paid to recurrence of jaundice.

Exercise can be undertaken within the limits of fatigue. Alcohol must be denied for 3 to 6 months. Diet can be unrestricted.

Hepatitis A virus

Hepatitis A accounts for 20–25% of clinical hepatitis in the developed world. It is largely asymptomatic in children under the age of 15 years. The causative agent of this infection is a small, spherical, positive-sense RNA virus, measuring 27 nm in diameter [13]. It belongs to the *picornaviridae* family of viruses, under the genus *hepatovirus* (Fig. 17.8).

The capsid (outer coat) consists of 60 capsomeres, each made up of the same four structural viral proteins, VP1, VP2, VP3 and VP4 [14]. The capsid encloses the RNA genome of the virus encoding its genetic information. The genome contains a single open reading frame which is translated into a polyprotein. This is cleaved by the viral protease enzyme to produce the four VP peptides and a number of non-structural peptides, which are important for the replication of the virus.

Sequencing studies have revealed that in the human population there are three circulating genotypes of the virus and each genotype is subdivided into two subgenotypes[15]. Only a single serotype has been identified.

The virus enters the body through the gastrointestinal tract, and in the marmoset there is suggestive evidence that it replicates here [16]. This is followed by a brief period of viraemia when the virus infects and replicates within the hepatocytes, which is the main site of virion production (Fig. 17.9). Cell uptake may involve attachment of the virus to the asialoglycoprotein receptor via IgA-virus complexes or the HAVCR1/TIM (T-cell immnunoglobulin mucin) receptor with its IgA1lambda ligand which has a synergistic effect on virus-receptor interaction [17]. The virus, possibly as an immune complex, is also seen in the Kupffer cells. Viral proteins are synthesized and HAV RNA replicated in the cytoplasm. Mature virus particles are packed into vesicles to be released into the bile.

The virus is not directly cytopathic and damage to liver cells is caused by T-cell-mediated immune responses.

The virus has been experimentally transmitted to marmosets and chimpanzees, and cultivated *in vitro* (Fig. 17.10).

A serum antibody (anti-HAV) appears as the stool becomes negative for virus, reaches a maximum in several months and is detectable for many years (Fig. 17.11). The appearance of serum IgM anti-HAV is diagnostic of acute infection. This antibody persists for only 2–6 months (Fig. 7.11) and rarely, in low titre, for up to 1 year. It gives way to IgG anti-HAV, which indicates immunity against the virus and long-term protection from re-infection.

PCR shows that faecal excretion of virus can persist for months [18]. A chronic carrier state has not been identified.

Epidemiology

The disease occurs sporadically or in epidemics and has an incubation time of 15–50 days. It is usually spread

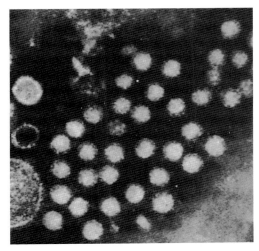

Fig. 17.8. Electron microscopy of hepatitis A virions in faeces. These are shown as 27-nm spheres. (×250 000.)

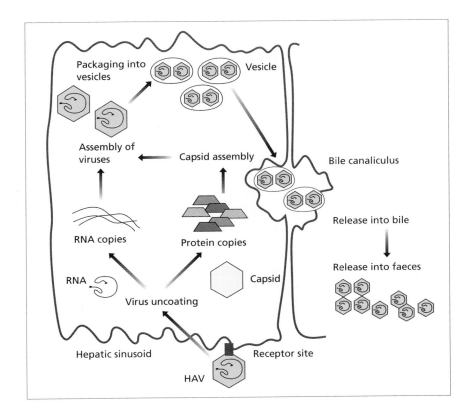

Fig. 17.9. The replication cycle of hepatitis A virus.

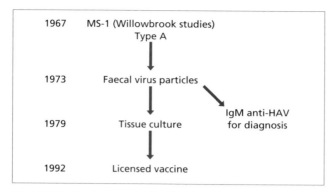

Fig. 17.10. Landmarks in the history of hepatitis A.

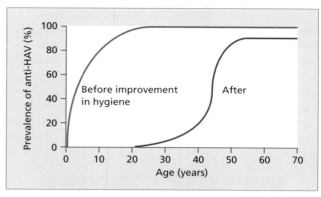

Fig. 17.12. Prevalence changes with improved hygiene. Fewer adults have immunity (IgG anti-HAV) to hepatitis A.

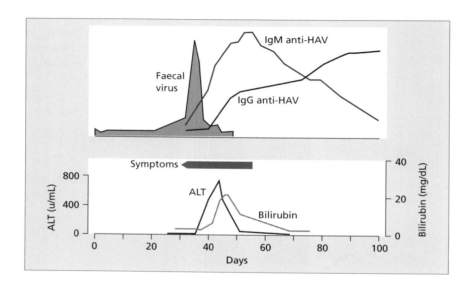

Fig. 17.11. The course of acute hepatitis A. ALT, alanine aminotransferase (serum glutamic pyruvic transaminase).

by the faecal–oral route. Parenteral transmission is extremely rare, but can follow transfusion of blood from a donor who is in the incubation stage of the disease [19].

The group most affected is aged 5–14 years, and adults are often infected by spread from children.

Spread is related to overcrowding, and to poor hygiene and sanitation. With improvements in these factors, the incidence is decreasing worldwide (Fig. 17.12). The annual incidence rate in the early 1990s varied from 5 per 100 000 population in Northern Europe and Japan to 9.1 in the USA and 60 per 100 000 in Africa and parts of South America [20,21]. The incidence has dropped dramatically in the USA and elsewhere in recent years as a result of vaccination programs in early childhood. In the USA, vaccination of children living in areas with consistently high HAV infection rates has led to a drop in the incidence of HAV infection in 2007 to 1.5 cases per 100 000 population, representing an 82% reduction since 1990 [21].

In developing countries, 90% of children have been infected and developed protective immunity by the age of 10 and clinical illness is uncommon. Adults, not previously exposed, visiting endemic areas and hospital staff in developed countries are at risk. As countries transition from underdeveloped to developed with less adults being immune to the virus, clinical illness may become more frequent.

Outbreaks have been reported among haemophiliacs receiving solvent–detergent-treated factor VIII concentrates [22]. Most sporadic cases follow person-to-person contact. Children in day-care centres and promiscuous homosexual men are at risk.

Explosive water-borne and food-borne epidemics have been described. Fruit-related epidemics are ascribed to poor hygiene in the handlers, to use of human sewage for soil fertilization or contaminated water for irrigation, rinsing or packaging [23].

Ingestion of raw clams and oysters from polluted waters has caused epidemics, including the one in

Shanghai, China, which affected over 292 000 people [24]. Contamination of shellfish beds with untreated sewage may lead to virus concentrations in shellfish tissues to levels 100-fold higher than those in surrounding waters. Steaming the clams may not kill the virus, for the temperature achieved inside the clams may not be sufficiently high.

Contamination during preparation has resulted in transmission via other foods, including sandwiches, orange juice, salads and meat. Recent outbreaks in developed countries have been traced to frozen raspberries and strawberries, fresh onions or tomatoes, and salsa. Local or imported produce has been implicated.

Clinical course

The hepatitis is usually mild, particularly in children where it is frequently subclinical or passed off as gastroenteritis. The disease is more serious and prolonged in adults. Cases requiring hospitalization were 22% among children younger than 5 to 52% among adults older than 60 (Centers for Disease Control, 2006). Pregnant women may require special attention. Fulminant hepatitis and death are rare complications (0.3% of cases in the USA in 2006) (Centers for Disease Control).

Needle liver biopsy in patients with acute hepatitis A shows a particularly florid portal zone lesion with expansion, marked cellular infiltration and erosion of the limiting plate and the presence of IgM plasma cells giving an appearance not dissimilar to autoimmune hepatitis [25]. IgM class anti-liver membrane antibodies (anti-LMA) have been described [26]. Cholestasis is marked. Hepatitis A may trigger *chronic autoimmune hepatitis type 1* in genetically predisposed individuals [27], but this is a rare event. This may be related to defects in suppressor T cells. Fibrin ring granulomas are described [28].

Cholestatic hepatitis A affects adults [29]. The jaundice lasts 42–110 days and itching is severe. The prognosis is excellent. A case can be made for cutting short the jaundice and relieving the itching by a short course of prednisolone 30 mg reducing to zero over about 3 weeks.

Nephrotic syndrome has been reported rarely [30].

Relapsing hepatitis A occurs in 3–20% of patients, after 30–90 days. The relapse resembles the original attack clinically and biochemically, and HAV is found in the stool [31]. The relapse may last several months but recovery eventually ensues [32]. IgM antibodies persist during this period but at lower levels. Rarely, the relapse can be associated with arthritis, vasculitis and cryoglobulinaemia [33].

Prognosis

This is excellent and recovery is usually full. Mortality in large epidemics is less than one per 1000 and HAV accounts for less than 1% of cases of fulminant viral hepatitis. In older people, however, the disease has considerable morbidity, mortality and treatment costs [20]. In non-hospitalized adults, the symptoms last about 34 days with 33 days' work loss. In a hospitalized patient, symptom duration is longer (68 days). Acute hepatitis A in persons with underlying chronic hepatitis C is more likely to have serious complications [9].

Follow-up of large epidemics in World War I [34] showed no long-term sequelae.

Prevention

The virus is excreted in the faeces for as long as 2 weeks before the appearance of jaundice. The anicteric patient may excrete the virus for a similar period. The virus is therefore disseminated before the diagnosis is made. For this reason, isolation of patients and contacts cannot be expected to influence significantly the spread of hepatitis.

HAV can persist in the environment for weeks. HAV can remain infectious after 1 month on environmental surfaces at ambient temperature. It can be inactivated by heating to over 85°C for longer than 1 min, by exposure to 2% glutaraldehyde or sodium hypochlorite (greater than 5000 ppm of free chlorine) and by microwaving.

Immune serum globulin (ISG) prophylaxis

Efficacy depends on the antibody concentration and hence the source of the plasma. ISG is being largely replaced by vaccine.

For pre-exposure prophylaxis, vaccine is preferred.

ISG must be given within 2 weeks following exposure (0.02 mL/kg IM). In this situation it is 80–90% effective. ISG may be given with the first dose of vaccine but the resultant HAV antibody titres may be reduced [35].

Hepatitis A vaccines

Viral particles generated in cell culture are inactivated with formaldehyde and mixed with alum used as adjuvant. There are two HAV vaccines, HAVRIX (GSK Biologicals) and VAQTA (Merck), whilst TWINRIX (GSK) is in combination with the hepatitis B vaccine. The vaccine is safe and immunogenic [14,36–38]. The only side effect is mild soreness of the arm, where it is administered. A single 1-mL dose of vaccine in adults is followed by a booster 6–12 months later (1440 EL.U of HAVRIX or 50 U of VAQTA). The single dose gives rapid protection within 1 month in 94–100% of those immunized. HAV vaccine is also shown to induce protective antibodies within 2 weeks, and so ISG is not needed even for those travelling shortly after the first dose of vaccine. If followed by the booster, 100% seroconversion ensues with long-lasting protection [39]. Prevaccination serum testing for anti-HAV is necessary only in those born after 1945, living in countries with low endemicity and who, presumably, have had a small chance of contracting the disease (Fig. 17.12). Children 12 months (minimum age) to 18 years of age receive 0.5 mL of the vaccine under the same immunization schedule (CDC recommendations).

In one dose the formol-inactivated vaccine was shown to be highly protective in children in a Jewish community in New York [37]. In a large study of children in Thailand, two doses protected against HAV for at least 1 year [40]. Protective levels of antibody persist for up to 12 years, whilst kinetic models indicate possible persistence for at least 25 years [41].

TWINRIX is licensed for use in persons aged 18 years and above. Primary immunization consists of three doses, administered on a 0-, 1-, and 6-month schedule. Antibody responses to both HAV and HBV in the vaccine are equivalent to those seen when the single-antigen vaccines are administered separately on standard schedules [42,43].

The use of the HAV vaccine versus ISG in an outbreak setting has recently been explored. The former was marginally less efficacious in preventing HAV infection [44]. This may be offset by the active and long-term immunity afforded by vaccination versus the temporary protection conferred by ISG.

Live attenuated HAV vaccine

This has been prepared from HAV in cell culture. It is inexpensive and has been widely used in developing countries such as China. Given subcutaneously, it seems safe and effective [45].

Indications for HAV vaccine (Table 17.2)

HAV vaccine is indicated for travellers to areas with poor hygiene standards. Unvaccinated, three to six visi-

Table 17.2. Groups for which the hepatitis A vaccine is recommended

Children in endemic areas or areas with high risk of infection
Travellers to or those working in endemic areas
Occupational exposure
Men who have sex with men
Intravenous drug users
Patients with clotting factor disorders
Military
Missionaries
Chronic liver disease (HCV)
? Immunosuppressed individuals

tors per 1000 per month will develop HAV. Children and staff in day-care units and their parents, and nurses, particularly those working in intensive care units, should be vaccinated. Global control will require early mass immunization in childhood (routine aged 1, catch-up aged up to 18, CDC recommendations) [46,47]. Eventually, vaccination will be combined with other paediatric vaccines. Such worldwide vaccination is a long way off, as the vaccine is expensive for countries in the third world [48].

Food handlers and sewage workers are candidates for vaccination. The military should be vaccinated, particularly if they are going to areas where hygiene is poor.

Promiscuous, homosexual males should be vaccinated.

HAV infection has a harmful effect on patients with chronic liver disease, especially HCV [9]. The HAV vaccine is effective in such patients [49]. It should probably be given to everyone with chronic liver disease, although there may be economic constraints. Prior HAV antibody testing should be done in those who may have been exposed, such as those originating from an area of high endemicity or older than 40 years of age.

Hepatitis E virus

Hepatitis E virus (HEV) has recently been assigned to a new family of viruses, namely the *hepeviridae,* under the genus *hepevirus.* Viral nucleotide sequences have been obtained from isolates from Burma [50], Mexico [51], Pakistan [52] and China [53]. There are marked variations in the nucleotide sequence of HEV strains isolated from all over the world. There are five genotypes of the virus; 1 and 2 are found in humans, 3 and 4 in humans and swine, and 5 is of avian origin. The mammalian genotypes are subdivided to several subtypes each ranging from 2 to 10 [54]. There is only one recognized serotype in the mammalian viruses (1-4).

The virus is 32–34 nm in diameter, with an outer capsid consisting of a single protein. It lacks an outer lipid envelope. The capsid encloses the RNA genome of the virus, which contains three open reading frames (ORFs). ORF 1 encodes the non-structural proteins of the virus, ORF2 the capsid protein and ORF3 a protein of unknown function [55].

HEV is excreted in the bile [56].

The virus causes sporadic cases and major epidemics of viral hepatitis in developing countries [56,57]. Many large epidemics of hepatitis, believed to be due to HAV, have now been identified as caused by HEV. As in the case of HAV, the disease is enterically transmitted, usually by sewage-contaminated water.

It is probably a non-cytopathic infection. Liver damage may be immune mediated. Immunity probably wanes and longevity of protective antibody is uncertain.

Clinical features

In general, hepatitis E resembles hepatitis A. It affects young adults and is rare in children [58]. It has a self-limited course. Human volunteer studies have indicated an incubation period of 22–46 days [59]. The onset is abrupt. The majority of clinical cases are jaundiced and there are no extrahepatic features. Chronicity is very rare but has recently been described in immunosuppressed patients who have received a liver transplant or are HIV infected.

Epidemic. Infection comes from drinking water contaminated by overflow of sewage. Monsoon seasons are associated with a high risk of epidemics. The mortality rate is high at 1%, and up to 20% in pregnant women.

Fulminant hepatic failure appears to be more common in Indian/ Asian pregnant women. The more severe outcome in pregnancy appears to be related to diminished cellular immunity and hormonal factors [60]. High virus levels have been detected in HEV RNA-positive pregnant women [61].

Sporadic. This is a common cause of acute viral hepatitis in endemic areas. It presents with moderate or severe symptoms, including acute liver failure, subacute liver failure and prolonged cholestatic hepatitis [62]. Mortality is 45% for fulminant or subacute liver failure. Unlike epidemic HEV, the mortality is not high in pregnant women [63].

Sporadic cases have in recent years been reported in industrialized countries in subjects who have not been to endemic areas of the world. These infections are associated with genotypes 3 and 4, are of swine origin and therefore represent zoonotic infections [56]. The disease is milder than with genotypes 1 and 2, possibly because of strain attenuation.

In Japan, HEV infection has also been documented through consumption of raw or undercooked deer and wild boar meat [64]. Contact with infected animals, whether wild or domestic, may also be another source of infection.

Seroepidemiological studies in western countries have indicated higher than expected prevalence of anti-HEV in blood donors and the general population. In the USA, anti-HEV was detected in an unexpectedly high percentage of homosexual men (15.9%) and IDUs (23.0%) as well as in blood donors (21.3%) [65].

Chronic infection has been observed in two post-liver transplantation patients [66,67]. In both cases, HEV RNA persisted for 5–7 years. Both patients were retransplanted and reinfection of the new liver graft occurred in one of them. The other developed antibodies. There was evidence of cirrhosis in one of the livers removed.

Diagnostic tests

Serum IgM and IgG antibodies are measured by ELISA using recombinant antigens or synthetic peptides prepared from cloned HEV [68]. These tests however vary greatly in sensitivity, making serodiagnosis less reliable than for other human hepatitis viruses. HEV RNA can be detected by RT-PCR in serum, but primarily in stool and the test is not readily available [69,70].

IgM anti-HEV appears with the onset of symptoms and disappears in the majority of cases by 6 months. IgG anti-HEV appears at about 10–12 days of illness and persists for years. Patients who had recovered from HEV infection remained anti-HEV positive for longer than 14 years, although durability of protection is unclear [71]. Viraemia is transient and HEV RNA is undetectable by 3 weeks.

Positive antibody tests have been reported from almost all parts of the developing world. They include Egyptian children [72], Kashmiris [63], Taiwanese [73] and migrant workers in Qatar [74].

Liver biopsy

This shows cholestasis, pseudoglandular formations, ballooning of hepatocytes and very prominent zone 1 infiltrates containing polymorphs (Fig. 17.13). Massive and submassive necrosis is seen in fulminant cases and bridging necrosis is the prominent feature of subacute hepatitis. Even after 5–10 years of follow-up cirrhosis is not seen.

Prevention

This is by provision of clean water, better sanitation and hygiene education.

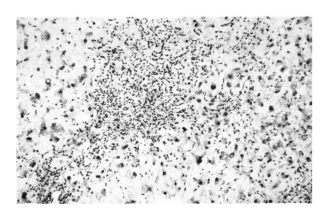

Fig. 17.13. Liver biopsy from a pregnant Arab girl suffering from acute hepatitis E showing cholestasis, pseudoglandular formations, ballooning degeneration of hepatocytes and very prominent portal zone cellular infiltrates. She recovered. (H & E, ×100.)

Studies in rhesus macaques indicated that a recombinant product based on the ORF2 expressed capsid protein elicited protective antibodies in immunized animals [75]. The capsid protein has been shown to be highly immunogenic and to elicit a neutralizing immune response which is protective. In addition, it appears to be a target of cell-mediated immunity [76].

A human vaccine based on a truncated form of the capsid protein (56 kDa) that retains the conformational neutralization epitope has been tested for efficacy in Nepal. It showed a 95.5% antibody response rate after 3 doses given at 0, 1 and 6 months, and an 87% efficacy rate [77].

Whether the vaccine becomes commercially available is dependent on its economic viability, since the demand, if any, in developed countries will be low.

References

1 Zuckerman AJ. The chronicle of viral hepatitis. *Bull. Hyg. Trop. Dis.* 1977; **54**: 113.

2 Dible JH, McMichael J, Sherlock SPV. Pathology of acute hepatitis. Aspiration biopsy studies of epidemic, arsenotherapy and serum jaundice. *Lancet* 1943; **ii**: 402.

3 Poulsen H, Christoffersen P. Abnormal bile duct epithelium in liver biopsies with histological signs of viral hepatitis. *Acta Path. Microbiol. Scand.* 1969; **76**: 383–390.

4 Tabor E. Guillain–Barré syndrome and other neurologic syndromes in hepatitis A, B, non-A, non-B. *J. Med. Virol.* 1987; **21**: 207–216.

5 Gordon SG, Reddy KR, Schiff L et al. Prolonged intrahepatic cholestasis secondary to acute hepatitis A. *Ann. Intern. Med.* 1984; **101**: 635–637.

6 Shaldon S, Sherlock S. Virus hepatitis with features of prolonged bile retention. *Br. Med. J.* 1957; **2**: 734–738.

7 Gimson AES, White YS, Eddleston ALWF et al. Clinical and prognostic differences in fulminant hepatitis type A, B, and non-A, non-B. *Gut* 1983; **24**: 1194–1198.

8 SK, Patel VM, Hollinger FB et al. Non-A, non-B fulminant hepatitis is also non-E, and non-C. *Am. J. Gastroenterol.* 1994; **89**: 57–61.

9 Vento S, Garafano T, Renzini C et al. Fulminant hepatitis associated with hepatitis A virus superinfection in patients with chronic hepatitis C. *N. Engl. J. Med.* 1998; **338**: 286–290.

10 Sherlock S, Walshe VM. The post-hepatitis syndrome. *Lancet* 1946; **ii**: 482.

11 Lyons DJ, Gilvarry JM, Fielding JF. Severe haemolysis associated with hepatitis A and normal glucose-6-phosphate dehydrogenase status. *Gut* 1990; **31**: 838–839.

12 Chan TK, Todd D. Haemolysis complicating viral hepatitis in patients with glucose-6-phosphate dehydrogenase deficiency. *Br. Med. J.* 1975; **i**: 131–133.

13 Feinstone SM, Kapikian AZ, Purcell RH. Hepatitis A: detection by immune electron microscopy of a virus-like antigen associated with acute illness. *Science* 1973; **182**: 1026–1028.

14 Martin A, Lemon SM. Hepatitis A virus: from discovery to vaccines. *Hepatology* 2006; **43**(Suppl. 1): S164–172.

15 Cristina J, Costa-Mattioli M. Genetic variability and molecular evolution of hepatitis A virus. *Virus Res.* 2007; **127**: 151–157.

16 Karayiannis P, Jowett T, Enticott M et al. Hepatitis A virus replication in tamarins and host immune response in relation to pathogenesis of liver cell damage. *J. Med. Virol.* 1986; **18**: 261–276.

17 Tami C, Silberstein E, Manangeeswaran M et al. Immunoglobulin A (IgA) is a natural ligand of hepatitis A virus cellular receptor 1 (HAVCR1), and the association of IgA with HAVCR1 enhances virus-receptor interactions. *J. Virol.* 2007; **81**: 3437–3446.

18 Yotsuyanagi H, Koike K, Yasuda K et al. Prolonged fecal excretion of hepatitis A virus in adult patients with hepatitis A virus as determined by polymerase chain reaction. *Hepatology* 1996; **24**: 10–13.

19 Hollinger FB, Khan NC, Oefinger PE et al. Post-transfusion hepatitis type A. *JAMA* 1983; **250**: 2313–2317.

20 Berge JJ, Drennan DP, Jacobs RJ et al. The cost of hepatitis A infections in American adolescents and adults in 1997. *Hepatology* 2000; **31**: 469–473.

21 Center for Disease Control. Prevention of hepatitis through active or passive immunization, recommendations of the Advisory Committee of Immunization Practices (ACIP). *MMWR* 1999; **48**: 1.

22 Mannuccio PM, Godvin S, Gringeri A et al. Transmission of hepatitis A to patients with haemophilia by factor VIII concentrates treated with organic solvent and detergent to inactivate viruses. *Ann. Intern. Med.* 1994; **120**: 1–7.

23 Hutin YJF, Pool V, Cramer EH et al. A multistate, food-borne outbreak of hepatitis. *N. Engl. J. Med.* 1999; **340**: 595–602.

24 Halliday ML, Kang LY, Zhou TK et al. An epidemic of hepatitis A attributable to the ingestion of raw clams in Shanghai, China. *J. Infect. Dis.* 1991; **164**: 852–859.

25 Teixeira MR Jr, Weller IV, Murray A et al. The pathology of hepatitis A in man. *Liver* 1982; **2**: 53–60.

26 Wiedmann KH, Bartholemew TC, Brown DJ et al. Liver membrane antibodies detected by immunoradiometric assay in acute and chronic virus-induced and autoimmune liver disease. *Hepatology* 1984; **4**: 199–204.

27 Vento S, Garofano T, Di Perri G et al. Identification of hepatitis A virus as a trigger for autoimmune chronic hepatitis type I in susceptible individuals. *Lancet* 1991; **337**: 1183–1187.

28 Ponz E, Garcia-Pagán JC, Bruguera M et al. Hepatic fibrin-ring granulomas in a patient with hepatitis A. *Gastroenterology* 1991; **100**: 268–270.

29 Gordon SC, Reddy KR, Schiff L et al. Prolonged intrahepatic cholestasis secondary to acute hepatitis A. *Ann. Intern. Med.* 1984; **101**: 635–637.

30 Zikos D, Grewal KS, Craig K et al. Nephrotic syndrome and acute renal failure associated with hepatitis A viral infection. *Am. J. Gastroenterol.* 1995; **90**: 295–298.

31 Sjögren MH, Tanno H, Fay O et al. Hepatitis A virus in stool during clinical relapse. *Ann. Intern. Med.* 1987; **106**: 221–226.

32 Glikson M, Galun E, Oren R et al. Relapsing hepatitis A. Review of 14 cases and literature survey. *Medicine (Baltimore)* 1992; **71**: 14–23.

33 Dan M, Yaniv R. Cholestatic hepatitis, cutaneous vasculitis and vascular deposits of immunoglobulin M and complement associated with hepatitis A virus infection. *Am. J. Med.* 1990; **89**: 103–104.

34 Cullinan ER, King RC, Rivers JS. The prognosis of infective hepatitis. A preliminary account of a long-term follow-up. *Br. Med. J.* 1958; **i**: 1315–1317.

35 Zaaijer HL, Leentvaar-Kuijpers A, Rotman H *et al.* Hepatitis A antibody titres after infection and immunization: implications for passive and active immunization. *J. Med. Virol.* 1993; **40**: 22–27.

36 Werzberger A, Kuter R, Nalin D. Six years follow-up after hepatitis A vaccination. *N. Engl. J. Med.* 1998; **338**: 1160.

37 Werzberger A, Mensch B, Kuter B *et al.* A controlled trial of a formalin-inactivated hepatitis A vaccine in healthy children. *N. Engl. J. Med.* 1992; **327**: 453–457.

38 Wasley A, Bell BP. Hepatitis A in the era of vaccination. *Epidemiol. Rev.* 2006; **28**: 101–111.

39 Sjögren MH, Hoke CH, Binn LN *et al.* Immunogenicity of an inactivated hepatitis A vaccine. *Ann. Intern. Med.* 1991; **114**: 470–471.

40 Innis BL, Snitbhan R, Kunasol P *et al.* Protection against hepatitis A by an inactivated vaccine. *JAMA* 1994; **271**: 1328–1334.

41 Van Damme P, Banatvala J, Fay O *et al.* Hepatitis A booster vaccination: is there a need? *Lancet* 2003; **362**: 1065–1071.

42 Knöll A, Hottenträger B, Kainz J *et al.* Immunogenicity of a combined hepatitis A and B vaccine in healthy young adults. *Vaccine* 2000; **18**: 2029–2032.

43 Czeschinski PA, Binding N, Witting U. Hepatitis A and hepatitis B vaccinations: immunogenicity of combined vaccine and of simultaneously or separately applied single vaccines. *Vaccine* 2000; **18**: 1074–1080.

44 Victor JC, Monto AS, Surdina TY *et al.* Hepatitis A vaccine versus immune globulin for postexposure prophylaxis. *N. Engl. J. Med.* 2007; **357**: 1685–1694.

45 Mao JS, Chai SA, Xic RY *et al.* Further evaluation of the safety and protective efficacy of live attenuated hepatitis A vaccine (H-2 strain). *Vaccine* 1997; **15**: 944–947.

46 Koff RS. Hepatitis A. *Lancet* 1998; **341**: 1643–1649.

47 Koff RS. The case for *routine* childhood vaccination against hepatitis A. *N. Engl. J. Med.* 1999; **340**: 644–645.

48 Teppakdee A, Tangwitoon A, Khemasuwan D *et al.* Cost-benefit analysis of hepatitis a vaccination in Thailand. *Southeast Asian J. Trop. Med. Public Health* 2002; **33**: 118–127.

49 Keeffe EB, Iwarson S, McMahon BJ *et al.* Safety and immunogenicity of hepatitis A vaccine in patients with chronic liver disease. *Hepatology* 1998; **27**: 881–886.

50 Reyes GR, Purdy MA, Jungsuh PK *et al.* Isolation of a cDNA from the virus responsible for enterically transmitted non-A, non-B hepatitis. *Science* 1990; **247**: 1335–1339.

51 Velázquez O, Stetler HC, Avila C *et al.* Epidemic transmission of enterically transmitted non-A, non-B hepatitis in Mexico, 1986–87. *JAMA* 1990; **263**: 3281–3285.

52 Bryan JP, Tsarev SA, Iqbal M *et al.* Epidemic hepatitis E in Pakistan: patterns of serologic response and evidence that antibody to hepatitis E virus protects against disease. *J. Infect. Dis.* 1994 ; **170**: 517–521.

53 Zhuang H, Cao XY, Liu CB *et al.* Epidemiology of hepatitis E in China. *Gastroenterol. Jpn.* 1991; **26** (Suppl.): 13513–1358.

54 Lu L, Li C, Hagedorn CH. Phylogenetic analysis of global hepatitis E virus sequences: genetic diversity, subtypes and zoonosis. *Rev. Med. Virol.* 2006; **16**: 5–36.

55 Tam AW, Smith MM, Guerra ME *et al.* Hepatitis E virus (HEV): molecular cloning and sequencing of the full-length viral genome. *Virology* 1991; **185**: 120–131.

56 Purcell RH, Emerson SU. Hepatitis E: An emerging awareness of an old disease. *J Hepatol* 2008; **48**: 494–503.

57 Aggarwal R, Naik SR. Epidemiology of hepatitis E past, present and future. *Trop. Gastroenterol.* 1997; **18**: 99–56.

58 Arankalle VA, Tsarev SA, Chadha MS *et al.* Age-specific prevalences of antibodies to hepatitis A and E viruses in Pune, India, 1982 and 1992. *J. Infect. Dis.* 1995; **171**: 447–450.

59 Chauhan A, Jameel S, Dilawari JB *et al.* Hepatitis E virus transmission to a volunteer. *Lancet* 1993; **341**: 149–150.

60 Jilani N, Das BC, Husain SA *et al.* Hepatitis E virus infection and fulminant hepatic failure during pregnancy. *J. Gastroenterol. Hepatol.* 2007; **22**: 676–682.

61 Kar P, Jilani N, Husain SA *et al.* Does hepatitis E viral load and genotypes influence the final outcome of acute liver failure during pregnancy? *Am. J. Gastroenterol.* 2008; **103**: 2495–2501.

62 Acharya SK, Dasarathy S, Kumer TL *et al.* Fulminant hepatitis in a tropical population, clinical course, aetiology and early predictors of outcome. *Hepatology* 1996; **23**: 1448–1455.

63 Khuroo MS, Rustgi VK, Dawson GJ *et al.* Spectrum of hepatitis E virus infection in India. *J. Med. Virol.* 1994; **43**: 281–286.

64 Takahashi K, Kitajima N, Abe N *et al.* Complete or near-complete nucleotide sequences of hepatitis E virus genome recovered from a wild boar, a deer, and four patients who ate the deer. *Virology* 2004; **330**: 501–505.

65 Thomas DL, Yarbough PO, Vlahov D *et al.* Seroreactivity to hepatitis E virus in areas where the disease is not endemic. *J. Clin. Microbiol.* 1997; **35**: 1244–1247.

66 Haagsma EB, van den Berg AP, Porte RJ *et al.* Chronic hepatitis E virus infection in liver transplant recipients. *Liver Transpl.* 2008; **14**: 547–553.

67 Aggarwal R. Hepatitis E: does it cause chronic hepatitis? *Hepatology* 2008; **48**: 1328–1330.

68 DeGuzman LJ, Pitrak DL, Dawson GJ *et al.* Diagnosis of acute hepatitis E infection using enzyme immunoassay. *Dig. Dis. Sci.* 1994; **39**: 1691–1693.

69 Ray R, Aggarwal R, Salunke PN *et al.* Hepatitis E virus genome in stools of hepatitis patients during large epidemic in North India. *Lancet* 1991; **338**: 783–784.

70 Nanda SK, Ansari IH, Acharya SK *et al.* Protracted viremia during acute sporadic hepatitis E virus infection. *Gastroenterology* 1995; **108**: 225–230.

71 Clayson ET, Myint KS, Snitbhan R *et al.* Viremia, fecal shedding, and IgM and IgG responses in patients with hepatitis E. *J. Infect. Dis.* 1995; **172**: 927–933.

72 Goldsmith R, Yarbough PO, Reyes GR *et al.* Enzyme-linked immunosorbent assay for diagnosis of acute sporadic hepatitis E in Egyptian children. *Lancet* 1992; **339**: 328–331.

73 Wu J-C, Sheen JJ, Chiang T-Y *et al.* The impact of travelling to endemic areas on the spread of hepatitis E virus infection: epidemiological and molecular analysis. *Hepatology* 1998; **27**: 1415–1420.

74 Shidrawi RG, Skidmore SJ, Coleman JC *et al.* Hepatitis E—an important cause of important non-A, non-B hepatitis among migrant workers in Qatar. *J. Med. Virol.* 1994; **43**: 412–414.

75 Purcell RH, Nguyen H, Shapiro M *et al.* Pre-clinicalimmunogenicity and efficacy trial of a recombinant hepatitis E vaccine. *Vaccine* 2003; **21**: 2607–2615.

76 Shata MT, Barrett A, Shire NJ *et al.* Characterization of hepatitis E-specific cell-mediated immune response using IFN-gamma ELISPOT assay. *J. Immunol. Methods* 2007; **328**: 152–161.

77 Shrestha MP, Scott RM, Joshi DM *et al.* Safety and efficacy of a recombinant hepatitis E vaccine. *N. Engl. J. Med.* 2007; **356**: 895–903.

CHAPTER 18
Hepatitis B

Anna S. F. Lok
University of Michigan, Ann Arbor, MI, USA

Learning points

- Patients with chronic HBV infection are at risk of developing cirrhosis, liver failure and hepatocellular carcinoma.

- Screening of at-risk persons is the first step in controlling HBV infection.

- Hepatitis B vaccines are safe and effective in preventing HBV infection and have been shown to prevent hepatocellular carcinoma.

- Persistent presence of HBeAg or persistently high serum HBV DNA levels is associated with an increased risk of cirrhosis, liver-related mortality and hepatocellular carcinoma.

- There are seven approved therapies for chronic hepatitis B: two formulations of interferon and five orally administered nucleos(t)ide analogues, lamivudine, adefovir dipivoxil, entecavir, telbivudine and tenofovir disoproxil fumarate.

- Antiviral treatment suppresses but does not eradicate HBV; in the absence of HBsAg loss most patients require long-term treatment. Long-term treatment of nucleos(t) ide analogues is associated with risks of antiviral drug resistance.

Introduction

In 1965, Blumberg *et al.* found an antibody in two multiply transfused haemophiliac patients that reacted with an antigen in a serum sample from an Australian aborigine [1]. Later, this antigen was found in other patients with serum hepatitis. Because of its discovery in an aboriginal serum, the antigen was initially called Australia antigen. The Australia antigen is now known to be the envelope of the hepatitis B virus (HBV) and has been renamed the hepatitis B surface antigen (HBsAg). In 1976, Blumberg was awarded the Nobel Prize for discovering the cause of hepatitis B.

HBV infection is a major global public health problem. It is estimated that over 2 billion people worldwide had been infected and 400 million are chronically infected. Chronic HBV infection can progress to cirrhosis, hepatic decompensation and hepatocellular carcinoma (HCC). Although most persons with chronic HBV infection will not develop these complications, 15–40% will and roughly 500 000 people die from these complications each year. The availability of safe and effective vaccines and several approved treatments have made hepatitis B a preventable, as well as a treatable, condition.

Hepatitis B virus

The hepatitis B virus belongs to the family of hepadnaviruses which also includes the duck hepatitis B virus (DHBV), ground squirrel hepatitis virus (GSHV) and woodchuck hepatitis virus (WHV). The hepatitis B virion (also known as the Dane particle) is a 42-nm particle with an outer envelope (HBsAg) surrounding a nucleocapsid that contains a small DNA genome (Fig. 18.1).

The HBV genome is a circular, partially double-stranded DNA of approximately 3200 base pairs. HBV DNA encodes four overlapping open reading frames (Fig. 18.2) [2]. The surface (S) gene codes for the small surface protein, HBsAg. The pre-S1 and pre-S2 regions along with the S gene code for the large and middle surface proteins, which may be involved in viral recognition by hepatocyte receptors. The core (C) gene codes for the hepatitis B core antigen (HBcAg). The polymerase (P) gene codes for a DNA polymerase/ reverse transcriptase. The X gene codes for the HBx protein, which has potent transcriptional transactivating function and may play a role in hepatocarcinogenesis. HBV is unique in that it produces a surplus of genome-free subviral 22-nm spheres or filaments. While all three envelope proteins, large, middle and small, are expressed on the surface of Dane particles, only the small surface protein is present in subviral particles.

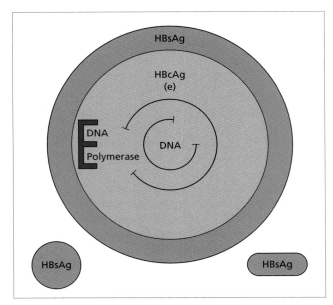

Fig. 18.1. Diagram of the hepatitis B virus (HBV). The complete virion (Dane particle) consists of a nucleocapsid, that expresses the hepatitis B core antigen (HBcAg), and an envelope, that expresses hepatitis B surface antigen (HBsAg). The nucleocapsid contains a partially double-stranded circular HBV DNA. Subviral particles comprising envelope protein only circulate in serum as spheres and tubules.

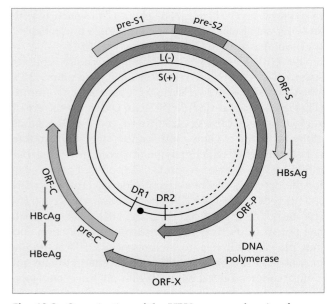

Fig. 18.2. Organization of the HBV genome showing four overlapping open reading frames (ORF): polymerase (P), surface (S), core (C) and X. The P gene encodes the polymerase protein which also functions as a reverse transcriptase. The S gene and the preceding pre-S1 and pre-S2 regions encode the large, middle and small surface proteins. The C gene and the preceding pre-C region encodes the core and e antigen.

Replication cycle

The replication cycle of HBV is illustrated in Fig. 18.3 [2]. After attachment and penetration of the hepatocyte, synthesis of the incomplete (+) strand HBV DNA occurs and the gap is closed, resulting in a fully double-stranded, covalently closed circular DNA (cccDNA). The cccDNA serves as a template for subgenomic viral RNA transcripts, which encode the envelope proteins as well as a greater than full length pregenomic RNA. The pregenomic RNA serves as a template for the transcription of the polymerase protein and the core protein and it is also encapsidated in the immature cytoplasmic core particles. Inside these immature core particles, the first (−) strand HBV DNA is synthesized by reverse transcription of the pregenomic RNA. Subsequently, the second (+) strand HBV DNA is replicated from the (−) strand HBV DNA, but this process is often incomplete, resulting in the secretion of virions with a partially double-stranded DNA molecule.

The cellular pool of cccDNA is maintained both by superinfection of the hepatocyte by additional virions and by import of nucleocapsids from the hepatocyte cytoplasm. Currently approved nucleos(t)ide analogues for the treatment of hepatitis B have very little or no direct inhibitory effect on cccDNA. The resistance of cccDNA to treatments that act primarily through inhibition of reverse transcription of the pregenomic RNA and the long half-life of infected hepatocytes (and hence cccDNA) account for the high rate of viral relapse when treatment is stopped.

HBV serotypes and genotypes

HBV has been classified into serotypes based on antigenic determinants on the small S protein. The common determinant is 'a'. In addition, there are two pairs of mutually exclusive allelic antigens: 'y' versus 'd' and 'w' versus 'r'. Thus, there are four possible major serotype combinations: ayw, ayr, adw and adr [3,4].

HBV has also been classified into eight genotypes (A–H) based on nucleotide sequences with varying distribution in different geographical regions (Fig. 18.4). HBV genotypes may play a role in determining the activity and risk of progression of liver disease, as well as response to interferon therapy [3].

HBV variants

HBV genome replicates via reverse transcription of the pregenomic RNA. Reverse transcriptase lacks proof reading ability. Therefore, there is a high error rate during HBV genome replication and HBV is present as a quasispecies (mixture of viral strains with variations in viral sequences) in chronically infected individuals.

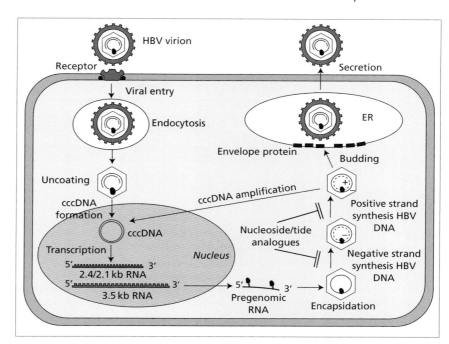

Fig. 18.3. HBV replication cycle. After entry of the virus into the hepatocyte, synthesis of the second-strand HBV DNA is completed. The covalently closed circular HBV DNA (cccDNA) serves as a template for the transcription of the pregenomic RNA as well as the translation of the core and polymerase proteins. The pregenomic RNA along with the core and polymerase proteins are packaged into core particles. Inside the core particle, the pregenomic RNA is reverse transcribed to the first (−) strand HBV DNA and then the second (+) strand HBV DNA. The core particle is coated with envelope proteins and secreted before the (+) stand HBV DNA synthesis is complete.

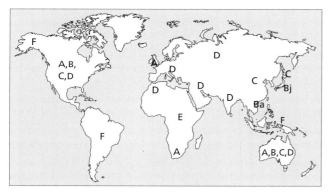

Fig. 18.4. Global distribution of HBV genotypes.

The predominant strain is selected for by endogenous factors such as the host immune response, replication fitness of the variant, and replication space as well as by exogenous factors such as antiviral (nucleos(t)ide analogues) or immune-based therapies (HBV vaccine and hepatitis B immune globulin; HBIG) [5].

Mutations in the precore and core promoter regions are the most common naturally occurring HBV mutations. The precore region is located upstream of the core region. The precore protein which is translated from an RNA that includes the precore and core regions is processed to a small soluble antigen, hepatitis B e antigen (HBeAg) (Fig. 18.5). The core promoter region upstream of the precore and core regions overlaps with the X gene and regulates the transcription of the pregenomic RNA and the precore mRNA and thereby HBV replication and HBeAg production.

The most common precore mutation is a point mutation at nucleotide 1896 of the HBV genome (G1896A) [6]. This mutation results in a premature stop codon, thus preventing the production of HBeAg (Fig. 18.5). It is most frequently found in association with HBV genotype D, and to a lesser extent in genotypes B, C and E, but rarely occurs in genotypes A, F or H. Initially, the precore stop codon variant was thought to be associated with fulminant hepatitis and severe forms of chronic liver disease but this variant can also be found in those who are in an inactive carrier state.

The most common core promoter variant encompasses a dual mutation, A1762T and G1764A, which down-regulate HBeAg production (Fig. 18.5). Core promoter variants can be found in all HBV genotypes, although they are most commonly associated with genotype C. Core promoter variants have been reported to be associated with an increased risk of HCC [7].

Immune response and mechanisms of hepatic injury

HBV is not directly cytopathic. The pathogenesis of HBV-related liver injury is determined by the interactions between the virus and the host immune response [8]. Although loss of HBsAg is often referred to as viral clearance, the rare but well documented re-emergence of viraemia in patients receiving immunosuppressive therapy demonstrates that complete viral clearance may never occur. Quiescent or inactive disease indicates that the virus is suppressed by the host immune response. In persons with chronic HBV infection, the different

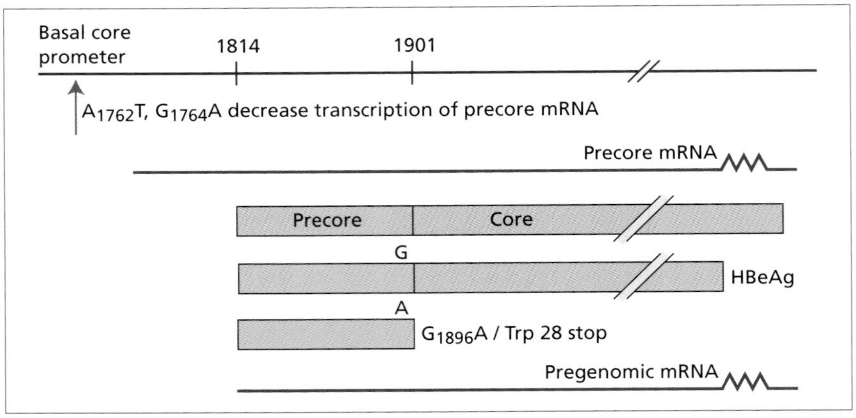

Fig. 18.5. Transcription and translation of HBV precore/core gene. The core promoter region regulates the transcription of precore messenger RNA (mRNA) and pregenomic RNA. The precore mRNA is translated into precore protein and then processed to the hepatitis B e antigen (HBeAg). The pregenomic RNA is reverse transcribed to HBV DNA and also translated to hepatitis B core antigen (HBcAg). HBcAg overlaps with HBeAg. The most common precore mutation is the substitution G1896A, which results in a change from tryptophan to a stop codon and prevents the production of HBeAg. Mutations in the core promoter region, notably A1762T and G1764A, down regulate the transcription of precore mRNA, thereby decreasing the production of HBeAg.

phases represent changes in balance between the host immune response and HBV replication.

In acute infection that resolves, there is a strong polyclonal and multispecific CD8+ T-cell response [8–10]. In chronically infected individuals, the T-cell responses are weak and poorly functional [11]. HBV-specific T cells are maintained in a dysfunctional state but not deleted. Increase in HBV-specific T-cell responsiveness has been observed in patients who undergo spontaneous or treatment-related HBeAg seroconversion [12]. It should be noted that while the host immune response in patients with chronic HBV infection may be ineffective in viral clearance, it can mediate liver damage [13]. Thus, the immune response can be a double-edge sword.

Epidemiology

HBV is transmitted by parenteral, percutaneous or sexual contact. The rate of chronic HBV infection varies from 0.1 to 20% in different areas of the world (Table 18.1) [14–17]. In low prevalence areas such as the USA, Western Europe, Australia and New Zealand, the rate is about 0.1 to 2%. In intermediate prevalence areas such as the Mediterranean countries, Eastern Europe, India and Singapore, the rate is approximately 3 to 5%. In high prevalence areas such as Southeast Asia and sub-Saharan Africa, the rate is 10 to 20%. The prevalence of current and past HBV infection is estimated to be 5% in the USA and close to 100% among adults in some parts of Southeast Asia and Africa. The worldwide incidence of HBV infection is decreasing but in many developed countries the decrease in incidence of acute HBV infec-

tion has not been paralleled by a decrease in the prevalence of chronic HBV infection due to immigration of carriers from endemic areas.

In most high endemic areas such as China, perinatal transmission is the major mode of spread but horizontal spread during the first 2 years of life is the predominant mode of transmission in African countries. Infection from mother to the neonate occurs at the time of birth and during close contact afterwards; *in utero* infection can occur but is uncommon. In intermediate prevalence areas, early childhood infection accounts for most cases of chronic infection. Infection probably occurs through close contacts within the household, abrasions, cuts, sharing of toothbrushes and razors and contaminated needles. In low prevalence areas, most infections are acquired in adult life through unprotected sexual intercourse or injection drug use. Infection is more common among homosexual men and those with multiple sexual partners. The risk of progression to chronic infection is inversely related to the age at infection; approximately 90% for perinatal infection, 25 to 50% for infection among toddlers, and very low (1–2%) for infection during adult life.

Modes of transmission

HBV is more easily spread than human immunodeficiency virus (HIV) or hepatitis C virus (HCV). This may be related to much higher levels of viraemia in some patients with chronic HBV infection (up to 12 $\log_{10}$ IU/mL compared to 5–7 $\log_{10}$ IU/mL in patients with HIV or HCV infection) as well as the ability of HBV to survive outside the human body for up to 7 days [18].

Table 18.1. Patterns of HBV infection

Characteristic	Pattern		
Prevalence	High	Intermediate	Low
Carrier rate	≥8%	2–7%	<2%
Geographical distribution	Southeast Asia	Middle East	United States and Canada
	China	Mediterranean basin	Western Europe
	Pacific Islands	Eastern Europe	Australia
	Sub-Saharan Africa	Central and South Asia	New Zealand
		Japan	
		Latin and South America	
Predominant age at infection	Perinatal and early childhood	Early childhood	Adult
Predominant mode of transmission	Maternal–infant, percutaneous	Percutaneous, sexual	Sexual, percutaneous

Blood transfusion is rarely a source of HBV infection nowadays. In some countries, blood donors are screened not only for HBsAg but also for hepatitis B core antibody (anti-HBc) and HBV DNA. The risk of transfusion-related hepatitis B from blood donors who test negative for HBsAg and anti-HBc is estimated to be 1 in 63 000 [19]. Addition of nucleic acid testing will detect a small number of donor units that may be associated with risk of transmitting HBV infection but the cost-effectiveness of nucleic acid testing is still debated [20].

Organ donors are routinely screened for HBsAg. Transmission of HBV infection has been reported after transplantation of non-hepatic organs such as kidneys and avascular tissues such as cornea from HBsAg-positive persons.

The role of anti-HBc screening is uncertain because of the potential loss of up to 5% of donors in low endemic areas and more than 50% of donors in high endemic areas. The likelihood of transmission from HBsAg-negative, anti-HBc-positive donors is very low for recipients of blood or non-hepatic organs such as kidneys but may be as high as 80% in liver recipients [21–23].

The health-care environment may provide a venue for spread of HBV. Transmission generally occurs from patient to patient or from patient to health-care personnel via contaminated surgical instruments or accidental needle stick; however, transmission from surgeons to patients through cuts in gloves had been reported [24]. In many countries, proof of immunity (through vaccination or past infection) is required of all surgeons and other medical staff performing invasive procedures and vaccination is offered to all staff that might come into contact with patients. Medical staff who are chronically infected with hepatitis B may not be allowed to perform invasive procedures unless they are HBeAg negative or have low or undetectable serum HBV DNA [25]. Vaccination programmes have greatly reduced the rate of infection among medical staff. Improved infection control, including segregation of HBsAg-positive patients and mandatory vaccination, have greatly reduced the incidence of HBV infection among haemodialysis patients.

The risk of maternal–infant transmission is related to the HBeAg and HBV DNA status of the mother [26,27]. Caesarean section has not been shown to eliminate the risk of perinatal HBV infection. Infants born to infected mothers may be breast fed if they have been vaccinated. The risk of transmission to the fetus during amniocentesis is low.

Sexual transmission remains the major mode of spread of HBV in developed countries. The risk is increased in persons with multiple sexual partners, sexually transmitted diseases or high-risk behaviours. Sexual transmission can be prevented by vaccination of spouses and steady sex partners in individuals with monogamous partners and safe sex practice, including use of condoms in those with multiple partners.

Prevention

Prevention of HBV infection is best achieved through education, instituting 'universal precaution' and vaccination [15,16].

Hepatitis B immune globulin

Hepatitis B immune globulin (HBIG) is a hyperimmune serum globulin with a high hepatitis B surface antibody (anti-HBs) titre. It is effective if given before or within hours of infection. HBV vaccine should always be given with HBIG, particularly if the subject is at risk of re-infection. HBIG is indicated for sexual contacts of persons with acute HBV infection, babies born to mothers infected with hepatitis B and victims of parenteral exposure (e.g. needle stick) to HBsAg-positive blood [15,16]. HBIG is also used to prevent HBV re-infection in patients who undergo liver transplantation for HBV-related liver disease.

HBV vaccines

Types of vaccines

There are two types of HBV vaccines, plasma-derived and recombinant. Plasma-derived vaccines are prepared by concentrating and purifying plasma from HBsAg carriers to produce 22-nm subviral particles that contain HBsAg alone. Plasma vaccines have been largely replaced by recombinant vaccines because of concerns about the potential to transmit blood-borne infections, although there are no data to support these concerns. Recombinant vaccines may be derived from yeast or mammalian cells. The yeast-derived vaccines contain small S protein only while the mammalian cell-derived vaccines contain small S protein with or without large and middle S proteins. The two most widely used HBV vaccines (Recombivax and Engerix-B) are yeast derived and do not contain thimerosal.

HBV vaccine is also available as combination vaccines with hepatitis A vaccine (Twinrix) and with diphtheria, tetanus and pertussis (DTP3) with or without *Haemophilus influenzae* type b (Hib) vaccines. These combination vaccines have similar efficacy and facilitate the incorporation of HBV vaccination into childhood immunization.

Indications for HBV vaccine (Table 18.2)

All newborns. Universal vaccination of all newborns regardless of maternal HBsAg status is necessary for global eradication of HBV infection. As of December 2007, 171 countries have introduced HBV vaccine into their national immunization programmes and more than 80% of infants have received the third dose of HBV vaccine. Countries that implemented universal HBV vaccination programmes early have begun to see a

Table 18.2. Indications for hepatitis B vaccination

All newborns*
All children and adolescents not vaccinated at birth
High risk adults:
Health-care workers
Men who have sex with men
Persons with multiple sexual partners
Injection drug users
Patients on haemodialysis
Institutionalized patients
Public safety workers
Spouse, sexual partners and household members of HBV carriers

*For infants born to mothers with chronic HBV infection, hepatitis B immune globulin (HBIG) should also be administered at birth.

benefit. In Taiwan, vaccination of newborns of mothers infected with hepatitis B was implemented in 1984 and universal vaccination of all newborns in 1986. Twenty years into the programme, the rate of chronic HBV infection among children and adolescents decreased from 9.8% to 1.2% and the risk of childhood HCC has decreased by 70% [28,29]. HBV vaccine was the first vaccine demonstrated to prevent cancer [30].

Neonates of HBsAg-positive mothers. This is the most important step toward the eradication of chronic HBV infection. These babies should receive HBIG and the first dose of vaccine at the same time at two different sites within 12 h of birth.

Catch-up vaccination. Children who were born before universal vaccination of newborns was implemented should be vaccinated before they reach adolescence when they are at risk of infection through sexual exposure and injection drug use.

High-risk adults. These include sexually active individuals with multiple sex partners and homosexual or bisexual men, household and sexual contacts of carriers, injection drug users, health-care workers, haemodialysis patients, patients requiring repeated blood or blood product transfusion and patients with chronic liver disease.

Prevaccination screening

The purpose of prevaccination screening is to identify individuals who have been exposed to HBV and who do not require vaccination. The cost-effectiveness of prevaccination screening depends on the prevalence of HBV infection in the community. Prevaccination screening is not necessary in non-endemic areas except for persons in high-risk groups but it should be performed in all adults in endemic areas. Screening can be performed by a single test for anti-HBc, which will detect individuals with past or current infection or by a combination of tests for HBsAg and anti-HBs. The advantage of the latter approach is that it will differentiate persons who are chronically infected from those who have immunity.

Dose schedule

HBV vaccine is usually administered in three doses at 0, 1 and 6 months (Table 18.3). For adults, the injections are given in the deltoid muscle whereas in newborns and young children the recommended site is the anterolateral thigh. Newborns of HBsAg carrier mothers should receive the first dose of HBV vaccine and HBIG within 12 h of birth. For patients on haemodialysis,

Table 18.3. Hepatitis B vaccines and dosage recommendations

Vaccine brand	Age group	Dose	Volume	Number of doses
Engerix-B	0–19 years	10 μg	0.5 mL	3
	≥20 years	20 μg	1.0 mL	3
Recombivax HB	0–19 years	5 μg	0.5 mL	3
	≥20 years	10 μg	1.0 mL	3
(Optional 2 doses)	11–15 years	10 μg	1.0 mL	2

For haemodialysis patients, recommended dose is 40 μg with each dose (Engerix-B 40 μg per 2.0 mL and Recombivax HB dialysis formulation 40 μg per 1.0 mL).

Table 18.4. Causes of non-response to HBV vaccine

Host factors
    Age > 40 years
    Obesity
    Smoking
    Genetics, certain HLA types
Other medical conditions
    Diabetes
    Cirrhosis
    Renal failure
    Conditions requiring immunosuppressive therapy
Unrecognized chronic HBV infection
Technical
    Subcutaneous administration
    Freezing of vaccine

higher doses of vaccine are needed. Some vaccines have also incorporated pre-S1 (large S) and/or pre-S2 (middle S) proteins to increase the immunogenicity and to circumvent vaccine escape mutants but these vaccines are not available in most countries.

Efficacy

A protective immune response defined as a hepatitis B surface antibody (anti-HBs) titre more than 10 mIU/mL is achieved in 90–95% of vaccine recipients. HBV vaccines have been shown to be effective in preventing HBV infection in homosexual men, haemodialysis patients, health-care workers and babies born to carrier mothers.

Postvaccination testing

Routine postvaccination testing to document anti-HBs seroconversion is unnecessary except in health-care workers, haemodialysis patients and persons who are at risk for recurrent exposure to HBV, such as spouse/sexual partner of an individual with chronic HBV infec-

tion and infants of HBV-infected mothers. Testing should be performed 1–2 months after completion of the three-shot primary vaccination series. For infants of mothers infected with hepatitis B testing should be performed at age 9–15 months. For haemodialysis patients, testing should be performed annually.

Management of non-responders

Table 18.4 summarizes reasons for non-response. The general recommendation for non-responders is to repeat a three-dose series; 50–75% will respond to the second course, and retesting for anti-HBs should be performed. Non-responders to the second course should be tested for HBsAg as some may have undiagnosed chronic HBV infection. For haemodialysis patients, response may be improved by using double-dose vaccine. Others have tried intradermal administration but this is technically difficult and inadvertent subcutaneous injections can result in diminished efficacy. Other methods that have been proposed to reduce the non-response rate include co-administration of interleukin-2, use of more potent adjuvants and addition of pre-S antigens.

Duration of protection

Roughly 50% of adolescents vaccinated as infants have protective anti-HBs titre after 20 or more years and 80% have anamestic response to booster vaccination [31–33]. Thus, while anti-HBs titres decrease with time, vaccine recipients may be protected even after anti-HBs titre has become undetectable. Breakthrough infections appear to occur mostly among those who did not have an initial response to vaccination. The need for booster for adolescents and young adults who were vaccinated at birth is controversial and the practice varies from country to country.

Safety

HBV vaccine is very safe and can be administered during pregnancy. The most common adverse reaction is soreness over the injection site. Other adverse reactions include low grade fever, malaise, headache, arthralgia and myalgia. Concerns about HBV vaccine and demyelinating central nervous system diseases including multiple sclerosis as well as autism have not been substantiated [34].

Vaccine escape mutants

Mutations in the surface protein, most commonly a glycine to arginine substitution at codon 145 (G145R), have been found in some children of mothers infected with hepatitis B who became infected despite vaccination

Table 18.5. Interpretation of HBV serological markers

HBsAg	HBV infection: acute or chronic
HBeAg	High levels of HBV replication and infectivity
Anti-HBe	Low levels of HBV replication and infectivity
Anti-HBc (IgM)	Recent HBV infection
Anti-HBc (IgG)	Recovered or chronic HBV infection
Anti-HBs	Immunity to HBV infection
Anti-HBc (IgG) + anti-HBs	Past HBV infection
Anti-HBc (IgG) + HBsAg	Chronic HBV infection

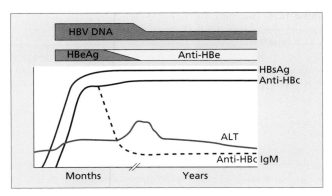

Fig. 18.7. Serological profile of chronic HBV infection. ALT, alanine aminotransferase; HBeAg, hepatitis B e antigen; HBsAg, hepatitis B surface antigen; HBc, hepatitis B core.

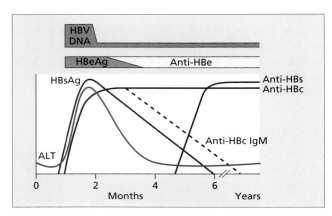

Fig. 18.6. Serological profile of acute HBV infection. ALT, alanine aminotransferase; HBeAg, hepatitis B e antigen; HBsAg, hepatitis B surface antigen; HBc, hepatitis B core.

[35]. These mutations decrease the binding of HBsAg to anti-HBs and are likely to have been selected to escape immune recognition. Although these mutants have been found in many parts of the world, the prevalence appears to be low and there is no indication that the efficacy of HBV vaccine is declining.

Diagnosis

Diagnosis of hepatitis B is based on clinical assessment and laboratory tests. Serological markers of HBV and quantitative serum HBV DNA levels are crucial for confirmation of the diagnosis of HBV infection and for determination of the stage of infection (Tables 18.5, 18.6 and Figs 18.6, 18.7). Most patients with chronic HBV infection do not have symptoms until their liver disease is at an advanced stage; therefore, screening of at-risk persons is critical in early diagnosis. Table 18.7 summarizes the Centers for Disease Control and Prevention Recommendations on who should be screened for hepatitis B [17].

Serological diagnosis

HBsAg and anti-HBs

HBsAg is the serological hallmark of HBV infection. It can be detected 1–10 weeks after an acute exposure to HBV, approximately 2–6 weeks before the onset of hepatitis symptoms or elevation of alanine aminotransferase (ALT). In patients who subsequently recover, HBsAg usually becomes undetectable after 4–6 months. Persistence of HBsAg for more than 6 months implies chronic infection. The disappearance of HBsAg is followed by the appearance of anti-HBs although in some patients there may be a window period of several weeks to months when neither HBsAg nor anti-HBs can be detected. In most patients who recovered from acute HBV infection, anti-HBs persists for life thus conferring long-term immunity.

As many as a third of HBsAg carriers have anti-HBs; in most instances, the antibodies are directed against one of the subtypic determinants and not the common 'a' determinant and are unable to neutralize the circulating virions. These persons are infected and should be managed similarly to other HBsAg-positive persons who do not have detectable anti-HBs.

HBcAg and anti-HBc

HBcAg cannot be detected in circulating blood but anti-HBc can. During acute infection, anti-HBc is predominantly of IgM class. IgM anti-HBc is an indicator of acute HBV infection and may be the sole marker during the window phase. IgM anti-HBc titre decreases during recovery while IgG anti-HBc titre increases. IgM anti-HBc persists at low titre in most patients with chronic HBV infection, titres increase during exacerbations of chronic hepatitis B making it sometimes difficult to differentiate from acute hepatitis B.

Table 18.6. Diagnosis of HBV infection

	HBsAg	HBeAg	Anti-HBc (IgM)	Anti-HBc (IgG)	Anti-HBs	Anti-HBe	HBV DNA	Interpretation
Acute HBV	+	+	+	−	−	−	+++	Early phase
Infection	−	−	+	+	−	+	+	Window phase
	−	−	−	+	+	+	+/−	Recovery phase
Chronic HBV	+	+	−	+	−	−	+++	HBeAg+ chronic hepatitis or
Infection								Immune tolerant phase
	+	−	−	+	−	+	+/−	Inactive carrier state
	+	−	−	+	−	+	++	HBeAg− chronic hepatitis
	+	+/−	+/−	+	−	+/−	++	Exacerbations of chronic hepatitis

Table 18.7. Recommendations on who should be screened for HBV

Individuals born in areas of high* or intermediate prevalence rates† for HBV including immigrants and adopted children‡§
    Asia: all countries
    Africa: all countries
    South Pacific Islands: all countries
    Middle East (except Cyprus and Israel)
    European Mediterranean: Malta and Spain
    The Arctic (indigenous populations of Alaska, Canada and Greenland)
    South America: Ecuador, Guyana, Suriname, Venezuela and Amazon regions of Bolivia, Brazil, Colombia and Peru
    Eastern Europe: all countries except Hungary
    Caribbean: Antigua and Barbuda, Dominica, Granada, Haiti, Jamaica, St. Kitts and Nevis, St. Lucia, and Turks and Caicos
    Central America: Guatemala and Honduras
Other groups recommended for screening
    US born persons not vaccinated as infants whose parents were born in regions with high HBV endemicity (≥8%)
    Household and sexual contacts of HBsAg-positive persons‡
    Persons who have ever injected drugs‡
    Persons with multiple sexual partners or history of sexually transmitted disease‡
    Men who have sex with men‡
    Inmates of correctional facilities‡
    Individuals with chronically elevated ALT or AST‡
    Individuals infected with HCV or HIV‡
    Patients undergoing renal dialysis
    All pregnant women
    Persons needing immunosuppressive therapy

ALT, alanine aminotransferase; AST, aspartate aminotransferase.
*HBsAg prevalence >8%.
†HBsAg prevalence 2–7%.
‡Those who are seronegative should receive hepatitis B vaccine.
§If HBsAg-positive persons are found in the first generation, subsequent generations should be tested.

IgG anti-HBc is present along with anti-HBs in persons who have recovered from HBV infection and with HBsAg in those who are chronically infected. Isolated presence of anti-HBc in the absence of HBsAg and anti-HBs may occur during the window period of acute hepatitis B when the anti-HBc is predominantly IgM class, many years after recovery from acute hepatitis B when anti-HBs has fallen to undetectable levels, or after many years of chronic HBV infection when HBsAg titre has decreased below the level of detection. In endemic countries and in those with high risk for HBV infection, isolated presence of anti-HBc is most often an indication of low-level HBV infection. HBV DNA is occasionally detected in serum, usually at low levels but HBV DNA is often present in the liver. Transmission of HBV infection has been reported from blood and organ donors with isolated anti-HBc, the risk being highest when livers from anti-HBc-positive donors are transplanted into seronegative recipients [21,23].

HBeAg and anti-HBe

HBeAg is a soluble protein derived from the processing of the precore protein. It is a marker of HBV replication and infectivity. Seroconversion from HBeAg to anti-HBe is usually associated with marked decrease in serum HBV DNA level and remission of liver disease. Some anti-HBe-positive patients continue to have active liver disease and high serum HBV DNA level; these patients often have precore or core promoter HBV variants that prevent or decrease the production of HBeAg [5].

HBV DNA

HBV DNA in serum is a marker of viraemia and infectivity. Real-time PCR assays are more sensitive with detection limits down to less than 10 IU/mL and have a wider range of linearity—up to 10^8 IU/mL. Using sensitive PCR assays, HBV DNA may be detected up to 2–3 weeks before the appearance of HBsAg in persons with acute HBV infection and HBV DNA may remain detectable after HBsAg seroconversion. HBV DNA levels fluctuate during chronic HBV infection; therefore, serial monitoring is important to determine which phase of infection the patient is in, to determine when antiviral treatment should be initiated and to monitor for virological response and breakthroughs during treatment.

Liver biopsy

The purpose of a liver biopsy is to assess the degree of necroinflammation and the extent of fibrosis. Sometimes, liver biopsies are performed to rule out other causes of liver disease. Liver biopsy is most useful in patients with chronic HBV infection who do not meet clear-cut criteria for treatment. Liver biopsy is not necessary for the diagnosis of HBV infection; however, immunohistochemical staining for HBsAg and HBcAg or PCR for HBV DNA including cccDNA may help in assessing efficacy of antiviral treatment.

Several studies showed that significant liver disease, moderate–severe inflammation and/or advanced fibrosis, can be found in patients with persistently normal ALT [36–38]. It should be pointed out that many of these studies defined persistently normal ALT based on two to three values over a 6-month period. In these studies, significant liver disease was mainly observed in older patients (>40 years) and in those with high serum HBV DNA levels.

Data on the accuracy of serum markers in predicting histological fibrosis in patients with chronic hepatitis B is limited [39]. Inflammation plays an important role in disease progression and response to antiviral therapy in patients with hepatitis B. Therefore, non-invasive tests of liver disease must be able to assess both inflammation and fibrosis. Liver stiffness measurement or elastography has been shown to correlate with fibrosis stages in patients with hepatitis C. Liver stiffness is influenced not only by fibrosis but also inflammation and oedema; indeed, several studies found that liver stiffness increased during exacerbations of hepatitis B and decreased after the exacerbations were resolved.

Clinical manifestations

The manifestations vary from subclinical hepatitis, anicteric hepatitis, icteric hepatitis to fulminant hepatitis during the acute phase; and from inactive carrier state to chronic hepatitis, cirrhosis, liver failure and HCC during the chronic phase. Perinatal or childhood infection is usually associated with little or no symptoms and a high rate of chronicity, whereas when adults become infected this is often associated with symptoms and a low risk of chronicity. Clinical manifestations, outcomes and treatment of patients coinfected with HIV or hepatitis D will be discussed in Chapters 19 and 22.

Acute HBV infection

Approximately 70% of patients with acute HBV infection have subclinical or anicteric hepatitis. The incubation period lasts 1–4 months. During the prodromal period, a serum sickness-like syndrome may develop. This is followed by malaise, anorexia, nausea, right upper quadrant discomfort and in some patients fever, vomiting and jaundice. Clinical symptoms and jaundice usually disappear after 1–3 months but some patients may have persistent fatigue even after ALT levels have returned to normal.

The most common findings on physical examination include soft, mildly tender hepatomegaly, jaundice and low-grade fever. Rarely, splenomegaly and spider nevi may be present.

Laboratory tests reveal acute hepatocellular injury with marked elevation in aspartate aminotransferase (AST) and ALT, with or without an increase in bilirubin. Persistent increase in bilirubin and prolongation of prothrombin time indicate severe liver injury.

Patients with acute hepatitis B test positive for HBsAg and IgM anti-HBc. During the early phase, HBeAg and

HBV DNA will also be present. Patients who present late in the course of illness may have seroconverted from HBeAg to anti-HBe with undetectable HBV DNA, and in some instances may have become HBsAg negative (Table 18.6 and Fig. 18.6) but will remain with detectable anti-HBc.

Chronic HBV infection

Many patients with chronic HBV infection have no symptoms while others may experience fatigue or right upper quadrant discomfort. Exacerbations of chronic hepatitis B may be asymptomatic or mimic acute hepatitis with fatigue, anorexia, nausea and jaundice and in rare instances hepatic decompensation.

Physical examination may be normal or there may be stigmata of chronic liver disease and mild hepatomegaly. In patients with cirrhosis the spleen may be palpable and there may be signs of liver failure: jaundice, leg oedema, ascites or encephalopathy. Stigmata of chronic liver disease such as spider nevi are rarely seen in patients with chronic hepatitis B.

Laboratory tests can be entirely normal even in patients with well compensated cirrhosis. Mild to moderate elevation in AST and ALT may be the only biochemical abnormality. ALT levels can be more than 1000 U/L during exacerbations and markers of impaired hepatic function (decreased albumin, increased bilirubin and prolonged prothrombin time) may be present. α-fetoprotein levels may be increased during exacerbations and may be as high as 5000 ng/mL. IgM anti-HBc titres are increased during exacerbations mimicking acute hepatitis B.

Patients with chronic HBV infection test positive for HBsAg and IgG anti-HBc (Table 18.6 and Fig. 18.7). During the early phases of chronic HBV infection, HBeAg and high levels of HBV DNA will also be present.

Extrahepatic manifestations

Serum sickness

Acute hepatitis is sometimes heralded by a serum sickness-like syndrome manifested as fever, skin rash and polyarthralgia.

Polyarteritis nodosa (PAN)

Approximately 10–30% of patients with PAN are found to be HBsAg positive [40]. The decline in HBV infection over the past decade has been associated with a decrease in frequency of HBV-related PAN. Immune complexes of HBV antigens and antibodies trigger injury of large, medium and small blood vessels. Vasculitis may affect cardiovascular, gastrointestinal, musculoskeletal, neu-

rological and dermatological systems. The course is variable and may be fatal.

Glomerulonephritis

HBV-related glomerulonephritis is rare and more often found in children. Membranous glomerulonephritis is most common especially among children but membranoproliferative, mesangiocapillary or focal proliferative glomerulonephritis, minimal change disease and IgA nephropathy have also been reported [41]. Severity of the renal disease does not correlate with HBV replication or severity of liver disease although antiviral therapy and HBeAg seroconversion have been associated with remission of renal and hepatic disease.

Essential mixed cryoglobulinaemia

Cryoglobulinaemia is more commonly associated with HCV infection than with HBV infection.

Papular acrodermatitis (Gianotti–Crosti disease)

Papular acrodermatitis is strongly associated with HBs antigenaemia in young children. It manifests as symmetrical, erythematous, maculopapular, non-itchy eruptions over the face, buttocks, limbs and occasionally the trunk.

Natural history

The natural course of HBV infection is determined by the interplay between: (1) the virus—HBV replication, HBV genotype and viral variants; (2) the host—age, gender, race/ethnicity, genetic make-up and immune response; and (3) the environment—alcohol, infection with other viruses such as hepatitis C, D or HIV, and carcinogens such as aflatoxin (Table 18.8) [42].

Acute HBV infection

Age at the time of infection and immune status of the host are the most important factors determining progression from acute to chronic HBV infection. Recovery from acute HBV infection is signified by loss of HBsAg and detection of anti-HBs. Using sensitive PCR assays, HBV DNA can be detected in the liver and sometimes also in the serum many years after 'recovery' from acute HBV infection [43]. It is now recognized that HBV persists at low levels, being held in check by the host immune response. This explains why reactivation of HBV replication has been observed in persons with serological markers of recovered HBV infection. Inability to eliminate HBV after 'immunological recovery' from transient acute HBV infection explains why virus eradication is

Table 18.8. Factors associated with increased risk of cirrhosis or hepatocellular carcinoma

Viral
    Persistent presence of HBeAg
    Persistently high HBV DNA
    HBV genotype C > B
    Core promoter mutations*
Host
    Male gender
    Older age
    Recurrent exacerbations
    Persistently elevated ALT
    Cirrhosis*
    Diabetes*
Environment
    Heavy drinking
    Cigarette smoking*
    Aflatoxin*
    HCV, HDV, HIV

ALT, alanine aminotransferase.
*Increased risk of hepatocellular carcinoma.

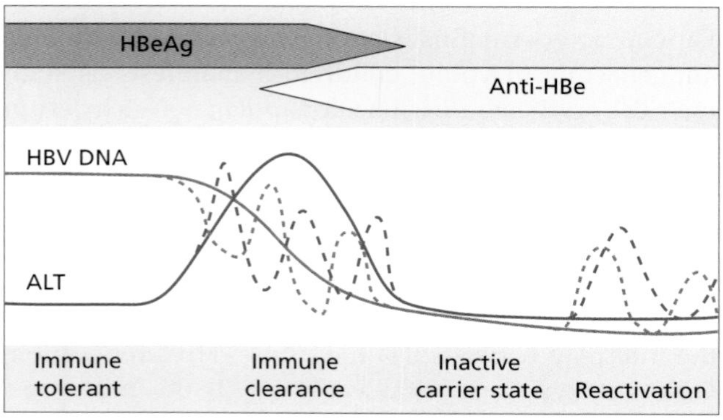

Fig. 18.8. Different phases of chronic HBV infection. ALT, alanine aminotransferase.

an unrealistic goal in patients receiving antiviral therapy for chronic HBV infection.

Chronic HBV infection

The course of chronic HBV infection consists of four phases (Fig. 18.8), although not every patient goes through all phases [42]. For example, the immune tolerant phase is short or absent in patients with childhood or adult acquired HBV infection that becomes chronic and many patients may never progress to the reactivation phase.

Immune tolerant phase

This phase is characterized by the presence of HBeAg, high serum HBV DNA levels and persistently normal ALT. Patients in this phase are typically young Asians with perinatally acquired HBV infection. The lack of liver disease despite high levels of HBV replication is believed to be due to immune tolerance to HBV.

The immune tolerant phase usually lasts 10–30 years, during which there is a very low rate of spontaneous HBeAg clearance. Most patients in the immune tolerant phase have minimal liver injury and prognosis is favourable during short-term follow-up, particularly in patients who undergo spontaneous HBeAg seroconversion before age 40. One study from Taiwan found that only 5% of patients progressed to cirrhosis and none developed HCC after a mean follow-up of 10.5 years [44]. The rate of progression to cirrhosis was low (less than 4%) in patients who underwent HBeAg seroconversion before age 40 but increased to 28% in those who did so after age 40 [45].

Immune clearance phase (HBeAg-positive chronic hepatitis)

This phase is characterized by the presence of HBeAg, high serum HBV DNA levels, persistent or intermittent elevation in ALT and active inflammation on liver biopsy.

A characteristic of the immune clearance phase is ALT flares which are believed to be manifestations of immune-mediated lysis of infected hepatocytes. Most ALT flares are asymptomatic but some are accompanied by symptoms of acute hepatitis and rarely jaundice and liver failure.

An important outcome of the immune clearance phase is HBeAg seroconversion. During this phase, spontaneous HBeAg seroconversion occurs at a much higher rate with rates as high as 10–20% per year. HBeAg seroconversion is frequently but not always accompanied by an ALT flare [46,47]. Not all ALT flares result in HBeAg seroconversion. In some cases, ALT flares are accompanied by marked decrease in serum HBV DNA but HBeAg remains positive. ALT flares are more common in men than women. The more frequent flares in men may account for the higher rates of cirrhosis and HCC in men.

Factors associated with HBeAg seroconversion include older age, higher ALT and ethnicity other than Asian. Studies in Asian countries showed that patients with HBV genotype B undergo HBeAg seroconversion at an earlier age and are more likely to have sustained biochemical and virological remission after HBeAg seroconversion than those with genotype C [48].

Inactive chronic hepatitis B

This phase is characterized by the absence of HBeAg, presence of anti-HBe, persistently normal ALT, and low or undetectable serum HBV DNA.

Patients who stay in this phase have a favourable prognosis, particularly if they had minimal liver injury during the preceding immune clearance phase. A study of Italian HBsAg-positive blood donors found no difference in mortality compared to uninfected controls after 23 years of follow-up [49]. However, some patients will revert back to HBeAg positivity and others will progress to HBeAg-negative chronic hepatitis. Inflammation and fibrosis have been found in the liver biopsies of HBeAg-negative patients with normal ALT; the risk is higher in older patients, those with high serum HBV DNA and those with intermittently abnormal ALT or ALT close to the upper limit of normal [36–38]. Patients should not be classified as inactive carriers until they have had HBV DNA and ALT testing on three to four occasions over a 12-month period documenting inactivity.

Reactivation phase (HBeAg-negative chronic hepatitis)

This phase is characterized by the absence of HBeAg, presence of anti-HBe, high HBV DNA, intermittent or persistently elevated ALT and continued necroinflammation. Whereas most patients reach this phase after a variable duration in the inactive carrier state, some progress directly from HBeAg-positive chronic hepatitis to HBeAg-negative chronic hepatitis. Patients in this phase are older and have more advanced liver disease because this represents a later stage in the course of chronic HBV infection.

Most patients have precore or core promoter HBV variants that prevent or decrease the production of HBeAg [5,6]. Although first described in Mediterranean countries, HBeAg-negative chronic hepatitis is seen all over the world and in many countries is more common than HBeAg-positive chronic hepatitis.

Spontaneous HBsAg clearance

Patients with chronic HBV infection may spontaneously clear HBsAg. The annual rate of HBsAg clearance has been estimated to be 1% per year but HBsAg clearance does not occur at a linear rate, being very uncommon during the early stages and increasing over time [50].

HBsAg clearance is generally accompanied by undetectable serum HBV DNA, normalization of ALT and improved liver histology [51]. However, low levels of HBV DNA may be detectable in some patients, more so in the liver than serum. The prognosis of patients who cleared HBsAg is excellent, particularly if HBsAg is cleared before age 50 and in those who have not progressed to cirrhosis [52,53]. HCC has been observed in patients who cleared HBsAg late.

Occult HBV infection

Occult HBV infection is defined as the detection of HBV DNA in the absence of HBsAg in serum [54]. HBV DNA is detected in the liver in most cases but HBV DNA is undetectable or present at low concentrations in the serum and lymphocytes. The vast majority of these patients are positive for anti-HBc indicating that they had prior infection with HBV. Occult HBV infection has been found in a higher percent of hepatitis C patients with HCC than those who do not have HCC, suggesting that past HBV infection or persistence of low-level HBV infection may contribute to HCC development.

Clinical outcomes

Clinical outcomes of chronic HBV infection include progression to cirrhosis, liver failure and HCC (Fig. 18.9). Host, viral and environmental factors contribute to the development of these outcomes (Table 18.8) [42]. Patients coinfected with HIV, HCV or HDV have increased risk of progression to cirrhosis and HCC.

Viral factors and clinical outcomes

Although HBV is not a cytopathic virus, recent studies found that high serum HBV DNA levels, delayed HBeAg seroconversion and HBV reactivation are associated with increased risk of cirrhosis, HCC and liver-related mortality [45,55–57]. These data indicate that persistently high level HBV replication is associated with increased risk of adverse outcomes. Because these studies were conducted in countries where the predominant mode of infection is maternal–infant transmission, the mean age of the participants was more than 40 years, and the participants were predominantly male, these results may not apply to persons with adult-acquired HBV infection who have been infected for a shorter duration or to persons with perinatal HBV infection who are younger than 40 years.

HBV genotype has also been found to be associated with clinical outcomes [3]. Studies in Asia showed that compared to genotype B, genotype C is associated with more rapid progression to cirrhosis and a higher rate of HCC [58]. The more aggressive course of genotype C may be related to the delay in HBeAg seroconversion and frequent association with core promoter mutations. The dual mutations A1762T and G1764A in the core promoter region are associated with more active hepatitis and have been shown to be associated with an increased risk of HCC [7]. Data correlating disease progression and other HBV genotypes are limited. A study in Spain found that deaths related to liver disease occurred more often in patients with genotype F and another study in Alaska natives showed that genotype F was associated with the highest incidence of HCC.

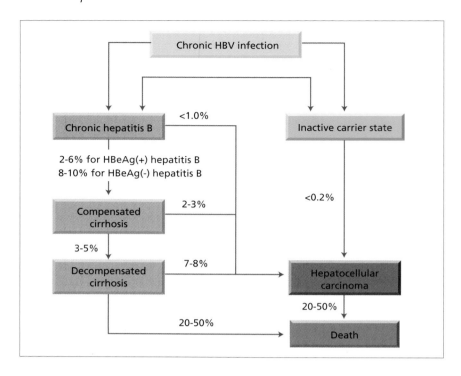

Fig. 18.9. Outcomes of chronic HBV infection.

Treatment

There has been substantial improvement in the treatment of chronic hepatitis B in the past 10 years. Currently, there are seven approved treatments, including five oral drugs. However, these drugs suppress but do not eradicate HBV; therefore, most patients require long-term and sometimes lifelong treatment to maintain clinical benefit.

Goals of treatment

The aims of hepatitis B treatment are to achieve sustained suppression of HBV replication and remission of liver disease. The ultimate goal is to prevent cirrhosis, liver failure and HCC. Parameters used to assess treatment response include decrease in serum HBV DNA, loss of HBeAg with or without seroconversion to anti-HBe, loss of HBsAg with or without seroconversion to anti-HBs, normalization in serum ALT and improvement in liver histology.

When to start (Table 18.9)

The decision whether to start or to defer treatment should balance the activity and stage of liver disease at presentation and the predicted risk of cirrhosis and HCC in the foreseeable future with the risks of treatment (adverse events, drug resistance and costs) [59–64]. Patients with life-threatening liver disease and those who are predicted to have a high risk of cirrhosis and

HCC within the next 10 years should be initiated on treatment while patients with mild disease and a low predicted risk of cirrhosis and HCC in the next 10 years may defer treatment. The latter patients should continue to be monitored so treatment can be instituted if they develop more active liver disease later on.

When treatment is strongly recommended

Patients with life-threatening liver disease, those with compensated cirrhosis and high HBV DNA levels, and those with medical conditions that require chemotherapy or immunosuppressive therapy should receive antiviral therapy.

Patients with acute liver failure and those with decompensated cirrhosis should receive antiviral therapy because there is much to gain and very little to lose. Treatment may stabilize or improve liver disease although clinical improvement may take a few months to be apparent [65]. Antiviral therapy has been shown to reverse liver failure, allowing patients to be removed from transplant waiting list and to improve survival compared to historical controls [66]. Antiviral therapy can also reduce the risk of HBV recurrence if these patients proceed to liver transplantation.

Patients with advanced fibrosis or compensated cirrhosis and high serum HBV DNA levels should receive antiviral therapy because treatment has been shown to prevent disease progression. In a landmark prospective, double-blind, randomized, placebo-controlled trial in patients who were HBeAg positive and/or had high

Table 18.9. Indications for hepatitis B treatment

Treatment strongly recommended
  Acute liver failure
  Decompensated cirrhosis and detectable serum HBV DNA
  Compensated cirrhosis and serum HBV DNA > 2000 IU/mL
  Severe exacerbations of chronic hepatitis B
Treatment should be considered
  HBeAg-positive chronic hepatitis, ALT persistently > 2 × ULN and HBV DNA > 20 000 IU/mL
  HBeAg-negative chronic hepatitis, ALT persistently > 2 × ULN and HBV DNA > 20 000 IU/mL
Treatment should be individualized
  HBeAg-positive, ALT 1–2 × ULN or age > 40
  HBeAg-negative, ALT 1–2 × ULN and/or HBV DNA 2000–20 000 IU/mL
Patients in whom treatment can be deferred
  Young patients in the immune tolerance phase or inactive carrier state

ALT, alanine aminotransferase; ULN, upper limit of normal.

serum HBV DNA levels (~150 000 IU/mL) with bridging fibrosis or cirrhosis, lamivudine treatment significantly decreased the rate of disease progression: 7.8 versus 17.7% (P = 0.001) and HCC: 3.9 versus 7.5% (P = 0.047) compared to untreated controls [67]. Professional guidelines recommended a lower threshold HBV DNA level (~2000 IU/mL) for initiating treatment because of recent findings that serum HBV DNA levels persistently higher than 2000 IU/mL are associated with increased risk of cirrhosis and HCC.

Prophylactic antiviral therapy is also recommended for HBsAg-positive persons who will be receiving cancer chemotherapy or immunosuppressive therapy for other medical conditions to prevent reactivation of HBV replication. Reactivation of HBV replication may manifest as increase in serum HBV DNA only, asymptomatic increase in ALT, symptomatic hepatitis, liver failure and death [68]. A systematic review of 14 studies on reactivation of hepatitis B during cancer chemotherapy found that the incidence of HBV reactivation was 24–88% with an average rate of 37%, liver failure attributed to HBV reactivation was seen in 13% and deaths related to HBV in 7% of patients [69]. Reactivation of hepatitis B was also associated with more frequent disruption of chemotherapy regimens and an increased rate of cancer-related deaths. Antiviral therapy initiated before or at the onset of chemotherapy or immunosuppressive therapy has been shown to reduce the incidence of HBV reactivation, HBV-related hepatitis, HBV-related liver failure and HBV-related death by 80–100% [69]. Reactivation of HBV replication with reappearance of HBsAg can also occur in patients with serological evidence of past infection (presence of anti-HBc with or without anti-HBs) but the incidence is lower. A study of 100 patients receiving chemotherapy for lymphoma found that biochemical hepatitis attributed to HBV occurred in 48% HBsAg-positive patients,

3.9% HBsAg-negative, anti-HBc-positive patients and 0% patients seronegative for HBV [70]. These data suggest that prophylactic antiviral therapy may not be necessary for all HBsAg-negative, anti-HBc-positive patients receiving chemotherapy or immunosuppressive therapy but prophylactic antiviral therapy should be considered for those receiving high-risk regimens such as chemotherapy for haematological malignancies, ablative therapy prior to bone marrow transplantation and regimens containing rituximab or steroids.

When treatment should be considered

Treatment should be individualized for patients who have compensated liver disease and have not progressed to cirrhosis. Those with persistently high serum HBV DNA levels and active liver disease should be treated. Patient age, HBeAg status, family history of HCC and patient preference should also be considered.

HBeAg-positive patients with ALT persistently more than two times the upper limit of normal (ULN) should be considered for treatment. Patients who are icteric or present with a severe flare may be considered for immediate treatment while other patients may be observed for 3–6 months and treatment initiated only in those who failed to achieve spontaneous HBeAg seroconversion. Activity of liver disease as determined by ALT and/or liver histology is used to guide treatment decision because patients with ongoing necroinflammation are at greater risk of adverse clinical outcomes. In addition, elevated baseline ALT is a strong predictor of treatment-related HBeAg seroconversion. In light of recent data indicating a strong association between adverse outcomes and persistently high serum HBV DNA levels or persistent presence of HBeAg, patients who remain HBeAg-positive as well as those with high serum HBV DNA and minimally elevated ALT after the age of 40 may also be treatment candidates, particularly if liver biopsies show evidence of moderate/ severe inflammation or advanced fibrosis.

HBeAg-negative patients with ALT more than two times ULN and serum HBV DNA more than 20 000 IU/ mL should be initiated on treatment. Patients who have mildly elevated ALT (one to two times ULN) and those with lower levels of serum HBV DNA (2000–20 000 IU/ mL) as well as those who have normal ALT and high levels of serum HBV DNA (>20 000 IU/mL) may be considered for treatment, particularly if their biopsies show evidence of moderate/ severe inflammation or advanced fibrosis or if they are above the age of 40.

When treatment may be deferred

Treatment may be deferred in young HBeAg-positive patients who are in the immune tolerant phase. Studies showed that the vast majority of these patients have no or minimal fibrosis on biopsy and favourable prognosis after 10 years of follow-up. Furthermore, the likelihood of treatment-related HBeAg seroconversion is low. Some of these patients will undergo spontaneous HBeAg seroconversion and enter the inactive carrier phase and may never require antiviral therapy while others may require treatment if they fail to undergo spontaneous HBeAg seroconversion after they enter the immune clearance phase (HBeAg-positive chronic hepatitis).

Treatment may also be deferred in patients who are truly in the inactive carrier phase. Categorization of inactive carrier phase should only be made after these patients have been observed for a year with at least three or four ALT and HBV DNA values to be certain they are not in the quiescent period of HBeAg-negative chronic hepatitis. Although HBV DNA can be detected in most of these patients and recrudescence of hepatitis may occur at a later stage, there is no evidence that treatment at this stage will alter the outcomes.

Because of the fluctuating course of chronic HBV infection, all patients with chronic HBV infection in whom treatment is deferred should continue to be monitored so treatment can be instituted at a later stage when HBV replication or liver disease becomes more active.

Other factors to consider

Other factors may influence the decision regarding when to initiate treatment. Age (a surrogate for the duration of infection) is an important consideration. Lower threshold for HBV DNA and ALT values may be used to guide treatment decision in older patients (>40 years) who have been infected for a longer duration.

An important consideration for young female patients is the immediacy of their plans to become pregnant.

Although two of the approved nucleos(t)ide analogues are listed as class B drugs (telbivudine and tenofovir), data on the safety of antiviral therapy during the first trimester of pregnancy are limited. Data in the Antiretroviral Pregnancy Registry showed that the prevalence of birth defects in babies who had been exposed to lamivudine or tenofovir in the first trimester was similar to population controls but only outcomes of live births were recorded and the impact of exposure to nucleos(t)ides on growth and development of the babies is unknown [71]. Data regarding the risk of birth defects associated with entecavir, adefovir, or telbivudine are limited because of the small number of live births reported. It has been suggested that antiviral therapy administered during the third trimester to pregnant mothers with high viraemia may reduce the risk of maternal–infant transmission. Although the rationale is sound, solid data to support the efficacy of this approach are lacking [72].

Familial clustering of HCC has been reported. There are no data to support the suggestion that antiviral therapy in patients who otherwise do not meet criteria for treatment will prevent HCC; however, thresholds for starting treatment may be lowered and decisions regarding when to start treatment should be individualized in patients with a family history of HCC.

Safety and efficacy of approved treatments

Currently, there are seven approved therapies: two formulations of interferon (IFN)—conventional and pegylated; and five nucleos(t)ide analogues—lamivudine, adefovir dipivoxil, entecavir, telbivudine and tenofovir disoproxil fumarate. Table 18.10 summarizes the response rates to these treatments in HBeAg-positive and in HBeAg-negative patients.

Interferon (IFN)

Interferon has both antiviral and immunomodulatory activity and was the first medication approved for hepatitis B. Pegylated IFN, which can be administered weekly, has largely superseded conventional IFN, which is administered daily or three times a week.

HBeAg-positive patients

A 1-year course of pegylated IFN resulted in HBeAg seroconversion in roughly 30% patients when assessed 24 weeks after cessation of treatment [73,74]. Addition of lamivudine led to a greater drop in serum HBV DNA during treatment but had no impact on HBeAg seroconversion or off-treatment HBV DNA suppression. Follow-up of patients in one trial for a mean of 3.5 years after completion of pegylated IFN with or without lamivu-

Table 18.10. Response rates to approved therapies for HBeAg-positive and HBeAg-negative chronic hepatitis B

	Response (%)							
	Lamivudine	Adefovir	Entecavir	Telbivudine	Tenofovir	Peginterferon*	Peginterferon + lamivudine*	Placebo
HBeAg-positive								
At week 48 or 52								
Histology improved	49–62	53–68	72	65	74	38	41	25
Undetectable HBV DNA	40–44	21	67	60	76	25	69	0–16
HBeAg seroconversion	16–21	12	21	22	21	27	24	4–6
HBsAg loss	<1	0	2	0	3	3	3	0
During extended treatment/follow-up								
Undetectable HBV DNA	na	39 (5)	94 (5)	79 (4)	72 (3)	13‡ (4.5)	26‡ (4.5)	na
HBeAg seroconversion	47 (3)	48 (5)	41 (5)	42 (4)	26 (3)	37%‡ (4.5)	36‡ (4.5)	na
HBsAg loss	0–3 (2–3)	2 (5)	5 (2)	1 (2)	8 (3)	8‡ (4.5)	15‡ (4.5)	na
HBeAg-negative								
At week 48 or 52								
Histology improved	60–66	64–69	70	67	72	48	38	33
Undetectable HBV DNA	60–73	51	90	88	93	63	87	0
HBsAg loss	<1	na	<1	<1	0	4	3	0
During extended treatment/follow-up†								
Undetectable HBV DNA	6 (4)	67 (5)	na	84 (4)	87 (3)	18‡ (4)	13‡ (4)	na
HBsAg loss	<1 (4)	5 (5)	na	<1 (2)	0 (3)	8‡ (4)	8‡ (4)	na

Histological improvement defined as a ≥2-point decrease in necroinflammatory score and no worsening of fibrosis score.
*Liver biopsy performed 24 weeks after stopping treatment.
†Timepoint in which response was assessed in years while on-treatment for nucleos(t)ide analogs and during off-treatment follow-up for peginterferon.
‡Assessment performed off treatment.
na, not available.

dine found that 37% had lost HBeAg and 11% had lost HBsAg [75]. The rate of HBsAg loss was significantly higher in patients with genotype A infection, 28%, compared to those with non-A infection, 3% (P <0.001). Among the initial responders, 81% had durable HBeAg loss and 30% had HBsAg loss.

HBeAg-negative patients

A 1-year course of pegylated IFN resulted in undetectable serum HBV DNA and normalization of ALT in 15% patients when assessed 24 weeks after cessation of treatment [76]. Addition of lamivudine led to a greater decline in serum HBV DNA during treatment but did not improve the rate of sustained virological response. Three years after completion of treatment, virological response (serum HBV DNA <10 000 copies/mL) was maintained in 22.6% versus 9.4%, biochemical response (ALT normalization) in 31.3% versus 18.9%, and HBsAg loss in 8.7% versus 0% of patients who received pegylated IFN with or without lamivudine versus lamivudine alone, respectively [77].

Predictors of response

In HBeAg-positive patients, the strongest predictor of IFN-induced HBeAg seroconversion is elevated pretreatment ALT level [78]. Other predictors include high histological activity index and low serum HBV DNA level. Recent studies showed that genotypes A and B are associated with a higher rate of HBeAg seroconversion than genotypes C and D and genotype A is associated with a higher rate of HBsAg loss [73–75]. It has also been suggested that decline in HBeAg and HBsAg titres during the first 12 or 24 weeks of pegylated IFN can predict long-term response. The utility of HBeAg and/or HBsAg monitoring in clinical practice needs to be validated in prospective studies.

There is no consistent predictor of sustained response among HBeAg-negative patients.

Side effects

The most common side effect of IFN is an initial 'flu-like illness. Other common side effects include fatigue, anorexia, weight loss, mild increase in hair loss, emotional lability (including anxiety, irritability and depression), bone marrow suppression and unmasking or exacerbation of autoimmune illnesses.

IFN is contraindicated in patients with decompensated cirrhosis because of the risk of sepsis and worsening of liver failure [79]. IFN should also be avoided in patients with HBV-related acute liver failure, severe exacerbations of chronic hepatitis B and in patients who require antiviral prophylaxis while receiving immunosuppressive or cancer chemotherapy.

Dose regimen

Pegylated IFN is administered for 48 weeks in both HBeAg-positive and in HBeAg-negative patients. The approved dose of pegylated IFN α-2a is 180 μg/week. Varying doses of pegylated IFN α-2b were used in clinical trials.

Nucleos(t)ide analogues

The five approved nucleos(t)ide analogues can be divided into three groups: L nucleosides, lamivudine and telbivudine; acyclic nucleoside phosphonates, adefovir dipivoxil and tenofovir disoproxil fumarate; and deoxyguanosine analogues, entecavir. These drugs act primarily by inhibiting the reverse transcription of the pregenomic RNA to HBV DNA. They do not have any direct inhibitory effect on cccDNA, the template for HBV DNA replication; therefore, viral relapse is common when treatment is withdrawn. Long-term treatment is associated with increasing risks of antiviral drug resistance, costs and side effects.

The selection of the initial treatment should be based on antiviral activity and risk of antiviral resistance. Table 18.10 compare the rates of response to the approved HBV nucleos(t)ide analogues. Entecavir, telbivudine and tenofovir have more potent antiviral activity followed by lamivudine and then adefovir. Entecavir and tenofovir are associated with the lowest rate of drug resistance, followed by adefovir, telbivudine and lamivudine.

HBeAg-positive patients

A 1-year course of nucleos(t)ide analogues resulted in very high rates of undetectable serum HBV DNA (21–76%) and histological improvement (49–74%), but only 12–22% of patients achieved HBeAg seroconversion and only 0–3% lost HBsAg [80–85]. Viral suppression was not sustained when treatment was stopped except in patients who lost HBeAg. For the latter patients, durability of HBeAg loss varied from 50 to 80%. Extending treatment for 12 months after confirmation of HBeAg seroconversion consolidates the response and reduces the likelihood of HBeAg reversion. Continuation of nucleos(t)ide analogue treatment beyond 1 year results in increasing rates of HBeAg seroconversion with 5-year rates of 40–50% [86–90].

HBeAg-negative patients

A 1-year course of nucleos(t)ide analogues resulted in extremely high rates of undetectable serum HBV DNA (51–93%) and histological improvement (60–72%), but less than 1% lost HBsAg [84,85,91,92]. Viral suppression was not sustained when treatment was stopped. Extending treatment of adefovir or tenofovir to 3–5 years resulted in a high rate of maintained viral suppression (67–87%) but the rate of HBsAg loss remained low (0–5%) [89,93,94].

Antiviral drug resistance

Antiviral drug resistance is a major limitation to the long-term use of nucleos(t)ide analogue therapy [95]. The first manifestation of antiviral resistance is virological breakthrough, which is defined as an increase in serum HBV DNA by more than 1 log from nadir or the redetection of HBV DNA in serum after its initial disappearance. Serum HBV DNA levels tend to be low initially because most antiviral drug-resistance mutants have decreased replication fitness compared to the wild-type virus but compensatory mutations that can restore replication fitness frequently emerge during continued treatment leading to a progressive increase in serum HBV DNA levels. Virological breakthrough may occur simultaneous with or precede biochemical breakthrough (ALT elevation in a patient who had normalized ALT). Antiviral resistance leads not only to loss of initial response but, in some instances, hepatitis flares and hepatic decompensation.

Monitoring of serum HBV DNA levels every 3–6 months is critical in determining virological response and in detecting virological breakthroughs. Virological breakthroughs are not always a result of antiviral resistance; non-adherence to medications is believed to account for 30–80% of breakthroughs. Counselling on medication adherence and retesting serum HBV DNA levels after 1–3 months should be performed before instituting rescue therapy unless the patient has decompensated liver disease or is experiencing a severe hepatitis flare. Results of antiviral drug resistance mutation testing can guide the selection of rescue therapy, particularly in patients who have been exposed to more than one nucleos(t)ide analogue.

Signature mutations in the reverse transcriptase region of the HBV polymerase gene associated with resistance to the approved nucleos(t)ide analogues are shown in Fig. 18.10 [95]. The most important mutation associated with resistance to lamivudine is a substitution of methionine for valine or isoleucine (M204V/I) in the tyrosine–methionine–aspartate–aspartate (YMDD) motif. The M204I but not the M204V mutation is also

associated with resistance to telbivudine. Mutations associated with resistance to adefovir include a substitution of alanine for threonine or valine (rtA181T/V) and a substitution of asparagine for threonine (rtN236T). These changes are also associated with a reduced susceptibility to tenofovir. The rtA181T mutation has also been shown to be associated with lamivudine resistance. Resistance to entecavir appears to occur through a two-hit mechanism. Selection of rtM204V/I mutation decreases susceptibility of the virus to entecavir slightly. Additional mutations at positions 184, 202 or 250 are necessary for the manifestation of entecavir resistance. Decreased activity of entecavir in viruses with rtM204V/I mutation explains why the rate of entecavir resistance is so much higher in patients with prior lamivudine resistance [96]. Mutations associated with resistance to tenofovir have not been fully characterized. Substitution of alanine for threonine (rtA194T) has been reported to be associated with resistance to tenofovir in a few patients [97] but this mutation has not been observed in patients in phase III clinical trials of tenofovir.

The incidence of genotypic resistance to the five approved nucleos(t)ide analogues varies from 0–25% at 1 year to 1–70% at 5 years (Table 18.11). It should be noted that resistance to one drug increases the risk of resistance to other drugs. Therefore, it is important to initiate treatment with a drug that has the least potential for drug resistance as sequential monotherapy may result in selection of multidrug resistance mutations [98].

Predictors of response

High pretreatment serum ALT is the strongest predictor of response, particularly among HBeAg-positive patients. Pooled data from four studies with a total of 406 HBeAg-positive patients who received lamivudine

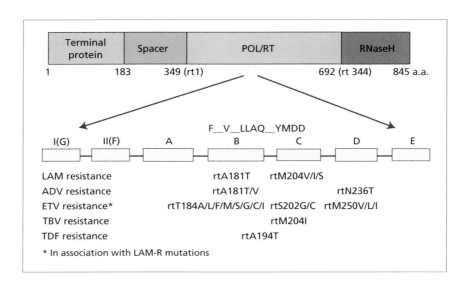

Fig. 18.10. Signature mutations in the HBV polymerase/ reverse transcriptase gene (POL/RT) associated with resistance to nucleos(t)ide analogue therapies. LAM, lamivudine ; ADV, adefovir dipivoxil; ETV, entecavir; TBV, telbivudine; TDF, tenofovir disoproxil fumarate.

Table 18.11. Incidence of genotypic resistance to approved HBV nucleos(t)ide analogues

	Incidence of genotypic resistance at year (%)				
	1	2	3	4	5
Nucleos(t)ide naïve patients					
Lamivudine	~20	45	55	71	65
Telbivudine	5–10	10–20	na	na	na
Adefovir dipivoxil	0	3	11	18	29
Entecavir	0	~1	1–2	1–2	1–2
Tenofovir disoproxil fumarate	0	0	0	na	na
Patients with lamivudine resistance					
Adefovir dipivoxil	~5	~20	na	na	na
Entecavir	6	15	36	46	51

na, not available.

Table 18.12. Approved doses of HBV nucleos(t)ide analogues

Lamivudine	100 mg daily
Adefovir dipivoxil	10 mg daily
Entecavir	0.5 mg daily (1.0 mg daily for patients with lamivudine resistance)
Telbivudine	600 mg daily
Tenofovir disoproxil fumarate	300 mg daily

for 1 year found that HBeAg seroconversion occurred in 2%, 9%, 21% and 47% of patients with ALT within normal, one to two times ULN, two to five times ULN, and more than five times ULN, respectively; the corresponding HBeAg seroconversion rates for 196 patients in the placebo group were 0%, 5%, 11% and 14%, respectively [78]. These data served as the basis for guideline recommendations of an ALT cut-off more than two times ULN for initiation of treatment. A correlation between pretreatment ALT and virological response and HBeAg seroconversion has also been observed with other nucleos(t)ide analogues. Response to nucleos(t)ide analogues across HBV genotypes is similar.

There is no consistent predictor of response in HBeAg-negative patients.

Side effects

Nucleos(t)ide analogues for hepatitis B are very well tolerated; however, like other nucleoside analogues there is a potential for mitochondrial toxicity. The need for vigilance is underscored by the withdrawal of clevudine because of mitochondrial toxicity and myopathy

[99] and a report of lactic acidosis in patients who received entecavir for severe liver failure [100]. Adefovir and tenofovir have been reported to be associated with nephrotoxicity manifesting as increase in serum creatinine in 3% of patients after 3–5 years of continuous treatment [86,90,93,94] as well as renal tubular dysfunction, including Fanconi's syndrome. Telbivudine has been reported to be associated with myopathy and peripheral neuropathy [89]. The risk of peripheral neuropathy was markedly increased in patients who received combination therapy of telbivudine and pegylated IFN.

Dose regimen

Nucleos(t)ide analogues for hepatitis B are administered as oral tablets once a day. Doses have to be adjusted in patients with impaired renal function. Table 18.12 lists the recommended doses for the five approved nucleos(t)ide analogues.

What should be the initial therapy?

The decision regarding nucleos(t)ide versus interferon therapy is based upon patient characteristics and preference. Table 18.13 summarizes the advantages and disadvantages of interferon and nucleos(t)ide analogue therapy. The main advantage of interferon is that it is administered for a finite duration. In addition, interferon appears to be associated with a higher rate of HBsAg loss although this benefit is mainly seen in patients with genotype A infection. Some studies found that interferon-induced HBeAg seroconversion is more durable than nucleoside-induced HBeAg seroconversion but direct comparison has not been performed. The main disadvantages of interferon are the need for parenteral administration and the side effects. Nucleos(t)

Table 18.13. Advantages and disadvantages of interferon and nucleos(t)ide analogue therapies

	Interferon	Nucleos(t)ide analogues
Route of administration	Parenteral	Oral
Duration of treatment	Finite, ~12 months	Indefinite, years
Antiviral activity	Modest, but has immunomodulatory effects	Potent: ETV / TDF / TBV > LAM > ADV
Antiviral resistance	None identified	Yes: LAM > TBV > ADV > ETV / TDF
Side effects	Frequent, may be serious	Negligible
		ADV / TDF nephrotoxicity
		TBV myopathy

ADV, adefovir dipivoxil; ETV, entecavir; LAM, lamivudine; TBV, telbivudine; TDF, tenofovir disoproxil fumarate.

ide analogues are administered orally and are very well tolerated but viral relapse is common when treatment is withdrawn, necessitating long durations of treatment with associated risks of antiviral drug resistance. In general, monotherapy with a nucleos(t)ide analogue or pegylated IFN is recommended as the initial therapy.

Nucleos(t)ide analogues are most appropriate for patients with decompensated liver disease, patients with contraindications to IFN and those who are willing to commit to long durations of treatment. Among the five approved medications, entecavir and tenofovir have the best profile regarding efficacy, safety and drug resistance. Entecavir is preferred in patients with other medical conditions that are associated with increased risks of renal insufficiency while tenofovir is preferred in young female patients who might be contemplating pregnancy and in those who might have been exposed to lamivudine in the past. Lamivudine and telbivudine should not be used as first-line therapy due to high rates of drug resistance while adefovir is largely superseded by tenofovir because of its weak antiviral activity.

Interferon therapy is not recommended for use in patients with hepatic decompensation, immunosuppression or medical or psychiatric contraindications. Interferon may be used in patients with compensated cirrhosis who have normal synthetic function and no evidence of portal hypertension. Interferon is most appropriate for young patients and those who are reluctant to commit to a long duration of treatment. Interferon is an attractive option for HBeAg-positive patients with genotype A infection because of the high rate of HBeAg seroconversion and HBsAg loss.

De novo combination therapy

De novo combination therapy has the potential for additive or synergistic antiviral activity and prevention of antiviral drug resistance; however, clinical studies showed that neither combination of lamivudine and pegylated IFN or lamivudine and another nucleos(t)ide

analogue had a clear advantage compared to monotherapy regarding speed or extent of viral suppression. The main advantage of these combination therapies was a reduction in the rate of lamivudine resistance. In view of the low rate of antiviral drug resistance associated with entecavir and tenofovir, the benefit of *de novo* combination of these two drugs or of either drug with pegylated IFN will be limited.

Compared to pegylated IFN alone, the addition of lamivudine to pegylated IFN resulted in more marked viral suppression during treatment but this difference was not maintained when treatment was stopped [73,74,76]. *De novo* combination of pegylated IFN and lamivudine was associated with a lower rate of lamivudine resistance compared to lamivudine monotherapy but it should be noted that lamivudine resistance was not encountered in patients who received pegylated IFN monotherapy.

Clinical trials of *de novo* combination of nucleos(t)ide analogues have shown that there is no additive or synergistic antiviral activity and resistance to lamivudine is reduced but not completely prevented. The lack of benefit of *de novo* combination therapy may be related to the fact that all the approved drugs share the same target. Furthermore, mutations associated with resistance to one drug may confer resistance to another drug. A phase II trial comparing combination of telbivudine and lamivudine versus telbivudine alone and lamivudine alone found that combination therapy was inferior to telbivudine alone [101]. Another trial comparing combination of lamivudine and adefovir to lamivudine alone in HBeAg-positive patients [102] found that decline in serum HBV DNA levels and HBeAg seroconversion in the two groups were comparable. At week 104, patients who received combination therapy had a significantly lower rate of lamivudine resistance of 15% versus 43% in the group that received lamivudine alone. The high rate of lamivudine resistance in the *de novo* combination therapy group was surprising and is probably related to the weak antiviral activity of adefovir.

When can treatment be stopped?

Ideally, antiviral therapy should be continued until HBsAg loss is confirmed; however, the likelihood that this will occur is low—approximately 3–6% after 3 years of nucleos(t)ide analogue therapy and roughly 5–10% after 4–5 years of completing a 1-year course of pegylated IFN therapy.

Pegylated IFN

Pegylated IFN is administered for a finite duration. The recommended duration of treatment is 48 weeks for both HBeAg-positive and HBeAg-negative patients.

Nucleos(t)ide analogues

Nucleos(t)ide analogues are administered until the desired endpoint is achieved. For patients who had decompensated cirrhosis, life-long treatment is recommended because of concerns for fatal flares when treatment is withdrawn. For patients who had compensated cirrhosis, life-long treatment is generally recommended but cessation of treatment may be considered in patients who are documented to have reversal of cirrhosis and in those who have confirmed HBsAg loss or HBeAg seroconversion provided that these patients are closely monitored so treatment can be promptly reinstituted if there is biochemical or clinical relapse.

For HBeAg-positive patients with precirrhotic liver disease, treatment should be continued until the patient has achieved HBeAg seroconversion (HBeAg negative, anti-HBe positive and undetectable serum HBV DNA) and completed at least 12 months of consolidation therapy. The validity of HBeAg seroconversion as a treatment endpoint has been questioned because some patients remain viraemic after HBeAg seroconversion and reversion to HBeAg positivity occurs in 30–50% of patients after treatment is stopped. These arguments indicate that many though not all patients will have inactive CHB and remain in that phase for months, years or decades after HBeAg seroconversion. Therefore, it is reasonable to discontinue treatment in patients who completed consolidation therapy after achieving HBeAg seroconversion as long as these patients continue to be monitored.

For HBeAg-negative patients with precirrhotic liver disease, the therapeutic endpoint is unclear. Preliminary data from one small study found that among 33 patients who discontinued treatment after 4–5 years of adefovir therapy and had undetectable serum HBV DNA for at least 3 years, 18 (55%) had long-term clinical remission and nine lost HBsAg during a 5-year post-treatment follow-up [103]. These data suggest that withdrawal of treatment may be possible in some patients who have had maintained viral suppression for a few years.

Management of patients with treatment failure

Management of patients with treatment failure is tailored to the type of treatment failure, the treatment that the patient is receiving, history of prior treatment and the pretreatment characteristics. For patients with strong indications for treatment, the general approach is to switch or add another therapy. For patients who do not have clear-cut indications for treatment, cessation of treatment and continued monitoring may be considered. Criteria for defining treatment failure have not been established for IFN treatment because response is more variable. Recent data suggest that monitoring HBsAg titre may be more accurate than monitoring serum HBV DNA levels in predicting long-term response to IFN therapy. These data need to be validated in prospective clinical studies.

Lack of initial response

Inadequate or slow decline in serum HBV DNA level during the first 12–24 weeks of nucleos(t)ide analogue therapy has been shown to be associated with increased risk of antiviral drug resistance during continued therapy [104]. These findings have led to the proposal that a second nucleos(t)ide analogue be added in patients with inadequate initial response. However, the data correlating initial response and subsequent antiviral resistance were derived from studies of lamivudine, adefovir or telbivudine. Studies of entecavir and tenofovir, which are more potent and have lower rates of drug resistance, found that serum HBV DNA levels continued to decline in patients who remained on treatment and overall rates of antiviral resistance were very low. These data indicate that most patients receiving entecavir or tenofovir may remain on the initial treatment provided that serum HBV DNA levels continue to decline.

Virological breakthrough after initial response

Virological breakthrough may be a result of antiviral resistance or medication non-adherence. Patients with virological breakthrough should be counselled regarding medication adherence and breakthrough confirmed by retesting for serum HBV DNA after 1–3 months. Rescue therapy should be started immediately in patients with decompensated liver disease or severe hepatitis flares and after confirmation of virological breakthrough in other patients. The choice of rescue therapy is dependent on the current and prior treatment if any, the pattern of resistance mutations if known and the susceptibility of these mutations to other nucleos(t)ide analogues. Table 18.14 summarizes the recommendations on rescue therapies. For patients with lamivudine resistance, tenofovir is the preferred treatment

Table 18.14. Rescue therapies for antiviral-resistant HBV

Types of resistance	Preferred treatment	Alternative treatment
Lamivudine/ telbivudine	Add or switch to tenofovir	Add adefovir
		Stop lamivudine/ telbivudine, switch to truvada
Adefovir	Switch to or add entecavir	Add lamivudine/ telbivudine
		Stop adefovir, switch to truvada
Entecavir*	Switch to or add tenofovir	Stop entecavir, switch to truvada
Tenofovir*	Switch to or add entecavir	Stop tenofovir, switch to truvada

Truvada, combination pill with emtricitabine and tenofovir, not approved for HBV.
*Limited clinical data.

because it has more potent antiviral activity compared to adefovir. Entecavir even at the higher dose of 1.0 mg is not an optimal rescue therapy because pre-existing presence of M204V/I mutation increases the risk of entecavir resistance. Initial studies showed that add-on adefovir is preferred to switching to adefovir mono-therapy in preventing subsequent adefovir resistance; whether continuation of lamivudine is necessary when tenofovir is used as rescue therapy remains to be determined.

References

1 Blumberg BS, Alter HJ, Visnich S. A 'new' antigen in leukemia sera. *JAMA* 1965; **191**: 541–546.
2 Ganem D, Prince AM. Hepatitis B virus infection—natural history and clinical consequences. *N. Engl. J. Med.* 2004; **350**: 1118–1129.
3 Fung SK, Lok AS. Hepatitis B virus genotypes: do they play a role in the outcome of HBV infection? *Hepatology* 2004; **40**: 790–792.
4 Norder H, Courouce AM, Coursaget P *et al.* Genetic diversity of hepatitis B virus strains derived worldwide: genotypes, subgenotypes, and HBsAg subtypes. *Intervirology* 2004; **47**: 289–309.
5 Chotiyaputta W, Lok AS. Hepatitis B virus variants. *Nat. Rev. Gastroenterol. Hepatol.* 2009; **6**: 453–462.
6 Carman WF, Hadziyannis S, McGarvey MJ *et al.* Mutation preventing formation of hepatitis B e antigen in patients with chronic hepatitis B infection. *Lancet* 1989: **2**: 588–591.
7 Yang HI, Yeh SH, Chen PJ *et al.* Associations between hepatitis B virus genotype and mutants and the risk of hepatocellular carcinoma. *J. Natl. Cancer Inst.* 2008; **100**: 1134–1143.
8 Guidotti LG, Chisari FV. Immunobiology and pathogenesis of viral hepatitis. *Annu. Rev. Pathol.* 2006; **1**: 23–61.
9 Ferrari C, Penna A, Bertoletti A *et al.* Cellular immune response to hepatitis B virus-encoded antigens in acute and chronic hepatitis B virus infection. *J. Immunol.* 1990; **145**: 3442–3449.
10 Ferrari C, Missale G, Boni C *et al.* Immunopathogenesis of hepatitis B. *J. Hepatol.* 2003; **39** (Suppl. 1): S36–42.
11 Ferrari C, Penna A, Bertoletti A *et al.* Cellular immune response to hepatitis B virus-encoded antigens in acute and chronic hepatitis B virus infection. *J. Immunol.* 1990; **145**: 3442–3449.
12 Rehermann B, Lau D, Hoofnagle JH *et al.* Cytotoxic T lymphocyte responsiveness after resolution of chronic hepatitis B virus infection. *J. Clin Invest.* 1996; **97**: 1655–1665.
13 Maini MKB, Lee C, Larrubia CK *et al.* The role of virus-specific CD8(+) cells in liver damage and viral control during persistent hepatitis B virus infection. *J. Exp. Med.* 2000; **191**: 1269–1280.
14 Lavanchy D. Hepatitis B virus epidemiology, disease burden, treatment, and current and emerging prevention and control measures. *J. Viral Hepatol.* 2004; **11**: 97–107.
15 Mast EE, Margolis HS, Fiore AE *et al.* A comprehensive immunization strategy to eliminate transmission of hepatitis B virus infection in the United States: recommendations of the Advisory Committee on Immunization Practices (ACIP) part 1: immunization of infants, children, and adolescents. *MMWR Recomm. Rep.* 2005; **54**: 1–31.
16 Mast EE, Weinbaum CM, Fiore AE *et al.* A comprehensive immunization strategy to eliminate transmission of hepatitis B virus infection in the United States: recommendations of the Advisory Committee on Immunization Practices (ACIP) Part II: immunization of adults. *MMWR Recomm. Rep.* 2006; **55**: 1–33.
17 Weinbaum CM, Williams I, Mast EE *et al.* Recommendations for identification and public health management of persons with chronic hepatitis B virus infection. *MMWR Recomm. Rep.* 2008; **57**: 1–20.
18 Bond WW, Favero MS, Petersen NJ *et al.* Survival of hepatitis B virus after drying and storage for one week. *Lancet* 1981; **1**: 550–551.
19 Dodd RY. Current viral risks of blood and blood products. *Ann. Med.* 2000; **32**: 469–474.
20 Roth WK, Weber M, Petersen D *et al.* NAT for HBV and anti-HBc testing increase blood safety. *Transfusion* 2002; **42**: 869–875.
21 Hollinger FB. Hepatitis B virus infection and transfusion medicine: science and the occult. *Transfusion* 2008; **48**: 1001–1026.
22 Wachs ME, Amend WJ, Ascher NL *et al.* The risk of transmission of hepatitis B from HBsAg(−), HBcAb(+), HBIgM(−) organ donors. *Transplantation* 1995; **59**: 230–234.
23 Dickson RC, Everhart JE, Lake JR *et al.* Transmission of hepatitis B by transplantation of livers from donors positive for antibody to hepatitis B core antigen. The National Institute of Diabetes and Digestive and Kidney Diseases Liver Transplantation Database. *Gastroenterology* 1997; **113**: 1668–1674.

24 Harpaz R, Von Seidlein L, Averhoff FM *et al.* Transmission of hepatitis B virus to multiple patients from a surgeon without evidence of inadequate infection control. *N. Engl. J. Med.* 1996; **334**: 549–554.

25 Gunson RN, Shouval D, Roggendorf M *et al.* Hepatitis B virus (HBV) and hepatitis C virus (HCV) infections in health care workers (HCWs): guidelines for prevention of transmission of HBV and HCV from HCW to patients. *J. Clin. Virol.* 2003; **27**: 213–230.

26 Wong VC, Ip HM, Reesink HW *et al.* Prevention of the HBsAg carrier state in newborn infants of mothers who are chronic carriers of HBsAg and HBeAg by administration of hepatitis–B vaccine and hepatitis-B immunoglobulin. Double-blind randomised placebo-controlled study. *Lancet* 1984; **1**: 921–926.

27 Wiseman E, Fraser MA, Holden S *et al.* Perinatal transmission of hepatitis B virus: an Australian experience. *MJA* 2009; **190**: 489–492.

28 Ni YH, Huang LM, Chang MH *et al.* Two decades of universal hepatitis B vaccination in taiwan: impact and implication for future strategies. *Gastroenterology* 2007; **132**: 1287–1293.

29 Chang MH, You SL, Chen CJ *et al.* Decreased incidence of hepatocellular carcinoma in hepatitis B vaccinees: a 20-year follow-up study. *J. Natl. Cancer Inst.* 2009; **101**: 1348–1355.

30 Chang MH, Chen CJ, Lai MS *et al.* Universal hepatitis B vaccination in Taiwan and the incidence of hepatocellular carcinoma in children. Taiwan Childhood Hepatoma Study Group. *N. Engl. J. Med.* 1997; **336**: 1855–1859.

31 Su FH, Cheng SH, Li CY *et al.* Hepatitis B seroprevalence and anamnestic response amongst Taiwanese young adults with full vaccination in infancy, 20 years subsequent to national hepatitis B vaccination. *Vaccine* 2007; **25**: 8085–8090.

32 McMahon BJ, Dentinger CM, Bruden D *et al.* Antibody levels and protection after hepatitis B vaccine: results of a 22-year follow-up study and response to a booster dose. *J. Infect. Dis.* 2009; **200**: 1390–1396.

33 Zanetti AR, Mariano A, Romano L *et al.* Long-term immunogenicity of hepatitis B vaccination and policy for booster: an Italian multicentre study. *Lancet* 2005; **366**: 1379–1384.

34 Demicheli V, Rivetti A, Di Pietrantonj C *et al.* Hepatitis B vaccination and multiple sclerosis: evidence from a systematic review. *J. Viral. Hepat.* 2003; **10**: 343–344.

35 Carman WF, Zanetti AR, Karayiannis P *et al.* Vaccine-induced escape mutant of hepatitis B virus. *Lancet* 1990; **336**: 325–329.

36 Kumar M, Sarin SK, Hissar S *et al.* Virologic and histologic features of chronic hepatitis B virus-infected asymptomatic patients with persistently normal ALT. *Gastroenterology* 2008; **134**: 1376–1384.

37 Lai M, Hyatt BJ, Nasser I *et al.* The clinical significance of persistently normal ALT in chronic hepatitis B infection. *J. Hepatol.* 2007; **47**: 760–767.

38 Nguyen MH, Garcia RT, Trinh HN *et al.* Histological disease in Asian-Americans with chronic hepatitis B, high hepatitis B virus DNA, and normal alanine aminotransferase levels. *Am. J. Gastroenterol.* 2009; **104**: 2206–2213.

39 Lok AS. Hepatitis B: liver fibrosis and hepatocellular carcinoma. *Gastroenterol. Clin. Biol.* 2009; **33**: 911–915.

40 Guillevin L, Lhote F, Gayraud M *et al.* Prognostic factors in polyarteritis nodosa and Churg-Strauss syndrome. A prospective study in 342 patients. *Medicine* (Baltimore) 1996; **75**: 17–28.

41 Lai KN, Lai FM, Chan KW *et al.* The clinico-pathologic features of hepatitis B virus-associated glomerulonephritis. *Q. J. Med.* 1987; **63**: 323–333.

42 Yim HJ, Lok AS. Natural history of chronic hepatitis B virus infection: what we knew in 1981 and what we know in 2005. *Hepatology* 2006; **43**: S173–181.

43 Rehermann B, Chang KM, McHutchinson J *et al.* Differential cytotoxic T-lymphocyte responsiveness to the hepatitis B and C viruses in chronically infected patients. *J. Virol.* 1996; **70**: 7092–7102.

44 Chu CM, Hung SJ, Lin J *et al.* Natural history of hepatitis B e antigen to antibody seroconversion in patients with normal serum aminotransferase levels. *Am. J. Med.* 2004; **116**: 829–834.

45 Chu CM, Liaw YF. Chronic hepatitis B virus infection acquired in childhood: special emphasis on prognostic and therapeutic implication of delayed HBeAg seroconversion. *J. Viral. Hepat.* 2007; **14**: 147–152.

46 Liaw YF, Chu CM, Su IJ *et al.* Clinical and histological events preceding hepatitis B e antigen seroconversion in chronic type B hepatitis. *Gastroenterology* 1983; **84**: 216–219.

47 Lok AS, Lai CL, Wu PC *et al.* Spontaneous hepatitis B e antigen to antibody seroconversion and reversion in Chinese patients with chronic hepatitis B virus infection. *Gastroenterology* 1987; **92**: 1839–1843.

48 Chu CJ, Hussain M, Lok AS. Hepatitis B virus genotype B is associated with earlier HBeAg seroconversion compared with hepatitis B virus genotype C. *Gastroenterology* 2002; **122**: 1756–1762.

49 Manno M, Camma C, Schepis F *et al.* Natural history of chronic HBV carriers in northern Italy: morbidity and mortality after 30 years. *Gastroenterology* 2004; **127**: 756–763.

50 Chu CM, Liaw YF. HBsAg seroclearance in asymptomatic carriers of high endemic areas: appreciably high rates during a long-term follow-up. *Hepatology* 2007; **45**: 1187–1192.

51 Ahn SH, Park YN, Park JY *et al.* Long-term clinical and histological outcomes in patients with spontaneous hepatitis B surface antigen seroclearance. *J. Hepatol.* 2005; **42**: 188–194.

52 Yuen MF, Wong DK, Fung J *et al.* HBsAg Seroclearance in chronic hepatitis B in Asian patients: replicative level and risk of hepatocellular carcinoma. *Gastroenterology* 2008; **135**: 1192–1199.

53 Chen YC, Sheen IS, Chu CM *et al.* Prognosis following spontaneous HBsAg seroclearance in chronic hepatitis B patients with or without concurrent infection. *Gastroenterology* 2002; **123**: 1084–1089.

54 Raimondo G, Allain JP, Brunetto MR *et al.* Statements from the Taormina expert meeting on occult hepatitis B virus infection. *J. Hepatol.* 2008; **49**: 652–657.

55 Yang HI, Lu SN, Liaw YF *et al.* Hepatitis B e antigen and the risk of hepatocellular carcinoma. *N. Engl. J. Med.* 2002; **347**: 168–174.

56 Iloeje U, Yang H, Su J *et al.* Predicting cirrhosis risk based on the level of circulating hepatitis B viral load. *Gastroenterology* 2006; **130**: 678–686.

57 Chen CJ, Yang HI, Su J *et al.* Risk of hepatocellular carcinoma across a biological gradient of serum hepatitis B virus DNA level. *JAMA* 2006; **295**: 65–73.

58 Yu MW, Yeh SH, Chen PJ *et al.* Hepatitis B virus genotype and DNA level and hepatocellular carcinoma: a prospective study in men. *J. Natl. Cancer Inst.* 2005; **97**: 265–272.

59 Sorrell MF, Belongia EA, Costa J *et al.* National Institutes of Health Consensus Development Conference Statement: management of hepatitis B. *Ann. Intern. Med.* 2009; **150**: 104–110.

60 European Association For The Study Of The Liver. EASL Clinical practice guidelines: management of chronic hepatitis B. *J. Hepatol.* 2009; **50**: 227–242.

61 Liaw YF, Leung N, Kao JH *et al.* Asian-Pacific consensus statement on the management of chronic hepatitis B: a 2008 update. *Hepatol. Int.* 2008; **2**: 263–283.

62 Lok AS, McMahon BJ. Practice guidelines: chronic hepatitis B. *Hepatology* 2007; **45**: 507–539.

63 Lok AS, McMahon BJ. Chronic hepatitis B: update 2009. *Hepatology* 2009; **50**: 661–662.

64 Degertekin B, Lok AS. Indications for therapy in hepatitis B. *Hepatology* 2009; **49**: S129–137.

65 Fontana RJ, Hann HW, Perrillo RP *et al.* Determinants of early mortality in patients with decompensated chronic hepatitis B treated with antiviral therapy. *Gastroenterology* 2002; **123**: 719–727.

66 Yao FY, Terrault NA, Freise C *et al.* Lamivudine treatment is beneficial in patients with severely decompensated cirrhosis and actively replicating hepatitis B infection awaiting liver transplantation: a comparative study using a matched, untreated cohort. *Hepatology* 2001; **34**: 411–416.

67 Liaw YF, Sung JJ, Chow WC *et al.* Lamivudine for patients with chronic hepatitis B and advanced liver disease. *N. Engl. J. Med.* 2004; **351**: 1521–1531.

68 Hoofnagle JH. Reactivation of hepatitis B. *Hepatology* 2009; **49**: S156–165.

69 Loomba R, Rowley A, Wesley R *et al.* Systematic review: the effect of preventive lamivudine on hepatitis B reactivation during chemotherapy. *Ann. Intern. Med.* 2008; **148**: 519–528.

70 Lok AS, Ma OC, Lau JY. Interferon alfa therapy in patients with chronic hepatitis B virus infection. Effects on hepatitis B virus DNA in the liver. *Gastroenterology* 1991; **100**: 756–761.

71 Fontana RJ. Side effects of long-term oral antiviral therapy for hepatitis B. *Hepatology* 2009; **49**: S185–195.

72 Chotiyaputta W, Lok AS. Role of antiviral therapy in the prevention of perinatal transmission of hepatitis B virus infection. *J. Viral. Hepatol.* 2009; **16**: 91–93.

73 Lau GK, Piratvisuth T, Luo KX *et al.* Peginterferon Alfa-2a, lamivudine, and the combination for HBeAg-positive chronic hepatitis B. *N. Engl. J. Med.* 2005; **352**: 2682–2695.

74 Janssen HL, van Zonneveld M, Senturk H *et al.* Pegylated interferon alfa-2b alone or in combination with lamivudine for HBeAg-positive chronic hepatitis B: a randomised trial. *Lancet* 2005; **365**: 123–129.

75 Buster EH, Flink HJ, Cakaloglu Y *et al.* Sustained HBeAg and HBsAg Loss after Long-Term Follow-up of HBeAg-Positive Patients Treated with Peginterferon a-2b. *Gastroenterology* 2008; **135**: 459–467.

76 Marcellin P, Lau GK, Bonino F *et al.* Peginterferon alfa-2a alone, lamivudine alone, and the two in combination in patients with HBeAg-negative chronic hepatitis B. *N. Engl. J. Med.* 2004; **351**: 1206–1217.

77 Marcellin P, Bonino F, Lau GK *et al.* Sustained response of hepatitis B e antigen-negative patients 3 years after treatment with peginterferon alpha-2a. *Gastroenterology* 2009; **136**: 2169–2179.

78 Perrillo RP, Lai CL, Liaw YF *et al.* Predictors of HBeAg loss after lamivudine treatment for chronic hepatitis B. *Hepatology* 2002; **36**: 186–194.

79 Perrillo R, Tamburro C, Regenstein F *et al.* Low-dose, titratable interferon alfa in decompensated liver disease caused by chronic infection with hepatitis B virus. *Gastroenterology* 1995; **109**: 908–916.

80 Dienstag JL, Schiff ER, Wright TL *et al.* Lamivudine as initial treatment for chronic hepatitis B in the United States. *N. Engl. J. Med.* 1999; **341**: 1256–1263.

81 Lai C, Chien R, Leung N *et al.* A one-year trial of lamivudine for chronic hepatitis B. Asia Hepatitis Lamivudine Study Group. *N. Engl. J. Med.* 1998; **339**: 61–68.

82 Marcellin P, Chang T, Lim SG *et al.* Adefovir dipivoxil for the treatment of hepatitis B e antigen-positive chronic hepatitis B. *N. Engl. J. Med.* 2003; **348**: 808–816.

83 Chang TT, Gish RG, de Man R *et al.* A comparison of entecavir and lamivudine for HBeAg-positive chronic hepatitis B. *N. Engl. J. Med.* 2006; **354**: 1001–1010.

84 Lai CL, Gane E, Liaw YF *et al.* Telbivudine versus lamivudine in patients with chronic hepatitis B. *N. Engl. J. Med.* 2007; **357**: 2576–2588.

85 Marcellin P, Heathcote EJ, Buti M *et al.* Tenofovir disoproxil fumarate versus adefovir dipivoxil for chronic hepatitis B. *N. Engl. J. Med.* 2008; **359**: 2442–2455.

86 Marcellin P, Chang TT, Lim SG *et al.* Long-term efficacy and safety of adefovir dipivoxil for the treatment of hepatitis B e antigen-positive chronic hepatitis B. *Hepatology* 2008; **48**: 750–758.

87 Gish RG, Lok AS, Chang TT *et al.* Entecavir therapy for up to 96 weeks in patients with HBeAg-positive chronic hepatitis B. *Gastroenterology* 2007; **133**: 1437–1444.

88 Liaw YF, Gane E, Leung N *et al.* 2-Year GLOBE trial results: telbivudine Is superior to lamivudine in patients with chronic hepatitis B. *Gastroenterology* 2009; **136**: 486–495.

89 Wang Y, Thongsawat S, Gane EJ *et al.* Efficacy and safety outcomes after 4 years of telbivudine treatment in patients with chronic hepatitis B (CHB). *Hepatology* 2009; **50**: 533A.

90 Heathcote EJ, Gane EJ, De Man RA *et al.* Three years of tenofovir disoproxil (TDF) treatment in HBeAg-positive patients (HBeAg+) with chronic hepatitis B (Study 103), preliminary analysis. *Hepatology* 2009; **50**: 533A–534A.

91 Hadziyannis SJ, Tassopoulos NC, Heathcote EJ *et al.* Adefovir dipivoxil for the treatment of hepatitis B e antigen-negative chronic hepatitis B. *N. Engl. J. Med.* 2003; **348**: 800–807.

92 Lai CL, Shouval D, Lok AS *et al.* Entecavir versus lamivudine for patients with HBeAg-negative chronic hepatitis B. *N. Engl. J. Med.* 2006; **354**: 1011–1020.

93 Hadziyannis S, Tassopoulos N, Heathcote E *et al.* Long-term therapy with adefovir dipivoxil for HBeAg-negative chronic hepatitis B for up to 5 years. *Gastroenterology* 2006; **131**: 1743–1751.

94 Marcellin P, Buti M, Krastev Z *et al.* Three years of tenofovir disoproxil fumarate (TDF) treatment in HBeAg-negative patients with chronic hepatitis B (Study

102); preliminary analysis. *Hepatology* 2009; **50**: 532A–533A.

95 Lok AS, Zoulim F, Locarnini S *et al.* Antiviral drug-resistant HBV: standardization of nomenclature and assays and recommendations for management. *Hepatology* 2007; **46**: 254–265.

96 Tenney DJ, Rose RE, Baldick CJ *et al.* Long-term monitoring shows hepatitis B virus resistance to entecavir in nucleoside-naive patients is rare through 5 years of therapy. *Hepatology* 2009; **49**: 1503–1514.

97 Amini-Bavil-Olyaee S, Herbers U, Sheldon J *et al.* The rtA194T polymerase mutation impacts viral replication and susceptibility to tenofovir in hepatitis B e antigen-positive and hepatitis B e antigen-negative hepatitis B virus strains. *Hepatology* 2009; **49**: 1158–1165.

98 Yim HJ, Hussain M, Liu Y *et al.* Evolution of multi-drug resistant hepatitis B virus during sequential therapy. *Hepatology* 2006; **44**: 703–712.

99 Fleischer RD, Lok AS. Myopathy and neuropathy associated with nucleos(t)ide analog therapy for hepatitis B. *J. Hepatol.* 2009; **51**: 787–791.

100 Lange CM, Bojunga J, Hofmann WP *et al.* Severe lactic acidosis during treatment of chronic hepatitis B with entecavir in patients with impaired liver function. *Hepatology* 2009; **50**: 2001–2006.

101 Lai CL, Leung N, Teo EK *et al.* A 1-year trial of telbivudine, lamivudine, and the combination in patients with hepatitis B e antigen-positive chronic hepatitis B. *Gastroenterology* 2005; **129**: 528–536.

102 Sung JJ, Lai JY, Zeuzem S *et al.* Lamivudine compared with lamivudine and adefovir dipivoxil for the treatment of HBeAg-positive chronic hepatitis B. *J. Hepatol.* 2008; **48**: 728–735.

103 Hadziyannis S, Sevastianos V, Rapti I. Outcome of HBeAg-negative chronic hepatitis B (CHG) 5 years after discontinuation of long term adefovir dipivoxil (ADV) treatment. *J. Hepatol.* 2009; **50**: S9, Abstract 18.

104 Yuen MF, Sablon E, Hui CH *et al.* Factors preceding hepatitis B virus DNA breakthrough in patients receiving prolonged lamivudine therapy. *Hepatology* 2001; **34**: 785–791.

CHAPTER 19
Hepatitis D

Patrizia Farci

National Institute of Allergy and Infectious Diseases, National Institutes of Health, Bethesda, MD, USA

Learning points

- HDV is a defective RNA virus that requires the helper function of HBV for virion assembly and transmission. As a consequence, HDV can only infect individuals who harbour HBV. Transmission of HDV occurs through the same routes as HBV.

- HDV transmission can occur by coinfection with HBV or by superinfection of a chronic HBsAg carrier. In coinfection, acute hepatitis D is usually self-limited because HDV cannot outlive the transient HBV infection, whereas in superinfection the underlying HBV infection supports the continuous replication of HDV.

- HDV causes acute and fulminant hepatitis as well as a rapidly progressive form of chronic viral hepatitis, leading to cirrhosis in 70 to 80% of cases. Cirrhosis may be a stable disease for many years but most patients die of liver decompensation or hepatocellular carcinoma unless they receive liver transplantation.

- Control of HBV infection by vaccination and better hygiene has resulted in a dramatic decline of HDV in developed countries. However, new foci of infection are emerging, especially in developing countries and immigration from endemic areas is causing a resurgence of HDV in Europe.

- Treatment of chronic hepatitis D is unsatisfactory. Interferon-α is the only licensed drug of proven benefit. It should be offered to all patients with well-compensated liver disease whereas it is contraindicated for patients with advanced cirrhosis, for which liver transplantation is the only valid therapeutic choice.

History

Hepatitis D virus (HDV) is one of the most interesting and unusual human pathogens, whose discovery originated from a fortuitous observation made by Rizzetto and colleagues in Turin, Italy in 1977 [1]. While examining liver biopsies from individuals with chronic hepatitis B, they discovered by immunofluorescence a new nuclear antigen that they named delta antigen and its antibody anti-delta. Initially thought to be a previously unrecognized hepatitis B antigen, it was later recognized as the expression of a novel human pathogen, the delta agent [2]. The association of HDV with hepatitis B virus (HBV) stems from the fact that HDV is a hybrid virus that incorporates the hepatitis B virus surface antigen (HBsAg) as its envelope protein. As a consequence, HDV can establish infection only in individuals who simultaneously harbour HBV. Infection with the delta agent is found worldwide and is associated with the most severe forms of acute, including fulminant, hepatitis and chronic liver disease in HBsAg-positive subjects. In 1983, the delta agent was renamed hepatitis delta virus (HDV) and the disease it causes hepatitis D.

Hepatitis D virus (Table 19.1)

HDV is a defective RNA virus that requires the helper function of HBV for virion assembly, release and transmission [3]. HDV does not resemble any known transmissible agent of animals, but shares similarities with plant viroids. Due to its uniqueness, it has been classified as the type species of a separate genus, *Deltavirus* [4]. HDV is the smallest animal virus, 35 to 37 nm in diameter, and the only one to possess a circular RNA genome, which contains a single-stranded negative RNA of about 1700 nucleotides (Fig. 19.1) [5]. The HDV genome encodes a single structural protein, the hepatitis delta antigen (HDAg). Within the virus particle is a nucleocapsid, a ribonucleoprotein complex formed by the RNA genome with the HDAg [3]. There are two related forms of HDAg, the short (HDAg-S; 195 amino acids) and the long (HDAg-L; 214 amino acids). HDAg-S is essential for viral replication, whereas HDAg-L is required for virus assembly and inhibits viral replication [3]. HDAg-L contains an isoprenylation motif at the C-terminus which plays an essential role in HDV assembly [6]. The virion is coated by HBsAg, which is the only

Sherlock's Diseases of the Liver and Biliary System, Twelfth Edition. Edited by James S. Dooley, Anna S.F. Lok, Andrew K. Burroughs, E. Jenny Heathcote.
© 2011 by Blackwell Publishing Ltd. Published 2011 by Blackwell Publishing Ltd.

Table 19.1. Characteristics of hepatitis D virus (HDV)

Classification:	genus deltavirus
Defective:	requires the helper function of HBV
Virion:	35–37 nm particle, coated by HBsAg
Genome:	1.7 kb single-stranded, circular RNA, negative polarity
Open reading frame:	one, encoding HDAg
Genotypes:	8
Pathogenicity:	high, acute and chronic hepatitis
Distribution:	worldwide, 15 million HBsAg carriers coinfected with HDV

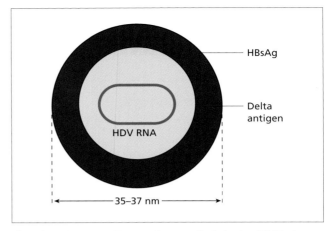

Fig. 19.1. Hepatitis D virus is a small, defective RNA virus coated by HBsAg provided by hepatitis B virus.

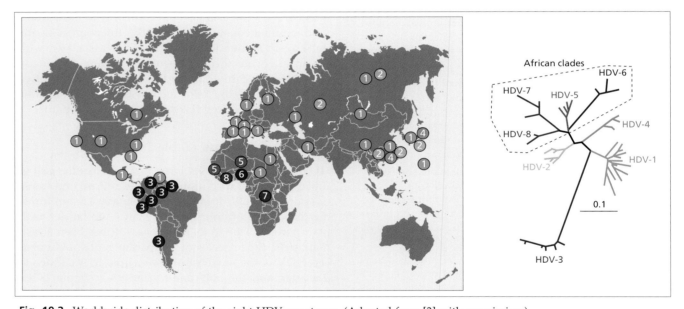

Fig. 19.2. Worldwide distribution of the eight HDV genotypes. (Adapted from [3] with permission.)

helper function provided by HBV. The HBsAg levels and the sequence of natural HBsAg variants influence the assembly and secretion of HDV [7].

The most distinctive aspect of the biology of this virus is its replication. Unlike all other RNA viruses, HDV lacks its own RNA polymerase. Thus, for replication HDV exploits a host cellular enzyme, the host RNA polymerase (Pol) II, which normally copies double-stranded DNA templates. HDV has the unique ability to redirect this cellular enzyme to transcribe the HDV RNA genome [8]. The only enzymatic activity that is inherent to HDV is mediated by RNA elements termed ribozymes (RNA enzymes), which cleave the circular

RNA genome producing a linear molecule [3]. The HDV ribozyme is the only catalytic RNA motif discovered in humans.

HDV genotypes

Like all RNA viruses, HDV is characterized by a high degree of genetic heterogeneity. Nucleotide sequences of HDV isolates obtained worldwide indicated the existence of eight genotypes, varying by as much as 38% over their entire genomic sequences [9,10]. The HDV genotypes differ in their geographic distribution (Fig. 19.2). While genotype 1 is detected worldwide, geno-

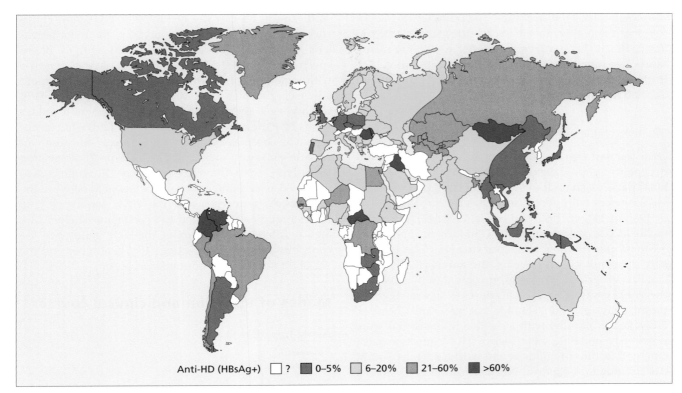

Fig. 19.3. Worldwide prevalence of HDV infection as measured by anti-HD in HBsAg carriers with acute or chronic hepatitis. (Adapted from [3] with permission.)

types 2, 3 and 4 are more geographically restricted. Genotypes 2 and 4 (previously termed IIa and IIb) are found primarily in the Far East; genotype 3 exclusively in the northern regions of South America. More recently, four new HDV genotypes have been detected in West and Central Africa (5, 6, 7 and 8) [9,10]. Evidence for a mixed HDV infection and HDV genome recombination has been recently described, providing a novel mechanism for HDV evolution [10].

Epidemiology

Transmission

HDV can be transmitted only to individuals who simultaneously harbour HBV. Persons with hepatitis B surface antibody (anti-HBs), being immune to HBV infection, are not susceptible to HDV. Transmission of HDV and HBV may occur simultaneously (coinfection) or HDV may infect a chronic HBsAg carrier (superinfection). The routes of HDV transmission are the same as for HBV, the most important being parenteral exposure to blood or blood products, either overtly or through the inapparent parenteral route involving interpersonal contacts. HDV can affect health-care workers, transfusion recipients and haemophiliacs. Intrafamily spread has been documented, both in adults and in children.

Sexual transmission may occur, particularly among sexually promiscuous groups, but HDV infection is infrequent in homosexual men. Vertical transmission is rare.

Geographic distribution

Infection with HDV has a global distribution with considerable geographic variation (Fig. 19.3). It has been estimated that 15 million HBsAg carriers are infected with HDV worldwide [11]. Seroepidemiological studies performed in the 1980s showed that the prevalence of HDV infection is high in the Mediterranean area, the Middle East, Central and Northern Asia, East Africa, the Amazon Basin and certain areas of the Pacific, whereas it is low in North America and Northern Europe, South Africa and Eastern Asia (Fig. 19.3) [3]. The high rate in Southern Europe is the result of a mixed epidemiological pattern characterized by endemic infection in the general population and epidemic outbreaks among intravenous drug users, whereas in industrialized countries HDV infection is mainly confined to intravenous drug users, although it can affect all groups that are at risk for HBV infection [3]. In developed countries, universal screening for HBsAg of blood and its derivatives has led to the virtual elimination of hepatitis D transmission through blood transfusion.

Epidemics of HDV infection, including outbreaks of fulminant hepatitis, have been reported in the Amazon Basin, Brazil (Labrea fever), Ecuador, Colombia (Santa Marta hepatitis), Venezuela and Equatorial Africa [12]. In these areas, children of the indigent population are affected and the mortality is high.

Changing epidemiology

Over the past two decades, there has been a significant decline in the prevalence of HDV infection along with HBV, particularly In Italy where the HDV prevalence in HBV carriers with liver disease has declined from 25% in 1987 to 14% in 1992 and 8% in 1997 [13]. Likewise, the incidence of acute hepatitis D in Italy dropped from 3.1 to 0.2 per 10^6 inhabitants per year [11]. This is probably the result of three events: the universal HBV vaccination programmes, the improvement in hygiene and the AIDS campaigns, which addresses the dangers of promiscuity and of shared syringes and needles. However, in parallel with a decline in areas that were previously endemic, new foci of HDV infection have emerged in other regions of the world, such as Southeastern Russia, Okinawa, Northern India and Albania (11). Moreover, immigration is posing a new threat for HDV resurgence in Europe. Recent epidemiological studies conducted in Germany [14], France [15], Italy [16] and England [17] have shown that the prevalence of HDV infection from the late 1990s has not further decreased in these countries. Overall, these epidemiological studies suggest that the reservoir of HDV in Europe is sustained by two different pools of HDV-infected individuals [13]. One is composed of individuals who survived the HDV epidemic in the 1970s and 1980s and the other is represented by young subjects who migrated to Europe from areas where HDV infection is endemic.

Pathogenesis

The liver is the only organ in which HDV can replicate. The virus is not directly cytopathic, and there is evidence that the liver damage is immunologically mediated [3]. The peak replication of HDV precedes the peak of the histopathological changes.

The mechanisms whereby HDV causes the most rapidly progressive form of liver fibrosis are unknown. Recently, it has been suggested that the long form of HDAg may play a role in HDV pathogenesis by inducing liver fibrosis through the regulation of transforming growth factor-β-induced signal activation [18]. This regulation is accomplished by isoprenylation of the long HDAg.

The role of the HDV genotypes in the pathogenesis of hepatitis D remains to be elucidated, although reported studies indicate that the genotype of HDV may influence the disease severity. Genotype 1, the most prevalent worldwide, has been associated with a broad spectrum of pathogenicity. In Taiwan, patients infected with genotype 1 had a lower remission rate and more adverse outcomes than those with genotype 2 [19]. Genotypes 2 and 4 have been associated with milder forms of acute and chronic hepatitis D [20], while genotype 3 has been associated with outbreaks of fulminant hepatitis in South America [21]. Genotype 3 is associated exclusively with the HBV genotype F, while a less restricted association has been documented between the other HDV genotypes and the HBV genotypes [10]. Further studies are needed to investigate whether biological differences exist among the HDV genotypes, the contribution of the coinfecting HBV genotypes and the variability of the host immune response.

Modes of infection and clinical course

Acute hepatitis D

Coinfection (Fig. 19.4)

The clinical expression of acute hepatitis D acquired by coinfection with HBV may range from mild to severe or even fulminant hepatitis. In most cases, acute hepatitis D is self-limited as HDV cannot outlive the transient HBs antigenaemia. The clinical picture is usually indistinguishable from acute hepatitis B alone. However, a biphasic rise in alanine and aspartate aminotransferases occurring a few weeks apart may be noted, the second rise being due to the acute effects of HDV. The outcome is a complete recovery, as typically seen in hepatitis B, and in only 2% of cases it progresses to chronicity [22]. The long-term outcome is therefore good.

Superinfection (Fig. 19.5)

In the superinfection pattern, the pre-existing HBV infection provides the ideal background for the full expression of HDV. This results in an overt, severe acute hepatitis, which may run a fulminant course. The acute clinical attack is usually marked by jaundice. It may present as an exacerbation of a pre-existing chronic hepatitis B, leading rapidly to liver failure, or as a new hepatitis in a previously asymptomatic HBsAg carrier. If the HBsAg state is unknown it may be misdiagnosed as acute hepatitis B [23]. Therefore, HDV infection should be considered in any HBsAg-positive subject with acute or fulminant hepatitis, the latter being more common in hepatitis D than in the other types of viral hepatitis [24]. Since the HBsAg-carrier state permits the continuous replication of HDV, superinfection of acute hepatitis D leads to chronic hepatitis D in over 90% of cases.

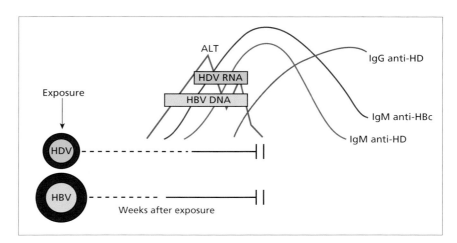

Fig. 19.4. Simultaneous infection with HBV and HDV results in acute hepatitis B with a rise in alanine transaminase (ALT) and the appearance of IgM anti-hepatitis B core. HDV infection follows with a second peak of ALT and the appearance of IgM anti-delta (anti-HD) in serum. Clearing of HBV is associated with clearing of HDV [11].

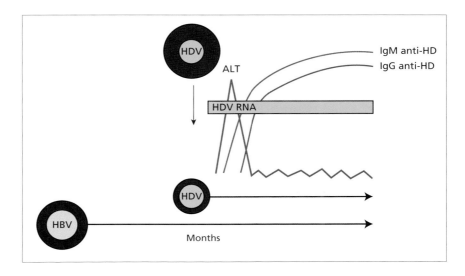

Fig. 19.5. HDV superinfection of a chronic HBsAg carrier results in an attack of acute hepatitis with the appearance of IgM anti-delta (anti-HD) followed by IgG anti-delta (anti-HD). The pre-existing HBV infection provides continuous support to HDV replication. This results in acute hepatitis progressing to chronicity in over 90% of the cases [11].

Chronic hepatitis D

The clinical presentation of chronic hepatitis D varies considerably. It may be virtually symptom free and discovered incidentally after a routine medical check, or it may present with symptoms. The most common is fatigue, but malaise, anorexia, right upper quadrant discomfort and dark urine can occur, especially if the disease is severe or advanced. Some may present with the complications of established cirrhosis with jaundice, encephalopathy, ascites or portal hypertension. There are no specific clinical features, although, at variance with chronic hepatitis B, half the patients with chronic hepatitis D report a history of a previous attack of acute hepatitis, which represents the time of superinfection with HDV. Many exhibit splenomegaly. The disease is severe at all ages, including children [25,26]. Typically, patients with chronic hepatitis D have persistently high serum aminotransferase levels, which tend to decrease

as the disease progresses to the late stage of cirrhosis. Most patients are hepatitis B e antibody (anti-HBe)-positive and have low or undetectable levels of serum HBV DNA, supporting the concept that the liver damage is caused by HDV. Chronic hepatitis D should always be suspected in HBsAg carriers with active liver disease and undetectable serum HBV DNA.

Laboratory test abnormalities in chronic hepatitis D are similar to those detected in chronic hepatitis B alone, with the exception in the former of higher levels of gammaglobulins. Patients with chronic hepatitis D may develop a variety of autoantibodies. About 5% of them show autoantibodies against the microsomal membrane of the liver and kidney (LKM-3) [11].

Hepatic histology

There are no distinctive histological features that differentiate hepatitis D from the other forms of viral

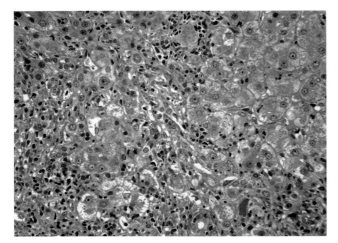

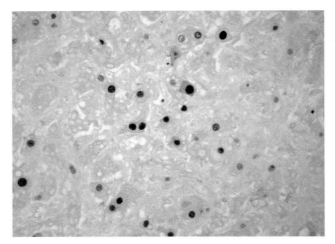

Fig. 19.6. Chronic hepatitis D showing marked periportal (interphase) and lobular inflammatory activity. Aggregates of Kuffper cells and lymphocytes are seen around hydropic and necrotic hepatocytes (H&E, × 200). (Courtesy of Dr Sugantha Govindarajan.)

Fig. 19.8. Immunoperoxidase staining showing hepatitis delta antigen in the hepatocyte nuclei (H&E, × 200). (Courtesy of Dr Sugantha Govindarajan.)

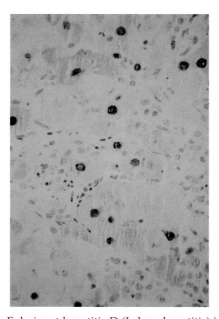

Fig. 19.7. Fulminant hepatitis D (Labrea hepatitis) in a 3-year-old girl from Northern Brazil who died after 3 days of symptoms. An autopsy liver sample shows microvesicular fatty change in large hepatocytes with central nucleus (Morular, plant-like cells). (Immunoperoxidase, × 500.)

acidophilic bodies in the parenchyma and portal tracts [27]. In the most severe cases, including fulminant hepatitis, confluent necrosis may involve dropout of most but not all hepatocytes (submassive necrosis) or virtually all hepatocytes (massive necrosis). In chronic hepatitis D, the degree of periportal necrosis (interface hepatitis) is usually more prominent than that seen in other forms of chronic viral hepatitis (Fig. 19.6) and it is often accompanied by active micronodular and macronodular cirrhosis.

A peculiar histological feature observed in epidemics of fulminant hepatitis D in the Amazon Basin is microvesicular steatosis of the hepatocytes which leads to the formation of morula cells (Fig. 19.7) [28]. Similar alterations, however, have also been observed in severe hepatitis D elsewhere, in Italy and Africa [3,11].

Detection of HDAg in the liver

Using immunofluorescence or immunohistochemistry, HDAg may be shown in the nuclei of hepatocytes (Fig. 19.8). The presence of HDAg increases from acute to chronic hepatitis but decreases as the disease progresses to the late stage of cirrhosis. Thus, it may give false-negative results in patients with advanced disease.

Course and prognosis

The course of chronic HDV infection varies considerably. Chronic hepatitis D is the least common but the most severe and rapidly progressive form of viral hepatitis at all ages. Cirrhosis develops in 70 to 80% of the cases within 5 to 10 years [29], and at a younger age, more than one decade earlier, than in HDV-negative

hepatitis, except that hepatitis D tends to be more severe. The morphological hepatic changes, consisting of hepatocellular necrosis and inflammation, are those typical of acute or chronic viral hepatitis. In acute hepatitis D, pathological changes are often focal with a prominent intralobular infiltration of inflammatory cells, mainly lymphocytes and macrophages, and a degenerative cytoplasmic eosinophilia leading to the formation of

HBV cirrhosis [30]. The risk of developing cirrhosis is about threefold higher in HDV-infected patients compared to those with HBV alone. Once established, HDV cirrhosis may be a stable disease for many years, but a high proportion of patients die of the complications of cirrhosis, end-stage liver disease and hepatocellular carcinoma (HCC), unless they receive liver transplantation. The proportion of patients who ultimately develop each of these complications is not well defined because of the difficulty in recruiting large cohorts of patients with chronic hepatitis D followed prospectively at regular intervals. Most of the data on complications rates have been inferred from retrospective studies; yet, they have provided an overall picture of the natural history of chronic hepatitis D. It has been estimated that the annual incidence of liver decompensation in HDV cirrhotic patients ranges from 2.6 to 3.6% and that of HCC from 2.6 to 2.8% [30,31]. In a recent longitudinal study conducted in Italy, liver decompensation was the most frequent cause of death in HDV cirrhosis [31]. In a longitudinal analysis of 200 Western European patients with compensated HBV cirrhosis, including 39 coinfected with HDV, the adjusted relative risk of HCC was threefold and that of decompensation and mortality twofold higher in HDV cirrhosis than in HBV cirrhosis during a median follow-up of 6.6 years. The cumulative 10-year survival free of liver transplantation is higher for patients with mild chronic hepatitis (100%) or severe chronic hepatitis (90%) than for those with histological (asymptomatic) cirrhosis (58%) or clinical cirrhosis (40%) [32]. As the disease progresses to end-stage liver disease, both alanine aminotransferase (ALT) levels and HDV replication tend to decrease. The mean interval between primary HDV infection and histological cirrhosis is about one decade, but once cirrhosis is established the disease is stable and compatible with a good quality of life for another decade. Thus, the mean interval between primary infection and liver decompensation is about two decades [32], although more rapidly progressive forms have been described [11].

In a minority of cases, HDV infection is marked by a non-progressive, benign course, as reported in some populations in endemic areas, such as the Greek community of Archangelos and the American Samoa [33]. Disease resolution may also occur spontaneously in the natural history of HDV infection, with a higher rate of spontaneous HBsAg clearance among HDV-positive than HDV-negative HBV carriers [34]. However, adverse clinical outcomes such as liver decompensation, HCC or death may occur if HBsAg clearance takes place after HDV disease has progressed to advanced stages.

As a consequence of a significant decline in HDV infection in developed countries, new, fresh forms of hepatitis D have become rare in Europe. The clinical scenario is now dominated by older patients who survived the clinical impact of hepatitis D at the time of the HDV epidemic between 1970 and 1980. These patients have a long-standing infection manifested either as advanced cirrhosis or, in a minority, as non-progressive, mild disease [32]. In recent years, however, there has been a resurgence of HDV infection in Europe and the number of florid HDV cases is on the rise again as a result of immigration from areas where HDV is endemic [14–17].

The interaction of HDV with other hepatitis viruses has been investigated. Whereas in patients with triple infection most reports have documented a suppressive effect of HDV on both HBV and HCV [17,35–37], studies from Taiwan have demonstrated a dominant suppressive role of HCV on HDV and HBV [38,39]. The titre of HBV DNA was significantly lower in patients with triple infection than in patients coinfected with HBV and HDV [39]. Coinfection with HIV does not seem to modify the course of chronic HDV disease [40,41], except in terms of a more elusive or absent antibody response to HDV leading to the reappearance of serum HDAg in some patients [42].

Diagnosis

Acute hepatitis D (Tables 19.2,19.3)

Coinfection (Fig. 19.4)

Coinfection is diagnosed by the simultaneous presence of serological markers of primary HBV and HDV infection. The most specific is the finding of serum IgM anti-HD in the presence of high-titre IgM anti-HBc. The latter precedes IgM anti-HD and appears concomitant with the clinical onset of acute hepatitis. IgM anti-HD appears within 1–2 weeks from the clinical onset, is gone by 5–6 weeks but it may last up to 12 weeks [43]. When serum IgM anti-HD disappears, serum IgG anti-HD is found. There may be a window period between the disappearance of one and the detection of the other. IgG anti-HD may appear only during convalescence and disappear within months to years after recovery [43]. Serum HD-Ag may be transiently detected before the appearance of IgM anti-HD, especially in the most severe forms. Loss of IgM anti-HD confirms the resolution of acute HDV infection, whereas persistence predicts chronicity. The serologic profile of primary HBV infection includes the detection of HBsAg, HBeAg or its antibody anti-HBe, as well as IgM and IgG anti-HBc. Anti-HBs becomes detectable later, during convalescence.

Superinfection (Fig. 19.5)

Superinfection with HDV almost invariably results in persistent HDV infection. The absence or presence of IgM anti-HBc at low titre distinguishes superinfection from coinfection [23]. The pre-existing HBV carrier state

Table 19.2. Hepatitis D: significance of serological and virological markers

Marker	Significance
IgM anti-HD	Acute or chronic infection with HDV
IgG anti-HD	Acute (low titre in coinfection, increasingly high titre in superinfection) or chronic infection (high titre with positive IgM anti-HD) Past HDV infection (low titre with negative IgM anti-HD)
HDV RNA	Active viral replication
	Acute (transient) and chronic infection (persistent)
HD-Ag	Active infection
	Acute infection (transient for a few days); undetectable in
	chronic infection because of immune complexes with anti-HD
	(can be detected in HIV-coinfected patients)

Table 19.3. Diagnosis of acute and chronic hepatitis D

	Acute hepatitis		Chronic hepatitis
	Coinfection	Superinfection	
HDV (serum)			
IgM anti-HD	+	+	+ (high titre)
IgG anti-HD	+	+	+ (high titre)
HDAg	+ (early, transient)	+ (early, transient)	−*
HDV RNA	+ (early, transient)	+	+
HDV (liver)			
HDAg	+	+	+
HDV RNA	+	+	+
HBV (serum)			
HBsAg	+ (transient)	+	+
IgM anti-HBc	+	−	−

*Undetectable in chronic infection because of immune complexes with anti-HD.

is indicated, besides HBsAg, by the finding of IgG anti-HBc and anti-HBe. HDV superinfection of an HBsAg carrier is marked by the early presence of HD antigenaemia and HDV RNA, along with increasing titres of IgM and IgG anti-HD in parallel with the progression to chronicity. Suppression of markers of HBV replication occurs during the acute phase.

Chronic hepatitis D

Chronic hepatitis D is diagnosed by the presence in serum of high titres of IgG and IgM anti-HD. IgM anti-HD is pentameric (19S) in primary infection and monomeric (7S) during chronic infection [11]. IgM anti-HD is a marker of HDV-induced liver damage. Testing for IgM anti-HD provides diagnostic as well as prognostic information. Its persistence predicts chronicity, whereas its decrease and disappearance predict impending resolution of chronic HDV disease, either spontaneous or induced by interferon therapy [44]. IgG and IgM anti-HD persist as do HDV RNA in serum and HDAg in the liver. The detection of HDAg in serum is not practical during the acute and chronic phase due to antigen sequestration in immune complexes with high-titre circulating antibodies.

Detection of HDV RNA

The detection of HDV RNA by reverse transcriptase polymerase chain reaction (RT- PCR) is the most reliable and sensitive method for the early diagnosis of HDV infection, before antibody seroconversion. It can detect 10 to 100 copies of the viral genome per mL of serum [43]. Recently, real-time RT-PCR assays to quantify HDV RNA have been developed [45,46]. These assays are important for investigating the molecular events during acute and chronic hepatitis D, as well as for monitoring the efficacy of antiviral therapy. However, a major problem is the lack of standardized and commercially available PCR assays, as detection and quantification of serum HDV RNA still relies on homemade assays [47].

Treatment

The aim of antiviral treatment is to eradicate HDV and HBV, and prevent the long-term sequelae of chronic hepatitis D, that is cirrhosis and hepatocellular carcinoma. However, these goals are not commonly achieved and treatment of chronic hepatitis D is still unsatisfactory [47]. The fact that HDV lacks a specific viral polymer-

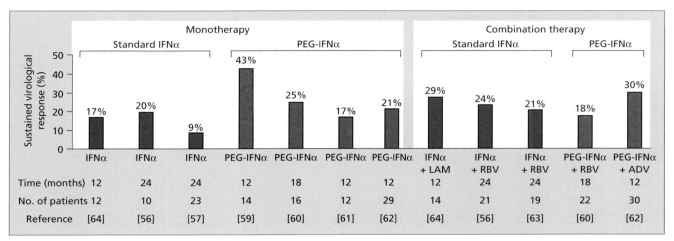

Fig. 19.9. Rate of sustained virological response in trials in which HDV RNA was assessed in serum using PCR assays with a sensitivity ranging from 10 to 1000 genome copies per mL. Patients with chronic hepatitis D were treated with standard or pegylated IFNα, alone or in combination with lamivudine or ribavirin. IFNα, standard interferonα; Peg-IFNα, pegylated interferon α; LAM, lamivudine; RBV, ribavirin. (Adapted from [47], with permission.)

ase along with its high pathogenic potential makes this virus a difficult target for antiviral therapy. There are at present no specific HDV inhibitors. Several antiviral agents have been tried [48], but only interferon-α (IFN-α) has proven to be beneficial in chronic hepatitis D.

Acute hepatitis D

There is no effective antiviral therapy for acute hepatitis D [48]. Patients should be closely monitored for clinical and biochemical parameters of liver function in order to diagnose as early as possible progression to fulminant hepatitis, for which liver transplantation is the only therapeutic choice. Patients with fulminant hepatic failure should be promptly transferred to a specialist liver unit with the facilities for liver transplantation.

Chronic hepatitis D

Interferon-α (IFN-α) monotherapy

IFN-α, the only licensed drug to treat chronic HDV infection, was first employed in the mid 1980s. Although the clinical evidence is mostly based on small and uncontrolled trials, the efficacy of IFN-α is related to the dose and duration of therapy. The usual regimen is 9 million units three times a week or 5 million units daily by injection for at least 1 year. In a controlled trial in Italy, 9 million units given thrice weekly for up to 1 year induced ALT normalization in about 50% of patients 6 months after stopping therapy [49]. This biochemical response correlated with an improvement in liver histology and a significant decrease (up to four log_{10}) in the levels of viraemia but not with a loss of HDV RNA, as

measured by sensitive PCR [50]. Overall, a 1-year course of standard IFN is associated with only a 10 to 20% chance of sustained HDV clearance when a sensitive PCR testing is used as the endpoint (Fig. 19.9), and 10% chance of HBsAg clearance [51]. Treatment response is poor in patients coinfected with HDV and HIV [52] as well as in those who are coinfected with HDV and HCV [53]. Treatment of chronic hepatitis D in children has been disappointing [54,55].

Studies on the long-term effects of IFN on the natural history of hepatitis D are limited. A prospective controlled trial of 36 patients followed for up to 20 years showed that 1-year treatment with high doses of IFN significantly improved the long-term clinical outcome and survival of patients with chronic hepatitis D, compared to those receiving 3 million units or no treatment [50]. Reversion of advanced hepatic fibrosis occurred in some patients with initially active cirrhosis.

Strategies to increase the efficacy of standard IFN have been explored, including longer duration of treatment [56,57] or even continuous therapy for up to 12 years [58], but most of the patients still failed to clear HDV and the rate of relapse is high. Moreover, these alternatives are poorly tolerated.

Pegylated IFN monotherapy

The efficacy and safety of the pegylated form of IFN (PEG-IFN) in chronic hepatitis D was evaluated in three small-size studies (Fig. 19.9) [59–61]. PEG-IFN-α2b was given at a dose of 1.5 μg/kg weekly for 12 months, and the virological response was measured with a sensitive PCR assay. In one trial [59], sustained virological response was reported in 43% of patients, even though most of them (85%) were previous non-responders to high doses of standard IFN. Results were less satisfactory in the other two trials, with sustained HDV RNA clearance in 25% [60] and 17% [61] of the patients, respectively. Clearance of HBsAg did not occur except in one patient [59], although the follow-up was presumably too short for such an event to occur. As seen with standard IFN-α [48], the response to PEG-IFN was better in patients with chronic hepatitis than in those with cirrhosis. Differences in disease duration and liver histology on entry into the trial may have contributed to the observed discrepancies in the rate of response. Similar results were obtained with PEG-IFN-α2a, with sustained HDV RNA clearance in 21% of the patients [62]. Despite their limitations, these studies have shown that PEG-IFN is well tolerated and more effective than standard IFN in both IFN-naïve patients and previous non-responders to standard IFN.

Combination therapy with standard or pegylated IFN

The efficacy of standard IFN-α in combination with ribavirin [63] or lamivudine [64,65] has been investigated in a few small-size trials (Fig. 19.9). These studies showed no significant advantages over IFN monotherapy in chronic hepatitis D. Similar results were obtained with the combination of PEG-IFN and ribavirin [60] or adefovir [62].

Interferon side effects

IFN is often poorly tolerated. Side effects, in particular psychiatric symptoms [66], are common especially with high doses and a prolonged course of therapy. Psychiatric symptoms, however, seem less frequent with PEG-IFN [60]. Continuous monitoring is mandatory for the early detection and management of medical and psychiatric complications. If IFN is administered for more than 1 year, the dose may need to be tailored according to the individual tolerance.

Nucleoside analogues and other agents

Despite the structural link of HDV with HBV, potent and specific inhibitors of HBV replication, such as nucleoside analogues, have no or limited effect on HDV replication [47]. This is probably due to the fact that these inhibitors have no effect on the expression of HBsAg, the only component provided by HBV to HDV. Lamivudine [67,68] and famciclovir [69] have no or limited effect on HDV replication or liver disease activity. Other antiviral agents including suramin, acyclovir and ribavirin, as well as immunomodulators such as steroids, thymosin, levamisole, thymic humoral factor-gamma 2, have been evaluated, but none was effective against HDV [48].

Monitoring antiviral therapy

In patients with chronic hepatitis D treated with standard or PEG-IFN, full blood counts and serum ALT levels should be monitored monthly. Serum HDV RNA should be quantified at baseline, 3, 6, 9 and 12 months of treatment, and at 6 months post-treatment. The major problem is the lack of commercial assays for the qualitative and quantitative assessment of HDV viraemia. Quantification of serum HBsAg levels provides an additional tool to improve treatment monitoring [70]. Continuous medical and psychiatric monitoring is mandatory.

Predictors of response to therapy

There are no baseline biochemical or virological variables that are predictive of a sustained virological response. Patients without cirrhosis are the most likely to respond, highlighting the importance of early diagnosis and treatment in chronic hepatitis D. Recent, but limited, studies of HDV RNA kinetics during treatment with pegylated IFN have shown that a negative PCR within 6 months of therapy is the best predictor of a sustained virological response [59,61]. In a minority, however, it fails to predict who will have a sustained viral loss or will relapse after termination of therapy [59]. HDV RNA kinetics might also help to adjust the duration of therapy by identifying slow responders who might benefit from a longer course of therapy. Larger studies are needed to better define the predictive value of a negative HDV RNA testing during the first 6 months of therapy.

Current recommendations

The superior results obtained with PEG-IFN suggest the use of this drug as a first-choice treatment for chronic hepatitis D [47]. The once-weekly administration of PEG-IFN provides better compliance for the long-term treatment of this disease. However, large controlled trials are still needed to determine the greater efficacy of pegylated versus standard IFN and to identify the best treatment schedule.

PEG-IFN should be offered to all IFN-naïve patients, as well as to previous non-responders to standard IFN. Therapy should be continued for at least 1 year before the patient is considered as a non-responder. Better results are obtained in chronic hepatitis D than in HDV-cirrhosis, which highlights the importance of starting treatment as soon as the diagnosis is made. The lesson learned from monitoring HCV RNA levels for guiding treatment decisions in chronic hepatitis C underline the need to develop standardized PCR assays for the detection and quantification of HDV viraemia. These assays will provide clinicians with important virological tools to assess an early response as well as to decide when treatment should be discontinued in patients with a delayed virological response and which patients might benefit from a longer course of therapy. Continuous clinical monitoring is essential for the early management of the side effects associated with IFN therapy.

Treatment with standard or PEG-IFN is contraindicated in patients with advanced or decompensated liver disease, for which liver transplantation is the only valid therapeutic choice. The risk of HDV reinfection of the graft is lower than that of ordinary HBV reinfection and can be prevented by the continuous administration of hepatitis B immunoglobulins (HBIG) and lamivudine [11]. Since the introduction of HBIG immunoprophylaxis, the risk of HDV reinfection has dropped to 10% and that of HBV reinfection to 30%. HDV reinfection of the graft may occur but, in the presence of low or undetectable levels of HBV DNA (detected only by sensitive PCR), liver disease does not recur (latent HDV infection). The addition of lamivudine before and after liver transplantation to HBIG has virtually abolished the risk of HDV reinfection of the graft [11].

Perspectives

New therapies are needed for the treatment of chronic hepatitis D because even with the use of pegylated interferon the overall rate of sustained virological response remains low and most of the patients relapse after discontinuation of therapy. The mechanisms for the poor response to IFN are not known although recent *in vitro* data suggest that HDV may impair the IFN-α stimulated JAK-STAT signalling pathway by blocking the Tyk2 activation [71].

Recent insights into the molecular biology of HDV may help to identify antiviral agents capable of interfering with the life cycle of this unique virus. Of greater promise is a novel class of antiviral agents, prenylation inhibitors, which block an essential step in the HDV assembly. *In vitro* studies have shown that inhibition of prenylation of HDAg-L, the only form of HDAg capable of mediating attachment to HBsAg for viral assembly, can abolish particle formation in a dose-dependent manner [72]. Using a novel transgenic mouse model for HBV that supports HDV replication, a prenylation inhibitor was shown to result in HDV clearance, thus opening the prospect of a clinical evaluation of this novel class of HDV inhibitors [73]. Other new molecular approaches include the use of antisense oligonucleotides [74], ribozymes [75] or small interfering RNA [76], but at present none of these approaches appears realistic. Until specific inhibitors of viral replication become available, HDV remains one of the most difficult targets for antiviral therapy.

Prevention

Vaccination against hepatitis B makes the recipient immune to HBV infection and thereby protects against HDV infection. Patients likely to contract HDV infection should be encouraged to receive the hepatitis B vaccine. The most effective measure to prevent HDV infection is universal vaccination of newborns against HBV. HBV carriers must be educated concerning the risks of acquiring HDV by continued intravenous drug use. Counselling should be provided also to HBsAg carriers living with HDV-infected patients to avoid the risk of HDV superinfection through sexual or household transmission.

References

1 Rizzetto M, Canese MG, Aricò S et al. Immunofluorescence detection of new antigen-antibody system (delta/anti-delta) associated to hepatitis B virus in liver and in serum of HBsAg carriers. *Gut* 1977; **18**: 997–1003.

2 Rizzetto M, Canese MG, Gerin JL et al. Transmission of the hepatitis B virus-associated delta antigen to chimpanzees. *J. Infect. Dis.* 1980; **141**: 590–602.

3 Taylor J, Farci P, Purcell RH. Hepatitis D (delta) virus. In: Knipe DM, Howley PM, eds. *Fields Virology*, 5th edn. Philadelphia: Lippincott, Williams and Wilkins, 2006, p. 3031–3046.

4 Mason WS, Burrell CJ, Casey J et al. Deltavirus. In: Fauquet CM, Mayo MA, Maniloff J, Desselberger U, Ball AL, eds. *Virus Taxonomy, Eighth Report of the International Committee on Taxonomy of Viruses*. London: Elsevier/Academic Press, 2005, p. 735–738.

5 Wang KS, Choo QL, Weiner AJ et al. Structure, sequence and expression of the hepatitis delta (delta) viral genome. *Nature* 1986; **323**: 508–514.

6 Glenn JS, Watson JA, Havel CM et al. Identification of a prenylation site in delta virus large antigen. *Science* 1992; **256**: 1331–1333.

7 Shih HH, Jeng KS, Syu WJ et al. Hepatitis B surface antigen levels and sequences of natural hepatitis B virus variants influence the assembly and secretion of hepatitis D virus. *J. Virol.* 2008; **82**: 2250–2264.

8 Lai MM. RNA replication without RNA-dependent RNA polymerase: surprises from hepatitis delta virus. *J. Virol.* 2005; **79**: 7951–7958.

9 Radjef N, Gordien E, Ivaniushina V et al. Molecular phylogenetic analyses indicate a wide and ancient radiation of African hepatitis delta virus, suggesting a delta virus genus of at least seven major clades. *J. Virol.* 2004; **78**: 2537–2544.

10 Dény P. Hepatitis delta virus genetic variability: from genotypes I, II, III to eight major clades? *Curr. Top. Microbiol. Immunol.* 2006; **307**: 151–171.

11 Rizzetto M, Smedile A. Hepatitis D. In: Schiff E, Sorrell M, Maddrey W, eds. *Diseases of the Liver*. Philadelphia: Lippincott, Williams and Wilkins, 2002, p. 863–875.

12 Torres JR. Hepatitis B and hepatitis delta virus infection in South America. *Gut* 1996; **38** (Suppl. 2): S48–55.

13 Rizzetto M. Hepatitis D: thirty years after. *J. Hepatol* 2009; **50**: 1043–1050.

14 Wedemeyer H, Heidrich B, Manns MP. Hepatitis D virus infection—not a vanishing disease in Europe! *Hepatology* 2007; **45**: 1331–1332.

15 Le Gal F, Castelnau C, Gault E *et al*. Hepatitis D virus infection—not a vanishing disease in Europe! Reply. *Hepatology* 2007; **45**: 1332–1333.

16 Gaeta GB, Stroffolini T, Smedile A *et al*. Hepatitis delta in Europe: vanishing or refreshing? *Hepatology* 2007; **46**: 1312–1313.

17 Cross TJ, Rizzi P, Horner M *et al*. The increasing prevalence of hepatitis delta virus (HDV) infection in South London. *J. Med. Virol.* 2008; **80**: 277–282.

18 Choi SH, Jeong SH, Hwang SB. Large hepatitis delta antigen modulates transforming growth factor-beta signaling cascades: implication of hepatitis delta virus-induced liver fibrosis. *Gastroenterology* 2007; **132**: 343–357.

19 Su CW, Huang YH, Huo TI *et al*. Genotypes and viremia of hepatitis B and D viruses are associated with outcomes of chronic hepatitis D patients. *Gastroenterology* 2006; **130**: 1625–1635.

20 Wu JC. Functional and clinical significance of hepatitis D virus genotype II infection. *Curr. Top. Microbiol. Immunol.* 2006; **307**: 173–186.

21 Casey JL, Brown TL, Colan EJ *et al*. A genotype of hepatitis D virus that occurs in northern South America. *Proc. Natl. Acad. Sci. U S A* 1993; **90**: 9016–9020.

22 Caredda F, Antinori S, Pastecchia C *et al*. Incidence of hepatitis delta virus infection in acute HBsAg-negative hepatitis. *J. Infect. Dis.* 1989; **159**: 977–979.

23 Farci P, Smedile A, Lavarini C *et al*. Delta hepatitis in inapparent carriers of hepatitis B surface antigen. A disease simulating acute hepatitis B progressive to chronicity. *Gastroenterology* 1983; **85**: 669–673.

24 Smedile A, Farci P, Verme G *et al*. Influence of delta infection on severity of hepatitis B. *Lancet* 1982; **2**: 945–947.

25 Farci P, Barbera C, Navone C *et al*. Infection with the delta agent in children. *Gut* 1985; **26**: 4–7.

26 Bortolotti F, Di Marco V, Vajro P *et al*. Long-term evolution of chronic delta hepatitis in children. *J. Pediatr.* 1993; **122**: 736–738.

27 Verme G, Amoroso P, Lettieri G *et al*. A histological study of hepatitis delta virus liver disease. *Hepatology* 1986; **6**: 1303–1307.

28 Buitrago B, Popper H, Hadler SC *et al*. Specific histologic features of Santa Marta hepatitis: a severe form of hepatitis delta-virus infection in northern South America. *Hepatology* 1986; **6**: 1285–1291.

29 Rizzetto M, Verme G, Recchia S *et al*. Chronic hepatitis in carriers of hepatitis B surface antigen, with intrahepatic expression of the delta antigen. An active and progressive disease unresponsive to immunosuppressive treatment. *Ann. Intern. Med.* 1983; **98**: 437–441.

30 Fattovich G, Giustina G, Christensen E *et al*. Influence of hepatitis delta virus infection on morbidity and mortality in compensated cirrhosis type B. The European Concerted Action on Viral Hepatitis(Eurohep). *Gut* 2000; **46**: 420–426.

31 Romeo R, Del Ninno E, Rumi M *et al*. A 28-year study of the course of hepatitis Delta infection: a risk factor for cirrhosis and hepatocellular carcinoma. *Gastroenterology* 2009; **136**: 1629–1638.

32 Rosina F, Conoscitore P, Cuppone R *et al*. Changing pattern of chronic hepatitis D in Southern Europe. *Gastroenterology* 1999; **117**: 161–166.

33 Hadziyannis SJ. Hepatitis delta: an overview. In: Rizzetto M, Purcell RH, Gerin JL *et al*., eds. *Viral Hepatitis and Liver Disease*. Torino: Minerva Medica, 1997, p. 283–289.

34 Niro GA, Gravinese E, Martini E *et al*. Clearance of hepatitis B surface antigen in chronic carriers of hepatitis delta antibodies. *Liver* 2001; **21**: 254–259.

35 Eyster ME, Sanders JC, Battegay M *et al*. Suppression of hepatitis C virus (HCV) replication by hepatitis D virus (HDV) in HIV-infected hemophiliacs with chronic hepatitis B and C. *Dig. Dis. Sci.* 1995; **40**: 1583–1588.

36 Arribas J, Gonzales-Garcia J, Lorenzo A *et al*. Single (B or C), dual (BC or BD) and triple (BCD) viral hepatitis in HIV-infected patients in Madrid, Spain. *AIDS* 2005; **19**: 1361–1365.

37 Heidrich B, Deterding K, Tillmann HL *et al*. Virological and clinical characteristics of delta hepatitis in Central Europe. *J. Viral Hepat.* 2009; **16**: 883–894.

38 Liaw YF. Role of hepatitis C virus in dual and triple hepatitis virus infection. *Hepatology* 1995; **22**: 1101–1108.

39 Lu SN, Chen TM, Lee CM *et al*. Molecular epidemiological and clinical aspects of hepatitis D virus in a unique triple hepatitis viruses (B, C, D) endemic community in Taiwan. *J. Med. Virol.* 2003; **70**: 74–80.

40 Buti M, Jardi R, Allende H *et al*. Chronic delta hepatitis: is the prognosis worse when associated with hepatitis C virus and human immunodeficiency virus infections? *J. Med. Virol.* 1996; **49**: 66–69.

41 Castellares C, Barreiro P, Martín-Carbonero L *et al*. Liver cirrhosis in HIV-infected patients: prevalence, aetiology and clinical outcome. *J. Viral Hepat.* 2008; **15**: 165–172.

42 Roingeard P, Dubois F, Marcellin P *et al*. Persistent delta antigenaemia in chronic delta hepatitis and its relation with human immunodeficiency virus infection. *J. Med. Virol.* 1992; **38**: 191–194.

43 Smedile A, Ciancio A, Rizzetto M. Hepatitis D. In: Richmann DD, Whitley RJ, Hayden FG, eds. *Clinical Virology: Hepatitis Delta Virus*. Washington DC: ASM Press, 2002, p. 1227–1240.

44 Borghesio E, Rosina F, Smedile A *et al*. Serum immunoglobulin M antibody to hepatitis D as a surrogate marker of hepatitis D in interferon-treated patients and in patients who underwent liver transplantation. *Hepatology* 1998; **27**: 873–876.

45 Yamashiro T, Nagayama K, Enomoto N *et al*. Quantitation of the level of hepatitis delta virus RNA in serum, by real-time polymerase chain reaction, and its possible correlation with the clinical stage of liver disease. *J. Infect. Dis.* 2004; **189**: 1151–1157.

46 Le Gal F, Gordien E, Affolabi D *et al*. Quantification of hepatitis delta virus RNA in serum by consensus real-time PCR indicates different patterns of virological response to interferon therapy in chronically infected patients. *J. Clin. Microbiol.* 2005; **43**: 2363–2369.

47 Farci P. Treatment of chronic hepatitis D: new advances, old challenges. *Hepatology* 2006; **44**: 536–539.

48 Niro GA, Rosina F, Rizzetto M. Treatment of hepatitis D. *J. Viral Hepat.* 2005; **12**: 2–9.

49 Farci P, Mandas A, Coiana A *et al*. Treatment of chronic hepatitis D with interferon alfa-2a. *N. Engl. J. Med.* 1994; **330**: 88–94.

50 Farci P, Roskams T, Chessa L *et al*. Long-term benefit of interferon alpha therapy of chronic hepatitis D: regression

of advanced hepatic fibrosis. *Gastroenterology* 2004; **126**: 1740–1749.

51 Battegay M, Simpson LH, Hoofnagle JH *et al.* Elimination of hepatitis delta virus infection after loss of hepatitis B surface antigen in patients with chronic delta hepatitis. *J. Med. Virol.* 1994; **44**: 389–392.

52 Puoti M, Rossi S, Forleo MA *et al.* Treatment of chronic hepatitis D with interferon alpha-2b in patients with human immunodeficiency virus infection. *J. Hepatol.* 1998; **29**: 45–52.

53 Weltman MD, Brotodihardjo A, Crewe EB *et al.* Coinfection with hepatitis B and C or B, C and delta viruses results in severe chronic liver disease and responds poorly to interferon-alpha treatment. *J. Viral Hepat.* 1995; **2**: 39–45.

54 Di Marco V, Giacchino R, Timitilli A *et al.* Long-term interferon-alpha treatment of children with chronic hepatitis delta: a multicentre study. *J. Viral Hepat.* 1996; **3**: 123–128.

55 Dalekos GN, Galanakis E, Zervou E *et al.* Interferon-alpha treatment of children with chronic hepatitis D virus infection: the Greek experience. *Hepatogastroenterology* 2000; **47**: 1072–1076.

56 Gunsar F, Akarca US, Ersoz G *et al.* Two-year interferon therapy with or without ribavirin in chronic delta hepatitis. *Antivir. Ther.* 2005; **10**: 721–726.

57 Yurdaydin C, Bozkaya H, Karaaslan H *et al.* A pilot study of 2 years of interferon treatment in patients with chronic delta hepatitis. *J. Viral Hepat.* 2007; **14**: 812–816.

58 Lau DT, Kleiner DE, Park Y *et al.* Resolution of chronic delta hepatitis after 12 years of interferon alfa therapy. *Gastroenterology* 1999; **117**: 1229–1233.

59 Castelnau C, Le Gal F, Ripault MP *et al.* Efficacy of peginterferon alpha-2b in chronic hepatitis delta: relevance of quantitative RT-PCR for follow-up. *Hepatology* 2006; **44**: 728–735.

60 Niro GA, Ciancio A, Gaeta GB *et al.* Pegylated interferon alpha-2b as monotherapy or in combination with ribavirin in chronic hepatitis delta. *Hepatology* 2006; **44**: 713–720.

61 Erhardt A, Gerlich W, Starke C *et al.* Treatment of chronic hepatitis delta with pegylated interferon-alpha2b. *Liver Int.* 2006; **26**: 805–810.

62 Wedemeyer H, Manns MP. Epidemiology, pathogenesis and management of hepatitis D: update and challenges ahead. *Nat. Rev. Gastroenterol. Hepatol.* 2010; **7**: 31–40.

63 Kaymakoglu S, Karaca C, Demir K *et al.* Alpha interferon and ribavirin combination therapy of chronic hepatitis D. *Antimicrob. Agents Chemother.* 2005; **49**: 1135–1138.

64 Canbakan B, Senturk H, Tabak F *et al.* Efficacy of interferon alpha-2b and lamivudine combination treatment in comparison to interferon alpha-2b alone in chronic delta hepatitis: a randomized trial. *J. Gastroenterol. Hepatol.* 2006; **21**: 657–663.

65 Yurdaydin C, Bozkaya H, Onder FO *et al.* Treatment of chronic delta hepatitis with lamivudine vs lamivudine + interferon vs interferon. *J. Viral Hepat.* 2008; **15**: 314–321.

66 Gaudin JL, Faure P, Godinot H *et al.* The French experience of treatment of chronic type D hepatitis with a 12-month course of interferon alpha-2B. Results of a randomized controlled trial. *Liver* 1995; **15**: 45–52.

67 Lau DT, Doo E, Park Y *et al.* Lamivudine for chronic delta hepatitis. *Hepatology* 1999; **30**: 546–549.

68 Niro GA, Ciancio A, Tillman HL *et al.* Lamivudine therapy in chronic delta hepatitis: a multicentre randomized-controlled pilot study. *Aliment. Pharmacol. Ther.* 2005; **22**: 227–232.

69 Yurdaydin C, Bozkaya H, Gürel S *et al.* Famciclovir treatment of chronic delta hepatitis. *J. Hepatol.* 2002; **37**: 266–271.

70 Manesis EK, Schina M, Le Gal F *et al.* Quantitative analysis of hepatitis D virus RNA and hepatitis B surface antigen serum levels in chronic delta hepatitis improves treatment monitoring. *Antivir. Ther.* 2007; **12**: 381–388.

71 Pugnale P, Pazienza V, Guilloux K *et al.* Hepatitis delta virus inhibits alpha interferon signaling. *Hepatology* 2009; **49**: 398–406.

72 Glenn JS, Marsters JC Jr, Greenberg HB. Use of a prenylation inhibitor as a novel antiviral agent. *J. Virol.* 1998; **72**: 9303–9306.

73 Bordier BB, Ohkanda J, Liu P *et al.* In vivo antiviral efficacy of prenylation inhibitors against hepatitis delta virus (HDV). *J. Clin. Invest.* 2003; **112**: 407–414.

74 Chen TZ, Wu JC, Au LC *et al.* Specific inhibition of delta antigen by in vitro system by antisense oligodeoxinucleotide: implications for translation mechanism and treatment. *J. Virol. Methods* 1997; **65**: 183–189.

75 Chia JS, Wu HL, Wang HW *et al.* Inhibition of hepatitis delta virus genomic ribozyme self-cleavage by aminoglycosides. *J. Biomed. Sci.* 1997; **4**: 208–216.

76 Chang J, Taylor JM. Susceptibility of human hepatitis delta virus RNAs to small interfering RNA action. *J. Virol.* 2003; **77**: 9728–9731.

CHAPTER 20
Hepatitis C

Geoffrey Dusheiko
Centre for Hepatology, University College London Medical School and Royal Free Hospital, London, UK

Learning points

- Hepatitis C is a potentially curable disease.
- Hepatitis C virus RNA testing enables direct testing and quantitation for the hepatitis C virus genome.
- The current standard of care for hepatitis C is pegylated interferon used in combination with ribavirin. Each genotype responds differently to treatment.
- A 24-week schedule for hepatitis C virus genotype 2 or 3 is sufficient whereas patients with genotype 1 require 48 weeks of therapy.
- Genetic variation in the immune response may contribute to the ability to clear the virus.

Introduction

Non-A, non-B hepatitis was formerly identified as hepatitis occurring after transfusion of blood products or intravenous drug use. There was evidence that the parenterally transmitted infection could lead to persistent infection and progress to chronic liver disease, cirrhosis and hepatocellular carcinoma (HCC). Recombinant DNA technological analysis of pools of plasma known to contain a relatively high titre of the putative agent enabled the molecular cloning of the genome of what is now known as hepatitis C virus (HCV) [1]. Antibodies derived from diagnosed non-A, non-B hepatitis patients were used to identify a cDNA clone encoding an immunodominant epitope within HCV non-structural protein 4. Subsequent intensive research demonstrated that HCV was the principal cause of parenterally transmitted non-A, non-B hepatitis worldwide.

Considerable progress has been made in our understanding of hepatitis C infection since its discovery. Treatments have also improved, so that more than half of patients with chronic hepatitis C can be cured. Newer, direct-acting antiviral therapies will further improve response rates.

Epidemiology

HCV infection is an important worldwide public health problem. Population prevalence data are unavailable for many countries, but it is believed that 2–3% of the world's population are persistently infected with HCV. Worldwide, up to 170 million individuals may be chronically infected, and are at risk of developing cirrhosis and HCC as a result of persistent infection [2]. Hepatitis C is one of the 10 leading causes of infectious disease deaths worldwide; perhaps 250 000 deaths per year are due to hepatitis C. HIV and hepatitis B coinfection are adding to the burden of disease. There are geographical differences in prevalence, which range from 0.6–22%. The highest prevalence has been reported from Africa (Egypt) and Asia, with a somewhat lower prevalence in industrialized countries in the West, although in countries such as Japan (2.3%) and Italy (2.2%) the prevalence is relatively high (Fig. 20.1). The prevalence in populous countries such as China and Indonesia may be as high as 3%. There are also differences in prevalence in various groups—up to 50% in some countries in intravenous drug users, but less than 0.04 % in blood donors in the UK, for example [3,4]. There are a number of difficulties in accurately determining the prevalence and a number of assumptions are made by epidemiologists relying on different strategies to compile the evidence. Until screening of blood donors was introduced, hepatitis C accounted for the vast majority of non-A, non-B post-transfusion hepatitis. The incidence of hepatitis C is falling in industrialized countries (Fig. 20.2). However, it is important to point out that the current burden of disease, that is the pool of existing cases of liver disease, is due to past infection as HCV was not identified until 1989 and by then had infected tens of millions of people worldwide. Hepatitis C is now the most common reason for a hepatology consultation and is the single leading indication for liver transplantation in Europe and North America (Table 20.1).

Sherlock's Diseases of the Liver and Biliary System, Twelfth Edition. Edited by James S. Dooley, Anna S.F. Lok, Andrew K. Burroughs, E. Jenny Heathcote.
© 2011 by Blackwell Publishing Ltd. Published 2011 by Blackwell Publishing Ltd.

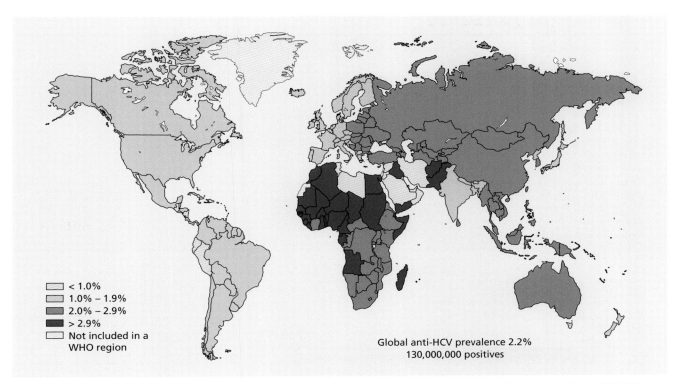

Fig. 20.1. Estimated HCV prevalence by region. (Source: Perz J *et al.*, unpublished data. Centers for Disease Control, 2002.)

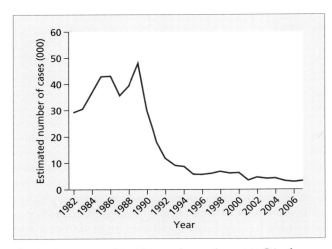

Fig. 20.2. Estimated incidence of acute hepatitis C in the USA, 1980–2007. (Source: Centers for Disease Control.)

Table 20.1. Number of liver transplants for HCV infection in the USA (Source Kim WR. The burden of hepatitis C in the United States. *Hepatology* 2002; **36**: S30–32.)

	Number of transplants per year		
	1991	1995	2000
HCV infection	343	1129	1679
All other	2588	2570	2900
HCV infection (%)	12	29	37

HCV can be transmitted via three routes: parenterally (usually by intravenous drug use or blood product transfusion), permucosally (usually sexually) or vertically. Parenteral transmission via intravenous drug use is the most common route, following the introduction of blood product screening for HCV. It is now estimated that intravenous drug use accounts for 80% of acute HCV infections. Acute HCV in HIV-positive individuals differs significantly from acute HCV monoinfection in its epidemiology, natural history, immunology and virology and is becoming an increasingly significant problem in HIV-infected persons. In contrast to the usual transmission of HCV, the majority of individuals in the reported HIV-positive cohorts describe possible permucosal transmission related to high-risk traumatic sexual practices, and perhaps parenteral transmission. In the past, in countries such as Italy, intrafamilial and sexual transmission of HCV undoubtedly contributed to the pool of infection. Nosocomial outbreaks of hepatitis C have been reported after lapses in infection control practices.

Table 20.2. Groups at risk of HCV infection

In developed and in developing countries, individuals at risk of HCV infection include:
   Injecting drug users (including past users)
   Health care workers with needlestick injury (0–10%)
   Individuals on haemodialysis, and after nosocomial outbreaks
   Those who engage in high-risk sexual practices
   Persons who received blood transfusion or infusion of factor concentrates before 1992
   HIV positive men who have sex with men
   Infants born to HCV-infected mothers (1–5%) particularly in mothers with high HCV RNA or HIV–HCV coinfection
In developing countries, additional sources of HCV infection include:
   Transfusions of unscreened blood
   Unsafe injections (including in health care settings) or other parenteral exposure to blood
   Use of blood-contaminated instruments for circumcision or surgery
   Traditional scarification
   Acupuncture
   Tattooing and ear piercing

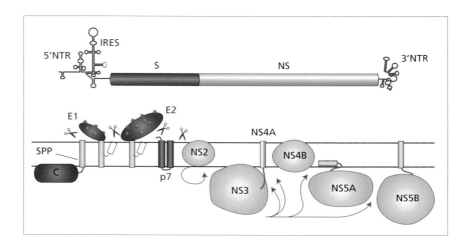

Fig. 20.3. HCV genome organization and polyprotein processing. S and NS correspond to regions coding for structural and non-structural proteins. (Reproduced from Penin F, Dubuisson J, Rey FA *et al. Hepatology* 2004; **39**: 5–19.)

Modes of infection and groups at risk differ in developed versus developing countries (Table 20.2).

Virology

HCV is a small, enveloped RNA virus and a member of the family Flaviviridae [5]. The genome of HCV resembles those of Flaviviridae, the pestiviruses and flaviviruses. The RNA genome contains around 9400 nucleotides of positive-sense RNA, comprising one long open reading frame encoding a polyprotein of 3010 to 3033 amino acids which is cleaved into functionally distinct polypeptides during or after translation. HCV has been designated the prototype of a third genus in the family Flaviviridae, hepacivirus. The nucleocapsid and envelope structural proteins are encoded at the 5′ end of the genome; the non-structural elements are downstream of this region (Fig. 20.3). Translation is mediated by an internal ribosome entry site in the 5′ untranslated region. The non-glycosylated capsid protein, C, com-

plexes with the genomic RNA to form the nucleocapsid. Two glycoprotein products, E1 or gp35 and E2 or gp70, are found in the viral envelope. There are hypervariable regions, particularly in the E1 and E2 domains; these regions (particularly those of the envelope glycoproteins) may be important antigenic sites and their variability may be important in persistence of infection and immunopathogenesis. Hepatitis C replicates via an error-prone RNA-dependent RNA polymerase. The rapid replication rate and turnover of HCV combined with the poor fidelity of the HCV RNA-dependent RNA polymerases, which lacks a proof-reading function, generates a population of viruses with closely related, but different, nucleotide sequences, or a 'quasispecies', in infected persons. Divergence may be enhanced by the induction of neutralizing antibodies targeted to the envelope proteins.

Cleavage at the carboxyl terminus of E2 generates a small protein, p7. The remainder of the non-structural region of the HCV genome is divided into regions NS2 to NS5 (Fig. 20.3). HCV encodes a protease at the NS2/ NS3 junction which cleaves this site. After cleavage, non-structural proteins remain associated with cellular membranes (the membranous web), forming a replication complex. NS3 has two functional domains, a protease, which is involved in cleavage of the remainder of the non-structural region of the polyprotein, and a helicase, which is assumed to be involved in RNA replication. The HCV protease, using NS4a as a cofactor, is a major target of specific protease inhibitor antiviral agents. HCV NS5 is cleaved to yield NS5a and NS5b. NS5b is a viral RNA-dependent RNA polymerase; NS5a also may be involved in genome replication [6].

HCV comprises six genotypes and hundreds of subtypes. Detailed investigation of HCV was previously hampered by the lack of an appropriate viral culture system, but this hurdle has been overcome with the development of the subgenomic HCV replicon system; these genomes, coupled to the non-structural region of the HCV genome, are able to replicate when transfected into Huh7 cells (derived from a human HCC) [7]. The production of infectious virus has been reported from full-length HCV RNA transfection into Huh-7 cells, using a JFH-1 strain isolated from a patient with fulminant hepatitis due to HCV genotype 2a [6,8].

Candidate receptors have been proposed; these include the tetraspannin CD81, the low density lipoprotein receptor, scavenger receptor class B type I (SR-BI) and heparin. Claudin-1 (a tight junction component) has been shown to be an important coreceptor [9].

Pathology and pathogenesis

In 15–40% of individuals, the acute disease resolves completely, with clearance of HCV RNA from serum, within 4 months. Thus the majority of patients infected with HCV progress to chronic infection. The pathogenic mechanisms that result in hepatitis are unknown. Lymphocytes are typically observed within the hepatic parenchyma, but the functional characteristics of these cells have not been fully defined.

Given the heterogeneous nature of the viral population that infects individuals, it is likely that a variety of strategies enable evasion of the host innate and adaptive immune response. Interferon-α (IFN-α) is induced by double-stranded RNA (present during viral replication); signalling pathways leading to type I IFN production are a first line of defence of the host to eradicate viruses. IFNs exert their antiviral function by binding to the IFN-α and -β receptors on the cell surface. The interaction triggers the JAK-STAT signalling cascade and induces expression of IFN-stimulated genes. The resulting innate antiviral response is a first line of immune defence against virus infection. HCV may inhibit the antiviral action of IFN-α and has evolved a mechanism

to interfere with type 1 IFN induction and signalling. For example HCV proteins E2 and NS3 may inhibit the action of the IFN-induced double-stranded-RNA-activated protein kinase, enabling the virus to abrogate the development of the adaptive immune response [10]. The retinoic-acid-inducible gene I and IFN regulatory factor 3 pathway of the innate antiviral response within infected hepatocytes are abrogated, thus enabling the evasion of innate immune defences within the infected cell [11].

HCV-specific HLA class I-restricted cytotoxic T lymphocytes that recognize epitopes in variable regions of the envelope or of non-structural proteins have been identified. A CD4+ proliferative T lymphocyte response to recombinant viral antigens has been found in infected individuals. There may be a correlation between the presence of CD4+ T-cell responses to HCV core and a benign course of infection in viraemic carriers with minimal hepatitis. Patients with self-limited hepatitis C display stronger virus-specific CD4+ IFN-γ cell reactivity. HCV-specific CD8+ cytotoxic T lymphocytes (CTL) are thought to play a key role in the elimination of HCV since the vigour of the HCV-specific CTL response during the incubation phase of acute HCV infection is greater in those who resolve infection than in those who progress to chronic infection.

There is an effect of viral mutation on T-cell recognition so that escape mutations leading to immune escape may favour persistence of the virus. The role of cell surface inhibitory receptors in recognition of HCV, and the development of antibodies that neutralize HCV infection require further study. A down-regulated cytotoxic activity of natural killer (NK) cells against HCV-infected liver cells has been postulated. Understanding the constitution of an effective immune response in the control of HCV may enable improved immunomodulatory therapies. The existence of multiple genotypes that differ by up to 20% at the amino acid level represents a major obstacle for immunological control and the development of prophylactic and therapeutic vaccines for HCV.

Once chronicity is established, HCV-specific CTL remain weakly detectable implying that the virus can persist despite the presence of these CTL and that it may be resistant to the effects of antiviral cytokines. T-cell exhaustion may be present. Owing to the lack of a proof-reading mechanism of the viral polymerase, mutations occur frequently in HCV and, if CTL are unable to clear the virus rapidly during early infection, the CTL response may select for T-cell escape mutants. Later, when the HCV-specific CTL response is weaker, there may be less selection pressure [12].

Fibrosis in chronic hepatitis C infection occurs as a result of the activation of hepatic stellate cells by cytokines and other signalling molecules induced by the inflammatory process. These produce and deposit extra-cellular matrix proteins. Fibrosis begins around the portal tracts and gradually extends out into the lobules towards the central veins. Factors shown to accelerate the progression to cirrhosis include older age at HCV acquisition, male gender, heavy alcohol intake and coinfection with either HBV or HIV. Steatosis may lead to advancing fibrosis.

There is no DNA intermediate in the replication of the HCV genome or integration of viral nucleic acid, and viral pathology may contribute to oncogenesis through cirrhosis and regeneration of liver cells. HCV infection rarely seems to cause acute liver failure.

Diagnostic tests for hepatitis C

Anti-HCV

Because detection of the viral antigen is difficult, measurement of antibodies to HCV by enzyme-linked immunosorbent assay has become important as an indication of past or present infection. Anti-HCV antibody titres may decline or disappear over time after resolved infection. Third-generation immunoassays include antigens from the nucleocapsid (C22) and other non-structural regions of the genome. The sequence of the HCV core protein is relatively highly conserved. Most patients with acute HCV infection are anti-HCV positive by the time serum alanine aminotransferase (ALT) levels peak but anti-HCV may be undetectable at presentation. IgM anti-HCV is not a reliable test for acute disease and is not readily available. Diagnosis of acute hepatitis C may require documentation of seroconversion to anti-HCV in an at-risk population.

Routine testing of blood donors occurs in most industrialized countries, and has greatly reduced the risk of transmission of HCV. Supplemental tests for antibody to HCV are required to confirm the specificity of an anti-HCV test in low-risk populations, including blood donors. The most widely used method is the recombinant immunoblot assay (RIBA) in which antibodies are sought to recombinant antigens of HCV coated on nitrocellulose strips. Samples are confirmed positive if antibodies to two or more HCV proteins are present, and are indeterminate if antibody to only one antigen is found. However, HCV RNA testing offers greater clinical utility to confirm or quantitate viraemia. A confirmed positive anti-HCV result in a patient negative for HCV RNA usually indicates past, resolved infection. Any unexplained raised serum aminotransferases, or a risk factor for hepatitis C, should prompt a test for anti-HCV.

New tests for HCV core antigen are in development. These tests may provide a more direct test for antigenaemia.

Serum HCV RNA

HCV RNA testing enables direct testing and quantitation for the HCV viral genome. Polymerase chain reaction (PCR) analysis provides a sensitive and specific assay for HCV RNA in blood and other tissues. PCR testing utilizes primers of known nucleotide sequence of HCV. Currently, the limit of detection for plasma HCV RNA by real time PCR is 10–15 IU/mL. HCV RNA has been detected within 1–2 weeks of transfusion in patients with hepatitis C. HCV RNA usually persists for decades in patients who develop chronic disease and there is little advantage in repeatedly quantitating HCV RNA in untreated patients, as there is generally no direct correlation with activity or progression of the disease. Accurate methods to quantify HCV RNA in serum have been developed and are of value in estimating viral concentrations before and during antiviral therapy. Several commercially available assays are in wide use. Individuals who test positive for anti-HCV should be tested for HCV RNA.

Genotyping

Variation in the genome sequence of HCV isolates has enabled classification into types and subtypes [13,14]. Several isolates of hepatitis C have been cloned. The sequence divergence of these isolates indicates that there are several major genotypes of hepatitis C, and component subtypes [15]. Six major genotypes and about 100 subtypes can be differentiated by restriction fragment length polymorphism, type-specific primers in PCR reactions or hybridization with type-specific probes. The definitive method for viral genotype is sequencing [16]. Geographic localization of these genotypes has been reported. Infections with types 1b and 1a are relatively common in Europe and the United States; infection with type 1b is frequent in Southern Europe. Epidemiological differences in age distribution of major types and the risk factors associated with particular genotypes have become apparent. In Europe, type 3a and 1a are relatively more common in young individuals with a history of intravenous drug use. Type 1b accounts for most infections in those aged 50 or more. Type 4 infection is the most prevalent infection in Egypt, and many parts of the Middle East and Africa. Genotype 5 was thought to be confined to South Africa but pockets of have been found in France, Spain, Syria and Belgium. Type 6 is prevalent in South East Asia, Asian Americans and Asian Australians.

Importantly, response to treatment is influenced by the infecting genotype. No inherently greater pathogenicity of type 1 HCV has been documented and several clinical investigations have documented severe and progressive liver disease after infection with each of the well-characterized genotypes.

Approaches to resistance testing after virological failure

Population and clonal sequencing are utilized. Other technologies are evolving, such as ultra deep pyrosequencing. The initial genetic characterization of resistance mutations following treatment with direct antiviral agents is population sequencing; sequencing of the coding region of the antiviral target is required.

Acute hepatitis C

The acute course of HCV infection is clinically mild, and typically unrecognized. Acute hepatitis C is thus only infrequently diagnosed. The mean incubation period of hepatitis C, defined as the time from exposure to the onset of symptoms, ranges from 2–12 weeks (average 7). It is shorter with large inoculae (e.g. following administration of factor VIII concentrate). The incidence of acute hepatitis C is falling in several industrialized countries as a result of blood screening, and perhaps the prevention of transmission of HCV during drug use. The diagnosis of acute hepatitis C is made by testing for anti-HCV and HCV RNA. HCV RNA becomes positive within 2 weeks of exposure. Most patients are anti-HCV positive within 8–10 weeks of exposure. Symptoms during the acute phase are non-specific and may include fatigue, lethargy, anorexia and right hypochondrial discomfort. Perhaps 25% of cases are icteric; patients with jaundice are more likely to clear the virus. Female gender and acute severe hepatitis associated with jaundice are associated with a higher chance of viral clearance. HIV coinfection is associated with viral persistence. Fulminant hepatitis is rare following hepatitis C infection, but has been reported, particularly following chemotherapy or withdrawal of chemotherapy. About 25% of patients have mildly elevated serum bilirubin. Peak serum ALT elevations are less than those encountered in acute hepatitis A or B. During the early clinical phase, serum ALT levels may fluctuate, and may become normal or near normal; HCV RNA may be intermittently negative during the acute phase, making determination of true convalescence somewhat difficult. Chronic hepatitis C infection is the major complication of acute hepatitis C. Higher rates of spontaneous recovery from acute hepatitis C have been observed in individuals with identified single nucleotide polymorphisms that lie in or near the *IL28B* gene on chromosome 19, which encodes IFN-λ3 [17]. The C/C genotype at rs12979860 strongly enhances resolution of HCV infection among individuals of both European and African descent, suggesting a primary role for *IL28B* in resolution of HCV infection.

Pathology

Most patients with well-documented acute hepatitis C do not require a liver biopsy. The pathological features that are constant in all types of acute viral hepatitis consist of parenchymal cell necrosis and histiocytic periportal inflammation [18]. The reticulin framework of the liver is usually well preserved, except in some cases of massive and submassive necrosis. The liver cells show necrotic changes that vary in form and intensity. The necrotic areas are usually multifocal, but necrosis tends to be frequently zonal, with the most severe changes occurring in the centrilobular areas. Individual hepatocytes often are swollen and may show ballooning but they can also shrink, giving rise to acidophilic bodies.

Dead or dying, rounded liver cells are extruded into the perisinusoidal space. There are variations in the size and staining quality of the nuclei. A monocellular infiltration, which is particularly marked in the portal zones, is the characteristic mesenchymal reaction. This is also accompanied by some proliferation of bile ductules.

Kupffer cells and endothelial cells proliferate and the Kupffer cells often contain excess lipofuscin pigment. In the icteric phase of typical acute hepatitis, the walls of the hepatic vein tributaries may be thickened and frequently are infiltrated, with proliferation of the lining cells in the terminal hepatic veins. Cholestasis may occur in the early stages of viral hepatitis, and plugs of bile thrombi may be found in the bile canaliculi.

Management

Early identification of acute hepatitis C is important, but may be difficult as the disease may be relatively silent; 75% of patients are not jaundiced and have non-specific symptoms. Management of acute sporadic hepatitis C includes conventional supportive treatment or specific antiviral therapy. Early spontaneous convalescence can be difficult to confirm; patients should be retested if HCV RNA becomes negative to differentiate transient versus sustained virus clearance [19]. Therapeutic trials of IFN-α have been undertaken. Recent studies have indicated that treatment benefits those patients who have been treated early. Early treatment of these individuals with IFN or combination pegylated IFN (PEG-IFN) and ribavirin (RBV) is usually advisable, but no consensus exists. In those who do not appear to be convalescing 2–4 months after onset of the disease, antiviral treatment (see below) should be considered, as a high percentage of patients (>80–90%) may respond, and the risk of chronic disease is high. Acute HCV monoinfection is far more responsive to treatment than chronic disease, and even IFN monotherapy has yielded very high (>90%) sustained virological responses (SVR), defined as HCV RNA negativity 6 months post-HCV treatment. In contrast, without specific HCV treatment only 20–50% of HIV-negative individuals will clear acute HCV infection.

The optimal timing and form of treatment for acute hepatitis C is not yet determined [20]. Studies are in progress to determine whether a wait and see strategy is detrimental, compared to immediate treatment. However, asymptomatic patients could be treated immediately as they appear to have a higher risk of chronic disease than those who present with acute symptomatic disease.

There needs to be increased surveillance for HCV, both to identify cases and assess the scope of the problem in at risk individuals. Generally, treatment should be given if the serum aminotransferases are elevated, and HCV RNA remains detected 2–4 months after first ascertainment, in a patient with apparent recent onset, to minimize the risk of chronicity. It is reasonable medical practice to recommend PEG-IFN and RBV although the need for RBV in this setting remains unclear. Treatment after an onset of 1 year is unsatisfactory, with results tantamount to the treatment of chronic infection. Immediate prophylactic intervention with IFN after a needlestick exposure, before the appearance of HCV RNA, is not justified. However, larger studies comparing immediate intervention after diagnosis versus delayed intervention, to avoid unnecessary treatment in those resolving the infection, have yet to be reported [21–26].

Chronic hepatitis C

Natural history

The acute phase and progression to chronic hepatitis C is usually silent. Thus the onset of chronic hepatitis C is often insidious and usually has gone unnoticed by the patient. The diagnosis of chronic hepatitis C is arbitrarily defined as the persistence of HCV RNA in serum for 6 months or longer. Self-limited infections may be associated with a delayed clearance of HCV RNA, albeit this is relatively uncommon [27]. Epidemiological risk factors, for example a past blood transfusion, intravenous drug use or sexual risk, can indicate a possible aetiology. Serum aminotransferase levels remain abnormal after 12 months in 60 to 85% of patients with type C post-transfusion or sporadic hepatitis; these patients have chronic hepatitis histologically. Serum aminotransferases decline from the peak values encountered in the acute phase of the disease, but typically remain abnormal by twofold to eightfold. Serum ALT concentrations may fluctuate over time, and may even be intermittently or consistently normal.

The chronic disease is generally slowly progressive; cirrhosis develops within 20 years in about 10–20% of patients with chronic disease, but can remain indolent for a prolonged period of time (Fig. 20.4) [28–30]. Variability in rates of progression of the disease makes the prediction of ultimate outcome difficult. The disease is not necessarily benign, however, and rapidly progressive cirrhosis can occur. HCV causes an estimated 8000 to 10 000 deaths annually in the USA [31].

Several interactive factors, including the age of acquisition, concomitant alcohol abuse, gender, coexisting viral disease particularly concurrent HBV or HIV infection and the host immune response, are aggravating factors that affect the morbidity of the disease (Table 20.3) [31–33]. A study of 2313 untreated patients reported that increasing age at infection was independently associated with disease progression. Two per cent of those infected before the age of 20 developed cirrhosis over a 20-year period compared to 6% of those infected between 31 and 40 years, 37% infected between the age of 41 and 50 years and 63% infected after the age of 50 [29]. HCV genotypes and HCV RNA viral load, although important determinants of the effectiveness of treatment, are not thought to influence the natural history of infection.

Older patients may present with complications of cirrhosis or HCC. HCC has been rarely observed in the absence of cirrhosis. During progressive disease, laboratory values become progressively more abnormal. Aspartate aminotransferase (AST) concentrations greater than ALT, a low serum albumin, a prolonged prothrombin time and low platelet counts suggest cirrhosis. Low levels of autoantibodies may be detected. A subset of patients with chronic hepatitis C infection may test positive for LKM1 antibody.

Anti-HCV persists for decades in chronic hepatitis C. HCV RNA is usually detectable in patients with abnormal serum aminotransferases and anti-HCV antibodies. Although most patients with raised serum ALT are HCV RNA-positive, the converse is not always true. Isolates of HCV in individual patients may show nucleotide substitutions over time, suggesting that HCV RNA mutates at a rate similar to that of other RNA viruses. A proportion of patients, perhaps 25–50% may have persistently normal serum ALT. However, 'normal serum aminotransferases' in patients with hepatitis C are frequently actually high relative to healthy individuals [34,35]. Low-grade hepatitis, and even low-grade fibrosis, may be present but fibrosis progression may be less rapid in females with low or normal ALT. In patients with 'normal ALT' who received antiviral therapy, further decline in ALT is observed in virological responders.

Extrahepatic manifestations

The infection can cause systemic disease, and may be associated with various systemic complications; these

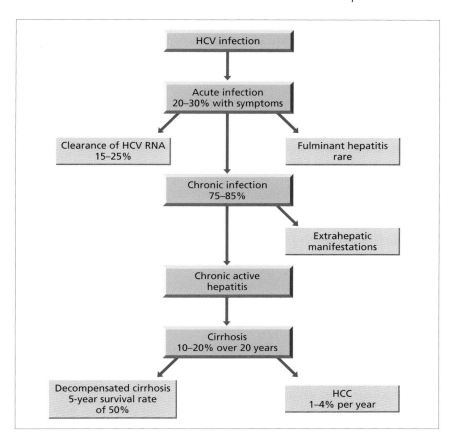

Fig. 20.4. Natural history of hepatitis C infection. (Reproduced from Chen SL, Morgan TR. The natural history of hepatitis C virus (HCV) infection. *Int. J. Med. Sci.* 2006; **3**; 47–52.)

Table 20.3. Factors adversely determining response to IFN

Baseline host and virus factors:
  Genetic polymorphism: IL28b rs12979860 TT
  African American ethnicity
  Age greater than 50 years
  High body mass index
  Hepatic steatosis
  High homeostasis model assessment index (HOMA)
  Advanced fibrosis or cirrhosis or advanced liver disease
  High baseline viral load
  Genotype 1 versus genotype 2 or 3
  Genotype 4, and probably 5 and 6
  HIV and HCV coinfection
On treatment:
  Poor adherence to therapy
  Excess alcohol
  Failure to achieve RVR
  Failure to achieve cEVR

include a form of autoimmune hepatitis, cryoglobuli-naemia, a vasculitis, lichen planus, porphyria cutanea tarda, lymphocytic sialoadenitis and membranous glomerulonephritis. There is an association between non-Hodgkin's lymphoma and hepatitis C infection [36–39].

Hepatitis C appears to induce insulin resistance; patients with hepatitis C have an increased prevalence of insulin resistance and type 2 diabetes mellitus. Molecular studies have shown that the HCV core protein can directly inhibit the insulin signalling pathway and increase reactive oxygen species production. There may be a direct genotype association (steatosis is more common in patients with genotype 3) that influences this metabolic effect, although this remains a contentious issue. Hepatitis C is commonly associated with hepatic steatosis. Replication of the virus is linked to lipid metabolism. The metabolic syndrome, that is obesity, insulin resistance or overt diabetes is associated with a poorer prognosis in patients with chronic hepatitis C. The clinical relevance is yet imperfectly understood but the interaction between steatosis, inflammatory processes, insulin resistance and impaired response to IFN may lead to an increased risk of hepatic fibrosis. The role of adjuvant therapies to improve insulin sensitivity or lipid-lowering agents to decrease cholesterol or triglyceride level is uncertain.

Pathology

The pathological features of HCV infection are quite characteristic, albeit not pathognomonic [18,40]. The presence of HCV RNA in serum tends to correlate with some degree of hepatitis and disappearance of HCV RNA, for example following successful IFN-α treatment, is followed by histological improvement. Typically, patients with chronic hepatitis C have mild portal tract inflammation with lymphoid aggregates or follicles and mild periportal piecemeal necrosis. Parenchymal steatosis, apoptosis and mild lobular inflammation are present and portal fibrosis or portal–central fibrosis may be present in later stages of disease. Bridging necrosis is not common. Rarely, granulomas can be observed. Although many of the lymphoid follicles are associated with bile ducts, ductopenia is not observed. Advanced disease, with cirrhosis or HCC is not generally associated with distinguishing features.

HCV antigens have been detected in scattered groups of cells, with granular cytoplasmic staining. The periportal lymphocytes around lymphoid follicles are mixed, but contain relatively large numbers of CD4 lymphocytes. A characteristic histological pattern of mild chronic hepatitis with portal lymphoid follicles and varying degrees of lobular activity is found in many patients with persistent hepatitis C infection. Fatty changes in the liver are usually not marked, but some steatosis can be observed in chronic HCV infection. Iron homeostasis may affect the outcome of hepatitis C. Hepcidin is the central regulator of systemic iron homeostasis. A positive correlation has been documented between serum hepcidin levels and both necroinflammation and fibrosis [41]. Others have found hepcidin levels to be lower in patients with chronic hepatitis C, suggesting that HCV may suppress this hormone, leading to liver iron accumulation [42].

Minor histological abnormalities, or degrees of hepatic fibrosis, in anti-HCV-positive, HCV RNA-negative individuals with normal serum ALT has been reported. The absence of HCV RNA in serum is evidence for, but not proof of, the absence of ongoing chronic hepatitis C as some reports have documented mild histological changes in some patients. The explanation and clinical significance of these abnormalities, and their prognosis, remains debated [43].

Management

Evaluation of liver disease

Treatment of hepatitis C has improved considerably over the last 10 years. A substantial proportion of patients with chronic hepatitis C can be cured although current treatments have limitations [44–46]. HCV RNA should be quantitated in all patients to confirm viraemia. If the test is reproducibly positive, serum aminotransferases, and bilirubin, alkaline phosphatase and prothrombin time should be measured to assess hepatic

function. The HCV genotype should be ascertained. In patients with risk factors for other forms of viral hepatitis, HBsAg and HIV infection must also be tested. Because autoimmune hepatitis is treated differently and because IFN can unmask or exacerbate autoimmune hepatitis, it is advisable to exclude this diagnosis by measuring titres of antismooth muscle and antiliver–kidney microsomal antibodies, even in patients with a positive anti-HCV test.

Liver biopsy and assessment of fibrosis

A liver biopsy is helpful in grading the degree of inflammation and staging the degree of fibrosis. Earlier guidelines recommended antiviral therapy for those patients with chronic hepatitis C who were deemed to be at highest risk of developing cirrhosis, that is patients with chronic hepatitis C who had persistently increased serum ALT levels, detectable levels of HCV RNA and histological evidence of portal or bridging fibrosis or inflammation and necrosis. However, recent guidelines suggest that potentially all patients with hepatitis C are candidates for treatment; a liver biopsy can be informative and provides unique clinical information but is not now considered mandatory for all patients. Liver biopsy has inherent sampling variability, but can be minimized by the inclusion of samples more than 25 mm in length. Interobserver variability has been found to occur.

Several non-invasive methods can be used to assess the stage of disease. Patients with hepatitis C can be appropriately studied by these markers of fibrosis, as these tests have been validated in this group. A calculation of aspartate aminotransferases to platelet ratio index (APRI) (aspartate aminotransferases (U/L)/ upper limit of normal × 100 divided by the platelet count (10^9/L)) can be used to indicate cirrhosis. Similarly, transient elastography (TE, fibroscan) which measures the speed of propagation of a shear wave in the liver, is a physical means of detecting cirrhosis. TE measures liver stiffness rather than fibrosis. Inflammation in the liver can contribute to tissue elasticity. The path of signal penetration is affected by obesity and ascites. Normal liver stiffness is in the range of 4–6 kilopascals, and cirrhosis is adjudged at levels of 12–14 kilopascals. A strong relationship between liver stiffness and the hepatic venous pressure gradient (HVPG) has been described. The Enhanced Liver Fibrosis (ELF™, Siemans) panel and Fibrotest (Biopredictive) are proprietary tests which utilize algorithms of biochemical tests and extracellular matrix components to estimate fibrosis.

APRI, Fibrotest, ELF, TE and ultrasound microbubble hepatic transit times (HTT) predict cirrhosis with relatively high diagnostic accuracies of 85–90%. These markers can reduce the need for liver biopsy. Non-invasive markers are desirable in patients with bleeding disorders (haemophilia) and hepatitis C. The markers may allow pragmatic decision making by clinicians, albeit that treatment of chronic hepatitis C is cost-effective in histologically mild, moderate and severe stages of precirrhotic disease. Low readings may allow a period of 'watchful waiting' prior to a decision on starting treatment and provide reassurance to patients or can be used in clinical practice as a tool for the confirmation of cirrhosis. However, the relative utility of these tests and the financial cost and capital outlay for non-invasive fibrosis evaluation require assessment in different centres. The APRI score is an inexpensive test which correctly predicts cirrhosis in 80–90% of patients [47–49]. ELF, TE and HTT are less widely available, and are more expensive, requiring capital outlay and operators. Despite high diagnostic accuracy, there is substantial overlap between groups, especially in the precirrhotic stage. Thus the diagnostic accuracy for cirrhosis of all current non-invasive tests is greater than that for the diagnosis of moderate to severe fibrosis. Two tests can provide concordance and where results are discordant, a biopsy is proposed. The clinical interpretation of TE results should be made by an expert clinician.

Patients with clinically overt cirrhosis do not require biopsy, but rather assessment of portal hypertension, including upper gastrointestinal endoscopy for varices and ultrasound for HCC surveillance.

General management

Careful clinical monitoring is suggested as an alternative to antiviral therapy for patients with less severe histological changes in whom cirrhosis may not develop. There is evidence that alcohol and hepatitis C may synergistically aggravate hepatic injury. Similarly coinfection with hepatitis B, HIV, obesity, hepatic steatosis, diabetes, male gender and older age at the time of acquisition of infection may increase the rate of fibrosis progression. Insulin resistance may develop. Patients with hepatitis C should be advised to minimize their intake of alcohol [50,51]. The patient should be advised not to donate blood. Patients can be told that the parenteral route is the most important route of transmission and that the virus is not easily transmitted except by this route. Those who are not immune should be vaccinated against hepatitis A and B. The risk of sexual transmission in monogamous partners is low.

Indications for treatment

All patients irrespective of the degree of fibrosis are potential candidates for treatment. Some patients with mild disease may not require immediate treatment however. Patients with psychiatric comorbidities which may be worsened with IFN treatment should be stabilized and treated jointly with psychiatrists [52–55]. Patients with compensated cirrhosis are candidates for treatment; successful clearance of HCV alters the natural history of the disease and reduces the risk of complications of cirrhosis. IFN-α is difficult to apply in decompensated cirrhosis and may precipitate deterioration. These patients should be considered for liver transplantation.

IFN-α and RBV treatment

Mechanisms of action

The current treatment of hepatitis C is PEG-IFN-α, given by subcutaneous injection once weekly, and oral RBV daily. The IFNs are a system of related proteins, derived from a multigene family. The IFNs have been classified into types, based on receptor specificity. Type 1 IFNs include IFN-α (leucocyte), IFN-β (fibroblast) and IFN-ω. Type II IFN is also known as immune IFN, IFN-γ. There is interest in the therapeutic potential of IFN-λ.

IFN act via species-specific, surface target-cell receptors. The cellular activities of IFN-α are mediated by the products of the IFN-inducible genes. IFNs interfere with several stages of the viral life cycle, although the actual mechanism varies with different viruses. IFNs thus induce several enzymes and proteins, the best characterized of which are the 2′5′ oligoadenylate synthetases (2′5′A synthetases), double-stranded RNA-dependent protein kinases, RNase L and the Mx protein GTPases. IFN is excreted in the urine, reabsorbed by the proximal tubules and undergoes lysosomal degradation in these cells. IFN-α is rapidly absorbed, with peak serum concentrations observed in 7–12 h, followed by a rapid decline. The terminal elimination half-life of IFN-α ranges from 3 to 8 h, with serum concentrations decreasing to below the limit of detection within 24 h of administration [56]. Plasma concentrations of recombinant IFN-α decrease to trough levels between each administration.

RBV is a guanosine nucleoside analogue. This agent shows only modest activity against hepatitis C but it increases the activity of IFN-α when the two agents are used in combination. The drug exerts its action after intracellular phosphorylation to mono, di- and triphosphate nucleotides. The precise mode of action probably includes perturbation of intracellular nucleoside triphosphate pools, interference with the formation of the 5′ cap structure of viral mRNA by competitive inhibition of both guanyltransferase and methyltransferase capping enzymes, direct inhibition of the viral mRNA polymerase complex and possibly enhancement of macrophage inhibition of viral replication. RBV may also

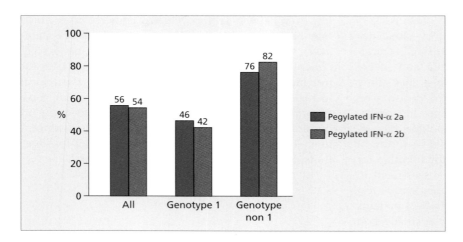

Fig. 20.5. Sustained virological response rates with pegylated IFN and ribavirin.

induce mutations in the hepatitis C genome affecting HCV replication.

Pegylated IFNs

Limitations in the effectiveness of IFN-α have been attributed to its rapid systemic clearance and short plasma elimination half-life of about 8 h. Subcutaneous formulations of PEG-IFN-α have been developed, which are produced by the covalent attachment of recombinant IFN-α to branched 40-kDa or 12-kDa polyethylene glycol moieties [57]. The PEG moieties are inert, long-chain, amphiphilic molecules produced by linking repeating units of ethylene oxide. These molecules protect the IFN protein from enzymatic degradation, reducing systemic clearance. Pegylation thus changes the pharmacokinetics and pharmacodynamics of IFN-αs; the improved drug concentrations and sustained exposure is clinically advantageous. The various PEG-IFN-αs extend the half-life to a similar degree, but other pharmacokinetic parameters are affected differently. The 40-kDa branched PEG-IFN-α 2a has a decreased volume of distribution compared to standard IFN. The 40-kDa IFN-α is associated with a greater reduction in renal clearance.

The sustained absorption and reduced clearance of subcutaneously administered PEG 40-kD and PEG 12-kDa allows for more convenient dosing, and results in higher SVR rates; 12-kDa PEG-IFN-α 2b and 40-kDa PEG-IFN-α 2a have been licensed for the treatment of hepatitis C.

Current treatment protocols

The aim of therapy is to achieve SVR. A sustained response is associated with reduction in inflammation and severity of fibrosis. PEG-IFN-α 2b is administered at a dose of 1.5 μg/kg per week by subcutaneous injec-

tion. RBV is administered according to body weight of the patient, for patients infected with genotypes 1–6. For patients less than 65 kg the dose of RBV is 800 mg/day orally. For patients between 65 and 85 kg the dose of RBV is 1000 mg/day. For patients more than 85 kg the dose of RBV is 1200 mg. PEG-IFN-α 2a is given at a fixed dose of 180 μg per week. RBV is given at a dose of 1000 mg if the patient weighs less than 75 kg or at a dose of 1200 mg for patients weighing more than 75 kg in patients with genotype 1 infection. However, patients with genotype 2 and 3 are treated with a dose of 800 mg/day of RBV.

The pivotal studies suggested that a 24-week schedule for HCV genotype 2 or 3 is sufficient whereas patients with HCV genotype 1 require 48 weeks of therapy. Thus patients with genotype 1 or 4 are treated for 12 months whereas patients with genotype 2 or 3 are treated for 6 months.

Sustained virological response rates

The efficacy of PEG-IFN-α 2a and 2b has been investigated in several controlled trials, and the outcome compared to standard IFN or IFN and RBV, based on virological, biochemical and histological responses. The combination of RBV and PEG-IFN-α has been shown to produce sustained virological responses in about 40 to 50% of patients overall [56] (Fig. 20.5). Large randomized controlled trials do not suggest that there are major differences in efficacy between these IFNs, although they have different pharmacokinetic profiles and molecular structures [58]. Forty-eight weeks of PEG-IFN-α 2b 1.5 μg/kg per week in combination with RBV 800 mg/day achieved a 54% SVR overall (42% for genotype 1, 80% for genotypes 2 and 3), in comparison with 47% for PEG-IFN-α 2b plus RBV. Analysis of response by patient weight demonstrated that the optimum dose of RBV is 10.6 mg/kg per day and those receiving this dose achieved SVR of 48% for genotype 1 and 88% for genotypes 2 and 3 [59].

Patients with genotype 1 who do not show an HCV RNA decline of at least 2 $\log_{10}$ after 12 weeks of therapy (early viral response, EVR) have little opportunity of achieving a SVR and therapy should be discontinued in these patients. Types of hepatitis C treatment response and their definitions are shown in Table 20.4 and Fig. 20.6. At week 24, HCV RNA should be measured by a sensitive qualitative PCR. Patients who are HCV RNA-positive at 6 months should stop therapy. For patients with genotype 2 or 3 it is unnecessary to check the viral load at 12 weeks. There may be benefit in prolonging therapy to 72 weeks in slow responders, that is those with a negative PCR after 24 weeks of treatment but who were detectable, with a more than 2 $\log_{10}$ decline at 12 weeks (pEVR). The efficacy of 72 weeks' treatment remains controversial and attrition rates are higher.

The response to treatment of genotype 4 is intermediate between genotype 1 and 2 or 3. A SVR is achieved in 43–70% with PEG-IFN and RBV. It is higher in Egyptians than Europeans and Africans. SVR rates increase to 80% with 24 weeks of therapy if a rapid virological response is achieved. There are limited published data on treatment outcome in patients with genotype 5—no prospective studies have been reported; SVR rates of 48% [60] and 66% have been reported in treated patients [61,62].

Table 20.4. Definition of responses

Response	Definition
Non-responders	No significant virological response occurs during treatment and the patient does not become HCV RNA negative at any point during treatment. Some investigators have differentiated between null responders showing little decline in HCV RNA (<1 log decline) and non-responders who show a decline in HCV RNA but did not become HCV RNA negative.
Relapsers	Virological response occurred; the patient became HCV RNA undetectable, and remained negative through the end of treatment, but relapse occurred after discontinuation of treatment.
Breakthroughs	Virological response occurred (before 24 weeks) but was not maintained at the end of treatment, i.e. the patient 'broke through'
Sustained virological response (SVR)	HCV RNA is undetectable at the end of 24 or 48 weeks of treatment (in patients treated appropriately depending on genotype) and remains undetectable 24 weeks after completion of treatment.
Rapid viral response (RVR)	HCV RNA becomes undetectable by 4 weeks of treatment.
Partial early viral response (pEVR)	HCV RNA levels remain detectable but decline by ≥2 logs by 12 weeks of treatment.
Complete early viral response (cEVR)	HCV RNA levels become undetectable by 12 weeks of treatment. Some studies have defined cEVR as negative at week 4 and 12 of treatment.
Slow responder	During treatment, the HCV RNA shows a decline, but does not become negative until after 12 weeks of treatment.

Fig. 20.6. Types of virological response. NR, non-responder; EVR, early viral response; RVR, rapid viral response. (Source: Davis G, Wong JB, McHutchison JG *et al.* Early virologic response to treatment with PEG IFN alfa-2b plus ribavirin in patients with chronic hepatitis C. *Hepatology* 2003; **38**: 645–652.)

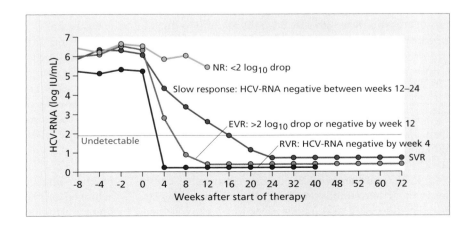

Relatively high treatment responses after 48 weeks of PEG-IFN and RBV have been reported (69–86%) in relatively small studies of genotype 6 [63,64].

Side effects of therapy

The major early side effects of IFN include influenza-like syndrome, chills, fever, malaise, muscle aches and headaches. These symptoms may be ameliorated by paracetamol (acetaminophen). Headaches, poor appetite, weight loss, increased need for sleep, psychological effects (irritability, anxiety, depression), hair loss, thrombocytopenia and leucopenia are also common side effects.

Unusual or severe side effects include seizures, acute psychosis, bacterial infections, autoimmune reactions and thyroid disease. Hyperthyroidism or thyroiditis is relatively common and can be seen in up to 5% of patients, particularly in those with pre-existing antithyroid antibodies. Thyroid function requires monitoring. Proteinuria, cardiomyopathy, skin rashes, and IFN antibodies may also occur. There have been reports of patients developing interstitial lung disease with IFN-α, or sarcoidosis. A neuroretinitis may occur, particularly in patients with diabetes. Neuroretinitis is a medical emergency and treatment must be stopped immediately if patients report visual symptoms or visual field abnormalities. Careful retinal examination is mandatory. There are rare reports of bone marrow suppression resulting in bone marrow aplasia. Idiopathic thrombocytopenia may be induced or activated by IFN.

The major side effects of RBV are haemolytic anaemia, myalgia, hyperuricaemia, some gastrointestinal upset or dyspepsia, cough or skin rash. Some patients also report irritability. Patients should be appropriately clinically monitored for the above side effects and white cells, haemoglobin and platelets, as well as AST, ALT, albumin and bilirubin should be measured every 4 weeks. It is necessary to monitor uric acid at intervals and thyroid function at 1 to 3-monthly intervals. Patients should be advised of the risk of teratogenicity with RBV, and the need for contraception (both patient and sexual partner) up to 6 months after completing treatment. Recently, it has been shown that genetic variants leading to inosine triphosphatase deficiency, a clinically unimportant condition, protect against haemolytic anaemia in hepatitis-C-infected patients receiving RBV [65].

Depression

Depression can be encountered or aggravated during IFN and RBV treatment for hepatitis C, and occurs in 20 to 40% of patients. Many patients receiving PEG-IFN and RBV treatment will experience depressive symptoms of at least moderate severity. Incident rates are high in the first 4 to 8 weeks and prevalence increases during the first 6 months of treatment. The most important premorbid patient characteristic is the presence of psychiatric symptoms before treatment. However, even patients with severe psychiatric disorders may be successfully managed with IFN, if they are stable psychiatrically before treatment. There are several case reports of suicide during IFN treatment.

The prevalence of depression is significantly higher in hepatitis C infected patients than amongst the general population. Psychiatric disorder can lead to higher risk behaviour, leading to a higher probability of hepatitis C via factors such as intravenous drug use. There thus may be a higher prevalence of depression through self-selection. There is an element of fear of discrimination or stigmatization that could influence this, and thus disease-related psychological burden may contribute. Hepatitis C may also affect the central nervous system. This is yet to be proven, but fatigue, neurocognitive symptoms and cognitive impairment have been reported. Cerebral magnetic resonance spectrometry has demonstrated elevated choline to creatinine ratios in patients infected with HCV compared with normal and hepatitis B virus infected individuals.

Depression can be modified by serotonin uptake inhibitors. Dose modifications may be necessary, particularly in patients with cirrhosis who have anaemia, low white cell counts and platelets due to portal hypertension. However, reductions in dose reduce response rates, and thus adherence to 80% of the dose for 80% of the time is encouraged, if possible.

Unfortunately, side effects frequently necessitate dose reductions, and discontinuation of therapy in 14–20%. It is important to motivate patients and to provide appropriate skilled support. Supportive therapies such as antidepressants, erythropoietin and granulocyte colony stimulating factor have been demonstrated to reduce the incidence of IFN-induced depression, anaemia and neutropenia, respectively, and enhance adherence to therapy but have not yet been shown to benefit the SVR rate. These treatments add to the expense of therapy.

The ideal outcome of treatment is a SVR, that is undetectable HCV RNA by real-time PCR 6-months after completing treatment. Some patients show a null response, others a partial response; unfortunately patients who have end of treatment response may relapse after cessation of treatment. The proportion of patients who show week 4 and 12 responses and later SVR responses in genotype 1 are shown in Fig. 20.7.

Abbreviated treatment

In the subgroup of patients with genotype 1 who achieved a rapid viral response (RVR) and had low baseline viral loads, SVR rates were comparable between

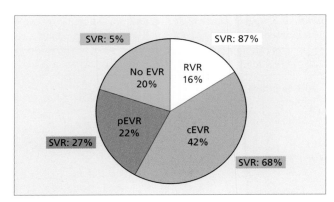

Fig. 20.7. The proportion of patients with genotype 1 infection, treated with PEG IFN-α 2a 180 μg/week plus ribavirin 1000–1200 mg/day for 48 weeks, who showed week 4 and 12 responses and later sustained viral response (SVR). n = 569. EVR, early viral response; cEVR, complete early viral response; pEVR, partial early viral response; RVR rapid viral response. (Source: Marcellin P *et al*. 58th AASLD, 2007, *Hepatology* 2007; **46** (Suppl. S1): Abstract 1308.)

groups who received standard treatment and shortened treatment. Thus abbreviated courses of treatment can be offered for patients with genotype 1 and low viral loads (600 000 IU/mL) and who show a RVR, that is are negative for HCV RNA by PCR at 1 month [66,67]. Similarly, it may be possible to stop treatment at 16 weeks for patients with genotype 2 and 3 who show a RVR [68–70]. Optimal dosing of RBV may be necessary to achieve an RVR and to prevent relapse in order to shorten treatment. High HCV RNA levels and cirrhosis in genotypes 3 are associated with a lower SVR rate.

Treatment of non-responders

A large number of patients have failed prior IFN treatment. Although the primary goal of treatment remains eradication of the virus, this goal may require the advent of new direct antivirals rather than re-treatment with PEG-IFN and RBV.

The overall SVR rates in retreated patients are in the region of 20%. Genotype, degree of fibrosis and prior treatment received are also important factors predictive of SVR; genotype 2 or 3 subjects respond better than genotype 1 subjects regardless of prior response [71].

A number of retreatment trials, including EPIC and HALT-C, have provided some evidence of the likelihood of response to retreatment of patients with advanced fibrosis or cirrhosis treated with PEG-IFN-α and RBV. EPIC3 and HALT-C have not shown a definite benefit of low-dose IFN in non-responders; the HALT-C trial did not show a difference in primary clinical outcomes, that is death, HCC, decompensation or histological progression (34.1 and 33.8% among PEG-IFN treated or observed groups). In the EPIC3, trial clinical events were not significantly reduced by maintenance IFN therapy versus observation overall, but maintenance therapy may delay progression of portal hypertension and variceal bleeding in a subset of patients [71–73].

Several retreatment trials have demonstrated that prior relapsers to IFN and RBV are more likely to respond to retreatment than non-responders [74]. In these studies week 12 HCV RNA was a good predictor of SVR; in EPIC, for example, 56% of those with undetectable HCV RNA at treatment week 12 (complete early viral response (cEVR) attained an SVR. Genotype, fibrosis stage and baseline viral load remain significant predictors of SVR after retreatment.

In non-randomized trials a slightly higher proportion of relapsed patients have responded to consensus IFN and RBV (50%) than to PEG-IFN-α 2 and RBV [75,76]. Higher discontinuation rates have been reported for extended duration of treatment. However, consensus IFN 15 μg/day is not approved in many countries and daily injections may be less appealing than weekly injections in clinical practice. The open-label REPEAT study investigated the efficacy of 48 versus 72 weeks of PEG-IFN-α 2a plus RBV for the retreatment of PEG-IFN-α 2b/RBV non-responders. This study also examined the role of induction dosing PEG-IFN 360 μg/week plus RBV during the first 12 weeks of therapy, followed by standard dosing for the remainder of the treatment period. SVR rate were significantly higher (but still low): 16% with 72 weeks of therapy versus 8% with 48 weeks. Premature withdrawal was more common in the longer-duration treatment groups [77,78].

Thus PEG-IFN plus RBV can be considered for non-responders or relapsers to either standard IFN plus RBV or PEG-IFN monotherapy. PEG-IFN plus RBV retreatment is of less value for patients without an SVR after a previous full course of PEG-IFN plus RBV. Treatment should be stopped if patients do not show an early viral response with re-treatment. Maintenance therapy is not recommended for patients with bridging fibrosis or cirrhosis who have failed a previous course of PEG-IFN plus RBV [79].

Patients with advanced fibrosis or cirrhosis are at risk of HCC and should undergo ultrasound and α-fetoprotein surveillance, with further imaging as necessary. Economic analysis favours retreatment of genotype 2 versus no antiviral treatment. Less value can be placed on the incurred costs of retreatment of genotype 1 or 4. It is important to note that patients requiring re-treatment for a prior failed treatment are older and may have more advanced disease. Thus there is an urgent need to develop therapies that improve responsiveness in naïve and prior non-responder patients.

Phase 2 and phase 3 trials are currently in progress evaluating the safety and efficacy of protease and polymerase inhibitors for treatment of prior non-responders.

Genetic determinants of treatment

There is considerable interest in gene expression profiles to predict response. Recent data from genome-wide association studies have tested the association of hundreds of thousands of single nucleotide polymorphisms (SNPs) in the human genome and response to PEG-IFN and RBV. An analysis of 1137 patients with hepatitis C enrolled in a clinical trial suggest that genetic responsiveness to IFN may be determined by a region upstream of the *IL28B* gene [80]. The advantageous polymorphism, a CC at rs12979860, was more common in patients that responded to IFN therapy than in non-responders. The effect of this gene variant on the function of the *IL28B* gene is unknown. The advantageous variant is more common in Caucasians and East Asians than in Black Americans but SVR rates were highest within each self-declared race group in patients with the cc allele (for example 69% of naïve Caucasians with genotype 1 infection and the *IL28B* cc allele had SVR compared to 27% of those with the tt allele). In Black Americans, 48% of those with the cc allele had SVR although the cc allele was present in only 14%. Approximately 90% of Chinese and Japanese carry a C allele at rs12979860. A more rapid antiviral response has been observed in those with the cc allele. The predictive value of the test and its clinical utility for decision making remains to be determined. Also, the role of this genetic determinant as a diagnostic test to determine response to newer direct antiviral agents with or without combination with IFN remains unknown until these data are analysed.

The treatment of patients with decompensated cirrhosis and of HIV–HCV coinfection is covered in Chapter 22.

New treatments on the horizon

The limitations of IFN and RBV treatment have necessitated a continuing search for improved therapies. Important progress is being made in the development of new treatments, in particular new specific inhibitors or direct antiviral agents active against hepatitis C. There is an urgent need to develop improved therapies for patients and to improve the outcomes in prior non-responders to treatment. New experimental data on IFN signalling in the liver, and refractoriness of STAT1 activation and IFN-induced responses in treatment non-responders also emphasize the therapeutic potential of new compounds.

A diverse range of targets are being exploited for anti-HCV drug development (Table 20.5). Several new NS3 protease inhibitors, NS5b nucleoside polymerase inhibi-

Table 20.5. Direct antiviral agents and novel agents in development

HCV inhibitors	Drug	Phase
NS3/4a protease inhibitors		
Linear class	Telaprevir	3
	Boceprevir	3
	Narlaprevir (SCH 900518)	2
Macrocyclic class	BI201335	2
	MK-7009	2
	TMC435	2
	R7227 (ITMN -191)	2
	BMS 650032	2
NS5B polymerase inhibitors		
Nucleos(t)ide analogue	IDX184	2
	PSI 7851	2
	RG7128	2
	INX 189	1
Non-nucleos(t)ide		
Palm	ABT-333	2
	ABT-072	2
	ANA598	2
	GS9190	2
	MK-3281	
Thumb	BI 207127	In development
	VCH 759	
	VCH -916	
	VX 222	
	Filibivur	
NS5A inhibitors	BMS-790052	2
Combinations	R7128 plus R7227 (ITMN-191)	2
	BMS-650032 plus BMS-790052	2
Cellular components		
Cyclophilin B inhibitors	NIM 811	2
	Debio 025	2
Immune modulators and novel IFNs	Albuferon	3
	PEG-IFN-λ	2
Other compounds	Viramidine	3
	Nitozoxanide	2
	Silybinin	2

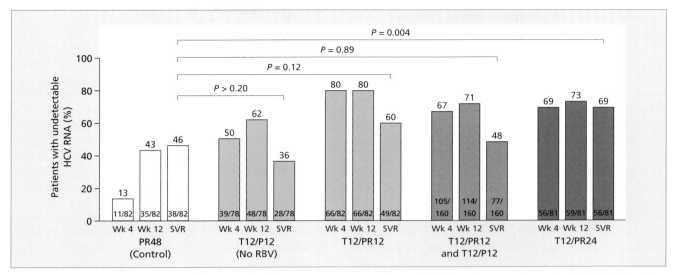

Fig. 20.8. PROVE 2 trial: analysis of result with telaprevir, PEG IFN and ribavirin showing rates of undetectable HCV RNA at week 4, week 12 and sustained viral response. Two-sided Fisher's exact test; *P* values shown for the comparison with PR at the same timepoint. P, PEG IFN-α 2a; R, ribavirin; T, telaprevir; Wk, week. Duration of treatment is expressed in weeks.

tors and non-nucleoside polymerase inhibitors are being assessed in phase 3 studies. Numerous compounds are being tested in phase 1 and 2 trials, so that the list is constantly changing.

Protease inhibitors in advanced study

VX-950 (telaprevir) is a peptidomimetic protease inhibitor of the hepatitis C NS3/4A protease. A median decrease in HCV RNA of 5.5 $\log_{10}$ in telaprevir plus PEG-IFN-α 2a, compared to 4.0 $\log_{10}$ HCV RNA drop in telaprevir monotherapy group has been observed.

Encouraging results in phase 2 and 3 studies have been reported. Genomic analysis of HCV sequences after a few weeks of monotherapy have shown that the emergence of resistance mutations develops relatively quickly. However, in phase 2 studies the combination of telaprevir, PEG-IFN and RBV improved SVR rates compared to PEG-IFN and RBV (69 versus 46%) in IFN naïve genotype 1 patients [81] (Fig. 20.8). Telaprevir has been dosed at 750 mg 8 hourly and 1125 mg 12 hourly, with both PEG-IFN-α 2a and 2b. Similar efficacy has been noted. A high percentage of patients (approximately 66–80%) achieve a rapid viral response (RVR), that is have undetectable HCV RNA with a triple combination of telaprevir, PEG-IFN and RBV by week 4; more than 80–90% of IFN naïve genotype 1 patients with undetectable HCV RNA at week 4 and 12 (extended RVR or eRVR) are cured after 6 months of therapy. RBV remains an essential component of treatment (Fig. 20.8). More recent results in pivotal trials have confirmed that a significantly higher proportion of naive genotype 1 patients have a SVR with 12 weeks of telaprevir, PEG

IFN alpha and RBV followed by additional (response guided therapy) 12 or 36 weeks of PEG IFN alpha and RBV than patients treated with 48 week of PEG IFN alpha and RBV for 48 weeks [82].

Among patients who achieve eRVR, i.e. are HCV RNA negative at weeks 4 and 12, 24-weeks of a telaprevir-based combination regimen gives similar results to 48-weeks of a telaprevir-based regimen [83]. Flu-like syndrome, nausea, diarrhoea, pruritus, rash, headache, insomnia and anaemia have been observed in telaprevir-treated patients. Moderate to severe rash and anaemia are observed in approximately 5% of patients. Antiviral resistance remains a limitation of the drug. Dose modifications of RBV or erythropoietin use are required. Severe rash has been noted in 5–7% of telaprevir recipients, and although some patients may respond to measures such as topical corticosteroids, severe generalized rash usually necessitates discontinuation of telaprevir. The pathogenesis of the rash is unknown, but eosinophilia has been noted. The median time to onset of moderately severe rash has been of the order of 7 weeks.

Phase 2–3 studies have been completed in prior nonresponders or relapsers. These groups require precise definition, but the results are encouraging. The PROVE 3 trial is a phase 2 study of telaprevir; 453 previous nonresponders infected with genotype 1 HCV were randomized to one of four treatment arms: 48 weeks of PEG-IFN and RBV (control); 24 weeks of PEG-IFN plus telaprevir (no RBV); 24 weeks of PEG-IFN plus RBV plus telaprevir followed by 24 weeks of PEG-IFN or RBV; or 12 weeks of PEG-IFN plus RBV plus telaprevir followed by 12 weeks of PEG-IFN and RBV. SVR was achieved in 51% of patients treated with 12 weeks of triple therapy and 53% of patients treated with 24 weeks of triple therapy; 69% of relapsed patients show an SVR. Patients who received PEG-IFN plus telaprevir without RBV achieved a relatively poor 24% SVR rate, further establishing the importance of RBV. The SVR rate among patients in the control arm was 14%. Similar encouraging results have been reported in phase 3 non responder trials [84].

Boceprevir is a small molecule inhibitor of the NS3/4a protease. Phase 2 studies in combination with PEG-IFN-α 2b and RBV in naïve and non-responder patients showed SVR rates of 74 versus 38% with 48 weeks of PEG-IFN and RBV therapy. Shorter treatment courses were less effective; SVR rates were 56%. Recently reported results have shown that SVR in Caucasian and Black patients after 48 weeks of PEG IFN alpha2b, RBV and boceprevir were significantly higher than controls with both response guided and fixed dose therapy; a lead in phase of PEG IFN and RBV has been utilised with boceprevir, but the clinical utility of the lead in is debated [85].

Boceprevir added to PEG IFN and RBV has now been shown to improve SVR rates in genotype 1 previous non-responders and relapsers. The effect in null responders is less clear [86]. Several other protease inhibitors are in development for the treatment of IFN naïve and experienced patients but the data are less mature at this time. The development of these and other agents raises new concerns regarding safety, tolerability, viral resistance, cost and cost effectiveness.

A compendium of other studies is in progress including large phase 3 studies in genotype 1 IFN naïve and non-responder patients. The benefit or otherwise of a lead in or delayed start comprised of 4 weeks of treatment with PEG-IFN and RBV followed by the protease inhibitor will require assessment. The ideal duration of treatment for different groups remains to be determined. Response-guided therapy lengthening for patients with slower responses may be important. Unfortunately, first generation peptidometic protease inhibitors do not appear to be active against genotype 3 infections and have variable activity against the remaining genotypes. Initial data indicate that RBV will remain an essential constituent of treatment with protease inhibitors for the time being.

Resistance

Resistant variants are present before treatment, as HCV exists as a mixed population of viruses, but most resistant viruses are relatively unfit compared to wild type virus and are undetectable with the sensitivities of current technologies. All antiviral drugs can select resistant variants; the nucleotide changes and amino acid changes that confer resistance to these drugs will require careful assessment. Patients with genotype 1a are more likely to develop resistance to protease inhibitors. Resistance mutations often result in loss of viral fitness, compared to wild type virus. These resistant variants, however, are selected during treatment and may result in treatment failure as they are enriched in the patient. Multiple nucleotide changes may be required to give rise to resistant variants explaining, for example, the differences in resistance observed between subtype 1a and 1b. Future treatments will require careful assessment of the efficacy of treatment, the risk of resistance and the clinical implications. The lack of cross resistance between PEG-IFN, RBV and combinations of antiviral agents of different classes may provide an opportunity for effective treatment of hepatitis C.

The NS3 escape mutation R155K appears be common to a variety of structurally diverse both linear and macrocyclic protease inhibitors if used in monotherapy. Other pathways to resistance have been reported. Cross resistance among protease inhibitors is likely to remain an important issue, making testing of these new agents in phase 1 somewhat problematical because of the risk of jeopardizing future therapy. The possibility of long persistence of resistance mutations within the NS3 protease (V36M/A, T54A/S, R155K) and the frequency of these mutations, as well as their clinical significance, requires careful study.

Replication inhibitors

The RNA-dependent RNA polymerase of HCV (NS5B) is an attractive target for drug development, as it is a key enzyme involved in HCV replication. The NS5B enzyme forms a replicase complex with other viral and cellular proteins in the perinuclear region. Two types of HCV polymerase inhibitors are in development: nucleoside and non-nucleoside (Table 20.6). HCV nucleoside

Table 20.6. Differences between protease and polymerase inhibitors

Protease inhibitors	Nucleoside analogues	Non-nucleoside inhibitors
Interact with the catalytic triad	Analogues of natural substrates	Five target sites at the polymerase
Genotype-dependent activity for some drugs	Need to be phosphorylated	Allosteric inhibition
Rapid selection of resistance	Inhibitory competition	Genotype-dependent activity
	Chain terminators	Rapid selection of resistance
	Similar activity against all genotypes	Polymorphisms may influence susceptibility
	High genetic barrier to resistance	

analogues block HCV replication by acting as chain terminators and thus stopping further elongation of the nascent RNA strand. Non-nucleosides interact with the polymerase outside the catalytic site, producing allosteric changes that compromise its function.

The HCV polymerase structure shares the same general right-handed configuration of HIV reverse transcriptase, which consists of finger, thumb and palm domains. At least five different sites (named A, B, C, D and E) have been shown to be targeted by non-nucleoside inhibitors. Mutations that confer resistance to an individual drug's binding sites do not cause cross-resistance to other drugs. As non-nucleoside inhibitors are allosteric blockers, different resistance patterns are observed. Polymerase inhibitors tend to work across genotypes; nucleoside inhibitors lead to slower resistance (Table 20.6). However, 1a/1b subtype profiling of polymerase inhibitors that bind at the known non-nucleoside binding sites has shown that inhibition might vary [87].

Silibinin A, silibinin B, both as water-soluble forms and as commercially available intravenous preparation, have been shown to inhibit the HCV RNA-dependent RNA polymerase function; intravenous silibinin may interfere with the NS5B–RNA interaction to inhibit HCV replication [88]. Silibinin A and silibinin B also inhibited HCV genotype 1b replicon replication and HCV genotype 2a strain JFH1 replication in cell culture [89].

Table 20.5 shows direct antiviral agents in development.

Many of the direct-acting antiviral agents show early promise, but it is not clear how treatment with these agents can be optimized. It is also not clear whether a lead-in strategy with PEG-IFN and RBV is important. Optimal dosing schedules also require further investigation, as does the safety and efficacy of 24 weeks' versus 48 weeks' combination therapies. There may be subtype differences in responsiveness and differing activity across genotypes 1 to 6 for new protease inhibitors.

A new array of side effects is being observed with these agents, which will require appropriate management. These have included rash, severe drug eruptions, gastrointestinal side effects, anaemia and bone marrow suppression, renal impairment and increase in serum aminotransferases. There may be an opportunity in the not too distant future for the use of combinations with all oral agents without PEG IFN for example NS3/4a protease with either NS5b polymerase inhibitors, or other combinations including NS5a inhibitors or cyclophilin inhibitors. It is to be hoped that such agents will prove synergistic and will reduce the potential for drug resistance thus providing a viable therapeutic option without IFN. There is nonetheless hope that protease inhibitors that are about to be licensed in 2011 will prove important additions to therapy. Oral treatments and agents with lower toxicity will improve treatment of HCV in the community and have a major societal impact on the existing burden of disease.

New immunomodulatory therapies, including T cell-inducing therapeutic vaccines, toll-like receptor agonists and entry inhibitors have also been developed and are being tested in patients. Liver-targeted prodrugs and novel glucosidase inhibitors or serine palmitoyltransferase inhibitors to interrupt HCV morphogenesis are being assessed. Cyclophilin inhibitors, including DEBIO-25, may possess additive antiviral efficacy and unique resistance profiles. New, long-acting IFNs are also being assessed. Pilot studies of nitazoxanide plus PEG-IFN and RBV have been completed.

Viramidine is a prodrug of RBV which may cause less haemolytic anaemia. Pharmacokinetic studies in animals have shown the drug to be preferentially taken up by the liver, with reduced exposure of RBV in plasma and red blood cells. Phase 3 studies have been completed; viramidine resulted in less anaemia than a weight-based dose of RBV but similar SVR rates [90].

Albuferon (alphaferon) is a novel 85.7-kDa protein consisting of IFN-α genetically fused to human serum albumin. The fusion with serum albumin extends the half life of the IFN. Albuferon may be dosed at intervals of 2 and possibly 4 weeks. Similar efficacy to that of PEG-IFN has been observed [91,92]. Cough was noted to be more frequent in albuferon-treated patients. Although apparently rare, and also reported in recipients of standard or PEG-IFN, interstitial lung disease has been reported in recipients of 1200 mg doses. PEG-IFN-λ is being tested. The type 3 IFN may have significantly less haematological toxicity but its antiviral efficacy requires assessment.

Vaccination

There are currently no vaccines for the prevention of HCV infection, and viral heterogeneity has made development of a vaccine a difficult task. A vaccine against hepatitis C seemed a remote possibility until recently. However, the outlook for hepatitis C vaccine has improved with advances in our understanding of the correlates of spontaneous immunity [93,94]. An early CD4 and CD8 T-cell response appears to be important. There are a number of intrinsic difficulties; HCV does not always stimulate a strong immune response and until recently there was difficulty in growing HCV in cell culture, although this has been overcome recently. Several new experimental approaches appear promising. These include protein-based, DNA-based approaches utilizing adjuvanted polypeptide to prime neutralizing antibody to the envelope glycoproteins or plasma DNA encoding envelope core and/or non-structural proteins. It is uncertain whether we can vaccinate to prevent initial infection; prophylaxis against chronic disease is a more realistic goal. A phase 1 safety

Table 20.7. Control of hepatitis C

Safe blood transfusion
Safe injections
Education
Preventing IV drug use
Clean needle programs
Treatment forms part of attempts to control the disease and requires appropriate treatment stratification
Other comorbid conditions or modifiable factors particularly alcohol obesity and coinfection with hepatitis B and HIV should be addressed
Future vaccination

and efficacy trial using an envelope E1–E2 vaccine has been completed.

Physicians should consider vaccinating patients with chronic hepatitis C against HAV and HBV.

There is an ongoing need for the information on the incidence of acute hepatitis C and the prevalence of chronic HCV infection and health-care costs relating to mortality and morbidity of hepatitis C. Primary prevention is important (Table 20.7) and hepatitis C vaccination would be a significant public health advance if the vaccine was available and marketed at an affordable price.

References

1 Choo QL, Kuo G, Weiner AJ *et al*. Isolation of a cDNA clone derived from a blood-borne non-A, non- B viral hepatitis genome. *Science* 1989; **244**: 359–362.

2 Shepard CW, Finelli L, Alter MJ. Global epidemiology of hepatitis C virus infection. *Lan. Infect. Dis.* 2005; **5**: 558–567.

3 Bellentani S, Miglioli L, Masutti F *et al*. Epidemiology of hepatitis C virus infection in Italy: the slowly unraveling mystery. *Microbe Infect.* 2000; **2**: 1757–1763.

4 Alter MJ. Epidemiology of hepatitis C. *Hepatology* 1997; **26**: 62S–65S.

5 Pawlotsky JM. Virology of hepatitis B and C viruses and antiviral targets. *J. Hepatol.* 2006; **44** (1 Suppl.): S10–S13.

6 Lindenbach BD, Rice CM. Unravelling hepatitis C replication from genome to function. *Nature* 2005; **436**: 933–938.

7 Lohmann V, Körner F, Koch JO *et al*. Replication of subgenomic hepatitis C virus RNAs in a hepatoma cell line. *Science* 1999; **285**: 110–113.

8 Wakita T, Pietschmann T, Kato T *et al*. Production of infectious hepatitis C in tissue culture from a cloned viral genome. *Nat. Med.* 2005; **11**: 791–796.

9 Evans MJ, von HT, Tscherne DM *et al*. Claudin-1 is a hepatitis C virus co-receptor required for a late step in entry. *Nature* 2007; **446**: 801–805.

10 Gale M Jr, Blakely CM, Kwieciszewski B *et al*. Control of PKR protein kinase by hepatitis C virus nonstructural 5A protein: Molecular mechanisms of kinase regulation. *Mol. Cell Biol.* 1998; **18**: 5208–5218.

11 Horner SM, Gale M Jr. Intracellular innate immune cascades and interferon defenses that control hepatitis C virus. *J. Interferon Cytokine Res.* 2009; **29**: 489–498.

12 Rehermann B, Nascimbeni M. Immunology of hepatitis B virus and hepatitis C virus infection. *Nat. Rev. Immunol.* 2005; **5**: 215–229.

13 Simmonds P, Holmes EC, Cha T-A *et al*. Classification of hepatitis C virus into six major genotypes and a series of subtypes by phylogenetic analysis of the NS-5 region. *J. Gen. Virol.* 1993; **74**: 2391–2399.

14 Simmonds P, Smith DB, McOmish F *et al*. Identification of genotypes of hepatitis C virus by sequence comparisons in the core, E1 and NS-5 regions. *J. Gen. Virol.* 1994; **75**: 1053–1061.

15 Simmonds P. Viral heterogeneity of the hepatitis C virus. *J. Hepatol.* 1999; **31**: 54–60.

16 Simmonds P, Bukh J, Combet C *et al*. Consensus proposals for a unified system of nomenclature of hepatitis C virus genotypes. *Hepatology* 2005; **42**: 962–973.

17 Thomas DL, Thio CL, Martin MP *et al*. Genetic variation in IL28B and spontaneous clearance of hepatitis C virus. *Nature* 2009; **461**: 798–801.

18 Dhillon AP, Dusheiko GM. Pathology of hepatitis C virus infection. *Histopathology* 1995; **26**: 297–309.

19 Jaeckel E, Cornberg M, Wedemeyer H *et al*. Treatment of acute hepatitis C with interferon alfa-2b. *N. Engl. J. Med.* 2001; **345**: 1452–1457.

20 Camma C, Almasio P, Craxi A. Interferon as treatment for acute hepatitis C—A meta-analysis. *Dig. Dis. Sci.* 1996; **41**: 1248–1255.

21 Wedemeyer H, Cornberg M, Wiegand J *et al*. Treatment duration in acute hepatitis C: the issue is not solved yet. *Hepatology* 2006; **44**: 1051–1052.

22 Malnick SD, Basevitch A. Peginterferon alfa-2b therapy in acute hepatitis C: impact of onset of therapy on sustained virologic response. *Gastroenterology* 2006; **131**: 683–684.

23 Kamal SM, Fouly AE, Kamel RR *et al*. Peginterferon alfa-2b therapy in acute hepatitis C: impact of onset of therapy on sustained virologic response. *Gastroenterology* 2006; **130**: 632–638.

24 Kurosaki M, Izumi N. Optimal timing of interferon treatment for acute hepatitis C. *Hepatol. Res.* 2006; **34**: 1–2.

25 Delwaide J, Bourgeois N, Gerard C *et al*. Treatment of acute hepatitis C with interferon alpha-2b: early initiation of treatment is the most effective predictive factor of sustained viral response. *Aliment. Pharmacol. Ther.* 2004; **20**: 15–22.

26 Wedemeyer H, Jackel E, Wiegand J *et al*. Whom? When? How? Another piece of evidence for early treatment of acute hepatitis C. *Hepatology* 2004; **39**: 1201–1203.

27 Cox AL, Netski DM, Mosbruger T *et al.* Prospective evaluation of community-acquired acute-phase hepatitis C virus infection. *Clin. Infect. Dis.* 2005; **40**: 951–958.

28 Poynard T, Ratziu V, Benmanov Y *et al.* Fibrosis in patients with chronic hepatitis C: Detection and significance. *Sem. Liver Dis.* 2000; **20**: 47–55.

29 Poynard T, Bedossa P, Opolon P. Natural history of liver fibrosis progression in patients with chronic hepatitis C. *Lancet* 1997; **349**: 825–832.

30 Poynard T, Ratziu V, Charlotte F *et al.* Rates and risk factors of liver fibrosis progression in patients with chronic hepatitis C. *J. Hepatol.* 2001; **34**: 730–739.

31 Alter HJ, Seeff LB. Recovery, persistence, and sequelae in hepatitis C virus infection: A perspective on long-term outcome. *Sem. Liver Dis.* 2000; **20**: 17–35.

32 Harris DR, Gonin R, Alter HJ *et al.* The relationship of acute transfusion-associated hepatitis to the development of cirrhosis in the presence of alcohol abuse. *Ann. Intern. Med.* 2001; **134**: 120–124.

33 Seeff LB, Hollinger FB, Alter HJ *et al.* Long-term mortality and morbidity of transfusion-associated non-A, non-B, and type C hepatitis: A national heart, lung, and blood institute collaborative study. *Hepatology* 2001; **33**: 455–463.

34 Snoeck E, Hadziyannis SJ, Puoti C *et al.* Predicting efficacy and safety outcomes in patients with hepatitis C virus genotype 1 and persistently 'normal' alanine aminotransferase levels treated with peginterferon alpha-2a (40KD) plus ribavirin. *Liver Int.* 2008; **28**: 61–71.

35 Zeuzem S, Alberti A, Rosenberg W *et al.* Review article: management of patients with chronic hepatitis C virus infection and 'normal' alanine aminotransferase activity. *Aliment. Pharmacol. Ther.* 2006; **24**: 1133–1149.

36 Ascoli V, Lo C, Artini M *et al.* Extranodal lymphomas associated with hepatitis C virus infection. *Am. J. Clin. Pathol.* 1998; **109**: 600–609.

37 Cohen P. Extrahepatic manifestations of the hepatitis C virus. *Presse Med.* 2000; **29**: 209–214.

38 Pozzato G, Mazzaro C, Crovatto M *et al.* Low-grade malignant lymphoma, hepatitis C virus infection, and mixed cryoglobulinemia. *Blood* 1994; **84**: 3047–3053.

39 Prati D, Zanella A, De Mattei C *et al.* Chronic hepatitis C virus infection and primary cutaneous B-cell lymphoma. *Br. J. Haematol.* 1999; **105**: 841.

40 Scheuer PJ, Ashrafzadeh P, Sherlock S *et al.* The pathology of hepatitis C. *Hepatology* 1992; **15**: 567–571.

41 Tsochatzis E, Papatheodoridis GV, Koliaraki V *et al.* Serum hepcidin levels are related to the severity of liver histological lesions in chronic hepatitis C. *J. Viral Hepat.*, in press.

42 Girelli D, Pasino M, Goodnough JB *et al.* Reduced serum hepcidin levels in patients with chronic hepatitis C. *J. Hepatol.* 2009; **51**: 845–852.

43 Hoare M, Gelson WT, Rushbrook SM *et al.* Histological changes in HCV antibody-positive, HCV RNA-negative subjects suggest persistent virus infection. *Hepatology* 2008; **48**: 1737–1745.

44 Dusheiko GM. Summary: antiviral treatment of hepatitis C virus. *Antiviral Res.* 1996; **29**: 77–82.

45 Dusheiko GM, Roberts JA. Treatment of chronic type B and C hepatitis with interferon alfa: An economic appraisal. *Hepatology* 1995; **22**: 1863–1873.

46 Hoofnagle JH. Management of hepatitis C: current and future perspectives. *J. Hepatol.* 1999; **31**: 264–268.

47 Wai CT, Greenson JK, Fontana RJ *et al.* A simple noninvasive index can predict both significant fibrosis and cirrhosis in patients with chronic hepatitis C. *Hepatology* 2003; **38**: 518–526.

48 Castera L, Le BB, Roudot-Thoraval F *et al.* Early detection in routine clinical practice of cirrhosis and oesophageal varices in chronic hepatitis C: comparison of transient elastography (FibroScan) with standard laboratory tests and non-invasive scores. *J. Hepatol.* 2009; **50**: 59–68.

49 Castera L, Vergniol J, Foucher J *et al.* Prospective comparison of transient elastography, Fibrotest, APRI, and liver biopsy for the assessment of fibrosis in chronic hepatitis C. *Gastroenterology* 2005; **128**: 343–350.

50 Sawada M, Takada A, Takase S *et al.* Effects of alcohol on the replication of hepatitis C virus. *Alcohol Alcohol.* 1993; **1B** (Suppl.): 85–90.

51 Miyakawa H, Sato C, Izumi N *et al.* Hepatitis C virus infection in alcoholic liver cirrhosis in Japan: its contribution to the development of hepatocellular carcinoma. *Alcohol Alcohol.* 1993; **1A** (Suppl.): 85–90.

52 Bonkovsky HL, Snow KK, Malet PF *et al.* Health-related quality of life in patients with chronic hepatitis C and advanced fibrosis. *J. Hepatol.* 2007; **46**: 420–431.

53 Johnson ME, Fisher DG, Fenaughty A *et al.* Hepatitis C virus and depression in drug users. *Am. J. Gastroenterol.* 1998; **93**: 785–789.

54 Miyaoka H, Otsubo T, Kamijima K *et al.* Depression from interferon therapy in patients with hepatitis C. *Am. J. Psychiatry* 1999; **156**: 1120.

55 Schaefer M, Hinzpeter A, Mohmand A *et al.* Hepatitis C treatment in 'difficult-to-treat' psychiatric patients with pegylated interferon-alpha and ribavirin: response and psychiatric side effects. *Hepatology* 2007; **46**; 991–998.

56 Khakoo S, Glue P, Grellier L *et al.* Ribavirin and interferon alfa-2b in chronic hepatitis C: assessment of possible pharmacokinetic and pharmacodynamic interactions. *Br. J. Clin. Pharmacol.* 1998; **46**: 563–570.

57 Kozlowski A, Charles SA, Harris JM. Development of pegylated interferons for the treatment of chronic hepatitis C. *BioDrugs* 2001; **15**: 419–429.

58 McHutchison JG, Lawitz EJ, Shiffman ML *et al.* Peginterferon alfa-2b or alfa-2a with ribavirin for treatment of hepatitis C infection. *N. Engl. J. Med.* 2009; **361**: 580–593.

59 Manns MP, McHutchison JG, Gordon SC *et al.* Peginterferon alfa-2b plus ribavirin compared with interferon alfa-2b plus ribavirin for initial treatment of chronic hepatitis C: a randomised trial. *Lancet* 2001; **358**: 958–965.

60 D'Heygere F, George C, Nevens F *et al.* Patients infected with HCV-5 present the same response rate as patients infected with HCV-1: results from the Belgian randomized trial for naive and relapsers (BERNAR-1). *J. Hepatol.* 2005; **42**: 203A.

61 Antaki N, Craxi A, Kamal S *et al.* The neglected hepatitis C virus genotypes 4, 5 and 6: an international consensus report. *Liver Int.* 2010; **30**: 342–355.

62 Antaki N, Hermes A, Hadad M *et al.* Efficacy of interferon plus ribavirin in the treatment of hepatitis C virus genotype 5. *J. Viral Hepat.* 2008; **15**: 383–386.

63 Fung J, Lai CL, Hung I *et al.* Chronic hepatitis C virus genotype 6 infection: response to pegylated interferon and ribavirin. *J. Infect. Dis.* 2008; **198**: 808–812.

64 Vutien P, Nguyen NH, Trinh HN *et al.* Similar treatment response to peginterferon and ribavirin in Asian and

Caucasian patients with chronic hepatitis C. *Am. J. Gastroenterol.* 2010; **105**: 1110–1115.

65 Fellay J, Thompson AJ, Ge D *et al*. ITPA gene variants protect against anaemia in patients treated for chronic hepatitis C. *Nature* 2010; **464**: 405–408.

66 Berg T, Weich V, Teuber G *et al*. Individualized treatment strategy according to early viral kinetics in hepatitis C virus type 1-infected patients. *Hepatology* 2009; **50**: 369–377.

67 Zeuzem S, Poordad F. Pegylated-interferon plus ribavirin therapy in the treatment of CHC: individualization of treatment duration according to on-treatment virologic response. *Curr. Med. Res. Opin.* 2010; **26**: 1733–1743.

68 Mangia A, Andriulli A. Tailoring the length of antiviral treatment for hepatitis C. *Gut* 2010; **59**: 1–5.

69 Diago M, Shiffman ML, Bronowicki JP *et al*. Identifying hepatitis C virus genotype 2/3 patients who can receive a 16-week abbreviated course of peginterferon alfa-2a (40KD) plus ribavirin. *Hepatology* 2010; **51**: 1897–1903.

70 Dai CY, Huang CF, Huang JF *et al*. Hepatitis C virus genotype 2/3 patients who can receive an abbreviated course of peginterferon/ribavirin: the important role of initial ribavirin doses. *Hepatology* 2010; **51**: 1861–1862.

71 Poynard T, Colombo M, Bruix J *et al*. Peginterferon alfa-2b and ribavirin: effective in patients with hepatitis C who failed interferon alfa/ribavirin therapy. *Gastroenterology* 2009; **136**: 1618–1628.

72 de Lope CR, Bruix J. Failure of interferon to prevent disease progression and liver cancer in hepatitis C virus infection: proof of absence or absence of proof? *Gastroenterology* 2010; **138**: 777–779.

73 Bruix J, Poynard T, Colombo M *et al*. Pegintron maintenance therapy in cirrhotic (metavir f4) HCV patients, who failed to respond to interferon/ ribavirn (ir) therapy: final results of the EPIC3 cirrhosis maintenance trial. European Association for the Study of the Liver Annual Meeting, 2009. *J. Hepatol.* 2009; **50** (Suppl. 1): Abstract 49.

74 Poynard T, Colombo M, Bruix J *et al*. Peginterferon alfa-2b and ribavirin: effective in patients with hepatitis C who failed interferon alfa/ribavirin therapy. *Gastroenterology* 2009; **136**: 1618–1628.

75 Kaiser S. [Consensus and peg-interferon in chronic hepatitis C. Therapy for refractory cases?] *MMW Fortschr. Med.* 2001; **143**: 36–37.

76 Kaiser S, Lutze B, Sauter B *et al*. Retreatment of HCV genotype 1 relapse patients to peginterferon/ribavirin therapy with an extended treatment regimen of 72 weeks with consensus interferon/ribavirin versus peginterferon alpha/ribavirin. AASLD Meeting, 2007. *Hepatology* 2007; **46** (Suppl. S1): Abstract 1310.

77 Jensen DM, Marcellin P, Freilich B *et al*. Re-treatment of patients with chronic hepatitis C who do not respond to peginterferon-alpha2b: a randomized trial. *Ann. Intern. Med.* 2009; **150**: 528–540.

78 Nelson DR, Davis GL, Jacobson I *et al*. Hepatitis C virus: a critical appraisal of approaches to therapy. *Clin. Gastroenterol. Hepatol.* 2009; **7**: 397–414.

79 Ghany MG, Strader DB, Thomas DL *et al*. Diagnosis, management, and treatment of hepatitis C: an update. *Hepatology* 2009; **49**: 1335–1374.

80 Ge D, Fellay J, Thompson AJ *et al*. Genetic variation in IL28B predicts hepatitis C treatment-induced viral clearance. *Nature* 2009; **461**: 399–401.

81 Hezode C, Forestier N, Dusheiko G *et al*. Telaprevir and peginterferon with or without ribavirin for chronic HCV infection. *N. Engl. J. Med.* 2009; **360**: 1839–1850.

82 Jacobson IM, McHutchison JG, Dusheiko, GM. Telaprevir in combination with peginterferon and ribavirin in genotype 1 HCV treatment naive patients. Final results of phase 3 Advance study. *Hepatol.* **52**: 4(Suppl) 427A.

83 Sherman KE, Flamm SL, Afdhal DR *et al*. Telaprevir in Combination with Peginterferon Alfa2a and Ribavirin for 24 or 48 weeks in Treatment-Naïve Genotype 1 HCV Patients who Achieved an Extended Rapid Viral Response: Final Results of Phase 3 ILLUMINATE Study. *Hepatol.* **52**: 4(Suppl) 401A.

84 McHutchison JG, Manns MP, Muir AJ *et al*.; PROVE3 Study Team. Telaprevir for previously treated chronic HCV infection. *N. Engl. J. Med.* 2010; **362**: 1292–1303. Erratum: Dosage error in article text. In: *N. Engl. J. Med.* 2010; **362**: 1647.

85 Poordad F, McCone J, Bacon BR *et al*. Boceprevir (BOC) Combined with Peginterferon alfa-2b/Ribavirin (P/R) for Treatment-Naïve Patients with Hepatitis C Virus (HCV) Genotype (G) 1: SPRINT-2 Final Results. *Hepatology* **52**: 4(Suppl) 402A.

86 Bacon BR, Gordon SC, Lawitz E *et al*. HCV RESPOND-2 Final Results: High Sustained Virologic Response Among Genotype 1 Previous Non-Responders and Relapsers to Peginterferon/Ribavirin when Re-Treated with Boceprevir Plus PEGINTRON (Peginterferon alfa-2b)/Ribavirin. *Hepatol.* 2011; **52**: 4(Suppl) 881A.

87 Nyanguile O, Devogelaere B, Vijgen L *et al*. 1a/1b subtype profiling of nonnucleoside polymerase inhibitors of hepatitis C virus. *J. Virol.* 2010; **84**: 2923–2934.

88 Ferenci P, Scherzer TM, Kerschner H *et al*. Silibinin is a potent antiviral agent in patients with chronic hepatitis C not responding to pegylated interferon/ribavirin therapy. *Gastroenterology* 2008; **135**: 1561–1567.

89 Ahmed-Belkacem A, Ahnou N, Barbotte L *et al*. Silibinin and related compounds are direct inhibitors of hepatitis C virus RNA-dependent RNA polymerase. *Gastroenterology* 2009; **138**: 1112–1122.

90 Marcellin P, Gish RG, Gitlin N *et al*. Safety and efficacy of viramidine versus ribavirin in ViSER2: Randomized, double-blind study in therapy-naive hepatitis C patients. *J. Hepatol.* 2010; **52**: 32–38.

91 Neumann AU, Pianko S, Zeuzem S *et al*. Positive and negative prediction of sustained virologic response at weeks 2 and 4 of treatment with albinterferon alfa-2b or peginterferon alfa-2a in treatment-naive patients with genotype 1, chronic hepatitis C. *J. Hepatol.* 2009; **51**: 21–28.

92 Nelson DR, Rustgi V, Balan V *et al*. Safety and antiviral activity of albinterferon alfa-2b in prior interferon nonresponders with chronic hepatitis C. *Clin. Gastroenterol. Hepatol.* 2009; **7**: 212–218.

93 Ferrari C. New perspectives for T-cell-based HCV vaccines. *J. Hepatol.* 2006; **45**: 163–165.

94 Folgori A, Capone S, Ruggeri L *et al*. A T-cell HCV vaccine eliciting effective immunity against heterologous virus challenge in chimpanzees. *Nat. Med.* 2006; **12**: 190–197.

CHAPTER 21
Hepatitis due to Non-A–E Viruses

Antonio Craxì[1] & Rosa Di Stefano[2]

[1]Gastroenterology and Hepatology, DIBIMIS, University of Palermo, Italy

[2]Virology, Dipartimento Scienze per la Promozione della Salute, University of Palermo, Italy

Learning points

- GBV-C, TTV and other viruses causing systemic infections (EBV, CMV, HSV, SARS, yellow fever) may cause acute hepatitis.

- Diagnosis of non-A–E hepatitis rests upon careful exclusion of infection with major hepatitis viruses and of hepatotoxins.

- Liver damage is usually mild (except for yellow fever and hepatitis caused by HSV), but occasionally jaundice can be present.

- Rarely, mostly in the immunocompromised patient, acute liver failure and death may ensue.

- Chronic hepatitis is not a consequence of acute non-A–E hepatitis.

General features of non-A–E hepatitides

A small number of patients who present with an acute elevation of aminotransferases have no known exposure to hepatotoxins and no evidence of hepatitis A, B, C, D or E virus (HAV, HBV, HCV, HDV or HEV) infection upon testing by sensitive serology or molecular assays. The exact frequency of such 'non-A–E' hepatitides is difficult to assess, due to the heterogeneity of risk factors for viral infections and also to the possibility that patients with conventional hepatitis may have false-negative results if tested only during the early phase of illness. The upsurge of acquired immunodeficiency syndrome (AIDS) has increased the incidence of hepatitis due to various unusual viruses. Non-A–E hepatitis is also important in those who are immunosuppressed, such as liver and bone marrow transplant recipients and patients receiving cancer chemotherapy. Non-A–E hepatitis may be seen in neonates and may follow a blood transfusion. Table 21.1 lists the non-A–E viral agents that can cause hepatitis.

Infection with viruses other than hepatitis A–E may be accompanied by alterations of liver tests, mostly elevations of aminotransferases. The biochemical pattern is usually that of mild hepatocellular damage, with alanine aminotransferase (ALT) no more than 10 times normal and no significant cholestasis, hyperbilirubinaemia or hypoalbuminaemia. Liver damage is usually transient and not associated with symptoms, and often goes undetected. Due to the usually mild and self-limiting course of disease, a liver biopsy is rarely needed. Pathology may show modest inflammatory infiltrates in the portal and periportal zone, single-cell acidophilic or spotty necrosis and Kupffer cell hyperactivity. Fibrosis is usually absent.

Rarely, mostly in the immunosuppressed host, non-A–E hepatitis, especially when caused by Epstein–Barr virus (EBV) or cytomegalovirus (CMV), may be symptomatic, severe and protracted. Specific antiviral treatment, where available, is needed only for severe cases.

The main clinical and diagnostic profiles of the relevant non-A–E viral agents are given in Table 21.2.

Hepatitis-associated aplastic anaemia

Hepatitis-associated aplastic anaemia (HAAA) is a syndrome in which an episode of hepatitis not linked to a major hepatotropic virus precedes the onset of severe anaemia due to bone marrow failure, possibly mediated by immunological mechanisms such as interferon-γ or the cytokine cascade. Although HAAA is a rare event, it occurs in 28% of young adults after liver transplantation for non-A–E hepatitis. Parvovirus B 19 has been isolated from the liver and the bone marrow of patients, mostly children, with HAAA, but its causal role is not established [1].

HAAA may be treated by immunosuppression with a response of 70% but relapses are frequent after treatment withdrawal and haematopoietic cell transplantation, with a reported survival of 82%.

Sherlock's Diseases of the Liver and Biliary System, Twelfth Edition. Edited by James S. Dooley, Anna S.F. Lok, Andrew K. Burroughs, E. Jenny Heathcote.
© 2011 by Blackwell Publishing Ltd. Published 2011 by Blackwell Publishing Ltd.

Table 21.1. Viral agents causing non-A–E hepatitis (only viruses with a relevant link to liver disease are discussed in text)

Hepatotropic viruses
  Flaviviridae other than hepatitis C virus:
    GBV-C/HGV
    Yellow fever virus (YFV)
  Circoviridae:
    Torque teno virus (TTV)
    Sanban, Yonban, SEN viruses, TTV-like mini virus (TTMV), TTV-like midi virus (TTMDV)
Systemic viral infections that cause transient liver involvement
  Herpesviridae:
    Epstein–Barr virus (EBV), cytomegalovirus (CMV), herpes simplex virus (HSV), varicella zoster virus (VZV), human herpesvirus 6 (HHV-6)
  Severe acute respiratory syndrome/ coronavirus (SARS/CoV)
  Parvovirus B19
  Measles virus
  Human immunodeficiency virus (HIV)
  Lassa, Marburg, Ebola

Table 21.2. Clinical patterns of infection with non-A–E viruses

Virus	Diagnostic tests	Liver damage	Other organ damage
Flaviviridae			
GBV-C/HGV	IgG (EIA)	None to mild	Lymphotropism
	Viral genome (nested RT-PCR)		no significant disease
Yellow fever virus (YFV) (FHF possible)	IgM (EIA)	Moderate to severe	None
Torquetenoviridae			
Torquetenovirus (TTV)	Viral genome (PCR)	Minimal, if any	None
Sanban, Yonban, SEN viruses and TTV-like minivirus	Viral genome (PCR)	Minimal, if any	None
Herpesviridae			
Epstein–Barr virus (EBV)	Monospot test	Mild to moderate	Infectious mononucleosis
	IgM anti-VCA (EIA)	(severe in immunosuppressed)	
Cytomegalovirus (CMV)	IgM (EIA)	Mild to moderate	Mononucleosis-like syndrome
	pp72 viraemia, pp65 antigenaemia	(severe in immunosuppressed)	
	Viral genome (PCR)		
Herpes simplex virus (HSV) (FHF possible)	Viral genome (PCR)	Mild to moderate	Generalized herpetic disease
Severe acute respiratory syndrome/ coronavirus (SARS-CoV)	Viral genome (RT-PCR)	Mild	Respiratory syndrome
Lassa	IgM (EIA)	Severe	Haemorragic fever
	Viral genome (RT-PCR)		

FHF, fulminant hepatic failure; EIA, enzyme immune assay; RT-PCR, real-time polymerase chain reaction.

Hepatotropic viruses

Flaviviridae other than HCV

GB virus C/ hepatitis G virus

Virology, pathogenesis and diagnosis

GB virus C (GBV-C) and hepatitis G virus (HGV) were described independently by Linnen *et al.* [2] and by Simons *et al.* [3] in patients with non-A–E hepatitis and were initially considered separate major aetiological agents of hepatitis. Sequence comparison of GBV-C and HGV subsequently showed them to be different isolates of one viral species, bearing a nucleotide and amino acid homology of 86 and 96%, respectively [4]. It is now referred to as GBV-C.

Based on sequence relatedness and overall genome structure, GBV-C is classified in the *Flaviviridae* family, like HCV and yellow fever virus (YFV). It has a linear, single-stranded RNA with positive polarity, containing approximately 9400 nucleotides, and one open reading frame (ORF), encoding a polyprotein of approximately 2840 amino acids. The GBV-C genome is similar to HCV in its organization. The ORF of GBV-C has a 30% amino acid sequence homology with HCV, with the greatest similarity in the NS3 and NS5b regions.

GBV-C is primarily a lymphotropic agent, which replicates in the bone marrow and spleen [5] but also in peripheral blood mononuclear cells and in the vascular endothelial cells [6]. Despite its association with hepatitis of unknown aetiology, the hepatotropism of GBV-C has been questioned [7]. Overall, it seems that GBV-C can replicate in the liver in a small proportion of infected patients and cause minor and transient liver damage.

Detection of GBV-C infection is performed by testing for antibodies against the E2 glycoprotein of GBV-C (anti-E2 antibodies) with an enzyme immunoassay. Confirmation of an active GBV-C infection is based on detection of viral genome by nested real-time polymerase chain reaction (RT-PCR) [8].

GBV-C viraemia may persist for years without hepatitis or other specific disease. However, spontaneous clearance of the virus occurs in 60 to 75% of immunocompetent subjects with seroconversion to anti-E2 antibodies. Most healthy individuals and patients with non-A–E acute hepatitis who are anti-GBV-C E2 positive are GBV-C RNA negative. Overall, the development of anti-E2 is an indication of previous infection and immunity.

Epidemiology

GBV-C infection has a worldwide distribution, with a prevalence 10-fold higher in African than in non-African countries. Phylogenetic analysis of GBV-C isolates demonstrated six genotypes [9,10].

The detection rate of GBV-C viraemia among healthy blood donors averages 2% (0.9–5.3%). Prevalence rates of anti-E2 antibodies (between 3.0 and 42.1% in different countries) are much higher than those of viraemia. Transmission via the blood-borne route and through sexual intercourse is the most common, although less frequently mother to child transmission occurs. High rates of active GBV-C infection are found in subjects with repeated parenteral exposures such as intravenous drug users (13 to 35%), in groups at high risk of exposure to blood and blood products (3.1 to 55% of patients on haemodialysis, 14 to 28% of those with haemophilia) and in sexually promiscuous individuals (13 to 63% of male homosexuals, 14 to 25% of female prostitutes).

Due to the common pathways of transmission, GBV-C RNA is also detected frequently among anti-HCV positive individuals, with a rate of coinfection of approximately 20%. The prevalence of GBV-C coinfection in patients infected with human immunodeficiency virus (HIV) varies between 14 and 45%, with a higher rate in male homosexuals and drug abusers [11].

Interaction with HIV

A first report [12] in a cohort of HIV-infected haemophilia patients suggested an improved survival in patients coinfected with GBV-C. Others studies have confirmed that coinfection with GBV-C and HIV is linked to a better outcome of HIV infection in terms of reduction in mortality rates and disease progression, together with higher CD4 cell counts and lower HIV viral load, independent of sex, age or race. Tillmann *et al.* [13] found that GBV-C viraemia was associated with better survival even after the development of acquired immunodeficiency syndrome (AIDS) and continued to be predictive of longer survival after the introduction of highly active antiretroviral therapy, and showed an inverse correlation between GBV-C and HIV viral loads. More recently, Williams *et al.* [14] found that GBV-C infection was detected in 85% of HIV-infected men in the Multicenter AIDS Cohort Study, and was associated with longer survival. Loss of GBV-C viraemia was a strong predictor of death, suggesting that survival benefit was dependent on the persistence of GBV-C viraemia in HIV-infected patients.

GBV-C may interact with HIV through a mechanism of viral interference. Other possible mechanisms could be the up-regulation of T-helper 1 (Th1) cytokine, down regulation of T-helper 2 (Th2) cytokine [15] or inhibition of the entry of HIV into target cells [16].

Clinical features

Although acute GBV-C infection rarely becomes chronic, the duration of GBV-C infection probably depends on the immune status of the host. Childhood acquisition of GBV-C commonly evolves into chronic infection, whereas sexual transmission in immunocompetent adults usually leads to rapid clearance of the virus [17]. HIV-infected subjects are less likely to clear GBV-C [18].

An active GBV-C infection can be detected in a high proportion of patients with non-A–E acute or chronic hepatitis, but no convincing evidence linking it directly to liver damage is available, regardless of the immune status of the patients [19,20].

Patients with chronic hepatitis B [21] or chronic hepatitis C [22] have a comparable severity of liver disease and response to treatment regardless of their GBV-C status. Similarly, the outcome of liver transplantation for hepatitis C is not affected by GBV-C [23].

No association between GBV-C and hepatocellular carcinoma has ever been reported.

Yellow fever virus (YFV)

Epidemiology and viral features

Yellow fever is a life-threatening, mosquito-borne flaviviral haemorrhagic fever characterized by severe hepatitis, renal failure, haemorrhage and rapid terminal events with shock and multiorgan failure [24–26]. Before the development of an effective vaccine it was among the most feared infectious diseases, and still affects as many as 200 000 persons annually in the two endemic regions of South America and equatorial Africa.

Yellow fever is transmitted in a cycle involving monkeys and mosquitoes in the jungle variety, but human beings can also serve as the viraemic host for mosquito infection in urban yellow fever. Recent increases in the density and distribution of the urban mosquito vector, *Aedes aegypti*, as well as the rise in air travel increase the risk of introduction and spread of yellow fever to North and Central America, the Caribbean and Asia.

YFV has a single serotype but, at the genome level, five genotypes can be distinguished (three in Africa and two in South America). The YFV positive-sense, single-stranded RNA genome contains a single open reading frame of 10 233 nucleotides, encoding three structural and seven non-structural proteins. The viral envelope (E) protein attaches to cell receptors and is a principal target for the immune response.

Pathology and pathogenesis

The hepatic injury of yellow fever has a typical midzonal pattern, with sparing of hepatocytes around the central vein and portal tracts. This could reflect low-flow hypoxia due to shock, but YFV antigens and YFV RNA have been observed principally in hepatocytes in the midzone, suggesting that these cells are most susceptible to virus infection. The infected hepatocytes undergo apoptotic cell death signalled by eosinophilic degeneration with condensed nuclear chromatin (Councilman bodies). Cell death by apoptosis rather than necrosis explains the reduced number of inflammatory cells in YFV hepatitis and the preservation of the reticulin framework. Intranuclear inclusions (Torres bodies) are diagnostic. With recovery, regeneration is complete without chronicity.

The pathogenesis of hepatic damage in YFV infection is controversial. Hypotension and shock mediated by cytokine dysregulation may cause ischaemic damage. Tumour necrosis factor-α (TNF-α) and other cytokines produced by Kupffer cells and splenic macrophages in response to direct virus injury and cytotoxic T cells involved in viral clearance might be responsible for hepatocyte injury.

Clinical features and diagnosis

Following an incubation period of 3–6 days, onset is sudden with fever, chills, headache, backache, prostration and vomiting, often of altered blood. The blood pressure falls, haemorrhages become widespread, jaundice and albuminuria are conspicuous and there is a relative bradycardia. Delirium proceeds to coma and death may occur within 9 days. With recovery, the temperature becomes normal and convalescence progresses rapidly. There are no sequelae and life-long immunity follows. The majority of infections are probably milder, with no detectable jaundice and only a few constitutional symptoms.

Laboratory confirmation is by demonstrating specific IgM antibodies to YFV. Yellow fever antigen may be detected in formalin-fixed, paraffin-embedded tissue cut from blocks made as long as 8 years before [27].

Prevention and treatment

Prevention consists of vaccination at least 10 days before arrival in an endemic area and by control of mosquitoes. A live, attenuated vaccine (YF 17D) has been in use for over 60 years but may cause a disease identical to wild-type virus at an incidence of 1 in 2.5 million [28].

Death in patients with YFV results principally from renal damage. The hepatic lesion is self-limited and short-lived and does not require special treatment. Some antivirals [26] have been evaluated but none have been shown to be effective. Studies on specific inhibitors of flaviviruses proteases and polymerases or with viral entry and assembly inhibitors are in progress.

The 'cytokine storm' represents also a potential target for therapeutic interventions with specific monoclonal antibodies.

Circoviridae: torque teno virus (TTV) and others

Virology, pathogenesis and diagnosis

The prototypic agent in this group was isolated in 1997 [29] from the blood of a Japanese patient with post-transfusion hepatitis of unknown aetiology, and was called TT virus (TTV) after the patient's initials. TTV is now know as torque teno virus, from the Latin *torques* (necklace) and *teno* (thin), thus maintaining the initial denomination TTV. It was the first human virus found to have a single-stranded circular DNA genome and was classified in the family *Circoviridae*, genus *Anellovirus*.

The TTV genome consists of a negative, single-stranded DNA with a circular structure and a total genomic length of approximately 3.8 kb. After the description of the original TTV isolate, many TTV-like variants were found in humans and were classified into five major phylogenetic groups (group 1 to 5), including SEN, Sanban and Yonban viruses. In 2000, Takahashi *et al.* [30] discovered a new group of viruses with a single-stranded, circular DNA that were termed TTV-like mini virus (TTMV), because of a genomic size of less than 2.9 kb. Later, two new TTV-like viruses were isolated from the blood of patients with acute viral infections and named small anellovirus 1 (SAV1) and small anellovirus 2 (SAV2) [31]. Finally, Ninomiya *et al.* [32] in 2007 isolated another agent with a genomic organization akin to that of TTV and TTMV and a full-length genome of 3.2 kb that was named torque teno midi virus (TTMDV).

The heterogeneous TTV group, including TTMV and TTMDV, is characterized by an extreme genetic diversity, not only due to genetic evolution but also to recombination between related isolates. Despite a marked divergence, there is a specific region of 130 nucleotides that is highly conserved, allowing the development of a PCR assay which can detect all members of the TTV group [33].

Infection with TTV is characterized by lifelong viraemia in up to 80% of subjects. Antibodies against TTV virions or recombinant ORF1 protein are detected in viraemic and non-viraemic individuals, suggesting that the humoral immune response is inadequate to clear the virus. The tissue tropism of TTV is rather broad. TTV genomes can replicate in the liver, bone marrow, spleen, lung and peripheral blood mononuclear cells.

Epidemiology and pathogenesis

TTV, TTMV and TTMDV infection have a worldwide distribution. Ninomiya *et al.* [33] reported extremely high prevalence rates of viraemia for TTV (100%), TTMV (82%) and TTMDV (75%) in the general population in Japan. The prevalence of TTV, TTMV and TTMDV infection increases with age and dual or triple infection is common. The detection of TTV and TTMV genomes in saliva, faeces and breast milk strongly suggest that the human *Anelloviridae* are transmitted by a horizontal route during early childhood.

TTV was originally described as a hepatitis agent. Shibata *et al.* [34] reported that TTV genotype 1 might be a cause of non-A, non-C fulminant hepatic failure. Japanese [35] and French researchers [36] found a direct relation between TTV infection, TTV viral load and various liver diseases but these findings were not confirmed by other investigators [37–40]. Although TTV is known to replicate in the liver, it does not fulfil the criteria for being a hepatitis virus, such as direct causal association between hepatic necroinflammation and TTV replication or an epidemiological association with acute or chronic liver disease [41]. There is even less evidence for hepatic pathogenicity of the other viral agents in this group.

Systemic viral infections that often cause transient liver involvement

Herpesviridae: EBV, CMV, HSV, VZV

Epstein–Barr virus

Epidemiology and clinical features

The Epstein–Barr virus (EBV), a member of the *Gammaherpesvirinae* subfamily, infects more than 90% of the world's population, thus representing one of the most prevalent human viral infections. EBV excites a generalized reticuloendothelial reaction [42] and causes infectious mononucleosis. Although mortality is minimal, liver failure is the cause of death in about half of the patients with fatal infectious mononucleosis [43].

Primary infection occurs in children through the oropharynx and is usually asymptomatic. EBV then spreads to other epithelial cells. Because the virus stimulates proliferation of B cells and a strong T-cell adaptive immune response, in immunocompetent hosts EBV infection is effectively contained. At this time the patient has the clinical syndrome of infectious mononucleosis, often accompanied by transient, self-limited elevation of aminotransferases [44]. Presentation, particularly in adults, may include fever and right upper quadrant abdominal discomfort. Pharyngitis and lymphadenopathy may be absent. In about 5 to 7% of patients, jaundice with a cholestatic pattern may be present [45,46]. Rarely, this may evolve into a vanishing bile duct syndrome [47]. Although uncommon, severe hepatitis with acute

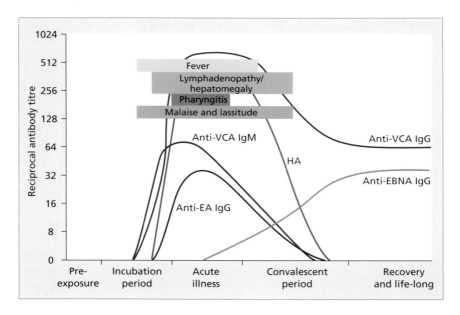

Fig. 21.1. Kinetics of EBV markers and symptoms in the course of primary infection in relation to clinical features. HA, heterophil antibodies; EA, early antigens; VCA, viral capsid antigens; EBNA, Epstein–Barr nuclear antigens.

or subacute liver failure may occur at the time of primary EBV infection even in immunocompetent individuals [43,48,49]. Chronic liver disease secondary to primary EBV infection manifesting as an autoimmune or 'cryptogenic' hepatitis have rarely been reported but the association is questionable [50].

Viral persistence is established by switching to latent infection [51]. A lifelong equilibrium follows between viral expression and host defence mechanisms. When this balance is disturbed, such as during immunosuppression, viral reactivation occurs, often accompanied by clinical manifestations including the development of hepatitis. Clinically significant EBV liver damage is mostly observed in the immunocompromised patients, including those with HIV infection, post-transplant patients and subjects with primary immunodeficiency disorders (Fig. 21.1).

Pathogenesis and hepatic histology

EBV-associated liver damage is characterized by lack of expression of EBV antigens in hepatocytes and abundant expression of EBV latency proteins in infiltrating lymphocytes. It is likely that cytotoxic T lymphocytes target EBV-infected B lymphocytes, causing collateral damage to liver cells. The changes are seen within 5 days and reach their peak between the 10th and 30th days. The sinusoids and portal tracts are infiltrated with large, mononuclear cells. Polymorphonuclear leucocytes and lymphocytes increase, and the Kupffer cells proliferate. The architecture of the liver is preserved. Zone 3 focal necroses may be randomly distributed with some lobular infiltrate. Later, binucleate liver cells and

mitoses are conspicuous. The regeneration is out of proportion to cell necrosis. The severity of the liver damage seems to be linked to the level of EBV viraemia and to CD8+ cells infiltrating the liver. After clinical recovery, abnormal T cells disappear, although this may take as long as 8 months. Chronic hepatitis and cirrhosis are not sequelae.

Diagnosis

Criteria to establish the diagnosis of EBV-associated hepatitis [52] include presence of suggestive histopathological features together with a virological profile compatible with EBV infection.

Aminotransferases are raised to about 20 times the normal in 80% of patients with infectious mononucleosis, but ALT values are usually lower than those found in the early stages of acute hepatitis A or B. Hyperbilirubinaemia is present in about one-half of patients. In about one-third the serum alkaline phosphatase value is increased, often more so than that of bilirubin. Occasionally, jaundice can be deep. Serum albumin level may be slightly decreased and the serum globulin value slightly elevated.

The monospot test is positive, indicating the presence of heterophilic antibodies, but this test is not specific for the diagnosis of primary EBV infection. EBV-associated conditions are diagnosed conclusively by an increase in serum IgM antibodies against viral capsid antigens, followed by an increase of IgG antibodies against viral capsid antigens. In the immunocompromised host, particularly with post-transplant lymphoproliferative disease, EBV antigens may be shown by immunofluorescence on liver biopsy. *In situ* hybridization and PCR assay are used for detection of EBV DNA in tissue samples [53].

Prevention and treatment

EBV rarely causes hepatitis after solid organ and bone marrow transplantation, but has been associated with post-transplantation lymphoproliferative disease. It is hence important to screen potential donors for EBV status and to apply pre-emptive antiviral therapy to the recipient where appropriate.

No specific treatment for EBV hepatitis exists. High-dose acyclovir reduces virus production in the throat, although it does not significantly alter the duration of the illness, probably because the symptoms are related to the immune response and not caused by virus infection of B lymphocytes.

Cytomegalovirus

Like EBV, cytomegalovirus (CMV) is a ubiquitous herpesvirus that infects the majority of humans. Seroepidemiological studies show an overall prevalence of CMV infection between 50 and 100% of the adult population, according to geographical region and socioeconomic status [54,55]. Exposure to the virus, through saliva, sexual contact, breastfeeding or placental transfer, occurs during the first two decades of life. After primary infection, CMV maintains a state of latency within the host because of its ability to escape the innate and adaptive immune response. As a consequence, clinical disease due to CMV infection may be the result of a primary infection or, more frequently, reactivation of latent infection.

As a rule, primary CMV infection in the normal host is clinically silent, although it may cause an acute mononucleosis-like syndrome in less than 10% of infected individuals [56]. Liver involvement is common, with raised aminotransferases in 90% and raised alkaline phosphatase in 60% of patients. Splenomegaly (33–53%) and hepatomegaly (0–53%) may be present. Jaundice, may occur and last 2–3 weeks. Fatal massive hepatic necrosis has rarely been reported. CMV infection is a rare cause of post-transfusion hepatitis.

Granulomatous hepatitis can develop in a previously normal adult with prolonged unexplained fever and without lymphadenopathy [57]. In these patients, liver biopsy shows non-caseating granulomas.

Occasionally, primary CMV infection in the immunocompetent host has been associated with severe multivisceral involvement, such as interstitial pneumonitis, hepatitis, haematological disorders, enteritis, encephalitis and myocarditis. Reactivation of the viral infection is common in healthy individuals, and it is usually asymptomatic but there is shedding of virus in saliva or urine.

Primary CMV infection and reactivation of latent virus in an immunocompromised host causes a disease that ranges from a self-limited febrile illness to a disseminated, severe, life-threatening disease. Cholangitis, papillary stenosis and sclerosing cholangitis can accompany CMV infections in patients with AIDS (Chapter 22).

CMV hepatitis is a major problem in adult and paediatric transplant recipients [58,59]. The infection is usually a primary one, rather than reactivation, and the donor is CMV antibody positive while the recipient is CMV antibody negative. However, reactivation of latent infection can occur in patients who had CMV infection previously.

Diagnosis of primary CMV infection depends on the demonstration of seroconversion from CMV-IgG antibodies negative to positive or on the detection of IgM antibodies, by enzyme immunoassay. The accuracy of diagnosis of recent primary infection has been improved by the IgG antibody avidity assay. Serology is not useful to identify CMV-associated disease in the immunocompromised host. The most valuable laboratory diagnostic tests are:
• Rapid CMV isolation from blood samples in human embryonic fibroblast monolayers
• Detection of tegument protein pp65 in leucocytes by immunostaining of cytocentrifuge preparations of blood cells (pp65 antigenaemia assay).
• Detection and quantification of CMV DNA by PCR assay—this is the most commonly used method in clinical practice.

Prevention and treatment

In immunocompetent adults, antiviral therapy is not necessary during mild CMV disease. In immunocompromised patients, such as liver transplant recipients, antiviral treatment is indicated to prevent CMV disease, through antiviral prophylaxis or pre-emptive therapy. Ganciclovir, a guanosine nucleoside analogue with a much longer intracellular half-life than that of acyclovir, and valganciclovir, a valine ester of ganciclovir that can be administered orally, has proved to be effective for treatment of CMV disease, in terms of clinical and virological response, and for reduction of incidence of CMV infection, after liver transplantation. Alternative agents include foscarnet and cidofovir.

Herpes simplex virus (HSV)

Human herpes virus types 1 and 2 (HSV-1 and HSV-2) affect all humans at some time during their lives. In infants, herpes hepatitis may be part of a generalized

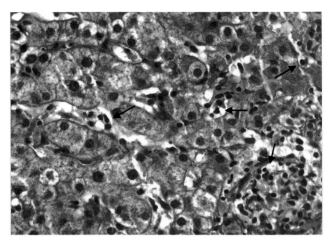

Fig. 21.2. Reactivation of latent HHV-6 in a liver transplant patient. Scanty portal and intralobular lymphoid infiltrates, the latter mainly with an intrasinusoidal distribution (arrows) with signs of pseudopeliosis. (Courtesy of Claudio Tripodo, MD, Department of Pathology, AOUP Palermo.)

herpetic disease. In adults, disseminated herpes simplex is very rare except in patients who are immunosuppressed.

HSV can cause acute hepatitis in immunosuppressed and also in immunocompetent persons. Herpetic mucocutaneous lesions are usually absent. The onset is with fever, prostration, marked elevation of aminotransferases and leucopenia. Jaundice is absent. Fulminant liver failure can develop [60].

Liver biopsy shows patchy areas of coagulative necrosis with surrounding hepatocytes containing viral inclusions. The virus can be seen on electron microscopy or by immunohistochemical staining. It can also be cultured from the liver tissue.

Diagnosis and treatment

PCR assays are used to confirm the diagnosis and for typing of HSV-1 and HSV-2.

Acyclovir or gancyclovir is curative and should only be used in severe cases.

Varicella zoster virus (VZV)

Varicella and varicella-zoster infection may be complicated by hepatitis in both normal and immunologically compromised individuals. In children, the picture must be distinguished from Reye's syndrome [61].

Human herpesvirus 6 (HHV-6)

Human herpesvirus 6 (HHV-6) infection occurs in almost all humans. Primary infection, in early childhood (asymptomatic or roseola infantum) leads to subclinical viral persistence and latency. Reactivation of latent HHV-6 is common after liver transplantation and may be due to reactivation of endogenous infection of the recipient or superinfection (reactivation in the transplanted organ). Most HHV-6 infections after liver transplantation are asymptomatic, but fever, rash and myelosuppression, hepatitis, pneumonitis and encephalitis may occur. Liver damage is mild and non-specific, consisting mostly of portal and perisinusoidal infiltrates, with minimal necrosis (Fig. 21.2). HHV-6 could enhance allograft rejection and increase severity of other infections including CMV, hepatitis C virus, and opportunistic fungi. Ganciclovir and valganciclovir are active against HHV-6 and may prevent its reactivation after transplantation. Established HHV-6 disease is treated with intravenous ganciclovir, cidofovir or foscarnet, complemented by reduction in the degree of immunosuppression [62].

Coronaviridae: SARS-coronavirus

Virology, pathogenesis and diagnosis

Severe acute respiratory syndrome (SARS) is a potentially lethal disease caused by a recently described coronavirus (SARS/CoV), which infects primarily the lung and the intestine [63]. Virus or viral products are also detected in other organs such as liver, kidney, and small intestine.

On the basis of phylogenetic analysis, SARS/CoV was designated as a member of the group 2b of the genus *Coronavirus*, of the *Coronaviridae* family. Similar to other *Coronavirus*, SARS/CoV is spherical with distinctive long, petal-shaped spikes composed of the S glycoprotein on the envelope. It is a positive-sense, single-stranded RNA virus with a genome size of almost 30 kb. The surface S protein is divided into two subdomains, S1 and S2. The amino acid sequences of the S1 domain are critical for establishing the target cell specificity and, consequently, the species tropism of SARS/CoV.

At least 5327 probable SARS cases, of whom 343 died, have been reported in China and the global toll probably exceeds 10 000 cases worldwide, with at least 1000 deaths [64]. Since the early reports of the disease, it became apparent that SARS is not merely a respiratory disease, as diarrhoea, a bleeding diathesis and liver damage with a cytolytic pattern were reported in patients infected by SARS-CoV [65].

Three major diagnostic methods available for SARS-CoV [66] include viral RNA detection by RT-PCR and virus-induced antibodies by immunofluorescence assay or by enzyme immunoassays. The receptor binding domain of the spike glycoprotein induces neutralizing antibodies, and thus is both a functional domain for cell receptor binding and a major neutralizing determinant. The genetically engineered, attenuated form of the virus or viral vector vaccine encoding the SARS-CoV spike glycoprotein has been shown to elicit protective immunity in vaccinated animals.

Clinical features and hepatic histology

Liver biopsy shows ballooning of hepatocytes and lobular lymphocytic infiltration together with marked accumulation of cells in mitosis and apoptosis [67]. Immunohistochemical studies revealed 0.5 to 11.4% of hepatocyte nuclei were positive for proliferative antigen Ki-67.

Altered liver tests were reported in 22 to 56% of patients at the time of hospital admission [65,68–70]. In a large series of 294 cases reported by Chan [71], 25% of patients had elevated ALT on admission and a further 45% had ALT elevation during the course of illness. In the majority of patients, ALT began to rise towards the end of the first week and peaked at the end of the second week. Most patients had transient ALT elevation, which normalized with the recovery of SARS. High peak ALT values predicted a more severe illness and a worse outcome. Pre-existent causes of liver disease, such as chronic infection with HBV, may worsen the outcome of SARS hepatitis.

SARS is a syndrome with a high death rate, mainly due to respiratory complications and to multiorgan failure. In this setting, SARS-CoV induced liver damage is of comparatively lesser relevance.

Treatment

Since the viral load in the affected organs directly correlates with the severity of symptoms and mortality, antiviral treatment should be beneficial. Shedding of SARS-CoV peaks at day 10 after the onset of symptoms, allowing time for antiviral treatment. The disease is characterized by uncontrolled replication of the virus and a prominent proinflammatory response. No randomized controlled trials with a specific anticoronavirus agent have been conducted with respect to therapy or prophylaxis. Reports using historical matched controls have suggested that treatment with interferon alfacon-1 combined with steroid, protease inhibitors together with ribavirin, or convalescent plasma containing neutralizing antibody, could be useful. No information is available on the specific efficacy of these measures for SARS-CoV induced liver damage [72].

Hepatitis due to exotic viruses

These very dangerous viruses have the liver as the primary target [73]. They include Marburg, Lassa and Ebola viruses.

Lassa fever is caused by an arenavirus transmitted from rodents to man or from man to man. It is largely found in West Africa. The case fatality rate is 36 to 67%, due to severe liver failure with massive coagulopathy. Diagnosis is made by demonstrating virus in the blood during the first few days and by IgM antibodies from the fifth day. It has been successfully treated with ribavirin [74].

Marburg virus disease is caused by an RNA virus transmitted by Vervet monkeys [75,76]. After an incubation period of 4–7 days the patients present with headache, pyrexia, vomiting, a characteristic rash, a haemorrhagic diathesis and central nervous system involvement. Serum aminotransferases are very high. Liver pathology shows single-cell acidophilic necrosis and Kupffer cell hyperactivity. This is followed by eccentric and radial extension of the necrosis, cytoplasmic inclusions and portal zone cellularity. Steatosis is noted in the severely affected. The virus can persist in the body for 2–3 months after initial infection.

Ebola virus infection resembles Marburg virus disease in clinical course and hepatic histology [77].

There is no specific treatment for these exotic virus infections. Symptomatic measures are used and very strict precautions are necessary to avoid spread through blood or body fluids from acutely infected humans to contacts.

References

1 Wong S, Young NS, Brown KE. Prevalence of Parvovirus B19 in liver tissue: non association with fulminant hepatitis or hepatitis- associated aplastic anaemia. *J. Infect. Dis.* 2003; **187**: 1581–1586.

2 Linnen J, Wages J Jr, Zhang-Keck ZY *et al.* Molecular cloning and disease association of hepatitis G virus: a transfusion-transmissible agent. *Science* 1996; **271**: 505–508.

3 Simons JN, Leary TP, Dawson GJ *et al.* Isolation of novel virus-like sequences associated with human hepatitis. *Nat. Med.* 1995; **1**: 564–569.

4 Alter H. The cloning and clinical implication of HGV. *N. Engl. J. Med.* 1996; **334**: 1536–1537.

5 Tucker TJ, Smuts HE, Eedes C *et al.* Evidence that GBV-C/hepatitis G virus is primarily a lymphotropic virus. *J. Med. Virol.* 2000; **61**: 52–58.

6 Handa A, Brown KE. GB virus C/hepatitis G virus replicates in human haematopoietic cells and vascular endothelial cells. *J. Gen. Virol.* 2000; **81**: 2461–2469.

7 Fan X, Xu Y, Solomon H *et al.* Is hepatitis G/GB virus C hepatotropic? Detection of hepatitis G/GB virus C RNA in liver and serum *J. Med. Virol.* 1999; **58**: 160–164.

8 Souza IE, Allen JB, Xiang J *et al.* Effect of primer selection on estimates of GB virus C (GBV-C) prevalence and response to antiretroviral therapy for optimal testing for GBV-C viremia. *J. Clin. Microbiol.* 2006; **44**: 3105–3113.

9 Tucker TJ, Smuts HE. GBV-C/HGV genotypes: proposed nomenclature for genotypes 1-5. *J. Med. Virol.* 2000; **62**: 82–83.

10 Muerhoff AS, Dawson GJ, Desai SM. A previously unrecognized six genotype of GB virus C revealed by analysis of 5′-untranslated region sequences. *J. Med. Virol.* 2006; **78**: 105–111.

11 Tillmann HL, Manns MP, Claes C *et al.* GB virus C infection and quality of life in HIV-positive patients. *AIDS Care* 2004; **16**: 736–743.

12 Toyoda H, Fukuda Y, Hayakawa T *et al.* Effect of GB virus C/hepatitis G virus coinfection on the course of HIV infection in hemophilia patients in Japan. *J. Acquir. Immune Defic. Syndr. Hum. Retrovirol.* 1998; **17**: 209–213.

13 Tillmann HL, Heiken H, Knapik-Botor A *et al.* Infection with GB virus C and reduced mortality among HIV-infected patients. *N. Engl. J. Med.* 2001; **52**: 83–90.

14 Williams CF, Klinzman D, Yamashita TE *et al.* Persistent GB virus C infection and survival in HIV-infected men. *N. Engl. J. Med.* 2004; **350**: 981–990.

15 Nunnari G, Nigro L, Palermo F *et al.* Slower progression of HIV-1 infection in person with GB virus C co-infection correlates wit an intact T-helper 1 cytokine profile. *Ann. Intern. Med.* 2003; **139**: 26–30.

16 Xiang J, George SL, Wunschmann S *et al.* Inhibition of HIV-1 replication by GB virus C infection through increases in RANTES, MIP-1 alpha, MIP-1 beta and SDF-1. *Lancet* 2004; **363**: 2040–2046.

17 Christensen PB, Fisker N, Mygind LH *et al.* GB virus C epidemiology in Denmark: different routes of transmission in children and low- and high-risk adults. *J. Med. Virol.* 2003; **70**: 156–162.

18 Clevenberg P, Durant J, Halfon P *et al.* High prevalence of GB virus C/hepatitis G virus infection in different risk groups of HIV-infected patients. *Clin. Microbiol. Infect.* 1998; **4**: 644–647.

19 Di Stefano R, Ferraro D, Bonura C *et al.* Are hepatitis G virus and TT virus involved in cryptogenic chronic liver disease? *Dig. Liver Dis.* 2002; **34**: 53–58.

20 Alter MJ, Gallagher M, Morris TT *et al.* Acute non–A-E hepatitis in the United States and the role of hepatitis G virus infection. *N. Engl. J. Med.* 1997; **336**: 741–746.

21 Yuen MF, Chan TM, Yip TP *et al.* Prevalence and significance of hepatitis GB virus-C/hepatitis G virus viremia in a large cohort of patients with chronic hepatitis B infection, with chronic hepatitis C infection, and on renal replacement therapy in Hong Kong. *Dig. Dis. Sci.* 2002; **47**: 432–437.

22 Campo N, Brizzolara R, Sinelli N *et al.* Hepatitis G virus infection in intravenous drug users with or without human immunodeficiency virus infection. *Hepatogastroenterology* 2000; **47**: 1385–1388.

23 Kallinowski B, Buhrmann C, Seipp S *et al.* Incidence, prevalence, and clinical outcome of hepatitis GB-C virus infection in liver transplant patients. *Liver Transpl. Surg.* 1998; **4**: 28–33.

24 Monath TP. Yellow fever: an update. *Lancet Infect. Dis.* 2001; **1**: 11–20.

25 Monath TP, Barrett ADT. Pathogenesis and pathophysiology of yellow fever. *Adv. Virus Dis.* 2003; **60**: 343–397.

26 Monath TP. Treatment of yellow fever. *Antiviral Res.* 2008; **78**: 116–124.

27 Hall WC, Crowell TP, Watts DM *et al.* Demonstration of yellow fever and dengue antigens in formalin-fixed, paraffin-embedded human liver by immunohistochemical analysis. *Am. J. Trop. Med. Hyg.* 1991; **45**: 408–417.

28 Barnett ED. Yellow fever: epidemiology and prevention. *Clin. Infect. Dis.* 2007; **44**: 850–856.

29 Nishizawa T, Okamoto H, Konishi K *et al.* A novel DNA virus (TTV) associated with elevated transaminase levels in post-transfusion hepatitis of unknown etiology. *Biochem. Biophys. Res. Commun.* 1997; **24**: 92–97.

30 Takahashi K, Iwasa Y, Hijikata M *et al.* Identification of a new human DNA virus (TTVlike mini virus, TLMV) intermediately related to TT virus and chicken anemia virus. *Arch. Virol.* 2000; **145**: 979–993.

31 Jones MS, Kapoor A, Lukashof VV *et al.* New DNA viruses identified in patient with acute viral infection syndrome. *J. Virol.* 2005; **79**: 8230–8236.

32 Ninomiya M, Nishizawa T, Takahashi M *et al.* Identification and genomic characterization of a novel human torque teno virus of 3.2 kb. *J. Gen. Virol.* 2007; **88**: 1939–1944.

33 Ninomiya M, Takahashi M, Nishizawa T *et al.* Development of PCR assays with nested primers specific for differential detection of three human Anelloviruses and early acquisition of dual or triple infection during infancy. *J. Clin. Microbiol.* 2008; **46**: 507–514.

34 Shibata M, Morizane T, Baba T *et al.* TT virus infection in patients with fulminant hepatic failure. *Am. J. Gastroenterol.* 2000; **95**: 3602–3606.

35 Tanaka H, Okamoto H, Luengrojanakul P *et al.* Infection with an unenveloped DNA virus (TTV) associated with posttransfusion non-A to G hepatitis in hepatitis patients and healthy blood donors in Thailand. *J. Med. Virol.* 1998; **56**: 234–238.

36 Tuveri R, Jaffredo F, Lunel F *et al.* Impact of TT virus infection in acute and chronic, viral and non viral-related liver diseases. *J. Hepatol.* 2000; **33**: 121–127.

37 Hsieh SY, Wu YH, Ho YP *et al.* High prevalence of TT virus infection in healthy children and adults and in patients with liver disease in Taiwan. *J. Clin. Microbiol.* 1999; **37**: 1829–1831.

38 Naoumov NV, Petrova EP, Thomas MG *et al.* Presence of a newly described human DNA virus (TTV) in patients with liver disease. *Lancet* 1998; **352**: 195–197.

39 Prati D, Lin YH, De Mattei C *et al.* A prospective study on TT virus infection in transfusion-dependent patients with beta-thalassemia. *Blood* 1999; **93**: 1502–1505.

40 Viazov S, Ross RS, Varenholz C *et al.* Lack of evidence for an association between TTV infection and severe liver disease. *J. Clin. Virol.* 1998; **11**: 183–187.

41 Okamoto H. History of discoveries and pathogenicity of TT viruses. *Curr. Top. Microbiol. Immunol.* 2009; **331**: 1–20.

42 Markin RS. Manifestations of Epstein–Barr virus-associated disorders in liver. *Liver* 1994; **14**: 1–13.

43 Pelletier LL, Borel DM, Romig DA *et al.* Disseminated intravascular coagulation and hepatic necrosis. Complications of infectious mononucleosis. *J. Am. Med. Assoc.* 1976; **235**: 1144–1146.

44 White NJ, Juel-Nelsen BE. Infectious mononucleosis hepatitis. *Semin. Liver Dis.* 1984; **4**: 301–306.

45 Kimura H, Nagasaka T, Hoshino Y *et al.* Severe hepatitis caused by Epstein–Barr virus without infection of hepatocytes. *Hum. Pathol.* 2001; **32**: 757–762.

46 Hinedi TB, Koff RS. Cholestatic hepatitis induced by Epstein–Barr virus infection in an adult. *Dig. Dis. Sci.* 2003; **48**: 539–541.

47 Kikuchi K, Miyakawa H, Abe K *et al.* Vanishing bile duct syndrome associated with chronic EBV infection. *Dig. Dis. Sci.* 2000; **45**: 160–165.

48 Jimenez-Saenz M, Perez-Pozo JM, Leal-Luna A *et al.* Lethal liver failure in an elderly patient with hepatitis B superinfected with Epstein–Barr virus. *Eur. J. Gastroenterol. Hepatol.* 2002; **14**: 1283–1284.

49 Cacopardo B, Nunnari G, Mughini MT *et al.* Fatal hepatitis during Epstein–Barr virus reactivation. *Eur. Rev. Med. Pharmacol. Sci.* 2003; **7**: 107–109.

50 Negro F. The paradox of Epstein-Barr virus-associated hepatitis. *J. Hepatol.* 2006; **44**: 839–841.

51 Tsurumi T, Fujita M, Kudoh A. Latent and lytic Epstein–Barr virus replication strategies. *Rev. Med. Virol.* 2005; **15**: 3–15.

52 Drebber U, Kasper HU, Krupacz J *et al.* The role of Epstein–Barr virus in acute and chronic hepatitis. *J. Hepatol.* 2006; **44**: 879–885.

53 Tsuchiya S. Diagnosis of Epstein-Barr virus-associated disease. *Crit. Rev. Oncol. Hematol.* 2002; **44**: 227–238.

54 Natali A, Valcavi P, Medici MC *et al.* Cytomegalovirus infection in a Italian population. antibody prevalence, virus excretion and maternal transmission. *New Microbiol.* 1997; **20**: 123–133.

55 Staras SA, Dollard SC, Radford KW *et al.* Seroprevalence of cytomegalovirus infection in the United States, 1988–1994. *Clin. Infect. Dis.* 2006; **43**: 1152–1153.

56 Wreghitt TG, Teare EL, Sule O *et al.* Cytomegalovirus infection in immunocompetent patients. *Clin. Infect. Dis.* 2003; **37**: 1603–1606.

57 Clarke J, Craig RM, Saffro *et al.* Cytomegalovirus granulomatous hepatitis. *Am. J. Med.* 1979; **66**: 264–269.

58 King SM, Petric M, Superina R *et al.* Cytomegalovirus infections in paediatric liver transplantation. *Am. J. Dis. Child.* 1990; **144**: 1307–1310.

59 Razonable RR. Cytomegalovirus infection after liver transplantation: current concepts and challenges. *World J. Gastroenterol.* 2008; **14**: 4849–4860.

60 Goodman ZD, Ishak KG, Sesterhenn IA. Herpes simplex hepatitis in apparently immunocompetent adults. *Am. J. Clin. Pathol.* 1986; **85**: 694–699.

61 Myers MG. Hepatic cellular injury during varicella. *Arch. Dis. Child.* 1982; **57**: 317–319.

62 Abdel Massih RC, Razonable RR. Human herpesvirus 6 infections after liver transplantation. *World J. Gastroenterol.* 2009; **15**: 2561–2569.

63 Guo Y, Korteweg C, McNutt MA *et al.* Pathogenetic mechanisms of severe acute respiratory syndrome. *Virus Res.* 2008; **133**: 4–12.

64 Feng D, de Vlas SJ, Fang LQ *et al.* The SARS epidemic in mainland China: bringing together all epidemiological data. *Trop. Med. Int. Health* 2009; **14** (Suppl. 1): 4–13.

65 Wong WM, Ho JC, Ooi GC *et al.* Temporal patterns of hepatic dysfunction and disease severity in patients with SARS. *JAMA* 2003; **290**: 2663–2665.

66 Suresh MR, Bhatnagar PK, Das D. Molecular targets for diagnostics and therapeutics of severe acute respiratory syndrome (SARS-CoV). *J. Pharm. Pharm. Sci.* 2008; **11**: 1s–13s.

67 Chau TN, Lee KC, Yao H *et al.* SARS-associated viral hepatitis caused by a novel coronavirus: report of three cases. *Hepatology* 2004; **39**: 302–310.

68 Lee N, Hui D, Wu A *et al.* A major outbreak of severe acute respiratory syndrome in Hong Kong. *N. Engl. J. Med.* 2003; **348**: 1986–1994.

69 Poutanen SM, Low DE, Henry B *et al.* Identification of severe acute respiratory syndrome in Canada. *N. Engl. J. Med.* 2003; **348**: 1995–2005.

70 Choi KW, Chau TN, Tsang O *et al.* Outcomes and prognostic factors in 267 patients with severe acute respiratory syndrome in Hong Kong. *Ann. Intern. Med.* 2003; **139**: 715–723.

71 Chan HL, Kwan AC, To KF *et al.* Clinical significance of hepatic derangement in severe acute respiratory syndrome. *World J. Gastroenterol.* 2005; **11**: 2148–2153.

72 Wong SS, Yuen KY. The management of coronavirus infections with particular reference to SARS. *J. Antimicrob. Chemother.* 2008; **62**: 437–441.

73 Howard CR, Ellis DS, Simpson DIH. Exotic viruses and the liver. *Semin. Liver Dis.* 1984; **4**: 361–374.

74 McCormick JB, King IJ, Webb PA *et al.* Lassa fever. Effective therapy with ribavirin. *N. Engl. J. Med.* 1986; **314**: 20–26.

75 Martini GA, Knauff HG, Schmidt HA *et al.* Uber eine bisher unbekannte von Affen eingeschleppte Infektions-krankheit: Marburg-Virus-Krankheit. *Dtsch. Med. Wschr.* 1968; **57**: 559–571.

76 Smith DH, Johnson BK, Isaacson M *et al.* Marburg-virus disease in Kenya. *Lancet* 1982; **1**: 816–820.

77 Ellis DS, Simpson IH, Francis DP *et al.* Ultra-structure of Ebola virus particles in human liver. *J. Clin. Pathol.* 1978; **31**: 201–208.

CHAPTER 22
HIV and the Liver

Marion G. Peters[1] & Vincent Soriano[2]

[1]Department of Gastroenterology, University of California, San Francisco, CA, USA
[2]Department of Infectious Diseases, Hospital Carlos III, Madrid, Spain

Learning points

- The liver is frequently affected in patients with HIV.
- Viral hepatitis is the second most common cause of death in HIV patients in North America and Western Europe.
- Liver fibrosis progression is more rapid in patients coinfected with HIV and viral hepatitis.
- Systemic opportunistic infections and neoplasms affecting the liver are seen in those with severe immunodeficiency and low CD4 counts.

Viral hepatitis and human immunodeficiency virus (HIV) infection

Chronic viral hepatitis B (HBV), C (HCV) and/or delta (HDV) comprise the most common liver diseases in HIV-infected individuals worldwide due to shared routes of transmission. Liver disease due to chronic HBV and HCV is the most frequent cause of non AIDS-related death among persons with HIV in Europe, the United States and Australia [1]. Serum aminotransferases are not good predictors of inflammation. Figure 22.1 shows the overlap of HIV, HBV and HCV epidemics.

Hepatitis A and B vaccination in HIV patients

All HIV patients should be tested for viral hepatitis and vaccinated against hepatitis A and B as early as possible if not immune (Table 22.1). HIV patients are less likely to respond to vaccination [2]. Response rates ranging from 17 to 56% have been reported in HIV patients, being especially impaired in those with lower CD4 counts [2]. No significant, distinctive, adverse clinical reactions to HBV vaccination have been described in HIV patients. Transient elevations in plasma HIV RNA lasting for several days to a few weeks have been spo-

radically reported [3]. The standard HBV vaccination schedule consists of three intramuscular doses of the hepatitis B vaccine at 0, 1 and 6 months. Hepatitis B vaccines are available as a single-antigen formulation and also in fixed combinations with inactivated hepatitis A vaccines. Anti-HBs titres should be checked 1 month after completion of the vaccine series to document response. If there is no response, revaccination can be considered.

HIV individuals are less likely to maintain sustained high and protective anti-HBs titres [4]. Breakthrough HBV infections have been reported in HIV patients when a decline in anti-HBs concentrations to less than 10 mIU/mL occurred. It may be difficult to distinguish between waning immunity and non-response in individuals with an unknown anti-HBs response following HBV immunization. The degree of anti-HBs response 4 to 12 weeks after a single booster dose may differentiate the two antibody response patterns. True non-responders will not elicit serum anti-HBs or show a minimal rise in titre. In contrast, those with waning immunity generally have a robust anamnestic response. Several re-immunization schedules for non-responders have been examined. Doubling the HBV vaccine dose may improve responses, at least in patients with higher CD4 counts and undetectable plasma HIV RNA. The use of adjuvants has not been proven to increase response rates to HBV vaccine.

A special situation is noted in patients positive for antibody to hepatitis B core (anti-HBc) but negative for both HBsAg and anti-HBs. This is infrequent in the general population, but common in HIV individuals [5]. It may reflect clearance of HBsAg but inability to mount an adequate anti-HBs response. Occasionally, an isolated anti-HBc may be a false-positive result, especially in low-risk populations [6]. Or it may reflect ongoing HBV viraemia with mutations in HBsAg. Following HBV booster vaccine, few HIV patients with isolated

Sherlock's Diseases of the Liver and Biliary System, Twelfth Edition. Edited by
James S. Dooley, Anna S.F. Lok, Andrew K. Burroughs, E. Jenny Heathcote.
© 2011 by Blackwell Publishing Ltd. Published 2011 by Blackwell Publishing Ltd.

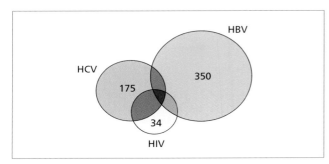

Fig. 22.1. Estimated number (millions) of individuals with HIV, HBV and HCV worldwide. Coinfection with HIV and HCV is estimated to be 7 million and with HBV 4 million.

anti-HBc exhibit an anamnestic response [7]. Therefore, the presence of isolated anti-HBc in HIV patients should not be interpreted as a surrogate marker of protection against HBV. Accordingly, these patients should be tested for HBV DNA. The patient should be treated as for chronic HBV if viraemic for HBV. If HBV DNA is not detectable, the patient should be vaccinated.

Hepatitis B and HIV

Epidemiology

Worldwide, there are an estimated 4 million individuals coinfected with HIV and HBV. Rates of coinfection with HBV vary throughout the world depending on the relative timing of exposure to both viruses [8]. In the USA and Western Europe, the rates of coinfection vary from 6 to 10%. Twenty per cent of HIV patients who are exposed to HBV as adults develop chronic HBV, compared to less than 5% of immunocompetent adults [9]. However, this is different in areas where HBV is endemic with a high rate of vertical and perinatal transmission (Asia and sub-Saharan Africa). Individuals usually develop chronic HBV infection as infants and then acquire HIV as adults. In endemic areas, the prevalence of HBV in HIV patients varies widely from 10 to 25%, depending on the country studied [8]. In the USA and Europe, genotype A is most common in HIV patients [10]. In endemic areas, the HBV genotype of the area predominates in HIV–HBV coinfected patients.

Diagnosis

All HIV positive patients should be tested for HBV (Table 22.1). If negative for all markers, the patient should be vaccinated. HIV patients with positive HBsAg require lifelong ongoing monitoring. If highly active antiretroviral therapy (HAART) is initiated, anti-HBV therapy is mandated (see below). Patients with evidence of past infection (anti-HBs and anti-HBc) or atypical

serology occasionally reactivate on HAART [8]. For this reason, HBV should be considered in the differential diagnosis of abnormal aminotransferases even if atypical serology is noted.

Pathogenesis

Hepatitis B is an immune-mediated infection. When HIV is uncontrolled, there is little inflammation in the liver. However, liver damage can occur after immune reconstitution with HAART. For this reason, physicians must know the status of HBV infection before initiating HAART and monitor the HBV status during HAART therapy. Patients with HIV and HBV coinfection have higher HBV DNA levels and lower serum alanine aminotransferase (ALT) levels than those with HBV alone. Liver fibrosis tend to be more advanced and the risk of end-stage liver disease is markedly increased in patients who are coinfected with HIV and HBV [11]. This risk is more pronounced in those with low CD4 counts or alcohol consumption. Despite the availability of HAART, including agents with potent anti-HBV activity, overall mortality and liver-related mortality is increased in HIV–HBV coinfected patients compared to HIV-monoinfected individuals [12]. Patients with elevated serum HBV DNA have lower CD4 counts at HAART initiation. They also have impaired CD4 restoration in response to HAART [13].

Treatment

Treatment endpoints for HBV in HIV patients remain the same as in those without HIV. However, loss of HBeAg or HBsAg as well as seroconversion to anti-HBe and anti-HBs is uncommon. The clinician must first decide whether the patient needs treatment for HIV alone, for HBV alone or for both viruses. If either HIV or both infections meet criteria for therapy, then treatment must include agents active against both viruses. Several nucleoside analogues have activity against both HIV and HBV so they cannot be used without HAART (Table 22.2). Recent guidelines from the USA and Europe recommend the use of two anti-HBV drugs as part of HAART in coinfected persons [14,15]. This is because therapy for HBV in HIV patients is usually lifelong, resistance to nucleoside analogues is common and flares with immune reconstitution can be life-threatening. The use of combination HBV therapy aims to decrease the development of resistance, even though there are limited data on combination therapy in either mono- or coinfected patients. Many HIV patients are lamivudine experienced. Development of lamivudine resistance to HBV is seen in 90% of patients at 4 years [16]. Entecavir has anti-HIV activity and should not be used without HAART [17]. Entecavir may be associated with high rate

Table 22.1. Approach to viral hepatitis in HIV patients

Test required by all HIV patients	Recommendation
Hepatitis A: HAV IgG	If negative: vaccinate
Hepatitis B: HBsAg, anti-HBs, anti-HBc	If negative: vaccinate
	If positive for HBsAg: manage as chronic HBV infection
	If only anti-HBc positive: check serum HBV DNA
	If HBV DNA negative: vaccinate against HBV
	If HBV DNA positive: manage as chronic HBV infection
Hepatitis C: Anti-HCV	If positive: test for HCV RNA, and for HCV genotype if viraemic

Table 22.2. HIV and HBV activity of current HBV medications

Drug	Antiviral activity			Recommended as part of antiretroviral therapy
	HBV wild type	HBV YMDD mutant	HIV	
Tenofovir	Yes	Yes	Yes	Yes
Entecavir	Yes	Yes at higher dose	Yes	No
Emtricitabine	Yes	No	Yes	Yes
Lamivudine	Yes	No	Yes	Yes
Adefovir	Yes	Yes	Not at 10 mg dose	No
Telbivudine	Yes	No	Yes*	No

*Limited data as yet.

of resistance if the HBV already has the YMDD mutation in its polymerase gene. Telbivudine may also have activity against HIV [18]. Combination therapy with tenofovir and emtricitabine (or lamivudine) is the preferred treatment at present for coinfected patients. HAART interruption may lead to a flare of HBV, which may be life threatening. For this reason patients should be warned against stopping drugs unless there is careful consultation and monitoring [19].

Treatment options are more limited if the patient does not meet criteria for HIV therapy. European guidelines recommend pegylated interferon (PEG-IFN) or adefovir [14]. PEG-IFN-α has not been well studied in the setting of HIV. It is most effective in immunocompetent patients with low viral load and high ALT, both rare in HBV–HIV coinfected patients. Patients with lower CD4 levels have poorer responses to interferon therapy. US guidelines recommend the early initiation of HAART in these patients because treatment options are limited and HBV disease progresses more rapidly in HIV patients [1,15].

There are multiple causes of abnormal ALT in patients with HIV and HBV (Table 22.3). Cell-mediated immunity plays a central role in the pathogenesis of chronic hepatitis B [20]. In an HIV–HBV coinfected patient with advanced immunosuppression, HBV replication is high but there is little liver inflammation. However, when HAART is initiated, improved cellular immunity can lead to recognition of virally infected hepatocytes and a flare in liver enzymes. Thus reactivation of HBV and

abnormal ALT may occur with improved immune response. If due to immune reconstitution, it often resolves with continued therapy. If HAART is initiated without anti-HBV agents then immune reconstitution usually occurs within 6–12 weeks and may be severe. If HAART is stopped, flares in HBV disease often occur. Flares in ALT may be due to the development of drug resistance (e.g. lamivudine) [8]. Abnormal ALT may be due to spontaneous HBV clearance. This occurs rarely in HIV patients. Finally, abnormal ALT may be due to drug toxicity or the development of other liver disease. Liver enzyme flares in HIV–HBV-coinfected patients on HAART therapy need to be carefully interpreted, with concomitant evaluation of serum HBV DNA, in order to correctly assign causality.

Hepatitis C and HIV

Epidemiology

Of the 35 million people living with HIV worldwide around 20% (approximately 7 million) have chronic hepatitis C. Risk factors for acquisition of both viruses are shared and include intravenous drug use and receipt of contaminated blood (e.g. haemophilia). As with HBV, patients with HIV infection and chronic hepatitis C have faster rates of liver fibrosis progression [21,22]. This is especially seen in those with low CD4 counts. Early introduction of HAART in these patients is encouraged.

Table 22.3. Causes of abnormal liver function tests in HIV patients

In all HIV patients
Acute hepatitis A, B or C
Acute hepatitis D if patient is HBsAg positive
Acute hepatitis B and D coinfection
Chronic hepatitis B or C
Chronic hepatitis B and D coinfection
Non-alcoholic fatty liver disease (NAFLD)
Alcoholic liver disease
Liver infections (e.g. tuberculosis, MAI)
Hepatotoxicity from drugs
HAART
Anti-infectives
Non-steroidal anti-inflammatory drugs
Neuropsychiatric medication
Over the counter medications, herbals, illicit drugs
Liver malignancy

In HIV–HBV coinfected patients
Reactivation of HBV with improved immune response
Immune reconstitution—continue therapy
HAART initiation without anti-HBV therapy—add HBV therapy
HAART stopped so patient not receiving HBV therapy—reinstitute HAART therapy
Development of HBV drug resistance
Spontaneous HBV clearance—occurs rarely in HIV patients
Other liver diseases

HAART, highly active antiretroviral therapy; MAI, *Mycobacterium avium* complex.

Outbreaks of acute hepatitis C in HIV patients

Outbreaks of hepatitis C among homosexual men have been reported in several large European and North American cities since year 2000 [23]. HCV is not efficiently transmitted by sexual contact, unlike HBV and HIV. High levels of sexual promiscuity, certain traumatic sex practices and concomitant ulcerative sexually transmitted diseases (e.g. syphilis), have all been associated with these HCV outbreaks. The increased level of HCV viraemia characteristically seen in HIV persons might further contribute to this enhanced infectivity [24]. HIV-infected patients progress to chronic HCV more frequently than HIV-negative individuals [25]. Response rates to interferon therapy are higher in acute HCV than for chronic HCV. Treatment should not be instituted before 12 weeks of estimated exposure, to allow for spontaneous HCV clearance to occur. A sustained virological response (SVR) to treatment in acute hepatitis C is lower in HIV patients compared to HIV-negative patients (60 versus 80%, respectively). It is unclear whether adding ribavirin to PEG-IFN offers any advantage when treating acute hepatitis C in HIV individuals. However, given the worse prognosis of HCV infection in HIV persons, many experts use both drugs for 24 weeks regardless of HCV genotype [26].

Pathogenesis

Progression to end-stage liver disease occurs more rapidly in this population [27]. The tolerance of antiretroviral agents is much poorer in the presence of underlying chronic hepatitis C, with higher rates of hepatotoxicity [28]. Successful treatment of chronic hepatitis C with clearance of HCV has been associated with a regression of liver fibrosis [29] and with a reduced risk of antiretroviral-related hepatotoxicity [30]. Liver fibrosis can be assessed by liver biopsy, serum markers or elastography. The non-invasive tools are generally accurate in discriminating lack of fibrosis and advanced fibrosis, and less precise with intermediate fibrosis stages [31]. Their predictive value is particularly good for advanced hepatic fibrosis and cirrhosis. However, serum fibrosis markers are generally less reliable in coinfected patients, given the inflammatory nature of HIV disease and/or the frequent use of drugs which may interfere with some fibrosis markers in the blood. This is the case for bilirubin elevations due to atazanavir, γ-glutamyl transpeptidase abnormalities with nonnucleoside reverse transcriptase inhibitors or cholesterol elevations using most ritonavir-boosted protease inhibitors. Patients with repeatedly normal serum ALT may benefit from HCV therapy. Serum ALT is not a good predictor of inflammation in HIV patients. Significant liver fibrosis has been reported in up to 25–40% of coinfected patients with normal ALT and even 'silent' cirrhosis in nearly 15% [32].

Treatment of HCV

All HIV persons with chronic HCV infection should be considered potential candidates for HCV therapy. The timing for HCV treatment should be decided on an individual basis. Severe neuropsychiatric disorders, alcohol and drug abuse are generally contraindication to HCV treatment. Host factors, including liver fibrosis stage, CD4 counts and patient motivation, are the most important variables that determine who will respond to HCV therapy (Table 22.4) [27]. HIV–HCV patients with *liver decompensation* (ascites, gastrointestinal bleeding, hepatic encephalopathy, etc.) should not be treated with PEG-IFN, given the higher risk of liver decompensation and serious side effects. These patients should be evaluated for liver transplantation. However, patients with compensated cirrhosis (Child–Pugh class A) may be treated with PEG-IFN plus ribavirin. These patients will benefit most from HCV clearance and potential reversal of severe liver fibrosis. Other predictors of response include estimated length of HCV infection, the severity of liver disease, the extent of HIV suppression, HCV genotype and viral load (Table 22.4). Genetic polymorphisms in the *IL28B* gene influence treatment response in HCV

Table 22.4. Factors associated with sustained virological response to HCV therapy in HIV patients

Host
Genetics (white ethnicity, *IL28b* polymorphisms)
Younger age
Minimal liver fibrosis
Low body mass index
No insulin resistance
No hepatic steatosis
Higher CD4 count
No polysubstance abuse
No psychiatric disease

Virus
Genotypes 2/3
Low baseline HCV RNA
Undetectable week 4 HCV RNA

Treatment
Adequate pegylated interferon dose
Weight-based ribavirin dose
Good adherence
No concurrent didanosine, zidovudine or abacavir
Haematopoietic growth factors as needed

monoinfected patients [33]. It has not been studied in coinfected patients yet. Treatment responses are inversely related to pretreatment baseline CD4 [14]. Insulin resistance is a negative predictor of response and is prevalent in coinfected patients, at least in part due to antiretroviral therapy including ritonavir-boosted protease inhibitors. Treatment compliance is critical. Adequate selection of treatment candidates, psychological and/or psychiatric support, and use of growth factors to avoid dose reductions of either PEG-IFN and/or ribavirin is required.

Toxicity of PEG-IFN and/or ribavirin and poorer response rates are more frequent in severely immune deficient patients. Interferon generally causes a decline in the absolute CD4 count which reverses after the end of treatment [34]. In drug-naïve coinfected patients with low CD4 counts, antiretroviral therapy should be initiated first. Once CD4 cells have improved and plasma HIV RNA is controlled, HCV therapy should be reassessed. Conversely, in antiretroviral-naïve individuals with good CD4 counts, hepatitis C should be treated first. These patients will further benefit from improved tolerance of antiretroviral drugs [30]. In patients with CD4 counts below 200 cells/mm^3 already on HAART, HCV treatment is usually deferred unless other favourable treatment predictors are present (e.g. HCV genotypes 2 or 3, low HCV load).

HCV kinetics is important in HIV patients. Virological responses can be assessed at early time points to identify who will and who will not respond to therapy. The best positive predictor of SVR is a negative HCV RNA after

4 weeks of therapy (RVR, rapid virological response). The best negative predictor is a less than 2 log decrease in HCV RNA after 12 weeks of therapy (EVR, early virological response) [35]. HIV patients have higher baseline HCV RNA levels and are less likely to have RVR and SVR [36].

Optimal PEG-IFN and ribavirin dosing and duration are currently under development. Adequate exposure to ribavirin is crucial to maximize responses to HCV therapy, particularly in HIV-coinfected patients. Weight-based ribavirin dosing is recommended [37]. Pharmacokinetic studies have shown a good correlation between ribavirin plasma levels and HCV RNA responses. This is rarely practical. Figure 22.2 shows the proportion of patients achieving SVR in pivotal trials as a function of distinct ribavirin doses and HIV status. There is no proven efficacy of higher doses of PEG-IFN in coinfected patients.

Guidelines recommended that duration of treatment in coinfected patients should be of 48 weeks regardless of HCV genotype (Fig. 22.3) [26,38]. Studies conducted in HCV-monoinfected patients have shown that RVR in patients treated with PEG-IFN–ribavirin is the best predictor of SVR. Attainment of RVR may permit a shorter duration of therapy. HIV–HCV coinfected patients with RVR also appear to have a high chance of SVR [39]. RVR is uncommon as HCV load is higher in HIV patients. But if HIV–HCV patients achieve RVR they may achieve SVR with a shorter duration of treatment [26]. Shorter periods of therapy (24 weeks) can be used in HIV patients with all of the following: (1) HCV genotype 2 and 3 with (2) RVR, (3) HCV load is low, (4) good adherence, (5) mild to moderate liver fibrosis and (6) weight-based ribavirin dosing [14,26]. For the remainder of HCV genotypes 2 and 3 patients, 48 weeks of therapy is recommended. In patients with HCV genotype 1 and 4, extension of treatment beyond 48 weeks is recommended in those with EVR but no RVR, as long as the medication is well tolerated. However, high drop-out rates limit the benefit of this strategy.

Antiretroviral drugs during HCV therapy

Nucleoside reverse transcriptase inhibitors (NRTIs) are the backbone of most current antiretroviral regimens. Interactions between antiretrovirals and ribavirin, a guanosine analogue are of concern. Didanosine (ddI) use is prohibited because of the potential increased risk of hepatic decompensation, pancreatitis and/or lactic acidosis in subjects on a combination of ddI and ribavirin [40]. Zidovudine should be used with caution because of its possible aggravation of ribavirin-induced anaemia. Where possible, adjustment of antiretroviral therapy to non-zidovudine-containing regimens prior

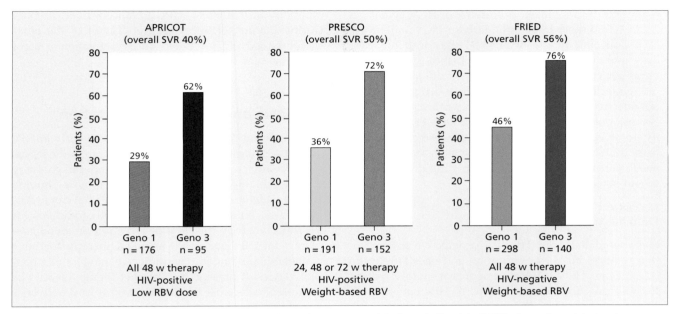

Fig. 22.2. Proportion of patients with sustained virological responses (SVR) in three large trials (APRICOT, PRESCO, FRIED) in HIV-positive and HIV-negative patients using low or weight-based ribavirin (RBV) doses (intent-to-treat analysis).

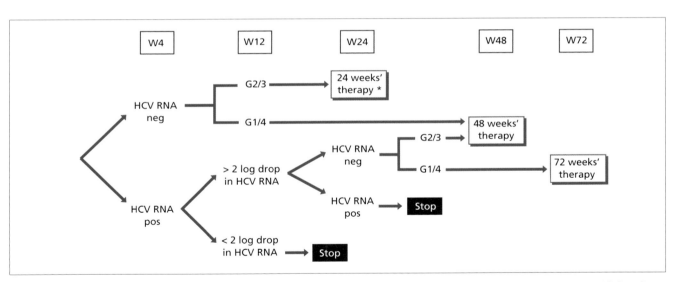

Fig. 22.3. Proposed optimal duration of HCV therapy in HCV–HIV-coinfected patients [14,26]. * Only in patients with baseline low viral load and minimal liver fibrosis.

to study entry should be strongly considered [8]. Abacavir use has also been discouraged in patients treated for hepatitis C given its potential interaction with ribavirin [41]. However, the use of weight-based ribavirin dosing may overcome this limitation. Current HIV treatment guidelines favour earlier initiation of HAART in HIV patients with chronic hepatitis C [14,15]. This is because the large benefit of HAART clearly outweighs its potential risks for liver toxicity [42].

Prospects of new HCV drugs in HIV/HCV coinfected patients

The advent of new antivirals against HCV is eagerly awaited by many HIV patients with chronic hepatitis C. Many patients are relatively young, show significant liver fibrosis and have already failed PEG-IFN–ribavirin. Baseline characteristics of hepatitis C in HIV patients differ from HIV-negative persons. HIV patients have higher viral load, greater prevalence of HCV genotypes 3 and 4, and more frequently harbour HCV-1a than -1b [43]. Concomitant use of HAART may lead to drug–drug interactions. Thus, the performance of direct antivirals for HCV in HIV patients may differ from HCV monoinfected patients. Many of these drugs are less or not effective against HCV genotypes other than HCV-1. Natural polymorphisms account for a lower susceptibility in HCV-1a than -1b viruses in the case of HCV protease inhibitors. However, these patients are in greatest need of therapy because of the more rapid progression to end-stage liver disease.

Delta hepatitis in HIV

Hepatitis delta virus (HDV) is a defective RNA virus that requires HBV for replication and uses HBsAg for its envelope. HDV is the most aggressive viral hepatitis. Its poor prognosis is accentuated in HIV patients [44]. The prevalence of HDV antibodies in HIV and HBV patients ranges from 15 to 50%, depending on geographical region and risk group category. In Western countries, HDV is more frequent in intravenous drug users than persons sexually infected with HIV. Most HIV patients seropositive for HDV are viraemic (HDV RNA$^+$). Treatment of chronic HDV in HIV patients with interferon is rarely effective [45], although no studies have examined the safety and efficacy of PEG-IFN for longer than 18 months, which has been shown to be relatively effective in HIV-uninfected persons.

HIV patients with multiple hepatitis viruses

The prevalence of multiple viral hepatitis (HBV–HCV, HBV–HDV, HCV–HBV–HDV) in HIV patients is below 5% in developed countries [46]. Replication of HDV uniformly predominates over other viruses. Low or undetectable HBV and/or HCV viraemia is noted with rapid progression to cirrhosis [47]. Patients carrying HBV–HCV infections exhibit reciprocal inhibition of virus replication. Which virus predominates may fluctuate with time [48]. In patients with severe immunosuppression, replication of all hepatitis viruses may occur simultaneously. In most HIV patients with relatively good immune status, viral interference favours HCV over HBV replication. Progression of liver disease is accelerated in HIV patients dually coinfected with HBV and HCV. These individuals are more prone to develop hepatocellular carcinoma [49]. Liver-related mortality is increased in HIV patients with multiple hepatitis viruses. This higher fatality is maintained even when HAART with anti-HBV activity is used. Treatment with PEG-IFN–ribavirin in HIV patients coinfected with HBV–HCV has been effective in small studies [50]. The treatment of all replicating viruses should be pursued, especially in patients with advanced liver fibrosis. During therapy of one virus, replication of the other should be actively monitored since reactivation of latent infections may occur [51].

Cirrhosis and liver transplantation

It is important that cirrhosis is recognized early in HIV patients. Routine screening of all cirrhotic patients for hepatocellular carcinoma should be undertaken every 6–12 months. Hepatocellular carcinoma is more common in HIV patients [49]. If cirrhotic patients have evidence of liver decompensation, they are not candidates for interferon therapy for HCV or HBV, but are good candidates for HBV nucleoside analogue therapy. Cirrhotic patients should undergo periodic screening for oesophageal varices. If present, beta blocker therapy should be instituted to decrease the heart rate by 10%. Prophylaxis for spontaneous bacterial peritonitis should be given to patients at high risk. This includes those with a prior episode of spontaneous bacterial peritonitis or with low ascitic fluid protein concentration. All patients with HIV who have end-stage liver disease are potential candidates for liver transplantation, as outlined in Chapter 37 [52].

HIV-associated opportunistic infections and the liver

Infections of the liver and biliary tract are common in patients with HIV infection who have severe immunodeficiency (<100 CD4$^+$ cell/μL) but rare in those with more preserved immune status. The most common pathogens are noted in Table 22.5. In severely immunosuppressed individuals, a variety of viruses, bacteria, fungi and parasites may affect the liver. These infections may be primary to the liver or secondary to a disseminated process. The typical presenting features are fever, right upper quadrant pain, hepatomegaly and cholestatic liver tests. Initial evaluation should include abdominal ultrasonography, which may identify focal lesions or dilated bile ducts. A liver biopsy may be indicated to detect the aetiological agent. An elevated serum alkaline phosphatase level is an indication for ultrasound or CT. Those patients with dilated bile ducts should proceed to endoscopic retrograde cholangiopancreatography (ERCP) to confirm biliary obstruction. Those patients with a focal non-vascular lesion should have a guided liver biopsy. In the absence of a focal or bile duct lesion, a liver biopsy should be performed. Special stains and culture must be requested to identify specific organisms. These should include bacterial and fungal stains as noted below.

Table 22.5. Hepatic involvement by opportunistic infections in HIV patients

Infections
Bacterial: tuberculosis, *Mycobacterium avium* complex, *Penicillium marneffei*, *Bartonella henselae*
Fungal: histoplasmosis, cryptococcosis, *Candida*, *Pneumocystis jiroveci*
Parasitic: toxoplasmosis, *Cryptosporidium*, *Microsporidia*
Viral: herpes viruses, varicela zoster, cytomegalovirus, Epstein–Barr virus

Neoplasms
Kaposi s sarcoma
Non-Hodgkin lymphoma

Bacterial infections

Tuberculosis may present with liver and/or splenic hypoechoic masses, and associated enlarged abdominal lymph nodes in patients with advanced immunodeficiency [53]. Multifocal abscesses may enlarge paradoxically following initiation of HAART, as an immune reconstitution inflammatory syndrome (IRIS). In addition to antituberculous drugs, corticosteroids may be helpful in treating IRIS. Hepatic tuberculosis may also present as miliary disease and granulomatous hepatitis. Overall, tuberculosis is a frequent cause of liver disease in HIV-infected individuals living in resource-limited countries. Empiric antituberculous treatment may be initiated in the presence of fever and abnormal liver enzymes. HIV patients with higher CD4 counts may have hepatic involvement as part of a disseminated infection.

Disseminated *Mycobacterium avium complex* infection generally occurs as granulomatous disease in the liver. Patients usually have very low CD4 counts (<50 cells/μL), weight loss, pancytopenia and prolonged fever. As in other granulomatous liver diseases, marked elevation of alkaline phosphatase is generally seen [54]. Diagnosis is made with liver biopsy and culture.

Bacillary peliosis hepatitis—the angioproliferative lesions in the liver resemble Kaposi's sarcoma. It is due to *Bartonella henselae*, a tiny Gram-negative organism which is difficult to culture. Systemic features include fever, lymphadenopathy, hepatosplenomegaly and cutaneous and bone lesions. It is treated by erythromycin.

Fungal infections

Fungal infections are usually part of late disseminated disease [55]. They include *Cryptococcus neoformans* where yeast can be shown in the liver. Similarly, histoplasmosis, coccidiomycosis and *Candida albicans* may involve the liver, almost always in patients with very low CD4 counts.

Histoplasmosis is a relatively common AIDS-defining illness in South and Central American countries. It generally occurs in HIV-infected persons with CD4 counts less than 100 cells/μL who are not receiving HAART.

Most patients present with fever, lymphadenopathy, pulmonary and gastrointestinal symptoms. Marked elevation in serum lactate dehydrogenase is typically seen. The diagnosis can be made by stain and culture of *Histoplasma capsulatum* of biopsies from bone marrow, lymph nodes or liver. If there is high clinical suspicion, empirical treatment with amphotericin B is often prescribed in endemic areas [56].

Disseminated infection by *Penicillium marneffei* is relatively common in HIV-infected patients with severe immunodeficiency living in India, China and Southeast Asia. The most common clinical manifestations are fever, weight loss, anaemia, papular skin lesions, hepatosplenomegaly and lymphadenopathy. Definite diagnosis requires culture of fungus from clinical specimens. Amphotericin B and itraconazole are effective treatments [57].

Parasitic infections

Although HIV-associated *toxoplasmosis* generally presents as multiple focal lesions in the central nervous system, extracerebral forms may appear in patients with very advanced immunodeficiency. In such cases, liver involvement occurs with neurological disease, but isolated hepatic toxoplasmosis has also been reported [58].

Viral infections

Herpesviruses may affect the liver, generally as part of disseminated disease. Varicella zoster, cytomegalovirus and Epstein–Barr may cause liver injury and ALT elevations in severely immunosuppressed HIV-infected persons. These infections may be life-threatening [59]. Specific antiviral therapy (e.g. acyclovir, gancyclovir) is recommended. HAART to improve the immune system and prevent relapses is warranted. *CMV* is a manifestation of late HIV and usually part of generalized disease. It is associated with fever and weight loss. Diagnosis is made by demonstrating nuclear and cytoplasmic inclusions in Kupffer cells, bile duct epithelium and occasionally hepatocytes. CMV can be quantitated by PCR in plasma.

AIDS cholangiopathy causes intra- and extrahepatic sclerosing cholangitis. It is associated with severe immunodeficiency with CD4 lymphocyte counts of less than 200 cells/µL. Cryptosporidia are the single most common pathogens identified. *Cryptosporidium parvum* is cytopathic for cultured human biliary epithelia via an apoptotic mechanism. *Microsporidia* or *cytomegalovirus* may be causative. The agent can be found in biliary or gallbladder wall and in bile. The patient presents with intermittent right upper abdominal pain and tenderness. Serum alkaline phosphatase may be strikingly high, but serum bilirubin is usually normal. Presentation may also be as painless cholestasis or as acute bacterial cholangitis. Those with low CD4 counts exposed to *Cryptosporidium* are at risk of biliary disease and death within 1 year.

Ultrasound is the best initial diagnostic tool. It shows bile duct thickening or biliary dilatation or both. ERCP is the diagnostic gold standard. Sphincterotomy during the procedure alleviates symptoms in most cases. Prognosis depends on the stage of immunosuppression and CD4 restoration under HAART.

HIV-associated neoplasms of the liver

In HIV the liver may be the site of primary cancer or metastatic disease (Table 22.5). Cancer is more common in HIV patients, especially those who are severely immune suppressed [60,61].

Primary *hepatocellular carcinoma* appears mainly in subjects with underlying chronic viral hepatitis, either B, C or delta having advanced liver fibrosis or cirrhosis. In the HIV setting, multiple lesions at presentation and worst outcome appear to occur more frequently than in HIV-negative individuals with hepatocellular carcinoma [49,62]. A quadruple phase CT or MRI is most useful for diagnosis. It usually shows early filling in the hepatic artery phase with washout in later phases [63]. In some cases biopsy of the lesion is required for diagnosis. Management of hepatocellular carcinoma in HIV should follow standard guidelines.

Non-Hodgkin's lymphoma is usually metastatic, but can be primary. It usually appears late, but may develop at any stage of the disease. Liver involvement may be the primary presentation. It presents as fever, weight loss, night sweats and abdominal pain, with a rise in serum ALT and especially serum alkaline phosphatase. Large hepatic lesions present with jaundice and pruritus. Ultrasound and CT show large, usually multifocal, solid, space-occupying lesions. Guided liver biopsy is diagnostic. Survival is generally short and response to chemotherapy poor. The prognosis depends on the degree of immunocompromise.

Kaposi's sarcoma largely affects homosexual men and is decreasing in prevalence. The patient is usually asymptomatic. It frequently involves the liver as purple–brown, soft nodules. Histology shows multifocal areas of vascular endothelial proliferation with pleomorphic spindle cells and extravasated erythrocytes. Ultrasound shows small hyperechoic nodules and dense peripheral bands. CT shows hypoattenuated lesions enhancing after contrast.

Antiretroviral-related liver injury in HIV

Prevention and management of antiretroviral-related liver injury have emerged as a major issue among HIV patients in the HAART era. Virtually every licensed antiretroviral medication has been associated with abnormal serum ALT, although certain drugs may cause liver injury more frequently than others [64,65]. In addition, comorbidities, such as chronic hepatitis B, C or D, predispose to injury [28,64]. Drug-induced liver injury (DILI) can lead to liver-related morbidity and mortality as well as discontinuation of HIV treatment. The AIDS Clinical Trials Group (ACTG) has defined a grading scheme against the patient's baseline aminotransferase levels [66]. In patients with a normal pretherapy ALT or AST, hepatic injury is graded as moderate or severe based on a 5-fold or 10-fold increase in aminotransferases, respectively. In patients with abnormal liver enzymes prior to therapy, a more than 3.5-fold or a 5-fold increase in ALT or AST is considered indicative of moderate or severe hepatotoxicity, respectively. Liver function test abnormalities require careful interpretation. Some drugs (e.g. nevirapine and less frequently efavirenz) increase γ-glutamyl transpeptidase serum levels. This laboratory result is often misinterpreted as a marker of liver damage, when isolated elevation of this enzyme actually reflects enzyme induction. Similarly, hyperbilirubinaemia alone should not be equated with liver injury, since it is frequently due to indirect hyperbilirubinaemia caused by medications such as indinavir or atazanavir [67]. This risk is increased in patients with underlying Gilbert's syndrome. On the other hand, drug-induced liver injury (DILI) that is associated with an elevated direct bilirubin and clinical jaundice portends a poor clinical outcome (Hy's law).

Clinical relevance of drug-induced liver injury

With the widespread use of HAART and the availability of new antiretroviral medications, DILI has gained prominent attention due to its negative impact on clinical outcomes [65]. DILI creates an economic burden on already strained medical budgets. Additional visits and hospital admissions are often required for appropriate patient care and management. Furthermore, HAART discontinuation interrupts maintenance of HIV suppression [68]. The severity of DILI may range from asymptomatic, the most common, to liver decompensation. The outcome may range from spontaneous resolution to liver failure and death [69]. Severe hepatotoxicity with acute hepatic necrosis is recognized in 2% of HIV patients dying from liver disease. In a large ACTG cohort of nearly 3000 patients initiating HAART, the most common grade 4 adverse events were liver-related; this risk was increased in patients with underlying chronic viral hepatitis [69]. Alcohol abuse has been associated with an increased risk of DILI. HIV patients are usually receiving multiple drugs as part of their care. Antibiotics, drugs for TB, fungi, non-steroidal anti-inflammatory drugs and neuropsychiatric medications all may cause DILI. Over the counter medications, including herbals and illicit drugs, ecstasy and cocaine, may be the culprit. Most ALT elevations resolve spontaneously, probably through a process called 'adaptation' [70].

After initiating HAART, the reported incidence of severe liver toxicity ranges from 2 to 18% [28,64]. Differences in study outcomes may be due to heterogeneity in patient populations, frequency of liver enzyme determinations, other potential exposures (e.g. alcohol), prevalence of chronic viral hepatitis and criteria used for defining severe hepatotoxicity. DILI is clearly more frequent in HIV-infected patients with underlying chronic hepatitis B and/or hepatitis C [71]. However, the vast majority of patients with chronic viral hepatitis tolerate HAART well, and the clinician should not be deterred from initiating antiretroviral therapy which is life saving

[42]. Risk factors for DILI include increase baseline ALT prior to initiating HAART, older age, female gender, advanced liver fibrosis and significant CD4 gains following HAART initiation [72,73,74]. DILI appears more common with first exposure to antiretroviral treatment.

Mechanisms of drug-induced liver injury in patients on HAART

There are a number of mechanisms involved in the development of hepatotoxicity associated with the use of antiretroviral medications (Table 22.6).

Hypersensitivity reactions. Metabolic host-mediated injury occurs when there is an excess of potentially harmful reactive drug metabolites. This is associated with genetic polymorphisms affecting critical metabolizing enzymes. The latency of onset is long (from 2 to 12 months), which poses problems for patient monitoring (Table 22.7). Patients on non-nucleoside reverse transcriptase inhibitors and the protease inhibitors may develop DILI via this mechanism [64]. Hypersensitivity reactions have been reported with nevirapine, abacavir and less frequently with amprenavir, both in HIV-infected patients and in subjects receiving HIV prophylaxis after potential exposure [75]. Allergic phenomena are idiosyncratic to the host. They have an intermediate onset of latency from a few days to 8 weeks. They are not dose related. The incidence of hypersensitivity

Table 22.6. Drug-related liver damage in HIV patients

Mechanisms	Drug class or coinfection	Comment
Mitochondrial toxicity	NRTI (especially ddl and d4T)	Tends to occur after prolonged exposure
Hypersensitivity	NNRTI: nevirapine NRTI: abacavir Protease inhibitor: amprenavir	Occurs early, usually within 12 weeks Often associated with rash HLA-linked; not favoured by HCV nor HBV
Direct toxicity intrinsic or idiosyncratic	NNRTI Protease inhibitors	Variable occurrence within class Dose-dependence for intrinsic damage
Immune reconstitution	Chronic hepatitis B unclear for HCV	Occurs within the first 1–3 months following initiation of HAART
Liver steatosis and steatohepatitis	NRTI: stavudine, didanosine, zidovudine PIs boosted with ritonavir (≥200 mg/day) Lipodystrophy, obesity, alcoholism	Producing mitochondrial damage in the liver Causing hypertrigliceridaemia
Non-cirrhotic portal hypertension	Didanosine association	Potentially life-threatening

ddI, didanosine; HAART, highly active antiretroviral therapy; NNRTI, non-nucleoside reverse transcriptase inhibitor; NRTI, nucleoside reverse transcriptase inhibitor; PI, protease inhibitor.

Table 22.7. Clinical presentation of antiretroviral-related liver toxicity

	Early onset	Late presentation
Interval	1–4 weeks	4–8 months
Mechanism	Immune-mediated	Direct toxicity, cumulative
Dose-related	No	Yes
Role of HCV	No	Yes
Role of CD4 counts	Yes	No
More common HIV drugs	Abacavir, nevirapine	Stavudine, didanosine, tipranavir

reactions is about 1 : 1000 in the general population, but is more common in patients with HIV [76]. Rechallenge should be avoided if drug hypersensitivity is suspected.

Mitochondrial toxicity. Chronic therapy with NRTIs for the treatment of HIV can also lead to mitochondrial toxicity after long-term exposure. NRTIs selectively inhibit DNA polymerase-γ, which is responsible for replication of mitochondrial DNA. Diminished mitochondrial function may lead to a decrease in oxidative phosphorylation, which in turn leads to aberrations in pyruvate metabolism and accumulation of lactate [75,77]. The spectrum of mitochondrial toxicity of NRTIs ranges from non-specific symptoms to lactic acidosis syndrome with fulminant hepatic failure. Symptoms include fatigue, abdominal bloating, anorexia and weight loss. Lactic acidosis syndrome is manifested by nausea, vomiting, and abdominal pain rapidly progressing to tachypnoea with severe acidosis. Liver function tests may be modestly elevated in this setting, often with AST more than ALT. Late recognition of this syndrome usually leads to a fatal outcome. The combination of didanosine and ribavirin may further enhance mitochondrial toxicity [40].

Hepatic steatosis and steatohepatitis. HIV-infected patients are at risk for hepatic steatosis. Steatosis is associated with insulin resistance, hyperlipidaemia and visceral adiposity [78]. This is noted in a high percentage of HIV-infected patients with the lipodystrophy syndrome [79]. Hepatic steatosis is highly prevalent in HIV seropositive patients, particularly in those with chronic hepatitis C and/or receiving NRTIs with high mitochondrial toxicity profiles (e.g. stavudine and didanosine) [80]. There is mild-to-moderate hepatic steatosis in many HIV patients with DILI [74]. HCV genotype 3 infection, which induces hepatic steatosis through a virally medi-

ated cytopathic effect, has been associated with an increased risk of DILI [81].

Non-cirrhotic portal hypertension. Severe liver disease in the absence of any recognizable aetiology has been reported occasionally in HIV individuals [82]. Patients may be found to have non-alcoholic fatty liver disease on liver biopsy [83]. Other HIV patients present with severe portal hypertension. This can be manifested clinically as gastrointestinal bleeding, pancytopenia, hypersplenism or varices on endoscopy. Liver biopsy in these cases has shown a variety of lesions, of which the most common is nodular regenerative hyperplasia [84] and hepatoportal sclerosis. These lesions are almost always noted in the absence of advanced liver fibrosis or cirrhosis. Characteristic histological lesions in the liver and prior exposure to didanosine are the main common features of this condition [82].

References

1 Weber R, Sabin CA, Friis-Moller N *et al.* Liver-related deaths in persons infected with the human immunodeficiency virus: the D: A: D study. *Arch. Intern. Med.* 2006; **166**: 1632–1641.

2 Overton ET, Sungkanuparph S, Powderly WG *et al.* Undetectable plasma HIV RNA load predicts success after hepatitis B vaccination in HIV-infected persons. *Clin. Infect. Dis.* 2005; **41**: 1045–1048.

3 Collier AC, Corey L, Murphy VL *et al.* Antibody to human immunodeficiency virus (HIV) and suboptimal response to hepatitis B vaccination. *Ann. Intern. Med.* 1988; **109**: 101–105.

4 Rivas P, Herrero MD, Puente S *et al.* Immunizations in HIV-infected adults. *AIDS Rev.* 2007; **9**: 173–187.

5 Hofer M, Joller-Jemelka HI, Grob PJ *et al.* Frequent chronic hepatitis B virus infection in HIV-infected patients positive for antibody to hepatitis B core antigen only. *Eur. J. Clin. Microbiol. Infect. Dis.* 1998; **17**: 6–13.

6 French AL, Lin MY, Evans CT *et al.* Long-term serologic follow-up of isolated hepatitis B core antibody in HIV-infected and HIV-uninfected women. *Clin. Infect. Dis.* 2009; **49**: 148–154.

7 Gandhi RT, Wurcel A, Lee H *et al.* Response to hepatitis B vaccine in HIV-1-positive subjects who test positive for isolated antibody to hepatitis B core antigen: implications for hepatitis B vaccine strategies. *J. Infect. Dis.* 2005; **191**: 1435–1441.

8 Koziel MJ, Peters MG. Viral hepatitis in HIV infection. *N. Engl. J. Med.* 2007; **356**: 1445–1454.

9 Hadler SC, Judson FN, O'Malley PM *et al.* Outcome of hepatitis B virus infection in homosexual men and its relation to prior human immunodeficiency virus infection. *J. Infect. Dis.* 1991; **163**: 454–459.

10 Peters MG, Andersen J, Lynch P *et al.* Randomized controlled study of tenofovir and adefovir in chronic hepatitis B virus and HIV infection: ACTG A5127. *Hepatology* 2006; **44**: 1110–1116.

11 Thio CL, Seaberg EC, Skolasky R, Jr *et al.* HIV-1, hepatitis B virus, and risk of liver-related mortality in the Multicenter Cohort Study (MACS). *Lancet* 2002; **360**: 1921–1926.

12 Hoffmann CJ, Seaberg EC, Young S *et al*. Hepatitis B and long-term HIV outcomes in coinfected HAART recipients. *AIDS* 2009; **23**: 1881–1889.

13 Idoko J, Meloni S, Muazu M *et al*. Impact of hepatitis B virus infection on human immunodeficiency virus response to antiretroviral therapy in Nigeria. *Clin. Infect. Dis.* 2009; **49**: 1268–1273.

14 Rockstroh JK, Bhagani S, Benhamou Y *et al*. European AIDS Clinical Society (EACS) guidelines for the clinical management and treatment of chronic hepatitis B and C coinfection in HIV-infected adults. *HIV Med.* 2008; **9**: 82–88.

15 Panel on Antiretroviral Guidelines for Adults and Adolescents. *Guidelines for the Use of Antiretroviral Agents in HIV-1-infected Adults and Adolescents*. Department of Health and Human Services, 2009.

16 Benhamou Y, Bochet M, Thibault V *et al*. Long-term incidence of hepatitis B virus resistance to lamivudine in human immunodeficiency virus-infected patients. *Hepatology* 1999; **30**: 1302–1306.

17 McMahon MA, Jilek BL, Brennan TP *et al*. The HBV drug entecavir - effects on HIV-1 replication and resistance. *N. Engl. J. Med.* 2007; **356**: 2614–2621.

18 Milazzo L, Caramma I, Lai A *et al*. Telbivudine in the treatment of chronic hepatitis B: experience in HIV type-1-infected patients naive for antiretroviral therapy. *Antivir. Ther.* 2009; **14**: 869–872.

19 Crane M, Oliver B, Matthews G *et al*. Immunopathogenesis of hepatic flare in HIV/hepatitis B virus (HBV)-coinfected individuals after the initiation of HBV-active antiretroviral therapy. *J. Infect. Dis.* 2009; **199**: 974–981.

20 Bertoletti A, Gehring AJ. The immune response during hepatitis B virus infection. *J. Gen. Virol.* 2006; **87**: 1439–1449.

21 Sulkowski MS, Mehta SH, Torbenson MS *et al*. Rapid fibrosis progression among HIV/hepatitis C virus-co-infected adults. *AIDS* 2007; **21**: 2209–2216.

22 Benhamou Y, Bochet M, Di MV *et al*. Liver fibrosis progression in human immunodeficiency virus and hepatitis C virus coinfected patients. The Multivirc Group. *Hepatology* 1999; **30**: 1054–1058.

23 Danta M, Brown D, Bhagani S *et al*. Recent epidemic of acute hepatitis C virus in HIV-positive men who have sex with men linked to high-risk sexual behaviours. *AIDS* 2007; **21**: 983–991.

24 Sherman KE, Rouster SD, Chung RT *et al*. Hepatitis C Virus prevalence among patients infected with Human Immunodeficiency Virus: a cross-sectional analysis of the US adult AIDS Clinical Trials Group. *Clin. Infect. Dis.* 2002; **34**: 831–837.

25 Thomas DL, Astemborski J, Rai RM *et al*. The natural history of hepatitis C virus infection: host, viral, and environmental factors. *JAMA* 2000; **284**: 450–456.

26 Soriano V, Puoti M, Sulkowski M *et al*. Care of patients coinfected with HIV and hepatitis C virus: 2007 updated recommendations from the HCV-HIV International Panel. *AIDS* 2007; **21**: 1073–1089.

27 Martin-Carbonero L, Benhamou Y, Puoti M *et al*. Incidence and predictors of severe liver fibrosis in human immunodeficiency virus-infected patients with chronic hepatitis C: a European collaborative study. *Clin. Infect. Dis.* 2004; **38**: 128–133.

28 Sulkowski MS, Thomas DL, Chaisson RE *et al*. Hepatotoxicity associated with antiretroviral therapy in adults infected with human immunodeficiency virus and the role of hepatitis C or B virus infection. *JAMA* 2000; **283**: 74–80.

29 Soriano V, Labarga P, Ruiz-Sancho A *et al*. Regression of liver fibrosis in hepatitis C virus/HIV-co-infected patients after treatment with pegylated interferon plus ribavirin. *AIDS* 2006; **20**: 2225–2227.

30 Uberti-Foppa C, De Bona A, Morsica G *et al*. Pretreatment of chronic active hepatitis C in patients coinfected with HIV and hepatitis C virus reduces the hepatotoxicity associated with subsequent antiretroviral therapy. *J. Acquir. Immune. Defic. Syndr.* 2003; **33**: 146–152.

31 de Ledinghen V, Douvin C, Kettaneh A *et al*. Diagnosis of hepatic fibrosis and cirrhosis by transient elastography in HIV/hepatitis C virus-coinfected patients. *J. Acquir. Immune. Defic. Syndr.* 2006; **41**: 175–179.

32 Sterling RK, Contos MJ, Sanyal AJ *et al*. The clinical spectrum of hepatitis C virus in HIV coinfection. *J. Acquir. Immune. Defic. Syndr.* 2003; **32**: 30–37.

33 Ge D, Fellay J, Thompson AJ *et al*. Genetic variation in IL28B predicts hepatitis C treatment-induced viral clearance. *Nature* 2009; **461**: 399–401.

34 Chung RT, Andersen J, Volberding P *et al*. Peginterferon Alfa-2a plus ribavirin versus interferon alfa-2a plus ribavirin for chronic hepatitis C in HIV-coinfected persons. *N. Engl. J. Med.* 2004; **351**: 451–459.

35 Torriani FJ, Rodriguez-Torres M, Rockstroh JK *et al*. Peginterferon Alfa-2a plus ribavirin for chronic hepatitis C virus infection in HIV-infected patients. *N. Engl. J. Med.* 2004; **351**: 438–450.

36 Torriani FJ, Ribeiro RM, Gilbert TL *et al*. Hepatitis C virus (HCV) and human immunodeficiency virus (HIV) dynamics during HCV treatment in HCV/HIV coinfection. *J. Infect. Dis.* 2003; **188**: 1498–1507.

37 Nunez M, Miralles C, Berdun MA *et al*. Role of weight-based ribavirin dosing and extended duration of therapy in chronic hepatitis C in HIV-infected patients: the PRESCO trial. *AIDS Res. Hum. Retroviruses* 2007; **23**: 972–982.

38 Alberti A, Clumeck N, Collins S *et al*. Short statement of the first European consensus conference on the treatment of chronic hepatitis B and C in HIV co-infected patients. *J. Hepatol.* 2005; **42**: 615–624.

39 Martin-Carbonero L, Nunez M, Marino A *et al*. Undetectable hepatitis C virus RNA at week 4 as predictor of sustained virological response in HIV patients with chronic hepatitis C. *AIDS* 2008; **22**: 15–21.

40 Ballesteros AL, Miro O, Lopez S *et al*. Mitochondrial effects of a 24-week course of pegylated-interferon plus ribavirin in asymptomatic HCV/HIV co-infected patients on long-term treatment with didanosine, stavudine or both. *Antivir. Ther.* 2004; **9**: 969–977.

41 Vispo E, Barreiro P, Pineda JA *et al*. Low response to pegylated interferon plus ribavirin in HIV-infected patients with chronic hepatitis C treated with abacavir. *Antivir. Ther.* 2008; **13**: 429–437.

42 Qurishi N, Kreuzberg C, Luchters G *et al*. Effect of antiretroviral therapy on liver-related mortality in patients with HIV and hepatitis C virus coinfection. *Lancet* 2003; **362**: 1708–1713.

43 Soriano V, Peters MG, Zeuzem S. New therapies for hepatitis C virus infection. *Clin. Infect. Dis.* 2009; **48**: 313–320.

44 Housset C, Pol S, Carnot F *et al*. Interactions between human immunodeficiency virus-1, hepatitis delta virus and

hepatitis B virus infections in 260 chronic carriers of hepatitis B virus. *Hepatology* 1992; **15**: 578–583.

45 Puoti M, Rossi S, Forleo MA *et al*. Treatment of chronic hepatitis D with interferon alpha-2b in patients with human immunodeficiency virus infection. *J. Hepatol.* 1998; **29**: 45–52.

46 Arribas JR, Gonzalez-Garcia JJ, Lorenzo A *et al*. Single (B or C), dual (BC or BD) and triple (BCD) viral hepatitis in HIV-infected patients in Madrid, Spain. *AIDS* 2005; **19**: 1361–1365.

47 Mathurin P, Thibault V, Kadidja K *et al*. Replication status and histological features of patients with triple (B, C, D) and dual (B, C) hepatic infections. *J. Viral Hepatol.* 2000; **7**: 15–22.

48 Raimondo G, Brunetto MR, Pontisso P *et al*. Longitudinal evaluation reveals a complex spectrum of virological profiles in hepatitis B virus/hepatitis C virus-coinfected patients. *Hepatology* 2006; **43**: 100–107.

49 Puoti M, Bruno R, Soriano V *et al*. Hepatocellular carcinoma in HIV-infected patients: epidemiological features, clinical presentation and outcome. *AIDS* 2004; **18**: 2285–2293.

50 Soriano V, Barreiro P, Martin-Carbonero L *et al*. Treatment of chronic hepatitis B or C in HIV-infected patients with dual viral hepatitis. *J. Infect. Dis.* 2007; **195**: 1181–1183.

51 Chakvetadze C, Bani-Sadr F, Le Pendeven C *et al*. Reactivation of hepatitis B virus replication during peginterferon-ribavirin therapy in an HIV/hepatitis C virus-co-infected patient with isolated anti-hepatitis B core antibodies. *AIDS* 2007; **21**: 393–394.

52 Roland ME, Stock PG. Liver transplantation in HIV-infected recipients. *Semin. Liver Dis.* 2006; **26**: 273–284.

53 Barnes PF, Bloch AB, Davidson PT *et al*. Tuberculosis in patients with human immunodeficiency virus infection. *N. Engl. J. Med.* 1991; **324**: 1644–1650.

54 Karakousis PC, Moore RD, Chaisson RE. Mycobacterium avium complex in patients with HIV infection in the era of highly active antiretroviral therapy. *Lancet Infect. Dis.* 2004; **4**: 557–565.

55 Centres for Disease Control and Prevention. Guidelines for Prevention and Treatment of Opportunistic Infections in HIV-Infected Adults and Adolescents. *MMWR* 2009; **58**: 1–207.

56 Huber F, Nacher M, Aznar C *et al*. AIDS-related Histoplasma capsulatum var. capsulatum infection: 25 years experience of French Guiana. *AIDS* 2008; **22**: 1047–1053.

57 Ustianowski AP, Sieu TP, Day JN. Penicillium marneffei infection in HIV. *Curr. Opin. Infect. Dis.* 2008; **21**: 31–36.

58 Rabaud C, May T, Amiel C *et al*. Extracerebral toxoplasmosis in patients infected with HIV. A French National Survey. *Medicine* (Baltimore) 1994; **73**: 306–314.

59 Keaveny AP, Karasik MS. Hepatobiliary and pancreatic infections in AIDS: Part one. *AIDS Patient Care STDS* 1998; **12**: 347–357.

60 Guiguet M, Boue F, Cadranel J *et al*. Effect of immunodeficiency, HIV viral load, and antiretroviral therapy on the risk of individual malignancies (FHDH-ANRS CO4): a prospective cohort study. *Lancet Oncol.* 2009; **10**: 1152–1159.

61 Monforte A, Abrams D, Pradier C *et al*. HIV-induced immunodeficiency and mortality from AIDS-defining and non-AIDS-defining malignancies. *AIDS* 2008; **22**: 2143–2153.

62 Brau N, Fox RK, Xiao P *et al*. Presentation and outcome of hepatocellular carcinoma in HIV-infected patients: a U.S.-Canadian multicenter study. *J. Hepatol.* 2007; **47**: 527–537.

63 Huang JS, Pan HB, Chou CP *et al*. Optimizing scanning phases in detecting small (<2 cm) hepatocellular carcinoma: whole-liver dynamic study with multidetector row CT. *J. Comput. Assist. Tomogr.* 2008; **32**: 341–346.

64 Nunez M, Soriano V. Hepatotoxicity of antiretrovirals: incidence, mechanisms and management. *Drug Saf.* 2005; **28**: 53–66.

65 Soriano V, Puoti M, Garcia-Gasco P *et al*. Antiretroviral drugs and liver injury. *AIDS* 2008; **22**: 1–13.

66 AIDS Clinical Trials Group. *Table for Grading Severity of Adult Adverse Experiences*. Rockville, MD: Division of AIDS, National Institute of Allergy and Infectious Diseases, 1996.

67 Lankisch TO, Moebius U, Wehmeier M *et al*. Gilbert's disease and atazanavir: from phenotype to UDP-glucuronosyltransferase haplotype. *Hepatology.* 2006; **44**: 1324–1332.

68 El-Sadr WM, Lundgren JD, Neaton JD *et al*. CD4+ count-guided interruption of antiretroviral treatment. *N. Engl. J. Med.* 2006; **355**: 2283–2296.

69 Reisler RB, Han C, Burman WJ *et al*. Grade 4 events are as important as AIDS events in the era of HAART. *J. Acquir. Immune. Defic. Syndr.* 2003; **34**: 379–386.

70 Kaplowitz N. Drug hepatotoxicity. *Sem. Liver Dis.* 1990; **10**: 234–235.

71 Torti C, Lapadula G, Puoti M *et al*. Influence of genotype 3 hepatitis C coinfection on liver enzyme elevation in HIV-1-positive patients after commencement of a new highly active antiretroviral regimen: results from the EPOKA-MASTER cohort. *J. Acquir. Immune. Defic. Syndr.* 2006; **41**: 180–185.

72 Nunez M, Lana R, Mendoza JL *et al*. Risk factors for severe hepatic injury after introduction of highly active antiretroviral therapy. *J. Acquir. Immune. Defic. Syndr.* 2001; **27**: 426–431.

73 Bonfanti P, Landonio S, Ricci E *et al*. Risk factors for hepatotoxicity in patients treated with highly active antiretroviral therapy. *J. Acquir. Immune. Defic. Syndr.* 2001; **27**: 316–318.

74 Aranzabal L, Casado JL, Moya J *et al*. Influence of liver fibrosis on highly active antiretroviral therapy-associated hepatotoxicity in patients with HIV and hepatitis C virus coinfection. *Clin. Infect. Dis.* 2005; **40**: 588–593.

75 Jain MK. Drug-induced liver injury associated with HIV medications. *Clin. Liver Dis.* 2007; **11**: 615–639, vii–viii.

76 Kaplowitz N. Drug-induced liver injury. *Clin. Infect. Dis.* 2004; **38** (Suppl. 2): S44–48.

77 Laguno M, Milinkovic A, de Lazzari E *et al*. Incidence and risk factors for mitochondrial toxicity in treated HIV/HCV-coinfected patients. *Antivir. Ther.* 2005; **10**: 423–429.

78 Sulkowski MS, Mehta SH, Torbenson M *et al*. Hepatic steatosis and antiretroviral drug use among adults coinfected with HIV and hepatitis C virus. *AIDS* 2005; **19**: 585–592.

79 Piroth L. Liver steatosis in HIV-infected patients. *AIDS Rev.* 2005; **7**: 197–209.

80 McGovern BH, Ditelberg JS, Taylor LE *et al*. Hepatic steatosis is associated with fibrosis, nucleoside analogue use, and hepatitis C virus genotype 3 infection in HIV-seropositive patients. *Clin. Infect. Dis.* 2006; **43**: 365–372.

81 Maida I, Babudieri S, Selva C *et al.* Liver enzyme elevation in hepatitis C virus (HCV)-HIV-coinfected patients prior to and after initiating HAART: role of HCV genotypes. *AIDS Res. Hum. Retroviruses* 2006; **22**: 139–143.

82 Maida I, Garcia-Gasco P, Sotgiu G *et al.* Antiretroviral-associated portal hypertension: a new clinical condition? Prevalence, predictors and outcome. *Antivir. Ther.* 2008; **13**: 103–107.

83 Ingiliz P, Valantin MA, Duvivier C *et al.* Liver damage underlying unexplained transaminase elevation in human immunodeficiency virus-1 mono-infected patients on antiretroviral therapy. *Hepatology* 2009; **49**: 436–442.

84 Mallet V, Blanchard P, Verkarre V *et al.* Nodular regenerative hyperplasia is a new cause of chronic liver disease in HIV-infected patients. *AIDS* 2007; **21**: 187–192.

CHAPTER 23
Autoimmune Hepatitis and Overlap Syndromes

Gideon M. Hirschfield & E. Jenny Heathcote
Liver Centre, Toronto Western Hospital, Toronto, ON, Canada

Learning points

- Autoimmune hepatitis remains a diagnosis reached after careful exclusion of other more common viral, metabolic and drug-induced liver disease.

- Patients may present with or without symptoms and classically have elevated transaminases, raised immunoglobulin G and positive autoantibodies (antinuclear and antismooth muscle antibodies).

- Careful histological evaluation remains important in establishing a diagnosis.

- Treatment with prednisone and azathioprine is generally very effective in the induction and maintenance of remission.

- Patients may demonstrate features of more than one autoimmune disease, so called overlap syndromes.

Introduction

Autoimmune hepatitis (AIH) is a poorly defined inflammatory liver disease, without a specific diagnostic marker. Clinically, serologically and histologically it represents a chronic relapsing hepatitis, associated with a plasma cell hepatic infiltrate, hypergammaglobulinaemia and positive autoantibodies. Exclusion of drug precipitants (prescribed or 'over the counter') and inherited metabolic liver disease in addition to confirmation of negative viral studies is required (Fig. 23.1).

Historical perspective. The concept of a 'chronic hepatitis' resulting in cirrhosis developed during the 20th century, with many proposed triggers including infections, alcohol, toxins or nutritional disease. A seemingly clinically distinct variant of chronic active hepatitis was recognized as affecting mostly women and children.

Appreciation for an autoimmune aetiology emerged in the 1940s as Waldenström [1] recognized the relevance of hypergammaglobulinaemia in chronic hepatitis, and Kunkel [2] described a persistent liver disease predominantly in young females with hypergammaglobulinaemia, alongside extrahepatic symptoms including rash, arthralgias, fever and amenorrhoea.

Serological testing in the 1950s supported an autoimmune aetiology for a proportion with chronic hepatitis. The lupus erythematous (LE) test was initially a diagnostic test for systemic lupus erythematosus (SLE), that later proved to be neither sensitive nor specific. Patients with active chronic liver disease and hypergammaglobulinaemia were found to have LE cells. The factor responsible for the phenomenon, noted when incubating the peripheral blood of a patient with LE cell factor, found in the bone marrow of patients with SLE, is a family of antinuclear antibodies (ANA) [3].

The laboratory findings suggestive of an immune-mediated disease prompted treatment with cortisone, and a marked symptomatic improvement was noted, suggesting an important inflammatory component to this disease. Prolonged immunosuppressive therapy with prednisolone and azathioprine, offered to patients from the 1960s onward, proved effective and remains standard therapy [4–6].

This presumed autoimmune liver disease was originally named lupoid hepatitis, a misleading label still occasionally used. Eventually, the term autoimmune hepatitis (AIH) was applied in 1965 by Cowling and Mackay, and endorsed globally in 1993.

Disease overview

Clinical manifestations. There is a broad spectrum of clinical manifestations, ranging from asymptomatic to fulminant hepatic failure with approaching 10% of patients presenting with acute liver failure. Although most patients present for medical attention at the onset

Sherlock's Diseases of the Liver and Biliary System, Twelfth Edition. Edited by James S. Dooley, Anna S.F. Lok, Andrew K. Burroughs, E. Jenny Heathcote.
© 2011 by Blackwell Publishing Ltd. Published 2011 by Blackwell Publishing Ltd.

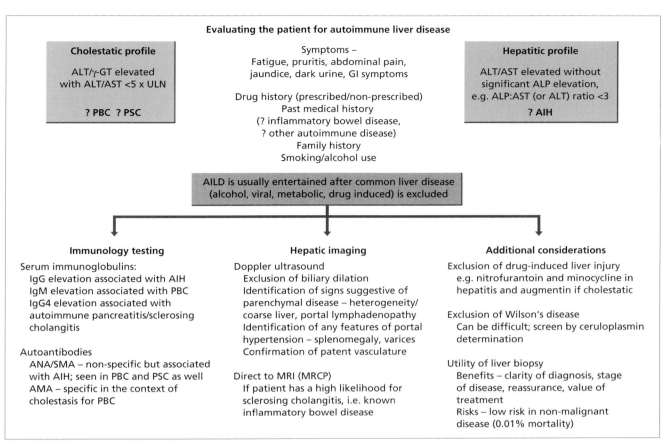

Evaluating the patient for autoimmune liver disease

Cholestatic profile

ALT/γ-GT elevated
with ALT/AST <5 x ULN

? PBC ? PSC

Symptoms –
Fatigue, pruritis, abdominal pain,
jaundice, dark urine, GI symptoms

Drug history (prescribed/non-prescribed)
Past medical history
(? inflammatory bowel disease,
? other autoimmune disease)
Family history
Smoking/alcohol use

Hepatitic profile

ALT/AST elevated without
significant ALP elevation,
e.g. ALP:AST (or ALT) ratio <3

? AIH

AILD is usually entertained after common liver disease
(alcohol, viral, metabolic, drug induced) is excluded

Immunology testing

Serum immunoglobulins:
IgG elevation associated with AIH
IgM elevation associated with PBC
IgG4 elevation associated with
autoimmune pancreatitis/sclerosing
cholangitis

Autoantibodies
ANA/SMA – non-specific but associated
with AIH; seen in PBC and PSC as well
AMA – specific in the context of
cholestasis for PBC

Hepatic imaging

Doppler ultrasound
Exclusion of biliary dilation
Identification of signs suggestive of
parenchymal disease – heterogeneity/
coarse liver, portal lymphadenopathy
Identification of any features of portal
hypertension – splenomegaly, varices
Confirmation of patent vasculature

Direct to MRI (MRCP)
If patient has a high likelihood for
sclerosing cholangitis, i.e. known
inflammatory bowel disease

Additional considerations

Exclusion of drug-induced liver injury
e.g. nitrofurantoin and minocycline in
hepatitis and augmentin if cholestatic

Exclusion of Wilson's disease
Can be difficult; screen by ceruloplasmin
determination

Utility of liver biopsy
Benefits – clarity of diagnosis, stage
of disease, reassurance, value of
treatment
Risks – low risk in non-malignant
disease (0.01% mortality)

Fig. 23.1. Evaluating a patient with autoimmune liver disease. ALP, alkaline phosphatase; ALT, alanine transaminase; AST, aspartate transaminase; ANA, antinuclear antibodies; AMA, antimitochrondial antibodies; MRCP, magnetic resonance cholangiopancreatography; MRI, magnetic resonance imaging; PBC, primary biliary cirrhosis; PSC, primary sclerosing cholangitis; γ-GT, γ-glutamyltransferase ; SMA, antismooth muscle antibodies.

of symptoms (fatigue, arthralgia, anorexia, jaundice), others are only found to have the disease incidentally. Whether all asymptomatic AIH progresses to symptomatic disease is not known, nor is there consensus on the significance in terms of outcome of the presence or absence of symptoms.

Clinical presentation and outcome varies between racial groups and geographical regions. Cirrhosis at presentation is more frequent in black North American patients with AIH than in white North Americans [7]. They are also younger at presentation, similar to patients from Brazil and Argentina. Africans, Asians and Arabs similarly have an earlier disease onset than patients from Northern Europe. Along with Alaskan natives, they additionally appear to have a higher frequency of cholestatic laboratory findings and of acute icteric disease.

The hepatitis may be chronic or present as intermittent episodes of apparently acute hepatitis.

Serology. Serological patterns of autoreactivity permit two major classifications of disease: type 1 is characterized by antinuclear (ANA) and/or antismooth muscle

(SMA) antibodies; type 2 by antiliver kidney microsomal type 1 (anti-LKM-1) antibodies. The identification of the antigen in type 2 disease, human cytochrome P450 2D6, has driven immunological dissection of the disease. Type 1 AIH lacks the same specificity, suggesting it comprises a number of different insults to the liver [8].

Epidemiology. Patients of all ages, both genders (female preponderance, with a ratio of about 4:1 for type 1 AIH, as compared to 9:1 for type 2 AIH) and all races may develop AIH. The prevalence of AIH is crudely estimated at 1.0–12 cases per 1 000 000 Caucasian Western European/North Americans; it appears to be markedly less common in Japan, whilst contemporary population-based estimates from Northern Europe (Sweden) estimates the annual incidence as 8.5 per 1 000 000 with a point prevalence of 107 per 1 000 000.

Natural history. Sherlock's follow-up study of 44 patients diagnosed between 1963 and 1967, who were randomly allocated into control and treatment (prednisolone) groups, provides stark natural history data for those

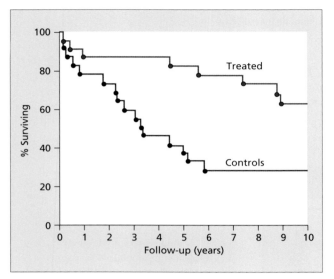

Fig. 23.2. Later results of the Royal Free Hospital trial of prednisolone in chronic autoimmune hepatitis. Note the improved survival in the treated group. (From [12].)

with severe disease. Ten-year survival data demonstrated a significantly improved survival in the treatment group, where 63% of patients were alive at 10 years (median survival 12.2 years) compared with only 27% (median survival 3.3 years) in the control group (Fig. 23.2). Untreated patients with mild hepatitis are said to have an approximately 1 in 5 chance of developing cirrhosis within 5 years and patients with mild-to-moderate laboratory disturbances have about a 50% chance of cirrhosis within 15 years but a 10-year survival of 90% [9–11,12].

Biological determinants of disease

Hepatic immunological tolerance is maintained in a number of ways, which include antigen priming in the liver, sinusoidal tolerance induction, induction of regulatory T cells and hepatic stellate cell-induced T-cell apoptosis. Loss of tolerance is precipitated as a result of a number of different events, which collectively culminate in a common final pathway towards liver injury. An interaction of host genetics and environmental triggers (infections, drugs, toxins) remains most probable. In animal studies the specific loss of tolerance to a known target autoantigen can be modelled by infection with hepatic adenovirus Ad5 expressing human cytochrome P450 2D6 [13].

Immunology. Data as a whole demonstrates a genetic predisposition, particularly associated with the HLA locus, systemic immunoregulatory changes notably affecting T regulatory (Treg) cell function and immune restricted responses to target antigens. Microscopic

evaluation of the liver demonstrates lymphocytes, macrophages, and plasma cells forming a portal mononuclear cell infiltrate that involves surrounding parenchyma to a varying degree (interface hepatitis). An antigen restricted immune-mediated injury is driven through a combination of cellular and antibody-dependent cytotoxicity. Patients have reduced numbers of peripheral Tregs, with decreased proliferative activity in response to stimulation. In patients with type 2 AIH, LKM antibody titres correlate with Treg numbers. Monocyte activation alongside this, also contributes to loss of tolerance and promotes chronicity [14].

Th1, Th2 and Th17 lymphocyte cell populations interact to generate disease; Th1 cells enhance expression of HLA class I and induce expression of HLA class II molecules on hepatocytes, Th2 cells favour autoantibody production by B lymphocytes and Th17 cells play a role in organ-specific autoimmune inflammation.

HLA loci and AIH. In European and North American Caucasians HLA-A1-B8, HLA-DRB1*0301 and HLA-DRB1*0401 are susceptibility loci. The alleles DRB1*0301 and DRB1*0401 encode a six-amino acid sequence at positions 67–72 in the DRβ polypeptide chain of the class II molecules of MHC. The amino acid lysine at position DRβ71 appears key [15]. Those over 60 years of age are more likely to have the HLA DRB1*04 allele, whilst the HLA A1-B8-DR3 haplotype is over-represented in men with AIH. The presence of HLA DRB1*03 has been shown as one of the characteristics associated with failure to respond to therapy [16].

As expected, HLA associations vary around the globe and may explain some of the differences in disease presentation; for example in Japan and Argentina, HLA-DRB1*0405 is associated with AIH, in Brazil, HLA-DRB1*1301 and DRB3*01 associate with disease whilst among Mestizo Mexicans, HLA-DRB1*0404 is predominant.

Non-HLA loci and AIH. Confident identification of non-HLA susceptibility loci will follow on from genomic analyses of large, well-characterized populations, studied in parallel to carefully chosen controls. The finding of other autoimmune diseases in patients and their relatives supports a genetic contribution to disease. Future studies may confirm already proposed candidate gene associations that are shared across autoimmune diseases such as type 1 diabetes, thyroid disease and primary biliary cirrhosis, for example the T-cell immunoregulatory receptor CTLA-4 [17].

Other immunoregulatory genes are probably based on the monogenetic association of AIH in the autoimmune polyglandular syndrome type 1 (APS1), which is a result of defects in a single gene, the autoimmune regulator type 1 (*AIRE-1*). This transcription factor

Table 23.1. Differential diagnosis for transaminitis

Drug-induced liver injury
Acute viral hepatitis
Chronic viral hepatitis (hepatitis B and C predominantly)
Steatohepatitis (alcoholic and non-alcoholic)
Autoimmune liver disease including overlap presentations
Coeliac disease
Hypothyroidism/ hyperthyroidism
Haemochromatosis
α-1-antitrypsin deficiency
Wilson's disease
Ischaemia (including Budd–Chiari)
Hepatic infiltration (malignant and non-malignant)

regulates clonal deletion of autoreactive T cells. Patients with APS1 suffer from mucocutaneous candidiasis and a number of organ-specific autoimmune diseases, including AIH [18].

Environmental and drug triggers. Environmental factors may include nutritional supplements/ herbal chemical compounds, drugs and viral infections. Drugs can induce both immunologically mediated hepatocellular and cholestatic liver disease.

Generally, liver injury results from the bioactivation of drugs to reactive metabolites, which may interact with cellular macromolecules, disrupt cellular signalling and lead to mitochondrial dysfunction. Phase 1 and 2 drug metabolism can induce immunological responses against haptens and autoepitopes of self-carrier proteins. Such injury occurs when enzyme–drug adducts migrate to the cell surface and form neoantigens, which become cytotoxic T-cell targets. The detection of antibodies that recognize drug-modified hepatic proteins in sera supports this, for example antibodies that recognize trifluoroacetate-altered hepatic proteins in the sera of patients with halothane-induced hepatitis [19]. Such drug-specific antibodies or autoantibodies that recognize native liver proteins have also been found in patients with liver injury caused by other drugs, including tienilic acid, dihydralazine and diclofenac [20].

In immunogenetically susceptible individuals, apoptosis of hepatocytes containing concentrated complexes of drug hapten-cytochrome P450, - UDP glucuronosyl transferase and/or other self-proteins facilitates effective presentation of autoantigens and loss of tolerance.

The *p-i* concept (*p*harmacological interaction of drugs/ chemicals with *i*mmune receptors) is also relevant and suggests certain drugs are able to bind to T-cell receptors, mimicking ligand–receptor interaction, so generating MHC-dependent T-cell activation. In patients who developed drug-induced hepatitis, drug-specific T cells have been detected and, in some cases, T-cell clones are generated (e.g. carbamazepine and halothane) [21].

Viral triggers. Viruses have repeatedly been shown to trigger autoimmune hepatitis, the best descriptions being following hepatitis A [22]. Careful history taking from patients can reveal viraemic symptoms prior to development of hepatitis. Sequence similarities between viral and self-proteins could trigger autoimmunity and the simultaneous presence of inflammatory cytokines during virus infection may add to the risk of developing self-perpetuating autoimmunity.

Disease presentation

General features. Since AIH presents at all ages, across men and women and in all races it needs to be considered in the differential of any hepatitis (Table 23.1).

Type 2 disease presents more acutely, at a younger age and immunoglobulin A deficiency is often noted, whereas symptoms, signs, family history, associated autoimmune diseases and treatment response are similar for both serological groups (Table 23.2) [23].

In childhood, sclerosing cholangitis with marked autoimmune features (called autoimmune sclerosing cholangitis by some), including interface hepatitis and serological features identical to type 1 AIH, is as common as AIH, but it affects boys and girls equally [24]. Differentiation relies on cholangiographic studies. It is not yet clear if these overlap cases have a worse outcome than AIH alone.

The fact that 30% of patients have cirrhosis at presentation, suggests clinically silent chronic hepatitis was probably present prior to diagnosis. Pathologists must be careful, however, not to mistake the acute collapse and architectural change of acute severe AIH (bridging necrosis) for cirrhosis.

Patterns of presentation. In a community study from California, approximately one-third had an acute onset of symptoms simulating acute viral hepatitis, half had chronic symptoms of greater than 6 months' duration, and the remaining patients were asymptomatic [25]. In an Italian study of just under 100 patients, two-thirds presented with a chronic pattern, one-quarter with an acute pattern, and a minority (1 in 20) were asymptomatic. All three groups though had a similar prevalence of moderate/ severe (versus mild) histological findings and liver cirrhosis [26].

The elderly may have an indolent progressive disease that is asymptomatic or masked by other concurrent conditions. There response to treatment is, however, the same.

Symptoms. When symptomatic, patients frequently note clinical jaundice, fatigue, arthralgias, arthritis, acne and amenorrhea. Acute presentations are often indistinguishable from a viral illness, and hepatic discomfort,

Table 23.2. Clinical differences between serological classifications of autoimmune hepatitis

	Type 1 AIH	Type 2 AIH
Relative prevalence	>80%	20% in Europe, 4% in USA
Autoantibodies commonly associated	ANA, SMA	LKM-1
Patient demographic	~70% women	Female predominance
Age of onset	Peak incidence 16–30 years, although 50% are older than 30 years	Average 10 years old but seen in adults, specifically in Europe
Other commonly associated autoimmune diseases	Prevalence of 17–48%: thyroid disease synovitis ulcerative colitis	Prevalence unclear: diabetes thyroid disease vitiligo pernicious anaemia IgA deficiency
Presentation	Acute onset rare	Frequently presents with cirrhosis in children and more aggressively
Response to treatment	Excellent response	May be more treatment resistant
Progression of disease	25% have cirrhosis at diagnosis; 45% develop cirrhosis	~80% develop cirrhosis

ANA, antinuclear antibodies; LKM-1, antiliver kidney microsomal type 1; SMA, antismooth muscle antibodies.

Table 23.3. Autoantibodies commonly associated with chronic liver disease

Autoantibody	Target	Notable association
Nucleus		
ANA	Nuclear membranes and DNA (general)	Type 1 AIH, PBC
Histones	Nucleosomes	Type 1 AIH, PBC
pANCA	Neutrophil granules	Type 1 AIH, PSC and PBC
Microsomal		
LKM-1	Mitochondrial enzyme CYP450 2D6	Type 2 AIH
Mitochondrial		
AMA	ATPase associated antigens of inner mitochondrial membrane	PBC, AIH
Smooth muscle		
SMA	Fibroblast actin, tubulin and intermediate filaments (general)	Type 1 AIH, PSC, PBC
Actin*	F-actin specifically	Type 1 AIH
Cytosol		
SLA/LP*	UGA repressor tRNA-associated protein	AIH
Liver cytosol-1*	Formiminotransferase cyclodeaminase	Type 2 AIH

*Cannot be measured outside research setting.
AIH, autoimmune hepatitis; ANA, antinuclear antibodies; AMA, antimitochrondial antibodies; SMA, antismooth muscle antibodies; LKM-1, antiliver kidney microsomal type 1; pANCA, perinuclear antineutrophil cytoplasmic antibody; PBC, primary biliary cirrhosis; PSC, primary sclerosing cholangitis; SLA/LP, soluble liver and pancreas antigen.

anorexia and nausea may be evident. Clinical features can range from firm hepatomegaly, splenomegaly (in which case a small liver is usually found) to other features of chronic liver disease including palmar erythema and telangiectasia.

Associated autoimmune diseases. Clinicians need to be aware of the possible association with other autoimmune disease that may be evident in as many as one in

three patients: Sjörgen's syndrome, autoimmune thyroid disease, autoimmune haemolysis, rheumatoid arthritis, ulcerative colitis and idiopathic thrombocytopenic purpura stand out. Coeliac disease can be coexistent, but care needs to be taken to ensure liver abnormalities are not secondary to coeliac disease itself.

Presentation after liver transplant. Autoimmune hepatitis can occur *de novo* after liver transplant (so called alloim-

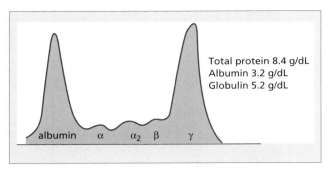

Fig. 23.3. Electrophoresis of the serum proteins. Note the very high γ-globulin.

mune hepatitis) or reoccur in those transplanted for AIH. Recurrences of autoimmune hepatitis, the development of an alloimmune phenomenon, or allograft dysfunction mimicking autoimmune hepatitis, are difficult to differentiate based on histological findings. Alloimmune hepatitis does not differ from recurrence of classic AIH based on serology, and they are treated similarly.

Laboratory features

Liver biochemistry and immunoglobulins. Elevated immunoglobulin G values (Fig. 23.3), commonly 1.2–3.0 times the upper limit, usually accompany a transaminitis, from minor elevations to levels in the thousands. In over 200 patients at one centre, aspartate aminotransferase levels at presentation were less than 2 times upper limit in just over 10%, 2 to 10 times upper limit in one-third and greater than 10 times the upper limit in just over half [27]. Elevated alkaline phosphatase values can be seen, but if greater than threefold, should prompt additional biliary investigation. Jaundice, coagulopathy and hypoalbuminaemia may be noted in very acute presentations. Haemolysis is a feature that should prompt exclusion of Wilson's disease.

Serology. Antinuclear antibodies and antismooth muscle antibodies categorize type 1 autoimmune hepatitis, whilst antibodies to liver and kidney microsome, mark the rarer, typically childhood-onset, type 2 autoimmune hepatitis (Table 23.3). Usual titres of serum autoantibodies are at or above 1 in 40–80, but found in isolation they have low positive predictive values since the prevalence of autoantibodies in healthy individuals exceeds the burden of disease; their presence also increases with age. Lower titres, at or above 1 in 20, are of significance only in children. Seronegative disease may also occur (Fig. 23.4).

Antinuclear antibodies. ANA are present alone (approximately 10%) or with SMA (approximately 50%) in two-

thirds of patients. ANA comprises antibodies with reactivity directed against nuclear membranes and DNA, although the target antigens are heterogeneous and incompletely defined, for example centromeres, ribonucleoproteins and cyclin A. Nuclear reactivity can be assessed by indirect immunofluorescence on Hep-2 cell lines or by enzyme-linked immunosorbent assay (ELISA) with recombinant or highly purified antigens. Classic AIH is associated with homogenous, speckled and nucleolar patterns. ANAs in AIH are not specific, unlike in primary biliary cirrhosis (PBC), and therefore assessment by immunofluorescence is preferable to use of ELISA-based automated assays.

Smooth muscle antibodies. SMA are directed against actin and non-actin components, including tubulin, vimentin, desmin and skeletin. SMA are present in approximately 90% of patients with AIH, either as the sole marker of the disease (approximately one-third) or in conjunction with ANA (approximately half). However SMA is very non-specific, and low titre antibody results are frequent in healthy individuals, particularly in those over 60 years of age, as well as those with an assortment of viral, autoimmune or malignant disease. Anti-F-actin antibodies, determined by ELISA, are more specific for type 1 AIH but assays are not universally available [28].

ANA and SMA levels fluctuate during the course of AIH and may disappear with corticosteroid therapy. Neither their titre at diagnosis nor their fluctuation during the course of illness predicts outcome in adult patients, and thus they are only of diagnostic value.

Microsomal antibodies. Different targeted autoantigens produce distinct microsomal immunofluorescence patterns leading to four subclassifications of LKM-1. LKM-1 (associated with type 2 AIH) reacts with the mitochondrial enzyme cytochrome P450 2D6 subtype (CYP2D6), inhibiting its activity *in vivo* [29]. CYP2D6 metabolizes several known medications, including antihypertensives and benzodiazepines, and is genetically polymorphic. LKM-2 reacts with CYP450 2C9 and has been associated with the hepatitis caused by the medication ticrynafen (tienilic acid), taken off the US market in 1982. LKM-3, which has affinity to uridine diphosphate glucuronosyl transferase, was previously associated with chronic hepatitis D, and LKM-4, which recognizes CYP1A2 and CYP2A6 (with an immunofluorescence pattern indistinguishable from LKM-1), has been described in patients with AIH associated with autoimmune polyendocrinopathy–candiasis–ectodermal dystrophy.

In practice, it is possible to misinterpret LKM-1 staining for antimitochrondial antibody (AMA), and recourse to an ELISA-based LKM-1 assay may be required.

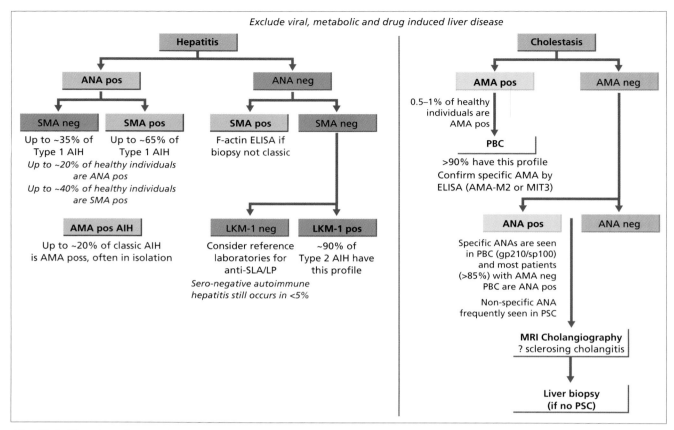

Fig. 23.4. Use of serology to distinguish patterns of autoimmune liver disease. ANA, antinuclear antibodies; AMA, antimitochrondial antibodies; ELISA, enzyme-linked immunosorbent assay; LKM-1, antiliver kidney microsomal type 1; PBC, primary biliary cirrhosis; PSC, primary sclerosing cholangitis; SMA, antismooth muscle antibodies.

Antibodies to LKM-1 are rare in the USA, occurring in only 4% of adults with AIH. They have been described mainly in paediatric patients in Europe, but 20% of patients with anti-LKM-1 in France and Germany are adults. Anti-LKM-1 and anti-LC-1 (liver cytosol) can occur alone or together in type 2 AIH. Anti-LC-1 recognizes formiminotransferase cyclodeaminase, a liver-specific 58-kDa metabolic enzyme [30].

Soluble liver and pancreas antigen. A third subtype of AIH (type 3) is occasionally described, based serologically on the presence of autoantibodies against soluble liver and pancreas antigen (SLA/LP). The two autoantibodies target the same antigen. Initially, individuals who were SLA/LP positive were classified as type 3 AIH, since it was observed first among patients negative for ANA, SMA and LKM. However three-quarters of patients with so-called type 3 AIH are also ANA and/or SMA positive, and clinically these individuals are indistinct from those with type 1 disease; conversely 10–30% of patients with type 1 AIH when tested are SLA/LP positive.

Anti-SLA/LP is a better marker of AIH than ANA or SMA, since normal individuals and those with non-hepatic disorders are invariably anti-LP negative. SLA/LP autoantibodies target a UGA-suppressor tRNA-associated protein, demonstrated to function as a selenocysteinyl-transfer RNA synthase [31].

Mitochondrial antibodies. Antimitochondrial antibodies may be found in AIH in as many as 20% of patients. They are usually lower in titre (≤1:40) and in some represent false positives misinterpreted by indirect immunofluorescence. The presence of AMA must not be directly taken to imply an AIH–PBC overlap syndrome. Long-term study of patients with AIH who are persistently AMA positive shows these individuals to have the same laboratory, histological and clinical features, as well as the same treatment outcomes compared to individuals who are AMA negative [32].

New markers remain to be identified and the advent of powerful tools such as proteomics has potential in this regard, for example the identification of phosphoglycerate mutase isozyme B as a putative target of autoantibodies in autoimmune hepatitis [33].

Imaging

Imaging is unlikely to help in the diagnosis of AIH but it is of use in excluding important differential diagnoses, in particular acute Budd–Chiari, infiltrative disease and unsuspected biliary processes. Doppler ultrasound is the initial investigation of choice as no radiation exposure is involved. In those with an acute/ subacute presentation of autoimmune hepatitis there is often marked histological architectural collapse. Radiologically, this may give a pseudocirrhotic appearance in the absence of true cirrhosis. Furthermore, in those with subacute liver failure, splenomegaly and ascites can be present without true chronic liver disease.

Biliary overlap is variably reported, more commonly in those presenting in childhood, suggesting that MR cholangiography should be routinely considered for those with AIH [34,35]. Careful interpretation is needed, as those with a cirrhotic liver may have peripheral secondary biliary changes consequent on architectural distortion, which resemble those of sclerosing cholangitis.

Periportal lymphadenopathy is a common finding in those with autoimmune liver disease and is rarely lymphoma, despite it commonly being raised by radiologists in the differential diagnosis. In those with a marked hepatitis, non-specific gallbladder wall thickening should not be mistaken for cholecystitis.

Cirrhosis regardless of aetiology is a risk factor for hepatocellular carcinoma [36], and those with biopsy proven cirrhosis or imaging highly suggestive after initial presentation may be considered for hepatocellular carcinoma surveillance programmes. However, hepatocellular carcinoma is generally considered uncommon in those with cirrhosis due to AIH (perhaps because patients are predominantly female and their disease is treated) and there are no data to demonstrate surveillance must be performed; individualized decisions remain reasonable.

Additionally, on treatment, imaging periodically is appropriate; historic data suggests 30% of patients progress histologically despite therapy [37]. A change in spleen size, alongside thrombocytopenia, is a useful parameter to evaluate when determining the need for variceal surveillance.

Liver biopsy and histological features

Few would be confident to diagnose and manage autoimmune hepatitis in the absence of histology.

Occasionally, there are scenarios where a presumptive diagnosis is made without a liver biopsy such as when overt contraindications to percutaneous biopsy exist or transjugular biopsy is not available. Generally, however, a liver biopsy should always be performed to identify features suggestive of AIH, to exclude alternative liver disease (in particular viral inclusions, vascular disease, steatohepatitis, alcoholic hepatitis, infiltration by lymphoma or adenocarcinoma, and for the potential to determine liver copper content), as well as to estimate fibrosis.

Those with access to laparoscopic biopsy have become aware that the disease is not necessarily homogenous. To minimize sampling error, care to obtain adequately sized liver specimens (≥2.5 cm) is essential as both parenchymal and biliary evaluation are important. Pretreatment histological findings may help predict outcomes [38] whilst liver biopsy is also used to confirm resolution of histological activity before stopping therapy with steroids. Histological activity commonly lags behind biochemical response by 3–6 months [6]. Portal plasma cell infiltrates, whilst on immunosuppressant therapy, are associated with relapse upon stopping treatment. However, an inactive biopsy does not equate with an absent risk of relapse.

Histological features. These include lymphoplasmacytic interface hepatitis (mononuclear cell infiltrate invading the limiting plate, i.e. the sharply demarcated hepatocyte boundary surrounding the portal triad), lobular hepatitis and centrilobular necrosis but the appearance of autoimmune hepatitis remains the same as that of chronic hepatitis, and although certain changes are common, no findings are specific (Figs 23.5–23.7). It is therefore usual for reports to conclude that the features are consistent with AIH, but viral and drug-induced liver injury cannot be excluded. Clinicians need to ensure that their pathologists pay close attention to biliary features, as it is not infrequent for patients with PBC to have interface activity and be initially reported as having autoimmune hepatitis.

Simplified grading. In a new, simplified scoring system, histology was graded atypical, compatible with AIH and typical. Interface hepatitis, lymphocytic/ lymphoplasmocytic infiltrates in portal tracts and extending into the lobule, emperipolesis (active penetration by one cell into

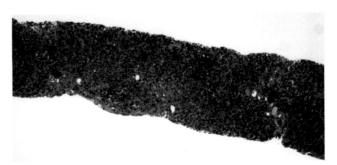

Fig. 23.5. Gross histological features of autoimmune hepatitis. (H & E, ×50.) Image provided by Dr Oyedele Adeyi, Staff Pathologist, Ass. Professor, Department of Laboratory Medicine & Pathobiology, University of Toronto.

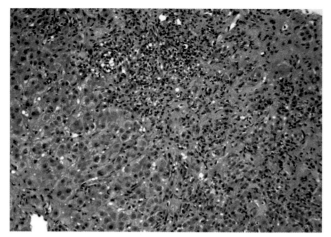

Fig. 23.6. Plasma-cell-rich hepatitis in acute autoimmune hepatitis. (H & E, ×100.) Image provided by Dr Oyedele Adeyi, Staff Pathologist, Ass. Professor, Department of Laboratory Medicine & Pathobiology, University of Toronto.

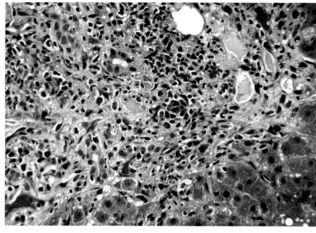

Fig. 23.8. Trichrome staining demonstrating marked interface hepatitis in acute autoimmune hepatitis, with plasma cell infiltration and incidental duct injury. (×200.) Image provided by Dr Oyedele Adeyi, Staff Pathologist, Ass. Professor, Department of Laboratory Medicine & Pathobiology, University of Toronto.

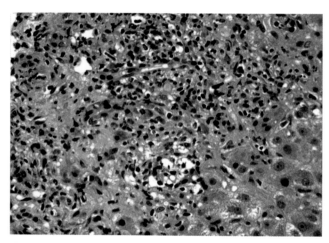

Fig. 23.7. Interface hepatitis, a characteristic lesion in autoimmune hepatitis. (H & E, ×200.) Image provided by Dr Oyedele Adeyi, Staff Pathologist, Ass. Professor, Department of Laboratory Medicine & Pathobiology, University of Toronto.

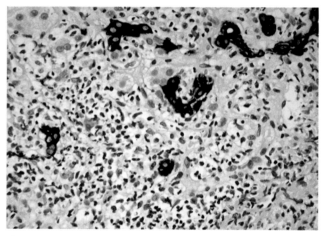

Fig. 23.9. Cytokeratin 7 stain demonstrating bile duct injury in acute-onset autoimmune hepatitis. Image provided by Dr Oyedele Adeyi, Staff Pathologist, Ass. Professor, Department of Laboratory Medicine & Pathobiology, University of Toronto.

and through a larger cell) and hepatic rosette formation were regarded as typical for the diagnosis of AIH. To be considered typical, each of the three features of classic AIH histology had to be present. Compatible features are a chronic hepatitis with lymphocytic infiltration without all the features considered usual. Histology was considered atypical when showing signs of another diagnosis, such as steatohepatitis, a condition that will increasingly coexist with AIH and confound evaluation [39].

Biliary lesions. The portal lesion generally spares the biliary tree but up to approximately 10% of biopsies may show duct destruction (not associated with detectable mitochondrial antibodies), and an additional approximately 10% show lymphocytic infiltration of bile duct

epithelium without ductopenia [40]. The histological pattern of injury may be indistinguishable from PBC. Just as the presence of antimitochondrial antibody does not mean the patient has PBC, nor are biliary changes synonymous with a diagnosis of an AIH–PBC overlap syndrome. All features need to be considered in the context of the presentation of the particular patient, including the severity of the underlying liver disease (Figs 23.8, 23.9).

Fibrosis and necroinflammatory activity. Some degree of fibrosis is almost always present. With disease progression, periportal fibrosis with formation of portal–portal and portal–central bridges and nodular regeneration results in cirrhosis. The severity of necroinflammatory activity is variable, ranging from mildly active hepatitis to bridging necrosis to massive hepatic necrosis (which should not be mistaken for cirrhosis). The degree of hepatocyte necrosis is not sufficiently reliable to determine prognosis, as sampling variation is common in those with an acute liver injury.

Ballooning degeneration, spotty hepatocyte necrosis, and apoptotic bodies are common but not specific. Syncytial multinucleated hepatocyte giant cells are seen in some, and giant cell hepatitis, seen more in children, is frequently, but not always, a variant of AIH. Giant cell hepatitis is also noted in atypical viral infections (reportedly paramyxoviral infection and human herpesvirus 6) as well as occasionally in PBC and drug-induced liver injury.

Surrogate markers of fibrosis. Non-invasive markers of liver fibrosis may have potential in the future. However validation will, be necessary and it will be important to evaluate the effects of active inflammation on any derived score. It should not be assumed that performance characteristics of non-invasive markers will be the same across diseases, genders and clinical scenarios. Liver stiffness is known to increase during hepatitic illnesses suggesting transient elastography during active hepatitis would potentially overestimate fibrosis stage at diagnosis in many patients.

Differential diagnosis

In the absence of a marker equivalent to a viral load, AIH is still a diagnosis of exclusion, and one traditionally confirmed by adequate response to treatment. Relapse off treatment can also be seen as confirmation of a correct diagnosis.

When evaluating the patient the clinician must remain vigilant for viral, drug and metabolic (e.g. Wilson's disease) presentations that can mimic AIH. The natural history of such insults can make it appear that the processes are steroid responsive if treatment is started on the assumption the disease is AIH. Re-evaluation of patients that do not respond to therapy as expected, is also important, although more often than not this is related to compliance rather than an alternative diagnosis.

Drug injury. It is not always possible to adequately exclude drug-induced liver injury, especially in those patients prescribed numerous simultaneous medications or taking unlicensed/ poorly defined herbal or nutritional supplements (see Chapter 24). Appropriate time must be given to charting all potential noxious agents, sometimes repeating the evaluation on more than one occasion, and asking patients to bring with them all substances taken. Perceptions of medications vary between patients and clinicians—apparently innocent use of cold and flu remedies may spark no concern

in a patient but still be relevant to the physician. Drug-related injury can mimic every clinical, biochemical, serological and histological feature of AIH. It is impossible to determine with complete certainty whether a drug or herbal apparently associated with AIH is responsible for precipitating the illness, or if the drug-induced illness is on a background of inherited predisposition. It is also possible that an individual previously had silent AIH that had remained undetected until evaluation.

Clinically, care must be taken to examine for significant lymphadenopathy, rash or neurological changes. Peripheral blood eosinophilia may suggest a drug injury; the so-called DRESS syndrome (drug rash with eosinophilia and systemic symptoms) includes a hepatitis in half of these cases.

The first implicated drug for a clear AIH like illness was the laxative DialosePlus®, with oxyphenisatin, a component proving to be the offending compound. Hepatotoxicity was noted as early as 1949 with later reports [41] demonstrating the association between the intake of oxyphenisatin and a marked increase in serum liver enzymes, serum bilirubin, globulin levels, positive ANA, SMA, LE cell test and a histological chronic hepatitis, which improved after drug withdrawal.

No list of potential hepatotoxic drugs can be complete (Tables 23.4, 23.5). Herbal and nutritional compounds are also reported to associate with an AIH-like liver disease, but the strength of the association may be hard to determine. The more common drugs reported to cause liver disease that resembles type 1 AIH include oxyphenisatin, nitrofurantoin, minocycline, α-methyldopa and clometacine. Drugs reported to cause liver disease that resembles type 2 AIH include dihydralazine, tienilic acid and halothane. New biological agents such as the anti-TNF monoclonal antibodies have also been reported to precipitate AIH, although the mechanism may differ, as the mode of activity of the drug probably alters normal immune function. Lists of further offending agents include atomoxetine (Strattera), benzarone,

Table 23.4. Drugs implicated in precipitating an autoimmune like hepatitis

Minocycline
Nitrofurantoin
Statins
Anti-TNF agents
Interferon-α
Indometacin
Ramipril
Terbinafine
Orlistat
Dihydralazine
Methyldopa
Halothane

Table 23.5. Herbal remedies noted to be associated with hepatotoxicity

Artemesia	Ma huang
Atractylis	Margosa oil
Black cohosh	Mistletoe
Callilepis	Noni (*Morinda citrifolia*)
Camellia sinensis (Chinese tea extracts)	Oil of cloves
Camphor	Onshido
Cascara sagrada	*Paeonia*
Chaparral leaf	Pennyroyal
Chaso	Plantango
Chrysanthemum	*Mentha pulegium*
Comfrey	Radix polygoni multiflori
Compositae	Radix tripterygii
Crotalaria	Red peony root
Dai-saiko-to	Rhizoma *Dioscorea bulbifera*
Fructus toosendan	Sassafras
	Saw palmetto
Fructus xanthii	*Scolopendra*
Gardenia	Semen cassiae
Germander	*Senecio* (groundsel)
Greater celandine	Senna
Hares' ear	Sho-saiko-to
Heliotropium (hathisunda)	Shou-wu-pian
Herba *Polygalae chinensis*	Skullcap
Hydroxycut	*Symphytum officinale*
Impila	*Teucrium chamaedrys*
Isabgol	*Teucrium polium*
Jin bu huang	*Tussilago farfara*
Kava Kava	Valerian root
LIV.52	

diclofenac, fenofibrate, 3-hydroxy-3-methyl-glutaryl-CoA reductase (HMG-CoA) reductase inhibitors (atorvastatin, rosuvastation, simvastatin), pemoline and phenprocoumon. Herbals may include dai-saiko-to, germander, 3,4-methylenedioxymetamphetamine ('ecstasy'), *Morinda citrifolia* (noni juice), black cohosh, *Echinacea* and chaparral leaf.

Viral hepatitis. Screening for hepatitis B and C is now universally available. Appropriate testing is necessary and for acute hepatitis B it is important to screen for HBsAg and anti-HBc IgM. Acute hepatitis C can be associated with fluctuating serology and repeat testing may be appropriate; serology (anti-HCV) can be negative, especially early after exposure, and HCV RNA is usually detected first. Immunocompromised patients may test negative for anti-HCV for much longer. Another unique characteristic of acute HCV infection is the fluctuation of HCV RNA levels, very low levels being frequently encountered. Consideration should also be given to hepatitis A, E, Epstein–Bar virus, adenovirus and parvovirus when screening for viral disease, particularly if clinically there is doubt as to the diagnosis. If giant cell changes are noted, testing for paramyxovirus or human herpes 6 virus should be considered. HIV status can be relevant, especially as immune reconstitution with highly active antiretroviral agents may lead to autoimmune disease, as well as reports of drug-induced AIH.

Wilson's disease. This autosomal recessive inherited liver disease of copper metabolism must be considered in all those with a transaminitis, histological hepatitis, steatohepatitis or cryptogenic cirrhosis if alternative aetiologies are not found. Previous assertions that age over 40 excludes Wilson's disease are now known to be incorrect. With an acute presentation of Wilson's disease all the features of AIH, including raised globulins, smooth muscle antibodies and an active histological hepatitis, may be observed. Identifying the best screening test for Wilson's disease is troublesome. Careful interpretation of urine copper excretion and liver copper estimation are most valuable; Kaiser–Fleischer rings are much less sensitive for liver disease than for neurological disease in those with Wilson's disease. Noting a relatively low alkaline phosphatase, particularly in those presenting with acute liver disease can help. Coexistent haemolysis is always a clear sign that Wilson's disease needs to be excluded. Genetic testing, can identify at least one mutation in 98% of patients, but is not usually accessible in a timely manner. Coexistent AIH and Wilson's disease has also been reported.

α-1-antitrypsin deficiency. This metabolic disease has a wide range of presentations including hepatitis, cholestasis and cirrhosis. In children it represents an additional differential diagnosis for autoimmune hepatitis; in adults an inactive cirrhosis is more usual. The combination of serum testing and typical histology (in particular the periportal red hyaline globules seen with periodic acid-Schiff stain) should rapidly confirm alpha 1 anti-trypsin deficiency.

Lupus. There is no such disease as lupoid hepatitis despite ongoing perceptions amongst some rheumatologists. SLE is commonly considered in patients with arthralgias in particular, but the presence of anti-dsDNA autoantibodies is a feature of AIH. In SLE the commonest reason for elevated liver enzymes is non-alcoholic fatty liver disease.

Alcohol. There is rarely any difficulty in distinguishing alcoholic hepatitis and autoimmune hepatitis, but regardless clinicians must document alcohol intake assiduously and pathologists must identify steatohepatitis and Mallory inclusions. However clinicians need not, expect their patients to be tee-total in the long term, although abstinence whilst symptomatic is of course sensible.

Diagnostic dilemmas

Autoantibody-negative patients. Approximately 10–20% of AIH patients are initially seronegative for the conventional autoantibodies, which may appear after a few weeks or even after immunosuppressive therapy is begun, or remain negative despite repeat testing. Evaluation for the highly specific anti-SLA/LP antibodies, if available, should be considered [42]. The presence of ANAs or SMAs does not correlate with the clinical or histological severity of AIH at diagnosis, but the degree of hypergammaglobulinaemia may do (rarely may not be present at diagnosis). Furthermore, no correlation exists between antibody status and response to immunosuppressive therapy exists. If patients meet the diagnosis of AIH based on other criteria, they should be considered for immunosuppressive therapy, regardless of antibody status [43].

Viral hepatitis. Twenty to forty per cent of patients with chronic HBV of HCV are persistently positive for various autoantibodies, usually, but not always, at low titres (1:20 or 1:40) [44]. Distinction of chronic viral hepatitis from AIH is important, because interferon therapy can potentially exacerbate autoimmune conditions, and corticosteroids can enhance viral replication. LKM was recognized as an antibody prevalent in HCV disease, which generated much debate. Though found in 50–86% of German and Italian patients with HCV, LKM has only been found in 1% of Western European and US patients with HCV infection. There is homology between the CYP450 2D6 and the HCV viral genome, possibly suggesting molecular mimicry. Patients with LKM-1 who are infected with HCV have less serological reactivity to recombinant CYP2D6 than do patients who are HCV negative. This suggests that the LKM antibodies in these two diseases are different. The fine specificities of LKM-1 antibodies in AIH have been shown to be different to those in HCV [45]. The

current general consensus is that interferon therapy is safe in patients with HCV with anti-LKM1 autoantibodies and/or ANA/SMA, and that serological features of autoimmunity are not related to interferon-related outcomes [46]. Where doubt remains, histological evaluation by a specialist hepatobiliary pathologist is valuable.

Coeliac disease. Gluten enteropathy is generally more common than previously recognized, with an estimated prevalence of approximately 1% in North America. It can be seen coincidentally with liver disease, or may itself be a cause of liver test abnormalities and liver dysfunction, with a prevalence of coeliac disease in those with cryptogenic cirrhosis estimated at 4% [47]. However, coeliac disease has been described in approximately 6% of individuals with AIH and in 3% with primary sclerosing cholangitis (PSC). The prevalence of PBC in coeliac disease is around 3%, whereas the prevalence of coeliac disease (diagnosed by small bowel biopsy) in PBC is approximately 6%. The false-positive rate of antitissue transglutaminase antibody testing has however been estimated to be nearly 50% in those with PBC and AIH, depending on the assay used. Therefore when testing for coeliac disease in patients with autoimmune liver disease, small bowel biopsy must follow a positive anti-tissue transglutaminase test.

Making a diagnosis in practice

In the absence of specific clinical and biochemical findings a diagnosis of AIH must be reached by a systematic and careful evaluation of the patient, and exclusion of alternative diagnoses, since diagnosis potentially commits a patient to lifelong immunosuppressive therapy. Clinical scoring systems (Tables 23.6, 23.7) can help although sometimes their origins relate to research driven concerns rather than routine clinical practice. No scoring system can replace the necessity to evaluate patients rigorously; all emphasize the importance of a liver biopsy (unless too unsafe to perform).

International Autoimmune Hepatitis Group (IAIHG). This is a group of clinicians who together created a diagnostic scoring system to objectively identify patients with either definite or probable AIH, and to exclude patients with biliary disease. The primary purpose was to allow research studies on well-defined patients, and not to generate a clinician friendly algorithm, as it included over 18 variables. It encompassed the varied disease onset, the wide spectrum of signs and symptoms, the variable serum aminotransferase levels and the inconsistency of autoantibodies. The presence of confounders such as alcohol, viruses and drug use is difficult to categorise. The original scoring system was shown to

Table 23.6. Revised diagnostic criteria for autoimmune hepatitis [48]

Category	Factor	Score
Gender	Female	+2
ALP: AST (or ALT) ratio	>3	–2
	<1.5	+2
Globulins or IgG (×upper limit of normal)	>2	+3
	1.5–2.0	+2
	1.0–1.5	+1
	<1.0	0
ANA, SMA or anti-LKM-1 titres	>1:80	+3
	1:80	+2
	1:40	+1
	<1:40	0
AMA	Positive	–4
Hepatotoxic drugs	Yes	–4
	No	+1
Alcohol	<25 g/day	+2
	>60 g/day	–2
Concurrent immune disease	Any non-hepatic disease of an immune nature	+2
Other autoantibodies	Anti-SLA/LP, actin, LC1, p-ANCA	+2
Histological features	Interface hepatitis	+3
	Plasma cells	+1
	Rosettes	+1
	None of above	–5
	Biliary changes	–3
	Atypical features	–3
HLA	DR3 or DR4	+1
Treatment response	Remission alone	+2
	Remission with relapse	+3
Pretreatment score		
Definite diagnosis		>15
Probable diagnosis		10–15
Post-treatment score		
Definite diagnosis		>17
Probable diagnosis		12–17

ALP, alkaline phosphatase; ALT, alanine transaminase; AST, aspartate transaminase; ANA, antinuclear antibodies; AMA, antimitochrondial antibodies; pANCA, perinuclear antineutrophil cytoplasmic antibody; SMA, antismooth muscle antibodies; LKM-1, antiliver kidney microsomal type 1; SLA/LP, soluble liver and pancreas antigen.

Table 23.7. Simplified criteria for diagnosing autoimmune hepatitis [39]

Variable	Cut-off	Points	Cut-off	Points
ANA or SMA	≥1:40	1	≥1:80	
LKM	–	–	≥1:40	2
SLA	–	–	Positive	
IgG	>ULN	1	>1.1 × ULN	2
Histology	Compatible	1	Typical	2
Absence of viral hepatitis	–	–	Yes	2

*Addition of points achieved for all autoantibodies (maximum, 2 points).
Probable AIH ≥ 6 points; definite AIH ≥ 7 points.

have a very high sensitivity, ranging from 97% to 100% for diagnosis of AIH in North America, Europe and Japan. The overall diagnostic accuracy of the scoring system is nearly 90%. A revised IAIHG score, published in 1999, did improve diagnostic accuracy for AIH, alongside exclusion of biliary disease, but remained unwieldy [48].

2008 Simplified Scoring System. A further simplified, clinically useful scoring system was published in 2008 [39] based on two cohorts of patients: a training set (n = 250) and a validation set (n = 109; including 10 'overlap patients'). Univariate analysis showed that immunoglobulin G levels, SMA and liver histology were good discriminators of AIH; immunoglobulin M (IgM), AMA and ANA titres and gender were less useful. Stepwise logistic regression identified the best predictors for AIH to be ANA and SMA titres, IgG levels and liver histology. When applied to a validation cohort this simplified system had an 88% sensitivity and 97% specificity (cut off ≥6) and 81% sensitivity and 99% specificity (cut off ≥7). Lack of standardization, particularly in autoantibody testing, remains a limitation for clinicians, as may access to experienced liver pathologists. Neither approach has formally taken Wilson's disease into account.

Management strategies

Corticosteroid therapy has been used since the 1950s, with an appreciation over time that steroids improve symptoms, biochemistry (serial monitoring of serum aspartate transaminase levels on treatment demonstrate rapid reductions in levels, often within hours) and survival. The relapsing course off steroids confirmed a need for long-term maintenance therapy using agents that spare steroid use, most commonly azathioprine or 6-mercaptopurine. The major trials evaluating immuno-suppressive therapy in AIH are relatively old, focus on treating advanced symptomatic disease but never-theless provide robust evidence that steroids give survival benefit [4–6]. Further follow-up data from randomized studies support sustained steroid-induced remission (normal transaminases, immunoglobulin G and inactive histology) [12] on maintenance with aza-thioprine, for over 90% of Type 1 patients [49–52]. Clinicians still face treatment conundrums for patients with less severe disease as there are evidence-based gaps to practice.

Who and how to treat AIH? The absolute indications for treatment are based on original studies of symptomatic patients and remain: (1) serum transaminases more than 10 times upper normal; or (2) transaminases more than fivefold elevated with a more than twofold elevation in IgG; or (3) histological evidence of bridging or multiaci-nar necrosis. These criteria represent a severe end of the disease spectrum, in which untreated patients have a mortality of over 1 in 3 within 6 months and a subse-quent 10-year survival of less than 1 in 3. The absence of fibrosis or cirrhosis is not a relevant guiding factor for starting treatment.

Patients outside the above criteria are still appropriate to treat but individual judgment is exercised, with a composite assessment of symptoms, liver biochemistry and histology. The literature suggests those with mild interface hepatitis have a normal 5-year survival and a 5-year progression to cirrhosis of around 20%, whilst mild–moderate laboratory abnormalities are associated with cirrhosis in 49% within 15 years but a 10-year sur-vival of 90% [10,11].

Just as the magnitude of biochemical changes do not correlate with histological injury, neither is there any distinguishing feature between those with and without symptoms. The hope in treating more mild disease is to prevent progression of disease and cirrhosis because corticosteroids may prevent and reverse fibrosis although this is not always the case. No treatment may be an option: a single centre experience showed that asymptomatic patients had lower serum aminotrans-ferase, total bilirubin and IgG values at baseline, and half received no therapy and their survival was no dif-ferent to those who did [53].

Patients with an inactive cirrhosis who may present with signs of liver failure and who are not candidates for medical therapy or who are progressing rapidly to acute liver failure, are candidates for liver transplanta-tion rather than steroids, which may only add to a risk of sepsis [54]. Such a fulminant presentation of AIH is still relatively uncommon, and can be hard to distin-guish from other causes of fulminant hepatitis. Classical features of AIH may not be present serologically, and histology can be unhelpful if necrosis is so severe as to be the only finding. Fulminant AIH does need to be distinguished from those presenting with active decom-pensated cirrhosis, in whom steroid therapy can lead to excellent results.

No trials have shown that azathioprine monotherapy is effective in inducing remission; its role is in mainte-nance therapy. Once remission has been obtained, the introduction of azathioprine permits the dose of corti-costeroids to be reduced. In one trial, azathioprine (75 mg/day) was stopped and prednisolone continued at a maintenance dose of 5–12.5 mg/day. The probability of relapse within 3 years was 32% in patients who stopped azathioprine compared with 6% in those who continued combination therapy [50]. In a further study, patients were randomized to high-dose azathioprine (2 mg/kg per day) after withdrawal of prednisolone or continued combination therapy (prednisolone 5–10 mg/ day and azathioprine 1 mg/kg per day). There were no significant differences between the two groups and no patient relapsed on azathioprine alone at 1-year follow up. Biochemical and histological remission was subse-quently sustained in 83% of patients on azathioprine over the longer term [52].

Treatment approaches. Two general treatment strategies have developed: (1) Prednisone monotherapy; and (2) combination therapy, either from the outset or with addition of azathioprine (or 6-mercaptopurine if pre-ferred) later (Table 23.8). Both strategies work but most now use a combination approach from the start, since this is associated with a lower occurrence of corticosteroid-related side effects (10% versus 44%) [49].

These two agents have side effects (Tables 23.9, 23.10) and the monitoring of patients is essential (Table 23.11). Particularly for azathioprine, clear communication must be maintained with the primary physician as regards regular monitoring of the full blood count. Hepatotoxicity with azathioprine is unusual, but should be borne in mind. Treatment with immunosuppressive therapy places patients at risk for sepsis, a particular concern for those with cirrhosis, in whom untreated infection can lead to rapid decompensation and death.

Ursodeoxycholic acid (UDCA) has been used for patients with mild disease in Japan, but this is not widely practiced elsewhere.

Steroid dose. Initial trials used 15 mg prednisolone daily, whilst others used prednisone monotherapy initiated at 60 mg daily, or prednisone 30 mg daily with azathio-prine 50 mg daily [4–6]. It is not possible to suggest with confidence a treatment regimen that suits all. Protocol-driven treatment is not logical, and it seems more sen-sible to tailor the treatment to the patient (including age,

Table 23.8. Broad overview of initial regimens for treating autoimmune hepatitis

	High dose monotherapy	Initial monotherapy with subsequent azathioprine		Combination therapy from outset	
	Prednisone (mg)	Prednisone (mg)	Azathioprine	Prednisone (mg)	Azathioprine (mg)
Week 1*	60	20–30	X	30	50
Week 2	40	20–30	X	20	50
Week 3	30	20–30	X	15	50
Week 4	30	20–30	1–2 mg/kg if responding and bilirubin <100 μmol/L	15	50
Early maintenance until end point agreed with patient	20	Tapering dose to 5–10 mg by 1 year		10	50

*Few specialists use monotherapy, and most favour reducing the steroid dose according to individual treatment response rather than per fixed protocol.

Table 23.9. Common practice pretreatment with steroids +/− azathioprine

Consider checking stools for ova and parasites
Start calcium (1000–1500 mg/day) and vitamin D supplementation (1000 IU/day)
Consider baseline bone mineral density +/− bisphosphonate prophylaxis
Check blood pressure and monitor on therapy periodically
Check blood glucose and urine glucose and monitor on therapy periodically
Screen for cataracts
Agree blood monitoring schedule for side effects
Discuss compliance strategies
Advise on prevention of infection, e.g. vaccinations, avoidance of bites in endemic areas
Screen for previous hepatitis B and consider monitoring/ intervention based on cAb status

comorbidities, severity of presentation) and the treatment response, in particular the falls in alanine transaminase (ALT) and IgG. One approach is 20 mg predniso(lo)ne daily with azathioprine 1–2 mg/kg per day either from the outset, or once treatment response is confirmed. Two to three months of 20 mg predniso(lo)ne daily is followed by therapy for 1–2 years at around 5–10 mg/day, the aim being to maintain normal liver biochemical tests and IgG values. Some prefer to initiate therapy at the higher dose of 30 mg, especially in the younger patient with more aggressive disease.

Treatment response. Response to immunosuppression therapy is assessed clinically, biochemically and possibly by repeat histological evaluation. In general, a biochemical response (a decrease in serum aminotransferase and globulins), occurs within 1–3 months. Resolution of inflammatory activity on liver biopsy is one clinical end point, but interim evaluation relies on serum transaminases and immunoglobulin measurement, as this reliably monitors activity and response to treatment [55]. When treatment is stopped even after 2 years of normal

tests approximately 80% of patients will relapse, 50% within 6 months.

A complete biochemical response is the aim, and a failure to see this should always lead to reappraisal (assuming compliance). Remission is considered normalization of transaminases, IgG and histological activity and around two-thirds of patients will enter remission within 18 months and nearly 90% will achieve this after 3 years of treatment. Histological remission lags behind clinical and biochemical remission by 3–6 months, explaining prolonged maintenance therapy and the use of histology by some as the final end point (Fig. 23.10).

In general, patients with mild or asymptomatic disease have better responses, although patients with established cirrhosis at presentation can achieve remission successfully with a 10-year life expectancy ranging from 60% [53] to more than 90% [56], the difference is probably due to variation in populations and reporting practices.

With remission, tapering of immunosuppression is appropriate, for example if by 2–3 months serum aminotransferase levels are normal, the prednisone dose can be decreased by 2.5–5 mg every 2–4 weeks. The precise strategy is clinician and patient specific, and in part relates to the initial dose of corticosteroid chosen, and the severity of disease at presentation. One typical approach has been to aim for complete clinical, biochemical and histological remission with prednisolone (e.g. 20 mg/day) and azathioprine (1 mg/kg per day; traditionally not initiated until the patient has a bilirubin <100 μmol/L). Steroids withdrawal is not normally completed until after at least 1 year of dual therapy.

Maintenance of remission. Long-term remission is maintained by low-dose corticosteroid alone, or in combination with azathioprine (1 mg/kg per day). Maintenance with azathioprine monotherapy is well established and once complete remission has been induced and sustained the majority of patients will remain in remission with azathioprine at a slightly higher dose (2 mg/kg) given alone. After a further period of remission it is possible to maintain remission at a dose of 1 mg/kg per day, and indeed many simply use 1 mg/kg from the outset. Some patients may need low-dose prednisone added back to the azathioprine.

Although a chronic relapsing disease, there is a natural desire for discontinuing treatment and there is no agreement as to how long to treat, particularly with azathioprine once prednisone has been withdrawn. Some of the factors that predict relapse are a failure to maintain consistently normal transaminases during therapy, time to

Table 23.10. Notable side effects of the common medications used in autoimmune liver disease

Drug	Side effect
Corticosteroids	Weight gain/ cushingoid Diabetes Cataract Hypertension/ fluid retention Poor wound healing Osteoporosis Adrenal suppression Impaired response to vaccination Susceptibility to infection
Azathioprine/ mercaptopurine *	Cytopenias Pancreatitis/ pneumonitis Nausea/ vomiting/ flu-like syndrome Hepatotoxicity Possible long-term malignancy risk
Mycophenolate mofetil *	Cytopenias Diarrhoea/ gastrointestinal upset Headache Rare colitis Possible long-term malignancy risk
Ursodeoxycholic acid	Weight gain Hair loss Diarrhoea Flatulence

*Monitoring including regular haematology and biochemistry required.

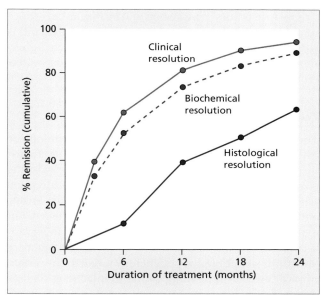

Fig. 23.10. The effect of prednisolone treatment in severe chronic autoimmune hepatitis.

Table 23.11. General measures in patients with autoimmune liver disease

Varices surveillance: screening by gastroscopy should be based on the presence of cirrhosis, or splenomegaly, or thrombocytopenia; in patients with biliary overlap presinusoidal portal hypertension may occur, and screening should be considered if platelets <200
Hepatocellular carcinoma surveillance: limited data upon which to guide but autoimmune hepatitis does not seem to be a high-risk disease for hepatocellular carcinoma development, although hepatocellular carcinoma has been reported in those with AIH
Vaccinations: routine hepatitis A and B vaccination for all patients; influenza and pneumococcal vaccinations periodically; appropriate evaluation pretravel by travel health clinic
Elective surgery: consider patient wearing medic-alert bracelet and educate as to risks associated with surgical procedures including drug toxicity, hypovolaemia, fluid management and analgesia

initial biochemical remission, high IgG at entry and marked portal plasma cell infiltrate [38]. Relapse is less likely if the aspartate transaminase (AST), gamma globulins and IgG are normal prior to withdrawal of treatment [57].

A main factor distinguishing patients who relapse is the duration of therapy preceding withdrawal of immunosuppression; in one small, non-randomized study sustained remission was obtained in 67% of patients treated for more than 4 years prior to cessation of therapy, in contrast to only 10% of those treated for 1–2 years [58]. Additionally, it is recognized that over 80% of patients on an indefinite azathioprine strategy (2 mg/kg) will remain in remission over a 5-year period [52]. Although relapse typically responds quickly and completely to retreatment, such patients are at increased risk of further relapse, and poorer outcomes, if drug withdrawal is reattempted [59]. Practice however varies, with some withdrawing therapy if a follow-up liver biopsy is reported as showing no inflammatory activity. There is limited evidence for an increase in lymphoma rate in patients with AIH, but no direct association with use of immunomodulatory agents [60].

If relapse occurs, prednisone will be needed to induce remission, and thereafter azathioprine (or equivalent) is usually given lifelong. Relapse if there underlying cirrhosis can precipitate liver failure, leading most to recommend indefinite azathioprine in this setting.

Pretreatment and on-treatment considerations

The side effect profiles of prednisone and azathioprine in particular are well known to all clinicians. Nevertheless in commencing a patient on immunosuppression the clinician must make an evaluation of the individual patient as regards monitoring for treatment side effects and educating patients, not just about compliance, but also about potential side effects. Such advice must also account for the location in which the physician practices (and the destinations the patient may travel to), as certain tropical areas will be more prone to infections such as strongyloides which thrive in the immunosuppressed. As a baseline, routine blood sugar determination, bone density and cataract screening should be considered, as well as screening for stool parasites if from an endemic area. On treatment advice should include education in prompt management of infections in particular.

Treatment challenges and alternative agents

Very few patients fail therapy assuming good compliance. Ethnicity, onset at an early age, hyperbilirubinaemia, HLA DRB1*03 and a presentation Model for Endstage Liver Disease (MELD) score of over 12 act as markers for treatment failure.

The choice of intervention in treatment 'resistant' patients is arbitrary, and not evidence based. As the numbers are small, data are limited, and sometimes extrapolated from studies focusing on new primary steroid-sparing treatments. Some try a higher dose of prednisone but alternative agents, such as calcineurin inhibitors, budesonide, mycophenolate mofetil and rapamycin have all been tried. Ciclosporin has been used successfully as primary treatment in paediatric and adult patients, and can act as a steroid-sparing agent. Similar studies have focused on the related agent tacrolimus. For both agents if chosen, the clinician must carefully appraise the risk from renal and neurological toxicity.

Budesonide. The potential for side effects from prednisone has driven interest in alternative steroid agents, particularly budesonide with its 90% first-pass hepatic metabolism. Clinicians must be aware that this is not the case in those with cirrhosis or portal hypertension. A large randomized trial of budesonide versus prednisone in new onset non-cirrhotic AIH showed budesonide to be superior in achieving a biochemical remission over the study period (60 versus 38.8%) with significantly fewer steroid side effects (72 versus 46.6%), and greater efficacy at achieving the primary endpoint of a complete response [61]. As the prednisolone comparison group was 40 mg, the baseline side-effect profile was probably higher than is generally seen. In contrast, the studies of budesonide for non-responders have been disappointing, although this population most probably will include patients with cirrhosis.

Mycophenolate mofetil. This agent is free of nephrotoxicity with its side effects being similar to azathioprine; in addition some report diarrhoea and headaches. For those intolerant of azathioprine it has a clear role, although it is less certain that it acts as a better immunosuppressant than azathioprine.

Monoclonal antibodies. Analogous to their use in other autoimmune/ transplant settings, agents such as the anti-CD20 monoclonal antibody rituximab may prove beneficial for selected patients but, as yet, no conclusive studies supporting this have been published.

Pregnancy and autoimmune hepatitis

For women with AIH, pregnancy and the consequences to maternal and fetal health is a frequent concern. Disease flares may occur during, but most often immediately after, pregnancy (4–12 weeks postpartum classically) [62], although no factors are predictive so monitoring is required for all (Table 23.12). Management is individualized in terms of the stage of disease and the

Table 23.12. Pregnancy and autoimmune hepatitis [76].

Counsel safety of medications and risk of relapse if treatment stopped
Arrange monitoring peri- and postpartum (monthly for 6 months)
Consider second trimester variceal surveillance if cirrhotic, and use of beta-blockers if significant varices present
Ensure baseline ultrasound includes Doppler studies (?splenic artery aneurysm)
Liaise closely with obstetrician: modify labour if cirrhotic with portal hypertension

degree of liver injury, but with one-third of patients having cirrhosis at diagnosis, particular note must be given to their obstetric management (ultrasound to look for splenic artery aneurysm, endoscopy in the second trimester if cirrhotic, and active involvement of the obstetrician to hopefully prevent a prolonged labour). In essence, ongoing use of either prednisone and/or azathioprine is considered acceptable and safe, when the risk of therapy are balanced by the benefits (Table 23.13). Stopping medication carries a risk of disease relapse with untoward consequences to the mother and fetus. There is a 3.4-fold risk of oral cleft palate with prednisone use in pregnancy according to one meta-analysis [63]. Budesonide appears to also be safe in pregnancy. Although azathioprine crosses the placenta there is a lack of teratogenicity in newborns and little evidence to suggest that there should be a dose reduction or drug withdrawal in patients who become pregnant while taking azathioprine. Mycophenoalte mofetil is, however, not considered safe during pregnancy, with reports of a characteristic phenotype associated with mycophenolate exposure during pregnancy. Supplemental or *de novo* prednisone use may be required but counter intuitively perhaps; most physicians shy away from *de novo* administration of azathioprine until after delivery. No convincing evidence exists to suggest mothers should not breast feed on steroids or azathioprine.

Contraception choices for patients with autoimmune hepatitis

Oral contraceptive use has been associated with a variety of liver disease, often documented in case reports rather than prospective studies. Cholestasis, peliosis hepatis and adenoma are most clearly identified as consequences of oestrogen-containing contraceptives. Vascular thromboses are also associated with oestrogen use, particularly in those with other thrombophilic tendencies. These events are, however, still rare. In patients with decompensated liver disease, or those early post-transplant (<1 year) it is generally advisable to avoid oestrogen-containing contraception. Similarly, for those with cholestatic liver disease, where oestrogens can promote further cholestasis, their use may need to be limited if cholestasis worsens. However,

this is not the case for those with other compensated chronic liver disease, or stable liver graft function, for whom low-dose oestrogen-containing contraceptives are well tolerated. If concern remains, progesterone-only contraceptive pills can be used, or non-hormonal barrier methods. Intrauterine contraceptive devices are appropriate and safe, and infective complications are extremely rare.

The elderly and autoimmune hepatitis

Autoimmune hepatitis affects all ages, and it is probably under-diagnosed in the elderly, because it is not always considered in the differential diagnosis [64]. A few reports have suggested that AIH may be less severe in the elderly but there are insufficient data available and experience confirms that AIH often presents in older patients, who have a higher chance of cirrhosis and who may present with severe disease. Active management of these patients, including biopsy to confirm the diagnosis, is appropriate as treatment responses are good and can lead to a normal life expectancy. Treatment failure seems less common in the elderly, perhaps because age-related changes in the cellular immune response may attenuate the disease and enhance its response to therapy. However, side effects of therapy must be more carefully managed, in particular steroid-induced diabetes and osteoporosis. Many choose a lower dose of prednisone when initiating treatment, and specialist guidelines often suggest bisphosphonate prophylaxis from the outset for those over the age of 65 commenced on steroids.

Childhood-onset autoimmune hepatitis

Subtle differences in treatment are noted for children. Most notably, it is very important to always consider Wilson's disease in children presenting with a hepatitis. Typically, recommended therapy begins with prednisolone 2 mg/kg per day (maximum 60 mg/day), which is gradually decreased over a period of 1–2 months alongside normalization of the transaminases. Maintenance therapy is usually 2.5–5 mg/day, a dose sufficient to sustain normal liver biochemistry. If normalization of liver biochemistry is not prompt, or side effects are prominent, azathioprine is added at a starting

Table 23.13. Safety of commonly used liver medications during pregnancy [76]

Drug	FDA risk assessment	Safety	Comments
Prednisone	C	Low risk: postulated increased cleft palate	Generally if required safe to use at lowest effective dose
Azathioprine	D	Data suggest low risk	Good safety record in IBD and AIH
Ciclosporin	C	Most safety data of all transplant immunosuppressants	Risk of precipitating acute/chronic rejection usually such that used without interruption in pregnancy; dose adjustment may be required
Tacrolimus	C	Probably safe, use as needed	As for CyA
Mycophenylate mofetil	C	Not recommended at present	
Sirolimus	C	Not recommended	Notable side effect is on wound healing therefore in absence of clear safety profile not used in pregnancy
Ursodeoxycholic acid	B	Low risk; used in intrahepatic cholestasis of pregnancy	Guidelines vary from stopping until third trimester if already using, to continuing without concern
Cholestyramine	C	Believed to be safe in pregnancy	Ensure vitamin supplementation as required
Rifampicin	C	Rifampicin should be used during pregnancy only if the potential benefit justifies the potential risk to the fetus	Best avoided in favour of other treatments for pruritus
Hydroxyzine	C		The use of hydroxyzine and cetirizine does not appear to be associated with increased teratogenic risk, although some studies suggest avoid in first trimester
Beta-blockers	C (1st trimester) D (2/3rd trimesters)	Fetal bradycardia; risk of intrauterine growth retardation	Routine variceal surveillance in the 2nd trimester is advisable and use of beta-blockers suggested on standard endoscopic assessment

The FDA-assigned pregnancy categories are one risk stratification tool:
Category A: adequate and well-controlled studies have failed to demonstrate a risk to the fetus in the first trimester of pregnancy (and there is no evidence of risk in later trimesters). Category B: animal reproduction studies have failed to demonstrate a risk to the fetus and there are no adequate and well-controlled studies in pregnant women. Category C: animal reproduction studies have shown an adverse effect on the fetus and there are no adequate and well-controlled studies in humans, but potential benefits may warrant use of the drug in pregnant women despite potential risks. Category D: there is positive evidence of human fetal risk based on adverse reaction data from investigational or marketing experience or studies in humans, but potential benefits may warrant use of the drug in pregnant women despite potential risks.

dose of 0.5 mg/kg per day, which, in the absence of signs of toxicity, is increased up to a maximum of 2–2.5 mg/kg per day until biochemical control is seen.

Non-adherence is the major concern for adolescents, playing significant roles in relapse. Furthermore, the risk of relapse is higher if steroids are administered on an alternate-day schedule compared to small daily doses which are better for disease control and helps avoid rescue courses of high-dose steroids, which are associated with side effects.

Treatment withdrawal is not usually attempted within 3 years from diagnosis or during/ immediately before puberty, when relapses are more common, most likely because of non-adherence.

Unlike adult practice, some monitor the response to treatment through the measurement of autoantibody titres as well as IgG levels, the fluctuation of which is correlated with disease activity. Sustained remission, achieved with prednisolone and azathioprine, can be maintained with azathioprine alone in many children with type 1 AIH, but this is not the case in type 2 AIH, a more aggressive hepatitis being frequently encountered. Some historic data suggest that the outcome over 10 years is poorer for those with type 2 AIH, as compared to type 1 disease [23].

For children with biliary involvement (routine magnetic resonance cholangiopancreatography (MRCP) being appropriate in all children with AIH) UDCA is commonly prescribed. However evidence to demonstrate benefit is not available.

Autoimmune hepatitis and liver transplantation

Treatment of AIH is very effective, so liver transplantation is needed for only a small number of patients.

As with cirrhosis from other aetiologies, liver transplantation is indicated principally for those with end-stage disease: a MELD score of more than 16 is a commonly threshold for potential transplant benefit. Other indications may be encephalopathy, ascites or recurrent variceal haemorrhage. Hepatocellular carcinoma is an uncommon indication in this group. For the small number of patients who present with acute or fulminant liver failure, steroid therapy is rarely helpful, can be dangerous in view of the risk for sepsis and therefore liver transplantation should be considered early [54].

Outcomes and disease recurrence. Results are as good as for any other indication although there is a risk of recurrence after transplantation. The broad criteria for the diagnosis of recurrent AIH include liver transplantation for autoimmune hepatitis, autoantibodies in significant titre (>1:40), sustained rises in serum aminotransferase activity (>2 times normal), elevated serum immunoglobulins, compatible liver histology (infiltration of portal tracts by plasma cells, piecemeal necrosis and bridging necrosis), corticosteroid dependency and exclusion of other causes of graft dysfunction (such as rejection and hepatitis C infection).

The reported recurrence is from about approximately 1 in 5 to approximately 1 in 2 at 5 years. The choice of immunosuppression does not appear to be a risk factor. Many clinicians adjust their immunosuppression protocols with recurrent disease in mind, by using long-term dual therapy from the outset, that is calcineurin inhibitor and azathioprine or mycophenolate.

Subsequent adjustment of immunosuppression often requires addition of prednisolone which is generally sufficient; steroid withdrawal may not always be possible.

De novo AIH. This clinical entity has features of a steroid-responsive AIH in patients transplanted for other non-immune indications and is characterized by a biochemical hepatitis, circulating autoantibodies, elevated immunoglobulins and an inflammatory infiltration with interface hepatitis [65]. Children are more at risk than adults, particularly those undergoing transplant for biliary atresia, but the condition is still relatively uncommon with an incidence of less than 1 in 20. There is usually a good response to additional immunosuppression with corticosteroids, but in some cases there is progression to cirrhosis and subsequent graft failure. Whether this is truly a *de novo* autoimmune phenomenon or merely a form of rejection is not clear.

Overlap syndromes

The effector arm of the immune system may lack precision and patients can have features that appear to overlap between hepatitic or biliary autoimmune liver disease. While combined criteria (biochemical, histological, immunological and cholangiographic) will discriminate the major 'autoimmune' liver diseases, individual components lack specificity and provide intrinsic scope for overlap (Table 23.14, Figs 23.11, 23.12).

This is a challenging area to study, with a history of varying definitions of different stringencies and a tendency to over diagnose (and report) what is perceived as an interesting entity. Additionally, to add confusion for the clinician is the diverse terminology used—for example autoimmune cholangitis has been used to refer to AMA-negative PBC, IgG4-associated sclerosing cholangitis, as well as childhood autoimmune hepatitis/ sclerosing cholangitis overlap.

There remains a need to carefully, and prospectively, characterize patients by a combination of serial laboratory, histological and radiological modalities over time, rather than make a 'snap shot' diagnosis. Clinical precision must be all the more certain if the label of overlap is to be used. An inadequately sized liver biopsy may give a misleading representation of inflammatory activity or biliary disease, and suboptimal magnetic resonance imaging (MRI) examination may over-call cholangiopathy, particularly in a patient with cirrhosis.

Definitions. The presence of the concurrent main characteristics of two autoimmune conditions at the same time or during the course of illness is generally the basis for defining an overlap syndrome. Autoimmune

Table 23.14. Summary features of autoimmune liver disease demonstrating traditional descriptions

	Autoimmune hepatitis	Primary biliary cirrhosis	Primary sclerosing cholangitis
Demographics	Female predominant (4:1) and all ages	Female predominant (9:1); usually postmenopausal at diagnosis	Male predominant (7:3); classically diagnosed in 40s, in association with inflammatory bowel disease
Symptoms	Asymptomatic commonly Alternatively acute jaundice, and upper abdominal pain Fatigue, acne, irregular menstruation	Commonly now asymptomatic; traditionally fatigue, pruritus, occasionally xanthoma	Often asymptomatic; may present with cholangitis, pruritus, abdominal pain or jaundice
Liver biochemical changes	Transaminases raised (ALT/AST)	Cholestatic profile predominates (raised ALP, γ-GT)	Cholestatic profile predominates (raised ALP, γ-GT)
Classical serum Ig elevation	IgG	IgM	Non-specific; IgG4 elevations may suggest a secondary aetiology
Autoantibodies	ANA, SMA (type 1 AIH) LKM (type 2 AIH)	AMA (Invariably ANA positive in AMA negative cases)	No specific associations, frequently ANA/SMA positive
Classic histology	Interface hepatitis Lobular hepatitis Necrosis/ collapse Fibrosis	Granulomatous lymphocytic destruction of interlobular bile ducts within portal triads with ductopenia and fibrosis	Periductal concentric fibrosis Ductopenia Ductular proliferation
Broad treatment	Prednisolone and Azathioprine as first line	UDCA (13–15 mg/kg)	No proven therapy except in secondary IgG4 associated sclerosing cholangitis (steroid responsive)
Usual basis for diagnosis	Combination of liver biochemistry, immunology and liver biopsy findings	Cholestatic liver tests in presence of AMA	Cholestasis with compatible imaging by MRCP/ERCP
Prognosis	Excellent long-term survival	UDCA biochemical responders have normal life expectancy	Once symptomatic ~50% chance of need for transplant over 15 years
Potential outlier features	Duct injury in 10%; antimitochondrial antibodies in up to 20%	Interface hepatitis and raised transaminases at presentation common	Interface hepatitis frequent; commonly ANA/SMA positive

ALP, alkaline phosphatase; ALT, alanine transaminase; AST, aspartate transaminase; ANA, antinuclear antibodies; AMA, antimitochrondial antibodies; ERCP, endoscopic retrograde cholangiopancreatography; γ-GT, γ-glutamyltransferase; pANCA, perinuclear antineutrophil cytoplasmic antibody; SMA, antismooth muscle antibodies; LKM, antiliver kidney microsomal; MRCP, magnetic resonance cholangiopancreatography; SLA/LP, soluble liver and pancreas antigen; UDCA, ursodeoxycholic acid.

hepatitis appears to be a common denominator, with overlap always involving this parenchymal process. Coincidental overlaps (e.g. HCV and AIH, AMA-positive hepatitis B) are not relevant to this discussion.

Autoimmune hepatitis/ primary biliary cirrhosis 'overlap'

Although bile duct destruction is generally not prominent in AIH, up to about 10% of biopsies may show duct destruction, and an additional approximately 10% show

lymphocytic infiltration of bile duct epithelium without ductopenia. The histological pattern of injury may be indistinguishable from PBC. Perhaps 10% of those with PBC will appear to clinically have an AIH overlap [40,66,67]. In PBC clinical trials the reported prevalence is lower, being less than 5% [68].

Criteria. An arbitrary French model for labelling this overlap has gained popularity and is based on patients having two of three criteria for both AIH and PBC. For a diagnosis of PBC the criteria are:

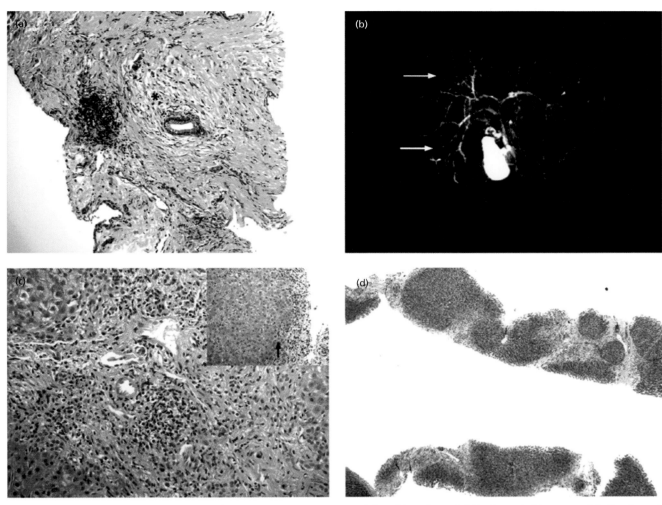

Fig. 23.11. Simultaneous development of autoimmune hepatitis in a patient with sclerosing cholangitis, accompanied by transient antimitochondrial antibody production. (A) Initial biopsy showing portal tract with periductal concentric oedema (*) (Masson trichrome). (B) Radial oblique thick slab magnetic resonance cholangiopancreatography image showing irregular 'beaded'

peripheral intrahepatic bile ducts (white arrows) indicative of sclerosing cholangitis. (C) Second biopsy showing portal tract with moderately dense lymphoplasmacytic inflammation (H & E); insert shows high power of portal tract with interface activity and several acidophilic bodies (arrow). (D) Low-power view of second biopsy showing cirrhosis with wide septa and small parenchymal nodules (Masson trichrome) [76].

1 alkaline phosphatase (ALP) ≥2 × upper limit of normal (ULN) or γ-glutamyltransferase (γ-GT) ≥5 × ULN
2 a positive test for AMA (>1 in 80) and
3 a liver biopsy specimen showing florid bile duct lesions.

For AIH the criteria are:
1 ALT ≥5 × ULN
2 IgG ≥2 × ULN or a positive test for SMA (>1 in 80) and
3 a liver biopsy showing moderate or severe periportal or periseptal lymphocytic piecemeal necrosis [69].

Both more and less stringent case definitions have been suggested by others, and there is no basis for accepting which definition to apply.

Presentation. The most frequent and the most readily identified presentation is represented by the simultaneous presence of features of both diseases at initial presentation. In some patients, features of AIH and PBC are temporally dissociated. Patients who clearly switch biochemically, serologically and histologically over time from one disease to another are rare. One series suggested 4.3% of patients with PBC over time were said to have developed AIH [67]. It has been claimed that anti-dsDNA antibodies are potentially a serological marker for AIH/PBC but this is speculative. Anti-dsDNA antibodies were detected in 60% of AIH/PBC overlap patients, but only in 4% of PBC patients and 26% of AIH patients [70]. Alternative aetiologies must be sought,

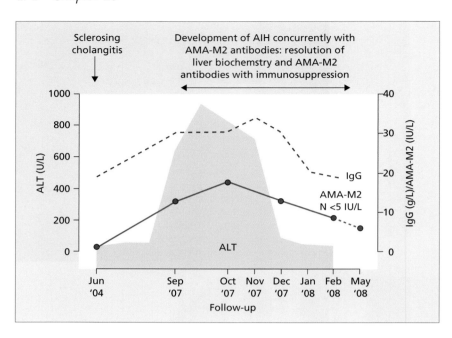

Fig. 23.12. Overlap features of autoimmune liver disease in the same patient described in Fig. 23.11. ALT, alanine transaminase; AMA, antimitochrondial antibodies [76].

and consideration always given to superimposed drug-induced liver injury.

Treatment. Therapeutic recommendations rely on the treatment strategies of either AIH or PBC, with the advice being always to treat the predominant process first. In a well-defined clinical trial cohort of 16 patients with AIH–PBC overlap syndrome, the response to UDCA therapy (13–15 mg/kg daily) and the survival of the patients was similar to patients with classical PBC [68]. Patients enrolled into clinical trials are not by definition a good reflection of general practice and thus others contradict this, showing a need for combination therapy, UDCA and steroids [71]. Generally, it is reasonable to start treatment with UDCA (13–15 mg/kg daily). If the patient does not achieve an adequate biochemical response (significant improvement in transaminases) in an appropriate time span (e.g. 3–6 months) steroids/azathioprine can be added. Some speculate that patients with overlap features in PBC have a poorer prognosis and there are data to support the concept that the degree of interface activity in PBC associates with outcome [72]. Additionally, some treatment response studies identify AST as a predictor of outcome in PBC [73].

Sclerosing cholangitis/ autoimmune hepatitis 'overlap' syndrome

AIH and PSC may be sequential in their occurrence. Use of the modified AIH score leads to a diagnosis of an overlap syndrome in between 8 and 10% of patients with PSC [74], whilst with dedicated liver MRI and liver histology, as many as 12% of adult patients with AIH may have detectable subtle cholangiophathies [34].

Criteria. There are no specific criteria for diagnosis and patients are expected to have features of both diseases on the basis of classic evaluation of imaging and liver biopsy. Routine serology alone is insufficient to diagnose an AIH/PSC overlap.

Treatment. A beneficial response to immunosuppressive therapy is frequently reported on the hepatitic component. UDCA is still widely administered in PSC (because of its favourable effect on liver biochemistry) although there is no survival benefit in either adults or children. Nevertheless, UDCA in combination with an immunosuppressive regimen is a common strategy. Survival has been suggested to be poorer if an overlap is found, even if treated.

Autoimmune sclerosing cholangitis. A prospective evaluation [24] found that half of children with AIH had bile duct changes diagnostic of SC at the time of presentation. All but one had serology of AIH type 1 and interface hepatitis and, in the absence of cholangiographic studies, at least a quarter would have been diagnosed as AIH type 1. This condition has been called 'autoimmune sclerosing cholangitis' (ASC). Interestingly, there is not the same degree of female predominance for those with ASC. Levels of alkaline phosphatase and γ-glutamyltransferase did not differ between the two groups, the only biochemical difference being a higher ratio between alkaline phosphatase over aspartate aminotransferase.

In both groups the parenchymal lesions responded to steroids, but half of the patients with ASC, also treated with 10 to 15 mg/kg UDCA, showed progression of bile duct disease on follow-up endoscopic retrograde cholangiopancreatography (ERCP). One patient (of 28) with AIH type 1 who had normal ERCP at presentation developed florid bile duct changes 8 years later. Inflammatory bowel disease was present in about 45% of children with ASC compared to about 20% of those with AIH and normal bile ducts on ERCP, and 90% of children with ASC had increased serum IgG levels as is seen with AIH.

IgG4-associated autoimmune hepatitis. Autoimmune pancreatitis is characterized by raised serum levels of IgG4 with IgG4-positive plasma cell infiltration histologically. It constitutes part of a systemic inflammatory disease process that can also in particular involve the larger bile ducts, resembling sclerosing cholangitis, as well as the kidneys, salivary glands, retroperitoneum, prostate and lung. Hepatic pseudotumours are part of the spectrum of disease and there are reports of hepatitis, mimicking classic autoimmune hepatitis. If patients with autoimmune pancreatitis have a liver biopsy, hepatic involvement is not infrequent [75] with the following patterns: (1) portal inflammation with or without interface hepatitis, (2) large bile-duct obstructive features, (3) portal sclerosis, (4) lobular hepatitis and (5) canalicular cholestasis. The disease occurs predominantly in older men and responds well to steroid therapy. Identification of patients is usually through measurement of IgG4 levels in the serum and, if available, immunostaining of biopsy material. Follow up for relapse is important, which may occur in a different site to that at presentation.

Conclusion

Autoimmune hepatitis and its overlapping syndromes are in need of a definitive diagnostic test. Proteomic, genomic and epigenetic analyses may be fruitful in this regard. Nevertheless, steroid use, with azathioprine to prevent relapse, is effective in inducing and maintaining remission, such that the 20-year life expectancy exceeds 80%.

References

1 Waldenstrom J. Leber, Blutproteine und Nahrungseiweiss. *Dtsch. Ges. Verda. Stoffwechselkr.* 1950; **15**: 113–119.

2 Kunkel HG, Ahrens EH, Eisenmenger WJ *et al.* Extreme hypergammaglobulinemia in young women with liver disease. *J. Clin. Invest.* 1951; **30**: 654.

3 Holborow EJ, Asherson GL, Johnson GD *et al.* Antinuclear factor and other antibodies in blood and liver diseases. *Br. Med. J.* 1963; **1**: 656–658.

4 Cook GC, Mulligan R, Sherlock S. Controlled prospective trial of corticosteroid therapy in active chronic hepatitis. *Q. J. Med.* 1971; **40**: 159–185.

5 Soloway RD, Summerskill WH, Baggenstoss AH *et al.* Clinical, biochemical, and histological remission of severe chronic active liver disease: a controlled study of treatments and early prognosis. *Gastroenterology* 1972; **63**: 820–833.

6 Murray-Lyon IM, Stern RB, Williams R. Controlled trial of prednisone and azathioprine in active chronic hepatitis. *Lancet* 1973; **1**: 735–737.

7 Verma S, Torbenson M, Thuluvath PJ. The impact of ethnicity on the natural history of autoimmune hepatitis. *Hepatology* 2007; **46**: 1828–1835.

8 Vergani D, Alvarez F, Bianchi FB *et al.* Liver autoimmune serology: a consensus statement from the committee for autoimmune serology of the International Autoimmune Hepatitis Group. *J. Hepatol.* 2004; **41**: 677–683.

9 Baggenstoss AH, Soloway RD, Summerskill WH *et al.* Chronic active liver disease. The range of histologic lesions, their response to treatment, and evolution. *Hum. Pathol.* 1972; **3**: 183–198.

10 Schalm SW, Korman MG, Summerskill WH *et al.* Severe chronic active liver disease. Prognostic significance of initial morphologic patterns. *Am. J. Dig. Dis.* 1977; **22**: 973–980.

11 De Groote J, Fevery J, Lepoutre L. Long-term follow-up of chronic active hepatitis of moderate severity. *Gut* 1978; **19**: 510–513.

12 Kirk AP, Jain S, Pocock S *et al.* Late results of the Royal Free Hospital prospective controlled trial of prednisolone therapy in hepatitis B surface antigen negative chronic active hepatitis. *Gut* 1980; **21**: 78–83.

13 Holdener M, Hintermann E, Bayer M *et al.* Breaking tolerance to the natural human liver autoantigen cytochrome P450 2D6 by virus infection. *J. Exp. Med.* 2008; **205**: 1409–1422.

14 Longhi MS, Mitry RR, Samyn M *et al.* Vigorous activation of monocytes in juvenile autoimmune liver disease escapes the control of regulatory T-cells. *Hepatology* 2009; **50**: 130–142.

15 Strettell MD, Donaldson PT, Thomson LJ *et al.* Allelic basis for HLA-encoded susceptibility to type 1 autoimmune hepatitis. *Gastroenterology* 1997; **112**: 2028–2035.

16 Czaja AJ, Strettell MD, Thomson LJ *et al.* Associations between alleles of the major histocompatibility complex and type 1 autoimmune hepatitis. *Hepatology* 1997; **25**: 317–323.

17 Agarwal K, Czaja AJ, Jones DE *et al.* Cytotoxic T lymphocyte antigen-4 (CTLA-4) gene polymorphisms and susceptibility to type 1 autoimmune hepatitis. *Hepatology* 2000; **31**: 49–53.

18 Vogel A, Strassburg CP, Obermayer-Straub P *et al.* The genetic background of autoimmune polyendocrinopathy-candidiasis-ectodermal dystrophy and its autoimmune disease components. *J. Mol. Med.* 2002; **80**: 201–211.

19 Vergani D, Mieli-Vergani G, Alberti A *et al.* Antibodies to the surface of halothane-altered rabbit hepatocytes in patients with severe halothane-associated hepatitis. *N. Engl. J. Med.* 1980; **303**: 66–71.

20 Beaune P, Dansette PM, Mansuy D *et al*. Human anti-endoplasmic reticulum autoantibodies appearing in a drug-induced hepatitis are directed against a human liver cytochrome P-450 that hydroxylates the drug. *Proc. Natl. Acad. Sci. U S A* 1987; **84**: 551–555.

21 Mauri-Hellweg D, Bettens F, Mauri D *et al*. Activation of drug-specific CD4+ and CD8+ T cells in individuals allergic to sulfonamides, phenytoin, and carbamazepine. *J. Immunol.* 1995; **155**: 462–472.

22 Singh G, Palaniappan S, Rotimi O *et al*. Autoimmune hepatitis triggered by hepatitis A. *Gut* 2007; **56**: 304.

23 Homberg JC, Abuaf N, Bernard O *et al*. Chronic active hepatitis associated with antiliver/kidney microsome antibody type 1: a second type of 'autoimmune' hepatitis. *Hepatology* 1987; **7**: 1333–1339.

24 Gregorio GV, Portmann B, Karani J *et al*. Autoimmune hepatitis/sclerosing cholangitis overlap syndrome in childhood: a 16-year prospective study. *Hepatology* 2001; **33**: 544–553.

25 Seo S, Toutounjian R, Conrad A *et al*. Favorable outcomes of autoimmune hepatitis in a community clinic setting. *J. Gastroenterol. Hepatol.* 2008; **23**: 1410–1414.

26 Ferrari R, Pappas G, Agostinelli D *et al*. Type 1 autoimmune hepatitis: patterns of clinical presentation and differential diagnosis of the 'acute' type. *Q. J. Med.* 2004; **97**: 407–412.

27 Al-Chalabi T, Underhill JA, Portmann BC *et al*. Effects of serum aspartate aminotransferase levels in patients with autoimmune hepatitis influence disease course and outcome. *Clin. Gastroenterol. Hepatol.* 2008; **6**: 1389–95, quiz 1287.

28 Czaja AJ, Cassani F, Cataleta M *et al*. Frequency and significance of antibodies to actin in type 1 autoimmune hepatitis. *Hepatology* 1996; **24**: 1068–1073.

29 Manns MP, Griffin KJ, Sullivan KF *et al*. LKM-1 autoantibodies recognize a short linear sequence in P450IID6, a cytochrome P-450 monooxygenase. *J. Clin. Invest.* 1991; **88**: 1370–1378.

30 Lapierre P, Hajoui O, Homberg JC *et al*. Formiminotransferase cyclodeaminase is an organ-specific autoantigen recognized by sera of patients with autoimmune hepatitis. *Gastroenterology* 1999; **116**: 643–649.

31 Wies I, Brunner S, Henninger J *et al*. Identification of target antigen for SLA/LP autoantibodies in autoimmune hepatitis. *Lancet* 2000; **355**: 1510–1515.

32 O'Brien C, Joshi S, Feld JJ *et al*. Long-term follow-up of antimitochondrial antibody-positive autoimmune hepatitis. *Hepatology* 2008; **48**: 550–556.

33 Lu F, Xia Q, Ma Y *et al*. Serum proteomic-based analysis for the identification of a potential serological marker for autoimmune hepatitis. *Biochem. Biophys. Res. Commun.* 2008; **367**: 284–290.

34 Abdalian R, Dhar P, Jhaveri K *et al*. Prevalence of sclerosing cholangitis in adults with autoimmune hepatitis: evaluating the role of routine magnetic resonance imaging. *Hepatology* 2008; **47**: 949–957.

35 Lewin M, Vilgrain V, Ozenne V *et al*. Prevalence of sclerosing cholangitis in adults with autoimmune hepatitis: a prospective magnetic resonance imaging and histological study. *Hepatology* 2009; **50**: 528–537.

36 Yeoman AD, Al-Chalabi T, Karani JB *et al*. Evaluation of risk factors in the development of hepatocellular carcinoma in autoimmune hepatitis: Implications for follow-up and screening. *Hepatology* 2008; **48**: 863–870.

37 Czaja AJ, Carpenter HA. Progressive fibrosis during corticosteroid therapy of autoimmune hepatitis. *Hepatology* 2004; **39**: 1631–1638.

38 Verma S, Gunuwan B, Mendler M *et al*. Factors predicting relapse and poor outcome in type I autoimmune hepatitis: role of cirrhosis development, patterns of transaminases during remission and plasma cell activity in the liver biopsy. *Am. J. Gastroenterol.* 2004; **99**: 1510–1516.

39 Hennes EM, Zeniya M, Czaja AJ *et al*. Simplified criteria for the diagnosis of autoimmune hepatitis. *Hepatology* 2008; **48**: 169–176.

40 Czaja AJ, Carpenter HA. Autoimmune hepatitis with incidental histologic features of bile duct injury. *Hepatology* 2001; **34**: 659–665.

41 Reynolds TB, Peters RL, Yamada S. Chronic active and lupoid hepatitis caused by a laxative, oxyphenisatin. *N. Engl. J. Med.* 1971; **285**: 813–820.

42 Kanzler S, Weidemann C, Gerken G *et al*. Clinical significance of autoantibodies to soluble liver antigen in autoimmune hepatitis. *J. Hepatol.* 1999; **31**: 635–640.

43 Czaja AJ. Behavior and significance of autoantibodies in type 1 autoimmune hepatitis. *J. Hepatol.* 1999; **30**: 394–401.

44 Cassani F, Cataleta M, Valentini P *et al*. Serum autoantibodies in chronic hepatitis C: comparison with autoimmune hepatitis and impact on the disease profile. *Hepatology* 1997; **26**: 561–566.

45 Sugimura T, Obermayer-Straub P, Kayser A *et al*. A major CYP2D6 autoepitope in autoimmune hepatitis type 2 and chronic hepatitis C is a three-dimensional structure homologous to other cytochrome P450 autoantigens. *Autoimmunity* 2002; **35**: 501–513.

46 Ferri S, Muratori L, Quarneti C *et al*. Clinical features and effect of antiviral therapy on anti-liver/kidney microsomal antibody type 1 positive chronic hepatitis C. *J. Hepatol.* 2009; **50**: 1093–1101.

47 Rubio-Tapia A, Murray JA. The liver in coeliac disease. *Hepatology* 2007; **46**: 1650–1658.

48 Alvarez F, Berg PA, Bianchi FB *et al*. International Autoimmune Hepatitis Group Report: review of criteria for diagnosis of autoimmune hepatitis. *J. Hepatol.* 1999; **31**: 929–938.

49 Summerskill WH, Korman MG, Ammon HV *et al*. Prednisone for chronic active liver disease: dose titration, standard dose, and combination with azathioprine compared. *Gut* 1975; **16**: 876–883.

50 Stellon AJ, Hegarty JE, Portmann B *et al*. Randomised controlled trial of azathioprine withdrawal in autoimmune chronic active hepatitis. *Lancet* 1985; **1**: 668–670.

51 Stellon AJ, Keating JJ, Johnson PJ *et al*. Maintenance of remission in autoimmune chronic active hepatitis with azathioprine after corticosteroid withdrawal. *Hepatology* 1988; **8**: 781–784.

52 Johnson PJ, McFarlane IG, Williams R. Azathioprine for long-term maintenance of remission in autoimmune hepatitis. *N. Engl. J. Med.* 1995; **333**: 958–963.

53 Feld JJ, Dinh H, Arenovich T *et al*. Autoimmune hepatitis: effect of symptoms and cirrhosis on natural history and outcome. *Hepatology* 2005; **42**: 53–62.

54 Ichai P, Duclos-Vallee JC, Guettier C *et al*. Usefulness of corticosteroids for the treatment of severe and fulminant forms of autoimmune hepatitis. *Liver Transpl.* 2007; **13**: 996–1003.

55 Luth S, Herkel J, Kanzler S *et al*. Serologic markers compared with liver biopsy for monitoring disease activity in autoimmune hepatitis. *J. Clin. Gastroenterol.* 2008; **42**: 926–930.

56 Roberts SK, Therneau TM, Czaja AJ. Prognosis of histological cirrhosis in type 1 autoimmune hepatitis. *Gastroenterology* 1996; **110**: 848–857.

57 Montano-Loza AJ, Carpenter HA, Czaja AJ. Improving the end point of corticosteroid therapy in type 1 autoimmune hepatitis to reduce the frequency of relapse. *Am. J. Gastroenterol.* 2007; **102**: 1005–1012.

58 Kanzler S, Gerken G, Lohr H *et al*. Duration of immunosuppressive therapy in autoimmune hepatitis. *J. Hepatol.* 2001; **34**: 354–355.

59 Montano-Loza AJ, Carpenter HA, Czaja AJ. Consequences of treatment withdrawal in type 1 autoimmune hepatitis. *Liver Int.* 2007; **27**: 507–515.

60 Werner M, Almer S, Prytz H *et al*. Hepatic and extrahepatic malignancies in autoimmune hepatitis. A long-term follow-up in 473 Swedish patients. *J. Hepatol.* 2009; **50**: 388–393.

61 Manns MP, Bahr MJ, Woynarowski M *et al*. Budesonide 3mg tid is superior to prednisone in combination with azathioprine in the treatment of autoimmune hepatitis. *J. Hepatol.* 2008; **2**: S369.

62 Buchel E, Van Steenbergen W, Nevens F *et al*. Improvement of autoimmune hepatitis during pregnancy followed by flare-up after delivery. *Am. J. Gastroenterol.* 2002; **97**: 3160–3165.

63 Park-Wyllie L, Mazzotta P, Pastuszak A *et al*. Birth defects after maternal exposure to corticosteroids: prospective cohort study and meta-analysis of epidemiological studies. *Teratology* 2000; **62**: 385–392.

64 Czaja AJ, Carpenter HA. Distinctive clinical phenotype and treatment outcome of type 1 autoimmune hepatitis in the elderly. *Hepatology* 2006; **43**: 532–538.

65 Kerkar N, Hadzic N, Davies ET *et al*. De-novo autoimmune hepatitis after liver transplantation. *Lancet* 1998; **351**: 409–413.

66 Czaja AJ. Frequency and nature of the variant syndromes of autoimmune liver disease. *Hepatology* 1998; **28**: 360–365.

67 Poupon R, Chazouilleres O, Corpechot C *et al*. Development of autoimmune hepatitis in patients with typical primary biliary cirrhosis. *Hepatology* 2006; **44**: 85–90.

68 Joshi S, Cauch-Dudek K, Wanless IR *et al*. Primary biliary cirrhosis with additional features of autoimmune hepatitis: response to therapy with ursodeoxycholic acid. *Hepatology* 2002; **35**: 409–413.

69 Chazouilleres O, Wendum D, Serfaty L *et al*. Primary biliary cirrhosis-autoimmune hepatitis overlap syndrome: clinical features and response to therapy. *Hepatology* 1998; **28**: 296–301.

70 Muratori P, Granito A, Pappas G *et al*. The serological profile of the autoimmune hepatitis/primary biliary cirrhosis overlap syndrome. *Am. J. Gastroenterol.* 2009; **104**: 1420–1425.

71 Chazouilleres O, Wendum D, Serfaty L *et al*. Long term outcome and response to therapy of primary biliary cirrhosis-autoimmune hepatitis overlap syndrome. *J. Hepatol.* 2006; **44**: 400–406.

72 Corpechot C, Carrat F, Poupon R *et al*. Primary biliary cirrhosis: incidence and predictive factors of cirrhosis development in ursodiol-treated patients. *Gastroenterology* 2002; **122**: 652–658.

73 Huet PM, Vincent C, Deslaurier J *et al*. Portal hypertension and primary biliary cirrhosis: effect of long-term ursodeoxycholic acid treatment. *Gastroenterology* 2008; **135**: 1552–1560.

74 van Buuren HR, van Hoogstraten HJE, Terkivatan T *et al*. High prevalence of autoimmune hepatitis among patients with primary sclerosing cholangitis. *J. Hepatol.* 2000; **33**: 543–548.

75 Umemura T, Zen Y, Hamano H *et al*. Immunoglobin G4-hepatopathy: association of immunoglobin G4-bearing plasma cells in liver with autoimmune pancreatitis. *Hepatology* 2007; **46**: 463–471.

76 Bhat M, Guindi M, Heathcote EJ, Hirschfield GM. Transient development of anti-mitochondrial antibodies accompanies autoimmune hepatitis-sclerosing cholangitis overlap. *Gut* 2009 Jan; **58**(1): 152–153.

CHAPTER 24
Drug-Induced Liver Injury

Leonard B. Seeff[1] & Robert J. Fontana[2]

[1] Formerly, National Institute of Diabetes and Digestive and Kidney Diseases, National Institutes of Health, Bethesda, MD, USA
[2] Department of Internal Medicine, University of Michigan Medical School, Ann Arbor, MI, USA

Learning points

- Hepatotoxicity may result not only from prescription and over-the-counter drugs but also from herbal products and dietary supplements.

- The worldwide epidemiology of drug-induced liver disease varies substantially, but its incidence is probably universally underestimated.

- Environmental factors as well as variation in host immune responses, drug metabolism and drug pharmacokinetics may all play a role in the molecular mechanisms of drug-induced liver injury.

- The clinical presentation and patterns of drug-induced liver injury can vary from asymptomatic laboratory abnormalities to life-threatening fulminant hepatitis.

- Approaches to case adjudication and causality assessment for hepatotoxicity are not standardized and require further improvement.

Introduction

The striking growth in the number of new prescription and over-the-counter drugs has greatly enhanced the therapeutic armamentarium, but at the expense of an increased risk and occurrence of adverse drug events. Furthermore, mounting public interest in herbal and weight-loss products, unregulated in many countries, has further added to this potentially serious problem [1,2]. Adverse reactions from conventional drugs are reported to account for 3 to 8% of all hospital admissions [3–5] and to have caused numerous fatalities [1,6,7]. Although adverse drug events can affect all body systems, the liver is especially vulnerable since most drugs undergo partial or complete metabolism and elimination through the liver.

Drug hepatotoxicity is most commonly classified into two broad categories: intrinsic hepatotoxicity (direct or predictable) and toxicity due to host idiosyncrasy (indirect or unpredictable) [8]. Examples of the former are inadvertent exposure to industrial or environmental chemicals and toxins such as carbon tetrachloride, phosphorus or certain mushrooms that cause dose-related liver injury in virtually all recipients. In contrast, 'idiosyncratic' hepatotoxicity from conventional drugs and herbal products cause liver injury in only a small number of recipients, ranging from 1 in 1000 to 1 in 100 000 or more, presumably through immunological [9], metabolic [10] or possibly genetically determined [11] mechanisms [12].

Liver injury from a drug generally begins weeks to months after commencing treatment, and the reaction usually subsides when the drug is discontinued but could advance if the drug is continued. If the drug is discontinued and restarted (rechallenged), the liver injury is more likely to recur after a shorter period of time and to be more severe [13].

Idiosyncratic hepatotoxicity is one of the most common reasons for an investigational drug not coming to market and the most common reason for an already approved drug being withdrawn or restricted [14,15] (Table 24.1). If liver injury is common or severe during drug development, this is generally recognized and the drug is never released. However, liver injury is sometimes not identified during the premarketing, phase III clinical trials because of its low frequency coupled with a study population of only several thousand patients insufficiently powered to detect rare adverse events [13]. Therefore, drug-induced liver injury is often first recognized after approval during postmarketing surveillance, when hundreds of thousands of patients receive the drug.

Frequency of drug-induced liver injury. Worldwide surveys indicate that drug-induced liver injury represents a relatively small fraction of all acute and chronic liver disease

---

Sherlock's Diseases of the Liver and Biliary System, Twelfth Edition. Edited by
James S. Dooley, Anna S.F. Lok, Andrew K. Burroughs, E. Jenny Heathcote.
© 2011 by Blackwell Publishing Ltd. Published 2011 by Blackwell Publishing Ltd.

Table 24.1. US and European regulatory actions due to drug-induced liver injury (1990–2009)

Withdrawals or not approved in the USA	Warnings
Iproniazid	Paracetamol (acetaminophen)
Ticrynafen	Leflunomide
Benoxaprofen	Nefazodone*
Nefazodone*	Isoniazid
Ibufenac	Labetolol
Perhexiline	Nevirapine
Dilevalol	Pyrazinimide/ rifampicin
Fipexide	Terbinafine
Benzarone	Valproic acid
Alpidem	Zifurlukast
Bendazac	Atomexitine
Chlormezanone	Saquinavir/ rifampicin
Pemoline	Interferon-α-1
Felbamate	Infliximab
Bromfenac	Telithromycin
Tolcapone	(Kava)
Trovafloxacin	(Lipokinex)
Troglitazone	
Ximelagatran	
Nimeluside	
(Hydroxycut)	

*The brand drug, Serzone, has been withdrawn both in the European and US market but a generic form is available in the USA with a black box warning. Items in parentheses are herbal products.

[16–23]. In one study from Switzerland, the frequency of prevalent hepatotoxicity on admission was 0.7%, whereas its incidence during hospitalization was 1.4% [24]. The true frequency of all forms of drug-induced injury is, however, uncertain [12,25,26], partly a result of poor reporting through physician ignorance, diffidence and insecurity [27]. Regarding *hepatotoxicity*, many cases first present with elevated serum aminotransferase or alkaline phosphatase levels without symptoms or jaundice, and thus may not be recognized at all or may be misdiagnosed. Moreover, raised aminotransferase levels may regress despite continuation of the drug, a situation referred to as 'adaptation' [28].

Worldwide epidemiology

Western countries. The true frequency of hepatotoxicity in the general population is poorly established because of the paucity of prospective population-based studies, its relatively low occurrence and the difficulty in making the diagnosis.

Retrospective database studies. Retrospective data have come largely from administrative claims databases and

from using International Classification of Diseases (ICD) coding that defines drug-induced liver injury [22–24,29–33]. Eight representative studies are shown in Table 24.2, five from the USA [23,29–32], two from the UK [22,33] and one from Switzerland [24]. The major limitation of retrospective data is the inability to confirm the validity of the diagnoses.

Data shown in Table 24.2 were accumulated over several years by evaluating between 732 and 1 636 792 individuals. The prevalence of hepatotoxicity, reported in five studies, ranged between 0.7 and 22.8%, although the latter percentage was an outlier. Estimated incidences, reported in three studies, were 1/100 000, 2.4/100 000 and 40.6/100 000. In one study, paracetamol (acetaminophen) hepatotoxicity exceeded the true idiosyncratic liver injury cases by a factor of 5 [29]. Another study focused on identifying specific drugs that cause liver injury (amoxicillin clavulanate, phenytoin, valproate and isoniazid) [32].

Prospective cohort and registry studies. Prospective studies involve gathering consecutive cases of drug-induced liver injury either at a single centre or through multicenter registries. One representative prospective study, performed at a Swedish University out-patient clinic, reported that 77 (6.6%) of 1164 successive patients with liver disease had possible drug-induced liver disease [34].

Three registry studies are shown in Table 24.3; two collect all cases of idiosyncratic drug-induced liver injury [35,36] while one accepts only cases of fulminant hepatic failure [37,38]. The Spanish Registry has been assembling cases over a 10-year period from 32 referral centres [35]. Among 570 cases submitted, 461 were considered *bona fide* instances of drug-induced liver injury; 49% were female, 71% were jaundiced, 51% were hospitalized and 7% died or required liver transplantation. The annual incidence of hepatotoxicity was 34.2 ± 10.7 cases per 100 000 inhabitants, and the annual incidence of severe drug-induced liver injury was 16.6 ± 6.7 cases per 100 000 inhabitants.

A second registry is part of the ongoing US Drug-Induced Liver Injury Network (DILIN) study, which recently reported findings in the first 300 consecutive cases collected [36]. The mean age of enrollees was 48 years, 60% were female and 7% were children. The median latency to liver injury was 42 days, and 54% were hospitalized. A single prescription drug was implicated in 73% of cases, 9% were attributed to herbals and dietary supplements and 18% had received more than one suspect medication. The most commonly implicated single drugs received were antimicrobials (45.5%), neuropsychiatric medications (15%) and immunomodulatory agents (5.5%). Among the 9% of patients requiring transplantation or who died, fewer than one-half died

Table 24.2. Retrospective database studies of drug-induced liver injury

Study [Ref.]	Beard [31]	Duh [30]	De Abajo [22]	Galan [23]	Meier [24]	Jinjuvadia [32]	Vuppalanchi [29]	Hussaini [33]
Years	77–81	92–93	94–99	93–02	96–02	94–04	99–03	98–04
Population size	280 000	NR	NR	NR	6383	1 485 500	NR	800
Number reviewed	28	170 000	1 636 792	4039	4209	7395	732	347
Methodology	ICD-9 codes (Inpatient)	ICD-9 codes (Inpatient/ outpatient)	Computer dx codes (Inpatient/ outpatient)	Manual review of records	ICD-10 codes	ICD-9 codes Inpatient/ outpatient	Manual review or EMR (Inpatient/ outpatient)	Manual review
Number with DILI (%)	12	50 (22.8%)	128	32 (0.8%)	88 (1.4%)	83 (1.1%)	5 (0.7%)	28 (8.1%)
DILI Incidence	1/100 000	40.6/100 000	2.4/100 000	NR	NR	NR	NR	NR
Mean age (years)	52	53	NR	52	56	39	36	Mostly elderly
Female (%)	92	47	NR	44	37	51	40	39
Outcome	All recovered	8% hospitalized	28% hospitalized, 1% transplanted	All recovered	Mostly recovered, 2 patients transplanted	12% death or transplanted	All recovered	One death, remainder recovered

ERM, electronic medical records; DILI, drug-induced liver injury; ICD, International Classification of Diseases; NR, not reported.

Table 24.3. Prospective registry studies of patients with drug-induced liver injury

Study [Reference]	Chalasani [36]	Andrade [35]	Ostapowicz/ Lee [37]*
Country	USA	Spain	USA
Years	04–07	94–04	98–07
No. of cases	300	461	119
Mean age (years)	48 + 18	53	43
% <18 years	7	NR	0
% Female	60	49	67
Injury at onset:			
% Hepatocellular	57	58	NR*
% Cholestatic	23	21	NR
% Mixed	20	21	NR
% Jaundice	73	71	NR
% Hospitalized	54	51	100
% Death/ transplanted	9	7	34 died, 40 transplanted
% Chronic injury	13	10	NR
Suspect drugs	45% Antibiotics	32 % Antibiotics	20% Antituberculosis
	15% Central nervous system	17% Central nervous system	12% Sulfa drugs
	5.5% Immunomodulatory	17% Musculoskeletal	10% Phenytoin
	5% Analgesics	10% Gastrointestinal	10% Herbals
	5% Antihypertensives		
	4% Anticancer		

*All patients had acute liver failure at entry with INR >1.5 and encephalopathy. The median alanine aminotransferase at presentation was 571 IU/mL.

of liver disease. Liver injury persisted beyond 6 months in 14% of the cases.

In the continuing US Acute Liver Failure Study Group registry, 40 (13%) of the first 308 reported cases from 23 referral centres consisted of idiosyncratic drug reactions, which included isoniazid, bromfenac and troglitazone [37]. The most commonly implicated drug, however, was paracetamol. In a follow-up report, 119 (11.5%) of 1033 consecutive cases of acute liver failure were attributed to idiosyncratic drug-related injury [38]. The mean age of patients was 43 years, 67% were female and only 26% survived without a transplant. The most commonly implicated medications in this follow-up report were antibiotics, which included antituberculosis drugs (20%), sulfa compounds (12%), phenytoin (10%) and herbals (10%).

Perhaps the most accurate data regarding the true incidence of hepatotoxicity come from a population-based prospective study conducted among 81 000 inhabitants of Northern France [16]. All potential cases of hepatotoxicity were referred to a central study team over a 3-year period. Ninety-five cases of hepatotoxicity were suspected, but only 34 were assessed as having probable hepatotoxicity. Their mean age was 50.9 years, 65% were female, and 6% died from liver injury. Only

30% had been referred to a gastroenterology specialist, indicating that the majority were managed by primary care physicians. Suspect medications included antibiotics (25%), psychotropics (22%), hypolipidaemics (12%) and non-steroidal anti-inflammatory drugs (10%). The annual incidence of drug-induced liver injury was estimated at 13.9 ± 2.4 episodes per 100 000 patient years and did not differ substantially by gender and age. This annual incidence of hepatotoxicity was over 16-fold higher than that reported to health authorities, signifying a high rate of under-reporting of drug-induced liver injury in the general population.

Asian countries. The epidemiology and risk factors for drug-induced liver injury have been less well studied in Asian than in Western countries. Available reports from Asia indicate, however, that implicated medications are more likely to be herbal and/or other traditional 'medicines' [39,40].

Expressions of hepatotoxicity

There is virtually no form of liver disease, acute or chronic, that drug-induced liver injury cannot simulate (Table 24.4) [41–43]. It is this fact that confounds the adjudication process.

Table 24.4. Expressions of drug-induced liver injury

Type of injury	Representative responsible drug(s)
Acute liver diseases	
Acute hepatocellular injury	Numerous drugs such as isoniazid, rifampicin, methyl dopa, telithromycin, ketoconazole, diclofanac
Mononucleosis-like	Sulfonamides, phenytoin, dapsone
Fulminant hepatitis	Paracetamol (acetaminophen)
Bland cholestasis	Anabolic/ androgenic steroids, ciclosporin
Cholestatic hepatitis	Chlorpromazine, erythromycin, amoxicillin–clavulanate, clarithromycin
Chronic liver diseases	
Chronic hepatitis	Methotrexate, lisinopril, trazodone, uracil
Autoimmune hepatitis	Nitrofurantoin, minocycline, methyldopa, oxyphenisatin
Macrovesicular hepatitis	Corticosteroids, methotrexate, asparaginase, alcohol, halothane
Microvesicular hepatitis	Valproic acid, tetracyclines, cocaine, amiodarone
Steatohepatitis	Amiodarone, griseofulvin, perhexillene maleate
Cirrhosis	Methotrexate, amiodarone
Granulomatous hepatitis	Allopurinol, rosiglitazone, sulfonamide, phenylbutazone, quinidine
Primary biliary cirrhosis-like	Chlorpromazine, erythromycin, amoxicillin–clavulanate, haloperidol
Peliosis hepatic	Anabolic steroids, oral contraceptives
Portal vein thrombosis	Oral contraceptives
Sinusoidal obstructive syndrome	Pyrrolozidine alkaloids, adriamycin, floxuridine, oncotherapy
Nodular transformation	Anabolic and contraceptive steroids
Adenoma	Anabolic and contraceptive steroids
Hepatocellular carcinoma	Thorotrast, anabolic and contraceptive steroids
Cholangiocarcinoma	Thorotrast
Angiosarcoma	Vinyl chloride, inorganic arsenicals

Acute liver diseases (Table 24.4). Drug-induced liver injury presents most commonly as acute liver disease, hepatocellular exceeding cholestatic injury. The injury may imitate acute viral hepatitis, including a mononucleosis-like picture, ranging from mild, asymptomatic illness to more severe injury, characterized by increased levels of both aminotransferases and serum bilirubin, and even fulminant hepatic failure. Hepatotoxicity may also simulate acute obstructive jaundice, presenting either as bland cholestasis with normal serum enzymes, or as cholestatic hepatitis, characterized by increases in both serum bilirubin and alkaline phosphatase. A third form of acute injury is macrovesicular and microvesicular steatosis.

Chronic liver diseases (Table 24.4). Drugs can also cause the entire spectrum of chronic liver diseases with histology resembling chronic viral or autoimmune hepatitis, macro- or microvesicular steatosis or steatohepatitis, and even fully established cirrhosis. Hepatotoxicity can also simulate chronic cholestatic diseases, presenting as chronic granulomatous liver disease or as a picture resembling primary biliary cirrhosis or sclerosing cholangitis, occasionally culminating in the vanishing bile duct syndrome. Drugs can also cause such vascular disorders as peliosis hepatis, hepatic vein thrombosis,

and the sinusoidal obstruction syndrome (previously veno-occlusive disease). Finally, drugs may induce hyperplasia such as nodular transformation, as well as benign (adenomas) and malignant (hepatocellular carcinoma, cholangiocarcinoma, angiosarcoma) neoplasms.

Classification of hepatotoxicity

Direct hepatotoxins typically cause dose-dependent liver damage and zonal hepatocyte necrosis, an effect readily reproducible in animals. Examples are carbon tetrachloride and paracetamol which cause centrilobular necrosis, yellow phosphorus which causes midzonal injury, and allyl alcohol which causes periportal injury (Fig. 24.1) [44–46]. Few direct hepatotoxins are available for routine public use with the notable exception of paracetamol. A recent study actually demonstrated that almost one-third of healthy volunteers administered a therapeutic dose of 4 g of paracetamol per day developed mild elevations in serum alanine aminotransferase (ALT) values together with detectable serum paracetamol-protein adducts [47].

'Idiosyncrasy' derives from a Greek word that means 'a mixture of one's own self' [13]. The term is applied to drugs that cause injury in a minority of individuals who appear uniquely susceptible due to alteration in host

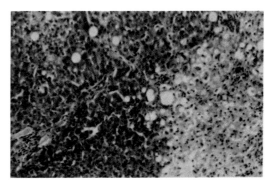

Fig. 24.1. Accidental carbon tetrachloride poisoning. To the right of the section, liver cells are necrotic and show hydropic degeneration and fatty change. Surviving cells to the left of the section show occasional fatty change. The portal zones are unaffected.

metabolism, uptake or processing of the drug. Unlike direct hepatotoxins, idiosyncratic hepatotoxicity does not present as a single type or pattern of liver injury. Generally, idiosyncratic liver injury is diffuse consisting of necrosis, cholestasis and/or steatosis that involves the entire lobule, accompanied by variable inflammatory cell infiltrates consisting of lymphocytes, plasma cells and eosinophils.

Idiosyncratic drug-induced liver injury may present with hypersensitivity or immunoallergic features in a minority of patients or as an autoimmune form of liver disease. The former is characterized by a generally short latency to liver injury onset with fever, rash, lymphadenopathy and arthralgias, together with eosinophilia and lymphocytosis [48]. Some drugs typically associated with this response include the sulfonamides, procainamide and the penicillins.

In some instances, circulating antibodies to liver and kidney endoplasmic reticulum (antiliver/kidney microsomal antibodies, anti-LKM) may develop. These antibodies result from an acquired immune response to a new antigen created by covalent binding between a reactive metabolite and a hepatocellular protein. Anti-LKM antibodies frequently react with cytochrome P450s (CYPs) but may also react with other drug-metabolizing enzymes [49,50]. Antienzyme antibodies have been found in hepatotoxicity caused by tienilic acid, dihydralazine and halothane [51–53]. The current concept is that a highly reactive metabolite binds covalently to or damages the enzyme that produced it [54]. Antibodies form if this enzyme is antigenic and advances outside the hepatocyte where it becomes attached to antigen-presenting cells. Because antibodies recognize different proteins from liver injury due to different drugs (i.e. bioactivating enzymes differ depending upon drug structure), antiliver antibodies should be useful in some instances in assessing causality. Aromatic anticonvul-

sants have been associated with antibodies to CYP3A11 and halothane has been associated with antibodies to the E2 subunit of pyruvate dehydrogenase. Most medications that cause hepatotoxicity, however, are not associated with a characteristic drug-metabolizing autoantibody profile.

Some drugs, such as aldomet, minocycline and nitrofurantoin, can cause an autoimmune form of liver injury characterized by a liver biopsy displaying prominent plasma cell infiltration, the presence of autoantibodies such as the antinuclear antibody (ANA) and smooth muscle antibody (SMA), and variable increases in serum immunoglobulin levels [55–57]. This poses the problem of distinguishing drug-induced from a pre-existing but unrecognized idiopathic form of autoimmune hepatitis. One clue to exclude pre-existing autoimmune hepatitis is that the liver injury resolves and the autoantibodies disappear after discontinuing the drug, although, in some instances, short- or long-term treatment with corticosteroids is necessary, particularly in those with jaundice, to induce remission of drug-induced autoimmune hepatitis.

Predictors of susceptibility and outcome in drug-induced liver injury

Type of presentation. It has long been assumed that drug-induced hepatocellular injury, particularly if accompanied by jaundice, is more likely than cholestatic liver disease to have a fatal outcome. This assumption is not supported by recent data from the Spanish, Swedish, and US registry studies that have found that both hepatocellular and cholestatic drug injury have a similar rate of mortality [35,36,58].

Female gender. There is also wide-spread belief that women are more likely than men to develop hepatotoxicity, especially with the use of herbal products or dietary supplements. The reasons offered for this include the lower body and liver weight of women, the greater use of and compliance with medication by women, and possible differences in drug-metabolizing enzyme activities. However, this view has been challenged by several reports [35,36,59]. In an analysis of Spanish Hepatotoxicity Registry patients, no difference in rates was found between men and women [35]. Similarly, in the ongoing Drug Induced Liver Injury Network (DILIN) prospective study, the frequency of drug-induced liver injury has been similar in men and women, although hepatocellular liver injury has occurred more frequently in women than men (65 versus 35%) [36].

Women may not be more susceptible to developing drug-induced liver injury but they do seem at increased risk for adverse outcomes. Data from the Acute Liver Failure study show a preponderance of women with paracetamol-related fulminant hepatitis as well as more severe idiosyncratic drug-induced liver disease [37,38]. Also, data from the Spanish Hepatotoxicity Registry indicated that more women than men required liver transplantation or died as a result of hepatotoxicity [60].

Age. The incidence of drug-induced liver injury is believed to increase with advancing age at exposure. The proposed reasons are that older people are more likely to use medications, especially multiple drugs, and that they are likely to have altered drug pharmacokinetics, accounting for reduced drug metabolism, distribution and elimination [61,62]. Some evidence supports an increased risk of hepatotoxicity with increasing age from drugs such as isoniazid and amoxicillin–clavulanate [63,64]. A study from Japan of 142 patients hospitalized for hepatotoxicity reported that persons older than 75 years of age were more likely than those under 75 to have higher levels of alkaline phosphatase and a cholestatic profile at presentation [65]. In addition, data from the Spanish registry indicates that subjects over age 60 are more likely to present with cholestasis [64]. Thus, older persons appear more prone than younger people to develop drug-induced cholestatic liver injury.

The frequency of hepatotoxicity is lower in children than adults, in part because they less commonly take medications, and rarely multiple drugs. Moreover, children appear less susceptible than adults to developing drug-induced liver injury, with a few exceptions. Children with viral infections have a relatively high predilection for developing Reye's syndrome when treated with aspirin [66]. They also appear more likely to develop a similar pattern of liver injury from treatment with valproate and erythromycin [67]. These effects may relate to age-related differences in P-450 gene expression, which is known to be markedly increased in children compared to adults.

Other potential predictors. Underlying chronic viral hepatitis, B or C, is believed to increase the risk of developing hepatotoxicity. This may be due to altered pharmacokinetics, up-regulated intrahepatic cytokine expression or alterations in drug metabolizing pathways. There are reports of an increased risk of drug-induced liver injury in persons with chronic viral hepatitis who are treated with isoniazid and rifampicin [68,69] as well as with ibuprofen and methimazole [70]. Also, there are multiple reports of an increased risk of hepatotoxicity in persons with human immunodeficiency (HIV) infection coinfected with hepatitis B or C treated with highly active antiretroviral therapy [71,72]. To further support a role for HCV infection is the evidence that the risk of hepatotoxicity is reported to decline with successful eradication of HCV RNA [71]. Additional prospective research of viral replication and immunological status is necessary, however, to ensure that the liver injury is not a result of viral flare.

Obesity and non-alcoholic fatty liver disease (NAFLD) do not appear to increase the risk of developing drug-induced liver injury. Numerous studies have shown that statins do not increase the risk of developing hepatotoxicity in persons with obesity and NAFLD [73–75]. Obesity is, however, associated with poorer outcomes in persons who develop acute liver failure, although the pattern, severity and outcome of drug-induced liver injury are not influenced by an increased body mass index measurement [35,58].

The poorer outcome may be the consequence of inapparent underlying obesity-related chronic liver disease, such as cirrhosis.

Alcohol. The role played by alcohol in enhancing hepatotoxicity requires additional study. There are reports indicating that the risk of isoniazid hepatotoxicity is increased in alcoholics [76]. Also, much attention has focused on determining whether alcohol augments paracetamol hepatotoxicity [77–79]. Indeed, it is theoretically plausible that chronic alcoholism increases the risk of paracetamol hepatotoxicity because alcohol induces hepatic CYP2E1, the enzyme responsible for converting paracetamol to its toxic metabolite, and because chronic alcoholism is associated with a reduction in protective glutathione and other essential nutrients [80]. There are even reports that chronic alcoholism enhances hepatotoxicity from receipt of low doses of paracetamol [79]. Challenging this view are data from the Acute Liver Failure study that showed a similar frequency of alcohol use among those with paracetamol hepatotoxicity regardless of whether the drug overdose was intentional or non-intentional [81]. Furthermore, the DILIN study found that an absence of alcohol consumption was associated with a poorer outcome [39].

Mechanisms of injury, drug metabolism and pharmacokinetics

Hepatic clearance of drugs given orally depends upon the efficiency of drug-metabolizing enzymes, intrinsic clearance, liver blood flow and the extent of plasma protein binding (Fig. 24.2). Drugs vary in their pharmacological effects based on these different pharmacokinetic factors [61].

Hepatic drug metabolism

Phase 1. The main drug-metabolizing system resides in the microsomal fraction of the hepatocyte, the smooth endoplasmic reticulum. Oxidation or hydroxylation of drugs, most commonly mediated through cytochrome (CYP) P450s, improves their solubility. Other drug-

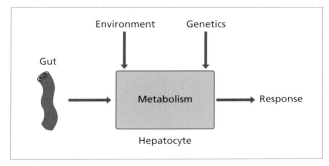

Fig. 24.2. The response of the liver to drugs depends on the interplay between absorption, environmental factors and genetics.

metabolizing reactions, such as conversion of alcohol to acetaldehyde by alcohol dehydrogenases, are present in the cytosolic fraction.

CYP enzymes are divided into gene families based upon 40% homology using Arabic numbers of 1 to 10; subfamilies are designated by a capital letter and specific isoforms are sequentially numbered. Currently, three CYP gene families (*CYP1, 2* and *3*) are identified as having a major role in drug metabolism (Fig. 24.3) [80]. Inducers of CYP metabolic pathways include barbiturates, alcohol, anaesthetics, hypoglycaemic and anticonvulsant agents, griseofulvin and rifampicin. Enzyme induction by these drugs may lead to slight liver enlargement.

Phase 2. Conjugation of a drug or its metabolite with a small endogenous molecule serves to further enhance solubility and elimination from the body. The enzymes concerned are usually not confined to the liver but are present there in high concentration (i.e. glucuronidation, sulfotransferases, acetyltransferases).

Phase 3. Active transport of drugs typically takes place at the biliary pole of the hepatocyte. Drug transport is energy dependent and can be saturated. Multiple factors determine whether the metabolized drug will be excreted in bile, urine or both. Highly polar parent drugs or metabolites as well as those with a molecular weight exceeding 200 Da are typically excreted in the bile. In contrast, the urinary route is more important with smaller molecules (Fig. 24.4). In humans, the multidrug resistant protein (MDR) is involved with transport of cationic drugs into bile. In addition, the multidrug resistance-associated proteins (MRPs) are involved in drug transport in the liver. The bile salt excretory protein (BSEP) and MDR3 are two other important canalicular transport proteins involved in drug excretion with a complex system involved in their regulation and function.

The cytochrome P450 system

Each CYP protein is encoded by a unique gene which has variable expression among individuals, accounting in part for the fourfold or higher difference in drug metabolism among healthy persons. Each CYP isoform has a unique 'substrate' binding site capable of binding some, but not all, drugs. Inter-individual differences in the expression and translation of CYP proteins may determine idiosyncratic reactions to drugs. An example is the poor metabolism of debrisoquine (an antiarrhythmic drug) due to abnormal expression of CYP2D6 [82], which can be identified by PCR amplification of parts of the mutant genes of CYP2D6. CYP2E1 is involved in the production of electrophilic metabolites of paracetamol. CYP3A is concerned with the metabolism of ciclosporin and many other drugs including erythromycin, statins and ketaconazole. CYP2C polymorphism affects the metabolism of mephenytoin, diazepam and many other drugs.

Enzyme induction and drug interactions. Induction of P450 enzymes may enhance the production of toxic metabolites. Ethanol induces CYP2E1 and may increase the toxicity of paracetamol via increased generation of *N*-acetylbenzoquinineimine (NAPQ1), a metabolite of paracetamol (Fig. 24.5). Similarly, paracetamol hepatotoxicity may increase in patients treated with isoniazid, which also induces CYP2E1 [83]. Ciclosporin, tacrolimus (FK506), erythromycin and ketoconazole compete for binding and metabolism by CYP3A4 and ciclosporin levels rise after they are given (Fig. 24.3).

Molecular mechanisms in drug-induced liver injury

The clinical manifestations of drug-induced liver injury are a consequence of hepatocyte death mediated by either apoptosis or necrosis [84]. Apoptosis involves cellular shrinkage and fragmentation into discrete bodies which maintain intact plasma membranes (Fig. 24.6). These apoptotic bodies are rapidly cleared by phagocytosis, leaving little substrate to induce a host immune response. In contrast, necrosis involves a profound loss of mitochondrial function with ATP depletion, leading to cellular swelling and lysis which then promotes a local inflammatory response.

The disassembly process in apoptosis is executed by intracellular caspases (cysteine-dependent aspartate-specific proteases), existing in hepatocytes as zymogens. The caspase cascade is activated by initiators and terminated or perpetuated by other intracellular proteins or events. Increased mitochondrial permeability may arise from extrinsic activation of hepatocytes which occurs at the cellular surface (e.g. extrinsic pathway) or within the cell itself (intrinsic pathway). The principal hepatic

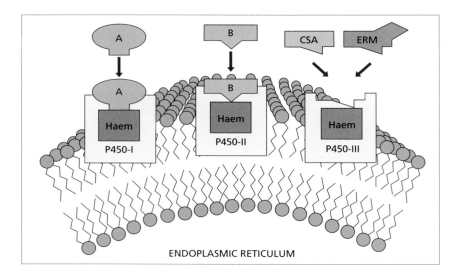

Fig. 24.3. P450s involved in drug metabolism are members of three gene families: P450-1, P450-2 and P450-3. Individual P450s have distinct catalytic properties. Ciclosporin (CSA) and erythromycin (ERM) bind to and are metabolized by P450s within the P450-3 family [80].

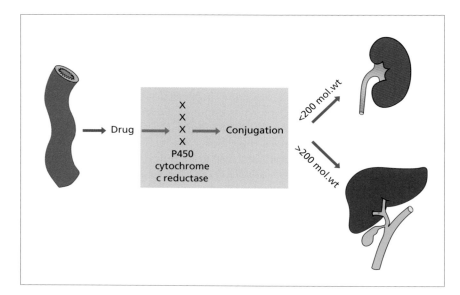

Fig. 24.4. Hepatic drug metabolism.

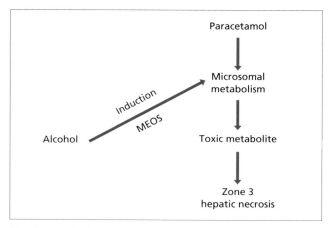

Fig. 24.5. Alcohol, as an enzyme-inducing agent, increases the production of toxic metabolites of paracetamol (acetaminophen), thus potentiating hepatic necrosis. MEOS: microsomal enzyme oxidizing system.

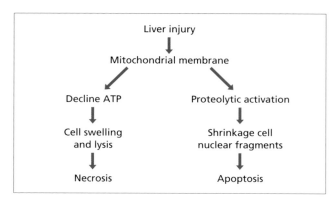

Fig. 24.6. Mechanism of hepatocyte death.

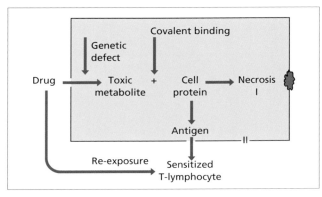

Fig. 24.7. The mechanisms of hepatotoxicity, direct metabolite-related and immunological hypersensitivity.

death receptors are tumour necrosis factor-1 (TNF-1) and Fas [85]. Drugs and their metabolites may either induce TNF production by Kupffer cells or natural killer cells of the innate immune system or help sensitize hepatocytes to the effects of TNF.

Drugs or their metabolites may also act as haptens and covalently bind hepatic proteins such as the CYP enzymes. Macrophages can then present these peptides on their cell surfaces bound to major histocompatability complex (MHC) class II. The adaptive immune system consisting of CD4 and CD8 T cells then contributes to apoptotic cell death mediated through Fas-ligand (Fig. 24.7). However, haptenization alone may be insufficient to trigger an immune response and a concomitant 'danger' signal such as mild background liver injury or a concomitant infectious or inflammatory condition may be required [86]. Important clinical correlates of intrahepatic and systemic danger signals include the increased risk of drug-induced liver injury and other adverse drug reactions in patients with AIDS [87].

Non-inflammatory or bland drug-induced cholestasis, as occurs with oral contraceptives or ciclosporin, may be due to inhibition of BSEP [88]. However, most clinically overt cholestatic reactions are associated with bile duct injury and a variable amount of inflammation. An hypothesis is that toxic drug metabolites undergo canalicular excretion and that exposed cholangiocytes are then injured as a result of an immune mediated reaction [89]. Interindividual differences in BSEP and MDR3 expression may play a role in drug-induced cholestasis [90].

Genetic polymorphisms in drug-induced liver injury

Like other complex diseases, different genes and environmental factors may contribute to both susceptibility and outcome in drug-induced liver injury [91,92]. Genes

involved may encode proteins with roles in several different pathways including drug metabolizing enzymes, drug transporters, apoptosis, acquired and innate immune responses and cellular repair and regeneration. Traditional studies have included candidate gene approaches with arbitrary selection of polymorphisms from genes of potential interest. For example, the slow acetylator genotype of *N*-acetyltransferase-2 (NAT-2) has been associated with an increased risk of isoniazid liver injury in some but not all studies [93–95]. Similarly, several studies have explored human leucocyte antigen (HLA) genotype polymorphisms and amoxicillin–clavulanate hepatotoxicity [96–98]. Two studies [96,97] involving 35 and 22 patients, respectively, identified a highly significant association of HLA DRB1*1501 with hepatotoxicity, a finding not confirmed in an independent cohort of 27 Spanish patients [98].

Commercial platforms containing probes for 500 000 and 1 000 000 single nucleotide polymorphisms (SNPs) typically present in 1 to 5% of the general population have also been proposed for genetic association studies of drug-induced liver injury [99]. With no specific *a priori* hypothesis, such extensive genotyping invariably identifies large numbers of associations by chance and therefore the threshold for significance in these studies is typically set at $P = 10^{-7}$ to 10^{-8}. Accordingly, it is now common to require duplication of a significant association in a second, independent cohort [100]. For example, the HLA-B*5701 haplotype was found to confer an 80-fold increased risk in susceptibility to flucloxacillin hepatotoxicity, a finding replicated in a second independent cohort of European patients [101]. However, since almost 5% of Caucasians have this haplotype, the absolute risk of developing drug-induced liver injury remains low in patients with this genotype (1 in 500). Nonetheless, knowing the HLA genotype could be helpful in establishing a diagnosis of drug-induced liver injury [102].

Diagnostic approaches and causality assessment of drug-induced liver injury

Diagnosing hepatotoxicity with certainty is problematic for several reasons. First, hepatotoxicity can simulate virtually every type of liver disease so that, in the absence of biomarkers or other specific tests [103], drug-induced liver injury is at present a diagnosis of exclusion [84]. It is therefore mandatory when assessing potential hepatotoxicity to exclude all causes of liver injury that it can mimic. Second, having access to all sequential clinical and biochemical data related to the injury, which is not always available, is key to defining the characteristics and pattern of the liver injury which aids in its diagnosis. Third, the medical condition for which the drug is given may itself cause liver dysfunction and thus confound the adjudication process. Fourth, because multiple drugs are commonly used, synergistic interactions may result as well as uncertainty about which drug is actually responsible for the injury. Finally, locating historical information that supports the potential for hepatotoxicity of a given drug can be challenging, especially in view of the innumerable drugs and herbals currently on the market.

Two primary methods are employed to assess causality in drug-induced liver injury—the use of general clinical acumen and utilization of numerical scoring systems [104,105]. The former involves applying careful judgment when clinical or biochemical evidence of liver injury appears linked to the use of a drug or herbal product. However, lacking a specific diagnostic test for hepatotoxicity, this approach to causality assessment is highly subjective, its accuracy depending upon the expertise of the interviewer and the intensity with which alternate causes are eliminated. Nevertheless, it is generally accepted as the 'gold standard' diagnostic approach; when undertaken by groups of experienced clinicians, the assessment is considered to be by 'expert opinion'.

A more objective means of assessing causality was proposed by international experts at a meeting of the Council for International Organizations of Medical Scientists (CIOMS) in 1989 [106,107]. The result was the development of a structured numerical scoring system to grade the likelihood of drug-induced liver injury. The meeting was supported by Roussel-Uclaf Pharmaceuticals, and hence the instrument was called RUCAM (Roussel-Uclaf Causality Assessment Method). This instrument is now regularly employed by field experts in hepatotoxicity and by pharmaceutical companies to evaluate suspected cases of drug-induced liver injury, but it is difficult to use and therefore has not achieved wide clinical acceptance, even among practicing hepatologists.

Other grading instruments proposed have included the M and V system (clinical diagnostic scale) and the Naranjo scale [108–110]. However, the former has been found to be less effective than RUCAM [111], as has the latter [112] which was developed originally for assessing *any* adverse drug reactions.

Clinical and biochemical presentations of drug-induced liver disease

Clinical presentation. Hepatocellular injury presents similarly to acute viral hepatitis, symptoms ranging from none at all to those typical of acute fulminant hepatitis. Generally, symptoms are non-specific, consisting of fatigue, myalgia, nausea and/or vomiting and, occasionally, mild right upper quadrant discomfort or pain. Depending upon the drug, symptoms may include mild fever, arthralgias and pruritus. Jaundice, together with marked pruritus, is a hallmark of cholestatic liver injury.

Biochemical presentation. Generally, the first indicator of drug-induced liver injury is detection of raised serum ALT and aspartate aminotransferase (AST) levels in *hepatocellular* injury and the alkaline phosphatase in *cholestatic* injury. The enzyme pattern with hepatocellular drug-induced liver injury resembles acute viral hepatitis, including an ALT increase that exceeds the AST increase. An uncertain issue is what the level of ALT elevation should be that triggers withdrawal of the potentially offending drug. This decision is usually based on the severity of the liver damage, the gravity of the disease being treated, and whether or not there is an alternative replacement drug. Some discontinue the drug if the ALT level exceeds three times the upper limit of normal (ULN) on two or more occasions, others when it exceeds five times ULN, and still others when it exceeds eight times ULN [113]. However, the level of ALT increase does not necessarily define current liver disease severity nor is it necessarily predictive of outcome [113]. A more robust indicator of liver disease severity is the addition of hyperbilirubinaemia (total bilirubin ≥2.5 mg/dL) or of overt jaundice, a combination that has been associated with a 10% or greater risk of liver-related mortality [35,58]. The US Food and Drug Administration (FDA) refer to this as 'Hy's rule', named for Dr Hyman J. Zimmerman, a pioneer in the study of hepatotoxicity [15,114]. Thus, if an affected person has debilitating clinical symptoms and/or increased levels of the total serum bilirubin, the drug should be discontinued even if the ALT elevation is only threefold elevated. Alkaline phosphatase is generally only slightly elevated in persons with hepatocellular injury, but is moderately to markedly increased with cholestatic injury. Bilirubin elevation is more common in cholestatic than in hepatocellular injury, but without necessarily having the same implications. This presentation, referred to as intrahepatic cholestasis, must be distinguished from jaundice of extrahepatic obstruction using imaging (e.g. ultrasonography) and/or other procedures (e.g. magnetic resonance cholangiopancreatography). Some drugs, such as oral contraceptives, may induce pure cholestasis, characterized by an increase only in the serum bilirubin level [88,115]. Serum enzymes less commonly assessed are γ-glutamyl transpeptidase and lactic dehydrogenase, although they can be moderately helpful in diagnostic evaluation.

Drug-induced liver disease may also present as *mixed hepatocellular/ cholestatic* liver disease, with significant increases in levels of both the aminotransferases and the alkaline phosphatase. Characterizing the presenting pattern of injury is important because drugs tend to be consistent in the type of injury they cause. However this is not always the case, because there may occasionally be deviation from the usual pattern or the pattern may change during the course of the injury, transitioning from hepatocellular to a mixed and even a cholestatic form over time [35].

For some drugs, the target is intracellular organelles such as mitochondria. Biochemical dysfunction in this situation ranges from mild to moderate elevations in bilirubin and aminotransferase levels to severe liver injury associated with an increase in the serum ammonia level and lactic acidosis.

Other laboratory tests. Other important tests are the prothrombin time (or INR), the complete blood count and differential, and tests for autoantibodies. The prothrombin time helps define disease severity, identifying eosinophilia helps to establish the injury as immunoallergic, while identifying increased levels of ANA, antismooth muscle antibodies (SMA) and antimicrosomal antibodies helps categorize it as of autoimmune origin. Finding antimitochondrial antibodies (AMA) helps distinguish drug-induced cholestatic liver disease from primary biliary cirrhosis, although transient AMA positivity may rarely be seen with hepatotoxicity, particularly if fulminant hepatitis develops.

Histological presentations. A biopsy is commonly not performed because it is problematic to routinely require an invasive procedure if there are no specific interventions to offer, and the biopsy may not be specifically diagnostic for drug-induced liver injury. While there are histological features that strongly suggest drug injury, such as zonal necrosis, eosinophilia and microvesicular steatosis, the biopsy is often most useful for identifying alternative diagnoses, including unanticipated cirrhosis, given the near epidemic of non-alcoholic fatty liver disease. Nevertheless, an astute and experienced pathologist who couples histopathology with clinical findings can provide extremely helpful diagnostic and at times, prognostic information [42,43,116].

Assessment of suspected drug-induced liver disease (Table 24.5)

The first step in evaluating a suspected case of hepatotoxicity is to exclude other more common causes of liver disease. With hepatocellular injury, conditions requiring exclusion are acute viral hepatitis, pre-existing autoimmune hepatitis, alcoholic liver disease, non-alcoholic fatty liver disease, acute congestive heart failure or other causes for hypotension [104,105]. Virus testing must include assays for hepatitis A (IgM anti-HAV), hepatitis B (HBsAg or IgM anti-HBc), and hepatitis C (anti-HCV and HCV RNA), and, preferably, hepatitis E, Epstein–Barr virus and cytomegalovirus infections. Measuring serum globulin levels and testing for autoantibodies helps exclude autoimmune hepatitis, while ultrasonography and cross-sectional imaging is used to screen for fatty liver and pancreaticobiliary disease such as gallstones or malignancy that may present with obstructive jaundice. Finally, complete evaluation requires excluding haemochromatosis, Wilson's disease and α-1-antitrypsin deficiency.

Important historical information includes alcohol use, cardiovascular disease and whether there had been an episode of acute hypotension. These factors may lead to hepatocellular injury, although their injury patterns are reasonably distinctive and separable from drug-induced liver injury.

With no alternative explanation for acute liver injury but receipt of a drug, the next step is to consider which drug might be responsible and to review the circumstances surrounding and features of the liver injury. A careful history must be taken of all medications (e.g. prescription, herbal, weight loss) received in the preceding 12 months, including their precise start and stop dates. Also important is whether there had been a previous episode of hepatotoxicity and, if so, what drug had been implicated. Defining features of the liver injury is helpful in implicating specific medications since most drugs that cause liver injury have a characteristic '*signature*'. Requirements include: establishing the time interval between start of the drug and onset of liver disease (*latency*); defining the *clinical pattern* of the liver injury (hepatocellular, cholestatic, mixed); and recording the time to recovery after drug discontinuation (*de-challenge*). Also important is to determine whether the drug responsible for the current injury had been received in the past, thus representing a *re-challenge*. The clinical pattern is defined using the R value equation [106,107]:

$$R \text{ value} = \frac{ALT \div ULN \text{ of } ALT}{\text{alkaline phosphatase} \div ULN \text{ of alkaline phosphatase}}$$

An R value ≥ 5 establishes hepatocellular; ≤ 2, cholestatic; and >2 but <5, a mixed pattern of injury.

Assessing causality for drug-induced liver disease

Assessment using clinical judgment. Once a specific drug is identified as potentially responsible for the liver injury, the final steps are to grade it for the likelihood of its implication as well as the severity of the liver injury. Various grading systems have been devised for this purpose. The US DILIN study group has developed enhanced grading systems for assessing both the likelihood and severity of the liver injury, as shown in Tables 24.6 and 24.7 [117].

Table 24.5. Evaluation of potential drug-induced liver injury

History	All drugs and herbals used in past 12 months
	Start and stop date(s) for all medications
	Past history of hepatotoxicity and use of implicated drug
	Symptoms at onset (fever, rash, fatigue, abdominal pain)
	Disease(s) for which medication taken
	Other disease(s), particularly cardiovascular
	Episode of acute hypotension
	Alcohol intake
Physical examination	Jaundice, rash, clinical evidence of pruritis
	Liver and spleen size
	Stigmata of chronic liver disease
Routine chemistries	Complete blood count and differential, platelets, total protein, albumin/ globulin
	Prothrombin time/ INR, creatinine
Liver chemistries	alanine aminotransferase, aspartate aminotransferase, alkaline phosphatase, total/ direct bilirubin, γ-GTP
Serologies	IgM anti-HAV, HBsAg, anti-HBc IgM, anti-HCV, HCV RNA, anti-HEV, anti-EBV, anti-CMV
Autoantibodies	antinuclear antibody, smooth muscle antibody, antimitochondrial antibody
Special tests	Serum iron, ferritin, ceruloplasmin, α-1-antitrypsin
Imaging	Ultrasound, CT, MRI (ERCP)

ERCP, endoscopic retrograde cholangiopancreatography; γ-GTP, γ-glutamyl transpeptidase.

Table 24.6. The Drug Induced Liver Injury Network (DILIN) grading system for causality assessment

Causality	Likelihood score (%)	Description
1 Definite	>95	Liver injury typical for drug or herbal; causality 'beyond a reasonable doubt'
2 Highly likely	75 to 95	Causality 'clear and convincing' but not definite
3 Probable	50 to 74	Causality supported by 'the preponderance of the evidence
4 Possible	25 to 49	Causality not supported by 'the preponderance of the evidence'
5 Unlikely	<25	Causality 'highly unlikely'
6 Insufficient evidence	Not applicable	

Adapted from [117].

Table 24.7. The Drug Induced Liver Injury Network (DILIN) grading system for liver disease severity

Score	Grade	Definition
1	Mild	ALT and/or alkaline phosphatase levels increased but total serum bilirubin <2.5 mg/ dL and INR <1.5
2	Moderate	ALT and/or alkaline phosphatase levels increased and total serum bilirubin ≥2.5 mg/ dL or INR ≥1.5
3	Moderate–Severe	ALT, alkaline phosphatase, bilirubin and/or INR increased and patient is hospitalized or ongoing hospitalization is prolonged because of drug-induced liver injury
4	Severe	ALT, alkaline phosphatase and total serum bilirubin is increased together with at least one of the following: (i) hepatic failure (INR ≥1.5, ascites or encephalopathy); or (ii) other organ failure due to liver injury
5	Fatal	Death or liver transplantation because of drug-induced liver injury

ALT, alanine aminotransferase.
Adapted from [117].

Follow-up of acute drug-induced liver injury. It is important to follow the affected person to resolution of the clinical symptoms and biochemical abnormalities. This provides important de-challenge information as well as information on whether the injury advanced to chronic liver disease [116]. Liver biopsy examination at this time helps categorize the status of the liver disease.

Assessment using RUCAM. The RUCAM, designed as an objective measure, confers points for clinical, biochemical, serological and radiological characteristics of liver injury [106,107]. Seven domains are included in the system:
- time to onset of the liver disease after starting the drug
- course of the liver disease
- risk factors for developing liver injury
- potential for hepatotoxicity of concomitant drugs
- exclusion of non-drug causes of liver injury
- previous information regarding hepatotoxicity of the implicated drug
- response to re-administration (i.e. re-challenge).

Each domain is awarded a positive or negative numerical score, the total ranging from −9 to +14. The scoring components differ somewhat according to the pattern of liver injury (hepatocellular, cholestatic/mixed).

Because RUCAM is an objective numerical scoring system, there should be little variation in scoring from one reviewer to another. However, contents of some of the seven domains are not clearly defined and therefore may be variably interpreted, even by expert reviewers [118]. Moreover, comparison of causality assessment between the 'expert opinion' approach and RUCAM shows a relatively poor correlation, RUCAM appearing to skew the results to a lower grade of likelihood [119]. Nevertheless, RUCAM retains popularity among some authorities because the expert opinion approach also has limitations [120]. Further efforts are needed to develop an improved RUCAM-like scoring instrument, preferably in a menu-driven electronic format.

Medical management

The primary management approach for hepatotoxicity is to immediately discontinue the offending medication. In most but not all situations, the liver injury will subside. When the injury presents as autoimmune hepatitis, and recovery fails even with drug discontinuation, corticosteroid treatment is commonly used, although with conflicting results [121,122]; two randomized controlled trials failed to demonstrate effectiveness of corticosteroid therapy in non-paracetamol-induced liver failure [123,124].

Antioxidants have been proposed as treatment for severe drug-induced liver injury [125,126], but a randomized controlled trial failed to demonstrate improvement except for those with low-grade encephalopathy [127]. Cholestyramine may benefit those with pruritus. Cholestyramine binds drug metabolites circulated enterohepatically with a half-life of 15 days and has been speculated to hasten recovery from leflunomide hepatotoxicity [128,129].

Liver injury from specific drugs

Numerous drugs are reported to cause liver injury, but the present review focuses only on those most commonly implicated in large drug registries.

Analgesics

Non-steroidal anti-inflammatory drugs (NSAIDs)

NSAIDs, including the cyclo-oxygenase-2 (COX-2) inhibitors, have caused hepatotoxicity with varying frequency. A survey in Denmark found that NSAIDs accounted for 9% of all instances of drug-induced liver injury between 1978 and 1987 [130]. One NSAID, bromfenac, has been withdrawn from use because of a high rate of severe hepatotoxicity.

Celecoxib. Surveys in multiple randomized controlled trials have identified extremely low rates of 'significant' aminotransferase elevations from celecoxib [131–133]. There are, nevertheless, reports of both acute hepatocellular and cholestatic injury occurring mostly in women up to 4 weeks after starting the drug, all of whom recovered [134–136]. Another selective inhibitor, rofecoxib, has been associated with a higher rate of liver injury [132], but has been withdrawn from use because of cardiotoxicity.

Nimesulide. Nimesulide was withdrawn from use in Spain, Italy and France because of hepatotoxicity, although the risk of severe liver injury (33.1/100 000 person years) has been found to be only slightly higher than in other NSAIDs [137]. There are, however, reports of both hepatocellular and cholestatic liver injury occurring within 15 weeks of drug administration, including death from liver failure [138–141].

Ibuprofen. Liver injury from this commonly used NSAID is rare although high drug doses have caused mild aminotransferase elevations, generally without symptoms. There are rare reports of serious and even fatal liver disease, presenting as immunoallergic hepatocellular injury, associated with the Stevens–Johnson syndrome; chronic cholestasis has also been seen, culminating in the vanishing bile duct syndrome [142–145]. One unsubstantiated report suggested that the risk for ibuprofen hepatotoxicity may be higher in persons with chronic hepatitis C infection [146].

Sulindac. This drug is commonly associated with hepatotoxicity [133,147,148]. A review of 91 cases reported to the FDA by 1993 revealed a variable pattern of liver injury, 43% presenting as cholestatic, 25% as hepatocellular and 22% as mixed injury [149]. Approximately three-quarters of affected person were female, and most were of advanced age. Some cases displayed features of hypersensitivity, including the Stevens–Johnson syndrome. Five per cent died as a result of liver disease.

Diclofenac. This frequently prescribed NSAID has been responsible for both mild, non-serious serum aminotransferase elevations as well as for several hundred instances of severe hepatotoxicity, including fatal cases [150,151]. A recent review identified diclofenac as among the top drugs responsible for hepatotoxicity worldwide, with an estimated incidence of 6.3 per 100 000 users [22,147,148]. The injury, generally occurring 3 to 6 months after beginning treatment, can present as hepatocellular or cholestatic liver disease or as autoimmune hepatitis [152,153]. Withdrawal of the drug leads to complete recovery in most instances. Diclofenac metabolism is mediated through CYP2C9, but the risk of hepatotoxicity is not associated with polymorphisms in this gene [154–156].

Antibacterials

Penicillins and cephalosporins

Amoxicillin–clavulanate. Amoxicillin–clavulanate is the most frequently reported antibiotic to cause drug-induced liver injury, although its overall rate of hepatotoxicity is estimated as less than 1 case per 100 000 patient years [157]. Most patients present with cholestasis and fever or rash 1 to 4 weeks after stopping therapy [158]. However, some patients may develop early hepatocellular liver injury and present as late as 8 weeks after ceasing therapy. Older men are at increased risk of augmentin hepatotoxicity, but younger adults and women may also be afflicted. Although most patients recover, some may experience prolonged cholestasis and a minority may develop ductopenia [159]. The clavulanate component of the drug is believed responsible for the toxicity but rare cases of severe liver injury have been reported with amoxicillin alone [160].

Cephalosporins. Cephalosporins share close structural homology with the penicillins and cross reactivity of acute hypersensitivity reactions are well reported. Despite their widespread use, cephalosporin-related hepatotoxicity is exceedingly uncommon. Typically, the presenting illness is cholestasis or granulomatous hepatitis with a latency of 1 to 4 weeks and abrupt onset of liver injury [161]. In most instances, recovery has been rapid with no residual liver injury [162]. Ceftriaxone, excreted predominantly in bile, has been associated with biliary sludge and pseudolithiasis due to the precipitation of a calcium salt of the drug [163].

Macrolides

Azithromycin and clarithromycin. Azithromycin, commonly prescribed to both children and adults, has a prolonged half-life that reaches high concentrations in the liver. Rare cases of self-limited cholestatic hepatitis have been reported after only a 5-day course of azithromycin [164]. In addition, some patients develop progressive ductopenia. Clarithromycin may also cause a similar liver injury, particularly in older individuals [165].

Erythromycin. This commonly used drug is well known to cause symptomatic cholestatic hepatitis with an incidence of 4 cases per 100 000 patient years [166]. Erythromycin estolate appears more likely than erythromycin succinate to cause this syndrome but progressive or fatal liver injury is rare [167,168]. Both ductopenia and vanishing bile duct syndrome have been reported [169].

Telithromycin. This semisynthetic macrolide derivative (i.e. ketolide) was approved for use in respiratory tract infections in 2004. Clinical trials demonstrated serum ALT elevations in 2% of treated patients and three cases of severe and rapid-onset hepatotoxicity with telithromycin were reported in 2006 [170]. In each instance, elevated liver chemistries and jaundice developed within 2 to 7 days and two of the patients died or underwent transplantation. A recent series of 42 cases confirmed a rapid onset of fever, abdominal pain and jaundice as well as the appearance of ascites in some cases which then resolved [171]. In 2007, restrictions on the applications of this drug were implemented.

Nitrofurantoin. Acute, self-limited hepatocellular, mixed, cholestatic, and even granulomatous reactions have been described with nitrofurantoin [172]. Most instances of acute hepatotoxicity occur within 6 weeks of treatment, often accompanied by fever, rash or eosinophilia. In addition, prolonged administration of nitrofurantoin for recurrent infections can lead to chronic hepatitis with serological and histological features simulating autoimmune hepatitis [55]. Most patients with the latter phenotype improve with drug cessation but some have required corticosteroids or even liver transplantation for long-term survival.

Quinolones

Quinolone antibiotics act by inhibiting bacterial DNA gyrase and DNA topoisomerase IV. They are generally well tolerated but all of them have been associated with hepatotoxicity that can be rapid in onset and potentially fatal [173].

Trovofloxacin appears to be particularly hepatotoxic, with over 150 cases of liver toxicity and 57 cases of acute liver failure reported up to 2006 [174]. Accordingly, severe restrictions have been placed on its use.

Sulfonamides and trimethoprim

A wide range of liver injury due to sulfonamide antimicrobials has been reported, including granulomatous hepatitis and progression to chronic liver disease [175]. The frequent presence of rash, fever and eosinophilia suggest an immunoallergic reaction, which is more commonly seen in HIV-positive individuals [176]. Co-trimoxazole (trimethoprim–sulfamethoxazole) is well known to cause cholestatic hepatitis which may rarely progress to acute liver failure. Co-trimoxazole has also been associated with a prolonged cholestatic illness with hepatic phospholipodois [177]. The sulfa component is believed responsible for most of these reactions but trimethoprim alone may cause cholestasis.

Tetracyclines

Intravenous administration of tetracycline has been associated with severe liver injury characterized by microvesicular steatosis with minimal or no hepatic necrosis. Clinically, mitochondrial toxicity is suspected with hypoglycaemia, renal failure, acidosis and pancreatitis [178]. However, this complication is now rare since high-dose intravenous administration has been abandoned.

Minocycline. Minocycline may lead to liver injury within 5 weeks of treatment, associated with eosinophilia and rash. Alternatively, some patients develop liver injury after only a year or more of treatment for acne with features of autoimmunity such as autoantibodies, arthritis and liver histology consistent with autoimmune hepatitis [179,180].

Doxycycline. This oral drug has rarely been associated with severe liver injury [181].

Antituberculosis agents

Drugs to treat tuberculosis can lead to significant liver biochemical abnormalities in up to 20% of those treated, particularly the elderly [182]. Possible risk factors include underlying viral hepatitis, HIV infection and alcoholism, which can also complicate causality assessment [183–185]. The use of multidrug therapy poses challenges in identifying the specific offending agent.

Isoniazid. Ten per cent or more of treated persons develop serum enzyme elevations which persist without toxicity or even regress despite continued use of the drug, a consequence of metabolic adaptation. However, isoniazid causes serious liver injury or jaundice in 1% of treated subjects. The rate of severe hepatotoxicity with isoniazid monotherapy for latent tuberculosis in children and young adults is probably lower at 1 in 1000 or less [186]. Most patients develop acute hepatocellular liver injury with focal necrosis and lobular and portal inflammation on biopsy [187]. In general, the hepatitis resolves with discontinuation of therapy but some may develop progressive liver failure.

Rifampicin. Given alone, rifampicin rarely causes hepatotoxicity but hyperbilirubinaemia may develop secondary to a drug-induced haemolysis. When rifampicin is combined with isoniazid, the risk of severe hepatotoxicity markedly increases, possibly due to induction of CYP enzymes involved in the metabolism of isoniazid [188,189].

Pyrazinamide. This drug causes dose-dependent hepatotoxicity. However, because it is usually combined with isoniazid and rifampicin, assigning causality and assessing the incidence has been difficult. Nonetheless, subjects receiving pyrazinamide-containing regimens may be at increased risk of hepatotoxicity and more severe liver injury [190].

Antifungal agents

Azole antibiotics. Azole antibiotics are potent inhibitors of CYP3A and have all been associated with hepatotoxicity. Ketoconazole treatment induces elevated liver-related chemistries in 10% of treated patients but significant injury occurs in only 1 in 15000 patient years [191]. Adverse reactions to ketoconazole are more frequent in women and people over the age of 40. Most develop acute hepatocellular injury with centrilobular necrosis but cholestatic hepatitis may also occur [192]. Itriconazole less commonly causes hepatotoxicity. Fluconazole may also cause mild liver biochemical abnormalities during treatment but significant liver injury is uncommon [193].

Terbinafine. This allyamine agent causes symptomatic hepatitis in up to 1 in 50 000 patient years [194]. Hepatotoxicity typically develops 4 to 6 weeks after commencing therapy for toenail or fingernail infections [195].

Antiretrovirals (Table 24.8)

The incidence of hepatotoxicity in patients receiving antiretrovirals ranges from 3 to 18% [196]. All protease inhibitors are metabolized by CYP3A4 and have been associated with hepatotoxicity, particularly high dose ritonavir which has a 3 to 9% risk of severe hepatotoxicity [197]. A black box warning was issued in 2006 regarding the increased risk of hepatitis in patients taking tipranavir and ritonavir, particularly in patients with HBV or HCV coinfection. Both indinavir and atazanavir have been associated with symptomatic increases in unconjugated hyperbilirubinaemia due to competitive inhibition of bilirubin uridine diphosphate-glucuronyltransferase [198]. It is recommended that patients receiving these drugs undergo serial liver biochemistry assessment with frequent monitoring if serum ALT is more than five times ULN and discontinuation

Table 24.8. Hepatotoxicity of the antiretroviral agents used to treat HIV infection

Drug	Precautions
Protease inhibitors	
Ritonavir (RTV, Norvir)	Hepatotoxicity with high-dose ritonavir (600 mg two times daily)
Lopinavir/ Ritonavir (Kaletra)	Avoid combination amprenavir–ritonavir (competing CYP3A4 substrates)
Amprenavir (APV, Agenerase)	Indirect hyperbilirubinaemia with indinavir and atazanavir (do not use
Saquinavir (SQV, Fortavase)	together)
Indinavir (IDV, Crixivan)	Severe hepatotoxicity with tipranavir has been reported; avoid use in
Fosamprenavir (FPV, Lexiva)	patients with underlying liver disease
Nelfinavir (NFV, Viracept)	
Atazanavir (ATV, Reyataz)	
Tipranavir (TPV, Aptivus)	
Darunavir (DRV, Prezista)	
Nucleoside reverse transcriptase inhibitors (NRTI)	
Zalcitabine (ddC, Hivid)	Lactic acidosis (especially with ddC, ddI, d4T) due to mitochondrial toxicity
Didanosine (ddI, Videx)	Increased risk of lactic acidosis with ribavirin in conjunction with ddI or d4T
Stavudine (d4T, Zerit)	Avoid ribavirin–ddI combination in HCV patients with advanced fibrosis due
Lamivudine (3TC, Epivir)	to risk of hepatic decompensation
Zidovudine (AZT, Retrovir)	Abacavir hypersensitivity more common in those with HLA B*5701 and
Abacavir (ABC, Ziagen)	pretreatment screening is recommended
Emtricitabine (FTC, Emtriva)	
Tenofovir (TFV, Viread)	
Abacavir/ iamivudine/zidovudine (Trizivir)	
Abacavir/ iamivudine (Epzicom)	
Zidovudine/ lamivudine (Combivir)	
Emtricitabine/ tenofovir (Truvada)	
Non-nucleoside reverse transcriptase inhibitors (NNRTI)	
Nevirapine (NVP, Viramune)	Nevirapine hepatotoxicity usually in first 6 weeks and more common with
Efavirenz (EFV, Sustiva)	HBV/HCV coinfection or in women with CD4 >250/mL or men with CD4 >400/
Delavirdine (DLV, Rescriptor)	mL
Fusion inhibitors	
Enfuvirtide (T-20, Fuzeon)	
Integrase inhibitors	
Raltegravir (RAL, Insentress)	Given subcutaneously
CCR5 antagonists	
Maraviroc (MVC, Salzentry)	Side-effect profile not well established.

if ALT is more than 10 times ULN, for jaundice, or clinical symptoms (Table 24.4) [199].

Nucleoside reverse transcriptase inhibitors are frequently associated with asymptomatic, low-level increases in lactic acid levels but significant liver injury is rare [200]. The mechanism of nucleoside reverse transcriptase inhibitor-associated lactic acidosis is believed to involve mitochondrial toxicity through inhibition of human mitochondrial polymerase-γ. *In vitro* studies demonstrate the strength of inhibition to be as follows: zalcitabine (ddC) > didanosine (ddI) > stavudine (d4T) > lamivudine (3TC) > zidovudine (AZT) > abacavir [201]. Current recommendations advise against coadministration of didanosine and stavudine due to an increased risk of lactic acidosis. In addition, administration of ribavirin in conjunction with didanosine or stavudine should be avoided in patients with HCV coinfection due to an increased risk of mitochondrial toxicity [202]. Finally, pretreatment screening for HLA-B*5701 is recommended to minimize, but not eliminate, the risk of an early hypersensitivity reaction with abacavir [203].

Nevirapine, a non-nucleoside reverse transcriptase inhibitor, is associated with a high rate of hepatotoxicity with hypersensitivity features and rash within a few weeks of starting treatment [204]. In addition, a cumulative dose may cause late-onset toxicity [205]. Risk factors for hepatotoxicity include HBV or HCV coinfection and higher CD4 counts. Efavirenz has been safely substituted in patients with prior nevirapine hepatotoxicity.

Cardiovascular drugs

Angiotensin-converting enzyme (ACE) inhibitors. ACE inhibitors rarely cause *bona fide* hepatotoxicity [206]. Captopril is most frequently reported to cause liver injury, but all ACE inhibitors can lead either to hepatocellular or cholestatic liver injury with symptoms of fever, myalgia and rash [207]. The angiotensin II receptor antagonists, also used to treat hypertension, infrequently cause cholestatic hepatitis [208,209].

α-*methyldopa.* Use of this antihypertensive agent has declined in recent years because of its numerous adverse effects, including hepatotoxicity [210]. Liver injury typically presents within a few months of starting treatment but hepatotoxicity occurring after many years of continuous treatment has also been reported. Such patients often present with detectable autoantibodies or a Coombs' positive haemolytic anaemia [211]. Liver biopsy may display feature of autoimmune hepatitis or characteristic pericentral inflammation while others may have severe necrosis. Most patients improve with drug cessation, although some may require steroids or even liver transplantation [212].

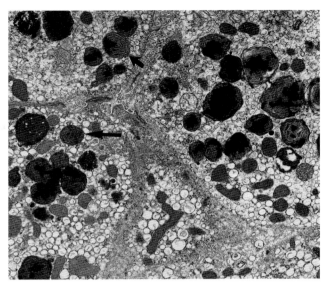

Fig. 24.8. Amiodarone hepatotoxicity: electron microscopy of the liver showing lysosomal lamellar bodies containing myelin figures (arrow).

Amiodarone. This commonly used antiarrhythmic leads to mild asymptomatic aminotransferase increases in 15 to 25% of treated patients [213]. Although overt hepatic injury is less common, it may be progressive and occasionally fatal. An acute hepatitis or cholestatic injury pattern may occur even after drug discontinuation. Also, some develop a chronic injury pattern with hepatic steatosis, fibrosis and Mallory bodies, simulating alcoholic liver disease [214]. Most of these patients have received high daily doses and develop a phospholipidosis in hepatic lysosomes presumably due to the prolonged drug half-life and lipophilicity (Fig. 24.8) [215]. Resolution of liver injury can be slow after drug discontinuation.

Beta-blockers. An uncommon, under-recognized side effect of labetalol, a selective α1- and β-adrenergic receptor, is acute hepatitis, which may be severe in some patients [216]. Hepatotoxicity with other selective and non-selective beta-blockers is very uncommon [217].

Calcium channel blockers. Nifedipine, verapamil and diltiazem are generally well tolerated but cases of rapid onset liver injury with immunoallergic features have been reported [218–220].

Hydralazine. Liver injury with this vasodilatory agent includes hepatitis, intrahepatic cholestasis, centrilobular necrosis and granulomatous hepatitis [221,222]. Markedly elevated serum aminotransferase levels with increased alkaline phosphatase levels and jaundice may develop within 6 months of starting therapy. Some patients may have increases in anticytochrome P-450 antibodies. Although most improve with drug cessation, fatal hepatotoxicity has been reported [223].

Central nervous system drugs

Anticonvulsants. The frequent use of these drugs in combination makes causality assessment particularly challenging. Carbamezapine causes mild increases in serum γ-glutamyl transpeptidase (γ-GTP), alkaline phosphatase and AST levels in up to 60, 15 and 22% of users, respectively, through microsomal enzyme induction [224]. Clinically significant liver injury, often associated with hypersensitivity features and less frequently with myelotoxicity, develops in 16 per 100 000 patient years [225]. Right upper quadrant pain resembling cholangitis sometimes occurs and many have granulomatous hepatitis on biopsy (Fig. 24.9) [226]. Time to liver disease onset is 1 to 16 weeks without obvious relationship to dose or serum level. Most patients improve with drug cessation and re-challenge is frequently positive [227].

Phenytoin is an aromatic anticonvulsant that frequently causes asymptomatic increases in γ-GTP and alkaline phosphatase levels and, less commonly, clinically significant liver injury [228]. Hepatic injury frequently accompanies the hypersensitivity reaction to phenytoin. Up to 60% of patients may have splenomegaly or lymphadenopathy which can mimic infectious mononucleosis [229]. In contrast to carbamazepine hepatitis, phenytoin liver injury occurs predominantly in adults and may be fatal [230].

Valproic acid is an anticonvulsant increasingly used in patients with bipolar disorder and migraine headaches. Clinical manifestations of hepatotoxicity may include hyperammonaemia and lactic acidosis in infants and children as well as severe hepatic necrosis and microvesicular steatosis [231]. Most liver injury occurs within 6 months of starting the drug, beginning with symptoms of lethargy and nausea and vomiting [232]. Retrospective studies indicate that patients under 2 years of age, those receiving multiple anticonvulsants and children with underlying developmental disorders and inborn errors of metabolism may be at increased risk. The latter observation suggests that potential inhibition of mitochondrial β-oxidation may explain the apparent improvement with l-carnitine therapy.

Lamotrigine is a broad-spectrum anticonvulsant associated with hypersensitivity skin rashes in 3 to 10% of treated patients, many of whom have mild liver biochemical abnormalities [233]. Additionally, some may develop acute liver failure [234].

Antidepressants

Many psychoactive drugs are lipophilic, requiring hepatic metabolism. It is therefore not surprising that many of them can cause hepatotoxicity. Tricyclic antidepressants can induce cholestatic liver injury and even prolonged cholestasis, as seen with amitriptyline or imipramine or, less frequently, hepatocellular injury [235,236]. Serotonin reuptake inhibitors are inhibitors of CYP isoenzymes and may lead to drug interactions. In addition, fluoxetine has been associated with hepatitis [237]. Paroxetine has also been implicated in both acute and chronic hepatitis and liver injury due to sertraline and venlafaxine have been reported [238–240].

The monoamine oxidase inhibitors phenelzine and trancypromine can also cause hepatotoxicity [241]. Nefazadone, which has mixed mechanisms of action, has caused subfulminant liver failure in multiple patients, prompting a recent label change and black-box warning [242,243]. Trazadone appears to be less hepatotoxic but cases of jaundice and chronic hepatitis have been reported [244]. Finally, bupropion has been associated with hepatitis and an autoimmune-like hepatitis [245,246].

Antidiabetic agents

Thiazolidinediones. These insulin sensitizing agents improve peripheral glucose uptake and help lower triglycerides. Troglitazone was withdrawn from the market in 2000 following 94 reported cases of liver failure [247]. In clinical trials, rates of elevated serum aminotransferase levels with rosiglitazone and pioglitazone were not different from placebo. Subsequent reports of hepatotoxicity with both pioglitazone and rosiglitazone have appeared including a single case of granulomatous hepatitis [248–251]. A recent review of the FDA database identified 21 cases of liver failure attributed to these agents, occurring after a median of 6 weeks; the estimated annual incidence was 2 cases per 100 000 patient years [252]. Patients with underlying liver disease are not at increased risk of hepatotoxicity, and these agents may benefit patients with non-alcoholic steatohepatitis, but long-term studies are needed [253,254].

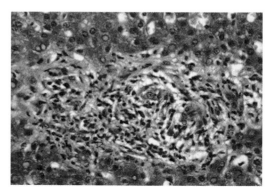

Fig. 24.9. Carbamazepine granulomatous hepatitis.

Other diabetic agents. Metformin is an oral biguanide hypoglycaemic agent. Both cholestatic and hepatocellular toxicity have rarely been described as well as lactic acidosis in patients with heart, liver and renal disease [255–257].

Hypolipidaemics

Fibrates. Administration of these drugs to animals is associated with hepatomegaly, peroxisome proliferation and tumours [258]. Mild aminotransferase elevations have been reported in humans, but serial liver biopsies have failed to demonstrate significant changes in subcellular organelles and peroxisomes when compared to untreated controls [259,260]. However, cases of hepatitis associated with fenofibrate have been reported [261].

Niacin. Niacin is well known to cause dose-dependent hepatotoxicity, particularly with doses exceeding 3 g per day. Severe hepatotoxicity and acute liver failure has been reported with the sustained-release formulation [262,263].

Statins. These HMG-CoA-reductase inhibitors, among the most commonly prescribed drugs worldwide, are rarely associated with severe hepatotoxicity. In clinical trials, statins were associated with mild serum ALT elevations in up to 3% of treated patients which were usually non-progressive despite continued treatment [264]. Additionally, up to 20% of patients may develop serum creatine phosphokinase elevations, associated with symptomatic myopathy in a minority of individuals, appearing to be linked to polymorphisms in the *SLC01B1* gene involved in statin uptake [265]. Despite differences in pharmacokinetics, lipophilicity, and degree of hepatic metabolism, all statins may cause rare but significant hepatotoxicity. In 40 published cases of statin hepatotoxicity, 57% were female, most were in their 50s or 60s and most had hepatocellular injury at presentation [266]. The reported duration of therapy prior to symptomatic hepatotoxicity ranged from 5 days to 4 years. An autoimmune-like hepatitis has been rarely reported in some patients with statin hepatotoxicity and may persist after drug discontinuation [267,268]. Multiple studies have demonstrated that statins are safe and effective in patients with NAFLD and compensated chronic liver disease [264].

Other hypolipidaemics. Ezetimibe inhibits intestinal uptake of cholesterol and has been used alone or in combination with other agents. Two non-fatal cases of hepatotoxicity with ezetimibe combined with simvistatin have been reported [269].

Inhalational anaesthetic agents

Halogenated anaesthetics were introduced in the 1950s as potent, fast-acting, non-irritant agents. However, infrequent cases of apparent severe hepatotoxicity associated with halothane led to decline in its use and the introduction of other safer agents. The incidence of halothane hepatotoxicity is 1 per 30 000, women and obese persons appearing to be more susceptible [270]. Most patients present with a fever and/or rash with myalgias days to weeks after repeated exposure. Centrilobular necrosis is a common histological feature but some patients have fatty infiltration or even granulomas in the liver (Fig. 24.10) [271]. Halothane hepatitis is commonly accompanied by peripheral eosinophilia, circulating autoantibodies to tissue antigens, and cellular and humoral immune sensitization to reactive-metabolite-modified liver neoantigens [272].

A review of 24 patients receiving enflurane demonstrated that this inhalational agent can also cause potentially severe hepatitis with a delay in onset of days to weeks after exposure [273]. However, the estimated incidence of 1 in 800 000 exposed patients is much lower than that observed with halothane. Numerous cases of liver injury attributable to isoflurane have also been reported but the projected incidence is even lower than that of enflurane [274,275]. Similarly, desflurane and sevoflurane have been associated with a similar profile of hepatotoxicity [276]. Patients with halogenated anaesthetic hepatotoxicity demonstrate similar autoantibodies

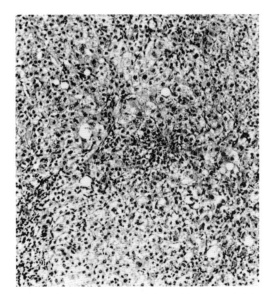

Fig. 24.10. Halothane-associated hepatitis. Hepatic histology shows cellular infiltration largely with mononuclear cell. Zone 3 areas show necrosis and cell swelling. Liver cell columns are disorganized. The appearances are virtually identical to those of acute viral hepatitis (H & E, ×96).

Table 24.9. Single herbal products and herbal mixtures reported to cause liver injury

Herbal	Type of liver injury
Atractylis gummifera	Diffuse hepatic necrosis
Black cohosh	Elevated serum enzymes, liver failure
Camphor	Elevated serum enzymes, Reye's syndrome
Cascara	Bridging fibrosis, bile duct proliferation
Chapparal	Cholestasis, zone 3 necrosis
Chaso and Onshido	Elevated serum enzymes, liver failure
Greater Celandine	Cholestasis
Germander	Zone 3 necrosis, cirrhosis
Impila	Hepatic necrosis
Ju bu huan	Periportal fibrosis, steatosis
Kava	Elevated serum enzymes, liver failure
Ma huang	Elevated serum enzymes, hepatic necrosis
Mistletoe (skullcap, valerian)	Elevated serum enzymes, acute hepatitis
Pennyroyal	Acute hepatitis, liver failure
Pyrrolizidine (comfrey, bush tea)	Sinusoidal obstruction syndrome
Sho-saiko-to (dai-saiko-to, TJ-9)	Bridging fibrosis, steatosis
Herbalife	Acute hepatitis, liver failure
Hydroxycut	Acute hepatitis, liver failure

Table 24.10. Herbal–drug interactions

Clinical effect	Herbal	Drug
Risk of bleeding	Danshen	Anticoagulants
Risk of bleeding	Dong quai	Anticoagulants
Risk of bleeding	Feverfew	Anticoagulants
Risk of bleeding	Garlic	Anticoagulants
Risk of bleeding	Ginkgo	Anticoagulants
Risk of clotting	Ginseng	Anticoagulants
Risk of bleeding	Papaya	Anticoagulants
Risk of clotting	St John's wort	Anticoagulants
Risk of bleeding	Tamarind	Anticoagulants
Purpura	Devil's claw	Anticoagulants
Risk of rejection	St John's Wort	Ciclosporin
Hepatotoxicity	Pyrrolizidines	CYP34A drugs
Hepatotoxicity	Germander	CYP34A drugs
Low prednisone concentration	Sho-saiko-to	Prednisone
Low spironolactone concentration	Liquorice	Spironolactone

and immunological profiles, suggesting a similar mechanism of liver injury as halothane hepatitis [277].

Herbals and weight-reduction products

Many consumers view herbal and weight-loss products as safe because they are 'natural' and because many have been used for centuries. Some consist of locally produced, single, traditional or ethnic botanicals, others are mixtures with multiple ingredients formulated and sold to enhance health and promote weight loss. The World Health Organization reports that 31 to 90% of populations in various countries, including those in the West, report having used herbals at least once [278]. The contribution of these products to the burden of hepatotoxicity is only now being defined. Approximately 10% of the first 300 adjudicated cases admitted to the US

DILIN prospective study were attributed to herbal or unregulated weight-loss products [39]. Similarly, a survey from Japan involving 1676 cases of drug-induced liver injury identified during a 10-year period found that 10% were attributed to dietary supplements and 7.1% to Chinese herbal drugs [40]. In contrast, 55% of all cases of hepatotoxicity reported from Singapore were accredited to traditional Chinese medications [41]. However, it is apparent that the frequency of liver injury from herbal products is seriously underestimated, either because their use is often not spontaneously reported by an affected person or because medical providers do not consider herbals and other over-the-counter products as potentially hepatotoxic [279,280]. Also concerning is that multiple herbal products are often used, commonly in the form of mixtures, making it difficult to identify the specific constituent responsible for the liver injury. Moreover, the injury may be caused by toxic contaminants, such as lead, mercury or arsenic [281,282].

Not only can herbals directly cause liver injury, but they may also modify the action of conventional medications being received simultaneously. Establishing herbal-induced hepatotoxicity, however, can be problematic because of the multiplicity of ingredients and the uncertain validity of reported contents. Shown in Table 24.9 is a listing of single herbals reported to cause liver injury [283], while Table 24.10 displays herbal–drug interactions [280].

Several commercially produced herbal combinations have also been reported to induce potentially fatal liver injury, including products marketed under the name of Herbalife, used for weight reduction [284–286]. Another is called Hydroxycut, also used for weight reduction as well as for body building. Following the identification of severe liver disease from its use, some cases culminating in death or requiring liver transplantation [287,288], the FDA required that the product be withdrawn from the market in 2009 [289].

References

1 Radimer K, Bindewald B, Hughes J *et al*. Dietary supplement use by US adults: data from the National Health and Nutrition Examination Survey: 1999–2000. *Am. J. Epidemiol.* 2004; **160**: 339–349.

2 Timbo BB, Ross MP, McCarthy PV *et al*. Dietary supplements in a national survey: prevalence of use and reports of adverse events. *J. Am. Diet. Assoc.* 2006; **106**: 1966–1974.

3 Pirmohamed M, James S, Meakin S *et al*. Adverse drug reactions as cause of admission to hospital: prospective analysis of 18,820 patients. *Br. Med. J.* 2004; **329**: 15–19.

4 McDonnell PJ, Jacobs MR. Hospital admissions resulting from preventable adverse reactions. *Ann. Pharmacother.* 2002; **36**: 1331–1336.

5 Budnitz DS, Pollock DA, Weidenbach KN *et al*. National surveillance of emergency department visits for outpatient adverse drug events. *JAMA* 2006; **296**: 1858–1866.

6 Wester K, Jonsson AK, Spigset O *et al*. Incidence of fatal drug reactions: a population based study. *Br. J. Clin. Pharmacol.* 2007; **65**: 573–579.

7 Leone R, Sottosanti L, Luisoa Iorio M *et al*. Drug-related deaths: an analysis of the Italian spontaneous reporting database. *Drug Saf.* 2008; **31**: 703–712.

8 Zimmerman HJ. *Hepatotoxicity: the Adverse Effects Of Drugs and other Chemical on the Liver*. New York: Appleton-Century-Crofts, 1978.

9 Liu ZX, Kaplowitz N. Immune-mediated drug-induced liver disease. *Clin. Liver Dis.* 2002; **6**: 755–774.

10 Lee WM. Drug-induced hepatotoxicity. *N. Engl. J. Med.* 2003; **349**: 474–485.

11 Ingelman-Sundberg M. Pharmacogenomic biomarkers for prediction of severe adverse drug reactions. *N. Engl. J. Med.* 2008; **356**: 637–639.

12 Navarro VJ, Senior JR. Drug-related hepatotoxicity. *N. Engl. J. Med.* 2006; **354**: 731–739.

13 Lee WM, Senior JR. Recognizing drug-induced liver injury: current problems, possible solutions. *Toxicol. Pathol.* 2005; **33**: 155–164.

14 Bakke OM, Mannochia MA, de Abajo F, Kaitin K, Lasagna. Drug safety discontinuations in the United Kingdom, the United States, and Spain from 1974–1993: a regulatory perspective. *Clin. Pharmacol. Ther.* 1995; **58**: 108–117.

15 Temple RJ, Himmel MH. Safety of newly approved drugs: implications for prescribing. *JAMA* 2002; **287**: 2273–2275.

16 Sgro C, Clinard F, Ouazir K *et al*. Incidence of drug-induced hepatic injuries: a French population-based study. *Hepatology* 2002; **36**: 451–455.

17 Bagheri H, Michel F, Lapeyre-Mestre M *et al*. Detection and incidence of drug-induced liver injuries in hospital: a prospective analysis from laboratory signals. *Br. J. Clin. Pharmacol.* 2000; **50**: 479–484.

18 Pillans PI. Drug associated hepatic reactions in New Zealand: 21 years experience. *N. Z. Med. J.* 1996; **109**: 315–319.

19 Friia H, Andreasen PB. Drug-induced hepatic injury: an analysis of 1100 cases reported to the Danish Committee on Adverse Drug Reactions between 1978 and 1987. *J. Intern. Med.* 1992; **232**: 133–138.

20 Olsson R, Brunlof G, Johansson ML, Persson M. Drug-induced hepatic injury in Sweden. *Hepatology* 2003; **38**: 531–532.

21 Garcia Rodriguez LA, Ruigomez A, Jick H. A review of epidemiologic research on drug-induced acute liver injury using the General Practice Research Database in the UK. *Pharmacotherapy* 1997; **17**: 721–728.

22 de Abajo F, Montero D, Madurga M, Garcia Rodriguez LA. Acute and clinically relevant drug-induced liver injury: a population based case-control study. *Br. J. Clin. Pharmacol.* 2004; **58**: 71–80.

23 Galan MV, Potts JA, Silverman AL, Gordon SC. Hepatitis in a United States tertiary referral center. *J. Clin. Gastroenterol.* 2005; **39**: 64–67.

24 Meier Y, Cavallaro M, Roos M *et al*. Incidence of drug-induced liver injury in medical inpatients. *Eur. J. Clin. Pharmacol.* 2005; **61**: 135–143.

25 Hazell L, Shakir SA. Under-reporting of adverse drug reactions: a systematic review. *Drug Saf.* 2006; **29**: 385–396.

26 Martin RM, Kapoor KV, Wilton LV, Mann RD. Under-reporting of suspected adverse drug reactions to newly marketed ('Black triangle') drugs in general practice. *Br. Med. J.* 1998; **317**: 119–120.

27 Lopez-Gonzalez E, Herdeiro MT, Fifueiras A. Determinants of under- reporting of adverse drug reactions: a systematic review. *Drug Saf.* 2009; **32**: 19–31.

28 Watkins PB. Idiosyncratic liver injury: challenges and approaches. *Toxicol. Pathol.* 2005; **33**: 1–5.

29 Vuppalanchi R, Liangpunsakul S, Chalasani N. Etiology of new-onset jaundice: how often is it caused by idiosyncratic drug-induced liver injury in the United States. *Am. J. Gastroenterol.* 2007; **102**: 558–562.

30 Duh MS, Walker AM, Kronlund KH Jr. Descriptive epidemiology of acute liver enzyme abnormalities in the general population of Massachusetts. *Pharmacoepidemiol. Drug Saf.* 1999; **8**: 275–283.

31 Beard K, Belic L, Aselton P *et al*. Outpatients drug-induced parenchymal liver disease requiring hospitalization. *J. Clin. Pharmacol.* 1986; **26**: 633–637.

32 Jinjuvadia, K, Kwan W, Fontana RJ. Searching for a needle in a haystack: use of ICD-9-CM codes in drug-induced liver injury. *Am. J. Gastroenterol.* 2007; **102**: 2437–2443.

33 Hussaini SH, O'Brien CS, Despott EJ, Dalton HR. Antibiotic therapy: a major cause of drug-induced jaundice in southwest England. *Eur. J. Gastroenterol. Hepatol.* 2007; **19**: 15–20.

34 de Valle MB, Av Klinteberg V, Alem N *et al*. Drug-induced liver injury in a Swedish University hospital out-patient hepatology clinic. *Aliment. Pharmacol. Ther.* 2006; **24**: 1187–1195.

35 Andrade RJ, Lucena MI, Fernandez MC *et al*. Drug-induced liver injury: an analysis of 461 incidences submit-

ted to the Spanish registry over a10–year period. *Gastroenterology* 2005; **129**: 512–521.

36 Chalasani N, Fontana RJ, Bonkovsky HL *et al.* Causes, clinical features and outcomes from a prospective study of drug-induced liver disease in the United States. *Gastroenterology* 2008; **135**: 1924–1934.

37 Ostapowicz G, Fontana RJ, Schiodt FV *et al.* Results of a prospective study of acute liver failure at 17 tertiary care centers in the United States. *Ann. Intern. Med.* 2002; **137**: 947–954.

38 Fontana RJ. Acute liver failure due to drugs. *Semin. Liver Dis.* 2008; **28**: 175–187.

39 Takikawa H, Murata Y, Horiike N *et al.* Drug-induced liver injury in Japan: an analysis of 1676 cases between 1997 and 2006. *Hepatol. Res.* 2009; **39**: 427–431.

40 Wai CT, Tan B-H, Chan C-L *et al.* Drug-induced liver injury at an Asian center: a prospective study. *Liver Int.* 2007; **27**: 465–474.

41 Zimmerman HJ. *Hepatotoxicity. The Adverse Effects of Drugs and Other Chemicals on the Liver*, 2nd edn. Philadelphia: Lippincott Williams & Wilkins, 1999.

42 Goodman ZD. Drug hepatotoxicity. *Clin. Liver Dis.* 2002; **6**: 381–397.

43 Ramachandran R, Kakar S. Histological patterns in drug-induced liver disease. *J. Clin. Pathol.* 2009; **62**: 481–492.

44 Recknagel RO. Carbon tetrachloride hepatotoxicity. *Pharmacol. Rev.* 1967; **19**: 145–208.

45 Diaz-Rivera RS, Collazo PJ, Pons ER *et al.* Acute phosphorus poisoning in man. A study of 56 cases. *Medicine* 1950; **29**: 269–298.

46 Rees KR, Tarlow MJ. The hepatotoxic action of allyl formate. *Biochem. J.* 1967; **104**: 757–761.

47 Watkins PB, Kaplowitz N, Slattery JT *et al.* Aminotransferase elevations in healthy adults receiving 4 grams of acetaminophen daily: a randomized controlled trial. *JAMA* 2006; **296**: 87–93.

48 Bonkovsky HL, Agrawal S, Fontana RB *et al.* Immunoallergic manifestations of drug-induced liver injury in the USA: results from the prospective study of the DILI network. *Gastroenterology* 2009; **136** (Suppl.1); Abstract 1590.

49 Robin MA, Le Roy M, Descatoire V, Pessayre D. Plasma membrane cytochromes P450 as neoantigens and autoimmune targets in drug-induced hepatitis. *J. Hepatol.* 1997; **26**: 23–30.

50 Manns MP, Obermayer-Straub P. Cytochromes P450 and uridine triphosphate-glucuronosyltransferase: model autoantigens to study drug-induced, virus-induced, and autoimmune liver disease. *Hepatology* 1997; **26**: 1054–1066.

51 Homberg JC, Andre C, Abuaf N. A new anti-liver-kidney microsome antibody (anti-LKM2) in tienilic acid-induced hepatitis. *Clin. Exp. Immunol.* 1984; **55**: 561–570.

52 Bourdi M, Larrey D, Nataf J *et al.* Anti-liver endoplasmic reticulum autoantibodies are directed against human cytochrome P-4501A2. A specific marker of dihydralazine-induced hepatitis. *J. Clin. Invest.* 1990; **85**: 1967–1973.

53 Nguyen C, Rose NR, Njoku DB. Trifluoroacetylated IgG4 ntibodies in a child with idiosyncratic acute liver failure after first exposure to halothane. *J. Pediatr. Gastroenterol. Nutr.* 2008; **47**: 199–202.

54 Beaune P, Dansette PM, Mansuy D *et al.* Human ant-endoplasmic reticulum autoantibodies appearing in a drug-induced hepatitis are directed against a human liver cytochrome P-450 that hyydroxylate the drug. *Proc. Natl. Acad. Sci. USA* 1987; **84**: 551–555.

55 Sharp JR, Ishak KG, Zimmerman HJ. Chronic active hepatitis and severe hepatic necrosis associated with nitrofurantoin. *Ann. Intern. Med.* 1980; **92**: 144–149.

56 Strader DB, Seeff LB. Drug induced chronic liver disease. *Clin. Liver Dis.* 1998; **2**: 501–522.

57 Gough A, Chapman S, Wagstaff K *et al.* Minocycline-induced autoimmune hepatitis and systemic lupus erythematosus-like syndrome. *Br. Med. J.* 1996; **312**: 169–172.

58 Bjornsson E, Olsson R. Outcome and prognostic markers in severe drug-induced liver disease. *Hepatology* 2005; **42**: 481–489.

59 Shapiro MA, Lewis JH. Causality assessment of drug-induced hepatotoxicity: promises and pitfalls. *Clin. Liver Dis.* 2007; **11**: 477–505.

60 Lucena MI, Andrade RJ, Kaplowitz N *et al.* Phenotypic characterization of idiosyncratic drug-induced liver injury: the influence of age and sex. *Hepatology* 2009; **49**: 2001–2009.

61 Schenker S, Bay M. Drug disposition and hepatotoxicity in the elderly. *J. Clin. Gastroenterol.* 1994; **18**: 232–237.

62 Pelkonen O, Turpeinin M, Hakkola J *et al.* Inhibition and induction of human cytochrome P450 enzymes: current status. *Arch. Toxicol.* 2008; **82**: 667–715.

63 Gronhangen RC, Hellstrom PE, Froseth B. Predisposing factors in hepatitis induced by isoniazid, rifampin treatment of tuberculosis. *Am. Rev. Respir. Dis.* 1978; **113**: 161–166.

64 Lucena MI, Andrade RJ, Fernandez MC *et al.* Determinants of the clinical expression of amoxicillin-clavulanate hepatotoxicity: a prospective series from Spain. *Hepatology* 2006; **44**: 850–856.

65 Onji M, Fujioka S, Takeuchi Y *et al.* Clinical characteristics of drug-induced liver injury in the elderly. *Hepatol. Res.* 2009; **39**: 546–552.

66 Hall SM. Reye's syndrome and aspirin: a review. *Br. J. Clin. Pract.* 1990; **70** (Suppl.): 4–11.

67 Maddrey WC. Drug-induced hepatotoxicity: 2005. *J. Clin. Gastroenterol.* 2005; **39**: 83–89.

68 Wong WM, Wu PC, Yuen MF *et al.* Antituberculosis drug-related liver dysfunction in chronic hepatitis B infection. *Hepatology* 2000; **31**: 201–206.

69 Wu JC, Lee SD, Yeh PF *et al.* Isoniazid-rifampin-induced hepatitis in hepatitis B carriers. *Gastroenterology* 1990; **98**: 502–504.

70 Gupta NK, Lewis JH. Review article: the use of potentially hepatotoxic drugs in patients with liver disease. *Aliment. Pharmacol. Ther.* 2008; **28**: 1021–1041.

71 Labarga P, Soriano V, Vispo ME *et al.* Hepatotoxicity of antiretroviral drugs is reduced after successful treatment of chronic hepatitis C in HIV-infected patients. *J. Infect. Dis.* 2007; **196**: 670–676.

72 Maida I, Babudieri S, Selva C *et al.* Liver enzyme elevation in hepatitis C virus (HCV): HIV-coinfected patients prior and after initiation of HAART: role of HCV genotypes. *AIDS Res. Hum. Retroviruses.* 2006; **22**: 139–143.

73 Chalasani N, Aljadhey H, Kesterson J *et al.* Patients with elevated liver enzymes are not at higher risk for statin hepatotoxicity. *Gastroenterology* 2004; **128**: 1287–1292.

74 Vuppalanchi R, Teal E, Chalasani N. Patients with elevated baseline liver enzymes do not have higher frequency

of hepatotoxicity from lovastatin than those with normal baseline liver enzymes. *Am. J. Med. Sci.* 2005; **329**: 62–65.

75 Lewis JH, Mortensen ME, Zweig S *et al.* Efficacy and safety of high-dose pravastatin in hypercholesterolemic patients with well-compensated chronic liver disease. Results of a prospective, randomized, double-blind, placebo-controlled multicenter trial. *Hepatology* 2007; **46**: 1453–1463.

76 Ozick LA, Jacob L, Comer GM *et al.* Hepatotoxicity from isoniazid and rifampin in inner-city AIDS patients. *Am. J. Gastroenterol.* 995; **90**: 1978–1980.

77 Whitcomb DC, Block GD. Association of acetaminophen hepatotoxicity with fasting and ethanol use. *JAMA* 1994; **272**: 1845–1850.

78 Seeff LB, Cuccherini BA, Zimmerman HJ *et al.* Acetaminophen hepatotoxicity in alcoholics. A therapeutic misadventure. *Ann. Intern. Med.* 1986; **104**: 399–404.

79 Zimmerman HJ, Maddrey WC. Acetaminophen (paracetamol) hepatotoxicity with regular intake of alcohol: analysis of instances of therapeutic misadventure. *Hepatology* 1995; **22**: 767–773.

80 Watkins PB. Role of cytochromes P-450 in drug metabolism and hepatotoxicity. *Semin. Liver Dis.* 1990; **10**: 235.

81 Larson AM, Polson J, Fontana RJ *et al.* Acetaminophen-induced acute liver failure: results of a United States multicenter, prospective study. *Hepatology* 2005; **42**: 1364–1372.

82 Shah RR, Oates NS, Idle JR *et al.* Impaired oxidation of debrisoquine in patients with perhexilene neuropathy. *Br. Med. J.* 1982; **284**: 295–299.

83 Murphy R, Swartz R, Watkins PB. *Severe acetaminophen toxicity in a patient receiving isoniazid. Ann. Intern. Med.* 1990; **113**: 799–800.

84 Abboud GM, Kaplowitz N. Drug-induced liver injury. *Drug Saf.* 2007; **30**: 277–294.

85 Faubion WA, Gores GJ. Death receptors in liver biology and pathobiology. *Hepatology* 1999; **29**: 1–4.

86 Uetrecht J. Idiosyncratic drug reactions: past, present and the future. *Chem. Res. Toxicol.* 2008; **21**: 84–92.

87 Gordin FM, Simon GL, Wofsy CB *et al.* Adverse reactions to trimethoprim-sulfamethoxazole in patients with the acquired immunodeficiency syndrome. *Ann. Intern. Med.* 1984; **100**: 495–499.

88 Stieger B, Fattinger K, Madon J *et al.* Drug- and estrogen-induced cholestasis through inhibition of the hepatocellular bile salt export pump (BSEP) of rat liver. *Gastroenterology* 2000; **118**: 422–430.

89 Lakehal F, Dansette PM, Becquemont L *et al.* Indirect cytotoxicity of flucloxacillin toward human biliary epithelium via metabolite formation in hepatocytes. *Chem. Res. Toxicol.* 2001; **14**: 694–701.

90 Lang C, Meier Y, Stieger B *et al.* Mutations and polymorphisms in the bile salt export pump and the multidrug resistance protein 3 associated with drug-induced liver injury. *Pharmacogenet. Genomics* 2007; **17**: 47–60.

91 Pachkoria K, Lucena MI, Molokhia M *et al.* Genetic and molecular factors in drug-induced liver injury: a review. *Curr. Drug Saf.* 2007; **2**: 97–112.

92 Harrill AH, Watkins PB, Su S *et al.* Mouse population-guided sequencing reveals that variants in CD4 contribute to acetaminophen-induced liver injury in humans. *Genome Res.* 2009; **19**: 1507–1515.

93 Huang YS, Chern HD, Su WJ *et al.* Polymorphism of the N-acetyltransferase 2 gene as a susceptibility risk factor for antituberculosis drug-induced hepatitis. *Hepatology* 2002; **35**: 883–889.

94 Cho HJ, Koh WJ, Ryu YJ *et al.* Genetic polymorphisms of NAT2 and CYP2E1 associated with antituberculosis drug-induced hepatotoxicity in Korean patients with pulmonary tuberculosis. *Tuberculosis* (Edinb) 2007; **87**: 551–556.

95 Bozok Centintas V, Erere OF, Kosova B *et al.* Determining the relation between N-acetyltransferase-2 acetylator phenotype and antituberculosis drug induced hepatitis by molecular biologic tests. *Tuberk. Toracs.* 2008; **56**: 81–86.

96 Hautekeete ML, Horsmans Y, van Waeyenberge C *et al.* HLA-association of amoxicillin-clavulanate-induced hepatitis. *Gastroenterology* 1999; **117**: 1181–1186.

97 O'Donohue J, Oien K, Donaldson P *et al.* Co-amoxiclav jaundice: clinical and histological features and HLA class II association. *Gut* 2000; **47**: 717–720.

98 Andrade RJ, Lucena MI, Alonso A *et al.* HLA class II genotype influences the type of liver injury in drug-induced idiosyncratic liver disease. *Hepatology* 2004; **39**: 1603–1612.

99 Hardy J, Singleton A. Genomewide association studies and human disease. *N. Engl. J. Med.* 2009; **360**: 1759–1768.

100 Kindmark A, Jawald A, Harbron CG *et al.* Genome-wide pharmacogenetic investigation of a hepatic adverse event without clinical signs of immunopathology suggests an underlying immune pathogenesis. *Pharmacogen. J.* 2008; **8**: 186–195.

101 Daly AK, Donaldson PT, Bhatnagar P *et al.* HLA-B*5701 genotype is a major determinant of drug-induced liver injury due to flucloxacillin. *Nat. Genet.* 2009; **41**: 816–819.

102 Molokhia M, McKeigue P. EUDRAGENE: European collaboration to establish a case-control DNA collection for studying the genetic basis of adverse drug reactions. *Pharmacogenomics* 2006; **7**: 633–638.

103 Davern TJ, James LP, Hinson JA *et al.* Measurement of serum acetaminophen-protein adducts in patients with acute liver failure. *Gastroenterology* 2006; **130**: 682–694.

104 Andrade RJ, Camargo R, Licena MI, Gonzalez-Grande R. Causality assessment in drug-induced hepatotoxicity. *Expert Opin. Drug Saf.* 2004; **3**: 329–344.

105 Seeff LB, Rockey DC. *Causality assessment for idiosyncratic drug-induced liver injury.* In: Andrade RJ, ed. *International Hepatology Updates.* Barcelona: Permanyer Publications, 2007, p. 89–99.

106 Benichou C. Criteria of drug-induced liver disorders: report of an International consensus meeting. *J. Hepatol.* 1990; **11**: 272–276.

107 Benichou C, Danan G, Flahault A. Causality assessment of adverse reactions to drugs II. An original model for validation of drug causality assessment methods: case reports with positive rechallenge. *J. Clin. Epidemiol.* 1993; **46**: 1331–1336.

108 Maria VA, Victorino RM. Development and validation of a clinical scale for the diagnosis of drug-induced hepatitis. *Hepatology* 1997; **26**: 664–669.

109 Aithal GP, Rawlins MD, Day CP. Clinical diagnostic scale: a useful tool in the evaluation of hepatotoxic adverse drug reactions. *J. Hepatol.* 2000; **33**: 949–952.

110 Naranjo CA, Busto U, Sellers EM *et al.* A method for estimating the probability of adverse drug reactions. *Clin. Pharmacol. Ther.* 1981; **30**: 239–245.

111 Lucena MI, Camargo R, Andrade RJ *et al.* Comparison of two clinical scales for causality assessment in hepatotoxicity. *Hepatology* 2001; **33**: 123–130.

112 Garcia-Cortes M, Lucena MI, Pachkoria K *et al.* Evaluation of naranjo adverse drug reactions probability scale in causality assessment of drug-induced liver injury. *Aliment. Pharmacol. Ther.* 2008; **37**: 780–789.

113 Senior JR. Monitoring for hepatotoxicity: What is the predictive value of liver 'function' tests? *Clin. Pharmacol. Ther.* 2009; **85**: 331–334.

114 Bjornsson E. Drug-induced liver injury: Hy's rule revisited. *Clin. Pharmacol. Therap.* 2006; **79**: 521–528.

115 Schaffner F. The effect of oral contraceptives on the liver. *JAMA* 1966; **198**: 1019–1021.

116 Aithal PG, Day CP. The natural history of histologically proved drug induced liver disease. *Gut* 1999; **44**: 731–735.

117 Fontana RJ, Watkins PB, Bonkovsky HL *et al.* Rationale, design and conduct of the Drug-Induced Liver Injury Network (DILIN) prospective study. *Drug Saf.* 2009; **32**: 55–68.

118 Rochon J, Protiva P, Seeff LB *et al.* Reliability of the Roussel Uclaf Causality Assessment Method for assessing causality in drug-induced liver injury. *Hepatology* 2008; **48**: 1175–1183.

119 Rockey DC, Seeff LB, Rochon J *et al.* Causality assessment in drug induced liver injury using a structured expert opinion process: comparison to RUCAM. *Hepatology* 2010; **51**: 2117–2126.

120 Arimone Y, Miremont-Salame G, Haramburu F *et al.* Inter-expert agreement of seven criteria in causality assessment of adverse drug reactions. *Br. J. Clin. Pharmacol.* 2007; **64**: 482–488.

121 Dechene A, Treicherl U, Gerken G *et al.* Effectiveness of a steroid and ursodeoxycholic acid combination therapy with drug-induced subacute liver failure. *Hepatology* 2005; **42**: A358.

122 Chalasani N, Fontana RJ, Davern T *et al.* Characteristics of patients with drug induced liver injury (DILI) who receive systemic steroids: preliminary results from the DILIN prospective study. *ACG annual meeting, October 2008, Las Vegas NV.*

123 Rakela J, Mosley JW, Edwards VM *et al.* A double-blind randomized trial of hydrocortisone in acute hepatic failure. *Dig. Dis. Sci.* 1991; **36**: 1223–1228.

124 European Association for the Study of the Liver Group. Randomized trial of steroid therapy in acute liver failure. *Gut* 1979; **20**: 620–623.

125 Walsh TS, Hopton P, Philips BJ *et al.* The effect of n-acetylcysteine on oxygen transport and uptake in patients with fulminant hepatic failure. *Hepatology* 1998; **27**: 1332–1340.

126 Sklar GE, Subramaniam M. Acetylcysteine treatment for non-acetaminophen induced acute liver failure. *Ann. Pharmacother.* 2004; **38**: 498–501.

127 Lee WM, Rossaro L, Fontana RJ *et al.* Intravenous n-acetylcysteine improves spontaneous survival in early stage non-acetaminophen liver failure. *Gastroenterology* 2009; **137**: 856–864.

128 Legras A, Bergemer-Fouquet AM, Jonville-Bera AP. Fatal hepatitis with leflunomide and itraconazole. *Am. J. Med.* 2002; **113**: 352–353.

129 Van Roon EN, Jansen TL, Houtman NM *et al.* Leflunomide for the treatment of rheumatoid arthritis in clinical practice: incidence and severity of hepatotoxicity. *Drug Saf.* 2004; **27**: 345–352.

130 Friis H, Andreasen PB. Drug-induced hepatic injury: an analysis of 1,100 cases reported to the Danish Committee on Adverse Drug Reactions between 1978 and 1987. *J. Intern. Med.* 1992; **232**: 133–138.

131 Maddrey WC, Maurath CJ, Verburg KM *et al.* The hepatic safety and tolerability of the novel cyclooxygenase-2 inhibitor celecoxib. *Am. J. Ther.* 2007; **7**: 153–158. (Erratum in *Am. J. Ther.* 2000; **7**: 341.)

132 Rostom A, Goldkind L, Laine L. Nonsteroidal anti-inflammatory drugs and hepatic toxicity: a systematic review of randomized controlled trial in arthritis patients. *Clin. Gastroenterol. Hepatol.* 2005; **3**: 489–498.

133 Sanchez-Matienzo D, Arana A, Castellsague J *et al.* Hepatic disorders in patients treated with COX-2 selective inhibitors or nonselective NSAIDs: a case/noncase analysis of spontaneous reports. *Clin. Therap.* 2006; **28**: 1123–1132.

134 Galan MV, Gordon SC, Silverman AL. Celecoxib-induced cholestatic hepatitis (letter). *Ann. Intern. Med.* 2001; **134**: 254.

135 Nachimuthu S, Volfinzon L, Gopal L. Acute hepatocellular and cholestatic injury in a patient taking celecoxib. *Postgrad. Med. J.* 2001; **77**: 548–550.

136 Grieco S, Miele L, Giorgi A *et al.* Acute cholestatic hepatitis associate with celecoxib. *Ann. Pharmacother.* 2002; **36**: 1887–1889.

137 Traversa G, Bianchi C, Da Cas R *et al.* Cohort study of hepatotoxicity associated with nimesulide and other non-steroidal anti-inflammatory drugs. *Br. Med. J.* 2003; **327**: 18–22.

138 Andrade RJ, Lucena MI, Fernandez MC, Gonzalez M. Fatal hepatitis associated with nimesulide. *J. Hepatol.* 2000; **32**: 174.

139 Tan H, Ong WMC, Lai SH, Chow WC. Nimesulide-induced hepatotoxicity and fatal hepatic failure. *Singapore Med. J.* 2007; **48**: 582–585.

140 Licata A, Calvaruso V, Capello M *et al* Clinical course and outcomes of drug-induced liver injury: Nimeluside as the first implicated medication. *Dig. Liver Dis.* 2010; **42**: 143–148.

141 Chitturi S, George J. Hepatotoxicity of commonly used drugs: non-steroidal anti-inflammatory drugs, antihypertensives, antidiabetic agents, anticonvulsants, lipid-lowering agents, psychotropic drugs. *Sem. Liver Dis.* 2002; **22**: 169–183.

142 Javier Rodriguez-Gonzales FJ, Montero JL, Puente J *et al.* Orthotopic liver transplantation after subacute liver failure induced by therapeutic doses of ibuprofen. *Am. J. Gastroenterol.* 2002; **97**: 2476–2477.

143 Laurent S, Rahier J, Geubel AP *et al.* Subfulminant hepatitis requiring liver transplantation following ibuprofen overdose. *Liver* 2000; **20**: 93–94.

144 Sternlieb P, Robinson RM. Stevens-Johnson syndrome plus toxic hepatitis due to ibuprofen. *NY State J. Med.* 1978; **78**: 1239–1243.

145 Allam I, Ferrell LD, Bass NM. Vanishing bile duct syndrome associated with ibuprofen use. *Am. J. Gastroenterol.* 1996; **91**: 1626–1630.

146 Riley TR 3rd, Smith JP. Ibuprofen-induced hepatotoxicity in patients with chronic hepatitis C: a case series. *Am. J. Gastroenterol.* 1998; **93**: 1563–1565.

147 Rodriguez LAG, Williams R, Derby LE *et al.* Acute liver injury associated with nonsteroidal anti-inflammatory drugs and the role of risk factors. *Arch. Intern. Med.* 1994; **154**: 311–316.

148 Aithal GP, Day CP. Non-steroidal anti-inflammatory drug-induced hepatotoxicity. *Clin. Liver Dis.* 2007; **11**: 563–575.

149 Tarazi EM, Harter JG, Zimmerman HJ *et al.* Sulindac-associated hepatic injury: analysis of 91 cases reported to the Food and Drug Administration. *Gastroenterology* 1993; **104**: 569–574.

150 Banks AT, Zimmerman HJ, Ishak KG, Harter JG. Diclofenac-associated hepatotoxicity: Analysis of 180 cases reported to the Food and Drug Administration as adverse reactions. *Hepatology* 1995; **22**: 820–827.

151 Breen EG, McNicholl J, Cosgrove E *et al.* Fatal hepatitis associated with diclofenac. *Gut* 1986; **27**: 1390–1393.

152 Scully LJ, Clarke D, Barr RJ. Diclofenac induced hepatitis. 3 cases with features of autoimmune chronic active hepatitis. *Dig. Dis. Sci.* 1993; **38**: 744–751.

153 Greaves RR, Agarwal A, Patch D *et al.* Inadvertant diclofenac rechallenge from generic and non-generic prescribing, leading to liver transplantation for fulminant liver failure. *Eur. J. Gastroenterol. Hepatol.* 2001; **13**: 71–73.

154 Aithal GP, Day CP, Leathart JB, Daly AK. Relationship of polymorphism in CYP2C9 to genetic susceptibility to diclofenac-induced hepatitis. *Pharmacogenetics* 2000; **10**: 511–518.

155 Bort R, Ponsoda X, Jover R *et al.* Diclofenac toxicity to hepatocytes: a role for drug metabolism in cell toxicity. *J. Pharmacol. Exp. Ther.* 1999; **288**: 65–72.

156 Daly AK, Aithal GP, Leathart JB *et al.* Genetic susceptibility to diclofenac-induced hepatotoxicity: contribution of UGT2B7, CYP2C8, and ABCC2 genotypes. *Gastroenterology* 2007; **132**: 272–281.

157 Larrey D, Vial T, Micaleff A *et al.* Hepatitis associated with amoxicillin-clavulanic acid combination: report of 15 cases. *Gut* 1992; **33**: 368–371.

158 Lucena MJ, Andrade RJ, Fernandez MC *et al.* Determinants of the clincial expression of amoxicillin-clavulanate hepatotoxicity: A prospective series from Spain. *Hepatology* 2006; **44**: 850–856.

159 Richardet JP, Mallat A, Zafrani ES *et al.* Prolonged cholestasis with ductopenia after administration of amoxicillin/clavunic acid. *Dig. Dis. Sci.* 199; **44**: 1997–2000.

160 Fontana RJ, Shakil AO, Greenson JK *et al.* Acute liver failure due to amoxicillin and amoxicillin/ clavulanate. *Dig. Dis. Sci.* 2005; **50**: 1785–1790.

161 Ammann R, Neftel K, Hardmeier T, Reinhardt M. Cephalosporin-induced cholestatic jaundice. *Lancet* 1982; **2**: 336–337.

162 Pacik PT. Augmentation mammaplasty: postoperative cephalosporin-induced hepatitis. *Plast. Reconstr. Surg.* 2007; **119**: 1136–1137.

163 Shiffman ML, Keith FB, Moore EW. Pathogenesis of ceftriaxone-associated biliary sludge. IN vitro studies of calcium-cetriaxone binding and solubility. *Gastroenterology* 1990; **99**: 1772–1778.

164 Chandrupatla S, Demetris AJ, Rabinovitz M. Azithromycin-induced intrahepatic cholestasis. *Dig. Dis. Sci.* 2002; **47**: 2186–2188.

165 Wallace RJ, Brown BA, Griffith DE. Drug intolerance to high-dose clarithromycin among elderly patients. *Diagn. Microbiol. Infect. Dis.* 1993; **341**: 251–252.

166 Derby LE, Jick H, Henry DA, Dean AD. Erythromycin-associated cholestatic hepatitis. *Med. J. Aust.* 1993; **158**: 600–602.

167 Bjornsson E, Kalaitzakis E, Olsson R. The impact of eosinophilia and hepatic necrosis on prognosis in patients with drug induced liver injury. *Aliment. Pharmacol. Ther.* 2007; **25**: 1411–1421.

168 Keeffe EB, Reis TC, Berland JE. Hepatotoxicity to both erythromycin estolate and erythromycin ethylsuccinate. *Dig. Dis. Sci.* 1992; **27**: 701–704.

169 Degott C, Feldmann G, Larrey D *et al.* Drug-induced prolonged cholestasis in adults: A histological semiquantitative study demonstrating progressive ductopenia. *Hepatology* 1992; **15**: 244–251.

170 Clay KD, Hanson JS, Pope SD *et al.* Brief communication: severe hepatotoxicity of telithromycin: three case reports and literature review. *Ann. Intern. Med.* 2006; **144**: 415–420.

171 Brinker AD, Wassel RT, Lyndly J *et al.* Telithromycin-associated hepatotoxicity: Clinical spectrum and causality assessment in 42 cases. *Hepatology* 2009; **49**: 250–257.

172 Stricker BH, Blok AP, Class FH *et al.* Hepatic injury associated with the use of nitrofurans: a clinicopathological study of 52 reported cases. *Hepatology* 1988; **8**: 599–606.

173 Jick SS, Jick H, Dean AD. A follow-up safety study of ciprofloxacin users. *Pharmacotherapy* 1993; **13**: 461–464.

174 Bjornsson E, Plsson R. Suspected drug-induced liver failures reported to the WHO database. *Dig. Liver Dis.* 2006; **38**: 33–38.

175 Alberti-Flor JJ, Hernandez ME, Ferrer JP *et al.* Fulminant liver failure and pancreatitis associated with the use of sulfamethaxazole-trimethoprim. *Am. J. Gastroenterol.* 1989; **84**: 1577–79.

176 van Der Ven AJ, Koopmans PP, Vree TB *et al.* Adverse reactions to co-trimoxazole in HIV infection. *Lancet* 1991; **338**: 431–433.

177 Munoz SJ, Martinez-Hernandez A, Maddrey WC. Intrahepatic cholestasis and phospholipodosis associated with the use of trimethoprim-aulfamethoxazole. *Hepatology* 1990; **12**: 342–347.

178 Shultz JC, Adamson JS, Workman WW *et al.* Fatal liver disease after intravenous administration of tetracycline in high dosage. *N. Engl. J. Med.* 1963; **269**: 999–1003.

179 Lawrenson RA, Seaman HE, Sundstrom A *et al.* Liver damage associated with minocycline use in acne: a systematic review of the published literature and pharmacovigilance data. *Drug Saf.* 2000; **23**: 333–340.

180 Knowles SR, Shapiro L, Shear NH. Serious adverse reactions induced by minocycline. Report of 13 patients and review of the literature. *Arch. Dermatol.* 1996; **132**: 934–939.

181 Bjornsson E, Lindberg J, Olsson R. Liver reactions to oral low-dose tetracyclines. *Scan. J. Gastroenterol.* 1997; **32**: 390–395.

182 Van Den Brande P, Van Steenbergen W, Vervoort G *et al.* Aging and hepatotoxicity of isoniazid and rifampin in

pulmonary tuberculosis. *Am. J. Respir. Crit. Care Med.* 1995; **152**: 1705–1708.

183 Devoto FM, Gonzalez C, Iannantuono R *et al.* Risk factors for hepatotoxicity induced by antituberculosis drugs. *Acta Phsiolo. Pharmacol. Ther. Lationaam* 1997; **47**: 197–202.

184 Wong WM, Wu PC, Yuen MF *et al.* Antituberculosis drug-related liver dysfunction in chronic hepatitis B infection. *Hepatology* 2000; **31**: 201–206.

185 Ungo JR, Jones D, Ashkin D *et al.* Antituberculosis drug-induced hepatotoxicity: The role of hepatitis C virus and the human immunodeficiency virus. *Am. J. Respir. Crit. Care Med.* 1998; **157**: 1871–1876.

186 Nolan CM, Goldberg SV, Buskin SE. Hepatotoxicity associated with isoniazid preventive therapy: A 7–year survey from a public health tuberculosis clinic. *JAMA* 1999; **281**: 1014–1018.

187 Pessayre D, Bentata M, Degott C *et al.* Isoniazid-rifampin fulminant hepatitis. A possible consequence of the enhancement of isoniazid hepatotoxicity by enzyme induction. *Gastroenterology* 1977; **72**: 284–289.

188 Steele MA, Burk RF, Des Prez RM. Toxic hepatitis with isoniazid and rifampicin: A meta-analysis. *Chest* 1991; **99**: 465–471.

189 Singh J, Arora A, Garg PK *et al.* Antituberculosis treatment induced hepatotoxicity: role of predictive factors. *Postgrad. Med. J.* 1995; **71**: 359–362.

190 Durand F, Bernuau J, Pessayre D *et al.* Deleterious influence of pyrazinamide on the outcome of patients with fulminant or subfulminant liver failure during antituberculosis treatment including isoniazid. *Hepatology* 1995; **21**: 929–932.

191 Lewis JH, Zimmerman HJ, Benson GD *et al.* Hepatic injury associated with ketoconazole therapy. Analysis of 33 cases. *Gastroenterology* 1984; **86**: 503–513.

192 Chien RN, Yang LJ, Lin PY *et al.* Hepatic injury during ketoconazole therapy in patients with onychomycosis: a controlled cohort study. *Hepatology* 1997; **25**: 103–107.

193 Gearhart MO. Worsening of liver unction with fluconazole and review of azole antifungal hepatotoxicity. *Ann. Pharmacother.* 1994; **28**: 1117–1181.

194 Hall M, Monka C, Krupp P *et al.* Safety of oral terbinafine: results of a post-marketing surveillance study in 25, 884 patients. *Arch. Dermatol.* 1997; **133**: 1213–1219.

195 Lazaros GA, Papatheodoridis GV, Delladetsima JK *et al.* Terbinafine induced cholestatic liver disease. *J. Hepatol.* 1996; **24**: 753–756.

196 Nunez M. Hepatotoxicity of antiretrovirals: incidence, mechanisms, and management. *J. Hepatol.* 2006: **44**: S132–139.

197 Wit FW, Weverling GJ, Weel J *et al.* Incidence of and risk factors for severe hepatotoxicity associated with antiretroviral combination therapy. *J. Infect. Dis.* 2002; **186**: 23–31.

198 Zucker SD, Qin X, Rouster SD *et al.* Mechanism of indinavir-induced hyperbilirubinemia. *Proc. Natl. Acad. Sci. USA* 2001; **98**: 12671–12676.

199 Kottilil S, Polis MA, Kovacs JA. HIV infection, hepatitis C infection, and HAART: hard clinical choices. *JAMA* 2004; **292**; 243–250.

200 Ogedegbe AE, Thomas DL, Diehl AM. Hyperlactaemia syndromes associated with HIV therapy. *Lancet Infect. Dis.* 2003; **3**: 329–337.

201 Kakuda TN. Pharmacology of nucleoside and nucleotide reverse transcriptase inhibitor-induced mitochondrial toxicity. *Clin. Ther.* 2000; **22**: 685–708.

202 Perronne C. Antiviral hepatitis and antiretroviral drug interactions. *J. Hepatol.* 2006: **44**: S119–125.

203 Zucman D, Truchis P, Majerholc C *et al.* Prospective screening for human leukocyte antigen B*5701 avoids abacavir hypersensitivity reaction in ethnically mixed French HIV population. *J. Acquir. Immune Defic. Syndr.* 2007: **45**: 1–10.

204 Baylor MS, Johann-Liang R. Hepatotoxicity associated with nevirapine use. *J. Acquir. Immune Defic. Syndr.* 2004; **15**: 538–539.

205 Sulkowski MS, Thomas DL, Mehta SH *et al.* Hepatotoxicity associated with nevirapine or efavirenz-containg antiretroviral therapy. Role of hepatitis B and C infections. *Hepatology* 2002; **34**: 182–189.

206 Hagley MT, Hulisz DT, Burns CM. Hepatotoxicity associated with angiotensin-converting enzyme inhibitors. *Ann. Pharmacother.* 1993; **27**: 228–231.

207 Rahmat J, Gelfand RL, Gelfand MC *et al.* Captopril-associated cholestatic jaundice. *Ann. Intern. Med.* 1985; **102**: 56–58.

208 Tabak F, Mert A, Ozaras R *et al.* Losartan-induced hepatic injury. *J. Clin. Gastroenterol.* 2002: **34**: 585–586.

209 Bosch X. Losartan-induced hepatotoxicity. *JAMA* 1997; **278**: 1572.

210 Maddrey WC, Boitnott JK. Severe hepatitis from methyldopa. *Gastroenterology* 1975; **68**: 351–360.

211 Neuberger J, Kenna JG, Nouri A *et al.* Antibody-mediated hepatocyte injury in methyl-dopa induced hepatotoxicity. *Gut* 1985; **26**: 1233–1239.

212 Pupppula AR, Steinheber FV. Fulminant hepatic failure associated with methyldopa. *Am. J. Gastroenterol.* 1977; **68**: 578–585.

213 Lewis JH, Ranard RC, Caruso A *et al.* Amiodarone hepatotoxicity: prevalence and clinicopathologic correlations among 104 patients. *Hepatology* 1989; **9**: 679–685.

214 Assy N, Schlesinger S, Hussein M. Severe cholestatic jaundice in the elderly induced by low-dose amiodarone. *Dig. Dis. Sci.* 2004; **49**: 450–452.

215 Guigui B, Perrot S, Berry JP *et al.* Amiodarone-induced hepatic phospholipidosis: a morphological alteration independent of pseudoalcoholic liver disease. *Hepatology* 1989; **8**: 1063–1068.

216 Clark JA, Zimmerman HJ, Tanner LA. Labetalol hepatotoxicity. *Ann. Intern. Med.* 1990; **113**: 211–213.

217 Larrey D, Henriol J, Heller F *et al.* Metoprolol-induced hepatitis: Rechallenge and drug oxidation phenotyping. *Ann. Intern. Med.* 1988; **108**: 67–68.

218 Shaw DR, Misan GMH. Johnson RD. Nifedipine hepatitis. *Aust. N. Z. J. Med.* 1987: **17**: 447–448.

219 Hare DL, Horowitz JD. Verapamil hepatotoxicity: A hypersensitivity reaction. *Am. Heart. J.* 1986; **11**: 610–611.

220 Shallcross H, Padley SP, Glynn MJ *et al.* Fatal renal and hepatic toxicity after treatment with diltiazem. *Br. Med. J.* 1987; **295**: 1236–1237.

221 Pariente EA, Pessayre D, Bernuau J *et al.* Dihydralazine hepatitis: report of a case and review of the literature. *Digestion* 1983; **27**: 47–52.

222 Jori GP, Peschile C. Hydralazine disease associated with transient granulomas in the liver. A case report. *Gastroenterology* 1973; **64**: 1163–1167.

223 Bourdi M, Gautier JC, Mircheva J *et al*. Antiliver microsomes autoantibodies and dihydralazine-induced hepatitis: specificity of autoantibodies and inductive capacity of the drug. *Mol. Pharmacol.* 1992; **42**: 280–285.

224 Pellock JM. Carbamazepine side effects in children and adults. *Epilepsia* 1987; **28**: S64–S70.

225 Askmark H, Wiholm B. Epidemiology of adverse drug reactions to carbamazepine as seen in a spontaneous reporting system. *Acta Neurol. Scand.* 1990; **81**: 131–140.

226 Levy M, Goodman MW, Van Dyre J *et al*. Granulomatous hepatitis secondary to carbamazepine. *Ann. Intern. Med.* 1981; **95**: 64–65.

227 William RJ, Ruppin DC, Grierson JM *et al*. Carbamazepine hepatitis: the clinicopathological spectrum. *J. Gastroenterol. Hepatol.* 1996; **1**: 159–168.

228 Aiges HW, Daum F, Olson M *et al*. The effects of phenobarbitol and diphenylhydantoin on liver function and morphology. *J. Pediatr.* 1980; **97**: 22–26.

229 Mullick FG, Ishak KG. Hepatic injury associated with diphenylhydantoin therapy: a clinicopathological study of 20 cases. *Am. J. Clin. Pathol.* 1980; **74**: 442–452.

230 Bryant AE, Dreifuss FE. Hepatotoxicity associated with antiepileptic drug therapy- avoidance , identification and management. *CNS Drugs* 1995; **4**: 99–113.

231 Zimmerman HJ, Ishak KG. Valproate-induced hepatic injury: analysis of 23 fatal cases. *Hepatology* 1982; **2**: 592–597.

232 Bryant AE, Dreifuss FE. Valproic acid hepatic fatalities. III. U.S. experience since 1986. *Neurology* 1996; **46**: 465–469.

233 Buchanan N. Lamotrigine: clinical experience in 200 patients with epilepsy and 4 year follow-up. *Seizure* 1996; **46**: 209–214.

234 Makin AJ, Fitt S, Williams R *et al*. Fulminant hepatic failure induced by lamotrigine. *Br. Med. J.* 1995; **311**: 292.

235 Morrow PL, Hardin NJ, Bonadies J. Hypersensitivity myocarditis and hepatitis associated with impipramine and its metabolite, desipramine. *J. Forens. Sci.* 1989; **34**: 1016–1020.

236 Biagi RW, Bapat BN. Intrahepatic obstructive jaundice from amitriptyline. *Br. J. Psychiatry* 1967; **113**: 1113–1114.

237 Capella D, Bruguera M, Figueras A *et al*. Fluoxetine-induced hepatitis: why is post-marketing surveillance needed? *Eur. J. Clin. Pharmacol.* 1999; **74**: 692–694.

238 Benbow SJ, Gill G. Drug points: Paroxetine and hepatotoxicity. *Br. Med. J.* 1997; **314**: 1387.

239 Hautekeete ML, Cole I, VanVlieberg H *et al*. Symptomatic liver injury probably related to sertraline. *Gastroenterol. Clin. Biol.* 1998; **22**: 364–365.

240 Horsmans Y, De Clercq M, Sempoux C. Venlaflaxine-associated hepatitis. *Ann. Intern. Med.* 1999; **130**: 944.

241 Bonkovsky HL, Blanchette PL, Schned AR. Severe liver injury due to phenelzine with unique hepatic deposition of extracellular material. *Am. Med. J.* 1986; **80**: 689–692.

242 Aranda-Michel J, Koehler A, Bejarano PA *et al*. Nefazodone-induced liver falure: report of three cases. *Ann. Intern. Med.* 1999; **130**: 285–288.

243 Eloubeidi MA, Gaede JT, Swaim MW. Reversible nefazadone-induced liver failure. *Dig. Dis. Sci.* 20000; **45**: 1036–1038.

244 Beck PL, Bridges RJ, Demetrick DJ *et al*. Chronic active hepatitis associated with trazadone therapy. *Ann. Intern. Med.* 1993; **118**: 791–792.

245 Hu KQ, Tiyyagura L, Kanel G *et al*. Acute hepatitis induced by bupropion. *Dig. Dis. Sci.* 2000; **45**: 1872–1873.

246 Humayun F, Shehab TM, Tworek J *et al*. A fatal case of bupropion (zyban) hepatotoxicity with autoimmune features: A case report. *J. Med. Case Reports* 2007; **1**: 88.

247 Graham DJ, Green L, Senior JR *et al*. Troglitazone-induced liver failure: A case study. *Am. J. Med.* 2003; **114**: 299–306.

248 Maeda K. Hepatocellular injury in a patient receiving pioglitazone. *Ann. Intern. Med.* 2001; **135**: 306.

249 Forman LM, Simmons DA, Diamond RH. Hepatic failure in a patient taking rosiglitazone. *Ann. Intern. Med.* 2000; **132**: 118–121.

250 Chase MP, Yarze JC. Pioglitazone-assocaited fulminant hepatic failure. *Am. J. Gastroenterol.* 2002; **97**: 502–503.

251 Dhawan M, Agrawal R, Ravi J *et al*. Rosiglitazone-induced granulmatous hepatitis. *J. Clin. Gastroenterol.* 2002; **34**: 582–584.

252 Floyd JS, Barbehenn E, Lurie P *et al*. Case series of liver failure associated with rosiglitazone and pioglitazone. *Pharmacoepi. Drug Saf.* 2009; **18**: 1238–1243.

253 Belfort R, Harrison SA, Brown K *et al*. A placebo-controlled trial of pioglitazone in subjects with nonalcoholic steatohepatitis. *N. Engl. J. Med.* 2006; **355**: 2297–2307.

254 Chalasani N, Teal E, Hall SD. Effect of rosiglitazone on serum liver biochemistries in diabetic patients with normal and elevated baseline liver enzymes. *Am. J. Gastroenterol.* 2005; **100**: 1317–1321.

255 Deutsch M, Kountouras D, Dourakis SP. Metfromin hepatotoxicity. *Ann. Intern. Med.* 2004; **140**: W25.

256 Desilets DJ, Shorr AF, Moran KA, Holtzmuller KC. Cholestatic jaundice associated with the use of metformin. *Am. J. Gastroenterol.* 2001; **96**: 2257–2258.

257 Misbin RI, Green L, Stadel BV *et al*. Lactic acidosis in patients with diabetes treated with metformin. *N. Engl. J. Med.* 1998; **338**: 265–266.

258 de la Iglesia FA, Farber E. Hypolipidemics carcinogenecity and extrapolation of experimental results for human safety assessments. *Toxicol. Pathol.* 1982; **10**: 152–174.

259 Blum CB. Comparison of properties of four inhibitors of 3–hydoxy-3-methylgultaryl-coenxyme A reductase. *Am. J. Cardiol.* 1994; **73**: 3D–11D.

260 de La Iglesia FA, Lewis JE, Buchanan RA *et al*. Light and electron microscopy of liver in hyperlipoproteinemic patients under long-term gemfibrozil treatment. *Atherosclerosis* 1982; **43**: 19–37.

261 Chatrenet P, Regimbeau C, Ramain JP *et al*. Chronic active cryptogenic hepatitis induced by fenofibrate. *Gastroenterol. Clin. Biol.* 1993: **17**: 612–613.

262 McKenney JM, Proactor JD, Harris S *et al*. A comparison of the efficacy and toxic effects of sustained vs immediate-release niacin in hypercholesterolemic patients. *JAMA* 1994; **271**: 672–677.

263 Gray DR, Morgan T, Chretine SD *et al*. Efficacy and safety of controlled-release niacin in dyslipoproteinemic veterans. *Ann. Intern. Med.* 1994; **121**: 252–258.

264 Chalasani N. Statins and hepatotoxicity: Focus on patients with fatty liver. *Hepatology* 2005; **41**: 690–695.

265 The SEARCH Collaborative Group. SLCO1B1 Variants and statin- induced myopathy—a genomewide study. *N. Engl. J. Med.* 2009; **359**: 1–11.

266 Russo MW, Scobey M, Bonkovsky HL. Drug-induced liver injury associated with statins. *Sem. Liver Dis.* 2009; **29**: 412–422.

267 Pelli N, Setti M, Ceppa P *et al*. Autoimmune hepatitis revealed by atorvastatin. *Eur. J. Gastroenterol. Hepatol*. 2003; **15**: 921–924.

268 Perger L, Kohler M, Fattinger K *et al*. Fatal liver failure with atorvastatin. *J. Hepatol*. 2003; **39**: 1096–1097.

269 Stolk MF, Becx MC, Kuypers KC, Seldenrijk CA. Severe hepatic side effects of ezetimibe. *Clin. Gastroenterol. Hepatol*. 2006; **4**: 908– 911.

270 Kenna JG, Neuberger J, Williams R. Specific antibodies to halothane-induced liver antigens in halothane-associated hepatitis. *Br. J. Anaesth*. 1987; **59**: 1286–1290.

271 Benjamin SB, Goodman ZD, Ishak KG *et al*. The morphologic spectrum of halothane-induced hepatic injury: analysis of 77 cases. *Hepatology* 1985; **5**: 1163–1171.

272 Kenna JG, Neuberger J. Immunopathogenesis and treatment of halothane hepatitis. *Clin. Immunother*. 1995; **3**: 108–124.

273 Lewis JH, Zimmerman HJ, Ishak KG *et al*. Enflurane hepatotoxicity: a clinicopthological study of 24 cases. *Ann. Intern. Med*. 1983; **98**: 984–992.

274 Sinha A, Clatch RJ, Stuck G *et al*. Isoflurane hepatotoxicity: a case report and review of the literature. *Am. J. Gastroenterol*. 1996; **91**: 2406–2409.

275 Turner GB, O'Rourke D, Scott GO *et al*. Fatal hepatotoxicity after re-exposure to isoflurane: a case report and review of the literature. *Eur. J. Gastroenterol. Hepatol*. 2000; **12**: 955–959.

276 Martin JL, Plevak DJ, Flannery KD *et al*. Hepatotoxicity after desflurane anesthesia. *Anesthesiology* 1995; **83**: 1125–1129.

277 Njoku D, Laster MJ, Gong DH *et al*. Biotransformation of halothane, enflurane, isoflurane, and desflurane to trifluoroacetylated liver proteins: association between protein acylation and hepatic injury. *Anesth. Analg*. 1997; **84**: 173–178.

278 World Health Organization. *Traditional Medicine*. Factsheet No. 134, 2008 Geneva: WHO. Available from: http://www.who.int/mediacentre/factsheets/fs134/en/index.html. (Accessed 13 Oct. 2010.)

279 Pittler MH, Ernst E. Hepatotoxic events associated with herbal medicinal products. *Aliment. Pharmacol*. 2003; **18**: 451–471.

280 Modi AA, Wright EC, Seeff LB. Complementary and alternative medicine (CAM) for the treatment of chronic hepatitis B and C: a review. *Antivir. Ther*. 2007; **12**: 285–295.

281 Ernst E. Heavy metals in traditional Indian remedies. *Eur. J. Clin. Pharmacol*. 2002; **57**: 891–896.

282 Saper RB, Phillips RB, Sehgal A *et al*. Lead, mercury, and arsenic in US- and Indian-manufactured Ayurvedic medicines sold over the internet. *JAMA* 2008; **300**: 915–923.

283 Strader DB, Seeff LB. Hepatotoxicity of herbal preparations. In: Boyer TD, Wright TL, Manns MP, eds. *Hepatology, a Textbook of Liver Disease*, 5th edn. Philadelphia: Elsevier, 2006, p. 551–560.

284 Elinav E, Pinsker G, Safadi R *et al*. Association between consumption of Herbalife® nutritional supplements and acute hepatotoxicity. *J. Hepatol*. 2007; **47**: 514–520.

285 Schoeffer AM, Engel A, Fattinger K *et al*. Herbal does not mean innocuous: ten cases of severe hepatotoxicity associated with dietary supplements from Herbalife® products. *J. Hepatol*. 2007; **47**: 521–526.

286 Seeff LB. Are herbals as safe as their advocates believe? *J. Hepatol*. 2009; **50**: 13–16.

287 Dara L, Hewett J, Lim JK. Hydroxycut hepatotoxicity: A case series and review of liver toxicity from herbal weight loss supplements. *World J. Gastroenterol*. 2008; **14**: 6999–7004.

288 Fong T-L, Klontz K, Canas-Coto A *et al*. Hepatotoxicity due to Hydroxycut®: a case series. *Am. J. Gastroenterol*. 2010; **105**: 1561–1566.

289 http://www.drugs.com/fda-consumer/warning-on-hydroxycut-products-14.html (Accessed Oct. 22 2010).

CHAPTER 25
Alcohol and the Liver

Stephen Stewart[1] & Chris Day[1,2]

[1] Liver Unit, Freeman Hospital, Newcastle upon Tyne, UK

[2] Faculty of Medical Sciences, Newcastle University, Newcastle upon Tyne, UK

Learning points

- In the absence of portal hypertension, a liver biopsy is required to determine the stage of alcoholic liver disease.

- Abstinence remains the cornerstone of treatment for alcoholic liver disease.

- For patients with acute severe alcoholic hepatitis, corticosteroid treatment is the standard of care.

- Patients with at least 3 months of abstinence that still have decompensated liver disease are unlikely to improve further and should be considered for liver transplantation assessment. Most transplant units, however, will not list patients for transplantation in most cases until there has been 6 months of abstinence.

Introduction

Worldwide, alcohol consumption is increasing. This is particularly notable in the UK where average alcohol consumption has more than doubled in the last 50 years. In France, however, the past 30 years has seen a decrease, perhaps due to government propaganda. In the USA, alcohol consumption, particularly of spirits, has also fallen, perhaps due to changing lifestyles.

The association of alcohol with cirrhosis was recognized by Matthew Baillie in 1793. In recent years, alcohol consumption has correlated closely with deaths from cirrhosis. Cirrhosis mortality has risen dramatically in the UK [1], where alcohol-related liver disease is now the fourth commonest cause of death in the under 65s.

Alcohol metabolism

Absorption and distribution

Alcohol is absorbed from the gastrointestinal tract by simple diffusion and peak blood alcohol concentrations are reached after 20 minutes. Most of the absorption occurs in the duodenum and upper jejunum. The rate of absorption is delayed following a meal and increases in proportion to the alcohol concentration of the drink consumed (Fig. 25.1).

Alcohol distribution is dependent on blood flow, with vascular organs such as the brain rapidly equilibrating with plasma levels. Alcohol is poorly soluble in lipids, possibly explaining the higher plasma concentrations found in females compared to males that have consumed the same amount of ethanol.

Alcohol cannot be stored and obligatory oxidation must take place, predominantly in the liver. The healthy individual cannot metabolize more than 160–180 g/day. Alcohol induces enzymes used in its catabolism, and the hazardous drinker, at least while the liver is relatively unaffected, can metabolize more.

Alcohol to acetaldehyde

Between 80 and 85% of ethanol oxidation is by initial conversion to acetaldehyde catabolized by alcohol dehydrogenase (ADH) (Fig. 25.2). This takes place in the cytosol. The resulting increase in the ratio of NADH/NAD, which is further increased by acetaldehyde oxidation, is partly responsible for the metabolic imbalances that occur following alcohol ingestion and has been considered to play a major role in the initial pathogenesis of alcohol-induced fatty liver.

Most of the remaining ethanol is metabolized by the microsomal ethanol-oxidizing system (MEOS) pathway, an accessory pathway that principally involves a specific alcohol-inducible form of cytochrome P450, designated CYP2E1 [2]. The induction of CYP2E1 in hazardous drinkers may explain their increased susceptibility to hepatotoxicity by other drugs that are converted to toxic metabolites by this enzyme system. An important example of this phenomenon is the increased susceptibility to the toxic effects of paracetamol (acetaminophen),

Sherlock's Diseases of the Liver and Biliary System, Twelfth Edition. Edited by James S. Dooley, Anna S.F. Lok, Andrew K. Burroughs, E. Jenny Heathcote.
© 2011 by Blackwell Publishing Ltd. Published 2011 by Blackwell Publishing Ltd.

where severe liver damage has been reported in dependent drinkers taking therapeutic doses [3].

Acetaldehyde to acetate

Most of the acetaldehyde formed from ethanol oxidation is further oxidized in the liver to acetate by aldehyde dehydrogenases (ALDHs). Acetate may be oxidized to carbon dioxide and water, or converted by the citric acid cycle to other compounds, including fatty acids. The inactive form of ALDH (ALDH2*2) is present in about 50% of Orientals. The accumulation of acetal-

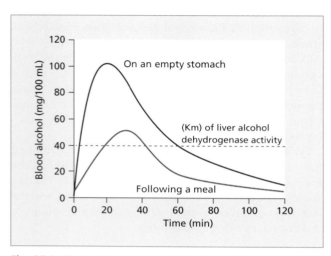

Fig. 25.1. Typical time course of blood alcohol concentration after ingestion of one unit either following a meal or on an empty stomach.

dehyde may account for the flushing seen with alcohol consumption in homozygotes.

Pathogenesis

Rodents given alcohol develop only a fatty liver. However, they cannot match the consumption achieved by humans, who may take 50% of total calories as alcohol. This level can be achieved in the baboon, which develops cirrhosis after 2–5 years of high alcohol consumption. Evidence for a direct hepatotoxic effect of alcohol, as opposed to an indirect effect related to the associated nutritional changes, comes from studies in human volunteers who, after 300–600 mL (10–20 oz) of 86% proof alcohol daily for 8–10 days, develop fatty change and electron microscopic abnormalities on liver biopsy [4].

Some of the pathways through which alcohol may cause liver injury are described below. Unfortunately, this improved knowledge of disease mechanisms has, to date, not led to a significant improvement in the therapy of alcoholic liver disease.

Pathogenesis of steatosis

The accumulation of triacylglycerol (TAG) within the liver is an early and reversible effect of alcohol consumption. Alcohol increases peripheral lipolysis and the altered liver redox potential increases fatty acid synthesis. This increase in substrate supply (glycerol and free fatty acids) enhances the rate of esterification, resulting in TAG accumulation. This is compounded by the

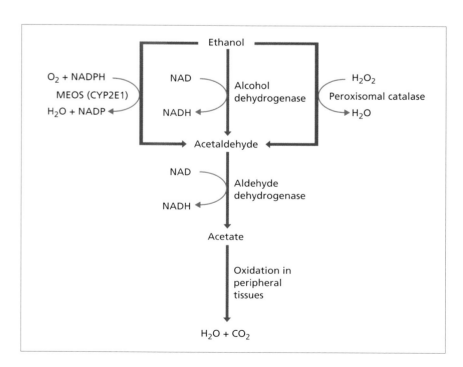

Fig. 25.2. The three pathways of alcohol oxidation. MEOS, microsomal ethanol oxidizing system; CYP2E1, cytochrome P4502E1.

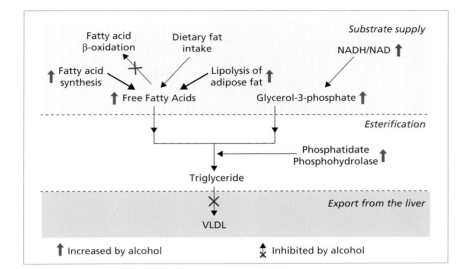

Fig. 25.3. The multiple mechanisms through which ethanol metabolism can lead to fatty liver. Ethanol causes fatty liver by increasing substrate supply, increasing fat esterification to triglyceride and reducing the export of very low density lipoprotein (VLDL) from the liver.

Table 25.1. Possible hepatotoxic effects of acetaldehyde

Induction of steatosis through altering the redox potential
Increasing sensitization to TNF-α mediated hepatocyte
   necrosis
Binding to host proteins:
   affecting folding and inducing endoplasmic reticular stress
   affecting function (e.g. microtubules)
   forming neoantigens

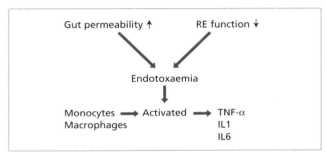

Fig. 25.4. Alcohol, endotoxinaemia and cytokine production. RE, reticuloendothelial; TNF, tumour necrosis factor; IL, interleukin.

alcohol-induced inhibition of the enzyme which controls TAG export from the liver, microsomal triglyceride transfer protein (MTP) [5] (Fig. 25.3).

Oxidative stress and lipid peroxidation

In alcohol-related liver disease (ALD) the generation of pro-oxidants overwhelms the endogenous antioxidant systems, resulting in lipid peroxidation. These pro-oxidants can come directly from ethanol metabolism or from activated phagocytes. Liver injury is compounded by the depletion of endogenous cellular, particularly mitochondrial, antioxidants in hazardous drinkers.

Acetaldehyde

Acetaldehyde is generated by both ADH and the MEOS systems and may account for many of the features of acute alcoholic hepatitis (Table 25.1). Acetaldehyde is extremely reactive and toxic; it binds to phospholipids, amino acid residues and sulphydryl groups. It can produce altered surface antigens and depolymerize proteins, altering their folding. When abnormally folded or unfolded proteins build up in the endoplasmic reticulum (ER), this results in a phenomenon known as 'ER

stress' [6]. ER stress induces further lipid synthesis, antioxidant depletion and ultimately apoptosis.

Endotoxin and cytokines

A complex relationship exists between endotoxin, Kupffer cell activation and the release of cytokines and chemokines. Endotoxin is increased in the blood of hazardous drinkers [7]. This is related to increased intestinal bacterial flora, increased gut permeability and reduced endotoxin scavenging by the reticuloendothelial system (Fig. 25.4). Endotoxin results in the release of cytokines and reactive oxygen species from Kupffer cells. In alcoholic hepatitis, tumour necrosis factor-α (TNF-α) and interleukin-8 (IL-8) production are particularly increased [8,9].

The biological effects of certain cytokines resemble the clinical and histological manifestations of ALD (Table 25.2). TNF-α can induce steatosis, the production of reactive oxygen species (ROS) and hepatocyte apoptosis. IL-8 is involved in the recruitment and activation of neutrophils.

Table 25.2. Biological effects of cytokines and clinical features of alcohol-related liver disease

Change	Alcohol-related liver disease	Cytokines
Fever	+	+
Anorexia	+	+
Muscle wasting	+	+
Hypermetabolism	+	+
Neutrophilia	+	+
Decreased albumin	+	+
Collagen disposition	+	+
Increased triglycerides	+	+
Decreased bile flow	+	+
Shock	+	+

Table 25.3. Alcohol and cancer

Mouth
Pharynx
Larynx
Oesophagus
Colon
Breast
Liver

Immunological liver damage

Protein adducts formed from ethanol metabolites and host proteins can act as neoantigens to incite humoral B-cell and cytotoxic T-cell lymphocyte responses in ALD. Antibodies can be shown against acetaldehyde protein adduct-derived epitopes [10] and hydroxyethyl radical–CYP2E1 adducts [11]. Antibodies can also be seen to native CYP2E1, suggesting that autoimmune mechanisms may play a role in alcohol-related liver disease [12]. The true importance of immunological mechanisms is not clear as they may represent an epiphenomenon whereby immune responses are generated to proteins released from hepatocytes damaged through other mechanisms.

Alcohol and fibrosis

The proliferation and activation of stellate cells in ALD is promoted by Kupffer cells and hepatocytes. Kupffer cells induce collagen synthesis through the production of transforming growth factor-β (TGF-β), TNF-α and ROS. Hepatocytes induce fibrosis through the production of ROS or through apoptosis. TGF-β is produced when apoptotic hepatocytes are phagocytosed and this in turn can activate stellate cells [13].

Alcohol and cancer

Alcohol consumption is associated with hepatocellular carcinoma and several extrahepatic cancers (Table 25.3).

The mechanisms are likely to be related to lipid peroxidation and DNA mutagenesis, reduced DNA methylation and immunosuppression.

Susceptibility

Environmental factors

Dose of alcohol

The average intake of alcohol in a large group of male dependent cirrhotic patients was 160 g/day for 8 years. The risk of developing ALD begins at 30 g/day of ethanol [14] but for most individuals the dose that confers a significant risk is greater than 80 g alcohol daily. The duration of consumption is also important. In one study, neither cirrhosis nor alcoholic hepatitis were seen in patients who consumed an average of 160 g of ethanol per day for less than 5 years, whereas 50% of patients consuming high levels of alcohol for an average of 21 years developed cirrhosis [15]. Liver injury appears to be unrelated to the type of beverage; reports that wine drinkers have a lower risk than beer and spirit drinkers and that drinkers of mixed beverages have a higher risk than those keeping to a single type of drink are probably explained by confounding lifestyle factors associated with particular drinking patterns. Continued daily imbibing is more dangerous than intermittent consumption when the liver is given the opportunity to recover; it is therefore recommended that individuals should have at least two alcohol-free days per week.

ALD and dependence do not necessarily go together. Those who develop alcohol-related liver damage are often not dependent on alcohol. Most dependent patients have normal liver function [16].

Diet

Cirrhosis mortality has been linked with diets high in pork (high in linoleic acid) consumption and unsaturated fats [17] and low in carbohydrate [18]. Obesity and associated hyperglycaemia increase the incidence of all stages of ALD in heavy drinkers [19,20].

Genetic factors

Gender

Hazardous drinking is increasing among women owing to a decline in the social stigma and the increased availability of alcohol. Women are less likely to be suspected of alcohol abuse; they present at a later stage, are more susceptible to liver injury and are more likely to relapse after treatment [21]. This may be related to the reduced volume of distribution of alcohol, or the fact that, in animal models at least, oestrogen increases gut permeability to endotoxin [22]. Women are more likely to progress from alcoholic hepatitis to cirrhosis even if they abstain [23].

Non-gender-linked genetic factors

Patterns of alcohol drinking are, at least partially, inherited; however, no specific genetic variants have been reproducibly associated with susceptibility in large studies. Susceptibility to liver disease may also have an inherited component. Concordance rates for alcohol-related cirrhosis are three times higher in monozygotic than in dizygotic twin pairs [24]. Alcohol-related liver damage is a polygenic disorder so multiple polymorphisms are likely to contribute. They are likely to be in genes controlling fat accumulation, oxidative stress, endotoxin-mediated release of proinflammatory cytokines and immunological damage [25].

Histological features

Fatty liver

Fat (steatosis) accumulates predominantly in zones 3 and 2 although in the more severely affected, the fatty change is diffuse. Typically the fat is in a macrovesicular (large droplet) form although it can also be in a microvesicular (small droplet) form.

Large fat droplets appear in hepatocytes within days of excess alcohol ingestion. Microvesicular fat probably reflects the presence of mitochondrial injury and resulting inhibition of fatty acid oxidation. In support, hepatic mitochondrial DNA deletion has been reported in patients with alcohol-related fatty liver. Fatty change can be quantified according to the proportion of hepatocytes that contain fat.

Alcoholic hepatitis

The full histological picture of a florid, acute alcoholic hepatitis is relatively rare. Typical features include some or all of the following:

Ballooning degeneration. Hepatocytes are swollen with granular cytoplasm often dispersed into fine strands. The nucleus is small and hyperchromatic. The ballooning is due to retention of water and to failure of the microtubular excretion of protein from the hepatocyte.

Acidophilic bodies. These represent hepatocyte apoptosis.

Mallory–Denk bodies. These are seen on haematoxylin and eosin stained sections as purplish-red intracytoplasmic inclusions. They may be more obvious with Masson's trichrome or chromophobe aniline blue stains. They consist of clumped organelles—largely intermediate filaments—and may target the hepatocyte for destruction. The Mallory-containing cell is surrounded by a satellite of polymorphs (Figs 25.5, 25.6).

Giant mitochondria. These form globular intracytoplasmic inclusions seen by light microscopy using a Masson trichrome stain.

Fibrosis. Collagen deposition is usually maximal in zone 3. The fibres are perisinusoidal and enclose normal or ballooned hepatocytes. The pericellular fibrosis is like lattice or chicken wire and has been termed 'creeping

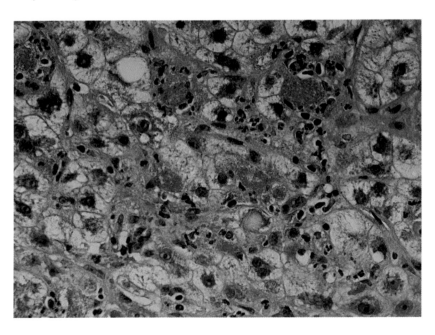

Fig. 25.5. Acute alcoholic hepatitis with ballooning degeneration, Mallory-Denk bodies and satellitosis (neutrophil polymorph infiltrate around hepatocytes). (H & E × 120). Photo provided courtesy of A.D. Burt.

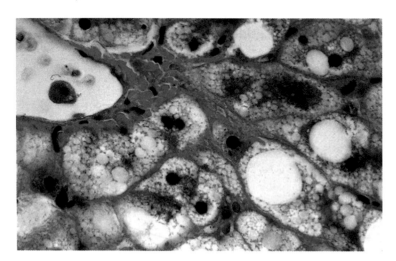

Fig. 25.6. Acute alcoholic hepatitis. Hepatocytes are ballooned and contain micro- and macrovesicular fat and clumps of purplish-red Mallory's alcoholic hyaline. (Chromophobe aniline blue, ×100.)

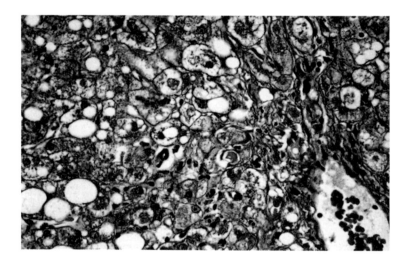

Fig. 25.7. Advanced zone 3 collagenosis with fatty change. A thickened hepatic vein can be seen bottom right. (Chromophobe aniline blue, ×100.)

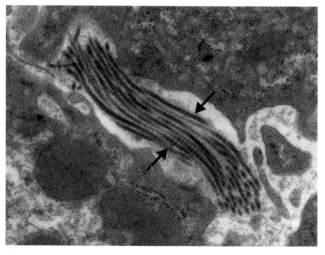

Fig. 25.8. Electron micrograph of liver in a patient with alcoholic liver disease. Note the deposition of collagen fibrils in Disse's space (arrowed). This could interfere with oxygen and metabolite exchange between blood and hepatocytes.

collagenosis' (Fig. 25.7) [26]. Collagenization of the space of Disse is shown by electron microscopy (Fig. 25.8) and is associated with a reduction in the porosity of the sinusoidal lining [27]. These changes interfere with the exchange of substances between plasma and the hepatocyte cell membrane and contribute to portal hypertension. Associated lesions in terminal and sublobular veins include lymphocytic phlebitis, gradual obliteration and eventual veno-occlusion [28].

Portal zone. Changes in the portal zone are inconspicuous and mild chronic inflammation is seen only in the advanced case. Zone 1 fibrosis if present is not now thought due to previous pancreatitis (Fig. 25.10) [29].

Cholestasis. Cholestasis in bile canaliculi is a feature of all types of alcohol-related liver disease. It is strongly associated with decreased survival.

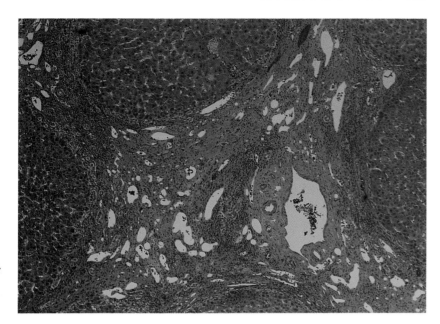

Fig. 25.9. End stage cirrhotic alcoholic liver disease. Established micronodular cirrhosis with areas of parenchymal extinction. (H & E, ×120.) Photo courtesy of A.D. Burt.

These histological patterns form a spectrum from minimal hepatitis to an advanced, probably irreversible, picture, where necrosis is more extensive and fibrosis is prominent. Alcohol-related hepatitis is a precursor of cirrhosis and in the majority of cases is superimposed on established cirrhosis.

Cirrhosis

Classical alcohol-related cirrhosis is micronodular (Fig. 25.9). No normal zonal architecture can be identified, and zone 3 venules are difficult to find. The formation of nodules is often slow because of an inhibitory effect of alcohol on hepatic regeneration. The amount of fat is variable and acute alcoholic hepatitis may coexist. With continuing necrosis and replacement by fibrosis, the cirrhosis may progress from a micro- to a macronodular pattern, and this is usually accompanied by a reduction in steatosis. When this end-stage picture is reached, an alcohol aetiology is difficult to confirm on histological grounds. Cirrhosis may follow pericellular fibrosis without apparent hepatic necrosis and inflammation.

Clinical features

History, examination and early recognition

Early recognition depends on a high index of suspicion. If hazardous drinking is suspected, the AUDIT questionnaire should be used (Table 25.4). Patients may present with non-specific digestive symptoms such as anorexia, nausea, diarrhoea, vague right upper abdom-

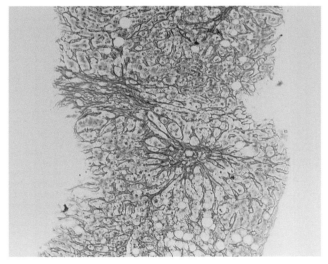

Fig. 25.10. Portal fibrosis in alcoholic liver disease. Gordon & Sweet's reticulin. Photo courtesy of A.D. Burt.

inal pain and tenderness or pyrexia. The patient may seek medical advice because of the more broad effects of alcohol dependence such as social disruption, poor work performance, accidents, violent behaviour, fits, tremulousness or depression. The diagnosis may be made when hepatomegaly, a raised serum transaminase or γ-glutamyl transpeptidase (γ-GT) level or macrocytosis are discovered at a routine examination, for instance at a life insurance check-up or during investigation of another condition. Physical signs may be non-contributory although tender hepatomegaly, prominent vascular spiders and associated features of chronic liver

Table 25.4. Alcohol use disorders identification test (AUDIT) questionnaire

Please circle the answer that is correct for you

1 How often do you have a drink containing alcohol?
  - Never
  - Monthly or less
  - 2–4 times a month
  - 2–3 times a week
  - 4 or more times a week

2 How many standard drinks containing alcohol do you have on a typical day when drinking?
  - 1 or 2
  - 3 or 4
  - 5 or 6
  - 7 to 9
  - 10 or more

3 How often do you have six or more drinks on one occasion?
  - Never
  - Less than monthly
  - Monthly
  - Weekly
  - Daily or almost daily

4 During the past year, how often have you found that you were not able to stop drinking once you had started?
  - Never
  - Less than monthly
  - Monthly
  - Weekly
  - Daily or almost daily

5 During the past year, how often have you failed to do what was normally expected of you because of drinking?
  - Never
  - Less than monthly
  - Monthly
  - Weekly
  - Daily or almost daily

6 During the past year, how often have you needed a drink in the morning to get yourself going after a heavy drinking session?
  - Never
  - Less than monthly
  - Monthly
  - Weekly
  - Daily or almost daily

7 During the past year, how often have you had a feeling of guilt or remorse after drinking?
  - Never
  - Less than monthly
  - Monthly
  - Weekly
  - Daily or almost daily

8 During the past year, have you been unable to remember what happened the night before because you had been drinking?
  - Never
  - Less than monthly
  - Monthly
  - Weekly
  - Daily or almost daily

9 Have you or someone else been injured as a result of your drinking?
  - No
  - Yes, but not in the past year
  - Yes, during the past year

10 Has a relative or friend, doctor or other health worker been concerned about your drinking or suggested you cut down?
  - No
  - Yes, but not in the past year
  - Yes, during the past year

Table 25.4. (*Continued*)

Scoring the audit

Scores for each question range from 0 to 4, with the first response for each question (e.g. never) scoring 0, the second (e.g. less than monthly) scoring 1, the third (e.g. monthly) scoring 2, the fourth (e.g. weekly) scoring 3, and the last response (e.g. daily or almost daily) scoring 4. For questions 9 and 10, which only have three responses, the scoring is 0, 2 and 4.

A score of 8 or more is associated with harmful or hazardous drinking, a score of 13 or more in women, and 15 or more in men, is likely to indicate alcohol dependence.

From: Saunders JB, Aasland OG, Babor TF *et al*. Development of the alcohol use disorders identification test (AUDIT): WHO collaborative project on early detection of persons with harmful alcohol consumption II. *Addiction* 1993; **88**: 791–803.

disease may be helpful. The clinical features do not reflect the hepatic histology and biochemical tests of liver function may be normal.

Laboratory investigations

Biochemical tests

Serum transaminase levels rarely exceed 300 IU/L. Aspartate aminotransferase (AST; serum glutamic oxaloacetic transaminase) is usually higher than the alanine aminotransferase (ALT; serum glutamic pyruvate transaminase) with the AST: ALT ratio usually exceeding 2:1. The serum γ-GT is a widely used screening test for hazardous drinking. The rise results mainly from enzyme induction, although hepatocellular damage and cholestasis may contribute. There are many false positives due to other factors, including enzyme-inducing drugs, and other diseases including non-alcoholic fatty liver disease. Serum carbohydrate-deficient (desialylated) transferrin levels may be a useful marker of excessive alcohol intake irrespective of liver disease but this test is not generally available [30].

Serum alkaline phosphatase may be markedly increased (greater than four times normal) especially in those with severe cholestasis and alcohol-related hepatitis. Serum IgA values may be very high. Blood and urinary alcohol levels can be used in the clinic to refute the individual with suspected ALD who denies imbibing. Non-specific abnormalities found in hazardous drinkers include elevations in uric acid, lactate and triglyceride, and reductions in glucose and magnesium. Hypophosphataemia is related to a renal tubular defect, independent of liver function impairment [31]. Hypophosphataemia can also be a result of the refeeding syndrome. Low serum tri-iodothyronine (T3) levels presumably reflect decreased hepatic conversion of thyroxine to T3 as levels correlate inversely with the severity of liver disease. Even sensitive biochemical methods may fail to reveal alcohol-related liver damage and liver biopsy is necessary in cases of doubt.

Table 25.5. Liver biopsy in alcohol-related liver disease

Diagnosis:

    rarely required to exclude other causes

    often required to differentiate alcohol-related hepatitis from decompensated cirrhosis

Prognosis / staging:

    useful to determine if steatosis or steatohepatitis

    gold standard to confirm or refute cirrhosis

Enforcing abstinence

Haematological changes

Macrocytosis is presumed to be due to a direct effect of alcohol on bone marrow. Deficiencies of folate and vitamin B_{12} can contribute in the malnourished. The combination of a raised mean cell volume and serum γ-GT will identify 90% of alcohol-dependent patients.

Imaging

Ultrasound may not detect mild steatohepatitis or early fibrosis. Even cirrhosis may be missed on ultrasound. Advanced disease can be seen if the liver is shrunken with an irregular edge or if there is portal hypertension with ascites and splenomegaly.

CT and MRI scanning are very useful in demonstrating fatty liver, an irregular liver surface, splenomegaly, portal collateral circulation, ascites and pancreatitis.

Liver biopsy

The diagnosis of alcohol-related liver injury can usually be made from the clinical history and the pattern of blood tests after excluding other causes of liver injury (Table 25.5). Staging the liver disease requires liver biopsy. This is important from a prognostic point of view, with fatty change less likely to progress to cirrhosis than alcoholic hepatitis or perivenular fibrosis [32].

Established cirrhosis can be confirmed and hepatocellular carcinoma and varices surveillance commenced if appropriate. A further advantage of liver biopsy is that other treatable liver diseases (reported to be present in up to 20% of heavy drinkers) can be excluded.

Clinical syndromes

Fatty liver

Patients with fatty liver alone are usually asymptomatic, the diagnosis being made when an enlarged, smooth, firm liver is discovered on examination or on ultrasonography. Liver function tests may be normal or the transaminases and alkaline phosphatase slightly increased. If the fatty liver is sufficiently severe to merit admission to hospital the patient has usually been drinking heavily for some time and may be anorexic. Symptoms may include nausea and vomiting with periumbilical, epigastric or right upper quadrant pain. Clinically, the fatty liver patient cannot be separated confidently from one with alcoholic hepatitis or even well compensated cirrhosis.

Acute alcoholic hepatitis

In the very mildest case, the diagnosis may be made only by a liver biopsy in an asymptomatic patient who is misusing alcohol and has shown abnormal serum enzyme tests and macrocytosis. Patients with more severe disease complain of fatigue, anorexia and weight loss. There is tender hepatomegaly and usually pyrexia. The patient may be obese, but some features of malnutrition are present in many patients.

Patients in the most severe categories have usually been drinking particularly heavily and not eating. The severe hepatic decompensation may be precipitated by vomiting, diarrhoea, an intercurrent infection or prolonged anorexia. The intake of quite modest and even therapeutic doses of paracetamol may precipitate a severe hepatitis in these patients (Fig. 25.11). In this situation, transaminase levels are very high [3].

Severe alcoholic hepatitis is typically associated with pyrexia, anorexia and jaundice. The patient may experience pain over an enlarged tender liver and an arterial bruit may be heard over the liver. Florid vascular spiders are usual. There may be signs of associated liver failure such as ascites, encephalopathy and a bleeding diathesis. The blood pressure is usually low with a hyperdynamic circulation. Signs of vitamin deficiencies may be found in the malnourished patient. When present, gastrointestinal haemorrhage is frequently from a local gastric or duodenal lesion, rather than related to portal hypertension.

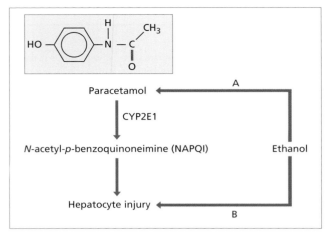

Fig. 25.11. The interaction between ethanol and paracetamol. Liver injury occurs when paracetamol is metabolized to the toxic intermediate *N*-acetyl-*p*-benzoquinoneimine (NAPQI) by the enzyme cytochrome P450 2E1 (CYP2E1). This will usually only occur when supratherapeutic doses are consumed. Liver injury can occur at therapeutic doses when toxicity is enhanced by ethanol through two mechanisms: (1) the induction of CYP2E1 and (2) the depletion of cytoplasmic and mitochondrial glutathione with a resulting increase in susceptibility to oxidative-stress-mediated hepatocyte apoptosis and necrosis.

Cirrhosis

Established cirrhosis can present without acute alcohol-related hepatitis, having been recognized clinically or histologically, and the picture can resemble any end-stage liver disease. Points suggesting alcohol as an aetiological agent include the history of alcohol abuse (which may be denied), the hepatomegaly and the extrahepatic features of hazardous drinking. Splenomegaly is a late feature.

Extrahepatic features

Bilaterally enlarged parotids are common and are analogous to those seen with other types of malnutrition. Gynaecomastia often appears after treatment and is a frequent complication of spironolactone therapy. The testes atrophy and sexual performance in men declines. Muscle mass wastes and falls may be complicated by fractures due to alcohol-induced osteoporosis. Dupuytren's contracture of the palmar fascia is related to alcohol and not to the cirrhosis [33].

Loss of memory and concentration, insomnia, irritability, hallucinations, convulsions ('rum fits') and tremor may be signs of dependence. These must be distinguished from early hepatic encephalopathy and withdrawal.

Hepatorenal syndrome seems particularly common in advanced liver disease caused by alcohol.

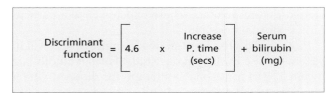

Fig. 25.12. Calculation of the discriminant function. P, prothrombin time. Serum bilirubin in μmol/L is divided by 17 to convert to mg/dL.

Arrhythmias, hypertension, cardiomyopathy and coronary artery disease are all associated with alcohol consumption.

Cancer of the oropharynx, oesophagus, colon and breast are more common in hazardous drinkers.

Prognosis

In ALD, liver histology is a good indicator of prognosis. Zone 3 fibrosis, perivenular sclerosis and alcohol-related hepatitis are all unfavourable histological features as they indicate a risk of progressing to cirrhosis [34]. Histological cholestasis is a bad prognostic indicator in alcohol-related hepatitis. In one study, 50% of patients with hepatitis developed cirrhosis after 10–13 years [32].

'Pure' fatty liver on biopsy can, however, also have serious implications. In a study of 86 patients followed for 10.5 years, nine developed cirrhosis and another seven developed fibrosis. A mixed pattern of steatosis, giant mitochondria and continued hazardous drinking predicted these serious developments [35].

Clinical and laboratory features with independent bad prognostic significance are encephalopathy, low serum albumin, increased prothrombin time, low haemoglobin level and large oesophageal varices [36]. Patients with encephalopathy, persistent jaundice and azotaemia are very liable to develop the hepatorenal syndrome.

Patients with acute alcoholic hepatitis often deteriorate during the first few days in hospital and 20–50% of the most severe cases die within 28 days of hospital admission. Those with a markedly prolonged prothrombin time, unresponsive to vitamin K, and with a high serum bilirubin have a particularly bad outlook [37]. Prothrombin time and bilirubin can be used to determine a *discriminant function* to estimate prognosis in alcohol-related hepatitis (Fig. 25.12). This score can then be used to inform treatment decisions [38,39]. The Glasgow Alcoholic Hepatitis Score uses INR, bilirubin, white cell count, urea and age to determine a score that is closely linked to survival and may be a better predictor than the discriminant function (Table 25.6) [40].

The outlook in alcohol-related cirrhosis is much better than that due to other causes. It depends on the ability

Table 25.6. The Glasgow Alcoholic Hepatitis Score

	Score		
	1	2	3
Age	<50	>50	–
White cell count (10⁹/L)	<15	>15	–
Urea (mmol/L)	<5	>5	–
Prothrombin time ratio	<1.5	1.5–2.0	>2.0
Bilirubin (μmol/L)	<125	125–250	>250

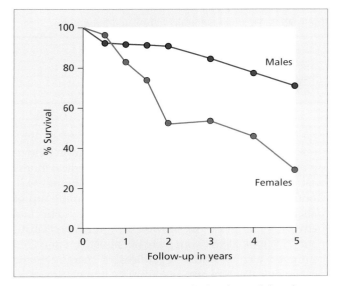

Fig. 25.13. The percentage survival of males and females with alcoholic cirrhosis.

of the patient to abstain, which in turn is related to family support, financial resources and socioeconomic state. Women with cirrhosis survive for a shorter time than men (Fig. 25.13). In a multicentre Veterans Hospital study, predictors of survival in patients with alcohol-related hepatitis and cirrhosis were age, grams of alcohol consumed, AST:ALT ratio and the histological and clinical severity of disease [41]. Those with poor nutrition were much more likely to die [42].

Treatment

Harmful drinking and dependence

The most important measure is to ensure total and immediate abstinence from alcohol. The development of a withdrawal syndrome (*delirium tremens*) should be treated with medication. Benzodiazepines, particularly chlordiazepoxide, are the usual first choice agent. This should ideally be delivered according to a symptom-triggered regimen. Patients with severe physical

Table 25.7. Treatments for alcohol dependence

Non-pharmacological
  Brief intervention
  Cognitive therapy
  Motivational enhancement therapy
  Psychotherapy
Pharmacological
  Acamprosate
  Naltrexone
  Disulfuram
  Baclofen

Table 25.8. Treatments for alcohol-related hepatitis

Abstinence
Corticosteroids
Pentoxifylline
Enteral nutritional support

problems are more likely to abstain than those who present with psychological issues. In a long-term follow-up of men attending a liver clinic, severe medical illness was critical in the decision to stop drinking [43]. Continued medical care is also essential. Follow-up of patients with ALD treated at the Royal Free Hospital between 1975 and 1990 showed 50% remained abstinent, 25% took alcohol but were not abusing it and 25% continued alcohol abuse regardless of therapy. Some psychological and pharmacological treatments are available to help abstinence and prevent relapse (Table 25.7). The less severely affected can receive *'brief interventional counselling'* from a doctor, nurse or similar person. This results in a 38% treatment benefit, albeit often temporary [44]. The more severely dependent patients will need psychiatric referral. Some patients may benefit from pharmacological therapy to help achieve abstinence and prevent relapse. Acamprosate and naltrexone are effective but contraindicated in severe liver disease [45]. Baclofen can be used in dependent patients with decompensated cirrhosis [46].

Acute alcohol-related hepatitis (Table 25.8)

Corticosteroids suppress the hepatic inflammatory response and are the most effective therapy. Conflicting results came from initial studies that included patients of all severities. A novel meta-analysis of the three largest trials showed steroids to associate with a significant survival benefit in the group of patients with a modified discriminant function of 32 or above [47]. This is now the standard of care. Active sepsis and bleeding are contraindications, but steroids can be started soon after these complications are controlled. A failure of the bilirubin to drop after 7 days of treatment identifies

steroid non-responders. These patients have a particularly poor prognosis [48].

Pentoxifyilline has been shown to improve survival in severe disease by 40% in one study. Further studies are awaited. It is a reasonable therapy for those in whom steroids are contraindicated [49].

Protein and calorie malnutrition must be corrected. Enteral nutritional supplementation may have a role in improving medium to long-term survival in patients with severe alcohol-related hepatitis. Which patients benefit most and the mechanism of action are still unclear [50].

Testosterone and *oxandrolone* are of no benefit.

Antioxidants (including *N*-acetylcysteine) have not been shown to improve survival [51,52].

Colchicine has failed to improve short-time survival in patients with alcohol-related hepatitis [49].

Pilot studies of the *molecular adsorbents recycling system (MARS)* and *anti-TNF antibodies* have showed promise but more rigorous studies have yet to show benefit for these treatments. When high-dose infliximab was combined with steroids, mortality was increased [53].

Cirrhosis

Cirrhosis is irreversible and therapy is usually directed at the complications. These include portal hypertension, encephalopathy and ascites. Drug metabolism is impaired and particular care must be taken, especially with sedatives. Consideration has been given to some agents aimed at improving the liver disease.

Propylthiouracil. Alcohol induces a hypermetabolic state which potentiates zone 3 anoxic liver injury. This is reduced by propylthiouracil in experimental animals. A long-term beneficial effect has been shown in patients with alcohol-related cirrhosis who continue to drink, but at lower levels [54]. This therapy has never gained general acceptance.

S-adenosyl-methionine (SAMe). A significant beneficial effect of SAMe treatment has been found in patients with Child's A and B cirrhosis in one study [55]. Further studies are awaited.

Phosphatidylcholine. This has been shown to attenuate ethanol-induced fibrosis in baboons [56]. A long-term trial in humans showed no benefit, most probably related to the dramatic reduction in drinking seen in the treated and placebo groups of patients [56].

Transplantation

Alcohol-related liver disease now accounts for 20–30% of all indications for liver transplant in the USA and UK.

In spite of initial concerns about comorbidities, initial graft and patient survival is similar to that found in other transplant recipients. The 5-year survival is increased with the greatest benefit seen in those with the most severe disease [57]. Nevertheless, transplantation for ALD remains controversial because of the risk of recidivism. Around 10–20% will drink excessively within the first 5 years, although this rarely leads to significant liver disease until 10 years post-transplant [58].

In reality, post-transplant recidivism is hard to predict. Patients should be monitored closely to detect relapse early and treat those that return to hazardous drinking. This is imperative to maintain the organ-donating public's support.

Six months' abstinence from alcohol is usually demanded by most units and has been found to be a predictor of post-transplant recidivism in some studies but not others. In some cases, the period may be reduced to 3 months if survival is unlikely beyond this. One of the main reasons for the period of abstinence is that many patients will recover and not need transplantation after this period. If recovery is not seen by 3 months abstinence, it is unlikely to occur [59].

Alcohol-related hepatitis is not an indication for liver transplantation.

References

1 Leon DA, McCambridge J. Liver cirrhosis mortality rates in Britain from 1950 to 2002: an analysis of routine data. *Lancet* 2006; **367**: 52–56.

2 Lieber CS, DeCarli LM. Ethanol oxidation by hepatic microsomes: adaptive increase after ethanol feeding. *Science* 1968; **162**: 917–918.

3 Zimmerman HJ, Maddrey WC. Acetaminophen (paracetamol) hepatotoxicity with regular intake of alcohol: analysis of instances of therapeutic misadventure. *Hepatology* 1995; **22**: 767–773.

4 Lane BP, Lieber CS. Ultrastructural alterations in human hepatocytes following ingestion of ethanol with adequate diets. *Am. J. Pathol.* 1966; **49**: 593–603.

5 Sugimoto T, Yamashita S, Ishigami M *et al.* Decreased microsomal triglyceride transfer protein activity contributes to initiation of alcoholic liver steatosis in rats. *J. Hepatol.* 2002; **36**: 157–162.

6 Kaufman RJ. Stress signaling from the lumen of the endoplasmic reticulum: coordination of gene transcriptional and translational controls. *Genes Dev.* 1999; **13**: 1211–1233.

7 Hoek JB. Endotoxin and alcoholic liver disease: tolerance and susceptibility. *Hepatology* 1999; **29**: 1602–1604.

8 McClain CJ, Cohen DA. Increased tumor necrosis factor production by monocytes in alcoholic hepatitis. *Hepatology* 1989; **9**: 349–351.

9 Bird G, Sheron N, Goka AK *et al.* Increased plasma tumour necrosis factor in severe alcoholic hepatitis. *Ann. Intern. Med.* 1990; **112**: 917–920.

10 Niemela O, Klajner F, Orrego H *et al.* Antibodies against acetaldehyde-modified protein epitopes in human alcoholics. *Hepatology* 1987; **7**: 1210–1214.

11 Clot P, Albano E, Eliasson E *et al.* Cytochrome P4502E1 hydroxyethyl radical adducts as the major antigen in autoantibody formation among alcoholics. *Gastroenterology* 1996; **111**: 206–216.

12 Vidali M, Stewart SF, Rolla R *et al.* Genetic and epigenetic factors in autoimmune reactions toward cytochrome P4502E1 in alcoholic liver disease. *Hepatology* 2003; **37**: 410–419.

13 Canbay A, Taimr P, Torok N *et al.* Apoptotic body engulfment by a human stellate cell line is profibrogenic. *Lab. Invest.* 2003; **83**: 655–663.

14 Bellentani S, Saccoccio G, Costa G *et al.* Drinking habits as cofactors of risk for alcohol induced liver damage. The Dionysos Study Group. *Gut* 1997; **41**: 845–850.

15 Lelbach WK. Cirrhosis in the alcoholic and its relation to the volume of alcohol abuse. *Ann. NY Acad. Sci.* 1975; **252**: 85–105.

16 Smith S, White J, Nelson C *et al.* Severe alcohol-induced liver disease and the alcohol dependence syndrome. *Alcohol* 2006; **41**: 274–277.

17 Nanji AA, French SW. Relationship between pork consumption and cirrhosis. *Lancet* 1985; **1**: 681–683.

18 Rotily M, Durbec JP, Berthezene P, Sarles H. Diet and alcohol in liver cirrhosis: a case-control study. *Eur. J. Clin. Nutr.* 1990; **44**: 595–603.

19 Naveau S, Giraud V, Borotto E *et al.* Excess weight risk factor for alcoholic liver disease. *Hepatology* 1997; **25**: 108–111.

20 Raynard B, Balian A, Fallik D *et al.* Risk factors of fibrosis in alcohol-induced liver disease. *Hepatology* 2002; **35**: 635–638.

21 Morgan MY, Sherlock S. Sex-related differences among 100 patients with alcoholic liver disease. *Br. Med. J.* 1977; **1**: 939–941.

22 Enomoto N, Takei Y, Kitamura T *et al.* Estriol enhances lipopolysaccharide-induced increases in nitric oxide production by Kupffer cells via mechanisms dependent on endotoxin. *Alcohol Clin. Exp. Res.* 2002; **26**: 66S–69S.

23 Pares A, Caballeria J, Bruguera M *et al.* Histological course of alcoholic hepatitis. Influence of abstinence, sex and extent of hepatic damage. *J. Hepatol.* 1986; **2**: 33–42.

24 Hrubec Z, Omenn GS. Evidence of genetic predisposition to alcoholic cirrhosis and psychosis: twin concordances for alcoholism and its biological end points by zygosity among male veterans. *Alcohol Clin. Exp. Res.* 1981; **5**: 207–215.

25 Wilfred de Alwis NM, Day CP. Genetics of alcoholic liver disease and nonalcoholic fatty liver disease. *Semin. Liver Dis.* 2007; **27**: 44–54.

26 Edmondson HA, Peters RL, Reynolds TB, Kuzma OT. Sclerosing hyaline necrosis of the liver in the chronic alcoholic. a recognizable clinical syndrome. *Ann. Intern. Med.* 1963; **59**: 646–673.

27 Horn T, Christoffersen P, Henriksen JH. Alcoholic liver injury: defenestration in noncirrhotic livers–a scanning electron microscopic study. *Hepatology* 1987; **7**: 77–82.

28 Goodman ZD, Ishak KG. Occlusive venous lesions in alcoholic liver disease. A study of 200 cases. *Gastroenterology* 1982; **83**: 786–796.

29 Morgan MY, Sherlock S, Scheuer PJ. Portal fibrosis in the livers of alcoholic patients. *Gut* 1978; **19**: 1015–1021.

30 Bell H, Tallaksen C, Sjaheim T *et al.* Serum carbohydrate-deficient transferrin as a marker of alcohol consumption in

patients with chronic liver diseases. *Alcohol Clin. Exp. Res.* 1993; **17**: 246–252.

31 Angeli P, Gatta A, Caregaro L *et al.* Hypophosphatemia and renal tubular dysfunction in alcoholics. Are they related to liver function impairment? *Gastroenterology* 1991; **100**: 502–512.

32 Sorensen TI, Orholm M, Bentsen KD *et al.* Prospective evaluation of alcohol abuse and alcoholic liver injury in men as predictors of development of cirrhosis. *Lancet* 1984; **2**: 241–244.

33 Bradlow A, Mowat AG. Dupuytren's contracture and alcohol. *Ann. Rheum. Dis.* 1986; **45**: 304–307.

34 Worner TM, Lieber CS. Perivenular fibrosis as precursor lesion of cirrhosis. *JAMA* 1985; **254**: 627–630.

35 Teli MR, Day CP, Burt AD *et al.* Determinants of progression to cirrhosis or fibrosis in pure alcoholic fatty liver. *Lancet* 1995; **346**: 987–990.

36 Gluud C, Henriksen JH, Nielsen G. Prognostic indicators in alcoholic cirrhotic men. *Hepatology* 1988; **8**: 222–227.

37 Maddrey WC, Boitnott JK, Bedine MS *et al.* Corticosteroid therapy of alcoholic hepatitis. *Gastroenterology* 1978; **75**: 193–199.

38 Carithers RL Jr, Herlong HF, Diehl AM *et al.* Methylprednisolone therapy in patients with severe alcoholic hepatitis. A randomized multicenter trial. *Ann. Intern. Med.* 1989; **110**: 685–690.

39 Ramond MJ, Poynard T, Rueff B *et al.* A randomized trial of prednisolone in patients with severe alcoholic hepatitis. *N. Eng. J. Med.* 1992; **326**: 507–512.

40 Forrest EH, Evans CD, Stewart S *et al.* Analysis of factors predictive of mortality in alcoholic hepatitis and derivation and validation of the Glasgow alcoholic hepatitis score. *Gut* 2005; **54**: 1174–1179.

41 Chedid A, Mendenhall CL, Moritz TE *et al.* Cell-mediated hepatic injury in alcoholic liver disease. Veterans Affairs Cooperative Study Group 275. *Gastroenterology* 1993; **105**: 254–266.

42 Mendenhall CL, Anderson S, Weesner RE *et al.* Protein-calorie malnutrition associated with alcoholic hepatitis. Veterans Administration Cooperative Study Group on Alcoholic Hepatitis. *Am. J. Med.* 1984; **76**: 211–222.

43 Patek AJ Jr, Hermos JA. Recovery from alcoholism in cirrhotic patients: a study of 45 cases. *Am. J. Med.* 1981; **70**: 783–785.

44 Wilk AI, Jensen NM, Havighurst TC. Meta-analysis of randomized control trials addressing brief interventions in heavy alcohol drinkers. *J. Gen. Intern. Med.* 1997; **12**: 274–283.

45 Schuckit MA. Alcohol-use disorders. *Lancet* 2009; **373**: 492–501.

46 Addolorato G, Leggio L, Ferrulli A *et al.* Effectiveness and safety of baclofen for maintenance of alcohol abstinence in alcohol-dependent patients with liver cirrhosis: ran-

domised, double-blind controlled study. *Lancet* 2007; **370**: 1915–1922.

47 Mathurin P, Mendenhall CL, Carithers RL *et al.* Corticosteroids improve short-term survival in patients with severe alcoholic hepatitis (AH): individual data analysis of the last three randomized placebo controlled double blind trials of corticosteroids in severe AH. *J. Hepatol.* 2002; **36**: 480–487.

48 Mathurin P, Abdelnour M, Ramond MJ *et al.* Early change in bilirubin levels is an important prognostic factor in severe alcoholic hepatitis treated with prednisolone. *Hepatology* 2003; **38**: 1363–1369.

49 Akriviadis E, Botla R, Briggs W *et al.* Pentoxifylline improves short-term survival in severe acute alcoholic hepatitis: a double-blind, placebo-controlled trial. *Gastroenterology* 2000; **119**: 1637–1648.

50 Cabre E, Rodriguez-Iglesias P, Caballeria J *et al.* Short- and long-term outcome of severe alcohol-induced hepatitis treated with steroids or enteral nutrition: a multicenter randomized trial. *Hepatology* 2000; **32**: 36–42.

51 Stewart SF, Prince M, Bassendine MF *et al.* A trial of antioxidant therapy alone or with corticosteroids in acute alcoholic hepatitis. *J. Hepatol.* 2002; **36** (Suppl. 1): 16.

52 Phillips M, Curtis H, Portmann B *et al.* Antioxidants versus corticosteroids in the treatment of severe alcoholic hepatitis: a randomised trial. *Hepatology* 2001; **34**: 250A.

53 Naveau S, Chollet-Martin S, Dharancy S *et al.* A double-blind randomized controlled trial of infliximab associated with prednisolone in acute alcoholic hepatitis. *Hepatology* 2004; **39**: 1390–1397.

54 Orrego H, Blake JE, Blendis LM *et al.* Long-term treatment of alcoholic liver disease with propylthiouracil. *N. Engl. J. Med.* 1987; **317**: 1421–1427.

55 Mato JM, Camara J, Fernandez de Paz J *et al.* S-adenosylmethionine in alcoholic liver cirrhosis: a randomized, placebo-controlled, double-blind, multicenter clinical trial. *J. Hepatol.* 1999; **30**: 1081–1089.

56 Lieber CS, Weiss DG, Groszmann R *et al*, For the Veterans Affairs Cooperative Study G. II. Veterans Affairs Cooperative Study of polyenylphosphatidylcholine in alcoholic liver disease. *Alcohol Clin. Exp. Res.* 2003; **27**: 1765–1772.

57 Poynard T, Barthelemy P, Fratte S *et al.* Evaluation of efficacy of liver transplantation in alcoholic cirrhosis by a case-control study and simulated controls. *Lancet* 1994; **344**: 502–507.

58 Pageaux GP, Bismuth M, Perney P *et al.* Alcohol relapse after liver transplantation for alcoholic liver disease: does it matter? *J. Hepatol.* 2003; **38**: 629–634.

59 Veldt BJ, Laine F, Guillygomarch A *et al.* Indication of liver transplantation in severe alcoholic liver cirrhosis: quantitative evaluation and optimal timing. *J. Hepatol.* 2002; **36**: 93–98.

CHAPTER 26
Iron Overload States

Paul Adams

University Hospital, London, Ontario, Canada

Learning points

- Haemochromatosis is a common genetic disease, which can usually be diagnosed with transferrin saturation, serum ferritin and genetic testing.

- Not all C282Y homozygotes will have biochemical evidence of iron overload.

- Not all C282Y homozygotes will demonstrate a progressive increase in total body iron overload over time.

- Liver biopsy has moved from a diagnostic test to a prognostic test in selected cases.

- Phlebotomy therapy is effective in preventing liver damage and is well tolerated in most patients.

The causes of iron overload can be broadly separated into those with a clear genetic mechanism, those associated with another pathology and a small group of intermediate conditions where there appears to be an interplay between genetic and acquired mechanisms (Table 26.1). There has been an explosion of information on classical genetic haemochromatosis (previously termed idiopathic or primary), which is now known to be due to a mutation in the *HFE* gene. These data have added much to the understanding of iron absorption from the intestine, to the identification of patients and family screening, and to the recognition of atypical patients. Inherited non-*HFE*-related iron overload is much less common than *HFE*-related genetic haemochromatosis.

Iron overload as a result of liver or haematological disease is not uncommon and genotyping for *HFE* mutations now allows these to be clearly separated from genetic haemochromatosis.

Normal iron metabolism

Absorption

The normal daily diet contains about 10–20 mg of iron (90% free; 10% bound in haem). Of this 1–1.5 mg is absorbed. This amount depends on body stores, more being absorbed as the need increases. The absorption process, sited in the duodenum and upper small intestine, is active and capable of transporting iron against a gradient.

The mechanism of absorption, although not fully understood, has gained much from the discovery of: (1) the *HFE* gene [1]; (2) the divalent metal transporter-1 (DMT-1); (3) the intracellular mechanisms for controlling the expression of transport and storage proteins, in particular iron regulatory proteins (IRPs); (4) the basolateral iron transporter (called IREG-1 or ferroportin); and (5) hepcidin, a polypeptide which plays a pivotal role in iron regulation [2].

In the intestinal lumen, ferric iron is reduced to ferrous iron by ferrireductase or ascorbic acid, following which the iron is transported by DMT-1 into the enterocytes of the villus. Expression of DMT-1 within these cells is regulated by the level of intracellular iron through an interaction between IRP-1 and the iron regulatory element (IRE) of DMT-1. The iron concentration within enterocytes is therefore important in determining the amount of iron absorbed from the intestinal lumen. Hypoxia inducible factor (HIF) plays a central role [3].

Ferroportin on the basolateral membrane of the enterocyte is responsible for the exit of iron from the cell. Once across the membrane, the iron has to be oxidized from ferrous to ferric to be available to bind and be carried by transferrin. Hephaestin and interestingly

Sherlock's Diseases of the Liver and Biliary System, Twelfth Edition. Edited by James S. Dooley, Anna S.F. Lok, Andrew K. Burroughs, E. Jenny Heathcote.
© 2011 by Blackwell Publishing Ltd. Published 2011 by Blackwell Publishing Ltd.

Table 26.1. Iron overload states

Inherited	
HFE mutation related	Genetic haemochromatosis (Type 1)
Non-*HFE* related	Juvenile haemochromatosis (Type 2)
	Transferrin receptor 2 (Type 3)
	Ferroportin disease (Type 4)
	Acaeruloplasminaemia
	Atransferrinaemia
Acquired	
Haematological disorders	Iron-loading anaemias
	thalassaemia major
	sideroblastic anaemia
	chronic haemolytic anaemia
	Parenteral iron overload
Chronic liver disease	End-stage cirrhosis
	Hepatitis C
	Alcoholic liver disease
	Non-alcoholic steatohepatitis
	Portacaval shunt
Dysmetabolic syndrome	
Dietary iron overload	
Inherited/acquired?	
African iron overload	
Neonatal haemochromatosis	
Associations	
Porphyria cutanea tarda	

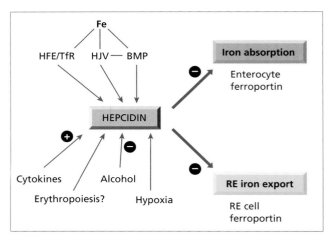

Fig. 26.1. Role of hepcidin in iron metabolism. TfR, transferrin receptor; HJV, haemojuvelin; BMP, bone morphogenetic protein; RE, reticuloendothelial.

caeruloplasmin subserve this oxidation. Dysfunction of ferroportin and also caeruloplasmin lead to iron accumulation in other cells where these proteins take part in iron transport.

The regulation of iron absorption appears to depend predominantly on changes in HIF and hepcidin (see below), which associates with ferroportin resulting in intracellular degradation and loss of function.

Regulation

After the discovery of the *HFE* gene, immunohistochemical studies showed particular localization of the protein to the crypt cells of the upper small intestine. Further studies showed that the HFE protein is expressed on the surface of cells [4] and that it interacts with the transferrin receptor TfR (1 and 2), reducing the affinity of the TfR for transferrin. The transferrin/TfR interaction is the major mechanism for uptake of iron into many cells. The expression of TfR is inversely related to intracellular iron levels. The mechanism by which HFE influences iron balance is still unclear despite the years of study since its discovery in 1996. More is known of other newly discovered polypeptides and transporters in particular hepcidin, haemojuvelin and bone morphogenetic proteins (BMPs).

Hepcidin, a polypeptide hormone produced in the liver, controls extracellular iron concentrations by binding to and inducing the degradation of the cellular iron exporter, ferroportin [2]. Levels of hepcidin are inversely related to iron absorption. Iron absorption is exquisitely sensitive to hepcidin levels and hepcidin holds a central pathogenic place in haemochromatosis, similar to that of insulin in diabetes [5].

The most potent known regulators of hepcidin synthesis are certain BMPs [6] that apparently act by binding to haemojuvelin (HJV = HFE2) as a coreceptor and signalling through Smad4, a transforming growth factor-β superfamily protein. Hepcidin production is also controlled by iron concentrations, hypoxia, anaemia, and inflammatory cytokines, especially interleukin-6 (Fig. 26.1).

Hepcidin, expressed in many cell types involved in iron transport, binds to ferroportin. The precise mechanism by which HFE protein, ferroportin and hepcidin interact is unclear. Normally, the response to excess body iron would be increased hepatic expression of hepcidin. The observed deficiency (absolute or relative to that expected) of hepcidin is a unifying explanation for increased iron absorption and iron overload observed in many hereditary forms of haemochromatosis, especially those associated with missense mutations in genes that encode HFE (*HFE*), transferrin receptor-2 (*TFR2*), hepcidin (*HAMP*) and haemojuvelin (*HJV*) [7,8].

Circulating iron

In the plasma, iron is bound to transferrin, a glycoprotein largely synthesized in the liver. Transferrin can bind two ferric iron molecules, and is responsible for the 'total iron-binding capacity' of serum of 250–370 μg/dL. This is normally around 20–40% saturated with iron. Physiological entry of iron into reticulocytes and hepatocytes depends upon transferrin receptors at the cell surface, which preferentially bind transferrin carrying iron. The receptor/iron transferrin complex is internalized and the iron released. This process is saturable. TfRs are down-regulated as the cell becomes replete with iron.

When serum transferrin is fully saturated, as in overt haemochromatosis, iron circulates also in 'non-transferrin bound' forms, associated with low-molecular-weight chelators. Iron in this form readily enters cells by a non-saturable process.

Storage of iron

Iron is stored in cells in ferritin, a combination of the protein apoferritin (H and L subunits) and iron. High concentrations of iron stimulate apoferritin synthesis. Up to 4500 atoms of iron can be stored within a single ferritin molecule. Aggregates of degraded ferritin molecules make up haemosiderin, which stains as blue granules with ferrocyanide. Lipofuscin, a yellow brown material may accumulate in association with iron overload, but does not contain iron.

Iron contained in cells as ferritin or haemosiderin is available for mobilization. The normal total body content of iron is about 4 g, of which 3 g is present in haemoglobin, myoglobin, catalase and other respiratory enzymes. Storage iron comprises 0.5 g; of this 0.3 g is in the liver but is not seen with the usual histological stains for iron. The liver is the predominant site for storage of iron absorbed from the intestine. When its capacity is exceeded, iron is deposited in other parenchymal cells, including the acinar cells of the pancreas, and the cells of the anterior pituitary gland. The reticuloendothelial system plays only a limited part in iron storage unless this is the result of transfusion, when it is concentrated particularly in the spleen.

Iron overload and liver damage

Fibrosis and hepatocellular damage are directly related to the iron content of the liver cell. The pattern of damage is similar irrespective of whether the overload is due to genetic haemochromatosis or to multiple transfusions. The severity of fibrosis is maximal in periportal areas where iron is particularly deposited.

When iron deposition is low it is stored as ferritin. As the load increases more is present as haemosiderin.

Removal of iron by venesection or chelation leads to clinical and biochemical improvement with reduction or prevention of hepatic fibrosis [9,10].

There are several processes by which iron can damage the liver. There is enhanced oxidative stress in patients with iron overload and this is associated with increased TGF-β1 expression. Oxidative stress causes lipid peroxidation of membranes of organelles leading to functional defects of lysosomes, mitochondria and microsomes. Mitochondrial cytochrome C oxidase activity is reduced. There is lysosomal membrane fragility and release of hydrolytic enzymes into the cytosol.

Hepatic stellate cells (lipocytes) are activated in genetic haemochromatosis and activation is reversed by iron removal. Stellate cell activation appears related to the release of cytokines and other substances from neighbouring cells rather than oxidant stress within stellate cells [11].

Genetic haemochromatosis

In 1865, Trousseau described the clinical syndrome of skin pigmentation, cirrhosis and diabetes now recognized as characteristic of late-stage genetic haemochromatosis. This is an autosomal recessive metabolic disorder in which there may be increased iron absorption over many years.

Molecular genetics

Sheldon in his classic monograph described idiopathic haemochromatosis as an inborn error of metabolism [12]. The discovery of genetic linkage of haemochromatosis to the HLA serotype allowed the inheritance to be defined as autosomal recessive, and placed the gene on chromosome 6.

In 1996, a positional cloning approach was successful in identifying the *HFE* gene approximately 6 megabases telomeric to the HLA-A locus on chromosome 6 [1] (Fig. 26.2). Eighty-five per cent of chromosomes from haemochromatosis patients contained a single mutation (C282Y, also designated Cys282Tyr) in the *HFE* gene compared with 3% of control chromosomes. In most populations of northern European origin, over 90% of haemochromatosis patients have been found to be homozygous for this mutation [13]. In southern European populations, the frequency of C282Y homozygosity is lower (65%) [14]. The high frequency of this mutation in genetic haemochromatosis points to individuals being descended from a single family or

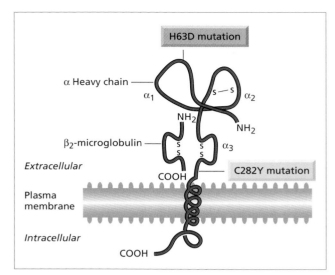

Fig. 26.2. Hypothetical model of the *HFE* protein based on homology with MHC molecules. The extracellular component has three α-domains, one of which binds to β2-microglobulin, a membrane spanning region and a short cytoplasmic tail. The C282Y mutation disrupts the disulphide bond in the α3-domain through the substitution of tyrosine for cysteine. The H63D mutation is in the α1-domains. (Modified from Feder JN *et al.* [1] with permission.)

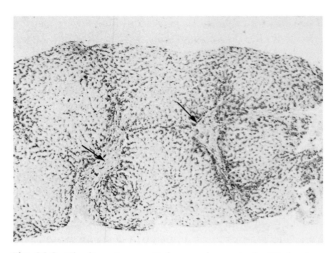

Fig. 26.3. The liver in genetic haemochromatosis. Cirrhosis is seen and hepatocytes are filled with blue-staining iron pigment. Fibrous tissue is also infiltrated with iron. The arrows indicate portal tracts. (Perls' strain, × 13.)

community (probably Celtic) in which the mutation initially occurred [15]. A second mutation described at the time of the discovery of the *HFE* gene (H63D; also known as His63Asp) is common in the normal population.

The frequency of C282Y homozygosity found in population screening studies is 1 in 200–300 [16–18]. This frequency, however, does not correspond to the frequency of clinically recognized haemochromatosis. Although biochemical penetrance (raised ferritin, transferrin saturation) is found in 50–80% of susceptible individuals, disease penetrance (i.e. symptoms, hepatic fibrosis/ cirrhosis) is low [19]. It has been demonstrated that approximately 28% of male C282Y homozygotes, but only 1% of female C282Y homozygotes, may have a haemochromatosis-related symptom [19].

The contribution of the H63D mutation to iron overload is unclear and the effect, if any, appears to have a low penetrance. Focus has mainly been on compound heterozygotes (C282Y/H63D) and H63D homozygotes, where it has been estimated that approximately 1.5% will develop significant iron overload [16].

Heterozygotes

The frequency of heterozygosity for the C282Y mutation in populations of Northern European origin is approximately 10%. Although heterozygotes have mean serum iron and transferrin saturation values higher than normal subjects, significant iron overload is extremely rare. However, since these individuals may have slight increases in intracellular iron it has been questioned whether this would enhance damage from other diseases. Hepatic fibrosis/cirrhosis due to hepatitis C or alcohol, however, has not been found to be worsened by heterozygosity for C282Y [20].

Pathology

The *liver* in the early stages may show only portal zone fibrosis with deposition of iron in the periportal liver cells and, to a lesser extent, in the Kupffer cells. Fibrous septa then surround groups of lobules and irregularly shaped nodules (*holly leaf appearance*). There is partial preservation of the architecture, although ultimately a macronodular cirrhosis develops (Fig. 26.3). Fatty change is unusual and the glycogen content of the liver cells is normal.

Cirrhotic patients with iron-free foci have a higher risk of developing hepatocellular carcinoma [21].

Iron deposition in organs beyond the liver is only seen with severe iron overload.

The *pancreas* may show fibrosis and parenchymal degeneration with iron deposition in acinar cells, macrophages, islets of Langerhans and fibrous tissue.

Heart muscle may be involved, muscle fibres being replaced by a mass of iron pigment within the sheath. Degeneration of the fibres is rare.

Spleen, bone marrow and duodenal epithelium do not show the iron overload seen elsewhere. *Brain* and *nervous tissue* are also usually free of iron.

Epidermal atrophy may reduce the *skin* to a flattened sheet. Hair follicles and sebaceous glands are inconspicuous. Characteristically, the melanin content of the basal layer is increased. Iron is usually absent from the epidermis but can often be seen deeper, especially in the basal layer.

Endocrine glands, including adrenal cortex, anterior lobe of pituitary and thyroid, may show varying amounts of iron and fibrosis.

The testes are small and soft with atrophy of the germinal epithelium without iron overload. There may be interstitial fibrosis and iron is found in the walls of capillaries.

Relation to alcoholism

In an experimental model of alcoholic liver disease, the addition of iron to the diet results in cirrhosis. In patients, the combination of haemochromatosis and excess alcohol intake results in more advanced liver disease [22]. Hepatic iron deposition is recognized in alcoholic liver disease (as well as other end-stage liver disease) and may be due to increased intestinal iron absorption in chronic alcohol abusers. Ethanol decreases hepcidin expression in both *in vitro* cellular studies and *in vivo* models [23], and this would be expected to increase iron absorption.

Clinical features

The classical picture is of a lethargic, middle-aged man with pigmentation, hepatomegaly, diminished sexual activity, loss of body hair and arthralgia; diabetes is common. This picture is seen in a minority of C282Y homozygotes. An asymptomatic patient is the most common scenario [24].

Diagnosis depends on a high degree of suspicion and should be considered in any patient with symptomless hepatomegaly and virtually normal biochemical tests of liver function [25]. In view of the C282Y homozygote frequency found in the community, the condition must be considerably more frequent than is recognized. There is a mean delay of 5–8 years between presentation and diagnosis [24].

Overt haemochromatosis is 10 times more frequent in males than females [26]. Women are spared by iron loss with menstruation and pregnancy. Female patients with haemochromatosis usually, but not always, have absent or scanty menstruation, have had a hysterectomy or are many years postmenopausal.

Haemochromatosis is rarely diagnosed before the age of 20, and the peak incidence is between 40 and 60 years.

The slate grey pigmentation when present is maximal in the axillae, groins, genitalia, old scars and exposed parts. It can occur in the mouth. The colour, due to increased melanin in the basal layer, appears through the atrophied, superficial epidermis. The skin is shiny, thin and dry.

Hepatic changes

The liver may be enlarged and firm. Abdominal pain, usually a dull ache with hepatic tenderness, is noted in 56% of cases [26].

Signs of hepatocellular failure are usually absent and ascites rare. The spleen is palpable but rarely large. Bleeding from oesophageal varices is unusual.

Primary liver cancer develops in 15–30% of cirrhotic patients [27–29]. It may be the mode of presentation, particularly in the elderly. It should be suspected if the patient shows clinical deterioration with rapid liver enlargement, abdominal pain and ascites. Serum α-fetoprotein may be increased.

Endocrine changes

At diagnosis, about 70% of cirrhotic patients, but only 17% of non-cirrhotic patients, have clinical diabetes [29]. This may be complicated by nephropathy, neuropathy, peripheral vascular disease and proliferative retinopathy. The diabetes may be easy to control or may be resistant to large doses of insulin. It could be related to a family history of diabetes, to cirrhosis of the liver which impairs glucose tolerance or to direct damage to the pancreas by iron deposition. In population screening studies of asymptomatic C282Y homozygotes, the prevalence of diabetes did not differ from the control population [16, 30].

Loss of libido or potency occurs in approximately 35% of patients and amenorrhoea in 15% of women [29]. Hypogonadism may be due to hypothalamic, pituitary or gonadal dysfunction or a combination of all three [31].

Pituitary function is impaired to a variable extent in about two-thirds of patients. This is related to iron deposition in the anterior pituitary. Gonadotrophin-producing cells are selectively affected. Hypogonadotrophic testicular failure is shown by impotence, loss of libido, testicular atrophy, skin atrophy and loss of secondary sexual hair. Plasma testosterone levels are subnormal. Testosterone levels increase following administration of gonadotrophins, suggesting that the testes are capable of responding.

Osteoporosis is seen particularly when hypogonadism is present [32].

Panhypopituitarism with hypothyroidism and adrenal corticodeficiency are rarer.

Cardiac changes

Changes on ECG are reported in 35% of patients presenting with haemochromatosis [29]. Echocardiographic abnormalities are also seen, are related to the degree of iron overload and improve with venesection [33]. Presentation with heart failure, particularly in younger subjects, is seen but is unusual. The picture is of progressive right-sided heart failure, sometimes with sudden death. The 'iron heart' is a weak one. Dysrhythmias are also seen.

Cardiac complications are presumably related to iron deposits in the myocardium and conducting system.

Arthropathy

In about two-thirds of patients, a specific arthropathy starts in the metacarpophalangeal joints (Fig. 26.4) [34]. Wrists and hips may also be affected [35]. It may be a presenting feature. Radiologically there is a hypertrophic osteoarthritis. Chondrocalcinosis is seen in the menisci and articular cartilage (Fig. 26.5). It is related to an acute crystal synovitis with calcium pyrophosphate.

Arthralgia is often the most difficult long-term clinical problem as it is resistant to conventional anti-inflammatory agents. It is present in 45% of patients at diagnosis. After depletion of body iron, 30% improve but in 20% symptoms worsen [29].

Special investigations

Transferrin saturation

In HFE-related haemochromatosis the serum iron is increased and the transferrin concentration/total iron binding capacity reduced, giving a high transferrin saturation. In those with an increased serum ferritin, this may be up to 100%. A normal transferrin saturation in the presence of a high serum ferritin should lead to consideration of other causes of hyperferritinaemia such as inflammation, metabolic syndrome with hepatic steatosis, alcohol excess and, rarely, non-HFE inherited iron overload, in particular ferroportin disease.

Serum ferritin

Ferritin is the major cellular iron storage protein. The form present in normal serum contains little iron. Its function there is uncertain. The serum concentration is proportional to body iron stores (Fig. 26.6). It is of value in assessing body iron stores [36–38], but can be unreliable in early diagnosis at the precirrhotic stage, and in patients with hepatic inflammation and a raised transaminase. It is useful in following treatment.

With hepatocellular necrosis, serum ferritin increases as it is released from liver cells [38]. High serum ferritin levels are also seen with inflammatory conditions, such as hepatitis, alcohol excess, fatty liver and some cancers.

Needle liver biopsy

Since the introduction of mutation analysis for the *HFE* gene, the indication for needle liver biopsy has changed. Previously, hepatic histology and iron quantification was important for diagnosis, giving an indication of the severity and pattern of iron deposition. Measurement of liver iron was important for calculation of the liver iron index (the liver iron concentration divided by the age of the patient), which was of diagnostic value in genetic haemochromatosis. Since mutation analysis confirms

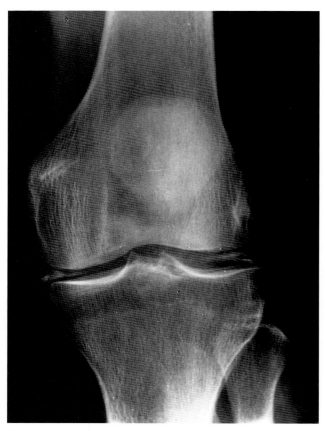

Fig. 26.5. Genetic haemochromatosis. Radiograph of the knee joint shows chondrocalcinosis in menisci and articular cartilage. (Courtesy of M. Barry.)

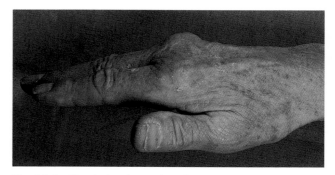

Fig. 26.4. Classical arthropathy of 1st and 2nd metacarpophalangeal joints in the hand.

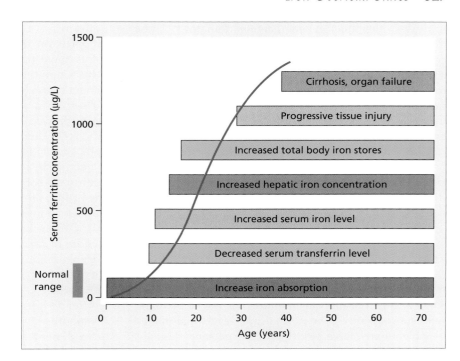

Fig. 26.6. Natural history of untreated genetic haemochromatosis. Relationship between the serum ferritin and the progression of events leading to the clinical syndrome [38].

the diagnosis in the majority of cases, liver biopsy is only necessary in C282Y homozygotes to assess whether there is severe fibrosis or cirrhosis (see Fig. 26.3), which determines the protocol for subsequent follow-up. Analysis of risk factors has shown that cirrhosis is unlikely in patients without hepatomegaly, with a normal alanine transaminase and a serum ferritin of less than 1000 µg/L [39]. The current recommendation is that in the absence of these features, liver biopsy is not necessary. If any of these features are present then liver biopsy is recommended since there is an approximate 50% chance of severe fibrosis or cirrhosis [40]. Hepatic elastography may be a useful tool for the non-invasive assessment of cirrhosis [41].

The liver section is stained with Perls' reagent. Visual scoring of the iron load (0–4+) depends upon the percentage of parenchymal cells with positive staining (0–100%). Chemical measurement of iron can be performed although it is recognized that the iron concentration varies between different samples from the same patient [42]. Iron can be measured on tissue extracted from the paraffin block if fresh tissue was not provided.

If mutation analysis does not show homozygosity for C282Y then liver biopsy is usually necessary to show whether or not there is iron overload and also the pattern of iron deposition, which may give an indication of the cause.

Liver biopsy is not necessary to follow de-ironing during treatment. Serum iron indices are sufficient. Follow-up liver biopsies have demonstrated a reduction in liver fibrosis [9].

Imaging

Using single-energy *CT scanning*, hepatic attenuation correlates with serum ferritin, but it is unable to detect hepatic iron overload less than five times the normal limit (40% of patients). The accuracy is greatly improved if dual-energy CT scanning is available.

MRI detects iron, which is a naturally occurring paramagnetic contrast agent. In overload states, marked decreases in T2 relaxation time are shown. Using special sequences, it is now possible to non-invasively obtain a measurement of hepatic iron concentration [43,44], which may be useful in selected patients such as the compound heterozygote (C282Y/H63D).

Differential diagnosis

Differentiation between classical genetic haemochromatosis and other causes of iron overload has been simplified by the introduction of genotyping for the C282Y mutation in the *HFE* gene. The differential diagnosis is usually with other chronic liver diseases associated with iron accumulation, haematological disease (not related to transfusion overload) and, more rarely, inherited but non-HFE-related iron overload. These include juvenile haemochromatosis and ferroportin disease. Acaeruloplasminaemia is exceptionally rare. African iron overload and neonatal haemochromatosis are specific to particular groups.

Serum iron and transferrin saturation, as well as serum ferritin, are sometimes increased in cirrhosis due to causes other than genetic haemochromatosis. These include alcohol and hepatitis C. The clinical picture may confuse, since the association of diabetes mellitus and cirrhosis is not uncommon, and patients with cirrhosis may become impotent, hairless and develop skin pigmentation. Hepatocellular failure, however, is unusual in haemochromatosis. The degree of iron overload with end-stage liver disease and juvenile haemochromatosis can be within the range of that seen in *HFE*-related haemochromatosis. Both are unrelated to mutations in *HFE*. A family history and clinical picture should make differentiation straightforward.

Prognosis

Much depends upon the amount and duration of iron overload. Early diagnosis and treatment is central to improving prognosis. Those treated in the precirrhotic stage and before diabetes mellitus has developed, and who subsequently have normal iron levels maintained by phlebotomy, have a normal life expectancy [29, 45]. This is important for patients applying for life insurance [46].

Cardiac failure worsens the outlook and such patients rarely survive longer than 1 year without treatment. Hepatic failure or bleeding oesophageal varices are rare terminal features.

The outlook is better than for cirrhosis in alcoholics who stop drinking. However, the patient with haemochromatosis who also abuses alcohol does worse than the abstinent patient.

The risk of developing hepatocellular carcinoma in haemochromatotic patients with cirrhosis is increased about 200 times [29] and is not reduced by de-ironing [47]. As in other cirrhotic groups, screening by ultrasound and α-fetoprotein at 6-monthly intervals is appropriate. A minority (approximately 15%) of hepatocellular carcinomas develop in non-cirrhotic haemochromatotic liver—as is found for hepatocellular carcinoma related to other aetiologies.

Treatment

Iron can be removed by venesection and can be mobilized from tissue stores at rates as high as 130 mg/day [48]. Blood regeneration is extraordinarily rapid, haemoglobin production increasing to six or seven times normal. Large quantities of blood must be removed, for 500 mL removes only 250 mg of iron, whereas the tissues contain up to 200 times this amount. Depending on the initial iron stores, the amount necessary to reduce them to normal varies from 2 to 45 g. Venesections of 500 mL are carried out weekly, or even twice weekly in particularly co-operative patients, and are continued until serum ferritin levels fall into the low normal range.

Transferrin saturation may remain elevated until the patient is on the verge of iron deficiency. Other endpoints have been the development of anaemia or a reduction in the mean cellular volume (MCV).

In an early study of the outcome of venesection, comparison of a venesection-treated with an untreated group showed a 5-year survival of 66% compared with 18% [47]. Venesection treatment results in increased well-being and gain in weight. Pigmentation and hepatosplenomegaly decrease. Liver function tests improve. Control of diabetes improves in some patients [29, 49]. The arthropathy is usually unaffected. Hypogonadism may lessen in men aged less than 40 years at diagnosis [50]. Cardiac function improves depending upon the severity of cardiac damage before venesection.

Hepatic fibrosis can improve following venesection but hepatic cirrhosis is generally regarded to be irreversible.

After de-ironing, venesection of 500 mL of blood every 3–6 months can prevent iron re-accumulation. However, many patients will not show rapid iron reaccumulation [51] and maintenance therapy can be tailored to the patient based on monitoring of post-treatment ferritin levels. A low iron diet is difficult to achieve and most patients remain on a normal diet with intermittent venesection.

Gonadal atrophy may be treated by replacement therapy with an intramuscular, depot testosterone. Human chorionic gonadotrophin (HCG) injections will increase testicular volume and sperm counts.

Diabetes should be treated by diet, oral hypoglycaemic agents and, if necessary, insulin.

Transplantation

The survival of patients with genetic haemochromatosis after liver transplant may be less than for other recipients (53 versus 81% survival at 25 months) [52,53]. The lower survival is related to cardiac complications and sepsis, emphasizing the need for early diagnosis and treatment.

Approximately one-third of patients undergoing liver transplantation unrelated to genetic haemochromatosis have hepatic iron deposition. Ten per cent have hepatic siderosis in the range of that seen in genetic haemochromatosis. *HFE* gene mutations are rare in this group. Patient survival after transplantation is significantly lower in those with hepatic iron overload [54]. Transplantation of the liver from a C282Y heterozygote is safe [55].

Whereas previous reports of the transplantation of a haemochromatotic liver into a normal recipient have not shown evidence of subsequent iron accumulation, this has been reported where the donor intestine as well as liver were derived from a C282Y homozygote [56].

Screening for early haemochromatosis in relatives

There are two ways of screening: biochemical tests for iron overload and mutation analysis (genotyping). Ideally, both are done since the results are complementary. If biochemical screening (transferrin saturation and serum ferritin) shows evidence for iron overload then genotyping for the C282Y mutation is done to show whether the individual is homozygous or heterozygous. If heterozygosity for C282Y is shown, H63D analysis is needed to detect the compound heterozygote (C282Y/H63D).

If the transferrin saturation and ferritin levels are very high in a Caucasian patient, then it is likely that the individual is homozygous for C282Y.

If there is only a mild elevation of transferrin saturation and ferritin, not unusual in the younger patient, it is not possible clinically to differentiate the C282Y homozygote from a heterozygote.

There had been concern that genetic testing may lead to insurance or employment discrimination but this has rarely been documented and did not occur in the Hemochromatosis and Iron Overload Screening (HEIRS) Study [46].

It is difficult at present to advise a C282Y homozygote who has no evidence of iron overload of the risk of developing iron overload (phenotypic penetrance) or disease (disease penetrance) [57]. There have been several studies in which a large cohort of healthy patients were followed for many years and had genetic testing for haemochromatosis 25 years later. In these studies, it has become apparent that not all C282Y homozygotes will have a progressive rise in ferritin and in many cases levels are not rising but even decreasing. These studies have provided a fascinating glimpse into the natural history of disease without treatment [58–60].

Children of a patient with genetic haemochromatosis should also be screened because of the 1 in 10 chance in northern European populations of the spouse being a carrier for the C282Y mutation. This would give a 1 in 20 chance of the child being affected. Screening (as for siblings) could be done but for young children below the age of consent this is not practical. An alternative approach is to perform mutation analysis in the spouse (C282Y and H63D) [61]. This would then give an indication of the possible genotypes in children and the need for later screening.

It is usually recommended that parents are also screened because of the possibility of unrecognized genetic haemochromatosis.

Population screening

Genetic haemochromatosis is a preventable condition and with early diagnosis and de-ironing life expectancy is normal. Hepatic fibrosis can reverse with phlebotomy therapy. These are powerful arguments for population screening of appropriate groups. Transferrin saturation for initial screening followed by DNA testing is a cost-effective strategy [62] but there is a significant biological variability in transferrin saturation that limits its reproducibility [63]. It has been found that use of a fasting sample gave no advantage either for sensitivity, specificity or positive predictive value [63].

Automated measurement of the unbound iron binding capacity (UIBC) is as effective and less expensive [64]. Population screening using C282Y genotyping first has the advantages of removing all of the false-positive cases with phenotyping [65]. The conclusions of the HEIRS study, which screened 101 168 participants in a multiethnic population, are summarized in Table 26.2.

Population screening has not been adopted by public health bodies because of the lack of information on the disease penetrance of genetic haemochromatosis [70].

Table 26.2. Lessons from the Haemochromatosis and Iron Overload Screening (HEIRS) study

Population screening as performed in the HEIRS study is not recommended
Genetic testing is well accepted with minimal risk of discrimination [46]
An elevated serum ferritin is very common, particularly in Asians; in the absence of C282Y homozygosity, this finding usually does not represent an increase of iron stores of >4 g [66]
Transferrin saturation has high biological variability which limits its role as a screening test [63]
Symptoms attributable to C282Y homozygosity are uncommon in individuals identified by population screening [67]
Mild increases in body iron stores in the range of 2–3 g were common in non *HFE*-C282Y homozygotes, but iron overload defined as iron stores >4 g was most common in C282Y homozygous men [68]
There may be a role for focused screening in a Caucasian population, with some debate about genotyping followed by phenotyping or phenotyping followed by genotyping [69]

Other iron storage diseases

Non-HFE-related inherited iron overload [7,8]

Not all patients with haemochromatosis have mutations in the *HFE* gene. These inherited non-HFE-related iron overload conditions are rare, but need to be considered based on clinical data.

Juvenile haemochromatosis. Patients present at an earlier age (second to fourth decade) with iron overload and cardiac and endocrine problems in particular. Cardiac disease may be life-threatening. The male to female ratio is equal. The condition is not linked to chromosome 6 [71]. These patients have been demonstrated to have mutations in the haemojuvelin or hepcidin genes [7]. Treatment is by venesection, although in patients with severe cardiac disease chelation therapy with desferrioxamine has also been used.

Ferroportin disease. This is autosomal dominant. Some patients have raised ferritin but normal transferrin saturation, with reticuloendothelial cell accumulation of iron and poor tolerance of venesection. Others are phenotypically closer to the picture of HFE-haemochromatosis [72]. These differences probably relate to the mutation responsible giving a loss or gain in protein function.

Acaeruloplasminaemia. This very rare syndrome due to a mutation in the caeruloplasmin gene is associated with excessive iron deposition, mainly in the brain, liver and pancreas. Serum ferritin is increased, but there is also anaemia and low serum iron and transferrin saturation. Liver copper concentration is normal, but iron concentrations are increased. Patients show extrapyramidal disorders, cerebellar ataxia and diabetes mellitus [73]. Venesection is not tolerated, but iron chelators have been used.

Others. These include iron overload due to mutations in the TfR type 2 gene [74], and in the iron-response element of H ferritin [75]. The latter is autosomal dominant. Transferrin deficiency has been found in a child with iron overload. The haematological picture was of severe iron deficiency although the tissues were loaded with iron.

Dysmetabolic syndrome

Iron overload may be associated with diabetes, obesity, hyperlipidaemia and hypertension. There is an elevated serum ferritin but normal transferrin saturation [76]. The condition does not appear to be familial and although some patients have *HFE* mutations there is no clear relationship.

Erythropoietic siderosis

Siderosis is associated with extremely high rates of erythropoiesis. The hyperplastic bone marrow may in some way direct the intestinal mucosa to take in excessive quantities of iron. This continues even in the presence of large iron stores. The iron is deposited first in the macrophages of the reticuloendothelial system and later in parenchymal cells of liver, pancreas and other organs.

Siderosis can therefore be expected in chronic haemolytic states, especially β-thalassaemia, sickle cell disease, congenital spherocytosis and hereditary dyserythropoietic anaemia. Iron overload may develop in mild sideroblastic anaemia without severe anaemia or transfusions. In individuals with haematological disease, the degree of iron overload seems more related to the underlying disorder than *HFE* mutations.

The siderosis is enhanced by *blood transfusions* as the iron given with the blood cannot be lost from the body. More than 100 units must have been transfused before siderosis is clinically recognizable. Misdirected iron therapy enhances the siderosis.

The siderosis is recognized clinically by increasing skin pigmentation and by hepatomegaly. Children fail to grow and to develop secondary sexual characteristics. Liver failure and frank portal hypertension are rare. The fasting blood glucose is raised, but clinical diabetes is excessively rare.

Although the amount of iron deposited in the heart is relatively small, myocardial damage is a major factor determining prognosis, especially in younger children. In children, symptoms arise when body iron reaches 20 g (100 units blood transfused); death from heart failure is likely when 60 g is reached.

Treatment is difficult. Splenectomy may reduce transfusion needs. A well-balanced, low-iron diet is virtually impossible. Twelve-hour overnight subcutaneous infusion of 2–4 g desferrioxamine given with a small syringe pump into the anterior abdominal wall is effective. Oral iron chelators such as deferasirox and deferiprone have been used in these patients [77].

Late-stage cirrhosis

Approximately 10% of explanted livers from patients having a transplant have a level of hepatic iron within the range for genetic haemochromatosis. In most cases this is not related to *HFE* mutations. Cryptogenic and alcoholic cirrhosis predominate [54]. The mechanisms of iron deposition are not fully understood although a low serum hepcidin may be a common disease mechanism.

Increased iron absorption is found in cirrhotic patients irrespective of aetiology. Cirrhotic patients with a large portal–systemic collateral circulation may absorb more. Interestingly, iron may accumulate rapidly in the liver of patients with surgical or spontaneous portal–systemic shunts, but in general the siderosis is slight and clinically insignificant.

Contributing factors to excess iron include alcoholic beverages with a high iron content, iron medications and haemolysis [78].

In the patient with alcoholic cirrhosis, hepatic histology shows the features of alcoholism as well as iron deposition. Iron deficiency follows limited venesection therapy suggesting that body iron stores are only moderately increased.

Chronic viral hepatitis

Nearly half of patients with chronic viral hepatitis (B and C) have an abnormal transferrin saturation and/or serum ferritin. *HFE* mutation analysis will identify those with genetic haemochromatosis. A high liver iron reduces the response rate to α-interferon in chronic hepatitis C. Removal of iron by venesection increases the end-of-treatment virological and histological response to short-term interferon therapy, but there is no significant benefit to the sustained response [79,80].

Non-alcoholic fatty liver disease

Serum iron indices are abnormal in around 50% of patients. In some populations increased hepatic iron is related to the C282Y mutation of *HFE*, and the presence of this mutation and increased hepatic iron correlates with the degree of hepatic fibrosis. This has not, however, been found in all populations [81,82].

Neonatal haemochromatosis

This very rare and fatal disorder is characterized by liver failure which starts *in utero*, together with hepatic and extrahepatic parenchymal iron overload which spares the reticuloendothelial system. Whether it represents a primary iron storage disorder, or the effect of liver disease of another cause superimposed on a liver already physiologically replete with iron, is not certain. In some cases it seems to be a disease associated with maternal–fetal alloimmunity and can be treated in pregnancy with high doses of immunoglobulin [83]. Liver transplantation, if successful, is curative.

African iron overload (Bantu siderosis)

This condition is seen in South African black people whose diet consists of porridge fermented in iron pots at an acid pH. Absorption is facilitated by the acid diet and by malnutrition. Traditional beer brewed in steel drums continues to cause iron overload in rural sub-Saharan Africa. Hepatic iron was considerably elevated (greater than $180\,\mu g/g$) in 5% of a study population [84]. The condition is not associated with mutations in *HFE*, but studies suggest that genetic as well as environmental factors affect the degree of iron overload [85,86].

Porphyria cutanea tarda (see Chapter 31)

Increased iron, one of the triggers for clinical expression, is associated with a high frequency of homozygosity and heterozygosity for the C282Y mutation of *HFE* although not in all populations [87,88]. Patients with evidence of iron overload are treated by venesection to remove the stimulus for attacks of photosensitivity.

References

1 Feder JN, Gnirke A, Thomas W *et al*. A novel MHC class I-like gene is mutated in patients with hereditary hemochromatosis. *Nat. Genet.* 1996; **13**: 399–408.

2 Nemeth E, Ganz T. The role of hepcidin in iron metabolism. *Acta Haematol.* 2009; **122**: 78–86.

3 Simpson RJ, McKie AT. Regulation of intestinal iron absorption: the mucosa takes control? *Cell Metabol.* 2009; **10**: 84–87.

4 Waheed A, Parkkila S, Zhou XY *et al*. Hereditary hemochromatosis: effects of C282Y and H63D mutations on association with beta2-microglobulin, intracellular processing, and cell surface expression of the HFE protein in COS-7 cells. *Proc. Natl. Acad. Sci. U S A* 1997; **94**: 12384–12389.

5 Pietrangelo A. Hemochromatosis: an endocrine liver disease. *Hepatology* 2007; **46**: 1291–1301.

6 Meynard D, Kautz L, Darnaud V *et al*. Lack of the bone morphogenetic protein BMP6 induces massive iron overload. *Nat. Genet.* 2009 Apr; **41**: 478–481.

7 Camaschella C, Poggiali E. Rare types of genetic hemochromatosis. *Acta Haematol.* 2009; **122**: 140–145.

8 Pietrangelo A. Hereditary hemochromatosis. A new look at an old disease. *N. Engl. J. Med.* 2004; **350**: 2383–2397.

9 Falize L, Guillygomarch A, Perrin M *et al*. Reversibility of hepatic fibrosis in treated genetic hemochromatosis: a study of 36 cases. *Hepatology* 2006; **44**: 472–477.

10 Powell LW, Dixon JL, Ramm GA *et al*. Screening for hemochromatosis in asymptomatic subjects with or without a family history. *Arch. Int. Med.* 2006; **166**: 294–301.

11 Ramm G, Ruddell R. Hepatotoxicity of iron overload: mechanisms of iron-induced hepatic fibrogenesis. *Semin. Liver Dis.* 2005; **25**: 433–449.

12 Sheldon JH. *Haemochromatosis*. Oxford Medical Publications, 1935, p. 164–340.

13 Bacon B, Powell LW, Adams PC *et al*. Molecular medicine and hemochromatosis: at the crossroads. *Gastroenterology* 1998; **116**: 193–207.

14 Piperno A, Sampietro M, Pietrangelo A *et al*. Heterogeneity of hemochromatosis in Italy. *Gastroenterology* 1998; **114**: 996–1002.

15 Distante S, Robson K, Graham-Campbell J *et al*. The origin and spread of the HFE-C282Y haemochromatosis mutation. *Hum. Genet.* 2004; **115**: 269–279.

16 Adams PC, Reboussin DM, Barton JC *et al*. Hemochromatosis and iron-overload screening in a racially diverse population. *N. Engl. J. Med.* 2005; **352**: 1769–1778.

17 Asberg A, Hveem K, Thorstensen K *et al*. Screening for hemochromatosis—high prevalence and low morbidity in an unselected population of 65,238 persons. *Scand. J. Gastroenterol.* 2001; **36**: 1108–1115.

18 Olynyk J, Cullen D, Aquilia S *et al*. A population-based study of the clinical expression of the hemochromatosis gene. *N. Eng. J. Med.* 1999; **341**: 718–724.

19 Allen KJ, Gurrin LC, Constantine CC *et al*. Iron-overload-related disease in HFE hereditary hemochromatosis. *N. Eng. J. Med.* 2008; **358**: 221–230.

20 Bataller R, North K, Brenner D. Genetic polymorphisms and the progression of liver fibrosis: a critical appraisal. *Hepatology* 2003; **37**: 493–503.

21 Deugnier YM, Charalambous P, Le Quilleuc D *et al*. Preneoplastic significance of hepatic iron-free foci in genetic hemochromatosis: a study of 185 patients. *Hepatology* 1993; **18**: 1363–1369.

22 Fletcher L, Dixon J, Purdie D *et al*. Excess alcohol greatly increases the prevalence of cirrhosis in hereditary hemochromatosis. *Gastroenterology* 2002; **122**: 563–565.

23 Harrison-Findik DD, Klein E, Crist C *et al*. Iron-mediated regulation of liver hepcidin expression in rats and mice is abolished by alcohol. *Hepatology* 2007; **46**: 1979–1985.

24 Adams PC, Kertesz AE, Valberg LS. Clinical presentation of hemochromatosis: a changing scene. *Am. J. Med.* 1991; **90**: 445–449.

25 Lin E, Adams PC. Biochemical liver profile in hemochromatosis. A survey of 100 patients. *J. Clin. Gastroenterol.* 1991; **13**: 316–320.

26 Moirand R, Adams PC, Bicheler V *et al*. Clinical features of genetic hemochromatosis in women compared to men. *Ann. Int. Med.* 1997; **127**: 105–110.

27 Deugnier YM, Guyader D, Crantock L *et al*. Primary liver cancer in genetic hemochromatosis—a clinical pathological and pathogenetic study of 54 cases. *Gastroenterology* 1993; **104**: 228–234.

28 Adams PC. Hepatocellular carcinoma in hereditary hemochromatosis. *Can. J. Gastroenterol.* 1993; **7**: 37–41.

29 Niederau C, Fischer R, Purschel A *et al*. Long-term survival in patients with hereditary hemochromatosis. *Gastroenterology* 1996; **110**: 1107–1119.

30 Acton RT, Barton JC, Passmore LV *et al*. Relationships of serum ferritin, transferrin saturation, and HFE mutations and self-reported diabetes in the Hemochromatosis and Iron Overload Screening (HEIRS) study. *Diabetes Care* 2006; **29**: 2084–2089.

31 Tweed MJ, Roland JM. Haemochromatosis as an endocrine cause of subfertility. *Br. Med. J.* 1998; **316**: 915–916.

32 Valenti L, Varenna M, Fracanzani AL *et al*. Association between iron overload and osteoporosis in patients with hereditary hemochromatosis. *Osteoporos. Int.* 2009; **20**: 549–555.

33 Cecchetti G, Binda A, Piperno A *et al*. Cardiac alterations in 36 consecutive patients with idiopathic hemochromatosis—polygraphic and echocardiographic evaluation. *Eur. Heart J.* 1991; **12**: 224–230.

34 Valenti L, Fracanzani AL, Rossi V *et al*. The hand arthropathy of hereditary hemochromatosis is strongly associated with iron overload. *J. Rheumatol.* 2008; **35**: 153–158.

35 Faraawi R, Harth M, Kertesz A, Bell D. Arthritis in hemochromatosis. *J. Rheumatol.* 1993; **20**: 448–452.

36 Brissot P, Bourel M, Herry D *et al*. Assessment of liver iron content in 271 patients: a reevaluation of direct and indirect methods. *Gastroenterology* 1981; **80**: 557–565.

37 Prieto J, Barry M, Sherlock S. Serum ferritin in patients with iron overload and with acute and chronic liver diseases. *Gastroenterology* 1975; **68**: 525–533.

38 Powell LW, Halliday JW, Cowlishaw JL. Relationship between serum ferritin and total body iron stores in idiopathic haemochromatosis. *Gut* 1978; **19**: 538–542.

39 Guyader D, Jacquelinet C, Moirand R *et al*. Non-invasive prediction of fibrosis in C282Y homozygous hemochromatosis. *Gastroenterology* 1998; **115**: 929–936.

40 Beaton M, Guyader D, Deugnier Y *et al*. Non-invasive prediction of cirrhosis in C282Y-linked hemochromatosis. *Hepatology* 2002; **36**: 673–678.

41 Adhoute X, Foucher J, Laharie D *et al*. Diagnosis of liver fibrosis using FibroScan and other noninvasive methods in patients with hemochromatosis: a prospective study. *Gastroenterol. Clin. Biol.* 2008; **32**: 180–187.

42 Villeneuve JP, Bilodeau M, Lepage R *et al*. Variability in hepatic iron concentration measurement from needle-biopsy specimens. *J. Hepatol.* 1996; **25**: 172–177.

43 Gandon Y, Olivie D, Guyader D *et al*. Non-invasive assessment of hepatic iron stores by MRI. *Lancet* 2004; **363**: 357–360.

44 St Pierre T, Clark P, Chua-anusorn W *et al*. Noninvasive measurement and imaging of liver iron concentrations using proton magnetic resonance. *Blood* 2005; **105**: 855–861.

45 Wojcik J, Speechley M, Kertesz A *et al*. Natural history of C282Y homozygotes for haemochromatosis. *Can. J. Gastroenterol.* 2002; **16**: 297–302.

46 Hall MA, Barton JC, Adams PC *et al*. Genetic screening for iron overload: no evidence of discrimination at one year. *J. Fam. Practice* 2007; **56**: 829–833.

47 Bomford A, Williams R. Long term results of venesection therapy in idiopathic haemochromatosis. *Q. J. Med.* 1976; **45**: 611–623.

48 Adams PC. Factors affecting rate of iron mobilization during venesection therapy for hereditary hemochromatosis. *Am. J. Hematol.* 1998; **58**: 16–19.

49 McClain D, Abraham D, Rogers J *et al*. High prevalence of abnormal glucose homeostasis secondary to decreased insulin secretion in individuals with hereditary haemochromatosis. *Diabetologia* 2006; **49**: 1661–1669.

50 Cundy T, Butler J, Bomford A, Williams R. Reversibility of hypogonadotrophic hypogonadism associated with genetic haemochromatosis. *Clin. Endocrinol.* 1993; **38**: 617–620.

51 Adams PC, Kertesz AE, Valberg LS. Rate of iron reaccumulation following iron depletion in hereditary hemochromatosis. Implications for venesection therapy. *J. Clin. Gastroenterol.* 1993; **16**: 207–210.

52 Kowdley K, Brandhagen D, Gish R *et al*. Survival after liver transplantation in patients with hepatic iron overload: the national hemochromatosis transplant registry. *Gastroenterology* 2005; **129**: 494–503.

53 Crawford D, Fletcher L, Hubscher S *et al*. Patient and graft survival after liver transplantation for hereditary hemo-

chromatosis: implications for pathogenesis. *Hepatology* 2004; **39**: 1655–1662.

54 Brandhagen D, Alvarez W, Therneau T *et al.* Iron overload in cirrhosis-HFE genotypes and outcome after liver transplantation. *Hepatology* 2000; **31**: 456–460.

55 Alanen K, Chakrabarti S, Rawlins J *et al.* Prevalence of the C282Y mutation of the hemochromatosis gene in liver transplant recipients and donors. *Hepatology* 1999; **30**: 665–669.

56 Adams PC, Alanen K, Preshaw R *et al.* Transplantation of haemochromatosis liver and intestine into a normal recipient. *Gut* 1999; **45**: 783.

57 Yamashita C, Adams PC. Natural history of the C282Y homozygote of the hemochromatosis gene (HFE) with a normal serum ferritin level. *Clin. Gastroenterol. Hepatol.* 2003; **1**: 388–391.

58 Gurrin LC, Osborne NJ, Constantine CC *et al.* The natural history of serum iron indices for HFE C282Y homozygosity associated with hereditary hemochromatosis. *Gastroenterology* 2008; **135**: 1945–1952.

59 Pankow JS, Boerwinkle E, Adams PC *et al.* HFE C282Y homozygotes have reduced low-density lipoprotein cholesterol: the Atherosclerosis Risk in Communities (ARIC) Study. *Translational Res.* 2008; **152**: 3–10.

60 Andersen RV, Tybjaerg-Hansen A, Appleyard M *et al.* Hemochromatosis mutations in the general population: iron overload progression rate. *Blood* 2004; **103**: 2914–2919.

61 Adams PC. Implications of genotyping of spouses to limit investigation of children in genetic hemochromatosis. *Clin. Genet.* 1998; **53**: 176–178.

62 Gagne G, Reinharz D, Laflamme N *et al.* Hereditary hemochromatosis: effect of mutation penetrance and prevalence on cost-effectiveness of screening modalities. *Clin. Genet.* 2007; **71**: 46–58.

63 Adams PC, Reboussin DM, Press RD *et al.* Biological variability of transferrin saturation and unsaturated iron binding capacity. *Am. J. Med.* 2007; **120**: 999.e1–e7.

64 Adams PC, Kertesz AE, McLaren C *et al.* Population screening for hemochromatosis: a comparison of unbound iron binding capacity, transferrin saturation and C282Y genotyping in 5,211 voluntary blood donors. *Hepatology* 2000; **31**: 1160–1164.

65 Delatycki M, Allen K, Nisselle A *et al.* Use of community genetic screening to prevent HFE-associated hereditary hemochromatosis. *Lancet* 2005; **366**: 316.

66 Harris EL, McLaren CE, Reboussin DM *et al.* Serum ferritin and transferrin saturation in Asians and Pacific Islanders. *Arch. Intern. Med.* 2007; **167**: 722–726.

67 McLaren GD, McLaren C, Adams PC *et al.* Clinical manifestations of hemochromatosis in HFE C282Y homozygotes identified by screening. *Can. J. Gastroenterol.* 2008; **11**: 923–930.

68 Gordeuk VR, Reboussin DM, McLaren CE *et al.* Serum ferritin concentrations and body iron stores in a multicenter, multiethnic primary-care population. *Am. J. Hematol.* 2008; **83**: 618–626.

69 Phatak PD, Bonkovsky HL, Kowdley KV. Hereditary hemochromatosis: time for targeted screening. *Ann. Int. Med.* 2008; **149**: 270–272.

70 Whitlock E, Garlitz B, Harris E *et al.* Screening for hereditary hemochromatosis: a systematic review for the U.S. Preventative Services Task Force. *Ann. Int. Med.* 2006; **145**: 209–223.

71 Papanikolaou G, Samuels M, Ludwig E *et al.* Mutations in HFE2 cause iron overload in chromosome 1q-linked juvenile hemochromatosis. *Nat. Genet.* 2004; **36**: 77–82.

72 Mayr R, Janecke AR, Schranz M *et al.* Ferroportin disease: a systematic meta-analysis of clinical and molecular findings. *J. Hepatol.* 2010; **53**: 941–949.

73 Xu X, Pin S, Gathinji M *et al.* Aceruloplasminemia: an inherited neurodegenerative disease with impairment of iron homeostasis. *Ann. N Y Acad. Sci.* 2004; **1012**: 299–305.

74 Camaschella C, Roetto A, Cali A *et al.* The gene TFR2 is mutated in a new type of haemochromatosis mapping to 7q22. *Nat. Genet.* 2000; **25**: 14–15.

75 Kato J, Fujikawa K, Kanda M *et al.* A mutation, in the iron-responsive element of H ferritin mRNA, causing autosomal dominant iron overload. *Am. J. Hum. Genet.* 2001; **69**: 191–197.

76 Moirand R, Mortaji A, Loreal O *et al.* A new syndrome of liver iron overload with normal transferrin saturation. *Lancet* 1997; **349**: 95–97.

77 Barton JC. Chelation therapy of iron overload. *Curr. Gastroenterol. Rep.* 2007; **9**: 74–82.

78 Wood MJ, Powell LW, Ramm GA. Environmental and genetic modifiers of the progression to fibrosis and cirrhosis in hemochromatosis. *Blood* 2008; **111**: 4456–4462.

79 Bonkovsky HL, Naishadham D, Lambrecht RW et al. Roles of iron and HFE mutations on severity and response to therapy during retreatment of advanced chronic hepatitis C. *Gastroenterology* 2006; **131**: 1440–1451.

80 Tung B, Edmond M, Bronner M *et al.* Hepatitis C, iron status, disease severity: relationship with HFE mutations. *Gastroenterology* 2003; **124**: 318–326.

81 Alla V, Bonkovsky H. Iron in non-hemochromatotic liver disorders. *Sem. Liver Dis.* 2005; **25**: 461–472.

82 Angulo P, Keach J, Batts K, Lindor K. Independent predictors of liver fibrosis in patients with nonalcoholic steatosis. *Hepatology* 1999; **30**: 1356–1362.

83 Whitington PF, Kelly S. Outcome of pregnancies at risk for neonatal hemochromatosis is improved by treatment with high-dose intravenous immunoglobulin. *Pediatrics* 2008; **121**: e1615–e1621.

84 Gangaidzo IT, Moyo VM, Saungweme T *et al.* Iron overload in urban Africans in the 1990s. *Gut* 1999; **45**: 278–283.

85 Gordeuk V, Mukiibi J, Hasstedt SJ *et al.* Iron overload in Africa. Interaction between a gene and dietary iron content. *N. Eng. J. Med.* 1992; **326**: 95–100.

86 Gordeuk V, Caleffi A, Corradini E *et al.* Iron overload in Africans and African-Americans and a common mutation in the SCL40A1 (ferroportin 1) gene. *Blood Cells Mol. Dis.* 2003; **31**: 299–304.

87 Ellervik C, Birgens H, Tybjaerg-Hansen A *et al.* Hemochromatosis genotypes and risk of 31 disease endpoints: Meta-analyses including 66,000 cases and 226,000 controls. *Hepatology* 2007; **46**: 1071–1080.

88 Cribier B, Chiaverini C, li-Youcef N *et al.* Porphyria cutanea tarda, hepatitis C, uroporphyrinogen decarboxylase and mutations of HFE gene. A case-control study. *Dermatology* 2009; **218**: 15–21.

CHAPTER 27
Wilson's Disease

Eve A. Roberts

Departments of Paediatrics, Medicine and Pharmacology, University of Toronto, Toronto, Ontario, Canada

Learning points

- Wilson's disease is a genetic disorder of copper handling which affects mainly the liver but also the brain, eyes and kidneys.

- Inheritance of Wilson's disease is autosomal recessive. Wilson's disease occurs in individuals who have mutations in both copies of the gene *ATP7B*; carriers have a mutation in only one copy.

- Wilson's disease can present as liver disease (hepatic form) or neuropsychiatric disease (neurological form).

- Anyone with Wilson's disease, whether symptomatic or not, requires lifelong treatment; carriers do not require treatment.

- The mainstay of initial treatment is with a chelator (D-penicillamine or trientine); liver transplantation is reserved for the acute liver failure presentation or for treatment failures.

This autosomal recessive disorder of copper metabolism is characterized mainly by liver and neurological disease. It is caused by mutations in the gene *ATP7B*, which encodes a copper-transporting P-type ATPase. In affected individuals copper accumulates in the liver, due to deficient caeruloplasmin synthesis and a marked reduction in biliary copper excretion.

Kinnier Wilson [1] first defined this condition, which he identified as familial and involving progressive neurological disease and cirrhosis. Copper deposited in the tissues is responsible for the hepatic and neurological changes, the greenish-brown pigmented rings in the periphery of the cornea (Kayser–Fleischer rings) and lesions in the kidneys and other organs. Tissue damage leads to cirrhosis of the liver and bilateral degeneration of the basal ganglia of the brain.

The typical daily dietary intake of copper is 2–5 mg, most of which is excreted in bile to maintain overall balance. Dietary uptake is not regulated and thus excretion is critically important. In Wilson's disease, daily copper excretion into bile is decreased by 80–90%. Hepatic copper overload develops. Excess copper leaches into the plasma and hence to other tissues.

Paradoxically, in the affected individual the serum copper level is almost always low (Fig. 27.1). Most plasma copper is normally found incorporated in caeruloplasmin. In Wilson's disease, serum caeruloplasmin levels are low because of lack of incorporation of copper into apocaeruloplasmin within the Golgi complex of the hepatocyte. Urinary copper excretion is increased, reflecting increased concentrations of non-caeruloplasmin-bound copper in the plasma. This exchangeable copper is loosely bound to albumin and certain amino acids, such as histidine. When serum copper levels are normal or elevated in Wilson's disease, it implies that plasma concentrations of non-caeruloplasmin-bound copper are exceedingly high.

Wilson's disease is found worldwide. The prevalence is approximately 1 in 30 000, with a carrier frequency of approximately 1 in 90 [3].

Molecular genetics: pathogenesis

The gene abnormal in Wilson's disease, *ATP7B*, is on the long arm of chromosome 13. Its gene product is a copper-transporting P-type ATPase, the 'Wilson ATPase', which has six copper-binding units [4]. Both the gene and the Wilson ATPase have been characterized extensively [5,6]. The *ATP7B* gene is expressed mainly in the liver.

In normal hepatocytes, the Wilson ATPase is predominantly located in the trans-Golgi network into which it transports copper for incorporation into caeruloplasmin (Fig. 27.2). When intracellular copper concentrations are increased, the Wilson ATPase redistributes to a vesicular compartment close to the bile canalicular membrane

Sherlock's Diseases of the Liver and Biliary System, Twelfth Edition. Edited by James S. Dooley, Anna S.F. Lok, Andrew K. Burroughs, E. Jenny Heathcote.
© 2011 by Blackwell Publishing Ltd. Published 2011 by Blackwell Publishing Ltd.

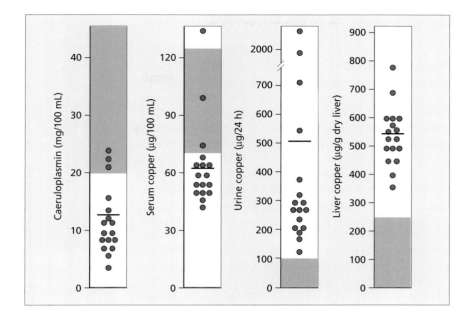

Fig. 27.1. Copper studies in 17 patients with Wilson's disease with chronic hepatitis resembling autoimmune hepatitis. Horizontal lines indicate mean values. Tinted areas represent the normal ranges for serum caeruloplasmin and serum copper and delineate the levels above which urine copper (>100μg/24h) and liver copper concentration (>250μg/g dry weight) are frequently found in Wilson's disease. Note that three patients had a normal serum caeruloplasmin level [2].

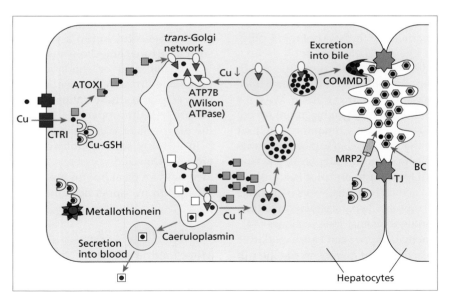

Fig. 27.2. Role of Wilson ATPase (ATP7B) in the hepatocellular disposition of copper. A doublet of hepatocytes is shown, with, on the right, the specialized bile canaliculus (BC) membrane located between two tight junctions (TJ). Starting at the left side of the diagram, copper (small red dots) is taken up across the sinusoidal plasma membrane by CTR1 (purple square), picked up and carried by ATOX1 (blue square) to the Wilson ATPase (yellow oval with arrow) in the trans-Golgi network. The Wilson ATPase either directs copper to production of caeruloplasmin or to excretion into bile, by a process which may also involve COMMD1. When intracellular copper concentrations are low or normal, the Wilson ATPase participates in production of holocaeruloplasmin (white square containing copper) in the Golgi apparatus; holocaeruloplasmin is then secreted into the blood. When intracellular copper concentrations are elevated, the Wilson ATPase expedites biliary excretion of copper. Glutathione (GSH; blue half circle) mediates other intracellular transfer, including incorporation into metallothionein and biliary excretion via MRP2. (Modified from Roberts EA, Sarkar B. *Am. J. Clin. Nutr.* 2008; **88**: 851S–854S.)

[7,8]. Mutations in the Wilson ATPase may interfere with some or all of its complex functions in hepatocytes.

Approximately 500 different mutations of *ATP7B* in Wilson's disease have been identified (http://www.wilsondisease.med.ualberta.ca/database.asp). Most are point or missense mutations in the transmembrane and ATPase regions. Ideally, alterations in *ATP7B* must be shown to cause protein dysfunction to be counted as disease-causing mutations. These numerous mutations make mutation analysis impractical as a routine diagnostic test, except in areas where one or two mutations predominate, such as Eastern Europe, Sardinia, Iceland and the Canary Islands.

Phenotype–genotype correlations are difficult because most patients are compound heterozygotes, with a different mutation on each chromosome. No clear relationship has been found between the individual mutations and clinical disease patterns. Mutations that interfere with expression of the Wilson ATPase are associated with early liver disease. Homozygosity for the most common mutation in European populations (His1069Gln) may be associated with onset in adulthood and neurological form [9]. Phenotypic variation within families carrying the same mutation may be due to genetic modifiers of *ATP7B*, variations in other proteins involved in the hepatocellular handling of copper, compensatory cytoprotective mechanisms or environmental factors affecting copper availability. Onset of symptoms is significantly delayed in patients with the ApoEε 3/3 polymorphism [10].

Several animal models for Wilson's disease exist. In mice, spontaneous point mutations in the murine *Atp7b* gene cause liver disease resembling human Wilson's disease [11]; an *Atp7b* knockout mouse has more severe liver disease [12]. The Long-Evans Cinnamon (LEC) rat has a large deletion in the rat *ATP7B*. Homozygous rats show marked hepatic copper accumulation in the first few months of life with low serum caeruloplasmin, and they develop severe acute hepatitis. Surviving rats progress to chronic hepatitis and hepatocellular carcinoma [13]. D-penicillamine protects against these changes [14].

Because it is redox-active, copper can cause oxidative injury in cells [15]. Toxic levels of copper in the liver in Wilson's disease cause alterations in hepatocellular mitochondria [16] and nuclei. Oxidative damage to mitochondria can be limited experimentally by vitamin E administration [17].

Pathology

Liver

The liver shows a spectrum of change from simple steatosis to periportal fibrosis to macronodular cirrhosis. With a fulminant hepatitis, submassive necrosis occurs.

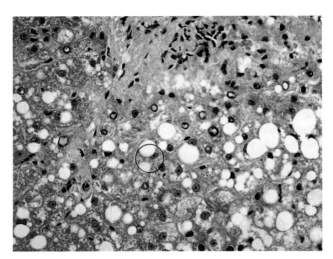

Fig. 27.3. Hepatolenticular degeneration (Wilson's disease). Liver cells adjoining a fibrous tissue band show gross vacuolation of their nuclei (glycogenic degeneration) and fatty change. (H & E, × 65.)

Liver cells are ballooned, show multiple nuclei, clumped glycogen and glycogenated nuclei (Fig. 27.3). Fatty change is usual. In some patients a particularly florid picture is seen with Mallory–Denk bodies, simulating acute alcoholic hepatitis. Alternatively, changes indicate chronic hepatitis (Fig. 27.4). Hepatic histology is not diagnostic, but in a young person with cirrhosis such a picture should always suggest Wilson's disease.

Rubeanic acid or rhodanine stains for copper are unreliable. In early disease, when copper is mainly in the cytoplasm, these stains do not detect any copper. Failure to stain copper on liver biopsy does not exclude the diagnosis of Wilson's disease.

In cirrhosis, some nodules are positive whereas others are not. Detected copper is usually periportal, associated with atypical lipofuscin deposits. It must be distinguished from copper accumulation due to cholestasis.

Electron microscopy

Mitochondria are large and pleiomorphic. They may contain 'dark bodies'. The most striking change is cystic dilatation of the tips of the mitochondrial cristae. Mitochondria may be abnormal even in asymptomatic patients.

Other organs

The *Kayser–Fleischer ring* is due to a copper-containing pigment deposited in Desçemet's membrane at the periphery of the posterior surface of the cornea.

The *kidney* shows fatty and hydropic change with copper deposition in the proximal convoluted tubules.

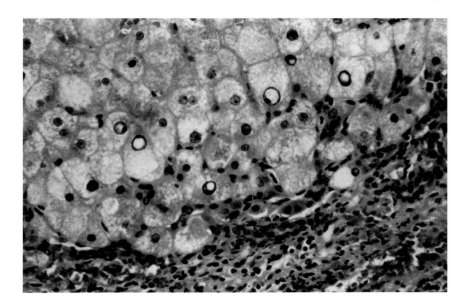

Fig. 27.4. Wilson's disease. In this example there is piecemeal necrosis and lymphocytic infiltration as in autoimmune hepatitis. Note the hepatocellular swelling due to finely divided fat, and vacuolization of nuclei. (H & E, × 350.)

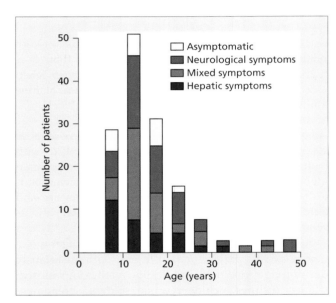

Fig. 27.5. Type of symptom complex at onset by age in 142 British and Chinese patients with Wilson's disease [18].

Clinical picture

Clinical presentation is highly variable. It differs with age (Fig. 27.5). Most children present with liver disease (*hepatic form*). Later on, neuropsychiatric changes become increasingly predominant (*neurological form*). Patients presenting after age 20 usually have neurological symptoms [18,19]. The two forms frequently overlap. Most patients have developed symptoms or have been diagnosed between 5 and 40 years old. Numerous reports, however, indicate that some patients are diagnosed in early childhood or in their 50s–60s [20,21].

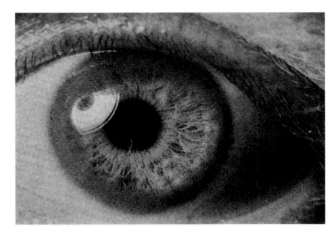

Fig. 27.6. Kayser–Fleischer ring. A brownish deposit is seen at the periphery of the cornea.

The *Kayser–Fleischer* ring (Fig. 27.6) is a greenish-brown corneal ring appearing near the periphery of the iris. The upper pole is first affected. Expert slit lamp examination is almost always necessary to show it. It is usually present with neurological abnormalities but may be absent in 40–60% of those with a hepatic form. A similar ring may rarely be found with prolonged cholestasis and cryptogenic cirrhosis [22].

Rarely, the posterior layer of the capsule of the lens may show greyish-brown 'sunflower' cataracts, which resemble those due to copper-containing foreign bodies.

Hepatic forms

Acute liver failure. This is characterized by progressive jaundice, ascites and hepatic and renal failure, usually in a child or young person. The liver cell necrosis is

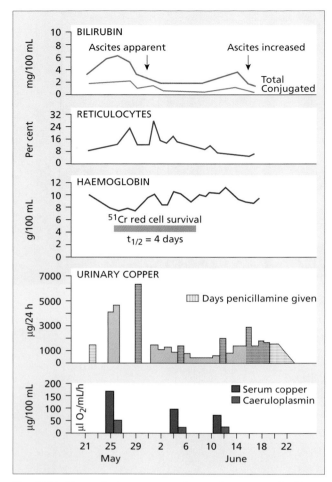

Fig. 27.7. Haemolytic crisis in Wilson's disease, marked by a rise in serum (mainly unconjugated) bilirubin and followed by reticulocytosis. The haemoglobin fell and red cell survival was reduced. Urinary copper was very high even without the administration of penicillamine. Serum copper was higher than that usually found in Wilson's disease. Ascites developed. The second episode of haemolysis, which was noted in June, was marked by a slight rise in serum bilirubin and a fall in haemoglobin [23].

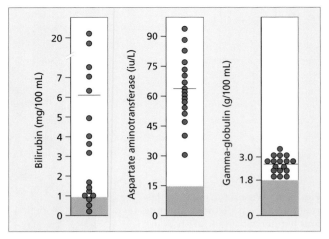

Fig. 27.8. Biochemical tests in 17 patients with Wilson's disease presenting as with chronic hepatitis resembling autoimmune hepatitis. Horizontal lines indicate mean values. Normal ranges are denoted by hatching (serum bilirubin 0.2–0.8 mg/dL; aspartate aminotransferase 4–15 IU/L; γ-globulin 0.7–1.8 g/dL) [2].

presumably related to accumulation of copper. Virtually all patients are already cirrhotic. Acute intravascular haemolysis is due to destruction of erythrocytes by a sudden flux of copper from the necrotic hepatocytes (Fig. 27.7) [23]. Haemolysis of similar type is reported in sheep with copper intoxication, and in humans in accidental copper poisoning.

Kayser–Fleischer rings may be absent. Urinary and serum copper levels are very high. Serum caeruloplasmin is usually low. However, it may be normal or raised since caeruloplasmin is an acute phase reactant, increased by active liver disease. Serum aminotransferases are inappropriately low for fulminant viral hepatitis and alkaline phosphatase may be very low [24]. In conventional American units, a low alkaline phos-

phatase to total bilirubin ratio (AP:TB less than 4) is highly suggestive of Wilson's disease, more so when associated with aspartate aminotransferase:alanine aminotransferase (AST:ALT) more than 2.2 [25].

Autoimmune hepatitis mimic. The condition presents at 10–30 years of age as an acute or chronic hepatitis with jaundice, elevated aminotransferases, hypergammaglobulinaemia and detectable non-specific autoantibodies (Fig. 27.8) [2,26]. Very rarely, Wilson's disease and autoimmune hepatitis are coincidental. All such patients require investigation for Wilson's disease.

Cirrhosis. The patient may present with insidiously developing cirrhosis, typically well-compensated. Clinical features include vascular spiders, splenomegaly, ascites and portal hypertension. Severe disease can exist without any neurological signs. Those showing evidence of hepatic decompensation may still respond well to medical treatment. Liver biopsy with measurement of hepatic copper concentration may be useful for diagnosis.

All children and younger adult patients with chronic liver disease should be screened for Wilson's disease. Those showing any deterioration in school or work performance, slurring of the speech, change in handwriting, early ascites or transient haemolysis require extensive investigation. Any with a family history of cirrhosis should also be screened.

Hepatocellular carcinoma is uncommon [27]. Induction of hepatic metallothionein by copper may be protective [28].

Neuropsychiatric forms

These broadly form subgroups according to the predominant features, and in order of incidence are: parkinsonian, pseudosclerotic, dystonic (dyskinetic) and choreic [29,30]. The neurological presentation may be acute and rapidly progressive. Early changes include a flexion–extension tremor of the wrists, grimacing, difficulty in writing, slurred speech and drooling. The limbs show a fluctuating rigidity. The intellect is fairly well preserved although patients with psychiatric disturbance usually present with a slow deterioration of the personality or depression. Approximately 15% of all patients present with psychiatric disturbance only.

Often the neurological changes are chronic. Onset is in early adult life with tremor, marked and of a wing-beating type, exaggerated by voluntary movement. Sensory loss and pyramidal tract signs are absent. The expression is vacant. Severely dystonic patients have a worse prognosis than other groups [31]. Among patients with neurological forms, 20% may only have minimal changes or steatosis on liver biopsy.

The electroencephalogram shows generalized non-specific changes which may also be seen in asymptomatic siblings. Presentation as a seizure disorder is rare.

Renal changes

Aminoaciduria, glycosuria, phosphaturia and uricosuria reflect renal tubular changes. These are presumably due to copper deposition in the proximal renal tubules.

Renal tubular acidosis is frequent and may be related to stone formation.

Other changes

Isolated episodes of haemolysis may occur; these resolve spontaneously. Rarely, the lunulae of the nails appear lavender due to increased copper. Skeletal changes include demineralization, premature osteoarthritis, sub-articular cysts and fragmentation of bone about the joints. Presenting symptoms may occasionally be limited to arthralgias and muscle weakness. Gallstones are related to haemolysis. Hypoparathyroidism is a rare association. Cardiac disease, in particular dysrhythmias, has been reported. Decreased fertility in women or repeated spontaneous abortions may occur.

Laboratory tests

Serum caeruloplasmin and copper levels are usually low [18,32–34]. Other causes of low caeruloplasmin include the genetic disorder acaeruloplasminaemia [35], advanced liver disease with synthetic failure and severe malnutrition. The caeruloplasmin level may be raised by inflammation, oestrogen administration, oral contraceptive drugs, biliary obstruction or pregnancy.

Basal 24-h urinary copper excretion is increased (>0.6 μmol/24 h). This highly informative test requires some attention to methodology. Wide-necked bottles with copper-free disposable polyethylene liners have been recommended. Simultaneous measurement of urinary creatinine validates completeness of collection. Up to three separate collections should be performed.

Incorporation of orally administered radio-copper into caeruloplasmin is no longer used for diagnosis.

Liver biopsy

The copper content should be measured although concentrations vary widely within a cirrhotic liver [36]. The biopsy can be extracted from the paraffin block for copper measurement [37]. Normal is less than 50 μg/g dry liver weight, and concentrations greater than 250 μg/g dry weight are typical in Wilson's disease (Fig. 27.9). Recent observations suggest that lower values, 70–100 μg/g dry weight, may occur in Wilson's disease [18,39]. Elevated hepatic parenchymal copper concentrations may be found in those with normal hepatic histology. Elevated values are also found with long-standing cholestasis and Indian childhood cirrhosis (Figs 27.1, 27.9).

Imaging

Cranial computed tomography scanning may show changes, including ventricular enlargement, before neurological changes appear. Magnetic resonance imaging is preferred as more sensitive. Dilatation of the third ventricle, focal lesions in the thalamus, putamen and pallidum are seen and bear a relationship to clinical subgroups [40].

Genetic strategies

Haplotype analysis (analysis of the alleles of microsatellite markers surrounding *ATP7B*) was an important strategy for cloning the gene abnormal in Wilson's disease. This technique retains some utility for diagnosing siblings of Wilson's disease patients (as affected, heterozygote or normal) when the mutation(s) cannot be identified in the affected proband [41]. Recently developed, high-throughput techniques permit sequencing of the entire *ATP7B* gene and thus are suitable for primary genetic diagnosis. These molecular techniques are expensive and not universally available, and they require expert interpretation by a knowledgeable geneticist.

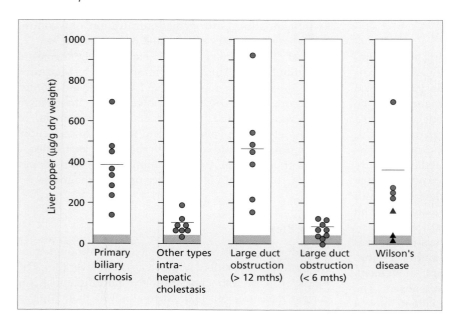

Fig. 27.9. Liver copper levels in patients with Wilson's disease and various types of cholestasis. Wilson's disease: purple triangle denotes heterozygote; black triangles denote siblings probably homozygous normal (these three patients not included in the calculation of the mean, black line); blue circles are affected patients. Normal ranges are denoted by shading [38].

Diagnostic difficulties

The combination of very low serum caeruloplasmin (<0.05 g/L) and presence of Kayser–Fleischer rings in a patient with hepatic or neurological disease establishes the diagnosis of Wilson's disease. However, many patients presenting with liver disease lack these characteristic features [33,34]. The need to pursue the diagnosis in patients where there is any clinical suspicion of Wilson's disease based on clinical, hepatic or neurological features must be emphasized. Basal 24-h urinary copper excretion should be measured. Urinary copper excretion after penicillamine challenge may be informative in children and adults [42,43]. Genetic diagnosis is absolute. Genotyping for a mutation known to be common in the local population can be helpful. Liver biopsy with estimation of liver copper concentration remains the cornerstone for clinical diagnosis, although sampling error may give a misleading result.

A diagnostic scoring system has been devised based on key clinical and laboratory features [44]. It has been subjected to preliminary validation in children [45].

Detection of symptom-free homozygotes

All siblings of individuals with Wilson's disease must be screened with physical examination, liver biochemistries, serum copper and caeruloplasmin and a basal 24-h urinary copper measurement. Slit-lamp examination for Kayser–Fleischer rings is worthwhile. A presymptomatic patient may appear entirely normal or have such features as hepatomegaly, splenomegaly or vascular spiders, and a slight rise in serum aminotrans-

ferase values. Kayser–Fleischer rings may be seen. Serum caeruloplasmin will usually be substantially less than 0.20 g/L. Basal 24-h urinary copper excretion is elevated. Liver biopsy with copper analysis is confirmatory.

Alternatively, if the mutation(s) of the index case are known, genetic diagnosis is the most efficient test in the siblings. Hepatic and neurological function needs to be investigated in siblings identified as affected. Every affected individual must be treated, even if symptom free. Heterozygotes do not require treatment.

Treatment (Table 27.1)

Early diagnosis is best, and treatment is lifelong. For the patient with symptomatic hepatic disease, chelation therapy is given. For patients with neurological disease, treatment options are less straightforward. Chelators or zinc can be effective, but close supervision is required because of possible neurological deterioration, especially with D-penicillamine.

After successful initial treatment, options for maintenance treatment include a reduction in the dose of chelator, or the substitution by zinc. Liver transplantation is indicated for the fulminant hepatic form and those with severe liver disease unresponsive to optimal medical management.

The initial phase of therapy is aimed at clinical improvement or stabilization. The front-line agents are D-penicillamine or trientine. D-penicillamine has been the mainstay of treatment since its therapeutic value was described by Walshe over 50 years ago. Despite its proven efficacy, it can have severe side effects; moreover,

Table 27.1. Treatment of Wilson's disease

Treatment	Indications	Side effects
Liver transplantation	Severe hepatic insufficiency/failure	Chapter 36
Chelators		
D-penicillamine	Initial therapy/maintenance	++
trientine	Initial therapy/maintenance	+/±
(tetrathiomolybdate)	(Under evaluation)	
Zinc (sulphate, gluconate or acetate)	Maintenance/presymptomatic?*	±

*Choice debatable, see text.

symptoms in a proportion of patients presenting with neurological disease may worsen initially. Trientine, developed for patients intolerant of D-penicillamine, is effective in such patients and it is also an excellent first-line therapy. It has fewer reported side effects than D-penicillamine. Zinc salts have a limited role as initial treatment. Ammonium tetrathiomolybdate is an investigational drug, which appears safe and effective as initial therapy of patients with neurological disease.

An important facet of all treatments is the absolute need for compliance, which is often a problem in patients constrained to take lifelong regular medication despite feeling perfectly well.

Penicillamine chelates copper and increases urinary excretion to as much as 15–45 μmol daily. Treatment in adults is started with 1–1.5 g D-penicillamine daily by mouth in three to four divided doses taken 1 h before meals. Improvement is slow and at least 6 months of continuous therapy should be given at this dose. If there is no improvement, the dose may be increased to 2 g daily for a limited time. Of patients with neurological disease, approximately 25% experience neurological deterioration before improvement is seen [31]. Improvement is marked by disappearance of the Kayser–Fleischer rings. Speech is clearer; tremor and rigidity lessen. Hand-writing is a good test of progress. Liver function improves. Liver biopsy, though not necessary clinically for follow-up, shows reversion to inactive cirrhosis. Failure to improve implies that irreparable tissue damage was present before treatment started or that there is a lack of compliance with treatment. Unless outright liver failure develops, treatment failure should not be declared until 1–2 years of optimal therapy has been given.

Success during this initial period of D-penicillamine therapy is judged by improvement in hepatic synthetic function. A brisk cupruria is expected. Serum non-caeruloplasmin-bound copper should return to normal but has not been validated as a clinical criterion. Whether the liver copper level returns to normal is controversial [46], but if it does, it takes many years of treatment. If

the expected improvement occurs after the initial period of treatment, the dose of D-penicillamine should be reduced to 750–1000 mg/day. Close follow-up is necessary to ensure continued improvement or stability and to monitor compliance. Evidence of excessive de-coppering is sought by estimating non-caeruloplasmin-bound copper concentration and measuring 24-h urinary copper output. A rapidly progressive hepatic deterioration may follow non-compliance of treatment in a previously well-controlled patient [46,47]. Patients on long-term D-penicillamine treatment require regular monitoring of bone marrow and renal function as long as they are taking this drug.

Adverse reactions to D-penicillamine occur in approximately 30% of patients with Wilson's disease [31]. These include hypersensitivity reactions within the first few weeks of treatment with fever and rash, leucopenia, thrombocytopenia and lymphadenopathy. This usually resolves when D-penicillamine is stopped. Treatment can be recommenced with slowly increasing doses of D-penicillamine along with prednisolone; however, switching to trientine is the better strategy. D-penicillamine may also cause proteinuria and a systemic lupus erythematosus (SLE)-like syndrome. It can cause aplastic anaemia. Skin changes include elastosis perforans serpiginosa and cutis laxa (progeric wrinkling). The latter is dose-related, so that long-term treatment with doses over 1 g/day is not recommended [3]. In the event of any serious or unremitting adverse effect of D-penicillamine, it should be discontinued and trientine should be substituted.

During the first 2 months of D-penicillamine treatment, white cell and platelet counts are done at least weekly, then monthly up to 6 months and thereafter at least annually. Urinalysis for proteinuria should be checked on these occasions. Clinical pyridoxine deficiency, a theoretical possibility, is exceedingly rare, but supplements of pyridoxine 25 mg daily are routinely used.

Trientine is a copper chelator initially introduced to treat patients intolerant of D-penicillamine [46,48]. It is very different chemically from D-penicillamine, which is perhaps why it can be used as an alternative treatment if D-penicillamine is not tolerated. Despite lower cupriuretic potency than D-penicillamine, it is clinically effective. The typical dose in adults is 1000–1200 mg daily divided into two doses, but total daily dose can be as high as 1800 mg. It can be a satisfactory first line of treatment for Wilson's disease [49–51]. Trientine has few side effects. Hypersensitivity reactions have not been reported although fixed drug reactions may occur. Pancytopenia has rarely been reported. Neurological deterioration in Wilson's disease patients is uncommon. Trientine should be stored in a refrigerator to prevent deterioration, and should be taken (as for penicillamine) on an empty stomach, preferably at least 1 h before eating.

Zinc inhibits gastrointestinal absorption of copper through the induction of intestinal metallothionein [52]. The dose for adults is 50 mg elemental zinc by mouth three times daily; the particular salt does not matter. Most long-term experience is in presymptomatic patients or those with neurological presentation. Its important advantage for treating the neurological form is that neurological deterioration seldom occurs [53]. Its efficacy as initial treatment in symptomatic patients remains disputed despite supportive data [54–56]. Hepatic decompensation has rarely been reported. Zinc is increasingly used for maintenance therapy in patients who have stabilized after initial treatment with chelators [52], but further experience is required to support its use as maintenance therapy. Zinc seems to have few adverse side effects, apart from nausea or gastric irritation. As with other treatments, compliance is essential. Zinc should be taken on an empty stomach.

Dimercaptopropanol (British Anti-Lewisite), the first available chelator therapy for Wilson's disease, is now used only very rarely, as an adjunct in patients with refractory neurological and/or psychiatric disease.

Tetrathiomolybdate is an investigational agent which has potent effects on copper disposition. In the intestine it prevents the absorption of copper. Absorbed drug complexes copper with albumin in the blood and thus interferes with copper damage to tissues. In initial treatment of patients with neurological disease, tetrathiomolybdate was infrequently associated with worsening of neurological symptoms as may occur with D-penicillamine [57]; a comparative study in the neurological presentation showed that tetrathiomolybdate plus zinc was more effective than trientine plus zinc [58].

Combination therapy (chelator plus zinc) should be reserved for patients with decompensated hepatic disease or a severe neurological form. The chelator dose (usually trientine 500 mg, in adults) is alternated with the zinc dose (50 mg elemental, in adults) throughout the day, with usually 5–6 hours between administration of either drug. Thus chelator is given at 6 AM and again 12 hours later (first and third doses), and zinc is given at noon and midnight (second and fourth doses of the day). This regimen requires a high degree of commitment from patient and/or the patient's family. If the treatment is successful, the patient can be switched to monotherapy (trientine or zinc) after 3 months. Patients with hepatic form who fail this regimen typically require liver transplantation. Although there are encouraging preliminary reports, this strategy remains investigational [59–61].

Physiotherapy is valuable for improving the patient's gait, writing and movement generally.

A low-copper diet is of no value as sole treatment, but copper-containing foods (liver, shellfish, nuts, chocolate and mushrooms) should be avoided. Alcoholic beverages should be excluded in the initial phase of treatment, but advice should be customized for each patient once clinical improvement and stability have been achieved. Vegetarians with Wilson's disease require supervision by a dietician.

Pregnancy in women with Wilson's disease is safe. Treatment is continued with the patient's normal medication. Prolonged interruption of treatment carries a major risk of hepatic insufficiency and possible death. Continued treatment with D-penicillamine [62], trientine [62] or zinc [63] has been well tolerated by mothers. It is difficult to quantify the potential risk to the infant; however, D-penicillamine is classified as a teratogen [64]. A daily dose of 750–1000 mg of either D-penicillamine or trientine, in well-controlled patients, has been used during the first two trimesters of pregnancy with reduction to 500 mg/day during the last trimester [62].

Hepatic transplantation may be indicated for the fulminant form (which is otherwise usually fatal), the young cirrhotic in severe hepatocellular failure who fails to improve after 2–3 months of optimal medical treatment, or the patient who develops severe liver failure after unwisely stopping therapy. Survival at 1 year is 79–87% [65–67]. The hepatic metabolic defect is corrected [68]. Although neurological features show improvement in some patients [69], this is not always the case and liver transplantation as treatment for neurological Wilson's disease remains highly controversial.

Before transplant, renal failure and haemolytic anaemia may be treated by albumin dialysis [70,71]. Acute haemolysis due to Wilson's disease has also been successfully treated by exchange transfusion [72].

Prognosis

Untreated Wilson's disease is progressive and fatal. The great danger is that the patient remains undiagnosed and dies untreated. This unfortunate outcome is likely in patients presenting with exclusively psychiatric symptoms, in whom positive family history or personal history of jaundice must be sought.

In hepatitis resembling autoimmune hepatitis, response to treatment can be poor, nine of 17 patients dying in one series before the era of liver transplantation [2]. Jaundice, ascites and a high serum bilirubin, elevated aminotransferases and coagulopathy time are ominous signs [73]. In children, a score composed of total serum bilirubin, AST, albumin, INR, and total white cell count appeared to have good predictive value for identifying need for urgent liver transplantation [60]. Liver transplantation is life saving in patients with the acute liver failure presentation of Wilson's disease.

In the acute neurological form the prognosis is poor, for cystic changes in the basal ganglia are irreversible. In the more chronic form the outlook depends on early diagnosis, preferably before symptoms have appeared [18]. The final prognosis also depends on the response to 6 months of continuous chelator treatment. Dystonia carries a poor prognosis, being little affected by chelation therapy.

Otherwise death is from chronic liver failure, variceal bleeding or intercurrent infections in those bedridden from neurological disability.

Patients diagnosed early in the disease course who adhere to their medical regimen faultlessly have a good prognosis.

Indian childhood cirrhosis

See Chapter 29.

References

1 Wilson SAK. Progressive lenticular degeneration: a familial nervous disease associated with cirrhosis of the liver. *Brain* 1912; **34**: 295–507.
2 Scott J, Gollan JL, Samourian S *et al.* Wilson's disease, presenting as chronic active hepatitis. *Gastroenterology* 1978; **74**: 645–651.
3 Scheinberg IH, Sternlieb I. *Wilson's disease*. Philadelphia: W B Saunders, 1984.
4 Bull PC, Cox DW. Wilson disease and Menkes disease: new handles on heavy-metal transport. *Trends Genet.* 1994; **10**: 246–252.
5 Fatemi N, Sarkar B. Structural and functional insights of Wilson disease copper- transporting ATPase. *J. Bioenerg. Biomembr.* 2002; **34**: 339–349.
6 Portmann R, Solioz M. Purification and functional reconstitution of the human Wilson copper ATPase, ATP7B. *FEBS Lett.* 2005; **579**: 3589–3595.
7 Schaefer M, Hopkins RG, Failla ML *et al.* Hepatocyte-specific localization and copper-dependent trafficking of the Wilson's disease protein in the liver. *Am. J. Physiol.* 1999; **276**: G639–646.
8 La Fontaine S, Mercer JF. Trafficking of the copper-ATPases, ATP7A and ATP7B: role in copper homeostasis. *Arch. Biochem. Biophys.* 2007; **463**: 149–167.
9 Stapelbroek JM, Bollen CW, van Amstel JK *et al.* The H1069Q mutation in ATP7B is associated with late and neurologic presentation in Wilson disease: results of a meta-analysis. *J. Hepatol.* 2004; **41**: 758–763.
10 Schiefermeier M, Kollegger H, Madl C *et al.* The impact of apolipoprotein E genotypes on age at onset of symptoms and phenotypic expression in Wilson's disease. *Brain* 2000; **123**: 585–590.
11 Roberts EA, Robinson BH, Yang S. Mitochondrial structure and function in the untreated Jackson toxic milk (tx-j) mouse, a model for Wilson disease. *Mol. Genet. Metab.* 2008; **93**: 54–65.
12 Huster D, Finegold MJ, Morgan CT *et al.* Consequences of copper accumulation in the livers of the Atp7b-/- (Wilson disease gene) knockout mice. *Am. J. Pathol.* 2006; **168**: 423–434.
13 Mori M, Hattori A, Sawaki M *et al.* The LEC rat: a model for human hepatitis, liver cancer, and much more. *Am. J. Pathol.* 1994; **144**: 200–204.
14 Togashi Y, Li Y, Kang JH *et al.* D-penicillamine prevents the development of hepatitis in Long-Evans Cinnamon rats with abnormal copper metabolism. *Hepatology* 1992; **15**: 82–87.
15 Seth R, Yang S, Choi S *et al.* In vitro assessment of copper-induced toxicity in the human hepatoma line, Hep G2. *Toxicol. In Vitro* 2004; **18**: 501–509.
16 Gu M, Cooper JM, Butler P *et al.* Oxidative-phosphorylation defects in liver of patients with Wilson's disease. *Lancet* 2000; **356**: 469–474.
17 Sokol RJ, McKim JM Jr, Devereau MW. [alpha]-Tocopherol ameliorates oxidant injury in isolated copper-overloaded rat hepatocytes. *Pediatr. Res.* 1996; **39**: 259–263.
18 Strickland GT, Frommer D, Leu ML *et al.* Wilson's disease in the United Kingdom and Taiwan. I. General characteristics of 142 cases and prognosis. II. A genetic analysis of 88 cases. *Q. J. Med.* 1973; **42**: 619–638.
19 Merle U, Schaefer M, Ferenci P *et al.* Clinical presentation, diagnosis and long-term outcome of Wilson's disease: a cohort study. *Gut* 2007; **56**: 115–120.
20 Wilson DC, Phillips MJ, Cox DW *et al.* Severe hepatic Wilson's disease in preschool-aged children. *J. Pediatr.* 2000; **137**: 719–722.
21 Ala A, Borjigin J, Rochwarger A *et al.* Wilson disease in septuagenarian siblings: Raising the bar for diagnosis. *Hepatology* 2005; **41**: 668–670.
22 Frommer D, Morris J, Sherlock S *et al.* Kayser-Fleischer-like rings in patients without Wilson's disease. *Gastroenterology* 1977; **72**: 1331–1335.
23 McIntyre N, Clink HM, Levi AJ *et al.* Hemolytic anemia in Wilson's disease. *N. Engl. J. Med.* 1967; **276**: 439–444.
24 Shaver WA, Bhatt H, Combes B. Low serum alkaline phosphatase activity in Wilson's disease. *Hepatology* 1986; **6**: 859–863.
25 Korman JD, Volenberg I, Balko J *et al.* Screening for Wilson disease in acute liver failure: a comparison of currently available diagnostic tests. *Hepatology* 2008; **48**: 1167–1174.
26 Milkiewicz P, Saksena S, Hubscher SG *et al.* Wilson's disease with superimposed autoimmune features: report of two cases and review. *J. Gastroenterol. Hepatol.* 2000; **15**: 570–574.
27 Walshe JM, Waldenstrom E, Sams V *et al.* Abdominal malignancies in patients with Wilson's disease. *Q. J. Med.* 2003; **96**: 657–662.

28 Polio J, Enriquez RE, Chow A *et al*. Hepatocellular carcinoma in Wilson's disease. Case report and review of the literature. *J. Clin. Gastroenterol.* 1989; **11**: 220–224.

29 Walshe JM, Yealland M. Wilson's disease: the problem of delayed diagnosis. *J. Neurol. Neurosurg. Psychiatry* 1992; **55**: 692–696.

30 Taly AB, Meenakshi-Sundaram S, Sinha S *et al*. Wilson disease: description of 282 patients evaluated over 3 decades. *Medicine (Baltimore)* 2007; **86**: 112–121.

31 Walshe JM, Yealland M. Chelation treatment of neurological Wilson's disease. *Q. J. Med.* 1993; **86**: 197–204.

32 Gibbs K, Walshe JM. A study of the caeruloplasmin concentrations found in 75 patients with Wilson's disease, their kinships and various control groups. *Q. J. Med.* 1979; **48**: 447–463.

33 Steindl P, Ferenci P, Dienes HP *et al*. Wilson's disease in patients presenting with liver disease: a diagnostic challenge. *Gastroenterology* 1997; **113**: 212–218.

34 Gow PJ, Smallwood RA, Angus PW *et al*. Diagnosis of Wilson's disease: an experience over three decades. *Gut* 2000; **46**: 415–419.

35 Harris ZL, Klomp LW, Gitlin JD. Aceruloplasminemia: an inherited neurodegenerative disease with impairment of iron homeostasis. *Am. J. Clin. Nutr.* 1998; **67** (Suppl.): 972S–977S.

36 Faa G, Nurchi V, Demelia L *et al*. Uneven hepatic copper distribution in Wilson's disease. *J. Hepatol.* 1995; **22**: 303–308.

37 Ludwig J, Moyer TP, Rakela J. The liver biopsy diagnosis of Wilson's disease. Methods in pathology. *Am. J. Clin. Pathol.* 1994; **102**: 443–446.

38 Smallwood RA, Williams HA, Rosenoer VM *et al*. Liver-copper levels in liver disease: studies using neutron activation analysis. *Lancet* 1968; **2**: 1310–1313.

39 Ferenci P, Steindl-Munda P, Vogel W *et al*. Diagnostic value of quantitative hepatic copper determination in patients with Wilson's Disease. *Clin. Gastroenterol. Hepatol.* 2005; **3**: 811–818.

40 Oder W, Prayer L, Grimm G *et al*. Wilson's disease: evidence of subgroups derived from clinical findings and brain lesions. *Neurology* 1993; **43**: 120–124.

41 Houwen RH, Roberts EA, Thomas GR *et al*. DNA markers for the diagnosis of Wilson disease. *J. Hepatol.* 1993; **17**: 269–276.

42 Martins da Costa C, Baldwin D, Portmann B *et al*. Value of urinary copper excretion after penicillamine challenge in the diagnosis of Wilson's disease. *Hepatology* 1992; **15**: 609–615.

43 Muller T, Koppikar S, Taylor RM *et al*. Re-evaluation of the penicillamine challenge test in the diagnosis of Wilson's disease in children. *J. Hepatol.* 2007; **47**: 270–276.

44 Ferenci P, Caca K, Loudianos G *et al*. Diagnosis and phenotypic classification of Wilson disease. *Liver Int.* 2003; **23**: 139–142.

45 Koppikar S, Dhawan A. Evaluation of the scoring system for the diagnosis of Wilson's disease in children. *Liver Int.* 2005; **25**: 680–681.

46 Scheinberg IH, Jaffe ME, Sternlieb I. The use of trientine in preventing the effects of interrupting penicillamine therapy in Wilson's disease. *N. Engl. J. Med.* 1987; **317**: 209–213.

47 Walshe JM, Dixon AK. Dangers of non-compliance in Wilson's disease. *Lancet* 1986; **1**: 845–847.

48 Walshe JM. Treatment of Wilson's disease with trientine (triethylene tetramine) dihydrochloride. *Lancet* 1982; **1**: 643–647.

49 Dahlman T, Hartvig P, Lofholm M *et al*. Long-term treatment of Wilson's disease with triethylene tetramine dihydrochloride (trientine). *Q. J. Med.* 1995; **88**: 609–616.

50 Dubois RS, Rodgerson DO, Hambidge KM. Treatment of Wilson's disease with triethylene tetramine hydrochloride (Trientine). *J. Pediatr. Gastroenterol. Nutr.* 1990; **10**: 77–81.

51 Arnon R, Calderon JF, Schilsky M *et al*. Wilson disease in children: serum aminotransferases and urinary copper on triethylene tetramine dihydrochloride (trientine) treatment. *J. Pediatr. Gastroenterol. Nutr.* 2007; **44**: 596–602.

52 Brewer GJ, Dick RD, Johnson VD *et al*. Treatment of Wilson's disease with zinc: XV long-term follow-up studies. *J. Lab. Clin. Med.* 1998; **132**: 264–278.

53 Brewer GJ, Yuzbasiyan-Gurkan V, Young AB. Treatment of Wilson's disease. *Semin. Neurol.* 1987; **7**: 209–220.

54 Czlonkowska A, Gajda J, Rodo M. Effects of long-term treatment in Wilson's disease with D-penicillamine and zinc sulphate. *J. Neurol.* 1996; **243**: 269–273.

55 Marcellini M, Di Ciommo V, Callea F *et al*. Treatment of Wilson's disease with zinc from the time of diagnosis in pediatric patients: a single-hospital, 10-year follow-up study. *J. Lab. Clin. Med.* 2005; **145**: 139–143.

56 Lee VD, Northup PG, Berg CL. Resolution of decompensated cirrhosis from Wilson's disease with zinc monotherapy: a potential therapeutic option? *Clin. Gastroenterol. Hepatol.* 2006; **4**: 1069–1071.

57 Brewer GJ, Hedera P, Kluin KJ *et al*. Treatment of Wilson disease with ammonium tetrathiomolybdate. III. Initial therapy in a total of 55 neurologically affected patients and follow-up with zinc therapy. *Arch. Neurol.* 2003; **60**: 379–385.

58 Brewer GJ, Askari F, Lorincz MT *et al*. Treatment of Wilson disease with ammonium tetrathiomolybdate. IV. Comparison of tetrathiomolybdate and trientine in a double-blind study of treatment of the neurologic presentation of Wilson disease. *Arch. Neurol.* 2006; **63**: 521–527.

59 Santos Silva EE, Sarles J, Buts JP *et al*. Successful medical treatment of severely decompensated Wilson disease. *J. Pediatr.* 1996; **128**: 285–287.

60 Dhawan A, Taylor RM, Cheeseman P *et al*. Wilson's disease in children: 37-Year experience and revised King's score for liver transplantation. *Liver Transpl.* 2005; **11**: 441–448.

61 Askari FK, Greenson J, Dick RD *et al*. Treatment of Wilson's disease with zinc. XVIII. Initial treatment of the hepatic decompensation presentation with trientine and zinc. *J. Lab. Clin. Med.* 2003; **142**: 385–390.

62 Sternlieb I. Wilson's disease and pregnancy. *Hepatology* 2000; **31**: 531–532.

63 Brewer GJ, Johnson VD, Dick RD *et al*. Treatment of Wilson's disease with zinc. XVII: Treatment during pregnancy. *Hepatology* 2000; **31**: 364–370.

64 Pinter R, Hogge WA, McPherson E. Infant with severe penicillamine embryopathy born to a woman with Wilson disease. *Am. J. Med. Genet.* 2004; **128**: 294–298.

65 Emre S, Atillasoy EO, Ozdemir S *et al*. Orthotopic liver transplantation for Wilson's disease: a single-center experience. *Transplantation* 2001; **72**: 1232–1236.

66 Pabon V, Dumortier J, Gincul R *et al*. Long-term results of liver transplantation for Wilson's disease. *Gastroenterol. Clin. Biol.* 2008; **32**: 378–381.

67 Martin AP, Bartels M, Redlich J *et al*. A single-center experience with liver transplantation for Wilson's disease. *Clin. Transplant.* 2008; **22**: 216–221.

68 Eghtesad B, Nezakatgoo N, Geraci LC *et al*. Liver transplantation for Wilson's disease: a single-center experience. *Liver Transpl. Surg.* 1999; **5**: 467–474.

69 Stracciari A, Tempestini A, Borghi A *et al*. Effect of liver transplantation on neurological manifestations in Wilson disease. *Arch. Neurol.* 2000; **57**: 384–386.

70 Kreymann B, Seige M, Schweigart U *et al*. Albumin dialysis: effective removal of copper in a patient with fulminant Wilson disease and successful bridging to liver transplanta-tion: a new possibility for the elimination of protein-bound toxins. *J. Hepatol.* 1999; **31**: 1080–1085.

71 Collins KL, Roberts EA, Adeli K *et al*. Single pass albumin dialysis (SPAD) in fulminant Wilsonian liver failure: a case report. *Pediatr. Nephrol.* 2008; **23**: 1013–1016.

72 Matsumura A, Hiraishi H, Terano A. Plasma exchange for hemolytic crisis in Wilson disease. *Ann. Intern. Med.* 1999; **131**: 866.

73 Nazer H, Ede RJ, Mowat AP *et al*. Wilson's disease: clinical presentation and use of prognostic index. *Gut* 1986; **27**: 1377–1381.

CHAPTER 28
Non-alcoholic Fatty Liver Disease and Nutrition

Stephen H. Caldwell & Curtis K. Argo
University of Virginia Health System, Charlottesville, Virginia, USA

Learning points

- Non-alcoholic fatty liver disease (NAFLD) is closely associated with obesity, insulin resistance and dyslipidaemia. Two broad types are recognized—simple steatosis is typically stable while non-alcoholic steatohepatitis (NASH) is characterized by significant cell injury and the potential for progression to cirrhosis.

- The prevalence of NAFLD and NASH is significantly influenced by ethnicity and familial factors. Both disorders can also occur in non-obese patients most of whom are physically deconditioned and thus can be said to be metabolically obese.

- Patients with NASH have an increased risk of death from vascular disease, non-hepatic malignancies and cirrhosis, which may be complicated by hepatocellular cancer. These disorders may also coexist, such as vascular disease in a patient with cirrhosis, presenting further clinical challenges.

- Excessive accumulation of hepatic lipid stores (steatosis) results from a combination of increased delivery of non-esterified fatty acids from uncontrolled lipolysis in other fat storage sites, increased *de novo* triglyceride synthesis from carbohydrates and increased delivery of diet-derived lipids. The mechanism of cell injury in NASH involves oxidative injury, especially to the phospholipid monolayer of small fat droplets and endoplasmic reticulum, free fatty acid induced changes in mitochondrial permeability and activation of apoptosis pathways (caspases), caspase-induced cytoskeletal injury evident as Mallory–Denk bodies and cell death by both necrosis and apoptosis (necroapoptosis). These processes result in activation of collagen-producing stellate cells, leading to fibrosis and ultimately to cirrhosis.

- Diet and exercise are cornerstones of optimal management. For patients with biopsy-proven NASH, pharmacological intervention may be appropriate to decrease the risks of cirrhosis, but therapy as yet is not effective. Thiazolidinediones are the most promising, but side effects will probably limit their wide application. Antioxidants will also probably play a significant role.

Introduction

Hepatic steatosis describes the accumulation of fat, mostly as triglyceride, cholesterol and phospholipids, in excess of 5–10% of liver weight. For many years, the discovery of fatty liver during a routine evaluation was not thought to have clinical significance. However, it was known that obese and diabetic patients could develop histological steatohepatitis similar to that seen with alcohol-induced liver disease [1]. The term 'NASH' or non-alcoholic steatohepatitis was introduced by Ludwig *et al.*, describing the lesion in various degrees of severity in patients without significant ethanol exposure [2]. The subsequent observation that NASH could progress over years to bland cirrhosis [3] was followed by others showing that NASH is a common cause of 'cryptogenic' cirrhosis, which accounts for 10–20% of all cirrhosis [3–6]. However, other early studies had shown that fatty liver is very often stable over a lifetime [7]. These issues came into sharper focus with recognition that non-alcoholic fatty liver disease (NAFLD) exists as a spectrum [8], from simple steatosis without evidence of cell injury, which tends to be stable over time, to steatohepatitis, which may progress to cirrhosis. In later stages, NASH-related cirrhosis loses diagnostic fatty infiltration and may have the appearance of 'cryptogenic' cirrhosis.

The emergence of a worldwide obesity epidemic has stimulated a great deal of ongoing research. The term 'NAFLD' was introduced as a means of grouping all of

Sherlock's Diseases of the Liver and Biliary System, Twelfth Edition. Edited by
James S. Dooley, Anna S.F. Lok, Andrew K. Burroughs, E. Jenny Heathcote.
© 2011 by Blackwell Publishing Ltd. Published 2011 by Blackwell Publishing Ltd.

the variants under one broad term. The names NAFLD and NASH have become established. NASH remains, by definition, a clinical–pathological diagnosis requiring both exclusion of ethanol (see below) as a major contributor, and the presence of cell injury, as evidenced by cellular ballooning, focal necrosis, fibrosis and inflammation. NAFLD and associated conditions have a substantial impact on health-care utilization and costs [9].

Further definitions, terminology and diagnosis

Although the diagnosis of NASH continues to require biopsy, the diagnosis of NAFLD can be made by imaging provided other diseases are excluded. Excluded disorders are those detected by serological evaluation—viral hepatitis, autoimmune liver disease, Wilson's disease, haemochromatosis and α_1-antitrypsin deficiency. However, drug-induced injury must be excluded; steatosis and steatohepatitis may coexist with these and other disorders and exposures (see below). In addition, NAFLD syndrome usually involves features related to insulin resistance typically in the setting of central or visceral adiposity, as discussed later.

Steatosis can be detected by a variety of imaging modalities, including ultrasound, computed tomography or magnetic resonance (MR) (Fig. 28.1). However, fatty infiltration of less than about 20% may not be detected [10]. Modifications and refinements, such as MR spectroscopy and three-point Dixon MR, can accurately detect reduced amounts and provide a numerical value for the estimated percentage of triglyceride content [11,12]. 'Presumed NAFLD' is a term usually used in larger epidemiological studies, such as NHANES (National Health and Nutrition Examination Survey), in which abnormal liver enzymes in the absence of other known or suspected liver disorders is presumed to be due to NAFLD. While useful from a research perspective, it is the least precise form of diagnosis.

The other key feature to make the diagnosis of NAFLD is the exclusion of ethanol exposure as a significant factor. This remains controversial, with little agreement between studies as to whether this means total abstinence or consumption below a threshold level. There are studies showing less or no apparent additional histological injury (and perhaps less injury) with modest alcohol consumption in NASH [13], and others showing obesity as a risk factor for alcohol-induced liver disease [14]. In general, daily consumption of less than 20 g in women and 30 g in men results in a low risk for the development of alcoholic liver injury, although this leaves a grey area for those with less modest daily consumption, but still below the ranges associated with alcohol-induced liver disease. Lifetime ethanol exposure rather than daily consumption suggest that about 10% of patients diagnosed with NASH may have a component of alcohol-related steatohepatitis (ASH) [15].

Liver biopsy, classification of non-alcoholic fatty liver disease and non-invasive markers of non-alcoholic steatohepatitis

Although non-invasive markers of histological injury are under study, the accurate diagnosis of NASH remains dependent on specific histological parameters in a biopsy. The key parameters include steatosis (usually mixed macro- and microvesicular), cellular ballooning, inflammation and fibrosis which ranges from slight perisinusoidal fibrosis to bridging and cirrhosis [16–18]. The major indicators of injury have been incorporated into a score commonly called the NAS (NAFLD Activity Score) and staging system of fibrosis, which currently is being used in most clinical trials [19]. These features have also been used to divide NAFLD into four types: (1) simple steatosis, (2) steatosis with inflammation alone, (3) steatosis with inflammation and ballooning, and (4) steatosis with inflammation and fibrosis [8]. In general, the latter two types constitute NASH (because ballooning and fibrosis usually parallel each other and are typically associated with inflammatory infiltrates). The first two types can be grouped into 'NNFL' (non-NASH fatty liver) [20]. The division of NAFLD into NASH and NNFL is significant because of their relationship to prognosis and appropriate therapy (Fig. 28.2 and Table 28.1).

Although liver biopsy remains the 'gold standard', there are practical limitations, including costs and risks. Importantly, sampling error is well recognized, and longer cores are needed for accurate fibrosis staging [21]. Minimal sizes are debated but most recommend

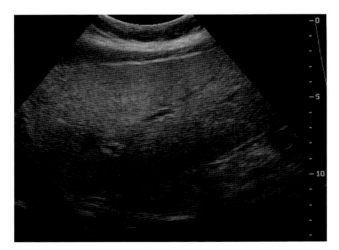

Fig. 28.1. Ultrasonographic image of a steatotic liver. The 'brightness' of the parenchyma (whitish shadowing) is characteristic of fatty liver. The histological correlate from this patient is shown in Fig. 28.8a,b.

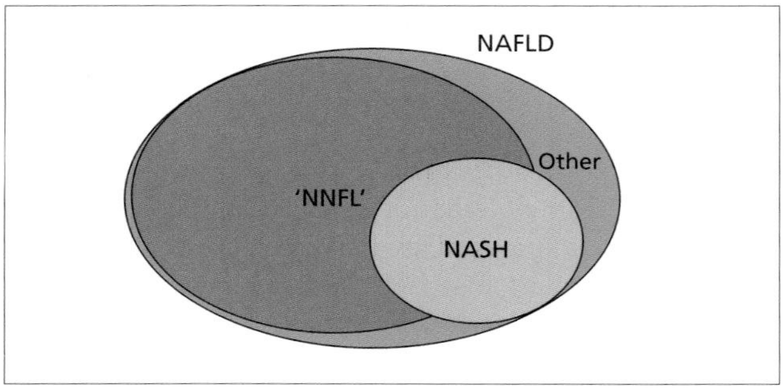

Fig. 28.2. Non-alcoholic fatty liver disease (NAFLD) exists as a spectrum that includes non-alcoholic steatohepatitis (NASH), which constitutes about one-third of cases. The remainder of the cases consist mostly of non-NASH fatty liver termed 'NNFL', and a small representation of other conditions such as storage diseases, discussed in the final section of this chapter.

Table 28.2. National Cholesterol Education Program: Adult Treatment Program III (NCEP ATP-III) Guidelines—metabolic syndrome components

Risk factor	Defining level
Abdominal obesity	Waist circumference
Men	>102 cm (>40 in)
Women	>88 cm (>35 in)
Triglycerides	≥150 mg/dL
HDL cholesterol	
Men	<40 mg/dL
Women	<50 mg/dL
Blood pressure	≥130/ ≥85 mmHg
Fasting blood glucose	≥110 mg/dL

Reaching the defining level for any three of the parameters satisfies the clinically applicable definition of metabolic syndrome.

Table 28.1. Working classification of non-alcoholic fatty liver disease

NNFL
Type 1 NAFLD: Steatosis with no inflammation or fibrosis
Type 2 NAFLD: Steatosis with non-specific lobular inflammation but absent of fibrosis or hepatocyte ballooning
NASH
Type 3 NAFLD: Steatosis with inflammation and fibrosis of variable levels (NASH)
Type 4 NAFLD: Steatosis, inflammation, hepatocyte ballooning, and fibrosis or Mallory–Denk bodies (NASH)

NNFL refers to non-NASH fatty liver and indicates the development of steatosis in the absence of significant ethanol exposure and without evidence of significant cell injury. Synonyms include simple steatosis and NAFL (non-alcoholic fatty liver). NASH, non-alcoholic steatohepatitis; NAFLD, non-alcoholic fatty liver disease.

2 cm or more. Non-invasive alternatives, which include a number of clinical scoring systems, as well as laboratory tests, cannot distinguish intermediate levels of injury [22]. However, these markers may eventually provide an accurate means of distinguishing NASH and NNFL, grading the severity of NASH and monitoring the response to therapeutic interventions. Promising parameters include collagen-related metabolites as indicators of fibrosis, adipocytokines as indicators of systemic fat metabolism and insulin signalling and cytokeratin 18 fragments as a measure of apoptosis pathways activation [23,24].

Clinical features

Most patients with NASH have insulin resistance and the metabolic syndrome (Table 28.2) with central or visceral obesity [25–28]. Insulin resistance can be demonstrated in the liver (failure to suppress glucose output), in skeletal muscle (diminished glucose uptake) and in adipose tissue (failure to suppress lipolysis and release of fatty acids). Indeed, resistance is likely to result from

systemic lipotoxicity (Table 28.3) [29,30]. Hypertension, hyperlipidaemia and type 2 diabetes, components of the metabolic syndrome, can cause confusion regarding possible drug-induced liver enzyme abnormalities in patients using antihypertensives, antidiabetic and anti-hyperlipidaemic agents, who are actually suffering from NASH.

Most patients also have impaired exercise tolerance (measured by oxygen consumption during graded exercise). These findings are consistent with 'metabolic obesity' even in those with relatively low body mass index (BMI) [31]. The average age for NASH patients is 40–50 years and for NASH-related cirrhosis it is 50–60 years. However, the emerging obesity epidemic has resulted in increasing numbers of children with this disease—sometimes with advanced fibrosis [32]. About 20% of patients report a family history of unexplained liver disease (see below). Other common associations include polycystic ovary syndrome, sleep apnoea and small bowel bacterial overgrowth [33,34]. The latter may explain the frequent association of vague abdominal symptoms seen in these patients. Many of these find-

Table 28.3. Key sites of insulin resistance

Tissue	Dysfunction
Adipose	Failure to suppress hormone-sensitive lipase activates release of FFA from triglyceride stores
Liver	Failure to suppress glucose production/ release from glycogenolysis and gluconeogenesis
Muscle	Failure in glucose uptake due to: decreased translocation of GLUT-4 transporter increased myocyte lipid stores impaired mitochondrial function

FFA, free fatty acids; GLUT-4 transporter, transmembrane insulin-responsive transporter found in adipose and muscle primarily responsible for glucose uptake from the circulation/ periphery.

ings, including hepatic dysfunction, can be unified under the concept of *systemic lipotoxicity*, which implicates toxicity related to excessive intracellular fatty acid accumulation which, in turn, alters cellular metabolism in many tissue types [35]. The occasional description of unexplained neurodegenerative disease in association with NASH also points towards the systemic nature of this disease [36]. The most common presentation of NAFLD is the detection of mildly abnormal aminotransferases during a routine clinical evaluation. However, there is a tendency for these levels to decline with progressive disease in parallel with decreasing steatosis, as fibrosis worsens. Thus it is important to examine the patient closely for stigmata of cirrhosis, including a firm, palpable liver and cutaneous signs such as palmer erythema and spider angiomata, as well as laboratory signs such as thrombocytopenia. Because NASH is often clinically silent during the early stages, it is not uncommon to make a diagnosis of cirrhosis 'by chance', for example during gall bladder surgery. Patients may also present with complications of portal hypertension, and occasionally with acutely decompensated, but previously unrecognized, disease [37]. Gastrointestinal bleeding from GAVE (gastric antral vascular ectasia) is sometimes seen.

Other physical findings include acanthosis nigricans (pigmentation and skin thickening in the axillae and posterior neck), which is more common in children. A prominent dorsal fat pad (buffalo hump) is common and has been associated with more severe histological disease [38]. Evidence of lipodystrophy should also be sought (see below).

Laboratory testing

Elevations of serum AST (aspartate aminotransferase) and ALT (alanine aminotransferase) are usually less than two times normal [39]. However, concentrations within the reference range may be associated with significant disease [40]. Aminotransferase patterns may be helpful in staging NASH, as an AST:ALT ratio greater than 1 suggests progression to more advanced fibrosis [41]. However, this pattern appears to be less reliable in patients on thiazolidinediones or statin medications. Serum IgA levels may be mildly elevated, possibly as a result of oxidative injury and the formation of neoantigens with a biliary mucosal B cell response, as previously suggested in alcohol-related liver disease [42,43]. Hyperuricaemia is common and thought to result from abnormalities in ATP metabolism resulting in ADP accumulation and excessive purine disposal. Antinuclear antibodies are detected in 25–30% of NASH patients. The mechanism for their development is not well understood. Disorders of the thyroid have also been associated with NAFLD.

Other laboratory abnormalities include abnormal lipoprotein profiles and markers of insulin resistance or diabetes. There are no consistent patterns of dyslipidaemia although hypertriglyceridaemia is usually found. Insulin resistance can be measured by the QUICKI test (quantitative insulin sensitivity check index) or the HOMA test (homeostasis model assessment) both of which are derived from the euglycaemic hyperinsulinaemic clamp test with mathematical modelling of fasting insulin and glucose levels. A modification of the QUICKI test can also be used as a measure of insulin resistance in adipose tissue.

Mitochondriopathies and lipodystrophy

Mitochondrial abnormalities similar to those seen in primary mitochondrial diseases have been observed in NASH [30,44]. The presence of ophthalmoplegia, neurodegenerative diseases, retinopathy, neural deafness or severe lipomatosis should raise suspicion of a primary disorder. Insulin resistance and dyslipidaemia are found in conditions resulting from mitochondrial DNA mutations such as symmetrical lipomatosis or Madelung's disease and the MIDD syndrome (maternally inherited diabetes and deafness) [45,46]. The lipodystrophies are linked to insulin resistance and to NASH [47]. Focal forms of these disorders are known, but how often these occur among otherwise typical NASH patients is not established—marked sparing of the limbs in an obese individual should raise suspicion.

Epidemiology of non-alcoholic fatty liver disease

The prevalence of NAFLD is remarkably high in populations of both industrialized and developing countries, although there is variation depending on the criteria used and the population studied [20,48]. In one study of adults based on histological findings, mild to severe steatosis was shown in 70% of obese patients compared to 35% of lean patients. Steatohepatitis was found in 18.5% of obese patients, compared to 2.7% of lean patients [49]. A relatively high prevalence has also been observed in countries with typically lower BMI such as in regions of Asia [50,51]. The annual incidence of NAFLD in prospectively followed adult populations is estimated to be about 3–5% [48]. NAFLD is also well documented in children. A US autopsy study of 742 children resulted in prevalence of 9.6% [52], and was more common in boys than girls (2 : 1 ratio). Other non-histology-based population studies in the USA, Europe and Asia have shown the prevalence in children to be approximately 2–3% [53–56]. Consistent with a strong familial component, there is a high prevalence of NAFLD among the adult relatives of affected children [57].

In the primary care setting, NAFLD accounts for at least one-third of cases of suspected chronic liver disease [58]. Among patients with abnormal liver enzymes, NAFLD accounts for 40–80% of cases, with its prevalence strongly influenced by the presence of coexisting obesity, diabetes and dyslipidaemia [59]. In severely obese patients (usually defined as BMI >35 kg/m^2), the prevalence of steatosis is over 90% from series of patients undergoing bariatric surgery [60]. About one-third of these patients have NASH, two-thirds have NNFL and 2–3% of patients have NASH-related cirrhosis. In another study, NAFLD was evident in 94% of obese patients (BMI ≥30 kg/m^2), 67% of overweight patients (BMI ≥25 kg/m^2), and 25% of normal-weight individuals [61].

From another perspective, three-quarters of type 2 diabetic patients have steatosis. The coexistence of diabetes in NAFLD patients more than doubles the prevalence of cirrhosis from 10 to 25% [62,63]. Among patients with hyperlipidaemia, at least two-thirds with hypertriglyceridaemia and one-third with hypercholesterolaemia have fatty liver by ultrasound imaging [64]. Refinement of the epidemiology of NAFLD in different forms of hyperlipidaemia is needed.

Ethnic variation in non-alcoholic fatty liver disease

The relationships between obesity, diabetes, hyperlipidaemia and NAFLD are influenced by ethnicity. People of African-American descent have significantly less hepatic steatosis in spite of a relatively high prevalence of obesity and diabetes [65]. In contrast, people of Hispanic-American descent have a higher prevalence, while those of primarily northern European and Asian-American descent have an intermediate prevalence of steatosis [66,67]. Although there is a constant relationship between liver triglyceride content and intraperitoneal fat (visceral adiposity) within ethnic groups, there is a substantial degree of dissociation between insulin resistance and both steatosis and visceral adiposity in some ethnic groups [68]. This unusual situation suggests the development of different forms of the metabolic syndrome based on the hypothesis of the 'thrifty genome' in ancient human evolution [69,70]. A possible genetic basis for ethnic variation has been identified based on genetic polymorphisms of a liver-expressed transmembrane phospholipase, PNPLA3 (patatin-like phospholipase domain-containing protein 3) [71].

Familial associations

Familial clustering of NASH and NAFLD could represent inherited genetic predisposition or common environmental factors such as dietary habits or activity levels [72–74]. The finding of impaired skeletal muscle mitochondrial metabolism and insulin resistance in the offspring of patients with type 2 diabetes suggests a genetic risk related to intracellular fat metabolism [75]. In a study of fatty liver by H^1 MR spectroscopy among siblings and parents of overweight probands with and without fatty liver, steatosis was detected in 17% of siblings and 37% of parents of the overweight group *without* fatty liver compared to 59% and 78% of siblings and parents respectively in the overweight group *with* fatty liver [52]. Taken together with studies of ethnic variation, these findings suggest a strong genetic component in the development of both NAFLD in general, and NASH in particular, although it remains to be seen whether the pattern of severity also follows predictable patterns.

Pathogenesis of non-alcoholic fatty liver disease and non-alcoholic steatohepatitis

Although the mechanism of hepatocellular injury in NASH can be encapsulated in the 'two hit' hypothesis [76]—accumulation of fat followed by oxidative injury—it is increasingly evident that the mechanism involves a complex cascade of events leading to hepatocellular injury, most evident as cellular ballooning and cell death (Fig. 28.3). Studies of the ballooned cell from various perspectives lead to an emerging concept of 'multiorganelle' failure, with impairment of critical organelles and inadequate compensatory pathways. These pathways are both driven by and contribute to systemic abnormalities, especially related to insulin resistance and disturbed energy homeostasis.

Mechanisms of steatosis

Lipid accumulation in the liver results from an imbalance between overall calorie intake and systemic calorie

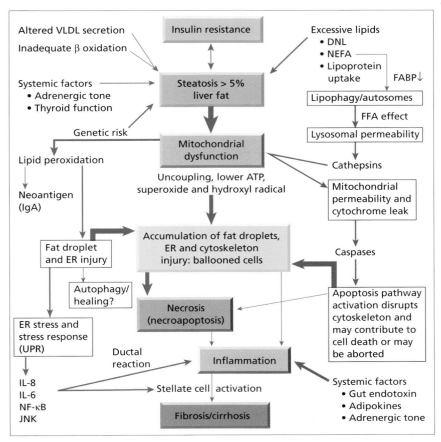

Fig. 28.3. Summary of the mechanism of non-alcoholic steatohepatitis (NASH) pathogenesis. VLDL, very low density lipoprotein; β oxidation, mitochondrial oxidation of fatty acids; DNL, *de novo* lipogenesis from carbohydrates such as glucose; NEFA, non-esterified fatty acids resulting from unrestrained lipolysis in adipose tissue. FABP is fatty acid binding protein, which is diminished in NASH (see text). FFA is free fatty acids, an excess appears to promote permeabilization of lysosomes and mitochondria with release of cathepsins and cytochrome C, inducing caspases which activate apoptosis pathways. ER is endoplasmic reticulum the dilation of which, along with accumulation of small fat droplets, contribute to cellular ballooning. UPR is the 'unfolded protein response' which defines a certain form of endoplasmic reticulum dysfunction. IL-8 and IL-6 refer to interleukins 8 and 6, which are increased in concert with JNK (c-Jun N-terminal kinase), and NF-κB (nuclear factor kappa-light-chain-enhancer of activated B cells) in the setting of ER dysfunction (see text). Ductal reaction refers to the activation of progenitor cells near the portal zones, which are likely to contribute to both portal inflammation and fibrosis. Stellate cells are the major collagen producing cells of the liver, which lead to fibrosis and eventually to cirrhosis.

utilization characteristic of the metabolic syndrome. Hepatic fat results from several possible mechanisms including synthesis of new fatty acids, especially from carbohydrate precursors (*de novo* lipogenesis), uptake of circulating free fatty acids (non-esterified fatty acids, NEFA) derived from adipose tissue lipolysis, uptake of diet-derived chylomicron remnants or uptake of very low density lipoprotein (VLDL)-derived low density lipoprotein (LDL) remnants. Liver fat can be disposed of by either oxidation or lipoprotein secretion especially as VLDL. NAFLD appears to be driven especially by NEFA uptake, *de novo* lipogenesis and altered lipid export. Recycling of lipids through the mechanisms of autophagy is an emerging aspect of pathogenesis, discussed below.

Regulation of lipid synthesis

Within the hepatocyte, lipid stores are primarily regulated by two main transcription factors: sterol regulatory element binding protein (SREBP), governed by insulin and dietary fatty acids, and carbohydrate response element binding protein (CREBP), governed by ambient glucose levels [77–79]. SREBP and CREBP stimulate nuclear transcription of the enzymes responsible for fatty acid synthesis, and subsequently their esterification into triglyceride, stored as triacylglycerides within cytosolic fat droplets, or exported as VLDL.

Biochemistry of de novo lipogenesis

At the molecular level, the synthesis of 16 carbon unsaturated palmitic acid (the initial end point of *de novo* lipogenesis), begins with translocation of carbohydrate-derived acetyl-CoA subunits as citrate, which pass through the mitochondrial membrane to the cytosol. ATP-dependent cytosolic condensation of acetyl-CoA subunits into palmitate depends on the activity of a key enzyme, acetyl CoA carboxylase, which is regulated by adrenaline (epinephrine), glucagon and insulin, and which activates formation of malonyl CoA from acetyl-CoA. Molecules of malonyl CoA then serve as the building blocks for assembly of the 16-carbon palmitic acid fatty acid, through a series of condensations catalysed by fatty acid synthase. Malonyl CoA also inhibits mitochondrial β-oxidation of fatty acids by blocking the carnitine shuttle, by which fatty acids destined for oxidation are moved into the mitochondrion.

Once formed, palmitate can undergo elongation in the endoplasmic reticulum to long-chain and very-long-chain fatty acids. Palmitate can also undergo desaturation and esterification to glycerol to form mono-, di- and triacylglycerols (triglycerides), which are incorporated into fat droplets in the endoplasmic reticulum or packaged through the activity of microsomal triglyceride transfer protein, in association with apolipoprotein B100 (apoB100), for secretion as VLDL [80].

Steatosis in humans

Based on studies using radiolabelled precursors, 59% of triglyceride synthesis in human NAFLD results from uptake of adipose-derived NEFA while *de novo* lipogenesis (driven by SREBP and CREBP) accounts for about 26% and dietary sources for 15% [81]. The high burden of NEFA appears to derive predominantly from visceral fat, and represents failure of insulin to suppress the activity of hormone-sensitive lipase at adipose stores (see insulin resistance below). Incorporation of NEFA into triglycerides and their contribution to steatosis appears from experimental work to depend on the activity of acyl CoA: diacylglycerol acyltransferase 1 (Dgat1) [82]. However, the other sources of fatty acids are also significant. Compared to normal, *de novo* lipogenesis is increased from 5 to 15–25%, and spill-over from intestinal-derived chylomicrons is increasingly recognized, and may also be a source of additional oxidative stress [83–85].

Opposing the accumulation of liver fat, VLDL secretion is increased in NAFLD but plateaus at a hepatic triglyceride content of 10%, indicating limited compensation for high circulating NEFA [86]. Moreover, the secretion of apoB100, a key component of normal VLDL, is impaired in human NAFLD and may correlate with the secretion of a larger VLDL particle with greater triglyceride relative to its apoB100 content [28,87].

Mitochondrial dysfunction

The accumulation of lipids in the liver is associated with an energy deficient state evidenced as diminished ATP content. This was shown experimentally over 50 years ago [88]. More recently, deficient hepatic ATP synthesis following intravenous fructose challenge in human NAFLD using ^{31}P MR spectroscopy has been shown [89]. The mitochondria appear to be both a target and a source of pro-oxidant free radicals (superoxide and hydroxyl radicals) the effects of which are key distinguishing features of NASH, as opposed to NNFL [90,91]. Mitochondrial morphological changes are readily evident in human NASH and include swelling and intramitochondrial crystals (Fig. 28.4). The crystalline structures appear to be phase transitions of cristae phospholipid bilayers [92].

Impaired function of the mitochondrial electron transport chain has been observed in both animal and human studies. It is due in part to over-expression of uncoupling protein and to dysfunction of components of the electron transport chain [93,94]. Electron transport chain activity is reduced to 40–70% of normal in all of the major complexes (I–V) in human NASH [95]. Although impairment of oxidative phosphorylation is evident, it is uncertain whether or not, overall net fatty acid oxidation is decreased or increased—some studies document a surprising net increase in mitochondrial β-oxidation [30,96]. A clearer consensus exists regarding changes in mitochondrial permeability, leading to release of mitochondrial cytochrome c and apoptosis signalling, as discussed below [97]. Increased mitochondrial cholesterol has been proposed as a mechanism contributing to mitochondrial dysfunction and associated changes in permeability [98,99].

Lipid composition in non-alcoholic fatty liver disease

Fat composition studies in NAFLD showed that most of the stored lipid is composed of triglyceride, with a lesser component of free fatty acids, although both were significantly increased compared to normal subjects [100]. Both macro- and microvesicular fat droplets are present in NAFLD, although smaller droplets are often less evident by conventional light microscopy without either specific fat stains (such as oil red O) or by osmium fixed specimens for electron microscopy. Recent lipidomic analysis of liver tissue in human NAFLD have shown significant differences in NASH versus NNFL [101].

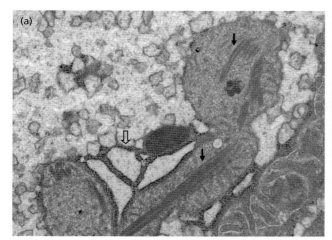

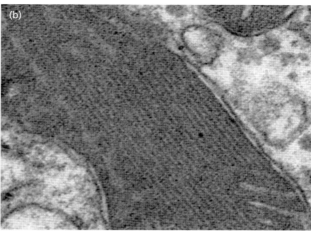

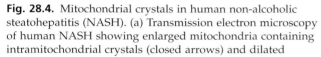

Fig. 28.4. Mitochondrial crystals in human non-alcoholic steatohepatitis (NASH). (a) Transmission electron microscopy of human NASH showing enlarged mitochondria containing intramitochondrial crystals (closed arrows) and dilated endoplasmic reticulum (open arrows). (b) Closer view of a mitochondrion containing intramitochondrial crystals (see text).

Stepwise increases in both triacylglycerol:diacylglycerol and free cholesterol:phosphotidylcholine ratios were noted from normal to NNFL to NASH subjects. Polyunsaturated fatty acids, such as eicosapentanoic acid and docosahexanoic acid, were relatively lower in NASH, leading to an elevated N6:N3 ratio, suggesting a relative excess of proinflammatory N6 fatty acids such as arachidonic acid. Interestingly, the level of hepatic free fatty acids, although higher compared to controls, were not different in NASH versus NNFL—this is another unresolved point of controversy (see below). Increased ceramide, a potentially toxic intermediary in sphingolipid metabolism, in peripheral white adipose tissue has been detected in obese patients with fatty liver versus those without [102].

Lipid peroxidation in non-alcoholic steatohepatitis

Ample evidence in humans indicates that cellular injury in a lipid-loaded hepatocyte is initiated by impaired control of aerobic metabolism resulting in oxidative stress and lipid peroxidation [103–107]. Although cytochrome p450 (ω-oxidation) or peroxisomal fatty acid oxidation may contribute to free radical formation, the superoxide radical is primarily derived from mitochondria. Once formed, it is metabolized via superoxide dismutase to hydrogen peroxide. Hydroxyl radicals result from decay of hydrogen peroxide, in the presence of Fe^{2+} via the Fenton or Haber–Weiss reactions. Unless detoxified by glutathione, hydroxyl radicals damage other cellular constituents, including membrane fatty acids, proteins and DNA through direct binding [108]. Injury to the fatty acids produces lipid peroxidation—a branching, chain reaction stimulated by a free radical attack on unsaturated fatty acids which produces another free radical and a lipid hydroperoxide. The latter degrades in a reaction catalysed by iron to form a second lipid-based free radical thus amplifying the process [109]. Oxidative injury to the phospholipid monolayer of small fat droplets, which contain insulin-sensitive lipases (PAT family proteins), and to the endoplasmic reticulum may be particularly relevant to development of cellular ballooning, impaired disposal of toxic free fatty acids and hepatic insulin resistance [105,110,111]. Other by-products of oxidative injury include metabolites of nitric oxide, particularly in macrophages, and neoantigen formation, which may explain a link to serum IgA elevation discussed earlier.

Autophagy, lysosomes, fatty acid induced injury and apoptosis

Disposal of accumulated and presumably injured fat droplets involves the process of lysosome-mediated autophagy (Fig. 28.5) [112,113]. Recent experimental work, mostly involving animal models or cell cultures, has indicated the relative stability of fat stored as triglycerides, compared to the potential toxicity of free fatty acids [114]. Impaired autophagy of small fat droplets, as well as diminished fatty acid binding protein shown in one human study, may contribute to accumulation of free fatty acids and cellular lipotoxicity [115]. Polymorphisms of the enzyme responsible for formation of triglycerides from diglycerides (Dgat or acyl-CoA: diacylglycerol acyltransferase) could also contribute to impaired disposal of free fatty acids [116]. Free fatty acids, in turn, alter lysosomal permeability leading to release of cathepsins (lysosomal proteases),

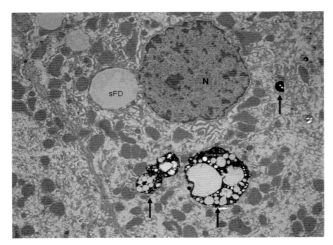

Fig. 28.5. Autophagosomes (arrows) containing ingested small fat droplets (sFD) in human NASH. N, nucleus.

which are associated with changes in mitochondrial permeability [117]. In cell culture models, this contributes to release of mitochondrial cytochrome C which activates caspases, leading to further activation of proapoptosis pathways, which are evident in human NASH [118,119]. Accumulation of palmitic acid has also been shown in cell culture to stimulate release of interleukin-8 from hepatocytes [120].

Endoplasmic reticulum stress, activation of inflammation, fibrosis and cell death

While final cell death may result from some combination of necrosis and apoptosis (necroapoptosis) [121], the activation of caspase 3 leads to fragmentation of cytokeratin 18. This is likely to contribute to formation of Mallory–Denk bodies, seen best in ballooned hepatocytes, and to cytokeratin 18 fragments detectable in blood [24,122]. Accumulation of free fatty acids and impaired function of endoplasmic reticulum (ER)-associated ApoB100 (an essential lipoprotein in ER-based VLDL synthesis) also contribute to ER stress with an accumulation of misfolded proteins within the ER [123,124]. ER stress, along with accumulation of free fatty acids and cell death, induce proinflammatory cytokines such as interleukin 8, through activation of transcription factors such as nuclear factor kappaB (NF-κB) and c-Jun N-terminal kinase (JNK) [120]. Importantly, this pathway appears to be active in human forms of the disease; the degree of activation of JNK related to ER stress distinguishes NASH from NNFL in human studies [125,126]. Modulation of this pathway also appears to improve antioxidant status in animal models [127]. Ultimately, activity in these pathways leads to accumulation of inflammatory infiltrates and activation of collagen-producing hepatic stellate cells (usually in

close association with cellular ballooning) characterized by transition from a vitamin A rich quiescent cell to a proliferating myofibroblast [128]. Activation of collagen-producing stellate cells is mediated, at least in part, by activation of the Toll-like receptor [129]. Progression of fibrosis may also depend on an altered repair process with impaired hepatocyte replication and increased activity of hepatic progenitor cells leading to a ductular reaction in the portal tracts [130].

The ballooned cell

Morphologically, the ballooned hepatocyte, identifiable by deficiency of intact cytokeratin [131], is most clearly associated with active steatohepatitis in human NASH. It consists of an accumulation of multiple, small fat droplets in association with distorted mitochondria, dilated ER and Mallory–Denk bodies, supporting a close link between each of these processes (Figs 28.6, 28.7). Because multiple pathways are undergoing simultaneous failure, the process can be described as multiorganelle failure. In this setting, the final event is most likely to be necrosis, although activation of apoptotic pathways plays a substantial role. This course is the likely explanation for the characteristic appearance of histological necrosis concurrent with activation of apoptosis leading to necroapoptosis.

Systemic factors

Hepatic fat is regulated by other systems involved with energy homeostasis including insulin/glucagon, the adipose organ, the adrenergic system and the thyroid axis. The demonstration of cold-activated brown adipose tissue in healthy men and its inverse relationship to obesity emphasizes the integration of energy management and thermoregulatory systems [132]. Adipose-derived cytokines and adipocytokines (such as adiponectin) play a role through modulation of insulin activity and the inflammatory response to fatty acid-induced injury. Noradrenergic modulation of the inflammatory infiltrate has also been demonstrated in animal models [133]. In human NAFLD, hepatic and extrahepatic insulin resistance is present in the majority of patients and is virtually inseparable from the pathophysiology of the disease.

Insulin resistance is primarily mediated by excessive free fatty acids and occurs in multiple insulin end-organs including adipose, skeletal muscle and the liver (Table 28.3) [30,134,135]. At the molecular level, insulin resistance is characterized by a shift from tyrosine phosphorylation in the insulin receptor substrate to serine phosphorylation, which blunts the anabolic effects of insulin in multiple downstream pathways, including both *metabolic pathways* (mediated by phosphatidyli-

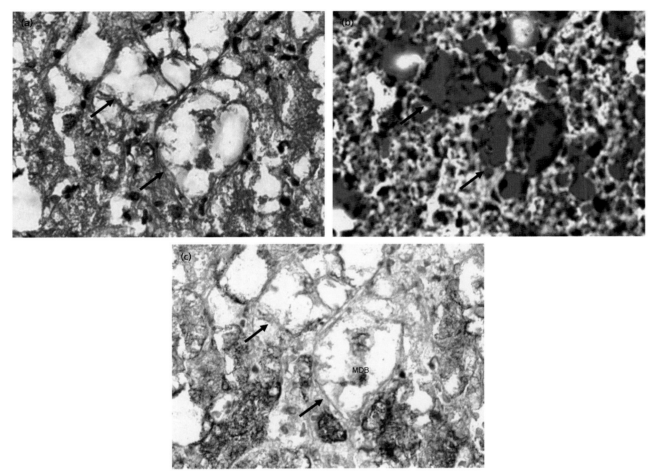

Fig. 28.6. Fat droplet accumulation and cytoskeletal injury in human non-alcoholic steatohepatitis (NASH). Serial images of (a) haematoxylin and eosin (H&E), (b) oil red O and (c) keratin 18 immunohistochemical (IHC) staining in human NASH. Arrows indicate ballooned cells detected by H&E and then by a fat stain using oil red O, showing accumulation of fat droplets, and then by IHC for cytokeratin 18 showing a deficiency of K18 and highlighting of a Mallory–Denk body (MDB; see text) indicating significant cytoskeletal injury. Lipid peroxidation is thought to underlie these processes.

nositol 3-kinase or PI 3-kinase, Akt, mTOR) and *mitogenic pathways* (mediated by Ras, Raf and mitogen-activated protein or MAP-kinase) pathways.

A complex set of interacting factors influence the shift from tyrosine to serine phosphorylation in the insulin receptor substrate. Inflammatory changes in adipose tissue, especially visceral stores, contribute to production of systemically active cytokines [136]. This process appears to be initiated by JNK activation, as a result of ER stress in the adipose tissue itself [137]. Resulting systemic tumour necrosis factor-α (TNF-α) and interleukins 6 and 8 have been implicated in insulin resistance through their effects on a modulator of cytokine activity known as SOCS (suppressor of cytokine signalling), which promotes a shift to serine phosphorylation in the insulin receptor substrate [138]. Changes in small bowel permeability also appear to contribute to activation of proinflammatory mediators through exposure to bacterial substances such as endotoxin [33]. The latter may partly explain the previously reported association between coeliac disease and NAFLD due to increased gut permeability in coeliac disease [139,140]. Adipose-derived adipokines, including adiponectin, leptin, resistin and visfatin, further modulate insulin signalling. Depressed production of adiponectin has a dominant role in NAFLD, as a result of diminished insulin-sensitizing effects when this substance declines. Normally, adiponectin binds to specific receptors to activate AMP kinase and promotes fatty acid oxidation in skeletal muscle and liver [141]. Increased production of adiponectin is one mechanism by which thiazolidinediones are thought to favourably affect NAFLD (see below). The newly described adipose-derived 'lipokines' such as C16:1n7-palmitoleate have also been

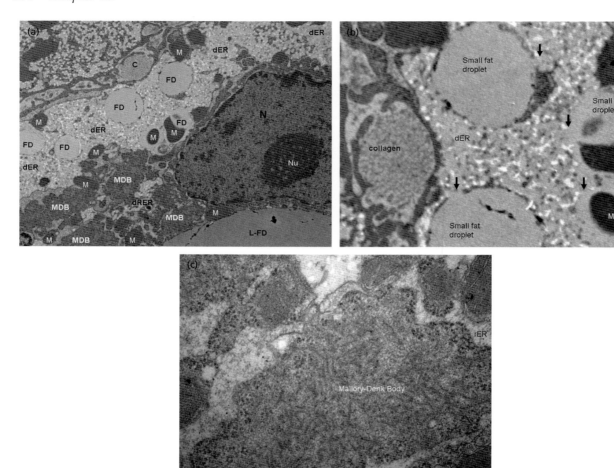

Fig. 28.7. Transmission electron microscopy in non-alcoholic steatohepatitis (NASH). (a) A closer view of a damaged hepatocyte shows: accumulation of fat droplets (FD) and a large fat droplet (L-FD); Mallory–Denk body (MDB), which represents collapse of the cytoskeleton; an extracellular bundle of collagen (C) as a marker of fibrosis; mitochondria (M) and dilated endoplasmic reticulum (dER) and rough endoplasmic reticulum (dRER). (b) Closer view of the fat droplets and associated endoplasmic reticulum dilation from the same sample. (c) Closer view of the MDB from the same sample.

proposed as modulators of liver fat content and muscle insulin activity [142].

The natural history of non-alcoholic fatty liver disease (non-alcoholic steatohepatitis and non-NASH fatty liver)

The contrasting clinical course of NASH versus NNFL indicates that these two conditions diverge early in the course of NAFLD although some patients probably transition from NNFL to NASH. Progression to cirrhosis is usually preceded by longstanding histological NASH and is infrequent in NNFL. In contrast, the risk for hepatocellular cancer appears to extend across both NASH and NNFL albeit less so in the latter [143,144]. NASH fibrosis staging is shown in Table 28.4.

Table 28.4. Fibrosis staging in non-alcoholic steatohepatitis

Stage 1: Pericentral vein or sinusoidal fibrosis (Zone 3)
Stage 2: Sinusoidal (Zone 3) and periportal fibrosis (Zone 1)
Stage 3: Bridging fibrosis between Zone 3 and Zone 1
Stage 4: Cirrhosis
NASH with cirrhosis
Cirrhosis with features suggestive of NASH
Non-specific (cryptogenic) cirrhosis

NASH, non-alcoholic steatohepatitis.

Cross-sectional and longitudinal histological studies

Cross-sectional, population-based, liver biopsy studies have demonstrated that older age, higher BMI, diabetes mellitus and abnormal aminotransferases are predictive of more severe histological injury in the initial diagnostic biopsies [145–147]. Longitudinal studies with serial

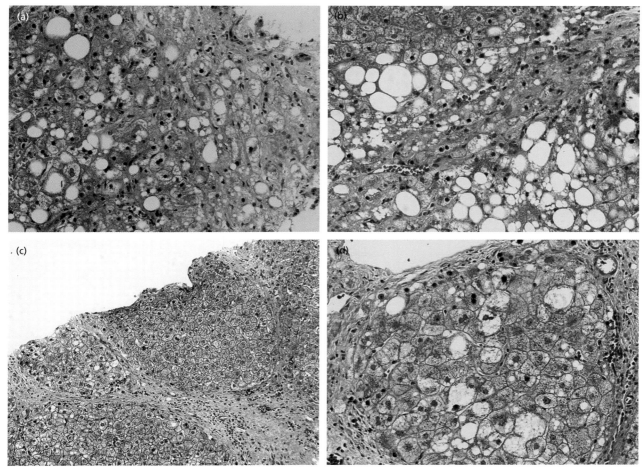

Fig. 28.8. Progression of non-alcoholic steatohepatitis (NASH) to cirrhosis. (a,b) Biopsies from 2004 from a 36-year-old female with obesity and type 2 diabetes who presented for evaluation with mild but persistent abnormal liver enzymes (see this patient's ultrasound from 2004, Fig. 28.1). The patient's mother previously passed away from cryptogenic cirrhosis. (c,d) Biopsy from the same patient in 2009. Note the overall loss of macrosteatosis (c) but the persistence of mild steatosis and ballooning in some cirrhotic nodules (d). This patient has progressed from NASH to a picture of 'cryptogenic cirrhosis' over 5 years. The strong family history is also characteristic of this disorder.

biopsies have shown that about one-third of NASH patients develop advanced fibrosis (stage 3 or 4 fibrosis) over 5–10 years from the time of the initial diagnosis (Fig. 28.8) [148]. Histological improvement is also seen in some patients, possibly due to adoption of lifestyle changes (exercise and diet) although progression occurs more frequently than improvement (38 versus 21%).

As fibrosis progresses, aminotransferases often decrease along with steatosis scores. Thus, it is not unusual for patients with cirrhosis to have aminotransferases within the normal reference range. Although usually relatively slow, progression to cirrhosis can occur in as little as 2–3 years [149]. Among patients diagnosed with NASH-related cirrhosis, the risk of developing a major complication of portal hypertension is 17, 23 and 52% at 1, 3 and 10 years, respectively [150]. A review of longitudinal, biopsy-based, natural history studies has shown that progression to advanced fibrosis was associated with age at the time of diagnosis and the degree of inflammation on the initial biopsy [148]. Although lobular inflammation was thought to be relatively more important, portal inflammation may be a marker for more advanced injury [151].

Outcomes and long-term survival

Clinical outcomes in NASH are strongly influenced by comorbid conditions associated with metabolic syndrome. As with the risk of developing cirrhosis, overall mortality diverges between NNFL and NASH. Existing long-term studies show several consistent patterns which impact on overall patient management. A compilation of available studies (Table 28.5) [152–155], shows that among patients with early stage NASH, overall

Table 28.5. Mortality outcomes in non-alcoholic fatty liver disease

	Adams 2005 [152]	Ekstedt 2006 [153]		Ong 2008 [154]	Rafiq 2009 [155]	
	NAFLD	NASH	NNFL	NAFLD	NASH	NNFL
Number	435	71	58	817	57	74
Age at diagnosis	49 ± 15	55 ± 12	47 ± 12	NC	54 ± 12	53 ± 25
Follow up (years)	7.6 ± 4	13.7 ± 1.3	13.7 ± 1.3	8.4	10.5 (median)	13 (median)
Deaths (total):	53 (12.6%)	19 (26.7%)	7 (12%)	80 (9.7%)	78 (45.1%)	
CAD	13 (2.9%)	11 (15.5%)	5 (8.6%)	20 (2.4 %)	7 (12.3)	15 (20.3)
Cancer	15 (3.4%)	4 (5.6%)	1 (1.7%)	19 (2.3 %)	5 (8.8)	9 (12.2)
Live	7 (1.6%)	2 (2.8%)	0	5 (0.6%)	10 (17.5%)	2 (2.7%)

Mortality studies of NAFLD consistently show an increased risk of liver-related death, but recent studies have also shown an increased risk for cardiovascular mortality compared to the general population. Ekstedt *et al.* showed that NASH patients have a 10 times increased risk of liver-related death, but also a two times increased risk of CAD-related mortality. Ong *et al.* and Rafiq *et al.* have shown a similarly increased level of risk for liver-related death in NASH.
NAFLD, non-alcoholic fatty liver disease referred to in this chapter as NNFL to indicate non-NASH fatty liver; NASH, non-alcoholic steatohepatitis; CAD, coronary artery disease; NC, not collected.

mortality over 10–15 years is about 10–12%, being significantly higher in NASH versus NNFL, compared to the general population. The risk of developing decompensated cirrhosis is 5–10% and for hepatocellular cancer it is 1–2%. There is a tenfold risk of cirrhosis relative to the general population. However, the leading causes of death in these studies were coronary artery disease (10%), extrahepatic malignancy (5%) and cirrhosis-related death (2%).

These results provide several clinical challenges. First, predicting those patients more likely to die from cirrhosis-related causes is essential to refine therapy but remains unresolved. Secondly, because the occurrence of cirrhosis is very much more common than liver-related death, many patients with NASH survive with coexisting cirrhosis and coronary disease and/or malignancy. Thus, the impact of anticoagulation following coronary stenting or the risks of surgical or pharmacological interventions in cancer is likely to be substantial. Finally, current outcomes studies reflect patient cohorts recruited in the 1980s and 1990s, and so may not reflect the effects of the burgeoning obesity epidemic and increasing prevalence of NAFLD in children.

Cryptogenic cirrhosis

The progression of NASH to a late stage of cirrhosis occurs with loss of the hallmark steatosis [3]. Epidemiological studies have shown that most patients with cryptogenic cirrhosis had significantly greater risks for NASH (obesity and diabetes) compared to control populations [4,5]. The association between NASH and cryptogenic cirrhosis has also been documented in post-transplantation studies (examining occurrence of NASH

in patients transplanted for cryptogenic cirrhosis) and more recently in 'look-back' histological studies [6,156] in which there are histological markers characteristic of prior NASH.

In past series, most patients with cryptogenic cirrhosis were female, about 60 years old, with a history of obesity and type 2 diabetes and minimal liver enzyme abnormalities [157]. The preponderance of females in these series probably represents attrition of males due to the greater burden of coronary vascular disease. There is often a history of fatty liver by imaging or histological NASH. However, loss of body fat in advanced cirrhosis can substantially obscure past obesity, which must be specifically sought in the history [158]. The mechanism of fat loss is uncertain, but may relate to changes in sinusoidal blood flow, lipoprotein metabolism or some more fundamental change in cellular metabolism. Hepatocellular cancer in this group tends to be diagnosed at a later stage, possibly due to inadequate surveillance [159].

Therapy of non-alcoholic fatty liver disease

Treatment trials of NASH may be influenced by lifestyle changes ranging from subtle changes in dietary composition, to improved physical conditioning *without* weight loss, to frank weight loss. These variables can spuriously obscure or enhance drug effects, if not adequately controlled for, and are likely to contribute to a strong placebo effect in pharmacological trials. Patient selection and stratification, endpoints of treatment and the relative risk–benefit of different interventions are among other challenging aspects of different treatment strategies.

Liver biopsy remains the gold standard for both defining populations at greatest risk for progression to cirrhosis (those with baseline NASH) and the best endpoint to define resolution. Composite surrogate markers, such as non-invasive measures of liver fat, fibrosis and cell injury, are emerging as potential alternatives. Because NASH is part of a systemic disease, endpoints of treatment may also include systemic markers such as indices of insulin resistance or adipocytokine production. Subset stratification based on predominant lipoprotein profiles (relative to apoB metabolism), cardiovascular risks or polymorphisms of key pathways such as local antioxidant mechanisms have yet to be adequately studied.

Exercise, calorie reduction and weight loss

NAFLD can be treated, at least in early stages, by conservative approaches such as dietary weight loss and increased physical conditioning. Two controlled trials of dietary weight loss with exercise in both adults and paediatric patients using histological endpoints demonstrated improved steatosis, inflammation and cell injury [160,161]. Less therapeutic effect was seen if fibrosis was present, but the short follow up may have limited the observation of a beneficial effect. Drastic calorie restriction can lead to decreased liver fat in as little as 11 weeks but this approach is not sustainable long term. Most common diet plans appear to be effective in achieving weight loss and the choice should be individualized [162]. Orlistat has some benefit in augmenting weight loss but does not offer a significant advantage overall [163,164].

The amount of weight loss and the frequency/ intensity of exercise needed to produce these effects is uncertain, but 10–15% weight reduction causes liver fat to dissipate [165]. Using waist circumference as a surrogate marker for visceral adiposity, more frequent and intense exercise is better [166]. Structured exercise programmes with professional contact also offer advantages [167]. Sustained exercise can improve glucose disposal in the mitochondria of skeletal muscle, which is known to be impaired in diabetes [168,169]. Exercise without weight loss can also alter hepatic histology [170–172]. This relationship supports the concept of the 'fit fat'—an important point to make with patients who may be discouraged if exercise doesn't produce quick weight loss [173,174]. Exercise testing to measure oxygen consumption or lactate levels (as a marker of the shift to anaerobic metabolism) can be useful tools in assessing this aspect of NAFLD but are not widely available.

Dietary composition

Some changes in dietary composition can be achieved with relatively little effort. For example, elimination of the high fructose corn syrup in sweetened beverages may be of benefit, as this sweetener in equal calorie amounts predisposes to accumulation of triglyceride in the liver of animals and humans [175–178]. Dietary histories in NASH patients suggest a deficit of the omega-3 fatty acids, and human lipidomic data has shown a high N6–N3 ratio in NASH liver samples suggesting that supplementation with omega-3 fatty acids may be of benefit [101,179].

Pharmacological intervention

Compliance with lifestyle recommendations is often limited. Pharmacological intervention could be considered in patients with active and potentially progressive disease who fail such measures. However, to date no specific pharmacological agent has been shown to be beneficial in treating NASH. Drugs can be categorized as cytoprotective and antioxidant, insulin-sensitizing, modulators of fat metabolism and more specific modulators of specific intracellular pathways.

Cytoprotective agents and antioxidants

Ursodeoxycholic acid (UDCA) is a tertiary bile acid, first tested in an early placebo-controlled trial in NASH [180]. Using about 15 mg/kg, similar improvements in aminotransferases, weight loss and histological parameters were seen in both treated groups, indicating no benefit. However changes in dietary composition and activity levels were not accounted for. A combination of UDCA and vitamin E supplements compared to double placebo, or vitamin E and placebo, showed reduction in steatosis, but no other improvement in other histological parameters in the end-of-treatment biopsies [181]. Another controlled study using UDCA at 30 mg/kg awaits full publication (Ratziu V, unpublished data). However another recent study using higher dose UDCA did not show clear benefit [182]. Taurine conjugates of UDCA have also undergone preliminary studies. Encouraging work with betaine (which replenishes glutathione stores and promotes secretion of fat as VLDL), S-adenosylmethionine and combination vitamin E and C have been reported [183–184]. A recent controlled trial showed positive results with high dose vitamin E (800 IU/day) compared with pioglitazone [185].

Insulin sensitizers

These have been the most promising pharmacological intervention in NASH. Pilot studies of metformin have had variable results although there may be a role in children (now in study) [186–188]. In contrast, the thiazolidinediones have resulted in a more consistent reduction in steatosis, inflammation and cell injury, but not fibrosis [189–198]. These agents, which act on the PPARγ receptor especially in adipose tissue, result in a shift of fat from the liver to the periphery, although the exact mechanism is uncertain. Mitochondrial changes suggest the occurrence of increased fatty acid oxidation as part of the effect [199]. Pioglitazone is the most consistently effective agent, although peripheral (adipose) weight gain is a significant problem with all of the thiazolidinediones. Weight gain can be significant and short courses are not effective; both problems are avoidable if increased exercise and dietary changes can be sustained during thiazolidinedione administration [200,201].

Lipid-modulating drugs

Despite the association of NASH and hyperlipidaemia, less is known about the role of fibrates (PPARα agonists favouring fatty acid oxidation) and statins (HMG CoA reductase inhibitors) in treating NASH. Fibrates were among the first agents to be tried with promising results. Prospective trials with histological endpoints have been conducted but await publication (Conjeevarum H, unpublished results).

Statins have only been studied using histological endpoints in small, uncontrolled studies and in only one controlled trial which lacked histological data. However, several consistent points have emerged from the literature [202]. First, in statin-treated NASH patients, the serum aminotransferases are not reliable indices to assess drug-induced benefit or injury. Minor fluctuations of the aminotransferases should not lead to stopping statin agents. Secondly, there may be a subpopulation of patients who have histological improvement, and also another group with increased risk of progressing to advanced fibrosis (stage 3 or 4 on biopsy). In a long-term observational study, steatosis and the mean fibrosis score decreased in a statin-treated cohort, but the percentage of patients with advanced stages of fibrosis increased in the statin-treated group [203]. However, a recent controlled trial showed no benefit from 12 months of simvastatin [204].

Other pharmacological agents

These include agents that modulate the angiotensin pathway (angiotensin receptor blockers) such as telmisartan, agents aimed at the grehlin–leptin (satiety) pathway, antiplatelet agents aimed at blocking profibrotic factors, agents which modulate ER stress, adenosine receptor blockers and TNF antagonists including pentoxifylline [205,206].

Bariatric surgery

Various forms of weight-reduction surgery ameliorate parameters of the metabolic syndrome, including NASH [207,208]. Surgery is usually reserved for severe obesity (BMI >40) or the presence of comorbidities such as sleep apnoea with BMI over 35. Portal hypertension in late-stage NASH (stage 3–4) increases operative risk as does advancing age, so that use of surgery requires an individual assessment of the risk–benefit balance.

Liver transplantation

The outcome of liver transplantation for NASH-related liver disease is difficult to interpret due to variation in nomenclature between institutions and overlap with cryptogenic cirrhosis. However, several studies have documented increased morbidity especially related to comorbidities such as obesity and diabetes [209,210]. One-year survival is as low as 50% in patients who are 60 years old or older with a BMI at or above 30, and a history of diabetes and hypertension [211]. Recurrence of NAFLD and NASH following transplantation for both NASH-cirrhosis and cryptogenic cirrhosis (see section on cryptogenic cirrhosis) is also well-documented and can be progressive [212–215].

Other forms of non-alcoholic fatty liver

NAFLD can be seen in a number of conditions where other mechanisms are involved although overlap with metabolic syndrome may be seen. For example, liver disease with steatosis is one of the most common and potentially severe side effects of total parenteral nutrition [216]. The amount and composition of the lipid infusion are related to the development of liver disease in this setting [217]. At the opposite end of the spectrum, severe fatty liver due to impaired lipoprotein synthesis is seen in the protein malnutrition of kwashiorkor [218].

Drug-induced forms of fatty liver disease are also well known. Liver toxicity due to methotrexate has many histological features in common with NASH and may represent an exacerbation of an underlying NASH-like process [219]. An acquired lipodystrophy with insulin resistance and potentially progressive steatohepatitis can also be seen in HIV-infected subjects in association with drug therapy (especially with stavudine and didanosine) [220]. Mitochondrial toxicity appears to play a significant role in this disorder [221]. Industrial substances have also been implicated in a form of toxin-associated steatohepatitis, which may be progressive and is reported to be independent of insulin resistance in some cases [222].

Steatosis can also be seen in a variety of inherited metabolic diseases including Wilson's disease (often with features of steatohepatitis), and childhood disorders such as glycogen storage diseases, galactosaemia, tyrosinaemia, hypobetalipoproteinaemia, abetalipoproteinaemia and the lipid storage diseases (cholesterol

Table 28.6. Other forms of non-alcoholic fatty liver disease (secondary non-alcoholic fatty liver disease)

Specific conditions associated with fatty liver
Lipodystrophies
Primary mitochondrial diseases
Weber–Christian disease
Wilson's disease
Bariatric surgery (weight loss surgery)
Jejunoileal bypass (no longer used)
Nutrition related disorders
Total parenteral nutrition
Kwashiorkor
Coeliac sprue
Medications
Amiodarone
Methotrexate
Nucleoside analogues (HAART, chemotherapy agents)
Tamoxifen
Toxins
Carbon tetrachloride (CCl_4)—fire extinguishers, refrigerants, dry cleaning pre-1940
Ethyl bromide (EtBr)—organic chemistry solvent
Perchloroethylene (C_2Cl_4)—dry cleaning, degreasing in automotive uses, paint stripping
Various petrochemicals

HAART, highly active antiretroviral therapy.

ester storage, Niemann–Pick, Tay–Sachs and Gaucher's disease), which reveal excessive fatty infiltration of the liver with cholesterol esters, sphingolipids, phospholipids, sphingomyelin, gangliosides or glucocerebrosides. The distribution of fat (predominantly in reticuloendothelial cells) and typical presentation in infancy (although not exclusively so) distinguish the lipid storage disorders from NAFLD/NASH (Table 28.6).

References

1 Zelman S. The liver in obesity. *Arch. Intern. Med.* 1958; **90**: 141–156.
2 Ludwig J, Viggiano TR, McGill DB, Ott BJ. Nonalcoholic steatohepatitis: Mayo Clinic experiences with a hitherto unnamed disease. *Mayo Clin. Proc.* 1980; **55**: 434–438.
3 Powell EE, Cooksley WG, Hanson R *et al.* The natural history of nonalcoholic steatohepatitis: a follow-up study of forty-two patients for up to 21 years. *Hepatology* 1990; **11**: 74–80.
4 Caldwell SH, Oelsner DH, Iezzoni JC *et al.* Cryptogenic cirrhosis: clinical characterization and risk factors for underlying disease. *Hepatology* 1999; **29**: 664–669.
5 Poonawala A, Nair SP, Thuluvath PJ. Prevalence of obesity and diabetes in patients with cryptogenic cirrhosis: A case-control study. *Hepatology* 2000; **32**: 689–692.
6 Maheshwari A, Thuluvath PJ. Cryptogenic cirrhosis and NAFLD: Are they related? *Am. J. Gastroenterol.* 2006; **101**: 664–668.
7 Teli MR, James OFW, Burt AD *et al.* The natural history of nonalcoholic fatty liver: A followup study. *Hepatology* 1995; **22**: 1714–1719.
8 Matteoni CA, Younossi ZM, Gramlich T *et al.* Nonalcoholic fatty liver disease: A spectrum of clinical and pathological severity. *Gastroenterology* 1999; **116**: 1413–1419.
9 Baumeister SE, Völzke H, Marschall P *et al.* Impact of fatty liver disease on health care utilization and costs in a general population: a 5-year observation. *Gastroenterology* 2008; **134**: 85–94.
10 Saadeh S, Younossi ZM, Remer EM *et al.* The utility of radiological imaging in nonalcoholic fatty liver disease. *Gastroenterology* 2002; **123**: 745–750.
11 Kovanlikaya A, Guclu C, Desai D *et al.* Fat Quantification Using Three-point Dixon Technique: In Vitro Validation. *Acad. Radiol.* 2005; **12**: 636–639.
12 Cassidy FH, Yokoo T, Aganovic L *et al.* Fatty liver disease: MR imaging techniques for the detection and quantification of liver steatosis. *Radiographics* 2009; **29**: 231–260.
13 Dunn W, Xu R, Schwimmer JB. Modest wine drinking and decreased prevalence of suspected nonalcoholic fatty liver disease. *Hepatology* 2008; **47**: 1947–1954.
14 Naveau S, Giraud V, Borotto E *et al.* Excess weight risk factor for alcoholic liver disease. *Hepatology* 1997; **25**: 108–111.
15 Hayashi PH, Harrison SA, Torgerson S *et al.* Cognitive lifetime drinking history in nonalcoholic fatty liver disease: some cases may be alcohol related. *Am. J. Gastroenterol.* 2004; **99**: 76–81.
16 Brunt EM, Janney CG, Di Bisceglie AM *et al.* Nonalcoholic steatohepatitis: A proposal for grading and staging the histologic lesions. *Am. J. Gastroenterol.* 1999; **94**: 2467–2474.
17 De la Hall MP, Kirsch R. Pathology of hepatic steatosis, NASH and related conditions. In: Farrell GC, George J, Hall MP de la, McCullough AJ, eds. *Fatty Liver Disease: NASH and Related Disorders*. Malden, MA: Blackwell Publishing, 2005, p. 13–22.
18 Yeh MM, Brunt EM. Pathology of nonalcoholic fatty liver disease. *Am. J. Clin. Pathol.* 2007; **128**: 837–847.
19 Kleiner DE, Brunt EM, Van Natta ML *et al.* Nonalcoholic Steatohepatitis Clinical Research Network. Design and validation of a histologic scoring system for NAFLD. *Hepatology* 2005; **41**: 1313–1321.
20 Argo CK, Caldwell SH. Epidemiology and natural history of non-alcoholic steatohepatitis. *Clin. Liver Dis.* 2009; **13**: 511–531.
21 Ratziu V, Charlotte F, Heurtier A *et al.* LIDO Study Group. Sampling variability of liver biopsy in nonalcoholic fatty liver disease. *Gastroenterology* 2005; **125**: 1898–1906.
22 Malik R, Chang M, Killimangalam B *et al.* The clinical utility of biomarkers and the nonalcoholic steatohepatitis CRN liver biopsy scoring system in patients with

nonalcoholic fatty liver disease. *J. Gastrol. Hepatol.* 2009; **24**: 564–568.

23 Younossi ZM, Jarrar M, Nugent C *et al.* A novel diagnostic biomarker panel for obesity-related nonalcoholic steatohepatitis (NASH). *Obes. Surg.* 2008; **18**: 1430–1437.

24 Feldstein AE, Wieckowska A, Lopez AR *et al.* Cytokeratin-18 fragment levels as noninvasive biomarkers for nonalcoholic steatohepatitis: A multicenter validation study. *Hepatology* 2009; **50**: 1072–1078.

25 Marchesini G, Bugianesi E, Forlani G *et al.* Nonalcoholic fatty liver, steatohepatitis, and the metabolic syndrome. *Hepatology* 2003; **37**: 917–923.

26 Nguyen-Duy T-B, Nichaman MZ, Church TS *et al.* Visceral and liver fat are independent predictors of metabolic risk factors in men. *Am. J. Physiol. Endocrinol. Metab.* 2003; **284**: E1065–E1071.

27 Machado M, Cortez-Pinto H. Non-alcoholic steatohepatitis and metabolic syndrome. *Curr. Opin. Clin. Nutr. Metab. Care* 2006; **9**: 637–642.

28 Fabbrini E, Magkos F, Mohammed BS *et al.* Intrahepatic fat, not visceral fat, is linked with metabolic complications of obesity. *PNAS* 2009; **106**: 15430–15435.

29 Taylor R. Causation of type 2 diabetes–the Gordian knot unravels. *N. Engl. J. Med.* 2004; **350**: 639–641.

30 Sanyal AJ, Campbell-Sargent C, Mirshahi F *et al.* Nonalcoholic steatohepatitis: Association of insulin resistance and mitochondrial abnormalities. *Gastroenterology* 2001; **120**: 1183–1192.

31 Wildman RP, Munter P, Reynolds K *et al.* The obese without cardiometabolic risk factor clustering and the normal weight with cardiometabolic risk factor clustering. *Arch. Intern. Med.* 2008; **168**: 1617–1624.

32 Schwimmer JB, Deutsch R, Rauch JB *et al.* Obesity, insulin resistance, and other clinicopathological correlates of pediatric nonalcoholic fatty liver disease. *J. Pediatr.* 2003; **143**: 500–505.

33 Miele L, Venanzio V, La Torre G *et al.* Increased intestinal permeability and tight junction alterations in nonalcoholic fatty liver disease. *Hepatology* 2009; **49**: 1877–1887.

34 Vanni E, Bugianesi E. The gut-liver axis in nonalcoholic fatty liver disease: Another pathway to insulin resistance? *Hepatology* 2009; **49**: 1790–1792.

35 Unger RH. Lipotoxic diseases. *Annu. Rev. Med.* 2002; **53**: 319–336.

36 Al-Osaimi AM, Berg CL, Caldwell SH. Intermittent disconjugate gaze: a novel finding in nonalcoholic steatohepatitis and cryptogenic cirrhosis. *Hepatology* 2005; **41**: 943.

37 Caldwell SH, Hespenheide EE. Subacute liver failure in obese females. *Am. J. Gastroenterol.* 2002; **97**: 2058–2062.

38 Cheung O, Kapoor A, Puri P *et al.* The impact of fat distribution on the severity of nonalcoholic fatty liver disease and metabolic syndrome. *Hepatology* 2007; **46**: 1091–1100.

39 Harrison SA, Neuschwander-Tetri B. Clinical manifestations and diagnosis of NAFLD. In: Farrell GC, George J, Hall P, McCullough AJ, eds. *Fatty Liver Disease; NASH and Related Disorders.* Malden, MA, USA: Blackwell Publishing, 2005, p. 159.

40 Mofrad P, Contos MJ, Haque M *et al.* Clinical and histological spectrum of nonalcoholic fatty liver disease associated with normal ALT values. *Hepatology* 2003; **37**: 1286–1292.

41 Sorbi D, Boynton J, Lindor KD. The ratio of aspartate aminotransferase to alanine aminotransferase: potential value in differentiating nonalcoholic steatohepatitis from alcoholic liver disease. *Am. J. Gastroenterol.* 1999; **94**: 1018–1022.

42 Nagore N, Scheuer PJ. Does a linear pattern of sinusoidal IgA deposition distinguish between alcoholic and diabetic liver disease? *Liver* 1988; **8**: 281–286.

43 Koskinas J, Kenna JG, Bird GL, Alexander GJM, Williams R. Immunoglobulin A antibody to a 200 kilodalton cytosolic acetaldehyde adduct in alcoholic hepatitis. *Gastroenterology* 1992; **103**: 1860–1867.

44 Caldwell SH, Swerdlow RH, Khan EM *et al.* Mitochondrial abnormalities in non-alcoholic steatohepatitis. *J. Hepatol.* 1999; **31**: 430–434

45 Feliciani C, Amerio P. Madelung's disease: Inherited from an ancient Mediterranean population? *N. Engl. J. Med.* 1999; **340**: 1481.

46 Guillausseau P-J, Massin P, Dubois-LaForgue D *et al.* Maternally inherited diabetes and deafness: A multicenter study. *Ann. Intern. Med.* 2001; **134**: 721–728.

47 Powell EE, Searle J, Mortimer R. Steatohepatitis associated with limb lipodystrophy. *Gastroenterology* 1989; **97**: 1022–1024.

48 Lazo M, Clark JM. The epidemiology of nonalcoholic fatty liver disease: a global perspective. *Semin. Liver Dis.* 2008; **28**: 339–350.

49 Wanless IR, Lentz JS. Fatty liver hepatitis (steatohepatitis) and obesity: An autopsy study with anlysis of risk factors. *Hepatology* 1990; **12**: 1106–1110.

50 Suzuki A, Angulo P, Lymp J *et al.* Chronological development of elevated aminotransferases in a nonalcoholic population. *Hepatology* 2005; **41**: 64–71.

51 Fan J-G, Farrell GC. Epidemiology of non-alcoholic fatty liver disease in China. *J. Hepatol.* 2009; **50**: 204–210.

52 Schwimmer JB, McGreal N, Deutsch R *et al.* Influence of gender, race, and ethnicity on suspected fatty liver in obese adolescents. *Pediatrics* 2005; **115**: e561–565.

53 Strauss RS, Barlow SE, Dietz WH. Prevalence of abnormal serum aminotransferase values in overweight and obese adolescents. *J. Pediatr.* 2000; **136**: 727–733.

54 Park HS, Han JH, Choi KM, Kim SM. Relation between elevated serum alanine aminotransferase and metabolic syndrome in Korean adolescents. *Am. J. Clin. Nutr.* 2005; **82**: 1046–1051.

55 Franzese A, Vajro P, Argenziano A *et al.* Liver involvement in obese children. Ultrasonography and liver enzyme levels at diagnosis and during follow-up in an Italian population. *Dig. Dis. Sci.* 1997; **42**: 1428–1432.

56 Tazawa Y, Noguchi H, Nishinomiya F, Takada G. Serum alanine aminotransferase activity in obese children. *Acta Paediatr.* 1997; **86**: 238–241.

57 Schwimmer JB, Celedon MA, Lavine JE *et al.* Heritability of nonalcoholic fatty liver disease. *Gastroenterology* 2009; **136**: 1585–1592.

58 Navarro VJ, St Louis T, Bell BZ, Sofair AN. Chronic liver disease in the primary care practices of Waterby, Connecticut. *Hepatology* 2003; **38**: 1062.

59 Daniel S, Ben-Menachem T, Vasudevan G *et al.* Prospective evaluation of unexplained chronic liver transaminase abnormalities in asymptomatic and symptomatic patients. *Am. J. Gastroenterol.* 1999; **94**: 3010–3014.

60 Machado M, Marques-Vidal P, Cortez-Pinto H. Hepatic histology in obese patients undergoing bariatric surgery. *J. Hepatol.* 2006; **45**: 600–606.

61 Bellentani S, Bedogni G, Miglioli L, Tiribelli C. The epidemiology of fatty liver. *Eur. J. Gastroenterol. Hepatol.* 2004; **16**: 1087–1093.

62 Younossi ZM, Gramlich T, Matteoni CA *et al.* Nonalcoholic fatty liver disease in patients with type 2 diabetes. *Clin. Gastroenterol. Hepatol.* 2004; **2**: 262–265.

63 Marchesini G, Brizi M, Morselli-Labate AM *et al.* Association of nonalcoholic fatty liver disease with insulin resistance. *Am. J. Med.* 1999; **107**: 450–455.

64 Assy N, Kaita K, Mymin D *et al.* Fatty infiltration of liver in hyperlipidemic patients. *Dig. Dis. Sci.* 2000; **45**: 1929–1934.

65 Caldwell SH, Harris DM, Hespenheide EE. Is NASH under diagnosed among African Americans? *Am. J. Gastroenterol.* 2002; **97**: 1496–1500.

66 Browning JD, Szczepaniak LS, Dobbins R *et al.* Prevalence of hepatic steatosis in an urban population in the United States: impact of ethnicity. *Hepatology* 2004; **40**: 1387–1395.

67 Weston SR, Leyden W, Murphy R *et al.* Racial and ethnic distribution of nonalcoholic fatty liver in persons with newly diagnosed chronic liver disease. *Hepatology* 2005; **41**: 372–379.

68 Guerrero R, Vega GL, Grundy SM, Browning JD. Ethnic differences in hepatic steatosis: An insulin resistance paradox? *Hepatology* 2009; **49**: 791–801.

69 Caldwell SH, Ikura Y, Iezzoni JC, Liu Z. Has natural selection in human populations produced two types of metabolic syndrome (with and without fatty liver)? *J. Gastroenterol. Hepatol.* 2007; **22** (Suppl. 1): S11–S19.

70 Harmon RC, Caldwell S. Propensity for non-alcoholic fatty liver disease: more evidence for ethnic susceptibility. *Liver Int.* 2009; **29**: 4–5.

71 Romeo S, Kozlitina J, Xing C *et al.* Genetic variation in PNPLA3 confers susceptibility to nonalcoholic fatty liver disease. *Nat. Genet.* 2008; **40**: 1461–1465.

72 Struben VM, Hespenheide EE, Caldwell SH. Nonalcoholic steatohepatitis and cryptogenic cirrhosis within kindreds. *Am. J. Med.* 2000; **108**: 9–13.

73 Willner IR, Waters B, Patil SR *et al.* Ninety patients with nonalcoholic steatohepatitis: insulin resistance, familial tendency, and severity of disease. *Am. J. Gastroenterol.* 2001; **96**: 2957–2961.

74 Abdelmalek MF, Liu C, Shuster J *et al.* Familial aggregation of insulin resistance in first-degree relatives of patients with nonalcoholic fatty liver disease. *Clin. Gastroenterol. Hepatol.* 2006; **4**: 1162–1169.

75 Petersen KF, Dufour S, Befroy D *et al.* Impaired mitochondrial activity in the insulin-resistant offspring of diabetes with type 2 diabetes. *N. Engl. J. Med.* 2004; **350**: 664–671.

76 Day CP, James OFW. Steatohepatitis: A tale of two hits. *Gastroenterology* 1998; **114**: 842–845.

77 Browning JD, Horton JD. Molecular mediators of hepatic steatosis. *J. Clin. Invest.* 2004; **114**: 147–152.

78 Tamura S, Shimomura I. Contribution of adipose tissue and de novo lipogenesis to nonalcoholic fatty liver diseases. *J. Clin. Invest.* 2005; **115**: 1139–1142.

79 Brown MS, Goldstein JL. The SREBP pathway: regulation of cholesterol metabolism by proteolysis of a membrane-bound transcription factor. *Cell* 1997; **89**: 331–340.

80 Harvey RA, Champe PC. *Biochemistry*, 3rd edn. Lippincott Williams and Wilkins, 2005.

81 Donnelly KL, Smith CI, Schwarzenberg SJ *et al.* Sources of fatty acids in liver and secreted via lipoproteins in patients with nonalcoholic fatty liver disease. *J. Clin. Invest.* 2005; **115**: 1343–1351.

82 Villanueva CJ, Monetti M, Shih M *et al.* Specific role for acyl coA: diacylglycerol acyltransferase 1 (Dgat1) in hepatic steatosis due to exogenous fatty acids. *Hepatology* 2009; **50**: 434–442.

83 Diraison F, Moulin P, Beylot M. Contribution of hepatic de novo lipogenesis and reesterification of plasma non esterified fatty acids to plasma triglyceride synthesis during non-alcoholic fatty liver disease. *Diabetes Metab.* 2003; **29**: 478–485.

84 Musso G, Gambino R, De Michieli F *et al.* Association of liver disease with postprandial large intestinal triglyceride-rich lipoprotein accumulation and pro/antioxidant imbalance in normolipidemic non-alcoholic steatohepatitis. *Ann. Med.* 2008; **40**: 383–394.

85 Barrows BR, Timlin MT, Parks EJ. Spillover of dietary fatty acids and use of serum nonesterified fatty acids for the synthesis of VLDL-triacylglycerol under two different feeding regimens. *Diabetes* 2005; **54**: 2668–2673.

86 Fabbrini E, Mohammed BS, Magkos F *et al.* Alterations in adipose tissue and hepatic lipid kinetics in obese men and women with nonalcoholic fatty liver disease. *Gastroenterology* 2008; **134**: 424–431.

87 Fujita K, Nozaki Y, Wada K *et al.* Dysfunctional very-low-density lipoprotein synthesis and release is a key factor in nonalcoholic steatohepatitis pathogenesis. *Hepatology* 2009; **50**: 772–780.

88 Dianzani MU. Uncoupling of oxidative phosphorylation in mitochondria from fatty livers. *Biochim. Biophys. Acta* 1954; **14**: 514–532.

89 Cortez-Pinto H, Chatham J, Chacko VP *et al.* Alterations in liver ATP homeostasis in human nonalcoholic steatohepatitis: A pilot study. *JAMA* 1999; **282**: 1659–1664.

90 Caldwell SH, Chang CY, Nakamoto RK, Krugner-Higby L. Mitochondria in nonalcoholic fatty liver disease. *Clin. Liver Dis.* 2004; **8**: 595–618.

91 Pessayre D, Fromenty B. NASH: A mitochondrial disease. *J. Hepatol.* 2005; **42**: 928–940.

92 Caldwell SH, de Freitas LA, Park SH *et al.* Intramitochondrial crystalline inclusions in nonalcoholic steatohepatitis. *Hepatology* 2009; **49**: 1888–1895.

93 Chen J, Schenker S, Frosto TA, Henderson GI. Inhibition of cytochrome c oxidase activity by 4-hydroxynonenal (HNE). Role of HNE adduct formation with the enzyme catalytic site. *Biochim. Biophys. Acta* 1998; **1380**: 336–344.

94 Diehl AM, Hoek JB. Mitochondrial uncoupling: role of uncoupling protein anion carriers and relationship to thermogenesis and weight control 'the benefits of losing control'. *J. Bioenerg. Biomembr.* 1999; **31**: 493–506.

95 Perez-Carrera M, Del Hoyo P, Martin MA *et al.* Defective hepatic mitochondrial respiratory chain in patients with nonalcoholic steatohepatitis. *Hepatology* 2003; **38**: 999–1007.

96 Schneider ARJ, Kraut C, Lindenthal B *et al*. Total body metabolism of 13C-octanoic acid is preserved in patients with non-alcoholic steatohepatitis, but differs between women and men. *Eur. J. Gastroenterol. Hepatol.* 2005; **17**: 1181–1184.

97 Ricci JE, Waterhouse N, Green DR. Mitochondrial functions during cell death, a complex (I-V) dilemma. *Cell Death Differ.* 2003; **10**: 488–492.

98 Caballero F, Fernández A, De Lacy AM *et al*. Enhanced free cholesterol, SREBP-2 and StAR expression in human NASH. *J. Hepatol.* 2009; **50**: 789–796.

99 Ma KL, Ruan XZ, Powis SH *et al*. Inflammatory stress exacerbates lipid accumulation in hepatic cells and fatty livers of apolipoprotein E knockout mice. *Hepatology* 2008; **48**: 770–781.

100 Mavrelis PG, Ammon HV, Gleysteen JJ *et al*. Hepatic free fatty acids in alcoholic liver disease and morbid obesity. *Hepatology* 1983; **3**: 226–231.

101 Puri P, Baillie RA, Wiest MM *et al*. A lipidomic analysis of nonalcoholic fatty liver disease. *Hepatology* 2007; **46**: 1081–1090.

102 Kolak M, Westerbacka J, Velagapudi VR *et al*. Adipose tissue inflammation and increased ceramide content characterize subjects with high liver fat content independent of obesity. *Diabetes* 2007; **56**: 1960–1968.

103 Fromenty B, Berson A, Pessayre D. Microvesicular steatosis and steatohepatitis: role of mitochondrial dysfunction and lipid peroxidation. *J. Hepatol.* 1997: **26** (Suppl. 1): 13–22.

104 Seki S, Kitada T, Sakaguchi H *et al*. In situ detection of lipid peroxidation and oxidative DNA damage in non-alcoholic fatty liver disease. *J. Hepatol.* 2002; **37**: 56–62.

105 Ikura Y, Ohsawa M, Suekane T *et al*. Localization of oxidized phosphatidyl-choline in nonalcoholic fatty liver disease: impact on disease progression. *Hepatology* 2006; **43**: 506–514.

106 Garcia-Monzon C, Martin-Perez E, Lo Iacono O *et al*. Characterization of pathogenic and prognostic factors of nonalcoholic steatohepatitis associated with obesity. *J. Hepatol.* 2000; **33**: 716–724.

107 Malaguarnera L, Madeddu R, Palio E *et al*. Heme oxygenase-1 levels and oxidative stress-related parameters in non-alcoholic fatty liver disease patients. *J. Hepatol.* 2005; **42**: 585–591.

108 Hruszkewycz AM. Evidence for mitochondrial DNA damage by lipid peroxidation. *Biochem. Biophys. Res. Commun.* 1988; **153**: 191–197.

109 Recknagle RO, Glende EA, Britton RS. Free radical damage and lipid peroxidation. In: RG Meeks, SD Harrison, RJ Bull, eds. *Hepatotoxicology*. Boca Raton, FL, USA: CRC Press, 1991, p. 401–436.

110 Bell M, Wang H, Chen H *et al*. Consequences of lipid droplet coat protein down regulation in liver cells: abnormal lipid droplet metabolism and induction of insulin resistance. *Diabetes* 2008; **57**: 2037–2045.

111 Puri V, Ranjit S, Konda S *et al*. Cidea is associated with lipid droplets and insulin sensitivity in humans. *PNAS* 2008; **105**: 7833–7838.

112 Harada M, Hanada S, Toivola DM *et al*. Autophagy activation by rapamycin eliminates mouse Mallory-Denk bodies and blocks their proteosome inhibitor-mediated formation. *Hepatology* 2008; **47**: 2026–2035.

113 Singh R, Kaushik S, Wang Y *et al*. Autophagy regulates lipid metabolism. *Nature* 2009; **458**: 1131–1135.

114 McClain CJ, Barve S, Deaciuc I. Good fat/bad fat. *Hepatology* 2007; **45**: 1343–1346.

115 Charlton M, Viker K, Krishnan A *et al*. Differential expression of lumican and fatty acid binding protein-1: new insights into the histologic spectrum of nonalcoholic fatty liver disease. *Hepatology* 2009; **49**: 1375–1384.

116 Kantartzis K, Machicao F, Machann J *et al*. The DGAT2 gene is a candidate for the dissociation between fatty liver and insulin resistance in humans. *Clin. Sci.* 2009; **116**: 531–537.

117 Li Z, Berk M, McIntyre TM *et al*. The lysosomal-mitochondrial axis in free fatty acid-induced hepatic lipotoxicity. *Hepatology* 2008; **47**: 1495–1503.

118 Feldstein AE, Canby A, Angulo P *et al*. Hepatocyte apoptosis and FAS expression are prominent features of human nonalcoholic steatohepatitis. *Gastroenterology* 2003; **125**: 437–443.

119 Ramalho RM, Cortez-Pinto H, Castro RE *et al*. Apoptosis and Bcl-2 expression in the livers of patients with steatohepatitis. *Eur. J. Gastroenterol. Hepatol.* 2006; **18**: 21–29.

120 Joshi-Barve S, Barve SS, Amancherla K *et al*. Palmitic acid induces production of proinflammatory cytokine interleukin-8 from hepatocytes. *Hepatology* 2007; **46**: 823–830.

121 Lemasters JJ. Dying a thousand deaths: Redundant pathways from different organelles to apoptosis and necrosis. *Gastroenterology* 2005; **129**: 351–360.

122 Amidi F, French BA, Chung D *et al*. M-30 and 4HNE are sequestered in different aggresomes in the same hepatocytes. *Exp. Mol. Path.* 2007; **83**: 296–300.

123 Su Q, Tsai J, Xu E *et al*. Apolipoprotein B100 acts as a molecular link between lipid-induced endoplasmic reticulum stress and hepatic insulin resistance. *Hepatology* 2009; **50**: 77–84.

124 Ohsaki Y, Cheng J, Suzuki M *et al*. Lipid droplets are arrested in the ER membrane by tight binding of lipidated apolipoprotein B-100. *J. Cell. Sci.* 2008; **121**: 2415–2422.

125 Ribeiro PS, Cortez-Pinto H, Solá S *et al*. Hepatocyte apoptosis, expression of death receptors, and activation of NF-kappaB in the liver of nonalcoholic and alcoholic steatohepatitis patients. *Am. J. Gastroenterol.* 2004; **99**: 1708–1717.

126 Puri P, Mirshahi F, Cheung O *et al*. Activation and dysregulation of the unfolded protein response in nonalcoholic fatty liver disease. *Gastroenterology* 2008; **134**: 568–576.

127 Marra F. Nuclear factor kB inhibition and nonalcoholic steatohepatitis: inflammation as a target for therapy. *Gut* 2008; **57**: 570–572.

128 Friedman SL. Hepatic stellate cells: Protean, multifunctional, and enigmatic cells of the liver. *Physiol. Rev.* 2008; **88**: 125–172.

129 Watanabe A, Hashmi A, Gomes DA *et al*. Apoptotic hepatocyte DNA inhibits hepatic stellate cell chemotaxis via toll-like receptor 9. *Hepatology* 2007; **46**: 1509–1518.

130 Richardson MM, Jonsson JR, Powell EE *et al*. Progressive fibrosis in nonalcoholic steatohepatitis: association with altered regeneration and a ductular reaction. *Gastroenterology* 2007; **133**: 80–90.

131 Lackner C, Gogg-Kamerer M, Zatloukal K *et al*. Ballooned hepatocytes in steatohepatitis: The value of keratin immunohistochemistry for diagnosis. *J. Hepatol.* 2008; **48**: 821–828.

132 van Marken Lichtenbelt WD, Vanhommerig JW, Smulders NM *et al*. Cold-activated brown adipose tissue in healthy men. *N. Engl. J. Med.* 2009; **360**: 1500–1508.

133 Li Z, Oben JA, Yang S *et al*. Norepinephrine regulates hepatic innate immune system in leptin-deficient mice with nonalcoholic steatohepatitis. *Hepatology* 2004; **40**: 434–441.

134 Roden M, Price TB, Perseghin G *et al*. Mechanism of free fatty acid-induced insulin resistance in humans. *J. Clin. Invest.* 1996; **97**: 2859–2865.

135 Saltiel AR, Kahn CR. Insulin signaling and the regulation of glucose and lipid metabolism. *Nature* 2001; **414**: 799–806.

136 Kintscher U, Hartge M, Hess K *et al*. T-lymphocyte infiltration in visceral adipose tissue: a primary event in adipose tissue inflammation and the development of obesity-mediated insulin resistance. *Arterioscler. Thromb. Vasc. Biol.* 2008; **28**: 1304–1310.

137 Hotamisligil GS. Inflammation and endoplasmic reticulum stress in obesity and diabetes. *Int. J. Obes.* 2008; **32**: S52–S54.

138 Farrell GC. Signaling links in the liver: knitting SOCS with fat and inflammation. *J. Hepatol.* 2005; **43**: 193–196.

139 Wigg AJ, Roberts-Thomson IC, Dymock RB *et al*. The role of small intestinal bacterial overgrowth, intestinal permeability, endotoxaemia, and tumour necrosis factor alpha in the pathogenesis of non-alcoholic steatohepatitis. *Gut* 2001; **48**: 206–211.

140 Bardella MT, Valenti L, Pagliari C *et al*. Searching for coeliac disease in patients with non-alcoholic fatty liver disease. *Dig. Liver Dis.* 2004; **36**: 333–336.

141 Yamauchi T, Kamon J, Minokoshi Y *et al*. Adiponectin stimulates glucose utilization and fatty-acid oxidation by activating AMP-activated protein kinase. *Nat. Med.* 2002; **8**: 1288–1295.

142 Cao H, Gerhold K, Mayers JR *et al*. Identification of a lipokine, a lipid hormone linking adipose tissue to systemic metabolism. *Cell* 2008; **134**: 933–944.

143 Guzman G, Brunt EM, Petrovic LM *et al*. Does nonalcoholic fatty liver disease predispose patients to hepatocellular carcinoma in the absence of cirrhosis? *Arch. Pathol. Lab. Med.* 2008; **132**: 1761–1766.

144 Paradis V, Zalinski S, Chelbi E *et al*. Hepatocellular carcinomas in patients with metabolic syndrome often develop without significant fibrosis: a pathological analysis. *Hepatology* 2009; **49**: 851–859.

145 Angulo P, Keach JC, Batts KP, Lindor KD. Independent predictors of liver fibrosis in patients with non-alcoholic steatohepatitis. *Hepatology* 1999; **30**: 1356–1362.

146 Dixon JB, Bhathal PS, O'Brien PE. Nonalcoholic fatty liver disease: predictors of nonalcoholic steatohepatitis and liver fibrosis in the severely obese. *Gastroenterology* 2001; **121**: 91–100.

147 Ratziu V, Giral P, Charlotte F *et al*. Liver fibrosis in overweight patients. *Gastroenterology* 2000; **118**: 1117–1123.

148 Argo CK, Northup PG, Al-Osaimi AM, Caldwell SH. Systematic review of risk factors for fibrosis progression in non-alcoholic steatohepatitis. *J. Hepatol.* 2009; **51**: 371–379.

149 Harrison SA, Torgerson S, Hayashi PH. The natural history of nonalcoholic fatty liver disease: A clinical histopathological study. *Am. J. Gastroenterol.* 2003; **98**: 2042–2047.

150 Hui JM, Kench JG, Chitturi S *et al*. Long-term outcomes of cirrhosis in nonalcoholic steatohepatitis compared with hepatitis C. *Hepatology* 2003; **38**: 420–427.

151 Brunt EM, Kleiner DE, Wilson LA *et al*; NASH Clinical Research Network. Portal chronic inflammation in nonalcoholic fatty liver disease (NAFLD): a histologic marker of advanced NAFLD—clinicopathologic correlations from the nonalcoholic steatohepatitis clinical research network. *Hepatology* 2009; **49**: 809–820.

152 Adams LA, Lymp JF, St Sauver J *et al*. The natural history of nonalcoholic fatty liver disease: a population-based cohort study. *Gastroenterology* 2005; **129**: 113–121.

153 Ekstedt M, Franzen LE, Mathiesen UL *et al*. Long-term follow-up of patients with NAFLD and elevated liver enzymes. *Hepatology* 2006; **44**: 865–873.

154 Ong JP, Pitts A, Younossi ZM. Increased overall mortality and liver-related mortality in non-alcoholic fatty liver disease. *J. Hepatol.* 2008; **49**: 608–612.

155 Rafiq N, Bai C, Fang Y *et al*. Long-term follow-up of patients with nonalcoholic fatty liver. *Clin. Gastroenterol. Hepatol.* 2009; **7**: 234–238.

156 Caldwell SH, Lee VD, Kleiner DE *et al*. NASH and cryptogenic cirrhosis: a histological analysis. *Ann. Hepatol.* 2009; **8**: 346–352.

157 Caldwell SH, Crespo DM. The spectrum expanded: cryptogenic cirrhosis and the natural history of non-alcoholic fatty liver disease. *J. Hepatol.* 2004; **40**: 578–584.

158 Crawford DHG, Shepherd RW, Halliday JW *et al*. Body composition in nonalcoholic cirrhosis: The effect of disease etiology and severity on nutritional compartments. *Gastroenterology* 1994; **106**: 1611–1617.

159 Giannini EG, Marabotto E, Savarino V *et al*. Hepatocellular carcinoma in patients with cryptogenic cirrhosis. *Clin. Gastroenterol. Hepatol.* 2009; **7**: 580–585.

160 Ueno T, Sugawara H, Sujaku K *et al*. Therapeutic effects of restricted diet and exercise in obese patients with fatty liver. *J. Hepatol.* 1997; **27**: 103–107.

161 Nobili V, Manco M, Devito R *et al*. Lifestyle intervention and antioxidant therapy in children with nonalcoholic fatty liver disease: a randomized, controlled trial. *Hepatology* 2008; **48**: 119–128.

162 Sacks FM, Bray GA, Carey VJ *et al*. Comparison of weight-loss diets with different compositions of fat, protein, and carbohydrates. *N. Engl. J. Med.* 2009; **360**: 859–873.

163 Zelber-Sagi S, Kessler A, Brazowsky E *et al*. A double-blind randomized placebo-controlled trial of orlistat for the treatment of nonalcoholic fatty liver disease. *Clin. Gastroenterol. Hepatol.* 2006; **4**: 639–644.

164 Harrison SA, Fecht W, Brunt EM, Neuschwander-Tetri BA. Orlistat for overweight subjects with nonalcoholic steatohepatitis: A randomized, prospective trial. *Hepatology* 2009; **49**: 80–86.

165 Harrison SA, Day CP. Benefits of lifestyle modification in NAFLD. *Gut* 2007; **56**: 1760–1769.

166 Irving BA, Davis CK, Brock DW *et al*. Effect of exercise training on abdominal visceral fat and body composition. *Med. Sci. Sports Exerc.* 2008; **40**: 1863–1872.

167 Hickman IJ. Obesity management in liver clinics: What's your style of lifestyle intervention? *J. Gastroenterol. Hepatol.* 2009; **24**: 327–328.

168 Phielix E, Schrauwen-Hinderling VB, Mensink M *et al.* Lower intrinsic ADP-stimulated mitochondrial respiration underlies in vivo mitochondrial dysfunction in muscle of male type 2 diabetic patients. *Diabetes* 2008; **57**: 2943–2949.

169 Schrauwen-Hinderling VB, Kooi ME, Hesselink MK *et al.* Impaired in vivo mitochondrial function but similar intramyocellular lipid content in patients with type 2 diabetes mellitus and BMI-matched control subjects. *Diabetologia* 2007; **50**: 113–120.

170 Lazo M, Caldwell SH. Is exercise an effective treatment for NASH? Knowns and unknowns. *Ann. Hepatol.* 2009; **8** (Suppl. 1): S60–66.

171 St George A, Bauman A, Johnston A *et al.* Steatohepatitis and metabolic liver disease. The independent effects of physical activity in patients with non-alcoholic fatty liver disease. *Hepatology* 2009; **50**: 68–76.

172 Johnson NA, Sachinwalla T, Walton DW *et al.* Aerobic exercise training reduces hepatic and visceral lipids in obese individuals without weight loss. *Hepatology* 2009; **50**: 1105–1112.

173 Stefan N, Kantartzis K, Machann J *et al.* Identification and characterization of metabolically benign obesity in humans. *Arch. Intern. Med.* 2008; **168**: 1609–1616.

174 Stevens J, Cai J, Evenson KR, Thomas R. Fitness and fatness as predictors of mortality from all causes and from cardiovascular disease in men and women in the lipid research clinics study. *Am. J. Epidemiol.* 2002; **156**: 832–841.

175 Ouyang X, Cirillo P, Sautin Y *et al.* Fructose consumption as a risk factor for non-alcoholic fatty liver disease. *J. Hepatol.* 2008; **48**: 993–999.

176 Tetri LH, Basaranoglu M, Brunt EM *et al.* Severe NAFLD with hepatic necroinflammatory changes in mice fed trans fats and a high-fructose corn syrup equivalent. *Am. J. Physiol.* 2008; **295**: G987–995.

177 Parks EJ. Dietary carbohydrates' effects on lipogenesis and the relationship of lipogenesis to blood insulin and glucose concentrations. *Br. J. Nutr.* 2002; **87** (Suppl. 2): S247–253.

178 Parks EJ, Skokan LE, Timlin MT, Dingfelder CS. Dietary sugars stimulate fatty acid synthesis in adults. *J. Nutr.* 2008; **138**: 1039–1046.

179 Cortez-Pinto H, Jesus L, Barros H *et al.* How different is the dietary pattern in non-alcoholic steatohepatitis patients? *Clin. Nutr.* 2006; **25**: 816–823.

180 Lindor KD, Kowdley KV, Heathcote EJ *et al.* Ursodeoxycholic acid for treatment of nonalcoholic steatohepatitis: results of a randomized trial. *Hepatology* 2004; **39**: 770–778.

181 Dufour J-F, Oneta CM, Gonvers J-J *et al,* Swiss Association for the Study of the Liver. Randomized placebo-controlled trial of ursodeoxycholic acid with vitamin E in nonalcoholic steatohepatitis. *Clin. Gastrol. Hepatol.* 2006; **4**: 1537.

182 Leuschner UF, Lindenthal B, Herrmann G, *et al.* NASH Study Group. High-dose ursodeoxycholic acid therapy for nonalcoholic steatohepatitis: a double-blind, randomized, placebo-controlled trial. *Hepatology.* 2010; **52**: 472–479.

183 Abdelmalek MF, Sanderson SO, Angulo P *et al.* Betaine for nonalcoholic fatty liver disease: results of a randomized placebo-controlled trial. *Hepatology* 2009; **50**: 1818–1826.

184 Harrison SA, Torgerson S, Hayashi P *et al.* Vitamin E and Vitamin C treatment improves fibrosis in patients with nonalcoholic steatohepatitis. *Am. J. Gastroenterol.* 2003; **98**: 2485–2490.

185 Sanyal AJ, Chalasani N, Kowdley KV, *et al.* NASH CRN. Pioglitazone, vitamin E, or placebo for nonalcoholic steatohepatitis. *N. Engl. J. Med.* 2010; **362**: 1675–85.

186 Bugianesi E, Gentilcore E, Manini R *et al.* A randomized controlled trial of metformin versus vitamin E or prescriptive diet in nonalcoholic fatty liver disease. *Am. J. Gastroenterol.* 2005; **100**: 1082–1090.

187 Caldwell SH, Argo CK, Al-Osaimi AM. Therapy of NAFLD: insulin sensitizing agents. *J. Clin. Gastroenterol.* 2006; **40** (Suppl. 1): S61–66.

188 Uygun A, Kadayifci A, Isik AT *et al.* Metformin in the treatment of patients with non-alcoholic steatohepatitis. *Aliment. Pharmacol. Ther.* 2004; **19**: 537–544.

189 Caldwell SH, Hespenheide EE, Redick JA *et al.* A pilot study of a thiazolidinedione, troglitazone, in nonalcoholic steatohepatitis. *Am. J. Gastrol.* 2001; **96**: 519–525.

190 Neuschwander-Tetri BA, Brunt EM, Wehmeier KR *et al.* Interim results of a pilot study demonstrating the early effects of the PPAR-γ ligand rosiglitazone on insulin sensitivity, aminotransferases, hepatic steatosis and body weight in patients with non-alcoholic steatohepatitis. *J. Hepatol.* 2003; **38**: 434–440.

191 Neuschwander-Tetri BA, Brunt EM, Wehmeier KR *et al.* Improved nonalcoholic steatohepatitis after 49 weeks of treatment with the PPAR-γ ligand rosiglitazone. *Hepatology* 2003; **38**: 1008–1017.

192 Sanyal AJ, Mofrad PS, Contos MJ *et al.* A pilot study of vitamin E versus vitamin E and pioglitazone for the treatment of nonalcoholic steatohepatitis. *Clin. Gastroenterol. Hepatol.* 2004; **2**: 1107–1115.

193 Promrat K, Lutchman G, Uwaifo GI *et al.* A pilot study of pioglitazone treatment for nonalcoholic steatohepatitis. *Hepatology* 2004; **39**: 188–196.

194 Tiikkainen M, Hakkinen A-M, Korsheninnikova E *et al.* Effects of rosiglitazone and metformin on liver fat content, hepatic insulin resistance, insulin clearance, and gene expression in adipose tissue in patients with type 2 diabetes. *Diabetes* 2004; **53**: 2169–2176.

195 Belfort R, Harrison SA, Brown K *et al.* A placebo-controlled trial of pioglitazone in subjects with nonalcoholic steatohepatitis. *N. Engl. J. Med.* 2006; **355**: 2297–2307.

196 Aithal GP, Thomas JA, Kaye PV *et al.* Randomized, placebo-controlled trial of pioglitazone in nondiabetic subjects with nonalcoholic steatohepatitis. *Gastroenterology* 2008; **135**: 1176–1184.

197 Ratziu V, Giral P, Jacqueminet S *et al.* LIDO Study Group. Rosiglitazone for nonalcoholic steatohepatitis: one-year results of the randomized placebo-controlled Fatty Liver Improvement with Rosiglitazone Therapy (FLIRT) Trial. *Gastroenterology* 2008; **135**: 100–110.

198 Idilman R, Mizrak D, Corapcioglu D *et al.* Clinical trial: insulin-sensitizing agents may reduce consequences of insulin resistance in individuals with non-alcoholic steatohepatitis. *Aliment. Pharmacol. Therapeut.* 2008; **28**: 200–208.

199 Caldwell SH, Patrie JT, Brunt EM *et al.* Neuschwander-Tetri BA. The effects of 48 weeks of rosiglitazone on hepa-

tocyte mitochondria in human nonalcoholic steatohepatitis. *Hepatology* 2007; **46**: 1101–1107.

200 Lutchman G, Modi A, Kleiner DE *et al*. The effects of discontinuing pioglitazone in patient with nonalcoholic steatohepatitis. *Hepatology* 2007; **46**: 424–429.

201 Argo CK, Iezzoni, JC, Al-Osaimi AM, Caldwell SH. Thiazolidinediones for the treatment in NASH: sustained benefit after drug discontinuation? *J. Clin. Gastroenterol.* 2009; **43**: 565–568.

202 Argo CK, Loria P, Caldwell SH, Lonardo A. Statins in liver disease: a molehill, an iceberg, or neither? *Hepatology* 2008; **48**: 662–669.

203 Ekstedt M, Franzen LE, Mathiesen UL *et al*. Statins in nonalcoholic fatty liver disease and chronically elevated liver enzymes: a histopathological follow-up study. *J. Hepatol.* 2007; **47**: 135–141.

204 Nelson A, Torres DM, Morgan AE *et al*. A pilot study using simvastatin in the treatment of nonalcoholic steatohepatitis: a randomized placebo-controlled trial. *J. Clin. Gastroenterol.* 2009; **43**: 990–994.

205 Satapathy SK, Sakhuja P, Malhotra V *et al*. Beneficial effects of pentoxifylline on hepatic steatosis, fibrosis and necroinflammation in patients with non-alcoholic steatohepatitis. *J. Gastroenterol. Hepatol.* 2007; **22**: 634–638.

206 Yokohama S, Yoneda M, Haneda M *et al*. Therapeutic efficacy of an angiotensin II receptor antagonist in patients with nonalcoholic steatohepatitis. *Hepatology* 2004; **40**: 1222–1225.

207 Mummadi RR, Kasturi KS, Chennareddygari S, Sood GK. Effect of bariatric surgery on nonalcoholic fatty liver disease: systematic review and meta-analysis. *Clin. Gastroenterol. Hepatol.* 2008; **6**: 1396–1402.

208 de Freitas AC, Campos AC, Coelho JC. The impact of bariatric surgery on nonalcoholic fatty liver disease. *Curr. Opin. Clin. Nutr. Metab. Care* 2008; **11**: 267–274.

209 Nair S, Verma S, Thuluvath PJ. Obesity and the effect on survival in patients undergoing orthotopic liver transplantation in the United States. *Hepatology* 2002; **35**: 105–109.

210 Burke A, Lucey MR. Non-alcoholic fatty liver disease, non-alcoholic steatohepatitis and orthotopic liver transplantation. *Am. J. Transplant.* 2004; **4**: 686–693.

211 Malik SM, deVera ME, Fontes P *et al*. Outcome after liver transplantation for NASH cirrhosis. *Am. J. Transplant.* 2009; **9**: 782–793.

212 Czaja AJ. Recurrence of nonalcoholic steatohepatitis after liver transplantation. *Liver Transpl. Surg.* 1997; **3**: 185–186.

213 Molloy RM, Komorowski R, Varma RR. Recurrent nonalcoholic steatohepatitis and cirrhosis after liver transplantation. *Liver Transpl. Surg.* 1997; **3**: 177–178.

214 Carson K, Washington MK, Treem WR *et al*. Recurrence of nonalcoholic steatohepatitis in a liver transplant recipient. *Liver Transpl. Surg.* 1997; **3**: 174–176.

215 Kim WR, Poterucha JJ, Porayko MK *et al*. Recurrence of nonalcoholic steatohepatitis following liver transplantation. *Transplantation* 1996; **62**: 1802–1805.

216 Cavicchi M, Beau P, Crenn P *et al*. Prevalence of liver disease and contributing factors in patients receiving home parenteral nutrition for permanent intestinal failure. *Ann. Intern. Med.* 2000; **132**: 525–532.

217 Kaminski DL, Adams A, Jellinek M. The effect of hyperalimentation on hepatic lipid content and lipogenic enzyme activity in rats and man. *Surgery* 1980; **88**: 93–100.

218 Quigley EM, Zetterman RK. Hepatobiliary complications of malabsorption and malnutrition. *Sem. Liver Dis.* 1988; **8**: 218–228.

219 Chitturi S, Farrell GC. Etiopathogenesis of nonalcoholic steatohepatitis. *Sem. Liver Dis.* 2001; **21**: 27–41.

220 Bongiovanni M, Tordato F. Steatohepatitis in HIV-infected subjects: pathogenesis, clinical impact and implications in clinical management. *Curr. HIV Res.* 2007; **5**: 490–498.

221 Lewis W, Dalakas MC. Mitochondrial toxicity of antiviral drugs. *Nat. Med.* 1995; **1**: 417–422.

222 Cotrim HP, Carvalho F, Siqueira AC *et al*. Nonalcoholic fatty liver and insulin resistance among petrochemical workers. *JAMA* 2005; **294**: 1618–1620.

CHAPTER 29
The Liver in the Neonate, in Infancy and Childhood

Deirdre A. Kelly
Birmingham Children's Hospital and University of Birmingham, Birmingham, UK

Learning points

- Two-thirds of children with liver disease present in the neonatal period. Infants who develop severe or persistent jaundice should be investigated to exclude haemolysis, sepsis or underlying liver disease. Neonatal jaundice, which persists beyond 14 or 21 days, should always be investigated even in breast-fed babies.

- Biliary atresia is the single commonest cause of neonatal liver disease and the main indication for liver transplantation in children under the age of 5 years. Palliative surgery performed before 8 weeks of age significantly improves survival with the child's native liver.

- Acute liver failure is a rare but fatal disease, with mortality of 70% without transplantation. The commonest causes are viral hepatitis or inherited metabolic liver disease. Referral to a specialist unit, supportive management and consideration for liver transplantation is essential.

- The commonest causes of chronic liver failure are extrahepatic biliary atresia or inherited metabolic liver disease in neonates, and autoimmune hepatitis and cystic fibrosis in older children. Nutritional support and management of hepatic complications have improved short-term outcome.

- Liver transplantation for acute or chronic liver failure achieves good quality life in over 80% of children long term.

Investigation of liver disease in children

The approach to the child with liver disease should be systematic and based on an accurate clinical history and a thorough physical examination. Investigating the liver in the infant relies on a multidisciplinary approach involving clinical chemistry, haematology, radiology, histopathology and microbiology. It is essential to recognize the effects of hepatic dysfunction on other body systems [1].

Biochemical tests

Biochemical liver function tests reflect the severity of hepatic dysfunction but rarely provide diagnostic information on individual diseases. Conjugated bilirubin is nearly always elevated in liver disease. Thus the most important investigation in neonates is the fractionation of bilirubin into unconjugated and conjugated *serum bilirubin* in order to differentiate between physiological or breast-milk jaundice and liver disease. Studies of normal neonates show that conjugated bilirubin should be less than 20 µmol/L and that the percentage of conjugated bilirubin of the total should be less than 20% [2]. Significantly elevated levels of unconjugated bilirubin (>300 µmol/L in term babies) may be associated with the development of kernicterus.

Aminotransferases are intracellular enzymes present in liver, heart and skeletal muscle. These enzymes reflect non-specific hepatic damage and may be normal in compensated cirrhosis. Elevated aspartate and/or alanine aminotransferase (AST, ALT) are also found in muscular dystrophy and this diagnosis should be excluded if there are no other signs of liver disease.

Serum alkaline phosphatase concentrations are higher in normal infants and children compared to adults. In paediatric liver disease, increased levels above normal indicate biliary epithelial damage, malignant infiltration, cirrhosis, or osteopenia secondary to vitamin D deficiency.

Serum γ-glutamyl transpeptidase (γ-GT) levels are useful as indicators of bile duct damage and in the diagnosis of familial intrahepatic cholestasis.

Extremely high levels of *serum cholesterol* may be found in prolonged cholestasis, particularly when intrahepatic as in Alagille's syndrome.

As in adults, the most useful tests of liver 'function' are *plasma albumin* concentration and *coagulation time*. Low albumin indicates chronicity of liver disease, while abnormal coagulation indicates significant hepatic dys-

Sherlock's Diseases of the Liver and Biliary System, Twelfth Edition. Edited by James S. Dooley, Anna S.F. Lok, Andrew K. Burroughs, E. Jenny Heathcote.
© 2011 by Blackwell Publishing Ltd. Published 2011 by Blackwell Publishing Ltd.

function, either acute or chronic. *Fasting hypoglycaemia* in the absence of other causes (e.g. hypopituitarism or hyperinsulinism) indicates poor hepatic function or metabolic disease and is a guide to prognosis in acute liver failure.

Bile acid metabolism

Bile acid secretion evolves during the final trimester of pregnancy and in the early neonatal period. In the infant, conjugation and pool size are reduced, as are secretion, intraluminal concentration and ileal active transport. Serum bile acids are increased. The main bile acid in neonates is glycocholic. After 1–3 months, glyco-chenodeoxycholic predominates.

Secretion of bile acids by the hepatocyte may be reduced and atypical bile acids produced, which may not be functionally adequate. A primitive pathway for the synthesis of fetal bile acids may be responsible for excretion of cholestatic bile acids during this period of immaturity of hepatic excretory function, which lasts in infants from birth until 3 months [3]. This picture of '*physiological cholestasis*' is enhanced in the low-birth-weight neonate. It may contribute to cholestasis produced by other factors, for example infection or prolonged parenteral nutrition.

Radiology

Ultrasound scanning of the abdomen provides information on the size and echogenicity of the liver and spleen, the size of the gallbladder and whether there are gallstones. It may identify tumours, haemangiomas, abscesses or cysts within the liver, and allows targeting of lesions for biopsy or aspiration. The gallbladder is best visualized after a 4 to 6-h fast. In the neonate, a small or absent gallbladder after fasting suggests either severe intrahepatic cholestasis or biliary atresia.

Radioisotope scanning is helpful in the differentiation of neonatal hepatitis (patchy uptake but good excretion) and biliary atresia (poor or absent excretion). Technetium trimethyl 1-bromoiminodiacetic acid (TEBIDA) is taken up well by hepatocytes despite elevated bilirubin levels. Pretreatment with phenobarbitone (5 mg/kg) for 3–5 days prior to the investigation improves hepatic uptake of isotope [1].

Liver size

Liver span in normal infants and children is measured by percussion of the upper border and percussion/ palpation of the lower border (Table 29.1) [4].

Circulatory factors and hepatic necrosis

In the fetus the right lobe of the liver is supplied largely by the portal vein whereas the left receives highly oxy-

Table 29.1. Approximate mean liver span of infants and children based on four studies on 470 subjects [4]

Age	Span (cm)
Birth	5.6–5.9
2 months	5
1 year	6
2 years	6.5
3 years	7
4 years	7.5
5 years	8
12 years	9

genated, placental blood. In the fetal mouse, expression of cytochrome P450 is greater in the left lobe [5]. This lobar heterogeneity disappears as the adult pattern of liver circulation develops. At the time of birth, loss of placental blood can be followed by atrophy of the left lobe.

Right-sided hepatic necrosis may be seen in post-mature infants dying around the time of birth. This is related to poor placental blood supply and anoxia at the time of delivery.

Disseminated midzonal necrosis is found with congenital cardiac defects. This may be due to a decrease in total hepatic blood flow. In others, the zone 3 changes of congestive heart failure may be seen. Cholestasis in the first week can be related to congenital cardiac defects and 'shock'.

Copper is increased in the fetal liver, more so in the left lobe than the right.

Localized necrosis of the liver may be due to herniation through defects of the anterior abdominal wall.

Neonatal jaundice

Almost two-thirds of children who have liver disease present in the neonatal period with persistent jaundice. Although physiological jaundice is common in neonates, infants who develop severe or persistent jaundice should be investigated to exclude haemolysis, sepsis or underlying liver disease. Neonatal jaundice that persists beyond 14 or 21 days should always be investigated, even in breast-fed babies.

Neonatal unconjugated hyperbilirubinaemia (Tables 29.2, 29.3).

The commonest causes of unconjugated hyperbilirubinaemia are physiological jaundice or breast-milk jaundice, although systemic disease, haemolysis from any cause or sepsis must be excluded.

Table 29.2. Investigations of the jaundiced newborn

Total and direct serum bilirubin
Blood group
Rhesus status
Coombs' test
Haematocrit
Blood smear for morphology
Blood culture
Blood glucose
Coagulation
Urine culture

Table 29.3. Unconjugated hyperbilirubinaemia in neonates related to time of onset

Birth to 2 days
   Haemolytic disease
3–7 days
   Physiological ± prematurity
      hypoxia
      acidosis
1–8 weeks
   Congenital haemolytic disorders
   Breast-milk jaundice
   Hypopituitarism
   Crigler–Najjar syndrome
   Hypothyroidism
   Perinatal complications: haemorrhage, sepsis
   Upper gastrointestinal obstruction

Physiological jaundice

Jaundice, reaching its peak within 2–5 days of birth and disappearing in 2 weeks, is common in normal infants. This is a benign self-limited process although it is more serious in low birth weight infants where it may persist for as long as 2 weeks. The urine contains both urobilinogen and bilirubin and the stools are paler than normal. Hepatic conjugating and transport systems for bilirubin are delayed in the neonate. Absorption of bilirubin from the intestine is increased. Bilirubin binding to albumin is reduced, particularly in premature infants. The jaundice is enhanced by factors that depress liver function, such as hypoxia and hypoglycaemia. Drugs such as water-soluble vitamin K analogues add to the jaundice.

Serum bilirubin levels may be *lower* in infants with circulatory failure, asphyxia and sepsis. Bilirubin may be a physiological antioxidant, providing protection against perinatal ischaemia–reperfusion tissue injury [6].

The bilirubinaemia is *not* physiological if the level exceeds 85 μmol/L (5 mg/dL) on the first day, 170 μmol (10 mg/dL) on the second day, or 205–220 μmol (12–13 mg/dL) at any time.

Unconjugated hyperbilirubinaemia in the neonatal period may be complicated by bilirubin encephalopathy (*kernicterus*, see below).

Management

Phototherapy. Unconjugated hyperbilirubinaemia may be prevented or controlled by exposure of the infant to light with a wavelength near 450 nm. The light converts bilirubin IXα photochemically to a relatively stable geometric isomer. Phototherapy is used if the total serum bilirubin exceeds or is equal to 290 μmol/L (17 mg/dL) during the first 48 h of life. It is discontinued after the serum bilirubin has decreased by more than 35 μmol (2 mg) or has fallen to 220 μmol (13 mg) or less.

Exchange transfusion. This may necessary in premature infants or those with haemolysis. It is indicated if the total serum bilirubin exceeds 340 μmol/L (20 mg/dL) by direct spectrophotometry, or a bilirubin rising at a rate greater than 17 μmol/L (1 mg/dL) per h despite phototherapy [7].

Breast-milk jaundice

Severe unconjugated hyperbilirubinaemia (serum bilirubin more than 205 μmol/L) associated with breast feeding is common, occurring in 0.5–2% of healthy newborn babies. Jaundice may develop after the fourth day of life (early pattern) or towards the end of the first week of life (late pattern) and usually peaks around the end of the second week of life. Jaundice may be protracted and last 1–2 months. It is commoner in boys. The aetiology is unknown. Infants who have Gilbert's syndrome may be at greater risk for breast-milk jaundice [8]. The diagnosis is clinical: an exclusively breast-fed infant with unconjugated hyperbilirubinaemia, normal conjugated bilirubin, haemoglobin and reticulocyte counts, no maternal blood group incompatibility and a normal physical examination except for jaundice.

Haemolytic disease of the newborn

Fetal–maternal incompatibility usually concerns the Rh blood factors and rarely the ABO or other blood groups. The prevalence is falling, now that anti-D immune globulin is given prophylatically to mothers.

Characteristically, the first-born escapes the disease unless the mother's blood has been sensitized by a previous transfusion of Rh-positive blood. The infant is jaundiced during the first 2 days of life. Serum unconjugated bilirubin is increased. The critical period is in the first few days when the more deeply jaundiced infants may develop *kernicterus*.

Diagnosis may be suspected by antenatal examination of the mother's blood for specific antibodies and confirmed by a positive Coombs' test in the infant and by blood typing on mother and child.

The risk of mental or physical impairment is low until the serum bilirubin increases well above 340 μmol/L (20 mg/dL).

Kernicterus

This grave condition complicates severe unconjugated hyperbilirubinaemia especially in prematurity, haemolytic disease or Crigler–Najjar syndrome. Management with phototherapy, exchange transfusion and phenobarbital has improved the outcome. Daily transcutaneous serum bilirubin estimations are valuable in management.

Kernicterus is related to circulating free bilirubin crossing the blood–brain barrier. Reduction of serum bilirubin–albumin binding may play a part and indeed albumin infusions have been used therapeutically.

Mechanisms of bilirubin toxicity and neurone damage are unknown. Kernicterus is potentiated by hypoxia, metabolic acidosis and septicaemia [9]. Organic anions, which compete for bilirubin binding sites on albumin, increase kernicterus although the serum bilirubin level falls. Such anions include salicylates, sulphonamides, free fatty acids and haematin.

Congenital haemolytic disorders

These can all lead to unconjugated hyperbilirubinaemia in the first 2 days of life. They include the red cell enzyme deficiencies (glucose-6-phosphate dehydrogenase and pyruvate kinase), congenital spherocytosis and pyknocytosis.

Glucose-6-phosphate dehydrogenase deficiency. Infants develop jaundice, usually on the second or third day of life. The precipitating haemolytic agent may be a drug such as salicylate, phenacetin or sulphonamides transmitted in the maternal breast milk. This condition is frequent in the Mediterranean area, in the Far East and in Nigeria [10].

Crigler–Najjar syndrome type I and II (see also Chapter 11)

Crigler–Najjar syndromes type l and II are autosomal recessive conditions, which lead to unconjugated hyperbilirubinaemia due to a deficiency of the enzyme bilirubin uridine diphosphate glucuronosyl transferase (UDPGT). In Crigler–Najjar type l, there is effectively no UDPGT present; in type 2, the defect is partial. They present in the first few days of life.

Type I is treated with either phototherapy or exchange transfusion. The aim of therapy is to maintain bilirubin levels low enough (<300 μmol/L) to prevent kernicterus. This may require up to 15 h of phototherapy a day [11]. Intercurrent infections with rapid increases in bilirubin should be managed with plasmapheresis or exchange transfusions.

Liver transplantation, including auxiliary transplantation, is a long-term option if damage to the nervous system has been avoided and may improve quality of life. It is the only effective method for preventing kernicterus. Hepatocyte transplantation has limited success [12,13].

In type II, treatment with phenobarbitone (5–10 mg/kg per day) may provide cosmetic improvement, but treatment is not usually required since kernicterus is rare.

Perinatal complications

Haemorrhage with release of blood into the tissues provides a bilirubin load which may exacerbate jaundice, particularly in the premature. Anaemia depresses hepatocellular function. Cephalohaematoma is a common association. The prothrombin time should be measured and vitamin K given.

Sepsis, whether umbilical or elsewhere, leads to unconjugated hyperbilirubinaemia in the first few days of life. Blood, urine and, if necessary, cerebrospinal fluid are cultured and appropriate antibodies given.

Upper gastrointestinal obstruction

About 10% of infants with congenital pyloric stenosis are jaundiced due to unconjugated bilirubin. The mechanism may be similar to that postulated for the increase in jaundice when patients with Gilbert's syndrome are fasted (Chapter 11).

Neonatal liver disease (conjugated hyperbilirubinaemia)

Conjugated hyperbilirubinaemia indicates liver disease, which may be due to the neonatal hepatitis syndrome, intrahepatic cholestasis or biliary atresia. The predictive value of conjugated hyperbilirubinaemia in the second week of life is a specific and sensitive marker of liver disease [14].

The neonatal liver responds in a similar way to different insults. Proliferation of giant cells is a common response and may reflect increased regenerative ability (Fig. 29.1). It is usually associated with extramedullary haemopoiesis. It may be found in most causes of neonatal liver disease such as viral infection and metabolic disease including galactosaemia (Fig. 29.1a). Familial cholestatic syndromes may be associated with a giant

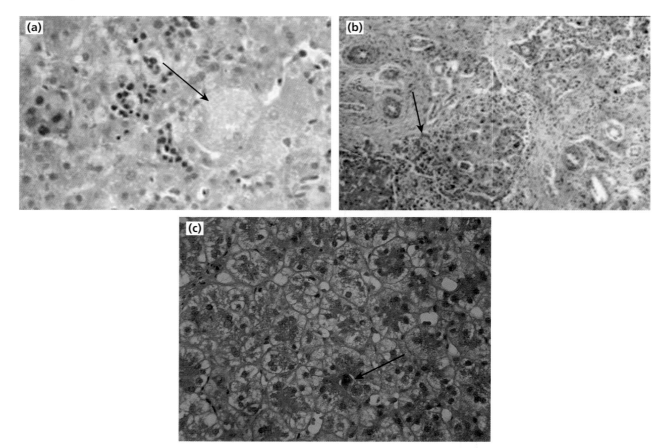

Fig. 29.1. Neonatal liver disease: histological appearances. (a) Development of giant cells (arrow) is a common response and may indicate regeneration. It is seen in most causes of neonatal liver disease such as viral infection and metabolic disease. Often there is extramedullary haemopoiesis. (b) With biliary obstruction, ductular proliferation (arrow) and bile canalicular plugging are usually seen, and fibrosis as in this biopsy from a child with biliary atresia. (c) Cholestasis due to parenteral nutrition. There are features of biliary obstruction, bile plugs (arrowed, with surrounding cholestatic rosettes of liver cells) and a giant cell reaction.

cell hepatitis but biliary obstruction is usually associated with ductular proliferation and bile canalicular plugging with or without a giant cell reaction (Fig. 29.1b). In all these conditions, the conjugated 'direct reacting' bilirubin is more than 20% of the total.

It is important to differentiate between those diseases that are self limiting, respond to therapy or require early surgery such as biliary atresia.

Clinical features and diagnosis (Table 29.4) [15]

Conjugated hyperbilirubinaemia may present at any time after birth. If it is detected in the first 24 h of life, sepsis must be excluded. Most causes of the neonatal liver disease have a similar presentation. The clinical history should include:
• details about the mother's pregnancy (drugs, alcohol, smoking, intercurrent illnesses, pruritis of pregnancy, hepatitis status and risk factors, e.g. drug abuse)
• Birth weight and gestational age

• Vitamin K administration
• Family history and consanguinity.

History of the present illness should include:
• Date of jaundice
• Colour of stools and urine
• Drug history, particularly parenteral nutrition
• Bleeding
• Petechiae or bruising
• Feeding history and weight gain
• Diarrhoea and vomiting.

The clinical features include:
• Jaundice, dark urine, pale yellow stools, failure to thrive or poor feeding
• Infants may be small for gestational age, especially those with Alagille's syndrome, metabolic liver disease and intrauterine infection
• Dysmorphic features in trisomy 18, trisomy 21, Alagille's syndrome, Zellweger's syndrome, and with certain congenital infections

Table 29.4. Conjugated hyperbilirubinaemia in neonates

Infection

   Viruses (cytomegalovirus, rubella, Coxsackie, herpes simplex) (Chapters 21)

   Syphilis

   Toxoplasmosis

   Bacteria (*Escherichia coli*)

Metabolic

   Galactosaemia

   α_1-Antitrypsin deficiency

   Tyrosinaemia type 1

   Cystic fibrosis

   Hereditary fructose intolerance

   Total parenteral nutrition

   Niemann–Pick C disease

   Progressive familial intrahepatic cholestasis 1,2,3

   Alagille's syndrome

Endocrine

   Hypopituitarism

   Hypothyroidism

Biliary atresia

Choledocal cyst

Miscellaneous

   Inspissated bile syndrome (erythroblastosis with cholestasis)

   Vascular causes

     'shock'

     congenital heart disease

• Hypoglycaemia in metabolic liver disease, hypopituitarism or severe liver disease

• Hypogonadism (in males) and optic dysplasia in hypopituitarism

• Hepatomegaly with or without splenomegaly

• Ascites is rare except in metabolic liver disease

• Bleeding from vitamin K deficiency (particularly if breast fed) or thrombocytopenia.

Investigations

Findings from biochemical liver function tests in conjugated hyperbilirubinaemia include:

• Total serum conjugated hyperbilirubin exceeds 20 μmol/L (1.2 mg/dL).

• Serum aminotransferases are usually elevated two to four times normal. Higher elevations suggest an infectious process.

• Serum alkaline phosphatase may be normal or only mildly elevated. High levels may indicate biliary obstruction or rickets.

• Serum γ-GT may be elevated. Normal or low γ-GT suggests certain bile canalicular transporter defects (Byler disease or progressive familial intrahepatic cholestasis).

• Serum albumin is usually normal unless there is severe prenatal disease.

• Serum cholesterol is usually elevated in children with severe cholestasis, for example in Alagille's syndrome or biliary atresia.

• Prothrombin and partial thromboplastin times are usually normal unless there is associated vitamin K deficiency (haemorrhagic disease of the newborn) or severe liver disease.

• Serum α_1-antitrypsin level and phenotype for the diagnosis of α_1-antitrypsin deficiency.

Serology for TORCH screen. Antibodies to herpes simplex, rubella, *Toxoplasma*, cytomegalovirus, adenovirus and Coxsackie viruses are estimated in both baby and mother and serology for syphilis. The serum is usually tested for hepatitis B surface antigen (HBsAg), IgM antihepatitis B core antigen (anti-HBcAg), IgM antihepatitis A virus (anti-HAV), antihepatitis C virus (anti-HCV) and HCV RNA, but these are rare causes of neonatal liver disease.

Urine tests. Cultures are taken for Gram-negative organisms and for cytomegalovirus infection. Aminoaciduria is noted. Reducing substances are sought if galactosaemia is suspected.

Metabolic tests. These include urinary reducing substances; the red cell enzyme galactose-1-phosphate uridyl transferase, urine and plasma amino acids and organic acids.

Endocrine tests. These include thyroid function tests and a 09.00 h cortisol level.

Bile salts. Urinary bile salts for assessment by fast atom bombardment mass spectrometry and tandem mass spectrometry may be required to identify primary bile salt deficiencies.

Other specific tests. These include measurement of carnitine and acyl carnitine in fatty acid oxidation disorders.

Abdominal ultrasound scan. This may be carried out (after 4-h fast) to detect gallbladder size. The gallbladder is usually present unless there is severe intrahepatic cholestasis or biliary atresia. Ultrasound can also diagnose choledochal cyst.

Radioisotope scan. This may be used to demonstrate hepatic uptake and biliary excretion (which may be delayed more than 4–6 h in neonatal hepatitis syndrome if there is severe cholestasis, and more than 24 h in biliary atresia).

Liver biopsy. Needle biopsy of the liver is easy and well tolerated in neonates, infants and children. It is required to determine the severity of hepatocellular injury and extent of fibrosis, evidence for infiltrative or storage disease and to differentiate intrahepatic cholestasis from extrahepatic obstruction. Portal zone duct proliferation and a biliary type of fibrosis are usually present in extrahepatic biliary atresia (Fig. 29.1b). A relative paucity of portal zone bile ducts supports the diagnosis of intrahepatic cholestasis. The PAS-positive bodies of α_1-antitrypsin deficiency may be seen after 2 months. Electron microscopy is essential if metabolic disease is suspected.

Percutaneous and endoscopic cholangiography. The percutaneous technique is of value when liver biopsy findings are equivocal and the TeBIDA suggests biliary atresia. Endoscopic cholangiography is employed using suitably sized instruments [16].

Family studies. At the onset it is valuable to test the blood of the mother, father and other siblings by appropriate methods and to store the sera for later use, or to collect DNA to examine for genetic diseases.

Neonatal hepatitis syndrome

This may be due to: (1) intrauterine infections, (2) endocrine causes such as hypothyroidism, or (3) inherited diseases including chromosomal abnormalities.

Intrauterine infection

Immunity is reduced in the neonate and virus infections are frequent and very liable to persist. Chronic hepatitis and cirrhosis may ensue. Similarly, older children with immunological deficits such as agammaglobulinaemia or who are receiving treatment with immunosuppressive drugs are at risk.

Toxoplasmosis, rubella, cytomegalovirus, herpes simplex (TORCH) infections

Congenital infections grouped under the acronym TORCH have similar clinical features: hepatosplenomegaly, jaundice, pneumonitis, petechial or purpuric rash, prematurity or poor intrauterine growth. Presentation with acute liver failure may occur with herpes simplex infection.

Cytomegalovirus

This is the commonest cause of intrauterine infection (Chapter 21). It is usually acquired placentally from an asymptomatic mother. It can also be transmitted in breast milk and from blood products. Many congenital infections are asymptomatic.

The disease may be fulminant with intense jaundice, purpura, hepatosplenomegaly, chorioretinitis, cataracts and pulmonary defects. Survivors may run a long course with persistent jaundice, hepatomegaly and disappearing bile ducts. The prognosis is good although 30% will develop cirrhosis requiring treatment by liver transplantation.

Intranuclear viral inclusions are seen in bile duct epithelium and rarely in hepatocytes. Diagnosis is made on urine or tissue *in situ* using PCR [17].

Herpes simplex

The liver may be involved in the course of a fulminating viraemia, contracted at birth from maternal genital herpes. Jaundice is due to viral involvement of the liver. Histologically, necrosis is seen with little or no inflammatory reaction. Giant cells are absent, but inclusion bodies may be found.

Treatment with i.v. ganciclovir is essential. Liver transplantation is usually contraindicated if there is multiorgan failure and the mortality is 70% [18].

Congenital rubella syndrome

This disease, if contracted in the first trimester of pregnancy, may cause fetal malformations. It may also persist through the neonatal period and into later life. The liver with the brain, lung, heart and other organs are involved in the generalized virus infection. Jaundice develops within the first 1 or 2 days with hepatosplenomegaly, cholestasis and slightly elevated serum transaminase levels.

Hepatic histology shows a typical giant cell hepatitis, with bile in swollen Kupffer cells and ductules with a focal hepatocellular necrosis and portal fibrosis. Erythroid haemopoietic tissue is relatively increased. The virus can be identified from the liver at necropsy or biopsy. Usually the hepatitis resolves completely.

Intrauterine *parvovirus* B19 can cause severe giant cell hepatic disease in the neonate, also fulminant liver failure and aplastic anaemia [19].

Congenital toxoplasmosis

Congenital toxoplasmosis is rare and results from maternal infection in the third trimester. Neonatal hepatitis is associated with central nervous system involvement with chorioretinitis (with large pigmented scars), hydrocephaly or microcephaly. The liver shows infiltration of portal zones with mononuclear cells. Extramedullary haemopoiesis with increased stainable iron is conspicuous. Histiocytes containing *Toxoplasma* may be present. It is diagnosed by finding *Toxoplasma* IgM antibodies and treated with spiramycin.

Congenital syphilis

Congenital syphilis is increasing again in frequency [20]. It causes a multisystem illness, with intrauterine growth retardation, failure to thrive, severe anaemia, thrombocytopenia, nephrotic syndrome, periostitis, nasal discharge ('snuffles'), skin rash, diffuse lymphadenopathy and hepatomegaly. Jaundice may be severe. Central nervous system involvement occurs in up to 30% of infants. Diagnosis involves serological testing, including the Venereal Disease Research Laboratory (VDRL) test and confirmatory testing for specific antitreponemal antibodies. Treatment is with penicillin.

Varicella

Varicella may occur in newborn infants if maternal infection occurs within 14 days of delivery. The disease is characterized by jaundice, extensive skin and multisystem involvement, especially pneumonia. In severe or fatal cases hepatic parenchymal involvement can be demonstrated [21]. Treatment is with aciclovir.

Human immunodeficiency virus (HIV) infection

Congenital HIV infection may present clinically as hepatitis with jaundice although later than in the neonatal period, typically at approximately 6 months of age [22]. Older children have a similar picture to adults with the same spectrum of infections, primary lymphoma and Kaposi's sarcoma. Hepatic histology shows more giant cell transformation and fewer granulomas [23]. Diffuse, lymphoplasmocytic infiltration is associated with lymphoid interstitial pneumonia.

Hepatitis A, B and C

Infections with these viruses in the neonate do not cause jaundice or neonatal hepatitis unless there is acute liver failure or severe hepatitis (see below).

Bacterial infection outside the liver

In the neonate, an immature reticuloendothelial system with decreased complement and opsonins impairs the ability of the liver and spleen to phagocytose bacteria. Conjugated hyperbilirubinaemia may occur with sepsis or localized extrahepatic infection, such as a urinary infection [24,25]. Serum aminotransferases may be slightly elevated, but hepatosplenomegaly is uncommon. Jaundice may also occur with streptococcal and staphylococcal infections and Gram-negative bacterial septicaemia.

Endocrine disorders

Hypothyroidism

Hypothyroidism is usually associated with an unconjugated hyperbilirubinaemia or the neonatal hepatitis syndrome and should be excluded in every patient. It is more common in girls than boys. Mild anaemia is common and the infant is sluggish. The diagnosis is confirmed by finding low serum thyroxine and triiodothyronine levels with high thyroid-stimulating hormone, and by observing the effects of therapy. The mechanism of the jaundice is unknown.

Hypopituitarism

Pituitary–adrenal dysfunction is associated with neonatal hepatitis syndrome in 30–70% of patients [26]. Clinical features include: conjugated hyperbilirubinaemia; hypoglycaemia in the perinatal period, septo-optic dysplasia [27] and hypoplasia of the optic nerves which is associated with hypopituitarism. There may also be midline facial abnormalities, nystagmus and microgenitalia in boys.

The diagnosis is made by identifying a low thyroid-stimulating hormone and a free thyroxine level with a low 9.00h cortisol value. It resolves with hormone replacement, thyroxine and hydrocortisone.

Chromosomal disorders

Trisomy 18

Trisomy 18 is associated with growth retardation, skeletal abnormalities and complex congenital heart disease. A giant-cell hepatitis has been reported [28,29].

Trisomy 21

The association between trisomy 21 and neonatal cholestasis or extrahepatic biliary atresia is reported. The neonatal hepatitis resolves spontaneously.

Idiopathic neonatal hepatitis

This is diagnosed after exclusion of known causes. The number of cases being diagnosed has diminished with the developments in molecular and genetic technology.

Neonatal hepatitis in preterm infants

Idiopathic neonatal hepatitis is a common referral in preterm babies, as many more premature infants survive. Most will have been given parenteral nutrition and are at risk of cholestasis. It is important to differentiate this condition from other known causes of neonatal hepatitis syndrome, parenteral nutrition-associated liver disease and biliary atresia which may have an atypical presentation in this age group. Examination of stools for pigment and a fasting ultrasound examination for gallbladder size are useful investigations to exclude biliary atresia. Liver biopsy is only indicated if there is persistent elevation of conjugated bilirubin and/or abnormal liver biochemistry. The prognosis is good.

Prolonged parenteral nutrition

The aetiology of parenteral nutrition-related liver disease is complex and is associated with prematurity, low birth weight and recurrent sepsis [30]. It is related to difficulties in enteral feeding, loss of the enterohepatic circulation of bile acids and consequent reduced bile formation, biliary stasis and sludging.

Infants have a gradual increase in serum conjugated bilirubin associated with elevation of transaminases, alkaline phosphatase and γ-GT. Liver biopsy shows nonspecific changes with features of extrahepatic biliary obstruction and bile in canaliculi (Fig. 29.1c). Biliary sludge and gallstones may develop. The disease is reversible if parenteral nutrition can be discontinued, but in infants with intestinal failure is the main indication for combined liver and bowel transplantation [30].

Inherited disease in the neonate

α₁-Antitrypsin deficiency

α_1-antitrypsin is synthesized in the rough endoplasmic reticulum of the liver. It comprises 80–90% of the serum α_1-globulin and is an inhibitor of trypsin and other proteases. Deficiency results in the unopposed action of these enzymes, in particular neutrophil elastase. The lungs are the major target, with damage to alveoli and resulting emphysema [31].

The gene for α_1-antitrypsin is on chromosome 14. There are about 75 different alleles at this locus, which can be distinguished by isoelectric focusing or agarose gel electrophoresis at acid pH, or by PCR analysis. M is the common, normal allele. Z and S are the most frequent abnormal alleles, which put the individual at risk of disease. One gene is derived from each parent. The combination results in normal, intermediate, low or zero serum α_1-antitrypsin levels. Protease inhibitor (Pi) MM gives a serum α_1-antitrypsin value of 20–53 μmol/L, the normal state. PiZZ results in a low concentration of 2.5–7 μmol/L and PiNull-Null gives zero levels. Both give a high risk of emphysema. PiSS and PiMZ give levels 50–60% of normal with no increased risk of lung disease. PiSZ gives α_1-antitrypsin levels of 8–19 μmol/L with a mildly increased risk [32,33].

Mutation of the gene can give deficiency of circulating α_1-antitrypsin by a number of mechanisms. Liver disease, however, only occurs with mutations where α_1-antitrypsin accumulates in hepatocytes. The classical type is PiZZ but the M_{malton} and M_{duarte} variants may do the same.

Pathogenesis of liver disease [33,34]. Only the PiZZ phenotype has been clearly associated with liver disease. This is not due to the low circulating levels of α_1-antitrypsin arriving at the liver, since other phenotypes with a low circulating levels do not develop hepatic damage. Intrahepatic accumulation of α_1-antitrypsin seems to be responsible. Studies of the molecular structure have shown that with the ZZ mutation there is polymerization of protein units. Normally, the reactive loop (Fig. 29.2) swings in between the β-helices of the so-called

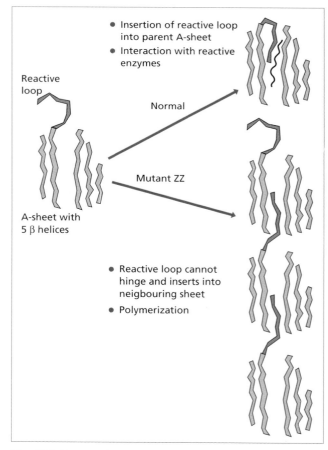

Fig. 29.2 Proposed mechanism of polymerization of ZZ α_1-antitrypsin.

A-sheet of the protein, where it interacts with elastase and other enzymes. In the ZZ mutant protein, the reactive loop cannot do this. It remains on the outside and is then available to insert into the A-sheet of an adjacent ZZ unit [35]. The polymers formed prevent export of most of the protein.

Accumulation of ZZ protein is thought to be responsible for liver damage but the mechanism is still unclear. Polymerization of ZZ protein occurs spontaneously or following minor perturbations such as a rise in temperature. However, the mutation of the α_1-antitrypsin protein is not the only reason for its retention. Cells from individuals with α_1-antitrypsin liver disease also have a reduction in the degradatory pathways in the endoplasmic reticulum [33]. The variation in clinical disease therefore appears to depend not only on the abnormal protein produced in PiZZ but also other cellular mechanisms as yet poorly understood.

Only a small proportion of individuals with α_1-antitrypsin deficiency ever develop liver disease, but it is the main cause of emphysema in early adulthood.

Clinical picture. α_1-antitrypsin deficiency is the commonest inborn error of metabolism to present with persistent neonatal jaundice, with an incidence of 1:7000 live births worldwide. Infants may present with intrauterine growth retardation, cholestasis, failure to thrive, hepatomegaly, or a vitamin K responsive coagulopathy. The latter is more likely in those infants who are not given prophylactic vitamin K at birth and who are being breast fed.

Liver biochemistry demonstrates a mixed hepatic/obstructive picture with elevated transaminases, alkaline phosphatase and γ-GT. Radiological investigations may indicate severe intrahepatic cholestasis with a contracted gallbladder on a fasting ultrasound, and delayed or absent excretion of radioisotope on hepatobiliary scanning. In homozygotes, the diagnosis is easily confirmed by detection of a low level of a$_1$-antitrypsin (<0.9 g/L).

Liver histology demonstrates giant cell hepatitis with characteristic periodic acid–Schiff (PAS), diastase resistant, positive granules of α_1-antitrypsin in hepatocytes, which may be detected by 6–8 weeks of age.

Management consists of nutritional support, fat-soluble vitamin supplementation and treatment of pruritus and cholestasis. Patients and parents should not smoke, and PiZZ individuals should be protected from passive smoking.

Parents are obligate heterozygotes. Thus there is a 25% chance of each subsequent fetus being affected. Antenatal diagnosis by chorionic villus sampling is now available using synthetic oligonucleotide probes specific for the M and Z gene or by restriction fragment length polymorphism [36].

Prognosis. The prognosis is variable. The long-term outlook for many infants with α_1-antitrypsin deficiency is good and in approximately 50% the liver disease resolves; 25% develop chronic liver disease [37], while the remainder require liver transplantation in the first year of life. Poor prognostic factors are prolonged jaundice, a higher AST at presentation and histology with severe bile duct reduplication, severe fibrosis with bridging septa and cirrhosis [38].

The few children with α_1-antitrypsin deficiency who present later in infancy or in childhood with hepatomegaly, but without any neonatal jaundice, usually are cirrhotic and have a poor prognosis.

Associations in later life. The incidence of liver disease in PiZZ individuals at age 50 years is about 15%, more frequent in males. Usually the changes in liver function are subtle, but the patient may present with complications of portal hypertension or ascites. Hepatocellular carcinoma may complicate cirrhosis.

Cystic fibrosis

Abnormalities of liver function tests or hepatic pathology are found in one-third of infants with cystic fibrosis. The spectrum of hepatic disorder is highly variable, but the clinical presentation is with jaundice, hepatomegaly, and failure to thrive and meconium ileus. Some infants have a giant-cell hepatitis. Extrahepatic bile duct obstruction may be due to inspissated bile actually plugging the common bile duct [39], which can be removed by choledochotomy. Occurrence of neonatal hepatitis syndrome in cystic fibrosis does not necessarily predict early development of cirrhosis.

Bile duct paucity syndromes

Alagille's syndrome (arteriohepatic dysplasia) [40]. This is an autosomal dominant condition with an incidence of 1:100000 live births worldwide. It is a multisystem disorder which is associated with cardiac, facial, renal, ocular and skeletal abnormalities. The condition is related to a deletion on the short arm of chromosome 20p, which has been identified in 60% of patients. It is related to mutations in the *Jagged 1* gene, which encodes a ligand of *Notch 1*, one of four members of a family of transmembrane receptor proteins [41]. The mutation is predominately sporadic [42].

Infants present with persistent cholestasis, severe pruritus, hepatomegaly and failure to thrive. The characteristic facial features are difficult to identify in infancy, but become prominent later in childhood. They include a triangular face with high forehead and frontal bossing, deep widely spaced eyes, saddle-shaped nasal bridge and pointed chin (Fig. 29.3). Cardiac abnormalities

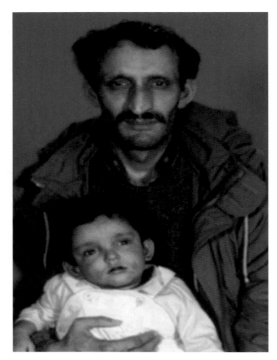

Fig. 29.3. In Alagille's syndrome, the characteristic facial features are difficult to identify in infancy, but become prominent later in childhood or in adult life (as in the father). They include a triangular face with high forehead and frontal bossing, deep widely spaced eyes, saddle-shaped nasal bridge and pointed chin.

include peripheral pulmonary stenosis, pulmonary and aortic valve stenosis and Fallot's tetralogy [40]. Hepatosplenomegaly is unusual unless there is progressive fibrosis, which is rare.

Skeletal abnormalities include abnormal thoracic vertebrae, 'butterfly' vertebrae and curving of the proximal digits of the third and fourth finger. Ocular abnormalities [43,44] include optic disease and papilloedema secondary to intra cranial hypertension, while posterior embryotoxin, which is detected on the inner aspects of the cornea near the junction of the iris, is demonstrated in 90% of patients by slit-lamp examination. Renal disease varies in severity from mild renal tubular acidosis to severe glomerular nephritis. Severe failure to thrive, which is complicated by gastrointestinal reflux and severe steatorrhoea secondary to fat malabsorption or pancreatic insufficiency is difficult to treat.

Liver biochemistry indicates severe cholestasis with: conjugated bilirubin above 100 μmol/L (6 mg/dL); raised alkaline phosphatase above 600 IU/L; γ-GT above 200 IU/L; raised transaminases; and plasma cholesterol above 6 mmol/L with normal triglycerides 0.4–2 mmol/L.

Tests of hepatic function such as albumin and coagulation are usually normal. Liver histology may be non-specific. The reduction in interlobular bile ducts is often difficult to identify in the neonatal period, particularly if cholestasis and giant cell hepatitis are also present. The histological appearance differs from extrahepatic biliary atresia because of the absence of portal fibrosis and biliary ductular proliferation.

Management. Intensive nutritional support is essential and pancreatic supplements may be required. Pruritus may be intractable and an indication for liver transplantation, although recent experience with the Molecular Reabsorbent Recirculating System (MARS) have produced relief for 6–12 months [45].

Prognosis is varied and depends on the extent of liver, cardiac or renal disease. Approximately 50% of children may regain normal liver function by adolescence while others require liver transplantation in childhood [40]. The 20 years predicted life expectancy is 75% for all patients, 80% for those not requiring liver transplantation and 60% for those who require liver transplantation [46]. The indications for liver transplantation are the development of cirrhosis and portal hypertension, intractable pruritus or severe decompensated growth failure. Pretransplant cardiac surgery or balloon dilatation may be indicated for severe pulmonary stenosis.

Genetic cholestatic syndromes

These diseases are related to defects in one of the members of ATP-binding cassette (ABC) transport superfamily (Table 29.5) (see also Chapter 11) [47]. They are concerned with the secretion of bile, but are important also in almost every cell organelle. The spectrum of disease caused by these defects is therefore diverse. Although usually familial with autosomal recessive inheritance, sporadic forms are identified.

Progressive familial intrahepatic cholestasis type 1

Progressive familial intrahepatic cholestasis type 1 (PFIC) was formerly called *Byler's disease* because of the association with the large numbers of an Amish kindred affected in Pennsylvania. The defect is now described from many parts of the world, including the Netherlands, Sweden and in Arab populations. Inheritance is autosomal recessive. It presents with cholestasis which eventually progresses to biliary fibrosis and cirrhosis. Liver transplantation is usually necessary in the first decade of life. Characteristically, serum γ-GT is low whereas alkaline phosphatase and serum primary bile acids are increased. Biliary bile acids are reduced.

The genetic defect has been mapped to the *FIC1* locus on chromosome 18q21–q22 to a region encoding a P-type ATPase (ATP8B1) involved in aminophospholipid trans-

Table 29.5. Genetic cholestatic syndromes

Disorder	Clinical	γ-GT	Chromosome	Genetic disorder
PFIC 1	Progressive	Normal	18q21–q22	P-type ATPase
BRIC	Recurrent jaundice, pruritus	Normal	18q21–q22	P-type ATPase
PFIC 2	Progressive	Normal	2q24	Canalicular bile acid transport
PFIC 3	Low phospholipids Bile ductular proliferation	High	7q21	Canalicular phospholipid transport (MDR3)
ARC	Renal dysfunction, cholestasis	Low	15q26	Snare trafficking defect
Dubin–Johnson	Conjugated hyperbilirubin	Normal	10q23q24	cMOAT (MRP2)

PFIC, progressive familial intrahepatic cholestasis; BRIC, benign recurrent intrahepatic cholestasis; γ-GT, γ-glutamyl transferase; MDR3, multiple drug resistance 3; MRP2, multidrug resistance protein 2; ARC, arthrogryphosis, renal dysfunction and cholestasis; cMOAT, canalicular multispecific organic anion transporter.

port between membrane leaflets [48]. There is defective bile acid transport at the canalicular membrane.

Liver transplantation is inevitable, but post-transplant diarrhoea is a significant problem.

Benign recurrent intrahepatic cholestasis

This presents with recurrent episodes of jaundice and pruritus, particularly in girls on the contraceptive pill [49]. The serum γ-GT is not elevated. The gene defect has been mapped to the *FIC1* locus, the same region as *PFIC1* 18q21–q22.

Progressive familial intrahepatic cholestasis type 2

This cholestatic disease is due to a mutation on chromosome 2 [50]. The gene encodes the human bile salt export pump (BSEP, ABCB11), an ATP-binding cassette transporter [51]. It does not involve the *PFIC1* locus but has been mapped to a locus on chromosome 2q24. This encodes the *BSEP* gene. The primary defect is a defective canalicular bile acid transport pump.

Patients present with cholestasis, giant cell hepatitis with fat malabsorption and pruritus. Serum γ-GT is normal and bile ductular proliferation is not seen. The disease has a variable progression to cirrhosis and liver transplantation.

Progressive familial intrahepatic cholestasis type 3

This form of neonatal cholestasis is marked by an elevated serum γ-GT and bile ductular proliferation. There is a mutation in the multiple drug-resistant gene (MDR3 or P glycoprotein 3) on chromosome 7q21 (Table 29.5). This moves phospholipid from the inner leaflet of the canalicular membrane to the outer leaflet, which faces the canalicular lumen [52]. Serum phospholipid is low. Bile acid transport is unimpaired as is bile flow, but in

the absence of phospholipid, the bile acids prove toxic to cholangiocytes and hepatocytes.

Treatment and outcome

Routine interventions for chronic cholestatic liver disease are required for all three forms. Treatment with ursodeoxycholic acid (20 mg/kg per day) may be helpful. Partial biliary diversion surgery is sometimes used successfully for PFIC 1 and 2 [53]. Although variability in the disease course is evident, liver damage usually progresses and many require liver transplantation during childhood. Early development of hepatocellular carcinoma in the first 5 years of life has been reported with PFIC 2 [54].

Abnormal bile acid synthesis

Defects in the synthesis of primary bile acids can cause decreased bile flow and abnormal transport and so cholestasis.

Bile acid synthesis defects may resemble PFIC type 2. *3β-hydroxy-C27-steroid dehydrogenase-isomerase deficiency* results in cholestasis without pruritus and with normal serum γ-GT and bile acids. Cholestasis has also resulted from *Δ4-3-oxosteroid-5β-reductase deficiency* [55].

Coprostanic acidaemia results from a defect in the conversion of coprostanic to varinic acid. It is associated with progressive cholestasis and death by 2 years of age.

Zellweger's cerebrohepatorenal syndrome is a fatal autosomal recessive condition with severe cholestasis. It is probably related to defective peroxisomal β-oxidation.

Treatment. Toxic intermediates are formed which cause cholestasis by interacting with hepatic bile acid transport. Replacement of exogenous bile acids results in the generation of bile acid-dependent flow and a decrease in the synthesis of toxic bile salts. The administration of chenodeoxycholic acid, ursodeoxycholic acid and cholic acid [56,57] effectively reduce pruritus and transaminases and serum bilirubin levels fall.

Dubin–Johnson syndrome (see also Chapter 11)

This is not a cholestatic disease, but is marked by a rise in serum conjugated bilirubin. It is caused by a mutation of an ABC transporter, canalicular multispecific organic anion transporter (cMOAT) [58].

Symptomatic treatment of cholestatic syndromes

The mainstay of treatment is intensive nutrition with adequate fat-soluble vitamin supplementation. Nutritional support is given by an increased energy intake of 120–150% of the estimated average, composed of 30–50% medium-chain triglyceride and high carbohydrate supplements. In severely malnourished infants, overnight or continuous nasogastric feeding may be required.

Fat-soluble vitamins are replaced orally by vitamin A 5000–15000 IU/day, vitamin D (α-calcidol) 50 ng/kg per day, vitamin K 2.5–5 mg/day and vitamin E 50–200 mg/day.

Pruritus is managed by a combination of phenobarbitone, ursodeoxycholic acid (10–20 mg/kg body weight), rifampicin (3 mg/kg) or by cholestyramine flavoured with apple purée, tomato juice or chocolate syrup [59].

Other causes of cholestatic jaundice

Neonatal lupus erythematosus syndrome

This presents as neonatal cholestasis and hepatitis [60]. Cutaneous lupus erythematosus and congenital heart block are associated.

Arthrogryphosis, cholestasis, renal tubular dysfunction (ARC)

This rare autosomal disorder presents with cholestasis, biliary hypoplasia, renal dysfunction and a low γ-GT. It is usually fatal and infants die of liver and renal failure within 12 months. The genetic defect is now known to be a disorder in a snare protein (VPS33B) involved in the regulation of vesicle and membrane fusion. It is the first human disorder associated with mutations in a gene involved in regulation of the SNARE-mediated mechanism of membrane tether and fusion and may lead to further understanding of the pathophysiology of biliary disorders [61].

Neonatal sclerosing cholangitis

This presents in early infancy with conjugated hyperbilirubinaemia which then resolves.

The aetiology is unknown but it may have a genetic basis [62]. The clinical picture includes: jaundice, development of hepatosplenomegaly, biliary cirrhosis and portal hypertension.

Laboratory investigations indicate elevated serum alkaline phosphatase and γ-GT. Endoscopic or percutaneous cholangiography demonstrates beaded irregularity of medium to large intrahepatic bile ducts in all patients and in extrahepatic ducts in 80%. Liver histology shows portal fibrosis with ductal proliferation developing into biliary cirrhosis. Surgical treatment is not indicated, but supportive management with nutrition is required. Most children require liver transplantation at some stage.

Structural abnormalities: biliary atresia and choledochal cyst

The commonest causes of extrahepatic or structural biliary obstruction in neonates are biliary atresia or choledochal cysts.

Biliary atresia

Extra hepatic biliary atresia is a disease of unknown aetiology with no proven genetic basis [63]. It is a rare disease which occurs with the frequency of approximately 1:15000 live births [64,65]. The disease affects both intra- and extrahepatic ducts with progressive destruction leading to cholestasis, fibrosis and cirrhosis. The disease is classified according to the extent of biliary damage. Type I biliary atresia affects the common bile duct with a cystic proximal bile duct; type II affects the common hepatic duct; type III, which is the most common, affects the whole of the extrahepatic biliary tree.

There appear to be two clinical phenotypes. There is a syndromic or embryonic form that accounts for 10–20% of cases and is distinguished by other congenital anomalies such as polysplenia, situs inversus, cardiac anomalies (e.g. atrial and ventricular septal defects), absence of the inferior cava etc. (biliary atresia splenic malformation syndrome) [66]. The perinatal or acquired form is more common and represents 80–90% of cases.

Developmental aspects

The biliary passages may fail to develop from the primitive foregut bud. The gallbladder may be absent or the biliary tract represented only by a gallbladder connecting directly with the duodenum. The more usual defect is failure of vacuolation of the solid biliary bud. This is usually partial and rarely extends throughout the biliary tree.

Pathogenesis

The underlying pathogenesis is unknown, but is likely to be multifactorial based on the interaction of genetic and environmental factors. Research to date has focussed on defects in morphogenesis, immunological dysregulation, viral infection such as reovirus or cytomegalovirus, or toxin exposure [67].

Pathology

The ducts may be absent or replaced by fibrous strands. Bile is absent from the extrahepatic biliary system including the gallbladder.

Clinical features

There are more females than males, and all races are affected. Infants are full term with a normal birth weight and present with persisting jaundice from the second day of life. Other features include pale stools, dark urine, failure to thrive and hepatomegaly. Splenomegaly may be found but is a late feature and implies significant hepatic fibrosis and early cirrhosis [68]. Occasionally, infants present with bleeding from vitamin K-responsive coagulopathy, which is more common in breast-fed infants who did not receive vitamin K perinatally. About 5% of all infants will have had an abnormal antenatal maternal ultrasound. This is due to the presence of a cyst within the otherwise obliterated biliary tree and is detectable from around 22 weeks of gestation.

The diagnosis is suggested by a serum conjugated bilirubin exceeding 100μmol/L (5mg/dL), a serum alkaline phosphatase exceeding 600IU/L, γ-GT exceeding 100IU/L. ALT and AST are between 100 and 200IU/L. Fasting ultrasound shows an absent or contracted gallbladder. Biliary scintigraphy with ^{99m}Tc-TEBIDA shows no excretion of isotope from liver into bowel 24h after administration. Liver histology shows fibrosis, cholestasis and proliferation of biliary ductules with a variable number of giant cells. There is paucity of interlobular ducts.

The diagnosis is usually confirmed at laparotomy with or without cholangiography in which the atretic biliary tree is shown. It is usual to carry out palliative surgery, the Kasai portoenterostomy. Some infants who present late (>100 days) with established cirrhosis may be candidates for liver transplantation as a primary procedure. The natural history of this disease without medical or surgical management treatment is that the majority of children die within 2 years of birth from end-stage liver failure.

Surgical management

The Kasai portoenterostomy is based on excision of the entire obliterated biliary tree to expose communicating biliary channels and create a Roux loop from the proximal jejunum which is anastomosed to the cut liver surface [69]. Restoration of biliary flow is considered the measure of success but depends on the age of surgery, the expertise of the surgeon and the extent of fibrosis at operation [65,70]. It is defined as normalization of serum bilirubin within 6 months of the procedure and in a recent UK report this was achieved in 57% of cases [71].

Age at surgery. Many studies have shown an improved outcome in terms of clearance of jaundice and native liver survival, the earlier the portoenterostomy is performed. Although the age at operation is an important factor, it may be a proxy for the extent of liver damage. Although initial results suggested that children operated on at 40 days of age did not show a significant survival advantage [72], recent data from Japan [73,74] suggest a clear advantage for those infants operated on earlier than 30 days of age, no difference in outcome in those operated on between 30 and 90 days, and a significant disadvantage only for those operated on later than 90 days.

Surgical expertise. The most important variable is the experience of the surgeon and the surgical centre. Recent studies have clearly demonstrated that the short and long-term outcome for children with biliary atresia is closely related to the experience of the surgeon and the centre [65,74,75]. These data led to the UK Department of Health directive to centralize surgery for all infants with suspected biliary atresia, which has been shown to improve the outcome [71].

Histology. Although it has been suggested that the extent of histological abnormality at operation [76] or the morphology of the extra hepatic biliary remnant influence both short and long-term outcome, this has not been found consistently [77].

Medical management

The important aspects of postsurgical management include prevention of complications, provision of nutritional and family support, requiring a multidisciplinary approach. This includes prevention of cholangitis, initially with intravenous antibiotics and subsequently with prophylactic low-dose oral antibiotics, which can be rotated at 8 or 12-week intervals (e.g. amoxycillin 125mg/day, cephalexin 125mg/day, trimethoprim 120mg/day) for 12 months as a minimum. Ursodeoxycholic acid (20mg/kg per day) may also be effective in encouraging bile flow and bile drainage. Nutritional support is essential to prevent malnutrition, overcome fat malabsorption and reduce the effect of excess catabolism. Fat-soluble vitamin supplementation should include vitamin A 5000–15000IU/day, vitamin D (alfacalcidol) 50 ng/kg per day, vitamin E 50–200 mg/day and vitamin K 2.5–5 mg/day.

The role of corticosteroids in improving biliary drainage is controversial. A number of small retrospective studies have suggested a beneficial effect with improved bile drainage and survival with native liver in children [69] but a prospective randomized placebo-controlled study in 71 infants found no significant effect on either native liver survival or proportion who cleared their jaundice [69].

Prognosis

Immediate complications include technical problems such as biliary leaks, exacerbation of ascites and ascending cholangitis. Longer-term complications include fat malabsorption and malnutrition, which leads to fat-soluble vitamin deficiency.

As the disease is progressive, all children will develop portal fibrosis, cirrhosis and portal hypertension, even if bile drainage has been established, which is more likely if there is recurrent cholangitis. However, 80% of children who have had a successful portoenterostomy are likely to survive more than 10 years with their native liver and achieve good quality of life [69,78]. Biliary atresia is the commonest indication for liver transplant in children. Currently, 76% of children under the age of 2 years who require transplantation have been born with biliary atresia (European Liver Transplant Registry 2005). The 15-year post-transplant survival is more than 80% [79].

Choledochal cyst (see also Chapter 14)

Choledochal cyst is a congenital malformation of the biliary system which may be identified in the fetus by antenatal ultrasound [80,81].

Clinical features and diagnosis

Choledochal cysts present with jaundice, abdominal mass and pain with acholic stools, but this is an unusual presentation in the neonatal period. There is a female predominance (female:male is 5:1). The diagnosis is made by identifying the choledochal cyst by ultrasound examination of the liver and confirmed by cholangiography, either percutaneous or endoscopic. Liver function tests are consistent with biliary obstruction and liver biopsy may demonstrate large bile duct obstruction and fibrosis, which is reversible after surgery.

Surgical treatment includes excision of all the affected ducts and re-establishment of biliary drainage by forming a hepaticojejunostomy. Drainage of the cyst into adjacent duodenum or jejunum is now contraindicated, because of the potential malignant transformation. The results of surgery are excellent, cholangitis is an occasional complication, and there is a 2.5% risk of malignancy in the residual biliary tree in adult life [82].

Spontaneous perforation of the bile ducts

This is a rare complication in which perforation occurs at the junction of the cystic and common hepatic ducts, perhaps due to a congenital weakness, inspissated bile or gallstones. Infants may present at any age from 2–24 weeks of age with abdominal distension, ascites, jaundice and acholic stools. Biliary peritonitis, with bile in hydroceles, hernial sacs and umbilicus may be obvious.

The diagnosis is confirmed by abdominal ultrasound, which may show free intraperitoneal fluid and dilated intrahepatic ducts. Biochemical liver function tests may be abnormal, with conjugated hyperbilirubinaemia and raised alkaline phosphatase and γ-GT. If the biliary leak is large, liver function tests may be virtually normal. Cholangiography shows the blocked cystic duct with the hepatic duct leak. Hepatobiliary scanning will demonstrate isotope into the peritoneal cavity. Treatment includes peritoneal drainage followed by repair of the perforation. The results of surgery are good.

Inspissated bile syndrome and cholelithiasis

Bile duct obstruction secondary to inspissated bile syndrome may be secondary to total parenteral nutrition, prolonged haemolysis and dehydration. It is more common in premature babies or those undergoing major surgery. The clinical picture is of biliary obstruction with pale stools, dark urine and abnormal liver function tests. The diagnosis is made by ultrasound, which demonstrates a dilated intra- and extrahepatic duct system with biliary sludge. Percutaneous transhepatic cholangiography will outline the anatomy and may be therapeutic with lavage of the biliary tree, but laparatomy and decompression of the biliary tree may be required. The use of ursodeoxycholic acid (20 mg/kg) and cholecystokinin may prevent the need for either surgical or radiological intervention.

Cholecystitis may occur in infants in association with gallstones from haemolysis or total parenteral nutrition, while acalculus cholecystitis may occur as part of generalized sepsis. Operative cholecystectomy (rather than laparoscopic) is the treatment of choice in this young age group for symptomatic cholecystitis in association with gallstones [83].

In older children, cholecystitis and gallstones may be associated with blood dyscrasias or congenital anomalies of the biliary tract, such as choledochal cysts or biliary atresia.

Acute liver failure in infancy

Acute liver failure in infancy usually presents with multisystem involvement. The diagnosis may initially be difficult as jaundice may be a late feature. Infants are usually small for gestational dates, with hypotonia, severe coagulopathy and encephalopathy. Neurological problems, such as nystagmus and convulsions, may be secondary to cerebral disease or encephalopathy. Renal tubular acidosis is common. Investigations include a search for multiorgan disease.

Galactosaemia

This rare autosomal disorder is secondary to a deficiency of galactose-1-phosphase uridyltransferase (GALT), essential for galactose metabolism, in the liver and red blood cells. It is inherited as an autosomal recessive with a frequency of between 1 in 10 000 and 1 in 60 000. There are more than 150 mutations reported in the *GALT* gene [84], and this genetic heterogeneity contributes to the wide phenotypic heterogeneity. A significant reduction of the transferase is found in heterozygotes.

Clinical picture

Acute illness results from the accumulation of the substrate galactose-1-phosphate (gal-1-P) following the introduction of milk feeds [85]. Infants present with collapse, sepsis, hypoglycaemia, and encephalopathy in the first few days of life or with progressive jaundice and liver failure. Ascites and hepatosplenomegaly may be noted. Cataracts are present. The disease may be complicated by Gram-negative sepsis, which stimulates a life-threatening severe bleeding diathesis.

The condition should be considered in all young patients with cirrhosis and even in the adult if there are suggestive features such as cataract.

Hepatic changes

Those dying in the first few weeks show diffuse hepatocellular fatty change. In the next few months, the liver shows pseudoglandular or ductular structures around the canaliculi which may contain bile. Regeneration is conspicuous, necrosis scanty and a macronodular cirrhosis results. Giant cells may be numerous (see Fig. 29.1a).

Diagnosis

The biochemical changes include galactosaemia, galactosuria, hyperchloraemic acidosis, albuminuria and aminoaciduria. The diagnosis is established by the detection of urinary reducing substances in the absence of glycosuria, and confirmed by reduced GALT enzyme activity in erythrocytes. Hepatic pathology demonstrates fatty change, periportal bile duct proliferation and iron deposition with extramedullary haematopoiesis. If galactose ingestion persists, hepatic fibrosis and cirrhosis may develop or be present at birth [86].

Prognosis and treatment

Liver function improves following exclusion of galactose from the diet unless liver failure or cirrhosis has developed. Galactose elimination is life-long, but efficacy may be limited by endogenous synthesis of gal-1-P, explaining the persistence of galactose metabolites despite compliance with dietary restriction [87].

The long-term outcome is disappointing. Learning difficulties and growth disturbance are described and are more common in girls, 75% of whom also develop ovarian failure.

Detection of galactosaemia in a neonatal screening program will lead to early detection, except for infants who present with fulminant hepatitis. Antenatal diagnosis is possible by chorionic villi sampling.

Neonatal haemochromatosis (NNH)

This disease is the commonest cause of acute liver failure in the neonate. It is characterized by the prenatal accumulation of intrahepatic iron, due either to a primary disorder of fetoplacental iron handling or a secondary manifestation of fetal liver disease.

There is no association with mutations in the genes for hereditary haemochromatosis or juvenile haemochromatosis [88]. NNH is extremely rare in first pregnancies, and once one affected child has been born the risk of recurrence in subsequent pregnancies is 80% but recurrence has never been reported in children born to the same father with different mothers. This pattern is strongly suggestive of a maternal alloimmune disorder, as recently reported [89].

Clinical features include intrauterine growth retardation, premature delivery, hypoglycaemia, jaundice and coagulopathy within the first 2 weeks. The outcome is fatal without treatment.

Biochemical liver function tests demonstrate an elevated bilirubin, and reduced transaminases and albumin. Serum iron binding capacity is low and hypersaturated (90–100%), with a grossly elevated ferritin level (>1000 µg/L). Diagnostic liver biopsy is not feasible because of the coagulopathy, but extrahepatic siderosis is found in minor salivary glands obtained by lip biopsy. Magnetic resonance imaging may confirm excess hepatic or extrahepatic iron.

Liver histology at autopsy demonstrates pericellular fibrosis, giant cell transformation, ductular proliferation and regenerative nodules. The distribution of siderosis is similar to adult hereditary haemochromatosis, with hepatocellular and extrahepatic parenchymal deposition and sparing of the reticuloendothelial system.

Medical management includes supportive therapy for acute liver failure and an 'antioxidant cocktail', which combines N-acetylcysteine (150 mg/kg per day), vitamin E (25 mg/kg per day), selenium (2–3 mg/kg per day), prostaglandin E1 (0.4–0.6 mg/kg per h), and desferrioxamine (30 mg/kg per day). Some children have responded to this regimen, but the majority require liver transplantation. Extrahepatic iron is mobilized following successful liver transplantation and does not recur [90].

Antenatal diagnosis is not possible, but the diagnosis may be suspected by the detection of non-specific abnormalities such as hydrops fetalis or intrauterine growth retardation. Prenatal iron accumulation may be detected by MRI, but the sensitivity is unknown. Treatment with immunoglobulin infusion from 16 weeks' gestation prevents recurrence in the majority, suggesting that this is an alloimmune disorder [91].

Disorders of mitochondrial energy metabolism

This group of disorders include a wide range of clinical phenotypes with any mode of inheritance: autosomal recessive, autosomal dominant or transmission through maternal DNA. A number of different defects involving the electron transport chain have been described. The pathological effects are secondary to dysfunction of the electron transport chain resulting in cellular ATP deficiency, impaired fat oxidation and the generation of toxic free radicals. Clinical symptoms vary, depending on the nature of the primary defect, the tissue or organ distribution and abundance, and the importance of aerobic metabolism in the affected tissue. The constituent proteins of the electron transport chain are encoded in two genomes, either nuclear DNA or mitochondrial DNA (mDNA), which is maternally inherited. In the context of liver failure, isolated deficiencies of the electron transport chain enzymes, mtDNA depletion syndromes and Alpers' syndrome are relevant [92].

Deficiencies of the electron transport chain enzyme

The most common isolated defects are complexes 4 and 1, although multiple deficiencies have been reported. Infants present with multisystem involvement with hypotonia, cardiomyopathy, and proximal renal tubulopathy and a severe metabolic acidosis. Relevant diagnostic investigations include elevated blood lactate, lactate/ pyruvate ratio more than 20, increased 3-OH-butyrate/ acetoacetate ratio above 2, or an increase in lactate, possible ketone bodies and, following a glucose load (2 g/kg), the detection of specific organic acids such as urinary 3-methyl-glutaconic acid or other Krebs' cycle intermediates. Coagulopathy is usually extreme, and may prevent liver or muscle biopsy, or cerebrospinal fluid examination. The diagnosis is based on demonstrating biochemical dysfunction of electron chain function in liver or muscle by histochemistry or enzyme analysis in fresh tissue. Demonstration of an elevated cerebrospinal fluid lactate compared with plasma lactate indicates neurological involvement [93].

Supportive management is usually the only option. Liver transplantation is only successful if the defect is confined to the liver, but is contraindicated if multisystem involvement is obvious as neurologic deterioration persists or may develop post-transplant.

Antenatal diagnosis is rarely possible as the underlying gene defects are unknown [94].

Mitochondrial DNA depletion syndromes

Mitochondria normally contain more than one copy of mDNA and replication is regulated by a number of factors encoded by nuclear genes. Mutations in these nuclear genes lead to a reduction in copy numbers of mDNA resulting in mitochondrial depletion. Mutations have been found in genes encoding the mitochondrial enzymes DNA polymerase-γ [95], thymidine kinase, deoxyguanosine kinase and succinyl CoA-ligase [93].

The clinical presentation and biochemical findings are similar to those of infants presenting with isolated electron transport chain deficiencies. Treatment is supportive as liver transplantation is contraindicated [95]. Antenatal diagnosis is possible if a mutation has been identified.

Alpers' syndrome. This is an autosomal recessive, developmental mtDNA depletion disorder characterized by degenerative brain and liver disease, which may be precipitated by valproate treatment [96]. Focal seizures usually precede liver disease. The clinical presentation is varied. Neurological features, lethargy and hypotonia are prominent. Hypertrophic cardiomyopathy and renal tubulopathy may develop. Hepatic involvement is unpredictable and includes isolated hepatomegaly, neonatal cholestasis and acute liver failure with coagulopathy.

The diagnosis is based on an elevated blood lactate, but this may be intermittent. Elevated cerebrospinal fluid/ plasma lactate ratio or elevated cerebrospinal fluid protein suggests central nervous system involvement.

Hepatic pathology is characterized by both micro- and macrovesicular steatosis, with hepatocyte degeneration and micronodular cirrhosis. Electron microscopy may reveal abnormal structure or number of mitochondria. Muscle histology may show increased lipid droplets. The presence of ragged red fibres on the Gomori stain are strongly suggestive of mtDNA abnormalities.

The definitive diagnosis is based on demonstrating dysfunction of electron transport chain function in affected tissue by histochemistry and direct measurement of enzyme activity combined with demonstration of reduced mtDNA copy number (<35% of control), usually in muscle [95].

Supportive management for acute liver failure is required with discontinuation of valproate. Transplantation is contraindicated if multisystem involvement is demonstrated. Antenatal diagnosis is occasionally possible if the underlying mutation is known

Tyrosinaemia type I

Tyrosinaemia type I is an autosomal recessive disorder due to a defect of fumaryl acetoacetase (FAA), which is the terminal enzyme in tyrosine degradation. The gene for FAA is on the short arm of chromosome 15. More than 40 mutations have been described to date [97], although in some populations a single mutation may be prevalent. There is a high lifetime risk of developing hepatocellular carcinoma, which historically is 40% [98].

Intermediate metabolites such as maleyl- and fumaryl-acetoacetate are highly reactive compounds that are locally toxic to the liver, while the secondary metabolite succinylacetone has both local and systemic effects, including cardiac, renal and neurological disease and inhibition of porphobilinogen synthase which is the cause of the neurological symptoms.

Clinical features are heterogeneous, even within the same family. Acute liver failure is a common presentation in infants between 1 and 6 months of age who present with mild jaundice, coagulopathy, encephalopathy and ascites. Hypoglycaemia is common, either due to liver dysfunction or hyperinsulinism from pancreatic islet cell hyperplasia.

In older infants, failure to thrive, coagulopathy, hepatosplenomegaly, hypotonia and rickets are common. Older children may present with chronic liver disease, a hypertrophic cardiomyopathy, renal failure or a porphyria-like syndrome with self-mutilation. Renal tubular dysfunction and hypophosphataemic rickets may occur at any age.

Biochemical liver function tests show an elevated bilirubin, transaminases, alkaline phosphatase and a reduced albumin. Plasma amino acids indicate a three-fold increase in plasma tyrosine, phenylalanine and methionine with grossly elevated α-fetoprotein levels. Urinary succinyl acetone is a pathognomonic but not an invariable finding. The diagnosis is confirmed by measuring FAA activity in fibroblasts or lymphocytes. Proximal tubular dysfunction is demonstrated by phos-

phaturia and aminoaciduria, and confirmed by a reduction in renal tubular absorption of phosphate (<80%).

Hepatic histology is non-specific with steatosis, siderosis and cirrhosis, which may be present in infancy. Hepatocyte dysplasia is associated with a risk of hepatocellular carcinoma.

Initial management is with a phenylalanine and tyrosine-restricted diet, which may improve overall nutritional status and renal tubular function but does not affect progression of liver disease. The discovery of 2(2-nitro-trifluoromethylbenzoyl)-1,3-cyclohexenedione (NTBC) or nitisinone, which prevents the formation of toxic metabolites, has altered the natural history of this disease in childhood. There is rapid reduction of toxic metabolites, normalization of tubular function, prevention of porphyria-like crises and improvement in both nutritional status and liver function, particularly in those who have acute liver failure [99].

The long-term outcome of children who have tyrosinaemia type I treated with nitisinone is unknown. These children require long-term monitoring and follow-up with 6-monthly abdominal ultrasound CT scans, or MRI and α-fetoprotein estimation for early detection of hepatocellular carcinoma. Liver transplantation is now only indicated for the development of acute or chronic liver failure unresponsive to NTBC, or suspicion of hepatocellular carcinoma.

Antenatal diagnosis is possible either by chorionic villus sampling which measures FAA directly, or from mutation analysis, or by measurement of succinyl acetone in the amniotic fluid. Prospective affected siblings may benefit from early NTBC therapy [100].

Liver disease in older children

Liver disease in children older than 6 months may be acute or chronic. As in infancy, there is a predominance of inherited disorders.

Acute viral hepatitis

All forms of acute viral hepatitis occur in children and include hepatitis A virus (HAV), HBV, post-transfusion HCV, epidemic hepatitis E virus (HEV), Epstein–Barr virus (EBV) and cytomegalovirus (CMV). In contrast to many adults, most children are asymptomatic and anicteric, and many episodes of hepatitis are subclinical.

Uncomplicated acute hepatitis is managed at home. Hospital admission is required only if the child has severe vomiting leading to dehydration, abdominal pain or lethargy, if coagulation parameters are prolonged or transaminase activity remains high. Fulminant hepatitis is a complication in less than 5% of paediatric cases. The main differential diagnoses are metabolic liver disease (e.g. Wilson's disease) or drug-induced liver disease.

Chronic liver disease

HBV and HCV are the commonest forms of viral hepatitis in childhood, but do not lead to serious liver disease until adolescence or adult life.

Hepatitis B virus infection [101]

Children are infected in childhood by: vertical transmission from a carrier mother; horizontal transmission from parents and other family members; by infected blood products; sexual abuse; or, in adolescents, drug abuse. Perinatal transmission occurs mainly through placental tears, trauma during delivery or contact of the infant mucous membrane with infected maternal fluid. Intrauterine transmission may occur. Hepatitis B virus carrier mothers, who are HBe antigen positive, have the highest infectivity with a 70–90% risk of transmission. Those mothers who are HBe antigen negative, but HBe antibody positive, may also transmit infection, and their infants are particularly at risk of developing fulminant liver failure, secondary to mutant HBV. Seventy per cent of infants infected perinatally will become chronic carriers unless immunized at birth.

Chronic carriers should be reviewed annually for evidence of seroconversion or progressive liver disease and/or hepatocellular carcinoma.

The indications for treatment in childhood are persistently raised serum aminotransferases, presence of HBe antigen with detectable HBV DNA in serum and features of chronic hepatitis on liver biopsy. There are no proven effective treatments. Interferon-α (5–10 million units/m^2 thrice weekly) by subcutaneous injection for 6 months has a sustained clearance rate of 40–50%. Children who have active histology, low HBV DNA levels (<1000 pg/mL), high serum aminotransferase enzymes and horizontal transmission are more likely to respond to interferon. Both lamivudine and adefovir have similar results in children as in adults with approximately 26% seroconversion after 12 months' treatment. Viral resistance is an issue, especially with lamivudine. Antivirals such as entecavir, telbivudine and tenofivir are under evaluation [102] (see Chapter 18).

The most important strategy to prevent HBV transmission in childhood includes routine antenatal screening of all women during pregnancy, with immunization of at-risk infants, or universal immunization of all infants. Protection persists for 10 years after vaccination in infancy [103].

Hepatitis C virus infection [104]

The importance of hepatitis C virus infection in children lies in later development of chronic liver disease. Children are infected with HCV either parenterally or vertically. Although now the commonest mode of infection, vertical transmission of HCV is unusual, ranging from 2–10% of offspring born to HCV-RNA-positive mothers. The risk of transmission is increased up to 48% by coexisting maternal HIV infection, and in those who have high HCV RNA titres. Breast feeding is not contraindicated.

Diagnosis is made by screening children at risk. Serum aminotransferases are typically normal or very slightly elevated, anti-HCV antibodies and HCV RNA are positive. The spontaneous seroconversion rate is 20% in children who have received blood products, and slightly less in perinatally infected children.

Children who have persistent positivity of HCV RNA and evidence of liver disease should be selected for therapy, which is best tolerated in younger children (3–5 years). The combination of pegylated interferon and ribavirin given for 12 months has a sustained viral response rate of 45% in genotype 1 and a 90% response rates in children with genotypes 2 and 3 when given for 6 months [105].

Autoimmune hepatitis [106]

Autoimmune hepatitis is a chronic inflammatory disorder affecting the liver, which is usually responsive to immunosuppressive drugs. It may affect children of any age from 6 months onwards, and there is a 3:1 female preponderance. Both forms of autoimmune hepatitis (type I—antinuclear antibodies and smooth muscle antibodies; and type II—liver, kidney microsomal antibodies) present in childhood.

Clinical features. In type I autoimmune hepatitis, the median age of onset is 10 years and the clinical presentation varies from acute hepatitis with autoimmune features to the insidious development of cirrhosis, portal hypertension and malnutrition. The association of multiorgan disease is higher in type I hepatitis with autoimmune thyroiditis, coeliac disease, inflammatory bowel disease, haemolytic anaemia and glomerulonephritis being the most common.

In type II autoimmune hepatitis, the age of onset is younger (median age 7.4 years); the clinical presentation is more likely to be acute, with fulminant hepatic failure in 11%. The diagnosis is made in the same way as in adults (Chapter 23).

Both forms of autoimmune hepatitis respond to immunosuppression with prednisolone 2 mg/kg per day (maximum 60 mg) in combination with azathioprine 0.5–2 mg/kg per day. About 90% of children will respond to the above regimen, but ciclosporin (2–4 mg/kg per day), tacrolimus (1–2 mg/day) or mycophenolate mofetil (20 mg/kg per day) may be helpful in inducing or maintaining remission. Discontinuation of corticosteroids and/or azathioprine may be considered if liver function tests have been normal for at least 1 year, but up to 80% of children relapse following discontinuation of treatment [106].

Sclerosing cholangitis may be secondary to ulcerative colitis, autoimmune hepatitis, histiocytosis X and immune deficiencies (Chapter 16).

Non-alcoholic steatohepatitis (NASH) (see also Chapter 28)

The increase in childhood obesity and the recognition of insulin resistance in a number of inherited disorders has lead to the diagnosis of this disorder in childhood. As in adults, children may have simple steatosis or steato-hepatitis which may progress to cirrhosis in childhood. The main difference is the frequent association with inherited syndromes associated with insulin resistance such as Alstrom's syndrome. NASH has also been reported after hypothalamic surgery, perhaps as a result of hyperphagia. The long-term outcome is not determined, but there may be a response to weight reduction and exercise. Therapeutic trials with metformin and other drugs have not been evaluated in childhood [107].

Congenital hepatic fibrosis (see Chapter 14)

This is a spectrum of disease which includes simple hepatic cysts, Caroli's syndrome and may be associated with either autosomal dominant or recessive polycystic renal disease. The main hepatic manifestations are cholangitis or portal hypertension. Liver transplantation is only required if hepatic decompensation develops or in association with renal transplantation.

Drug-induced liver disease

The mechanisms leading to drug-induced liver damage are similar in adults and children (see Chapter 24), although there is less risk of adverse drug reactions in younger children. However, in childhood there is a specific increased risk of valproate hepatotoxicity in children less than 3 years of age (see above) [108].

Paracetamol (acetaminophen) poisoning

Paracetamol toxicity is the most common cause of drug-induced fulminant liver failure. It leads to a direct dose-dependent hepatotoxic effect. In childhood, paracetamol toxicity may develop in children aged under 3 years of age, either by deliberate paracetamol poisoning by carers, long-term chronic ingestion of paracetamol or deliberate overdose in adolescents. Children have a lower incidence of liver failure with paracetamol over-dose than adults (unless taken with alcohol), perhaps because the rate of glutathione resynthesis is higher.

Aspirin

Aspirin gives rise to dose-dependent hepatotoxicity that is mild, asymptomatic and reversible. Adverse effects are associated with levels exceeding 15 mg/dL in 90%, which may occur in children treated for juvenile chronic arthritis. Hepatic features include an asymptomatic elevation in transaminases with a normal bilirubin level, which usually occurs 6 days after initiation of treatment. In less than 5% of children, severe hepatocellular injury may ensue with prompt recovery on withdrawal of treatment.

Metabolic disease in older children

Metabolic disease in older children presents with hepatomegaly often without jaundice, with or without splenomegaly or neurological involvement. The main causes of metabolic liver disease in older children include α_1-antitrypsin deficiency (see above), cystic fibrosis, Gaucher's disease, tyrosinaemia type I, glycogen storage diseases, hereditary fructose intolerance and Wilson's disease.

Wilson's disease (see Chapter 27)

Wilson's disease is an autosomal recessive disorder with an incidence of 1 : 30 000 live births. The Wilson's disease gene is on chromosome 13 and encodes a copper transporting P-type ATPase (ATP7B) [109] (see Chapter 27).

Clinical features in childhood include hepatic dysfunction (40%) and psychiatric symptoms (35%). Children under the age of 10 years usually present with hepatic symptoms. The hepatic presentation of Wilson's disease is similar to adults with hepatomegaly, vague gastrointestinal symptoms, subacute or fulminant hepatitis, and chronic hepatitis or cirrhosis. Neurological symptoms may be non-specific. Children may present with deteriorating school performance, abnormal behaviour, lack of coordination and dysarthria. Renal tubular abnormalities, renal calculi and haemolytic anaemia are associated features. The characteristic Kayser–Fleischer rings are rare before the age of 7 years and may be absent in up to 80% of older children.

Biochemical liver function tests indicate chronic liver disease with low albumin (<35 g/L), minimal transaminitis and a low alkaline phosphatase (<200 U/L). The diagnosis is established by detecting a low serum copper (<10 μmol/L), a low serum caeruloplasmin (<200 mg/L), excess urine copper (>1 μmol/24 h), particularly after penicillamine treatment (20 mg/kg per day), and an elevated hepatic copper (>250 mg/g dry weight of liver).

Approximately 25% of children may have a normal or borderline caeruloplasmin since it is an acute phase protein.

Histological features of Wilson's disease depend on the clinical presentation. There may be microvesicular steatosis, chronic hepatitis, hepatocellular necrosis, multinucleated hepatocytes and Mallory's hyaline, hepatic fibrosis and cirrhosis. In children who have fulminant hepatitis, the histological features are those of severe hepatocellular necrosis with cirrhosis.

Management is with a low-copper diet and penicillamine (20 mg/kg per day), or trientine 25 mg/kg per day. Oral zinc may be used under particular circumstances (see Chapter 27). In asymptomatic children or in those who have minimal hepatic dysfunction, the outlook is excellent, although fulminant hepatic failure with haemolysis may occur if treatment is discontinued. Liver transplantation is essential for children who present with subacute or fulminant hepatitis and in children with advanced cirrhosis and portal hypertension.

It is essential for siblings to be screened in order to treat asymptomatic patients and to detect heterozygotes. Mutation analysis is now more reliable than measurement of serum copper and caeruloplasmin [110] if the mutations in the proband are known.

Non-Wilsonian copper-related cirrhosis in childhood

There are a number of rare diseases related to copper toxicoses, in which there is progressive fatal liver disease caused by excessive copper ingestion. These are now rare due to changes in cooking techniques. They include: Indian childhood cirrhosis, in which copper was acquired from milk which had been heated in brass utensils [111]; Tyrolean childhood cirrhosis, in which copper was acquired from diluted sweetened milk which had been boiled in copper utensils, although an underlying genetic defect has also been described [112]; and sporadic childhood copper-related cirrhosis, in which copper was acquired from water used to make up infant feeds, usually from private wells.

Cystic fibrosis liver disease

Cystic fibrosis is a common autosomal recessive disease, with an incidence of approximately 1 in every 3000 live births worldwide [113]. The gene responsible for cystic fibrosis [114] encodes the cystic fibrosis transmembrane regulator (CFTR), a large protein of 1480 amino acids which belongs to the ATP-binding cassette family and is expressed in the apical membrane of biliary epithelial cells. Although the main clinical manifestations are with lung or pancreatic disease, liver disease is recognized in 4.5–20%, depending on age and the definition of significant liver disease. Despite advances in the understand-

ing of the genetic defects in cystic fibrosis, no definite genetic mutation has been associated with the development of liver disease.

Clinical features

Most children who have cystic fibrosis and liver disease are asymptomatic in the early stages. In infants, cholestatic neonatal hepatitis may be a presenting feature (see above), but more commonly the presentation is with hepatosplenomegaly or the complications of portal hypertension. Biliary disease includes asymptomatic gallstones in 20% and microgallbladder on ultrasound in 10–40%, but biliary strictures are uncommon [115].

Early detection of liver disease is unsatisfactory. There are transient abnormalities of alkaline phosphatase in up to 50% of patients (increases in γ-GT in 30% of males and 60% of females) while bilirubin levels and coagulation times are normal until late in the disease. Ultrasonography detects increased echogenicity in 41% of patients, but does not differentiate fatty infiltration from fibrosis. Microgallbladder with or without gallstones is found in 25% of patients [116,117].

Liver histology includes fatty infiltration, focal biliary cirrhosis and multilobular cirrhosis. Non-specific mild inflammation around the portal tracts is found in association with chemical cholangitis (granular eosinophilic secretions in bile ducts in association with ductal proliferation of bile ducts). Fibrosis develops initially around the portal tracts and gradually extends between portal tracts until cirrhosis has developed. Cholestasis is rarely identified. Liver biopsy should be performed to establish the extent and severity of liver disease and is indicated when there is persistent transaminitis, hepatic echogenicity on ultrasound, hepatomegaly and/or splenomegaly, or evidence of hepatic dysfunction [118].

Treatment consists of intensive nutritional support and the prevention and management of hepatic complications. Nutritional support includes: an energy intake to 150% of average requirements by carbohydrate supplements, such as glucose polymer, or by increasing the percentage of fat; increasing the proportion of medium chain triglyercides to 50% of the fat content; and supplementation with fat-soluble vitamins, including vitamin A (5–15000 IU/day), vitamin E (100–500 mg/day), vitamin D (50 ng/kg) and vitamin K (1–10 mg/day).

The use of ursodeoxycholic acid (10–20 mg/kg) is accepted despite the absence of clinical trials. There is some evidence that treatment with ursodeoxycholic acid improves the biochemical indices of liver function, and may prevent progression if prescribed before the development of significant liver disease [118].

The main hepatic complication is the development of portal hypertension and bleeding oesophageal varices. Prophylactic therapy is not recommended, but band

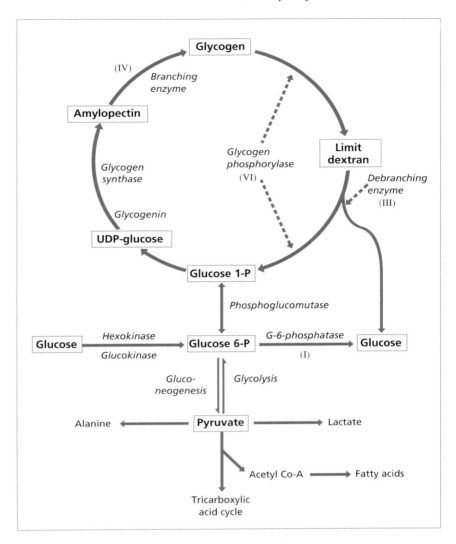

Fig. 29.4. Metabolic pathways in glycogen metabolism. Roman numerals indicate the defect in glycogen storage diseases. (Modified from [122].)

ligation is effective if variceal haemorrhage develops. A useful alternative is the insertion of a transjugular intrahepatic portal systemic shunt (TIPSS), which can be performed in children more than10 kg.

Cystic fibrosis liver disease usually progresses to cirrhosis and portal hypertension. Indications for liver transplantation include the development of end-stage liver failure with jaundice, ascites and coagulopathy, or intractable portal hypertension. It is important to consider transplantation before the development of significant pulmonary complication (<50% of normal function) in order to prevent the necessity for heart, lung and liver transplantation. The use of pulmonary DNAse preoperatively is recommended. Perioperative antibiotics should be based on the sensitivity of colonized pulmonary bacteria. The outcome following liver transplantation is similar to that in children transplanted for other causes of liver disease. Lung function may improve or stabilize after transplantation [119].

Glycogen storage disease [120,121]

The hepatic glycogen storage disorders (GSDs) are a group of inherited disorders affecting the metabolism of glycogen to glucose leading to excessive and/or abnormal glycogen in the tissues (Fig. 29.4). The frequency is approximately 1 in 25 000 live births. There are many variants with different enzymatic or structural defects (Table 29.6). In the hepatic forms diagnosis is usually in infancy or early childhood with hypoglycaemia, massive hepatomegaly, poor physical growth, a tendency to increased fat deposition, particularly in the cheeks, and biochemical abnormalities. Type V (muscle phosphorylase) and VII (phosphofructokinase) involve only muscle, or muscle and erythrocyte, respectively [120].

The critical abnormality is usually insufficient glucose production by the liver (Fig. 29.4) which results in hypoglycaemia when the blood glucose level is not supported by an inflow of glucose from the intestinal tract.

Table 29.6. The hepatic glycogen storage diseases

Type	Enzyme defect	Tissues involved
Ia	Glucose-6-phosphatase	Liver, kidney
I non-a	Glucose-6-phosphatase transporter	Liver
II	Lysosomal α-1,4-glucosidase (acid maltase)	Generalized
III	Amylo-1,6-glucosidase (debranching enzyme)	Liver, muscle, white blood cells
IV	Amylo-1,4,1,6-transglucosidase (branching enzyme)	Generalized
VI	Liver phosphorylase	Liver, white blood cells
IXa, IXb	Phosphorylase kinase	Liver, white blood cells, red blood cells
XI	GLUT2 transporter	Liver, kidney, pancreas

The other abnormalities follow from this defect and from the metabolic reactions to hypoglycaemia

The diagnosis is based on demonstrating the respective enzyme deficiency and confirming the genetic defect. Antenatal diagnosis is available for all genetically defined disorders. All are autosomal recessive, except for phosphorylase kinase deficiency which is X-linked.

Glycogen storage disease type I

Glycogen storage disease type I (GSD I) is due to defective breakdown of glucose-6-phosphate, resulting in decreased hepatic production of glucose and accumulation of glycogen in liver, kidney and intestine. There are two subtypes: GSD 1a, due to glucose-6-phosphatase deficiency, and GSD non-a (previously Ib, Ic, Id) due to defects of the glucose-6-phosphatase transporter.

Glycogen storage disease type Ia: glucose-6-phosphatase deficiency, Von Gierke's disease

GSD Ia is inherited as an autosomal recessive trait. The glucose-6-phosphatase gene has been mapped to chromosome 17q21. Over 70 mutations have been identified [121].

Infants usually present with hypoglycaemic seizures, hepatomegaly and failure to thrive. Biochemical investigations reveal fasting hypoglycaemia (<1.5 g/L) with lactic acidosis (>5 mmol/L), hyperlipidaemia (cholesterol >6 mmol/L and triglycerides >3 mmol/L), and

hyperuricaemia. Hepatic transaminases are usually normal or mildly elevated.

Hepatic changes. The liver is enlarged, smooth and brown. Liver histology reveals steatosis and glycogen storage. In formol-fixed material, glycogen is washed out leaving an appearance of clear, plant-like cells. Excess fat is usually present. Pericellular zone 3 fibrosis and Mallory bodies have been described in type Ia glycogenesis [120]. The glycogen is usually stable, persisting many days post-mortem and despite severe ketosis or prolonged anaesthesia. Histochemical stains for glucose-6-phosphatase are negative and the enzyme is not detected in liver. Cirrhosis does not develop. Hepatocellular adenomas and, rarely, carcinomas are late developments [123].

Treatment. This is based on providing a continuous supply of exogenous glucose to maintain normal blood sugar. In infants, this is achieved by frequent day-time feeding, use of oral (slow release) uncooked corn starch, or continuous nocturnal enteral glucose feeds. In older children, frequent calorie supplements and the use of corn starch is usually sufficient. If dietary control is effective, normal growth and development can be expected, although hepatomegaly and hyperlipidaemia persist [124].

Long-term complications. These include hypoglycaemic brain damage, poor growth, osteoporosis, renal dysfunction and calculi, and hepatic adenomata which may undergo malignant transformation [125]. Puberty may be delayed and females have ultrasound evidence of polycystic ovaries [126]. Liver transplantation corrects the metabolic defect, but is not indicated for metabolic control. Chronic renal failure occurs in older patients whose disease has been ineffectively treated. Type I glycogenosis can present in adults as hypoglycaemic symptoms and/or hepatomegaly [127].

Glycogen storage disease type I non-a (previously known as Ib, Ic, Id).

In this disorder glucose-6-phophatase is normal, but dysfunctional. It is due to a defect in glucose-6-phosphate transport into the microsome which has been localized to chromosome 11q23. Several mutations have been reported [128].

The clinical and biochemical features are similar to GSD type Ia, but neutropenia with recurrent infections and inflammatory bowel disease occur. Management of GSD I non-a patients is the same as in GSD Ia except that G-CSF (granulocyte colony stimulating factor) or GM-CSF (granulocyte-macrophage colony stimulating factor) is required to correct neutropenia and improve chronic inflammatory bowel disease [128,129].

Glycogen storage disease type II (Pompe's disease)

This primary lysosomal disease is due to deficiency of lysosomal acid α-1,4-glucosidase which normally degrades glycogen within lysosomes. It is not associated with liver disease.

There is weakness of skeletal muscle, cardiomegaly, hepatomegaly and macroglossia. Mental development is normal. Infantile, childhood and adult-onset forms exist. The infantile form is the most severe. Glucagon and adrenaline tests are normal and hypoglycaemia does not occur. Hyperlipidaemia is conspicuous.

All organs show vacuolated cells due to the enlarged lysosomes, which contain the glycogen. Vacuolated lymphocytes are found in peripheral blood and marrow. The liver cells at autopsy show particularly prominent vacuoles.

Glycogen storage disease type III (Cori's disease)

The inheritance of GSD III is autosomal recessive. The gene is located at chromosome 1p21 and several mutations have been reported. The defect is expressed in both liver and muscle. There is deficiency in the debrancher enzyme or amylo-1-6-glucosidase deficiency. The metabolic defect is mild as other routes of gluconeogenesis are intact and there is no renal involvement.

The clinical presentation is similar to GSD type I, without renal involvement but with peripheral myopathy and cardiomyopathy. Patients who have muscle involvement may develop progressive skeletal myopathy and wasting, progressing to severe muscle weakness later in life. As the abnormally structured residual glycogen is fibrogenic, hepatic fibrosis and cirrhosis are identified [130,131].

Liver histology is similar to GSD I apart from the presence of fibrosis and little steatosis. Diagnosis is confirmed by identifying the deficient enzyme in leucocytes or hepatic tissue or by DNA analysis.

Dietary treatment is similar to that of GSD type I, but a higher protein intake is recommended due to the demand of gluconeogenic amino acids. Most metabolic abnormalities diminish at puberty and long-term outcome is determined by the development of myopathy, cardiomyopathy or cirrhosis. Hepatic adenomas occur in 25% of patients, less often than that found in type I [125].

Glycogen storage disease type IV (Andersen's disease)

This rare disease is due to a defect in the enzyme required for normal branching of the glycogen molecule (α1,4-glycan-6-glycosyltransferase). Accumulation is generalized and occurs in liver, heart, muscle, skin, intestine, brain and peripheral nervous system.

Inheritance is autosomal recessive. The hepatic and neuromuscular forms of GSD IV are caused by mutations in the same gene, which has been localized to chromosome 3p12 [132].

It usually presents with evidence of severe liver disease in late infancy but there may be cardiac, muscle and neurological involvement. Hypoglycaemia is rare except as a feature of liver failure.

Hepatic histology demonstrates cirrhosis and accumulation of abnormally shaped glycogen that is diastase resistant. Dietary treatment is as for other forms of GSD. There is rapid development of cirrhosis necessitating liver transplantation in the first 5 years of life. Progression of extrahepatic disease has been reported post-transplantation [133].

Glycogen storage disease types VI and IX

These variants are due to defects in hepatic phosphorylase and phosphorylase kinase, respectively. The liver phosphorylase gene is located on chromosome 14q21-22. The genetics of the phosphorylase kinase system is complex as the enzyme consists of four subunits encoded on different genes (X chromosome as well as autosomes), which are differentially expressed in different tissues. The clinical expression of individual enzyme deficiencies and isoforms is variable and depends on the severity and distribution of the enzyme defect [134].

The phenotype of both GSD types VI and IX is milder than in other forms of GSD. Children present with hepatomegaly and growth failure, but hypoglycaemia is rare. Hyperlipidaemia and ketosis may occur. Hepatic transaminases are often slightly raised, but progression to cirrhosis is unusual.

Liver histology reveals distension of hepatocytes with fibrosis and small fat droplets.

Dietary treatment other than nocturnal corn starch is rarely necessary and spontaneous catch-up growth occurs before puberty. Neither cardiomyopathy nor myopathy have been recognized, and the long-term outlook is excellent.

Glycogen storage disease type XI

This rare disorder is associated with glycogen accumulation in liver and kidney, fasting hypoglycaemia, postprandial hyperglycaemia and hypergalactosaemia. It is due to defective function of the GLUT2 transporter in hepatocytes, pancreatic β-cells, enterocytes and renal tubular cells, leading to a reduction in the import and export of glucose and galactose in affected tissues. Hypoglycaemia occurs secondary to the reduction in glucose transport from the liver and defective renal reabsorption of glucose and galactose. Hepatic and renal glycogen accumulation lead to impaired tubular function, Fanconi nephropathy and rickets. The GLUT2 gene has been localized to chromosome 3q26.1–q26.3, and 34 different mutations have been reported [135].

The main clinical features are hepatomegaly and renal tubular dysfunction. Infants present with vomiting, fever, failure to thrive and hypophosphataemic rickets. Older children have short stature, protuberant abdomen, hepatomegaly, moon-shaped facies and fat deposition around the shoulders and abdomen. Fasting hypoglycaemia is common. Chronic diarrhoea due to sugar malabsorption may occur. Rickets and osteoporosis lead to pathological fractures. Mild abnormalities of liver function are common but hepatic adenomas and malignancies have not been reported.

The diagnosis is confirmed by DNA mutation analysis. Antenatal diagnosis has not been reported.

Treatment is supportive, and includes replacement of water and electrolytes, alkalinization with Shohl's or bicarbonate solutions, vitamin D and phosphate supplementation, galactose restriction and frequent small meals. Fructose is an alternative carbohydrate source as its absorption is not mediated by GLUT2.

The prognosis is good, with stabilization in adult life.

Hereditary fructose intolerance (HFI)

This autosomal recessive disorder is due to the absence or reduction of fructose-1-phosphate aldolase B in liver, kidneys and small intestine. The incidence is 1 : 23 000 live births [136]. The gene for has been mapped to chromosome 9q22.3. About 20 mutations are known.

The clinical presentation is related to the introduction of fructose or sucrose in the diet. Vomiting is a prominent feature with failure to thrive, hepatomegaly and coagulopathy. Occasionally, infants may present with acute liver failure with jaundice, encephalopathy and renal failure. Older children demonstrate aversion to fructose-containing food.

Biochemical liver function tests indicate raised hepatic transaminases, hypoalbuminaemia and hyperbilirubinaemia. Plasma amino acids may be elevated secondary to liver dysfunction and there may be hyperuricacidaemia and hypoglycaemia. Haematological abnormalities such as anaemia, acanthocytosis and thrombocytosis are associated. Urinary investigations will indicate fructosuria, proteinuria, amino aciduria and organic aciduria in association with a reduction in the tubular reabsorption of phosphate. Diagnosis is suggested by reducing substances in the urine and confirmed by a reduction or absence of enzymatic activity in liver or intestinal mucosal biopsy or by mutation analysis. Hepatic pathology varies from complete hepatic necrosis to diffuse steatosis and periportal intralobular fibrosis which may progress to cirrhosis if fructose is continued.

Fructose elimination from the diet reverses hepatic and renal dysfunction, and growth and development are normal if diagnosed early enough. Fulminant hepatic failure may develop on the reintroduction of fructose, sucrose or sorbitol. Hepatoma has been reported [137]. Antenatal diagnosis is possible by chorionic villus sampling or mutation analysis.

Fructose-1,6-bisphosphatase deficiency

Fructose-1,6-bisphosphatase deficiency is an autosomal recessive disorder resulting in impaired gluconeogenesis from all precursors including fructose. Liver and muscle express distinct enzymes. The liver enzyme has been mapped to chromosome 9q22.2-22.3, and several mutations have been described [138]. Hypoglycaemia occurs with lactic acidosis, but there is no liver disease.

Glutaric aciduria type II

This disturbance of organic acid metabolism presents in infants or adults as recurrent hypoglycaemia with elevated serum free fatty acid. There may be hepatomegaly. The liver often shows fatty change. Periportal fibrosis and hypoplastic extrahepatic ducts are reported [139].

Lysosomal storage disorders (see Chapter 4)

Lysosomal storage disorders are due to specific enzyme deficiencies resulting in abnormal storage of partially degraded macromolecules in the lysosomes. The clinical spectrum ranges from prenatal hydrops fetalis to mild disease in adulthood [140]. The liver and spleen are important sites for abnormal lysosomal storage, hence hepatosplenomegaly is a frequent finding. Most are associated with neurological deterioration, but Gaucher's disease, Niemann–Pick disease, Wolman's disease and cholesterol ester disease have significant liver disease.

Gaucher's disease

Gaucher's disease is the most frequent lysosomal storage disorder, and is commoner in Ashenazi Jews (see also Chapter 4). This autosomal recessive disorder is secondary to a deficiency of glucosyl-ceramide-β-glucosidase which is deficient in leucocytes, hepatocytes and amniocytes. The gene has been localized to chromosome 1q21 and over 160 mutations have been described [141].

It may present in infancy with acute liver failure, but is more usual in late childhood with hepatosplenomegaly, and respiratory, neurological and bone disease. The diagnosis is suggested by the identification of large multinucleated Gaucher cells in bone marrow aspirate and liver (see Fig. 4.8), and is confirmed by enzyme assay. Hepatic fibrosis may be severe leading to cirrhosis.

Recent therapy for Gaucher's disease includes recombinant enzyme replacement, substrate deprivation for the non-neuronopathic form, bone marrow or liver transplantation [142].

Niemann–Pick disease (NPD)

Niemann–Pick disease is a group of storage disorders associated with sphingomyelin storage. There are three forms: types A, B and C [143].

Types A and B disease (NPA and NPB) are autosomal recessive disorders caused by deficiency of the lysosomal enzyme sphingomyelinase. The sphingomyelinase gene has been localized to chromosome 11p15.4, and about 20 mutations are known. NPA is associated with infantile neurodegeneration, failure to thrive and multiorgan involvement, whereas NPB has no neurological involvement, but presents with hepatosplenomegaly with survival into adulthood. Enzyme replacement therapy is now available [144].

Niemann–Pick disease type C is caused by a defect of intracellular lipid trafficking and is clinically, biochemically and genetically distinct from NPA and NPB. It is an autosomal recessive disorder. The defective gene (*NPCI*) has been localized to chromosome 18q11-12 in more than 95% of patients [145]. Over 100 mutations have been described. The disease presents with neonatal cholestasis or with hepataosplenomagaly and neurological deterioration. Supranuclear vertical gaze palsy is pathognomonic for this disorder. Death is in early adolescence with dementia and respiratory problems [145,146].

Occasionally, the disease presents with acute liver failure in infancy, but liver transplantation is contraindicated as the neurological disease persists. Enzyme replacement therapy is being evaluated.

Wolman's disease and cholesteryl ester storage disease

These two rare disorders are caused by a recessively inherited deficiency of lysosomal acid lipase, resulting in accumulation of cholesterol esters and triglycerides in most body tissues. There is increased cholesterol synthesis, up-regulation of LDL-receptor gene expression and increased lipoprotein production, which is more severe in Wolman's disease.

The gene has been localized to chromosome 10q22.2-22.3, and over 20 mutations described [147,148]. Antenatal diagnosis is possible by direct enzyme assay in chorion villus cells or by mutation analysis.

Liver histology reveals vacuolated hepatocytes and Kupffer cells and foamy histiocytes [149]. Periportal fibrosis and cirrhosis may be evident. Foam cells are also be seen in bone marrow aspirates, spleen and lymph nodes. In Wolman's disease, small intestinal biopsy demonstrates infiltration of the lamina propria with foamy histiocytes.

Wolman's disease. Patients present in the first few weeks of life with vomiting and diarrhoea, malabsorption, failure to thrive and hepatosplenomegaly [148]. Jaundice, low-grade pyrexia, anaemia, abdominal distension and leucopenia may be present. Adrenal calcification is seen on X-ray; other diagnostic features are vacuolated lymphocytes in peripheral blood films and foam cells in bone marrow aspirates. Treatment with intravenous nutrition, plasma infusion, corticosteroids and dietary supplements is ineffective [149]. Bone marrow transplantation may play a role [150]. Most patients die before 6 months of age.

Cholestyl ester storage disease. The clinical features are less severe. Hepatomegaly may be present from childhood or diagnosed in adult life [148]. Liver dysfunction, splenomegaly, hyperlipidaemia and xanthelesma are often present. Liver failure may occur. Treatment with HMG CoA reductase inhibitors, cholestyramine, a low cholesterol diet and fat-soluble vitamin supplements is helpful [151], while successful liver transplantation has been reported [152].

Mucopolysaccharidoses

These lysosomal storage diseases, are due to deficiencies of the enzymes involved in the degradation of dermatin sulphate, heparin sulphate, chondroitin sulphate or keratin sulphate. Many variants are described and although hepatosplenomegaly is a feature, liver disease is not associated [153].

Hurler's syndrome (gargoylism) is inherited as an autosomal recessive and is characterized by deficiency of the lysosomal degrading enzyme, α-L-iduronidase, in liver, cultured skin fibroblasts and leucocytes. It is characterized by coarse facial features, dwarfism, limitation of joint movement, deafness, abdominal hernias, hepatosplenomegaly, cardiac abnormalities and mental retardation.

The liver is large and firm. Microscopically, liver cells are swollen and together with Kupffer cells accumulate glycosaminoglycan, demonstrated by colloidal iron stain. Electron microscopy shows characteristic membrane-bound inclusions in hepatocytes and Kupffer cells. This lysosomal storage material disappears in the majority of patients after bone marrow transplantation [154].

Diagnosis may be made by finding increased urinary or leucocyte mucopolysaccharides. Culture of skin biopsies shows fibroblasts containing mucopolysaccharides.

Familial hypercholesterolaemia

This is an autosomal dominant disease due to absence of a gene that codes for the LDL receptor on cell membranes [155]. The liver contains 60% of such receptors. Children are usually identified as part of family screening, unless they are homozygotes. They have increased plasma total cholesterol and LDL from birth, cutaneous xanthomas develop and most homozygotes die from coronary artery disease before the age of 30 years.

Hypercholesterolaemia is controlled by reduction in dietary saturated fats and administration of bile acid sequestrants such as cholestyramine or apheresis [156]. Statins are now routine even for children [157]. Homozygotes may require combined heart and liver transplantation for the coronary disease and to provide normal LDL receptors in liver [158].

Gene therapy, using 'transplant' of autologous hepatocytes genetically corrected with recombinant retroviruses carrying the LDL receptor, has been successful although hepatocyte transplantation is also a possibility [159].

Cirrhosis and portal hypertension

Any form of chronic or metabolic liver disease in the neonate or child may lead to cirrhosis and portal hypertension. *Cardiac cirrhosis* is unusual in childhood unless secondary to constrictive pericarditis.

Hepatic decompensation occurs when there is loss of hepatic synthetic function and the development of complications such as malnutrition, bleeding oesophageal varices, ascites, encephalopathy and hepatorenal failure. The clinical features include palmar and plantar erythema, telangiectasia, malnutrition, hypotonia and hepatosplenomegaly with ascites. Jaundice may be absent.

Management includes nutritional support to prevent malnutrition (see above) and the prevention of complications. Metabolic bone disease may be severe with pathological fractures. Treatment with infusions of bisphosphonates are beneficial.

Oesophageal or rectal varices develop inevitably with increasing hepatic fibrosis and portal hypertension. Variceal haemorrhage is managed in a similar way to adults; resuscitation with albumin, fresh frozen plasma, red cell transfusions; H$_2$ blockers or proton pump inhibitors; intravenous octreotide (3–5 μg/kg per h) and/or glypressin (0.3–1 unit/kg per h) or vasopressin (0.2–0.4 unit/kg per hour); therapeutic sclerotherapy or band ligation as required.

In children with intractable variceal bleeding, haemorrhage may be controlled by insertion of a transhepatic portal vein stent (TIPSS). The success rate is 80–100% and may control bleeding and allow time for consideration for transplantation. Complications include occlusion of the stent, infection and development of encephalopathy.

The use of TIPSS to control portal hypertension in children with compensated liver disease such as cystic fibrosis is an increasing indication for this procedure [160]. The use of propranolol or band ligation as prophylactic therapy remains unproven in children.

Sepsis is common and may precipitate encephalopathy. Treatment with appropriate broad-spectrum antibiotics, such as cefuroxime (20 mg/kg per dose t.d.s.), amoxicillin (25 mg/kg per dose t.d.s.) and metronidazole (8 mg/kg per dose t.d.s.), are useful first-line drugs until bacterial cultures are positive.

Salt and water retention leading to ascites and cardiac failure should be effectively managed with diuretics and salt and water restriction.

Chronic encephalopathy is difficult to detect in children, but may present with regression in school work, lack of energy and drowsiness. It is best treated with lactulose, although protein restriction (2 g/kg) may be necessary

Liver transplantation

Indications

The indications for liver transplantation include acute or chronic liver failure, metabolic liver disease or inborn errors of metabolism with extrahepatic disease and unresectable liver tumours. Over the last 20 years, the success of paediatric liver transplantation has altered the prognosis for many infants and children. The main factors in improving survival in this age group include advances in preoperative management such as the treatment of hepatic complications and nutritional support. The developments in innovative surgical techniques to expand the donor pool have extended liver transplantation to the neonatal age group, while improvements in postoperative management including immunosuppression have led not only to increased survival, but also improved quality of life.

As in adults, most children are transplanted for chronic liver failure. Biliary atresia remains the commonest indication for children transplanted under the age of 5 years [79]. The indications for liver transplantation for children with acute liver failure depend on the aetiology and the extent of multisystem disease. Children who have a poor prognosis include those who have: non-A–G hepatitis; rapid onset of coma with progression to grade III or IV hepatic coma; diminishing liver size; and falling serum transaminases associated with increasing bilirubin (>300 μmol/L (>18 mg/dL)) and persistent coagulopathy (>50 s). Liver transplantation is contraindicated for children who have evidence of multisystem involvement (e.g. mitochondrial disease) or irreversible brain damage from cerebral oedema or hypoglycaemia [161].

Inborn errors of metabolism

Liver transplantation is indicated for inborn errors of metabolism if the hepatic enzyme deficiency leads to irreversible liver disease or liver failure and/or hepatoma (e.g. tyrosinaemia type I, Wilson's disease) or severe extrahepatic disease (e.g. primary oxalosis or Crigler–Najjar syndrome) [162].

Indications for transplantation for liver tumours include either unresectable benign tumours causing hepatic dysfunction or unresectable malignant tumours without evidence of extrahepatic metastases [163].

Surgical approach, immunosuppressive regimens and outcome

In these days of organ donor shortage, most children will receive a split liver transplant. Postoperative management and immunosuppression are similar to adults (Chapter 36). Most children now receive induction immunosuppression with monoclonal antibodies, tacrolimus with or without steroids and mycophenolate.

Postoperative complications are also similar, but children have a low rate of rejection (<30%), a higher rate of hepatic artery thrombosis (10%) and are more likely to develop primary EBV infections as 65% of children undergoing liver transplantation will be EBV-negative. It is important to diagnose primary EBV infection as early as possible so that immunosuppression may be reduced to prevent further progression to lymphoproliferative disease.

Side effects of immunosuppression are similar in children and adults. The major difference is the effect of corticosteroids on growth and ultimate height. Hirsutism and gingival hyperplasia, which are well-known side effects of ciclosporin, have an important effect on quality of life, particularly in adolescents. The prevention of nephrotoxicity, which is common to both ciclosporin and tacrolimus, needs careful monitoring of immunosuppressive levels to minimize this long-term effect and transfer to renal sparing agents such as sirolimus or mycophenolate mofetil [164].

Current results from international units indicate that 1-year survival after paediatric liver transplantation is 90%, while long-term survival rates (10–15 years) are more than 80% [165].

Children who survive the initial 3-month post-transplant period without major complications should achieve a normal lifestyle, despite the necessity for continuous immunosuppressive monitoring. Prospective studies have indicated a rapid return to normal nutritional status in over 80% of children within 1 year post-transplant. Linear growth may be delayed between 6 and 24 months post-transplant, which is directly related to corticosteroid dosage and to malnutrition and preoperative stunting.

Early studies of neuropsychological development pre- and post-transplant demonstrated that the rate of improvement post-transplant is related to the extent of motor or psychological developmental delay pretransplant, thus highlighting the necessity for early transplantation, particularly for infants who have chronic liver disease [166]. Prospective studies have shown that there is an initial deterioration in psychosocial development post-transplant, which is maybe related to the prolonged hospitalization, and to stress of the transplant operation [167]. Long-term studies have shown that children surviving liver transplantation enter puberty normally, girls will develop menarche, and both boys and girls will have pubertal growth spurts. Successful pregnancies have been reported. Non-compliance with immunosuppressive therapy is a significant problem in adolescents and a major cause of graft loss [168].

Tumours of the liver

See also Chapter 34 and 35. Primary tumours in infants and children are rare; two-thirds are diagnosed before the second year of life. They may arise from liver cells and/or from supporting structures. Secondary tumours are extremely rare and are usually associated with a neuroblastoma of the adrenals.

Diagnosis

Biochemical tests may be normal. The most usual abnormality is an increase in serum γ-GT and $α_2$-globulin levels. Serum α-fetoprotein may be increased. The site and extent of the tumour must be defined by ultrasound, CT, MRI and, if necessary, angiography. Guided liver biopsy is usually a safe method of confirming the diagnosis

Hamartomas

These benign, congenital lesions present as an abdominal mass in the first 2 years of life. They may be an incidental finding at autopsy and must be distinguished from malignant tumours. They consist of abnormal arrangements of all the cells of the normal liver, particularly bile ducts and fibroblasts. They contain central veins and are nearly always cystic. They require no treatment.

Mesenchymal hamartoma

This is a rare developmental anomaly, largely of bile ducts, seen in children less than 2 years old. It is treated conservatively, or if necessary by surgical excision.

Malignant mesenchymoma (undifferentiated sarcoma)

This is seen in older children (6–12 years). Histology is that of sarcoma with PAS-positive intracytoplasmic pink globules. The tumour should be resected surgically with subsequent chemotherapy.

Adenomas

These rare tumours do not become malignant, and over the years may even regress. They consist of sheets of liver cells and have a fibrous capsule. They should be treated conservatively.

Hepatoblastoma

This is the commonest tumour in children under the age of 3 years Tumours are classified as: fetal, embryonal, macrotrabecular and small-cell undifferentiated. Children usually present with an enlarged liver and a grossly elevated α-fetoprotein. Other associations include: hemihypertrophy, Wilms' tumour, precocious puberty and familial adenomatosis coli. The prognosis is now excellent with a combination of chemotherapy, surgery or liver transplantation [163].

Hepatocellular carcinoma

This is rare in childhood, but is associated with tyrosinaemia type 1, Hepatitis B or C and has recently been reported with PFIC2 usually present after 5 years of age [54]. Males are more frequently affected than females. The tumours are often single, large and metastasize late. Cirrhosis may be absent.

The patients present with weight loss, abdominal swelling in the right upper quadrant, pain, ascites and jaundice. Calcification in the tumour may be noted. α-fetoprotein is usually negative.

Treatment. Surgical resection is rarely possible. However, following lobectomy, growth and development are normal. Chemotherapy may be useful in reducing tumour size before resection. The fibro-lamellar form has a much better prognosis and resection is more often possible [169]. Transplantation is sometimes indicated in small tumours with no extrahepatic spread.

Infantile haemangioendothelioma

This, usually benign, vascular tumour of infancy consists of endothelium-lined channels of capillary size. It may be associated with skin haemangiomas. It presents before 6 months of age as an abdominal mass. Cardiac failure may be related to arteriovenous shunts within the tumour. A systolic bruit may be heard in the epigastrium. Severe anaemia and thrombocytopenia have been attributed to microangiopathic haemolysis related to the abnormal, tortuous, narrow vessels within the tumour [170].

The diagnosis is made by CT and MRI [170]. Treatment includes managing cardiac failure, and hepatic arterial embolization for refractory heart failure .The prognosis is usually good [171].

References

1 Kelly DA, Green A. Investigation of paediatric liver disease. *J. Inherit. Metab. Dis.* 1991; **14**: 531–537.
2 Keffler S, Kelly DA, Powell JE *et al.* Population screening for neonatal liver disease: A feasibility study. *J. Pediatr. Gastroenterol. Nutr.* 1998; **27**: 306–311.
3 Kimura A, Yamakawa R, Ushijima K *et al.* Fetal bile acid metabolism during infancy: analysis of 1β-hydroxylated bile acids in urine, meconium and faeces. *Hepatology* 1994; **20**: 819–824.
4 Naveh Y, Berant M. Assessment of liver size in normal infants and children. *J. Pediatr. Gastroenterol. Nutr.* 1984; **3**: 346–348.
5 Chianale J, Dvorak C, Farmer DL *et al.* Cytochrome P-450 gene expression in the functional units of the fetal liver. *Hepatology* 1988; **8**: 318–326.
6 Benaron DA, Bowen FW. Variation of initial serum bilirubin rise in new born infants with type of illness. *Lancet* 1991; **338**: 78.
7 Tan KL. Comparison of the effectiveness of phototherapy and exchange transfusion in the management of non-hemolytic neonatal hyperbilirubinemia. *J. Pediat.* 1975; **87**: 609–612.
8 Monaghan G, McLellan A, McGeehan A *et al.* Gilbert's syndrome is a contributory factor in prolonged unconjugated hyperbilirubinemia of the newborn. *J. Pediatr.* 1999; **134**: 441–446.
9 Hansen TWR. Bilirubin in the brain. Distribution and effects on neurophysiological and neurochemical processes. *Clin. Pediatr.* 1994; **33**: 452–459.
10 Kaplan M, Beutler E, Vreman HJ *et al.* Neonatal hyperbilirubinemia in glucose-6-phosphate dehydrogenase-deficient heterozygotes. *Pediatrics* 1999; **104**: 68–74.
11 Strauss KA, Robinson DL, Vreman HJ *et al.* Management of hyperbilirubinemia and prevention of kernicterus in 20 patients with Crigler-Najjar disease. *Eur. J. Pediatr.* 2006; **165**: 306–319.
12 Fox IJ, Chowdhury JR, Kaufman SS. Treatment of the Crigler–Najjar syndrome type I with hepatocyte transplantation. *N. Engl. J. Med.* 1998; **338**: 422–426.
13 Dhawan A, Mitry RR, Hughes RD. Hepatocyte transplantation for liver-based metabolic disorders. *J. Inherit. Metab. Dis.* 2006; **29**: 431–435.

14 Powell JE, Keffler S, Kelly DA *et al*. Population screening for neonatal liver disease: potential for a community-based programme. *J. Med. Screen.* 2003; **10**: 112–116.

15 Kelly DA. The approach to the child with liver disease. In: Kelly DA ed. *Diseases of the Liver and Biliary System in Children*, 3rd edn. Oxford: Wiley-Blackwell, 2008, p. 21–34.

16 Brown CW, Werlin SL, Geenen JE *et al*. The diagnostic and therapeutic role of endoscopic retrograde cholangiopancreatography in children. *J. Pediatr. Gastroenterol. Nutr.* 1993; **17**:19–23.

17 Chang M-H, Huang HH, Huang ES *et al*. Polymerase chain reaction to detect human cytomegalovirus in livers of infants with neonatal hepatitis. *Gastroenterology* 1992; **103**: 1022–5.

18 Marret S, Buffet-Janvresse C, Metayer J *et al*. Herpes simplex hepatitis with chronic cholestasis in a newborn. *Acta Paediatr.* 1993; **82**: 321–323.

19 Langnas AN, Markin RS, Cattral MS *et al*. Parvovirus B19 as a possible causative agent of fulminant liver failure and associated aplastic anaemia. *Hepatology* 1995; **22**: 1661–1665.

20 Yarlagadda S, Acharya S, Goold P *et al*. A syphilis outbreak: recent trends in infectious syphilis in Birmingham, UK, in 2005 and control strategies. *Int. J. STD AIDS* 2007; **18**: 410–412.

21 Yu HR, Huang YC, Yang KD. Neonatal varicella frequently associated with visceral complications: a retrospective analysis. *Acta Pediatr. Taiwan* 2003; **4**: 25–28.

22 Persaud D, Bangaru B, Greco MA *et al*. Cholestatic hepatitis in children infected with the human immunodeficiency virus. *Pediatr. Infect. Dis. J.* 1993; **12**: 492–498.

23 Jonas MM, Roldan EO, Lyons HJ *et al*. Histopathologic features of the liver in paediatric acquired immune deficiency syndrome. *J. Pediatr. Gastroenterol. Nutr.* 1989; **9**: 73–81.

24 Hamilton JR, Sass-Kortsak A. Jaundice associated with severe bacterial infection in young infants. *J. Pediat.* 1963; **63**: 121–132.

25 Garcia FJ, Nager AL. Jaundice as an early diagnostic sign of urinary tract infection in infancy. *Pediatrics* 2002; **109**: 846–851.

26 Spray CH, McKiernan P, Waldron KE *et al*. Investigation and outcome of neonatal hepatitis in infants with hypopituitarism. *Acta Paediatr.* 2000; **89**: 951–954.

27 Fahnehjelm, KT, Fischler B, Jacobson L *et al*. Optic nerve hypoplasia in cholestatic infants: a multiple case study. *Acta Ophthalmol .Scand.* 2003; **81**: 130–137.

28 Alpert LI, Strauss L, Hirschhorn K. Neonatal hepatitis and biliary atresia associated with trisomy 17–18 syndrome. *N. Engl. J. Med.* 1969; **280**: 16–20.

29 Ikeda S, Sera Y, Yoshida M *et al*. Extrahepatic biliary atresia associated with trisomy 18. *Pediatr. Surg. Int.* 1999; **15**: 137–138.

30 Beath SV, Needham SJ, Kelly DA *et al*. Clinical features and prognosis of children assessed for isolated small bowel (ISBTx) or combined small bowel and liver transplantation (CSBLTx). *J. Pediatr. Surg.* 1997; **32**: 459–461.

31 Crowther DC, Belorgey D, Miranda E *et al*. Practical genetics: alpha-1-antitrypsin deficiency and the serpinopathies. *Eur. J. Hum. Genet.* 2004; **12**: 167–172.

32 Fairbanks KD, Tavill AS. Liver disease in alpha 1-antitrypsin deficiency: a review. *Am. J. Gastroenterol.* 2008; **103**: 2136–2141.

33 Perlmutter DH. Pathogenesis of chronic liver injury and hepatocellular carcinoma in alpha-1-antitrypsin deficiency. *Pediatr. Res.* 2006; **60**: 233–238.

34 Teckman JH. Alpha1-antitrypsin deficiency in childhood. *Sem. Liver Dis.* 2007; **27**: 274–281.

35 Lomas DA. Loop-sheet polymerization: the structural basis of Z α1-antitrypsin accumulation in the liver. *Clin. Sci* 1994; **86**: 489.

36 Povey S. Genetics of alpha 1-antitrypsin deficiency in relation to neonatal liver disease. *Mol. Biol. Med.* 1990; **7**:161–172.

37 Volpert D, Molleston JP, Perlmutter DH. Alpha1-antitrypsin deficiency-associated liver disease progresses slowly in some children. *J. Pediatr. Gastroenterol. Nutr.* 2000; **31**: 258–263.

38 Francavilla R, Castellaneta SP, Hadzic N *et al*. Prognosis of alpha-1-antitrypsin deficiency-related liver disease in the era of paediatric liver transplantation. *J. Hepatol.* 2000; **32**: 986–992.

39 Davies CA, Daneman A, Stringer DA. Inspissated bile in a neonate with cystic fibrosis. *J. Ultrasound. Med.* 1986; **5**: 335–337.

40 Alagille D, Estrada A, Hadchouel M *et al*. Syndromic paucity of interlobular bile ducts (Alagille syndrome or arteriohepatic dysplasia): review of 80 cases. *J. Pediat.* 1987; **110**: 195.

41 Li L, Krantz ID, Deng Y *et al*. Alagille syndrome is caused by mutations in the human Jagged 1, which encodes a ligand for Notch 1. *Nat. Genet.* 1997; **16**: 243–251.

42 Oda T, Elkahloun AG, Pike BL *et al*. Mutations in the human Jagged 1 gene are responsible for the Alagille syndrome. *Nat .Genet.* 1997; **16**: 235–242.

43 Brodsky MC, Cunniff C. Ocular anomalies in the Alagille syndrome (arteriohepatic dysplasia). *Ophthalmology* 1993; **100**: 1767.

44 Narula P, Gifford J, Steggall MA *et al*. Visual loss and idiopathic intracranial hypertension in children with Alagille Syndrome. *J. Pediatr. Gastroenterol. Nutr.* 2006; **43**: 348–352.

45 Narula P, Dell Olio D, van Mourik IDM *et al*. Experience with molecular absorbent recirculating system (MARS) in a single centre. *J. Pediatr. Gastroenterol. Nutr.* 2004; **39**: S159.

46 Lykavieris P, Hadchouel M, Chardot C *et al*. Outcome of liver disease in children with Alagille syndrome: a study of 163 patients. *Gut* 2001; **49**: 431–435.

47 Liu C, Aronow BJ, Jegga AG *et al*. Novel resequencing chip customized to diagnose mutations in patients with inherited syndromes of intrahepatic cholestasis. *Gastroenterology* 2007; **132**: 119–126.

48 Bull LN, van Eijk MJ, Pawlikowska L *et al*. A gene encoding a P-type ATPase mutated in two forms of hereditary cholestasis. *Nat. Genet.* 1998; **18**: 219–224.

49 van Ooteghem NA, Klomp LW, van Berge-Henegouwen GP *et al*. Benign recurrent intrahepatic cholestasis progressing to progressive familial intrahepatic cholestasis: low GGT cholestasis is a clinical continuum. *J. Hepatol.* 2002; **36**: 439–443.

50 Strautnieks SS, Bull LN, Knisely AS *et al*. A gene encoding a liver-specific ABC transporter is mutated in progressive

familial intrahepatic cholestasis. *Nat. Genet.* 1998; **20**: 233–238.

51 Jansen PL, Strautnieks SS, Jacquemin E *et al.* Hepatocanalicular bile salt export pump deficiency in patients with progressive familial intrahepatic cholestasis. *Gastroenterology* 1999; **117**: 1370–1379.

52 Jacquemin E. Role of multidrug resistance 3 deficiency in pediatric and adult liver disease: one gene for three diseases. *Sem. Liver Dis.* 2001; **21**: 551–562.

53 Kurbegov AC, Setchell KD, Haas JE *et al.* Biliary diversion for progressive familial intrahepatic cholestasis: improved liver morphology and bile acid profile. *Gastroenterology* 2003; **125**: 1227–1234.

54 Knisely AS, Strautnieks SS, Meier Y *et al.* Hepatocellular carcinoma in ten children under five years of age with bile salt export pump deficiency. *Hepatology* 2006; **44**: 478–486.

55 Daugherty CC, Setchell KDR, Heubi JE *et al.* Resolution of liver biopsy alterations in three siblings with bile acid treatment of an inborn error of bile acid metabolism (Δ4-3-oxosteroid 5β-reductase deficiency). *Hepatology* 1993; **18**: 1096–1101.

56 Clayton PT, Mills KA, Johnson AW *et al.* Delta 4–3-oxosteroid 5β-reductase deficiency: failure of ursodeoxycholic acid treatment and response to chenodeoxycholic acid plus cholic acid. *Gut* 1996; **38**: 623–628.

57 Suchy FJ. Bile acids for babies? Diagnosis and treatment of a new category of metabolic liver disease. *Hepatology* 1993; **18**: 1274–1277.

58 Paulusma CC, Kool M, Bosma PJ *et al.* A mutation in the human canalicular multispecific organic anion transporter gene causes the Dubin–Johnson syndrome. *Hepatology* 1997; **25**: 1539–1542.

59 Kaufman SS, Murray ND, Wood RP *et al.* Nutritional support for the infant with extrahepatic biliary atresia. *J. Pediat.* 1987; **110**: 679–686.

60 Rosh JR, Silverman ED, Groisman F *et al.* Intrahepatic cholestasis in neonatal lupus erythematosus. *J. Pediatr. Gastroenterol. Nutr.* 1993; **17**: 310–312.

61 Gissen P, Tee L, Johnson CA *et al.* Clinical and molecular genetic features of ARC syndrome. *Hum. Genet.* 2006; **120**: 396–409.

62 Hadj-Rabia S, Baala L, Vabres P *et al.* Claudin-1 gene mutations in neonatal sclerosing cholangitis associated with ichthyosis: a tight junction disease. *Gastroenterology* 2004; **127**:1386–1390.

63 Hartley J, Davenport M, Kelly DA. Biliary atresia. *Lancet* 2009; **374**: 1704–1713.

64 Livesey E, Cortina Borja M, Sharif K *et al.* Epidemiology of biliary atresia in England and Wales (1999–2006). *Arch. Dis. Child. Fetal Neonatal. Ed.* 2009; **94**: F451–F455.

65 McKiernan PJ, Baker AJ, Kelly DA. The frequency and outcome of biliary atresia in the UK and Ireland. *Lancet* 2000; **355**: 25.

66 Davenport M, Tizzard S, Underhill J *et al.* The biliary atresia splenic malformation syndrome: a 28-year single-center retrospective study. *J. Pediat.* 2006; **149**: 393–400.

67 Bezerra JA. The next challenge in pediatric cholestasis: deciphering the pathogenesis of biliary atresia. *J. Pediatr. Gastroenterol. Nutr.* 2006; **43**: S23–29.

68 Roberts EA. The jaundiced baby. In: Kelly DA, ed. *Diseases of the Liver and Biliary System in Children*, 3rd edn. Oxford: Wiley-Blackwell, 2008, p. 57–105.

69 Kelly DA, Davenport M. Current management of biliary atresia. *Arch. Dis. Child.* 2007; **92**: 132–135.

70 Mieli-Vergani G, Howard ER, Portman B *et al.* Late referral for biliary atresia—missed opportunities for effective surgery. *Lancet* 1989; **1**: 421–423.

71 Davenport M, de Ville de Goyet J, Stringer MD *et al.* Seamless management of biliary atresia in England and Wales (1999–2002). *Lancet* 2004; **363**:1354–1357.

72 Davenport M, Kerkar N, Mieli-Vergani G *et al.* Biliary atresia: the King's College Hospital experience. *J. Pediatr. Surg.* 1997; **32**: 479–485.

73 Nio M, Ohi R, Miyano T *et al.*; Japanese Biliary Atresia Registry. Five- and 10-year survival rates after surgery for biliary atresia: a report from the Japanese Biliary Atresia Registry. *J. Pediatr. Surg.* 2003; **38**: 997–1000.

74 Petersen C, Harder D, Abola Z *et al.* European biliary atresia registries: summary of a symposium. *Eur. J. Pediatr. Surg.* 2008; **18**: 111–116.

75 Chardot C, Carton M, Spire-Bendelac N *et al.* Prognosis of biliary atresia in the era of liver transplantation: French National Study from 1986 to 1996. *Hepatology* 1999; **30**: 606–611.

76 Gautier M, Jehan P, Odievre M. Histologic study of biliary fibrous remnants in 48 cases of extrahepatic biliary atresia: correlation with postoperative bile flow restoration. *J. Pediat.* 1976; **89**: 704–709.

77 Tan CEL, Davenport M, Driver M *et al.* Does the morphology of the extrahepatic biliary remnants in biliary atresia influence survival? A review of 205 cases. *J. Pediatr. Surg.* 1994; **29**: 1459–1464.

78 Lykaveris P, Chardot C, Sokhn M *et al.* Outcome in adulthood of biliary atresia; a study of 63 patients who survived for over 20 years with their native liver. *Hepatology* 2005; **41**: 366–372.

79 European Liver Transplant Registry. www.eltr.org (accessed 3 Nov. 2010).

80 Bancroft JD, Bucuvalas JC, Ryckman FC *et al.* Antenatal diagnosis of choledochal cyst. *J. Pediatr. Gastroenterol. Nutr.* 1994; **18**: 142–145.

81 Stringer MD, Dhawan A, Davenport M *et al.* Choledochal cysts: lessons from a 20 year experience. *Arch. Dis. Child* 1995; **73**: 528–531.

82 de Vries JS, de Vries S, Aronson DC *et al.* Choledochal cysts: age of presentation, symptoms, and late complications related to Todani's classification. *J. Pediatr. Surg.* 2002; **37**: 1568–1573.

83 Reif S, Sloven DG, Lebenthal E. Gallstones in children. Characterization by age, aetiology, and outcome. *Am. J. Dis. Child.* 1991; **145**: 105–108.

84 Tyfield L, Reichardt J, Fridovich-Keil J *et al.* Classical galactosemia and mutations at the galactose-1-phosphate uridyl transferase (GALT) gene. *Hum. Mutat.* 1999; **13**: 417–430.

85 Gitzelmann R. Galactose-1-phosphate in the pathogenesis of galactosemia. *Eur. J. Pediatr.* 1995; **154** (Suppl. 2): S45–49.

86 Monk AM, Mitchell AJH, Milligan DW *et al.* Diagnosis of classical galactosaemia. *Arch. Dis. Child.* 1977; **52**: 943–946.

87 Berry GT, Nissim I, Lin Z *et al.* Endogenous synthesis of galactose in normal men and patients with hereditary galactosemia. *Lancet* 1995; **346**: 1073–1074.

88 Kelly AL, Lunt PW, Rodrigues F *et al.* Classification and genetic features of neonatal haemochromatosis: a study of 27 affected pedigrees and molecular analysis of genes implicated in iron metabolism. *J. Med. Genet.* 2001; **38**: 599–610.

89 Whitington PF, Malladi P. Neonatal hemochromatosis: is it an alloimmune disease? *J. Pediatr. Gastroenterol. Nutr.* 2005; **40**: 544–549.

90 Flynn DM, Mohan N, McKiernan P *et al.* Progress in treatment and outcome for children with neonatal haemochromatosis. *Arch. Dis. Child. Fetal Neonatal Ed.* 2003; **88**: F124–F127.

91 Whitington PF, Hibbard JU. High-dose immunoglobulin during pregnancy for recurrent neonatal haemochromatosis. *Lancet* 2004; **364**: 1690–1698.

92 Leonard JV, Schapira AH. Mitochondrial respiratory chain disorders II: neurodegenerative disorders and nuclear gene defects. *Lancet* 2000; **355**: 389–394.

93 Valnot I, Osmond S, Gigarel N *et al.* Mutations of the SCO1 gene in mitochondrial cytochrome c oxidase deficiency with neonatal-onset hepatic failure and encephalopathy. *Am. J .Hum. Genet.* 2000; **67**:1104–1109.

94 Sokal EM, Sokol R, Cormier V *et al.* Liver transplantation in mitochondrial respiratory chain disorders. *Eur. J. Pediatr.* 1999; **158** (Suppl. 2): S81–S84.

95 Thomson M, McKiernan P, Buckels J *et al.* Generalised mitochondrial cytopathy is an absolute contraindication to orthotopic liver transplant in childhood. *J. Pediatr. Gastroenterol. Nutr.*1998; **26**: 478–481.

96 Nguyen KV, Ostergaard E, Ravn SH *et al.* POLG mutations in Alpers syndrome. *Neurology* 2005; **65**: 1493–1495.

97 Heath SK, Gray RG, McKiernan P *et al.* Mutation screening for tyrosinaemia type I. *J. Inherit. Metab. Dis.* 2002; **25**: 523–524.

98 Weinberg AG, Mize CE, Worthen HG. The occurrence of hepatoma in the chronic form of hereditary tyrosinemia. *J. Pediatr.* 1976; **88**: 434–438.

99 Lindstedt S, Holme E, Lock EA *et al.* Treatment of hereditary tyrosinaemia type I by inhibition of 4-hydroxyphenylpyruvate dioxygenase. *Lancet* 1992; **340**: 813–817.

100 McKiernan PJ. Nitisinone in the treatment of hereditary tyrosinaemia type 1. *Drugs* 2006; **66**: 743–750.

101 Shah U, Kelly D, Chang MH *et al.* Management of chronic hepatitis B in children. *J. Pediatr. Gastroenterol. Nutr.*2009; **48**: 399–404.

102 Kelly DA. Current status of treatment of hepatitis B in children. *Adv. Exp. Med. Biol.* 2010; **659**: 121–128.

103 Boxall EH, Sira J, El-Shukri N *et al.* Long-term persistence of immunity to hepatitis B after vaccination during infancy in a country where endemicity is low. *J. Infect. Dis.* 2004; **190**: 1264–1269.

104 Harris HE, Mieli-Vergani G, Kelly D *et al.* A national sample of individuals who acquired their hepatitis C virus infections in childhood/adolescence—risk factors for advanced disease. *J. Pediatr. Gastroenterol. Nutr.* 2007; **45**: 335–341.

105 Wirth S, Pieper-Boustani H, Lang T *et al.* Peginterferon alfa-2b plus ribavirin treatment in children and adolescents with chronic hepatitis C. *Hepatology* 2005; **41**: 1013–1018.

106 Mieli-Vergani G, Heller S, Jara P *et al.* Autoimmune hepatitis. *J. Pediatr. Gastroenterol. Nutr.* 2009; **49**: 158–164.

107 Rashid M, Roberts EA. Nonalcoholic steatohepatitis in children. *J. Pediatr. Gastroenterol. Nutr.* 2000; **30**: 48–53.

108 Murray KF, Hadzic N, Wirth S *et al.* Drug-related hepatotoxicity and acute liver failure. *J. Pediatr. Gastroenterol. Nutr.* 2008; **47**: 395–405.

109 Frydman M, Bonne-Tamir B, Farrer LA *et al.* Assignment of the gene for Wilson disease to chromosome 13: linkage to the esterase D locus. *Proc. Natl. Acad. Sci. USA* 1985; **82**: 1819–1821.

110 Tanner S. Disorders of copper metabolism. In: Kelly DA, ed. *Diseases of the Liver and Biliary System in Children*, 3rd edn. Oxford: Wiley-Blackwell, 2008, p. 328–348.

111 Tanner MS. Role of copper in Indian childhood cirrhosis. *Am. J. Clin. Nutr.* 1998; **67**:1074S–1081S.

112 Tanner MS. Indian childhood cirrhosis and Tyrolean childhood cirrhosis. Disorders of a copper transport gene? *Adv. Exp. Med. Biol.* 1999; **448**: 127–137.

113 Rowe SM, Miller S, Sorscher EJ. Mechanisms of disease. Cystic fibrosis. *N. Engl. J. Med.* 2005; **352**: 1992–2001.

114 Riordan JR, Rommens JM, Kerem B *et al.* Identification of the cystic fibrosis gene: cloning and characterization of complementary DNA. *Science* 1989; **245**: 1066–1073.

115 Colombo C. Hepatobiliary disease in cystic fibrosis. In: Kelly DA, ed. *Diseases of the Liver and Biliary System in Children*, 3rd edn. Oxford: Wiley-Blackwell, 2008, p. 270–288.

116 Potter CJ, Fishbein M, Hammond S *et al.* Can the histologic changes of Cystic Fibrosis-associated hepatobiliary disease be predicted by clinical criteria? *J. Pediatr. Gastroenterol. Nutr.* 1997; **25**: 32–36.

117 Patriquin H, Lenaerts C, Smith L *et al.* Liver disease in children with cystic fibrosis: US and biochemical comparison in 195 patients. *Radiology* 1999; **211**: 229–232.

118 Colombo C, Crosignani A, Assaisso ML *et al.* Ursodeoxycholic acid therapy in cystic fibrosis associated liver disease: a dose-response study. *Hepatology* 1992; **16**: 924–930.

119 Melzi M, Colledan M, Strazzabosco M *et al.* Liver transplant in cystic fibrosis: a poll among European centres. A study from the ELTR (European Liver Transplant Registry). *Transpl. Int.* 2006; **19**: 726–731.

120 Burchell A. Glycogen storage diseases and the liver. *Bailliere's Clin. Gastroenterol.* 1998; **12**: 337.

121 Chen YT. Glycogen storage diseases. In: Scriver CR, Beaudet AL, Sly WS, Vall D, eds. *The Metabolic and Molecular Bases of Inherited Disease.* New York: McGraw-Hill, 2001, p. 1521–1551.

122 Wolfsdorf JI, Holm IA, Weinstein DA. Glycogen storage diseases. Phenotypic genetic and biochemical characteristics and therapy. *Endocrinol. Metabol. Clin. N. Am.* 1999; **28**: 801–823.

123 Bianchi L. Glycogen storage disease I and hepatocellular tumours. *Eur. J. Pediatr.* 1993; **152** (Suppl. 1): S63–70.

124 Smit GP. The long-term outcome of patients with glycogen storage disease type Ia. *Eur. J. Pediatr.* 1993; **152** (Suppl. 1): S52–S55.

125 Labrune P, Trioche P, Duvaltier I *et al.* Hepatocellular adenomas in glycogen storage disease type I and III: a series of 43 patients and review of the literature. *J. Pediatr. Gastroenterol. Nutr.* 1997; **24**: 276–279.

126 Lee PJ, Patel A, Hindmarsh PC *et al.* The prevalence of polycystic ovaries in the hepatic glycogen storage dis-

eases: its association with hyperinsulinism. *Clin. Endocrinol. (Oxf)* 1995; **42**: 601–606.

127 Talente GM, Coleman RA, Alter C *et al.* Glycogen storage disease in adults. *Ann. Intern. Med.* 1994; **120**: 218–226.

128 Veiga-da-Cunha M, Gerin I, Chen YT *et al.* A gene on chromosome 11q23 coding for a putative glucose- 6-phosphate translocase is mutated in glycogen-storage disease types Ib and Ic. *Am. J. Hum. Genet.* 1998; **63**: 976–983.

129 Visser G, Rake JP, Fernandes J *et al.* Neutropenia, neutrophil dysfunction, and inflammatory bowel disease in glycogen storage disease type Ib: results of the European Study on Glycogen Storage Disease type I. *J. Pediat.* 2000; **137**:187–191.

130 Coleman RA, Winter HS, Wolf B *et al.* Glycogen storage disease type III (glycogen debranching enzyme deficiency): correlation of biochemical defects with myopathy and cardiomyopathy. *Ann. Intern. Med.* 1992; **116**: 896–900.

131 Shen J, Bao Y, Liu HM *et al.* Mutations in exon 3 of the glycogen debranching enzyme gene are associated with glycogen storage disease type III that is differentially expressed in liver and muscle. *J. Clin. Invest.* 1996; **98**: 352–357.

132 Bao Y, Kishnani P, Wu JY, Chen YT. Hepatic and neuromuscular forms of glycogen storage disease type IV caused by mutations in the same glycogen-branching enzyme gene. *J. Clin. Invest.* 1996; **97**: 941–948.

133 Selby R, Starzl TE, Yunis E *et al.* Liver transplantation for type IV glycogen storage disease. *N. Engl. J. Med.* 1991; **324**: 39–42.

134 Burwinkel B, Shiomi S, Al Zaben A *et al.* Liver glycogenosis due to phosphorylase kinase deficiency: PHKG2 gene structure and mutations associated with cirrhosis. *Hum. Mol. Genet.* 1998; **7**:149–154.

135 Santer R, Steinmann B, Schaub J. Fanconi-Bickel syndrome–a congenital defect of facilitative glucose transport. *Curr. Mol. Med.* 2002; **2**: 213–227.

136 Ames CL, Rellos P, Ali M *et al.* Neonatal screening for hereditary fructose intolerance: frequency of the most common mutant aldolase B allele (A149P) in the British population. *J. Med. Genet.* 1996; **33**: 837–841.

137 Odièvre M, Gentil C, Gautier M *et al.* Hereditary fructose intolerance in childhood. Diagnosis, management, and course in 55 patients. *Am. J. Dis. Child.* 1978; **132**: 605–608.

138 Kikawa Y, Inuzuka M, Jin BY *et al.* Identification of genetic mutations in Japanese patients with fructose-1,6-bisphosphatase deficiency. *Am. J. Hum. Genet.* 1997; **61**: 852–861.

139 Wilson GN, De Chadarevian J-P, Kaplan P *et al.* Glutaric aciduria type II: review of the phenotype and report of an unusual glomerulopathy. *Am. J. Med. Genet.* 1989; **32**: 395–401.

140 Rohrbach M, Clarke JT. Treatment of lysosomal storage disorders: progress with enzyme replacement therapy. *Drugs* 2007; **67**: 2697–2716.

141 Cox TM. Gaucher disease: understanding the molecular pathogenesis of sphingolipidoses. *J. Inherit. Metab. Dis.* 2001; **24** (Suppl. 2): 106–121.

142 Brady RO. Enzyme replacement for lysosomal diseases. *Annu. Rev. Med.* 2006; **57**: 283–296.

143 Schuchman EH, Desnick RJ. Niemann-Pick diseases types A and B: acid sphingomyelinase deficiencies. In: Scriver CR, Beaudet AL, Sly WS, Vall D, eds. *The Metabolic and Molecular Bases of Inherited Disease.* New York: McGraw-Hill, 2001, p. 3589–3609.

144 Verot L, Chikh K, Freydiere E *et al.* Niemann-Pick C disease: functional characterization of three NPC2 mutations and clinical and molecular update on patients with NPC2. *Clin. Genet.* 2007; **71**: 320–330.

145 Imrie J, Dasgupta S, Besley GT *et al.* The natural history of Niemann-Pick disease type C in the UK. *J. Inherit. Metab. Dis.* 2007; **30**: 51–59.

146 Kelly DA, Portmann B, Mowat AP *et al.* Niemann-Pick disease type C: diagnosis and outcome in children, with particular reference to liver disease. *J. Pediat.* 1993; **123**: 242–247.

147 Anderson RA, Bryson GM, Parks JS. Lysosomal acid lipase mutations that determine phenotype in Wolman and cholesterol ester storage disease. *Mol. Genet. Metab.* 1999; **68**: 333–345.

148 Assmann G, Seedorf U. Acid lipase deficiency: Wolman disease and cholesteryl ester storage disease. In: Scriver CR, Beaudet AL, Sly WS, Vall D, eds. *The Metabolic and Molecular Bases of Inherited Disease.* New York: McGraw-Hill, 2001, p. 3551–3571.

149 Wolman M. Wolman disease and its treatment. *Clin. Pediatr. (Phila)* 1995; **34**: 207–212.

150 Krivit W, Peters C, Dusenbery K *et al.* Wolman disease successfully treated by bone marrow transplantation. *Bone Marrow Transpl.* 2000; **26**: 567–570.

151 Rassoul F, Richter V, Lohse P *et al.* Long-term administration of the HMG-CoA reductase inhibitor lovastatin in two patients with cholesteryl ester storage disease. *Int. J. Clin. Pharmacol. Ther.* 2001; **39**:199–204.

152 Arterburn JN, Lee WM, Wood RP *et al.* Orthotopic liver transplantation for cholesteryl ester storage disease. *J. Clin. Gastroenterol.* 1991; **13**: 482–485.

153 Wraith JE. The mucopolysaccharidoses: a clinical review and guide to management. *Arch. Dis. Child.* 1995; **72**: 263–267.

154 Resnick JM, Krivit W, Snover DC *et al.* Pathology of the liver in mucopolysaccharidosis: light and electron microscopic assessment before and after bone marrow transplantation. *Bone Marrow Transpl.* 1992; **10**: 273–280.

155 Brown MS, Goldstein JL. Lipoprotein receptors in the liver: control signals for plasma cholesterol traffic. *J. Clin. Invest.* 1983; **72**: 743–747.

156 Palcoux JB, Atassi-Dumont M, Lefevre P *et al.* Low-density lipoprotein apheresis in children with familial hypercholesterolemia: follow-up to 21 years. *Ther. Apher. Dial.* 2008; **12**: 195–201.

157 Baumer JH, Shield JP. Hypercholesterolaemia in children guidelines review *Arch. Dis. Child .Educ. Pract. Ed.* 2009; **94**: 84–86.

158 Bilheimer DW, Goldstein JL, Grundy SM *et al.* Liver transplantation to provide low-density-lipoprotein receptors and lower plasma cholesterol in a child with homozygous familial hypercholesterolemia. *N. Engl. J. Med.* 1984; **311**: 1658–1664.

159 Nguyen TH, Mainot S, Lainas P *et al.* Ex vivo liver-directed gene therapy for the treatment of metabolic diseases: advances in hepatocyte transplantation and retroviral vectors. *Curr. Gene Ther.* 2009; **9**: 136–149.

160 Johnson SP, Leyendecker JR, Joseph FB *et al.* Transjugular portosystemic shunts in pediatric patients awaiting liver transplantation. *Transplantation* 1996; **62**: 1178–1181.

161 Bonatti H, Muiesan P, Connolly S *et al.* Liver transplantation for acute liver failure in children under 1 year of age. *Transpl. Proc.* 1997; **29**: 434–435.

162 Kayler LK, Rasmussen CS, Dykstra DM *et al.* Liver transplantation in children with metabolic disorders in the United States. *Am. J. Transpl.* 2003; **3**: 334–339.

163 Pimpalwar AP, Sharif K, Ramani P *et al.* Strategy for hepatoblastoma management. Transplant versus non-transplant surgery. *J. Pediatr. Surg.* 2002; **37**: 240–245.

164 Arora-Gupta N, Davies P, McKiernan P *et al.* The effect of long term calcineurin inhibitor therapy on renal function in children after liver transplantation. *Pediatr. Transpl.* 2004; **8**: 145–150.

165 Busuttil RW, Farmer DG, Yersiz H *et al.* Analysis of long-term outcomes of 3200 liver transplantations over two decades: a single-center experience. *Ann. Surg.* 2005; **241**: 905–916.

166 Van Mourik IDM, Beath D, Kelly D. Long term nutrition and neurodevelopmental outcome of liver transplantation in infants aged less than 12 months. *J. Pediatr. Gastroenterol. Nutr.* 2000; **30**: 269–276.

167 Krull K, Fuchs C, Yurk H *et al.* Neurocognitive outcome in pediatric liver transplant recipients. *Pediatr. Transpl.* 2003; **7**: 111–118.

168 Molmenti E, Mazariegos G, Bueno T *et al.* Noncompliance after pediatric liver transplantation. *Transpl. Proc.* 1999; **31**: 408.

169 Shah SA, Cleary SP, Tan JC *et al.* An analysis of resection versus transplantation for early hepatocellular carcinoma: defining the optimal therapy at a single institution. *Ann. Surg. Oncol.* 2007; **14**: 2608–2614 .

170 Selby DM, Stocker JT, Waclawiw MA *et al.* Infantile haemangioendothelioma of the liver. *Hepatology* 1994; **20**: 39–45.

171 Stanley P, Geer GD, Miller JH *et al.* Infantile hepatic haemangiomas. Clinical features, radiologic investigations, and treatment of 20 patients. *Cancer* 1989; **64**: 936–949.

CHAPTER 30
The Liver in Pregnancy

Andrew K. Burroughs[1] & E. Jenny Heathcote[2]

[1] Royal Free Sheila Sherlock Liver Centre, Royal Free Hospital and University College, London, UK

[2] Liver Centre, Toronto Western Hospital, Toronto, ON, Canada

---

Learning points

- Liver disease must be distinguished as incidental to pregnancy, as pre-existing liver disease or specific to pregnancy.

- Herpes hepatitis can occur in normal pregnancy and needs to be looked for as it is treatable with aciclovir.

- Acute fatty liver of pregnancy, pregnancy toxaemias, including HELLP syndrome, present in the last trimester; they may have overlapping clinical and laboratory features, and may lead to an acute liver failure syndrome. Early diagnosis, with consideration of early delivery of the fetus, is imperative to improve fetal and maternal outcomes.

- Ursodeoxycholic acid is indicated as therapy for intrahepatic cholestasis of pregnancy as it improves maternal well being, relieves itching and improves fetal outcomes.

Normal pregnancy

Physical examination may show palmar erythema and vascular spiders. The liver is impalpable.

Gallbladder motility decreases while the lithogenic index of bile increases [1]. Haematocrit, serum urea, uric acid, albumin and total protein values decrease, and the presence of placental and bone isoenzymes generates an increase in alkaline phosphatase [2]. Cholesterol and triglyceride levels increase, while aminotransferase concentrations remain unchanged. Total and free bilirubin concentrations are lower in all trimesters, while conjugated bilirubin and γ-glutamyl transferase (γ-GT) levels are reduced only in the second and third trimesters [3].

Needle liver biopsy in normal pregnancy gives virtually normal histological appearances. Electron microscopy shows some increase in endoplasmic reticulum.

Liver blood flow is within the normal range [4]. In pregnancy, blood volume and cardiac output increase. The liver blood flow comprises 35% of the cardiac output in non-pregnant females and only 28% of the cardiac output in pregnancy. The excess blood volume is shunted through the placenta.

Liver disease in pregnancy

It is useful to classify liver diseases in pregnancy into one of three categories (Table 30.1):
- Those specific to pregnancy
- Those coincidental with pregnancy
- Those that are already established.

Diseases specific to pregnancy

Hyperemesis gravidarum

In the first trimester of a normal pregnancy, nausea and vomiting frequently occur and are associated with faster-than-usual gastric dysrhythmias [5]. If atypically prolonged, these symptoms may lead to intense weight loss, dehydration and mild jaundice, which is termed hyperemesis gravidarum. This occurs in between 1 and 20 per 1000 pregnancies [6]. Transient hyperthyroidism may occur in 60% owing to the thyroid-stimulating activity of human chorionic gonadotropin [6]. In addition, aminotransferase levels may be raised, usually to no more than 250 IU/L [6]. Liver biopsy is normal or may have mild fatty change.

Hyperemesis gravidarum is associated with age (<20 years), nulliparity, obesity, pre-existing diabetes and non-smoking status [7]. It is rare for it to recur [6]. Liver enzymes return to normal when dehydration and malnutrition are corrected. Steroids [8] and ondansetron [6] are effective. Birth weight may be reduced.

Sherlock's Diseases of the Liver and Biliary System, Twelfth Edition. Edited by James S. Dooley, Anna S.F. Lok, Andrew K. Burroughs, E. Jenny Heathcote.
© 2011 by Blackwell Publishing Ltd. Published 2011 by Blackwell Publishing Ltd.

Table 30.1. Liver disease in pregnancy

Disease	Notes
Peculiar to pregnancy	
Acute fatty liver	Rare, presents vomiting, variable prognosis
Toxaemias	Hepatic haemorrhage may be a complication
HELLP syndrome	Haemolysis, elevated serum, liver enzymes, low platelet count
Recurrent cholestasis	Good prognosis, familial, recurs, fetal wastage
Hyperemesis	Rare cause of jaundice
Intercurrent	
Viral hepatitis	Prognosis as in non-pregnant
	A—no effect on fetus
	B—rarely transmitted to fetus
	C—anti-HCV positive check HCV RNA
	E—often fatal in Africa and Asia
Gallstones	Rare cause of jaundice, ultrasound diagnosis
Underlying chronic liver disease	Rare to become pregnant, prognosis variable, stillbirths increased

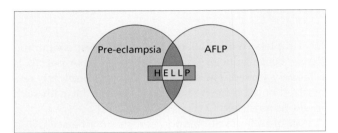

Fig. 30.1. Venn diagram showing the overlap between pre-eclampsia, acute fatty liver of pregnancy (AFLP) and the HELLP syndrome.

Table 30.2. Clinical and laboratory features of 12 patients with acute fatty liver of pregnancy (data from [9])

Feature	Number of patients
Nausea/ vomiting	12
Severe heartburn	4
Abdominal pain	7
Jaundice	11
Leucocytosis	12
Thrombocytopenia	9
Proteinuria	7
Oedema	7
Hypertension	8
Serum urea increased	9

Rare complications include oesophageal rupture, Wernicke's encephalopathy, central pontine myelinolysis, retinal haemorrhage and spontaneous pneumomediastinum [6].

Diseases of late pregnancy

The three pregnancy-related diseases are fatty liver of pregnancy, pre-eclampsia or eclampsia and the HELLP syndrome. There is considerable overlap between them (Fig. 30.1), for instance 40% of sufferers from acute fatty liver of pregnancy show evidence of eclampsia (hypertension, proteinuria and oedema) [9].

The diseases are of unknown cause, they are commoner in twins and there is no chronicity.

Acute fatty liver of pregnancy

The first description is usually attributed to Sheehan [10] who, in 1940, described obstetric acute liver atrophy as a cause of jaundice in pregnancy. It affects approximately 1:14 000 pregnancies [11].

Clinical features

The onset is usually between the 34th and 36th week and is marked by nausea, repeated vomiting and abdominal pain followed by jaundice (Table 30.2). Earlier presentation is so exceptional that alternative diagnoses should be considered. It is commoner with twins and male births and in primiparae [9].

In those severely affected, the course is marked by encephalopathy, renal failure, pancreatitis, oesophagitis, haemorrhages, disseminated intravascular coagulation and pulmonary emboli. Ascites may be found.

Polydipsia and polyuria with transient diabetes insipidus have been reported [9,12]. Signs of pre-eclampsia are found in 50% [9]. The differential diagnosis lies between acute viral or drug induced hepatitis and toxaemia of pregnancy, including HELLP syndrome. Obstetric causes of renal failure, such as haemolytic uraemic syndrome and thrombotic thrombocytopenic purpura, must also be considered—a blood film can help in the differential diagnosis, as well as careful attention to the antecedent history.

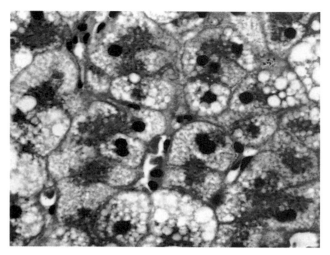

Fig. 30.2. Acute fatty liver of pregnancy. Hepatocytes have a foamy appearance with a central dense nucleus. (H & E, ×120.)

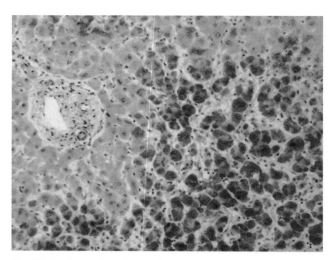

Fig. 30.3. Acute fatty liver of pregnancy: zone 3 hepatocytes are full of microvesicular fat droplets. Portal zones are normal and inflammation is minimal. (Oil red, ×40.)

Serum biochemical changes

Serum ammonia and amino acid levels are increased, reflecting mitochondrial failure. This is also suggested by lactic acidosis. High serum uric acid levels are usual and may be related to the tissue destruction and lactic acidosis [9]. Plasma urea, uric acid and creatinine are usually elevated, even with mild jaundice. Uric acid concentrations rise days before symptoms [9].

Hypoglycaemia can be profound. Hyponatraemia and hyperkalaemia can occur.

Hyperbilirubinaemia is 90% conjugated, without haemolysis in contradistinction to pregnancy toxaemia where jaundice is rare except when there is haemolysis. Serum transaminase values are variable, rarely above 500 IU/L and may be normal [13]. Total serum gamma-globulin is not elevated and can help distinguish acute fatty liver from acute or chronic hepatitis [9].

Haematological findings

Leucocytosis and thrombocytopenia are common but the blood film may be leucoerythroblastic [9]. Prothrombin time and partial prothrombin time are increased. Fibrinogen levels are decreased. Severe bleeding is frequent, but disseminated intravascular coagulation is found in only 10% [9].

Liver histology

Liver biopsy is not usually necessary, as often the obstetric management regarding delivery takes precedence over the precise diagnosis of the liver dysfunction, but can be performed by the transjugular route. The histological picture is of microvesicular and macrovesicular

fat droplets with ballooned hepatocytes containing dense, central nuclei (Fig. 30.2). Zone 1 (periportal) is relatively spared. The microvacuoles may be clearly recognized only on fresh sections stained for fat with such methods as oil red O (Fig. 30.3) [9,13,14].

Foci of inflammation and necrosis may be seen; also cholestasis with bile canalicular plugs and bile-stained Kupffer cells. Liver architecture is normal.

Electron microscopy confirms vacuoles and may show a honeycomb appearance in the smooth endoplasmic reticulum. Mitochondria are large and pleomorphic with paracrystalline inclusions [12].

Multiorgan involvement is shown by fatty infiltration of the renal tubules and renal lesions typical of pre-eclampsia. Fatty infiltration of the pancreas and the heart have been reported [13].

Ultrasonography of the liver may show a diffuse increased echogenicity which is very suggestive of acute fatty liver of pregnancy (AFLP). A normal sonogram does not exclude the diagnosis. CT shows a low attenuation value in 30% [15].

Course and prognosis

Early recognition with prompt treatment has allowed diagnosis of milder cases and the current maternal mortality is 0–18% [16]. The fetal mortality (9–23%) remains high [16], in part related to inherited enzyme defects of long chain fatty acid metabolism described below.

Death is usually due to extrahepatic causes, such as disseminated intravascular coagulation with massive haemorrhage, including subcapsular haematoma and rupture and to renal failure. These features are not seen in the less-severe cases.

Table 30.3. The mitochondrial cytopathies

Causes
  Acute fatty liver of pregnancy
  Reye's syndrome
  Genetic defects in mitochondrial function
  Drug-related
Features
  Vomiting and apathy
  Lactic acidosis
  Hypoglycaemia
  Hyperammonaemia
  Microvesicular fat in organs

Recurrences are extremely rare and related in part to genetic predisposition [17].

Management

The management of the average, mild case is careful observation of the mother and fetus in hospital. If the mother's status deteriorates (intractable vomiting, increased jaundice and features of a coagulopathy), the pregnancy should be delivered.

Coagulopathy, renal failure, hypoglycaemia and infections are treated. The prognosis is relatively favourable if intensive care is adequate [18]. Intra-abdominal haemorrhage may necessitate laparotomy for clot evacuation. The intensive care must continue post-partum and intra-abdominal haemorrhage may follow caesarean section. Hepatic transplantation is rarely necessary [18,19].

The baby may need corticosteroids to treat lung immaturity.

Oesophagitis with bleeding is a frequent complication [9] and omeprazole or a similar drug should be given.

Aetiology

AFLP can be regarded as a member of the *mitochondrial cytopathy family* (Table 30.3) [20]. Members include Reye's syndrome, genetic defects in mitochondrial enzymes and drug reactions, especially to sodium valproate and nucleoside analogues.

Apart from the breakdown of carbohydrate, nearly all the reactions involved in energy production take place in mitochondria. Some oxidative phosphorylation includes the oxidation of fuel molecules by oxygen and simultaneous energy transduction into ATP. Fatty acids are broken down in the mitochondria into shorter, derivative fatty acids and acyl-CoA. This cycle of repeated fatty acid cleavage requires a series of specific enzymes.

The mitochondrial cytopathies are marked by vomiting and weakness. Lactic acidosis and metabolic acidosis are related to defective mitochondrial energy supply and defects in oxidative phosphorylation. Hypoglycaemia may be related to failure of mitochondrial citric acid cycle function. Raised blood ammonia relates to defects in mitochondrial Krebs' cycle enzymes. Microvesicular fat is seen in the organs.

Several cases of AFLP are associated with homozygous long-chain 3-hydroxyacyl-coenzyme A dehydrogenase (LCHAD) deficiency in a fetus who has a heterozygote mother for LCHAD deficiency, whereby the latter cannot metabolize the extra free fatty acids that are not metabolized by the fetus [21,22]. However, several factors appear to contribute to this fetal–maternal interaction [21]. LCHAD deficiency is caused by a genetic defect of mitochondrial trifunctional protein [23]. Careful observation of children born to mothers with AFLP is warranted as they may be homozygous for LCHAD deficiency. These children are at risk of hypoglycaemia, fatty liver, dilated cardiomyopathy, progressive neuromyopathy and sudden infant death syndrome [24,25]; thus, early diagnosis and dietary intervention could be lifesaving. Fortunately, prenatal diagnosis is possible [26]. AFLP is also associated with HELLP (haemolysis, elevated liver enzymes, low platelet count) syndrome [27]. The G1528C mutation resulting in the conversion of glutamic acid to glutamine (E474Q), has been found to be present in 20% of AFLP cases [28]. Short-chain acyl-CoA dehydrogenase deficiency has also been associated with AFLP [29].

Pregnancy *per se* may affect mitochondrial function. The mode of initiation of the mitochondrial cytopathies, apart from the genetic enzyme defects, is uncertain. It might be viral, or due to drugs such as aspirin which has been implicated in the development of Reye's syndrome. It might be toxic and AFLP has followed exposure to toluene [30]. Nutritional factors have also been suggested.

AFLP should be regarded as part of a systemic mitochondrial dysfunction affecting particularly liver, muscle, nervous system, pancreas and kidneys. The mother should be investigated for mitochondrial dysfunction, especially if the baby dies *in utero* or exhibits failure to thrive.

Pregnancy toxaemias

These conditions are characterized by hypertension, proteinuria and fluid retention. The term 'pregnancy toxaemia' includes a spectrum of conditions (Table 30.4). The target organs are the uterus, kidney and brain. Hepatic damage is only seen in patients with severe pre-eclampsia and eclampsia.

The aetiology of pre-eclampsia is unknown. It is marked by generalized vasospasm with increased systemic vascular resistance and enhanced pressor responses to endogenous vasoconstrictors. Endothelial

Table 30.4. Spectrum of pregnancy toxaemias

Pre-eclampsia
HELLP syndrome
Infarction
Bleeding and rupture

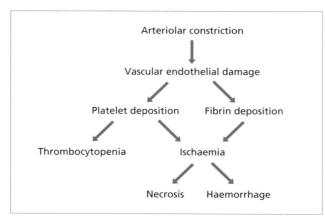

Fig. 30.4. The liver in eclampsia. Hepatocellular necrosis and haemorrhage follow ischaemia related to vascular endothelial damage.

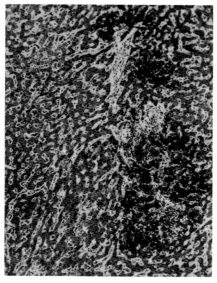

Fig. 30.5. The liver in eclampsia. Focal periportal necrosis of liver cells; the lesion contains fibrin. (Mallory's phosphotungstic acid, ×80.)

cell injury may decrease endothelial-dependent vasodilators and increase production of vasoconstrictors coming from both endothelial cells and platelets. Serum from pre-eclamptic patients contains factors that increase endothelial cell permeability [31]. The vascular endothelium may be a target for blood-borne products of reduced placental perfusion [32].

Vascular endothelial damage leads to platelet deposition, thrombocytopenia and fibrin deposition in sinusoids. The resultant ischaemia accounts for the focal and diffuse hepatocellular necrosis and haemorrhages in zone 1 (Fig. 30.4).

In mild cases, increases in serum alkaline phosphatase and transaminase values are frequent [33]. Minor signs of disseminated intravascular coagulation, such as a reduction in platelets, are also common.

Jaundice is infrequent and often terminal. It is usually haemolytic with disseminated intravascular coagulation. Failure of renal bilirubin excretion may contribute. Serum bilirubin is less than 6 mg/dL (100 μmol/L).

Severe pre-eclampsia or toxaemia may present with epigastric pain, nausea, vomiting, hypertension, right upper quadrant tenderness due to infarction [34] or haematoma [35,36].

Hepatic histology shows periportal (zone 1) fibrin deposits [37] and haemorrhage, which progress to small necrotic foci, infarcts and haematomas. Zone 3 necrosis and haemorrhage represent shock. An inflammatory reaction is characteristically absent (Fig. 30.5). Capillary and hepatic arterial thrombi and, rarely, intrahepatic portal venous thrombi may be noted. *Serum transaminases* are usually more than 10 times elevated.

Rupture of the liver is associated with shock and accounts for 15% of deaths [37].

Ultrasound and CT show focal filling defects, or haematomas.

The *treatment* of both mild and severe toxaemia is by delivering the pregnancy and by supportive care.

The HELLP syndrome

This is a rare variant of pre-eclampsia [38,39]. It consists of haemolysis, elevated liver enzymes and low platelet count [40]. It often affects multipara. The blood pressure may be normal and proteinuria may be absent.

Liver histology shows fibrin deposition [41]. This suggests severe pre-eclamptic liver disease and calls for immediate delivery. The laboratory results do not reflect hepatic histology [41]. Perinatal mortality is 10–60% and the maternal mortality 1.5–5% [42].

Management is delivery of the fetus and supportive therapy for the mother, as for eclampsia. Rarely, liver transplantation has been used [43].

Women heterozygous for factor V Leiden have an increased risk of developing HELLP syndrome [44], while placental CD95 ligand (CD95L) has been shown to act systemically to cause liver damage in patients with HELLP syndrome, and blockade of CD95L results in reduced liver damage via inhibition of apoptotic mechanisms [45]. This finding may eventually lead to new therapies, although the relationship between HELLP syndrome and defects in fatty acid oxidation requires further evaluation [46].

Table 30.5. Acute fatty liver of pregnancy and toxaemias contrasted: overlaps exist

	Acute fatty liver	Toxaemia
Abdominal pain	50%	100%
Jaundice	100%	40%
Serum transaminases (× normal)	<10	>10
Scans	Diffuse change	Focal abnormalities
Liver biopsy	Microvesicular fat	Fibrin (perisinusoidal)
Liver failure	Present	Absent

Overlap between AFLP and hypertension-associated liver dysfunction of pregnancy

Many patients with AFLP show signs of pre-eclampsia [9,47] (Table 30.5); therefore, the two conditions may form part of the same disease spectrum, or may be associated with the same metabolic defect, namely LCHAD deficiency. Indeed, both older [48] and newer [38] studies have found fatty livers in a significant proportion of patients with eclampsia. One study involving 41 consecutive patients with pre-eclampsia with or without liver dysfunction revealed that all women had a significant amount of microvesicular fat upon oil red O staining [49].

Although the association between AFLP and HELLP syndrome or pre-eclampsia is suggested by the frequency with which both conditions occur in mothers of infants who have LCHAD deficiency [27], this apparent connection may in fact be due to misdiagnosis of AFLP as HELLP syndrome [9,50]. Some sources recommend monitoring platelet counts, as these levels decrease just before HELLP syndrome and AFLP become manifest [51].

Hepatic infarcts, haematomas, and liver rupture in pregnancy are associated with severe pre-eclampsia or eclampsia in 80% of cases [52] and, to a lesser degree, with HELLP syndrome and AFLP [52], often in association with disseminated intravascular coagulation. Liver rupture presents as sudden abdominal pain associated with nausea and vomiting, and shock may develop very quickly [53]. The initial treatment of choice is the conservative management of hepatic haematomas; however, facilities for urgent laparotomy should be available. Arterial embolization and surgery are needed for rupture. Liver transplantation may be successful [54], but rarely needed.

Hepatic adenomas, often with peliosis hepatis, and often associated with oral contraceptives, may rupture during pregnancy (see Chapters 24 and 34).

Cholestasis of pregnancy

In its mildest form, pruritus is the only abnormality [55]. It usually commences in the last trimester, but can start as early as the second or third month. Jaundice is rarely deep and usually follows after 2 weeks of pruritus, rarely exceeding 100 μmol/L [55]. The urine is dark and the stools pale. General health is preserved and there is no pain. Weight loss may be great. The liver and spleen are impalpable. After delivery, jaundice disappears and within 1–2 weeks the pruritus has ceased. The condition usually recurs with subsequent pregnancies. Consecutive pregnancies in multiparous patients are associated with variability in the severity and in the time of onset.

Laboratory changes

Serum shows an increase in conjugated bilirubin and alkaline phosphatase values. Serum transaminases are normal or slightly increased, rarely surpassing 250 IU/L [55]. These changes return to normal after delivery. Serum bile acids are increased (>10 μmol/L) [56], and the primary bile acids (cholic and chenodeoxycholic acids) predominate [57]. γ-GT concentrations may be normal.

Steatorrhoea is usual. It correlates with the severity of the cholestasis.

The prothrombin time is prolonged due to vitamin K deficiency. Cholestyramine enhances the hypoprothrombinaemia.

Hepatic histology shows mild focal and irregular cholestasis. Electron microscopy shows the changes in the microvilli of the bile canaliculi common to all forms of cholestasis.

Aetiology

Multiple factors probably interact with the genetic predisposition to alter the canalicular and hepatic membranes so changing their transport of sex steroids. Hormonal factors are suggested by worsening with multiple pregnancies and recurrences with menstruation or oestrogen therapy. The administration of progesterone has been reported shortly before the development of cholestasis [58].

At least 10 different *MDR3* mutations associated with intrahepatic cholestasis of pregnancy (ICP) have been identified [16], and are present in 30% of ICP cases in the UK [58]. One report has shown that certain *MDR3* gene variants (*ABCB4*) are associated with a severe form of ICP [59]. Another study demonstrated that splicing mutations in the *MDR3* gene result in ICP (although γ-GT levels were normal), and may be associated with stillbirths and gallstone disease [60]. *MDR3* mutations are also found in progressive familial intrahepatic cholestasis [61].

The condition is particularly common in Scandinavia, northern Europe, Chile, Bolivia and China. It is very rare in Asiatic or Black women [55].

Appropriate nutritional support is essential. Vitamin K supplements given at least 6 hours before delivery are necessary as the risk of post-partum haemorrhage is increased.

Treatment with dexamethasone 12 mg/day for 1 week (then tapered over the subsequent 3 days) may improve pruritus by suppressing fetoplacental oestrogen synthesis [53]. Although dexamethasone aids fetal lung maturation [62], its effectiveness in ICP remains debatable. However, it is less effective than ursodeoxycholic acid (UDCA) [63], which, when administered at or above 1 g/day (up to 2 g/day), is safe, modifies the bile acid pool (possibly via post-transcriptional mechanisms), relieves pruritus and improves liver function within 2 weeks [64,65]; and also reduces fetal mortality [64]. Studies have demonstrated that UDCA is also more effective than S-adenosyl-L-methionine and cholestyramine [66,67], and it is at present the first-line treatment for ICP.

Epidemiology

Cholestasis of pregnancy is often familial, and has been reported in mothers, sisters and daughters, some of whom develop pruritus when given oral contraceptives. Male family members may show the cholestatic tendency when given oestrogens [56]. Findings support a Mendelian dominant inheritance.

In Chile, cholestasis is associated with Araucarial Indian descent, rather than with Chilean Caucasians [55].

Diagnosis

In the first pregnancy, the differentiation from viral hepatitis and other conditions causing jaundice may be difficult. Absence of constitutional symptoms, prominent pruritus and biochemical tests suggesting cholestasis are helpful. Ultrasound helps to exclude obstruction to main bile ducts. Liver biopsy is rarely necessary, but the appearances are diagnostic. Failure of the pruritus to stop after delivery, with continuing high serum alkaline phosphatase values, suggests underlying primary biliary cirrhosis, and serum mitochondrial antibody tests should be performed and obtaining a liver biopsy considered. Alternatively, a familial cholestatic disorder may be present. After delivery, the woman may show a cholestatic response to small doses of oestrogen, which may preclude subsequent use of oral contraceptives.

Prognosis and management

Prognosis for the mother is excellent. The fetus, however, is at increased risk of miscarriage, premature labour,

distress, prematurity and death [68]. The fetus must be carefully monitored and termination is indicated for distress [65]. The mother should be delivered at 38 weeks, or at 36 weeks if the cholestasis is severe [68]. Fetal outcomes are improved if the mother has taken UDCA [64].

The mother is warned that the condition will usually return in a subsequent pregnancy and that she may develop pruritus if she takes oral contraceptive drugs.

Budd–Chiari syndrome (Chapter 9)

Pregnancy is a procoagulant state as shown by increased fibrinogen levels and increased values for factor VIII, factor IX (Christmas) and factor XII (Hagemann). Rarely, venous thrombosis, particularly the Budd–Chiari syndrome and hepatic microthrombi, complicate pregnancy, especially in patients having an underlying defect in blood coagulation. This may be the lupus anticoagulant and anticardiolipin antibodies, which favour repeated abortions [69], antithrombin III deficiency or factor V Leiden mutation [70]. Factors precipitating the actual thrombosis are unclear but may be infections. A thrombophilia screen must be performed. Anticoagulation may be necessary [71], and transjugular intrahepatic portosystemic shunt (TIPS) can be performed. Liver transplantation has been performed [72]. The fetus is rarely affected, but maternal mortality is increased [73].

Pregnancy in those with acute or chronic liver disease

Viral hepatitis

Viral hepatitis causes about 50% of jaundice in pregnancy [74]. It is particularly serious in developing countries with a mortality ranging from 10 to 45%. In developed countries, the course and mortality of acute hepatitis in pregnancy are about the same as in the non-pregnant. Fetal abnormalities are not recorded, but stillbirths may be increased.

Hepatitis A

The disease is passed to the mother by contact with the excreta of older children attending nursery schools. Pregnant women exposed should receive immunoglobulin and vaccine immediately. The course is similar to that in the non-pregnant even in the last trimester. It is rarely transmitted to the fetus.

Hepatitis B

Pregnant women in close contact with persons carrying hepatitis B must receive hepatitis B vaccine, which is safe in pregnancy, and also hepatitis B immunoglobulin. An acute attack of hepatitis B usually runs the same course in the pregnant as in the non-pregnant woman. The chances of the disease progressing to chronic hepatitis are less than 10%. In underdeveloped countries, the mortality is high and fetal wastage and stillbirths are increased. The effect on the baby of a mother carrying hepatitis B is very serious (Chapter 18).

Screening of mothers for hepatitis B viral markers should be universal and not simply directed to those in high risk groups.

The *hepatitis delta virus* can be transmitted to the fetus from a mother who is carrying both hepatitis B and delta. This results in more serious hepatitis. A baby vaccinated against hepatitis B immediately after birth and with concomitant administration of hepatitis B immune globulin (HBIG) and follow up vaccination and 1 month and 6 months of age, ensures protection in most.

Indications for therapy for chronic hepatitis B are based on the severity of the underlying liver damage and serum HBV-DNA concentrations. Postmarketing surveillance has shown lamivudine is safe in the first trimester and telbivudine or tenofovir have been given in the second and third trimester, enabling rapid reductions in HBV DNA loads. The baby must receive immediate vaccination at delivery. As with some other immune-mediated diseases, the pregnant state can be associated with less activity whereas following delivery a significant flare up of chronic hepatitis B may occur. For HIV-infected patients, combivir (lamivudine plus zidovudine) is safe. In those with a low CD4 count, lopinavir or nevirapine are advised. Prophylactic oral antiviral agents in the last trimester, in immune-tolerant mothers with HBV DNA more than $10 \times 7\,IU/mL$, are used in some centres but good evidence of their value is not available.

Hepatitis C

The chances of a hepatitis C carrier mother transmitting the disease to her baby are very small [75]. Routine Caesarean section is not indicated. The risk of transmission is increased if the mother has a high titre of circulating hepatitis C virus RNA or is HIV positive. Maternal blood hepatitis C virus RNA should be checked if the mother is antibody positive. Vertical transmission was not reported in a study from Egypt [76]. Antibody to hepatitis C virus passes the placenta and values may be positive for 6 months, the lifespan of circulating maternal antibody. The infant should be checked by measuring serum hepatitis C virus RNA at 1 month after birth and a year later as viral clearance is not unusual in a neonate. Breast feeding has not been associated with vertical transmission of hepatitis C virus infection [76].

Interferon and ribavirin are contraindicated during pregnancy.

Hepatitis E

Hepatitis E is associated with up to a 30% maternal and up to 50% fetal mortality, reported mostly in the developing world where there is poor access to clean drinking water [77]. The mother presents with acute liver failure regardless of the stage of pregnancy. A correlation with viral titre and liver disease severity is observed [78]. Maternal mortality related to hepatitis E is much higher in certain parts of the world, for example India, and may be due to infection with genotypes 1 or 2.

Herpes simplex virus (HSV type II)

This infection is usually reported in the immunocompromised, but is reported in pregnant women [79,80]. This might be related to a defect in cell-mediated immunity thought to exist in pregnancy. The hepatitis can mimic AFLP but is marked by very high serum transaminase levels but without jaundice. This enzyme pattern should alert the clinician to the diagnosis. Herpetic lesions can often be detected on the vulva or cervix. Liver biopsy shows extensive hepatocellular necrosis and intranuclear herpetic inclusions (Fig. 30.6). CT often shows multiple, low-density areas of necrosis. The treatment is with aciclovir [78,80]. Late diagnosis even despite treatment is associated with a high fatality rate.

Biliary tract disease

During pregnancy the bile becomes more lithogenic and gallbladder emptying is impaired [1]. Gallstones form [81]. Immediately post-partum, gallbladder ultrasound examinations have shown sludge in 26.2% and gallstones in 5.2%. One year later, only two of 45 patients with sludge and 13 of 15 with gallstones still had abnormal ultrasound findings. In spite of these observations, symptoms of gallbladder disease during pregnancy are rare.

Patients with choledocholithiasis can be successfully relieved by endoscopic retrograde cholangiopancreatography (ERCP) and sphincterotomy. This may be performed as early as the second trimester [82]. Cholecystectomy, whether by open operation [83] or the laparoscopic technique [84], is safe during pregnancy.

Hepatotoxic drugs and the pregnant woman

The pregnant woman can react to drugs causing jaundice in a similar fashion to the non-pregnant. Drugs may potentiate jaundice or kernicterus in the newborn. In

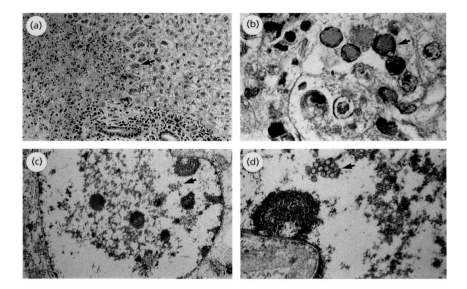

Fig. 30.6. Herpes simplex hepatitis in the third trimester of pregnancy. (A, B) Light microscopy: (A) shows moderate portal inflammation with periportal necrosis. Both (A) and (B) (high power) show classic Cowdry A inclusions in nuclei (arrows). (C, D) Electron micrographs show aggregates of 106-nm viral particles (arrows) in the nucleus of an infected hepatocyte. The biopsy grew herpes simplex. (Courtesy of Dr Caroline Riely.)

particular, drugs such as sulfonamides, which displace bilirubin from its binding site to serum, albumin should be avoided. Drugs such as phenacetin given to the mother may precipitate jaundice in an infant with glucose-6-phosphate dehydrogenase deficiency.

Pre-existing liver disease

Pregnancy in women with cirrhosis carries an increased risk of fetal and/or maternal morbidity and mortality. Liver disease per se is not an indication for termination. Cirrhosis may now be identified at an early asymptomatic stage and may not always have been diagnosed prior to conception. Both maternal and fetal outcome is better than previously reported [85] but the odds for poor outcome remain high (OR 42.5) thus the obstetrician needs to be aware of the diagnosis. The patient should be monitored simultaneously by their obstetrician and their hepatologist. The early diagnosis of cirrhosis allows preventive strategies for untoward complications, for example variceal haemorrhage. In mothers who are HBsAg positive effective treatments exist, which may be given to prevent viral transmission during delivery. Ultrasound and advanced radiologic techniques allow rapid diagnosis, particularly if there is biliary disease. Nevertheless, all pregnant mothers with known liver disease should be managed in a high-risk pregnancy unit, better still close to a liver transplant centre with dual management by an obstetrician and a hepatologist.

Variceal haemorrhage may be promoted by the increase in blood volume which starts early in the second trimester. It can be effectively prevented either medically, by prescribing prophylactic non-selective beta-blockers (which are safe throughout pregnancy), and/or banding of varices—before or during pregnancy. Thus all mothers with cirrhosis require an endoscopy to check for varices, if not previously diagnosed, during the second trimester of their pregnancy.

Variceal haemorrhage may also complicate portal vein thrombosis or other causes of non-cirrhotic portal hypertension where the beneficial effect of beta-blockade is less certain and prophylactic variceal banding can be the preferred therapy. Such patients generally have massive splenomegaly so both anaemia and thrombocytopenia can be present; both threaten outcome.

Chronic cholestatic liver disease

The introduction of routine screening of liver biochemistries in adults has meant that most cholestatic liver disease is diagnosed earlier in its course, when the patient is asymptomatic, non-cirrhotic and fertile. There are no reports of fetal toxicity in mothers taking ursodeoxycholic acid, an agent frequently taken by those with cholestasis.

Children with both syndromic (Alagille) and other genetic and idiopathic chronic cholestatic liver diseases now live to be fertile adults, as do those with a successful Kasai procedure for biliary atresia. If cholestasis is not accompanied by pruritus prior to pregnancy, a woman may remain asymptomatic until term, but those with pruritus present prior to pregnancy can develop severe pruritus, starting as early as the first trimester. If pruritus is poorly responsive to unabsorbed antipruritic therapy, that is anion exchange resin, regular plasmapheresis may be required until the fetus is of sufficient maturity to be safely delivered [86].

Autoimmune hepatitis

This disease predominantly affects females regardless of age. At least one-third have cirrhosis at time of presentation (even if the diagnosis is made in childhood). A diagnosis of asymptomatic autoimmune hepatitis (AIH), once thought rare, is now diagnosed with increasing frequency. Abnormal liver enzymes may be noted for the first time during pregnancy, although the pregnant state most often induces inactive AIH. Those taking prednisone and/or azathioprine prior to pregnancy can safely stay on either or both. Treatment should not be stopped but doses can often be reduced during pregnancy as many (70%) go into remission. The placenta is a relative barrier to azathioprine and metabolites [87]. Flare ups post-partum occur in 30–50% and should be anticipated, that is blood checks should be carried out 4–12 weeks after delivery [86,87]. Breastfeeding is allowed even if the mother is taking corticosteroids or azathioprine [88–90].

Serious maternal complications are reported in 7.8–9% of mothers with cirrhosis, with fetal loss close to 30% [90]. In 35 Scandinavian women with AIH who had 63 pregnancies, there were no significant differences from control mothers in the number of still births or malformations. Preterm delivery is not unusual.

Wilson's disease

This disease has protean presentations, most often in childhood, and cirrhosis is common. Appropriate chelation therapy with D-penicillamine or trientine reverse any liver failure but life-long therapy is needed. Young women, as long as they do not stop their chelation therapy, do not have an increased maternal or fetal mortality [91]. Birth defects are described when D-penicillamine is given in high dose (1.5–2.0 g/day) for management of cysteinosis but not with lower doses or with trientine. Hypothyroidism and low zinc levels requiring supplements may be observed in the offspring of mothers who take D-penicillamine during pregnancy [92]. Zinc, an alternative therapy for Wilson's disease which increases intestinal metallothionien and thus binds copper in the gut, is also safe to use during pregnancy [93]. Breast feeding is not recommended whilst taking chelation theapy

Pre-existent Budd-Chiari syndrome

A recent report of 24 pregnancies in 16 women, indicated that nine had received prior therapy (surgical or radiological); in 17 of the 24 pregnancies, mothers were anticoagulated throughout to delivery [94]. The fetal mortality prior to week 20 was 29% [94]. Excessive bleeding related to treatment with anticoagulation may occur. Anticoagulation must be with low molecular weight heparin or vitamin K antagonists as warfarin is teratogenic.

Pregnancy in liver transplant recipients

A delay to conception is recommended of at least 1 year post-transplant, and until the condition of the graft is stable. Successful outcomes are frequent [95], but the pregnancy must be regarded as high risk [96]. Immunosuppression must be continued and monitored particularly carefully. There is a high risk of gestational hypertension and other material complications as well as premature delivery and of low birth weight infants. Congenital anomalies are not increased. Breast feeding whilst taking immunosuppression is not recommended. Liver transplantation during pregnancy has been reported [97].

References

1 Feingold KR, Wiley T, Moser AH *et al*. De novo cholesterogenesis in pregnancy. *J. Lab. Clin. Med.* 1983; **101**: 256–263.
2 Adeniyi FA, Olatunbosun DA. Origins and significance of the increased plasma alkaline phosphatase during normal pregnancy and pre-eclampsia. *Br. J. Obstet. Gynaecol.* 1984; **91**: 857–862.
3 Bacq Y, Zarka O, Brechot J-F *et al*. Liver function tests in normal pregnancy: a prospective study of 103 pregnant women and 103 matched controls. *Hepatology* 1996; **23**: 1030–1034.
4 Munnell EW, Taylor HC Jr. Liver blood flow in pregnancy—hepatic vein catheterization. *J. Clin. Invest.* 1947; **26**: 952–956.
5 Maes BD, Spitz B, Ghoos YF *et al*. Gastric emptying in hyperemesis gravidarum and non-dyspeptic pregnancy. *Aliment. Pharmacol. Ther.* 1999; **13**: 237–243.
6 Kuscu NK, Koyuncu F. Hyperemesis gravidarum: current concepts and management. *Postgrad. Med. J.* 2002; **78**: 76–79.
7 Fell DB, Dodds L, Joseph KS *et al*. Risk factors for hyperemesis gravidarum requiring hospital admission during pregnancy. *Obstet. Gynecol.* 2006; **107**: 277–284.
8 Safari HR, Fassett MJ, Souter IC *et al*. The efficacy of methylprednisolone in the treatment of hyperemesis gravidarum: a randomized, double-blind, controlled study. *Am. J. Obstet. Gynecol.* 1998; **179**: 921–924.
9 Burroughs AK, Seong NH, Dojcinov DM *et al*. Idiopathic acute fatty liver of pregnancy in 12 patients. *Q. J. Med.* 1982; **51**: 481–497.
10 Sheehan HL. The pathology of acute yellow atrophy and delayed chloroform poisoning. *J. Obstet. Gynaecol. Br. Emp.* 1940; **47**: 49.
11 Pockros PJ, Peters RL, Reynolds TB. Idiopathic fatty liver of pregnancy: findings in 10 cases. *Medicine (Baltimore)* 1984; **63**: 1–11.
12 Reyes H, Sandoval L, Wainstein A *et al*. Acute fatty liver of pregnancy: a clinical study of 12 episodes in 11 patients. *Gut* 1994; **35**: 101–106.

13 Rolfes DB, Ishak KG. Acute fatty liver of pregnancy: a clinicopathologic study of 35 cases. *Hepatology* 1985; **5**: 1149–1158.

14 Bernuau J, Degott C, Nouel O *et al*. Non-fatal acute fatty liver of pregnancy. *Gut* 1983; **24**: 340–344.

15 Mabie WC, Dacus JV, Sibai BM *et al*. Computed tomography in acute fatty liver of pregnancy. *Am. J. Obstet. Gynecol.* 1988; **158**: 142–145.

16 Hay JE. Liver Disease in Pregnancy. *Hepatology* 2008; **47**: 1067–1076.

17 Schoeman MN, Batey RG, Wilcken B. Recurrent acute fatty liver of pregnancy associated with a fatty-acid oxidation defect in the offspring. *Gastroenterology* 1991; **100**: 544–548.

18 Pereira SP, O'Donoghue J, Wendon J *et al*. Maternal and perinatal outcome in severe pregnancy-related liver disease. *Hepatology* 1997; **26**: 1258–1262.

19 Ockner SA, Brunt EM, Cohn SM *et al*. Fulminant hepatic failure caused by acute fatty liver of pregnancy treated by orthotopic liver transplantation. *Hepatology* 1990; **11**: 59–64.

20 Sherlock S. Acute fatty liver of pregnancy and the microvesicular fat diseases. *Gut* 1983; **24**: 265–269.

21 Wilcken B, Leung K-C, Hammond J *et al*. Pregnancy and fetal long-chain 3-hydroxyacylcoenzyme A dehydrogenase deficiency. *Lancet* 1993; **341**: 407–408.

22 Treem WR, Shoup ME, Hale DE *et al*. Acute fatty liver of pregnancy, hemolysis, elevated liver enzymes, and low platelets syndrome, and long chain 3-hydroxyacyl-coenzyme A dehydrogenase deficiency. *Am. J. Gastroenterol.* 1996; **91**: 2293–2300.

23 Rajasri AG, Srestha R, Mitchell J. Acute fatty liver of pregnancy (AFLP)—an overview. *J. Obstet. Gynaecol.* 2007; **27**: 237–240.

24 Ibdah J, Bennett M, Rinaldo P *et al*. A fetal fatty-acid oxidation disorder as a cause of liver disease in pregnant women. *N. Engl. J. Med.* 1999; **340**: 1723–1731.

25 Gutierrez Junquera C, Balmaseda E, Gil E *et al*. Acute fatty liver of pregnancy and neonatal long-chain 3-hydroxyacylcoenzyme A dehydrogenase (LCHAD) deficiency. *Eur. J. Pediatr.* 2009; **168**: 103–106.

26 Nada MA, Vianey-Saban C, Roe CR *et al*. Prenatal diagnosis of mitochondrial fatty acid oxidation defects. *Prenat. Diagn.* 1996; **16**: 117–124.

27 Yang Z, Zhao Y, Bennett MJ *et al*. Fetal genotypes and pregnancy outcomes in 35 families with mitochondrial trifunctional protein mutations. *Am. J. Obstet. Gynecol.* 2002; **187**: 715–720.

28 Yang Z, Yamada J, Zhao Y *et al*. Prospective screening for pediatric mitochondrial trifunctional protein defects in pregnancies complicated by liver disease. *JAMA* 2002; **288**: 2163–2166.

29 Bok LA, Vreken P, Wijburg FA *et al*. Short-chain Acyl-CoA dehydrogenase deficiency: studies in a large family adding to the complexity of the disorder. *Pediatrics* 2003; **112**: 1152–1555.

30 Paraf F, Lewis J, Jothy S. Acute fatty liver of pregnancy after exposure to toluene. A case report. *J. Clin. Gastroenterol.* 1993; **17**: 163–165.

31 Haller H, Hempel A, Homuth V *et al*. Endothelial-cell permeability and protein kinase C in pre-eclampsia. *Lancet* 1998; **351**: 945–949.

32 Roberts JM, Redman CWG. Pre-eclampsia: more than pregnancy-induced hypertension. *Lancet* 1993; **341**: 1447–1451.

33 Sibai B, Dekker G, Kupferminc M. Pre-eclampsia. *Lancet* 2005; **365**: 785–799.

34 Kronthal AJ, Fishman EK, Kuhlman JE *et al*. Hepatic infarction in pre-eclampsia. *Radiology* 1990; **177**: 726–728.

35 Manas KJ, Welsh JD, Rankin RA *et al*. Hepatic haemorrhage without rupture in pre-eclampsia. *N. Engl. J. Med.* 1985; **312**: 424–426.

36 Riely CA, Romero R, Duffy TP. Hepatic dysfunction with disseminated intravascular coagulation in toxaemia of pregnancy: a distinct clinical syndrome. *Gastroenterology* 1981; **80**: 1346.

37 Rolfes DB, Ishak KG. Liver disease in toxemia of pregnancy. *Am. J. Gastroenterol.* 1986; **81**: 1138–1144.

38 Fletcher JP. Eclampsia and microangiopathic haemolytic anaemia. *Med. J. Aust.* 1971; **1**: 1065–1066.

39 Weinstein L. Syndrome of haemolysis, elevated liver enzymes, and low platelet count: a severe consequence of hypertension in pregnancy. *Am. J. Obstet. Gynecol.* 1982; **142**: 159–167.

40 Saphier CJ, Repke JT. Hemolysis, elevated liver enzymes, and low platelets (HELLP) syndrome: a review of diagnosis and management. *Semin. Perinatol.* 1998; **22**: 118–133.

41 Barton JR, Riely CA, Adamec TA *et al*. Hepatic histopathologic condition does not correlate with laboratory abnormalities in HELLP syndrome (haemolysis, elevated liver enzymes, and low platelet count). *Am. J. Obstet. Gynecol.* 1992; **167**: 1538–1543.

42 Sibai BM, Taslimi MM, El-Nazer A *et al*. Maternal–perinatal outcome associated with the syndrome of haemolysis, elevated liver enzymes, and low platelets in severe preeclampsia-eclampsia. *Am. J. Obstet. Gynecol.* 1986; **155**: 501–509.

43 Shames BD, Fernandez LA, Sollinger HW *et al*. Liver transplantation for HELLP syndrome. *Liver Transpl.* 2005; **11**: 224–228.

44 Muetze S, Leeners B, Ortlepp JR *et al*. Maternal factor V Leiden mutation is associated with HELLP syndrome in Caucasian women. *Acta Obstet. Gynecol. Scand.* 2008; **87**: 635–642.

45 Strand S, Strand D, Seufert R *et al*. Placenta-derived CD95 ligand causes liver damage in hemolysis, elevated liver enzymes, and low platelet count syndrome. *Gastroenterology* 2004; **126**: 849–858.

46 Ibdah J. Acute fatty liver of pregnancy: an update on pathogenesis and clinical implications. *World J. Gastroenterol.* 2006; **12**: 7397–7404.

47 Sibai BM. Imitators of severe pre-eclampsia/eclampsia. *Clin. Perinatol.* 2004; **31**: 835–852, vii–viii.

48 Sheehan H, Lynch J. *Pathology of Toxaemia of Pregnancy*. Edinburgh: Churchill Livingstone, 1973.

49 Minakami H, Oka N, Sato T *et al*. Preeclampsia: a microvesicular fat disease of the liver? *Am. J. Obstet. Gynecol.* 1988; **159**: 1043–1047.

50 Zucker SD. Is it HELLPful to consider the hanging LCHAD in pregnancy-associated liver disease? *Gastroenterology* 2003; **124**: 1548–1550.

51 Minakami H, Yamada H, Suzuki S. Gestational thrombocytopenia and pregnancy-induced antithrombin deficiency: progenitors to the development of the HELLP syndrome

and acute fatty liver of pregnancy. *Semin. Thromb. Hemost.* 2002; **28**: 515–518.

52 Minuk GY, Lui RC, Kelly JK. Rupture of the liver associated with acute fatty liver of pregnancy. *Am. J. Gastroenterol.* 1987; **82**: 457–460.

53 Neerhof MG, Zelman W, Sullivan T. Hepatic rupture in pregnancy. *Obstet. Gynecol. Surv.* 1989; **44**: 407–409.

54 Hunter SK, Martin M, Benda JA *et al.* Liver transplant after massive spontaneous hepatic rupture in pregnancy complicated by preeclampsia. *Obstet. Gynecol.* 1995; **85**: 819–822.

55 Reyes H. The enigma of intrahepatic cholestasis of pregnancy: lessons from Chile. *Hepatology* 1982; **2**: 87–96.

56 Glantz A, Marschall HV, Mattson LA. Intrahepatic cholestasis of pregnancy: relationships between bile acid levels and fetal complication rates. *Hepatology* 2004; **40**: 467–474.

57 Bacq Y, Myara A, Brechot M-C *et al.* Serum conjugated bile acid profile during intrahepatic cholestasis of pregnancy. *J. Hepatol.* 1996; **22**: 66–70.

58 Milkiewicz P, Gallagher R, Chambers J *et al.* Obstetric cholestasis with elevated gamma glutamyl transpeptidase: incidence, presentation and treatment. *J. Gastroenterol. Hepatol.* 2003; **18**: 1283–1286.

59 Wasmuth HE, Glantz A, Keppeler H *et al.* Intrahepatic cholestasis of pregnancy: the severe form is associated with common variants of the hepatobiliary phospholipid transporter gene ABCB4. *Gut* 2007; **56**: 265–270.

60 Schneider G, Paus TC, Kullak-Ublick GA *et al.* Linkage between a new splicing site mutation in the MDR3 alias ABCB4 gene and intrahepatic cholestasis of pregnancy. *Hepatology* 2007; **45**: 150–158.

61 Trauner M, Fickert P, Wagner M. MDR3 (ABCB4) defects: a paradigm for the genetics of adult cholestatic syndromes. *Semin. Liver Dis.* 2007; **27**: 77–98.

62 Hirvioja ML, Tuimala R, Vuori J. The treatment of intrahepatic cholestasis of pregnancy by dexamethasone. *Br. J. Obstet. Gynaecol.* 1992; **99**: 109–111.

63 Glantz A, Marschall HU, Lammert F *et al.* Intrahepatic cholestasis of pregnancy: a randomized controlled trial comparing dexamethasone and ursodeoxycholic acid. *Hepatology* 2005; **42**: 1399–1405.

64 Palma J, Reyes H, Ribalta J *et al.* Ursodeoxycholic acid in the treatment of cholestasis of pregnancy: a randomized, double-blind study controlled with placebo. *J. Hepatol.* 1997; **27**: 1022–1028.

65 Davies MH, da Silva RC, Jones SR *et al.* Fetal mortality associated with cholestasis of pregnancy and the potential benefit of therapy with ursodeoxycholic acid. *Gut* 1995; **37**: 580–584.

66 Kondrackiene J, Beuers U, Kupcinskas L. Efficacy and safety of ursodeoxycholic acid versus cholestyramine in intrahepatic cholestasis of pregnancy. *Gastroenterology* 2005; **129**: 894–901.

67 Roncaglia N, Locatelli A, Arreghini A *et al.* A randomised controlled trial of ursodeoxycholic acid and S-adenosyl-l-methionine in the treatment of gestational cholestasis. *Br. J. Obstet. Gynaecol.* 2004; **111**: 17–21.

68 Rioseco AJ, Ivankovic MB, Manzur A *et al.* Intrahepatic cholestasis of pregnancy: a retrospective case–control study of perinatal outcome. *Am. J. Obstet. Gynecol.* 1994; **170**: 890–895.

69 Pelletier S, Landi B, Piette JC *et al.* Antiphospholipid syndrome as the second cause of non-tumorous Budd–Chiari syndrome. *J. Hepatol.* 1994; **21**: 76–80.

70 Senzolo M, Cholongitas E, Patch D *et al.* Update on the classification, assessment of prognosis and therapy of Budd-Chiari syndrome. *Nat. Clin. Pract. Gastroenterol. Hepatol.* 2005; **2**: 1–9.

71 Fickert P, Ramschak H, Kenner L *et al.* Acute Budd–Chiari syndrome with fulminant hepatic failure in a pregnant woman with factor V Leiden mutation. *Gastroenterology* 1996; **111**: 1670–1673.

72 Grant WJ, McCashland T, Botha JF *et al.* Acute Budd-Chiari syndrome during pregnancy: surgical treatment and orthotopic liver transplantation with successful completion of the pregnancy. *Liver Transpl.* 2003; **9**: 976–979.

73 Khuroo MS, Datta DV. Budd-Chiari syndrome following pregnancy. Report of 16 cases, with roentgenologic, hemodynamic and histologic studies of the hepatic outflow tract. *Am. J. Med.* 1980; **68**: 113–121.

74 Simms J, Duff P. Viral hepatitis in pregnancy. *Semin. Perinatol.* 1993; **17**: 384–393.

75 Roberts EA, Yeung L. Maternal infant transmission of hepatitis C virus infection. *Hepatology* 2002; **36** (5 Suppl. 1): S106–113.

76 Mostafa M, Sharaf S, Hashem M *et al.* Prospective cohort study of mother-to-infant infection and clearance of hepatitis C in rural Egyptian villages. *J. Med. Virol.* 2009; **81**: 1024–1031.

77 Patra S, Kumar A, Trivedi SS *et al.* Maternal and fetal outcomes in pregnant women with acute hepatitis E virus infection. *Ann. Intern. Med.* 2007; **147**: 28–33.

78 Kar P, Jilani N, Husain SA *et al.* Does hepatitis E viral load and genotypes influence the final outcome of acute liver failure during pregnancy? *Am. J. Gastroenterol.* 2008; **103**: 2495–2501.

79 Klein NA, Mabie WC, Shaver DC *et al.* Herpes simplex virus hepatitis in pregnancy: two patients successfully treated with acyclovir. *Gastroenterology* 1991; **100**: 239–244.

80 Allen RH, Tuomala RE. Herpes simplex virus hepatitis causing acute liver dysfunction and thrombocytopenia in pregnancy. *Obstet. Gynecol.* 2005; **106**: 1187–1189.

81 Everson GT. Pregnancy and gallstones. *Hepatology* 1993; **17**: 159–161.

82 Baillie J, Cairns SR, Putnam WS *et al.* Endoscopic management of choledocholithiasis during pregnancy. *Surg. Gynecol. Obstet.* 1990; **171**: 1–4.

83 Swisher SG, Schmit PJ, Hunt KK *et al.* Biliary disease during pregnancy. *Am. J. Surg.* 1994; **168**: 576–579.

84 Morrell DG, Mullins JR, Harrison PB. Laparoscopic cholecystectomy during pregnancy in symptomatic patients. *Surgery* 1992; **112**: 856–859.

85 Shaheen AA, Myers RP. The outcomes of pregnancy in patients withy cirrhosis: a population based study. *Liver Int.* 2009; **30**: 275–283

86 Alallam A, Barth D, Heathcote EJ. Role of plasmapheresis in the treatment of severe pruritus in pregnant patients with primary biliary cirrhosis: case reports. *Can. J. Gastroenterol.* 2008; **22**: 505–507.

87 de Boer NK, Jarbandhan SV, de Graaf P *et al.* Azathioprine use during pregnancy: unexpected intrauterine exposure to metabolites. *Am. J. Gastroenterol.* 2006; **101**: 1390–1392.

88 Buchel E, Van Steenbergen W, Nevens F, Fevery J. Improvement of Autoimmune hepatitis during pregnancy followed by flare-up after delivery. *Am. J. Gastroenterol.* 2002; **97**: 3160–3165.

89 Terrabuio DR, Abrantes-Lemos CP, Carrilho FJ, Cançado EL. Follow-up of pregnant women with autoimmune hepatitis: the disease behavior along with maternal and fetal outcomes. *J. Clin. Gastroenterol.* 2009; **43**: 350–356.

90 Werner M, Björnsson E, Prytz H *et al.* Autoimmune hepatitis among fertile women: strategies during pregnancy and breastfeeding? *Scand. J. Gastroenterol.* 2007; **42**: 986–991.

91 Sinha S, Taly AB, Prashanth LK *et al.* Successful pregnancies and abortions in symptomatic and asymptomatic Wilson's disease. *J. Neurol. Sci.* 2004; **217**: 37–40.

92 Sternlieb I. Wilson's disease and pregnancy. *Hepatology* 2000; **31**: 531–532.

93 Brewer GJ, Johnson VD, Dick RD *et al.* Treatment of Wilson's disease with zinc. XVII: treatment during pregnancy. *Hepatology* 2000; **31**: 364–370.

94 Rautou PE, Angermayr B, Garcia-Pagan JC *et al.* Pregnancy in women with known and treated Budd-Chiari syndrome: maternal and fetal outcomes. *J. Hepatol.* 2009; **51**: 47–54.

95 Coffin CS, Shaheen AA, Burak RW *et al.* Pregnancy outcomes among liver transplant recipients in the United States: a nationwide case control analysis. *Liver Transpl.* 2010; **16**: 56–63.

96 Murthy SK, Heathcote EJ, Nguyen GC. Impact of cirrhosis and liver transplant on maternal health during labour and delivery. *Clin. Gastroenterol. Hepatol.* 2009; **7**: 1367–1372.

97 Hamilton MI, Alcock R, Magos L *et al.* Liver Transplantation during pregnancy. *Transpl. Proc.* 1993; **25**: 2967–2968.

CHAPTER 31
The Liver in Systemic Disease

Humphrey J. F. Hodgson
Centre for Hepatology, Royal Free Campus, UCL Medical School, London, UK

Learning points

- In many systemic diseases there are unimportant alterations in the results of biochemical tests of liver function that fluctuate with disease activity.
- Drugs for treating systemic disease often alter the results of liver function tests.
- Granulomatous liver disease, diagnosed on histology, often prompted by an elevated serum alkaline phosphatase level, is a manifestation of many different immunological and infectious processes.
- Acute hepatic porphyrias, presenting with neurological symptoms including severe abdominal pain, may be difficult to diagnose; urine testing for porphyrins in the acute state is vitally important.

The liver may be involved in systemic infections, collagen-vascular and autoimmune disorders, haematological malignancies and endocrine disorders. Involvement varies from florid to the asymptomatic, although in the latter instance investigations such as liver biopsy prompted by abnormal liver biochemistry can be a valuable diagnostic approach.

Collagen-vascular and autoimmune disorders

Systemic lupus erythematosus

The clinical manifestations of systemic lupus erythematosus (SLE) are most commonly in joints, skin, kidney and central nervous system. Diagnosis is confirmed by a characteristic autoantibody pattern, notably anti-double stranded DNA (dsDNA), which may overlap with the autoantibody profile seen in autoimmune hepatitis. However, whilst liver function test abnormalities are common in SLE (~60%), only in one-third do the tests fluctuate with disease activity. Typically, these biochemical changes are mild disturbances in serum alkaline phosphatase and transaminases. Drug therapy for SLE, particularly non-steroidals, including aspirin, often explains these abnormal tests [1]. Remember also that corticosteroid therapy and other immunosuppressive drugs used for SLE and other collagen-vascular diseases may reactivate HBV, leading to overt HBV-associated liver disease. Prophylactic antivirals can prevent this (see Chapter 18).

Clinical manifestations are very rare, apart from mild hepatomegaly. Significant histopathological findings have been reported in 8–20% of patients, including a few patients with advanced fibrosis or cirrhosis, fatty change and granulomas, but these may often be chance associations [2–4]. Both reactive hepatitis and mild centrilobular necrosis, however, seem to be associated with SLE, and, as with other collagen-vascular diseases, there are a few patients with nodular regenerative hyperplasia [5–7]. The term 'lupoid hepatitis' was coined to refer to patients with florid autoimmune hepatitis, not patients with SLE, and should be discontinued. Whilst in children there is a clinical association between SLE and autoimmune hepatitis, this is rare in adults [8].

Anticardiolipin syndrome

This syndrome, with antiphospholipid antibodies and/or lupus anticoagulant in the serum, may occur as a primary disorder or associated with autoimmune disorders (not only SLE). Amongst the systemic manifestations (arterial and venous thromboembolism, recurrent abortions, livedo reticularis, migraine and thrombocytopenia), the liver may be involved with Budd–Chiari syndrome, focal ischaemia, portal hypertension

Sherlock's Diseases of the Liver and Biliary System, Twelfth Edition. Edited by James S. Dooley, Anna S.F. Lok, Andrew K. Burroughs, E. Jenny Heathcote.
© 2011 by Blackwell Publishing Ltd. Published 2011 by Blackwell Publishing Ltd.

attributed to microvascular thombosis and possibly autoimmune cholangiopathy [9,10]. Long-term anticoagulation may be required. A few patients have come to liver transplantation.

Rheumatoid arthritis and Felty's syndrome

Usually, the liver is asymptomatic in rheumatoid arthritis, although minor changes in liver function tests, particularly alkaline phosphatase, are common—up to 50% of cases—and may mirror disease activity [11]. Changes in γ-glutamyl transpeptidase (γ-GT) are less frequent, and some serum alkaline phosphatase is derived from bone. Liver histology appearances are generally nonspecific, such as mild fatty infiltration, focal necroses, sinusoidal dilatation or complicating amyloidosis. Kupffer cells are hyperplastic. Nodular regenerative hyperplasia is a clear association, and in some patients (generally with florid arthritis and extra-articular manifestations) criteria for Felty's syndrome (rheumatoid arthritis, splenomegaly and leucopenia) are fulfilled [12,13]. The nodular regenerative hyperplasia is related to obliterative vasculitis of small portal veins [6], leading to portal hypertension. Drug therapy may affect liver function tests (e.g. non-steroidals [14], steatosis with corticosteroid therapy, cholestasis with gold [15], and more recently hepatitis with ant-TNF biologicals [16]); methotrexate therapy is a particular issue due to its fibrotic potential, particularly after the total doses exceed 1.5 g [17].

Sjögren's syndrome

Primary Sjögren's (keratoconjunctivitis sicca, xerostomia, salivary gland enlargement), as well as secondary (associated with rheumatoid arthritis) are often associated with non-specific changes in liver function tests. Ten per cent of patients with primary Sjögren's and up to 40% with secondary may have serum antimitochondrial antibodies [18], and the latter if biopsied are likely to show histopathology characteristic for primary biliary cirrhosis (generally stage 1) [19–21]. An apparent association of Sjögren's syndrome and HCV infection may well represent extrahepatic manifestations of HCV [22].

Scleroderma

In the limited form of scleroderma—characteristically the CREST syndrome (subcutaneous calcinosis, Raynaud's, oesophageal dysmotility, sclerodactyly and telangiectasia)—the liver is usually unaffected. In systemic sclerosis, prospective studies have reported a low incidence of significant liver involvement, but there is undoubtedly overlap with primary biliary cirrhosis (PBC) [23]; 25% of patients with scleroderma have antimitochondrial antibodies, and 25% of patients with PBC have the anticentromere antibodies characteristic of scleroderma; 5–10% of PBC patients have scleroderma clinically in some series [23].

Polyarteritis nodosa and other vasculitides

Polyarteritis nodosa involving medium or large arteries (and portal vein) may in extreme cases lead to hepatic infarction and massive necrosis [24]. HBV infection may be present in 10–20% of cases, and the immunosuppression required to control the vasculitis should be combined with antiviral therapy (see Chapter 18). Other medium and small vessel vasculitides, including microscopic polyarteritis, Churg–Strauss syndrome, giant-cell arteritis and polymyalgia rheumatica, are often associated with abnormal liver function tests during disease activity, but usually do not affect the liver clinically [25]. The vasculitis of Behçet's disease may initiate hepatic venous occlusion and Budd–Chiari syndrome.

Hepatic granulomas

Hepatic granulomas are aggregates of macrophages, often transformed to an epithelioid appearance, in the liver parenchyma. Their significance varies from a nonspecific, asymptomatic, incidental finding in a liver biopsy, to the hallmark of a disease, generally infectious or immune in nature. There are many causes (Table 31.1) [26,27]. Granulomas are found in 4–10% of needle liver biopsies [28]. Such a finding initiates a diagnostic path [29] (Table 31.1), but does not necessarily lead to definition of a condition requiring treatment. In 10%, no cause is found even after full histological characterization, staining for possible causative organisms and culture [27].

Granulomas usually represent a response to antigenic stimuli. The liver is particularly involved because the large number of sinusoidal cells, including *Kupffer cells* (resident macrophages) endocytosing old cells, foreign particles, tumour cells and micro-organisms, and presenting antigens to lymphocytes. *Endothelial cells* also clear macromolecules and small particles by receptor-mediated endocytosis. The antigenic stimuli fall into common categories: drugs, infections, chemicals and a group where the antigen is unrecognized, including sarcoidosis, PBC and granulomatous hepatitis.

Granulomas are of varying size, between 50 and 300 μm in diameter, occurring anywhere in the liver, but most frequently near portal tracts. They are sharply defined and do not disturb the normal pattern of the liver. Classically, they consist of pale-staining, epithelioid cells with surrounding lymphocytes (Fig. 31.1). Giant cells, central caseation and necrosis may be present. Older lesions may be surrounded by a fibrous

Table 31.1. Differential diagnosis of some diseases with hepatic granulomas

Disease	Diagnostic aids
Sarcoidosis	Chest X-ray, serum angiotensin-converting enzyme, bronchoalveolar lavage
Tuberculosis	Tuberculin skin test, bronchoalveolar lavage, isolation of organism, acid-fast staining
Brucellosis	Blood culture, agglutinin titre
Berylliosis	Industrial exposure, chest X-ray
Syphilis	*Treponema* test
Leprosy	Race, lepromin skin test
Histoplasmosis	Complement fixation test, chest X-ray
Infectious mononucleosis	Blood film, monospot, IgM EBV antibodies
AIDS	Poorly formed granulomas, acid-fast and fungal stains
Primary biliary cirrhosis	Mitochondrial antibody
Lymphomas	Chest X-ray, lymph node biopsy, CT scan
Drug reaction	History
HCV	Anti-HCV and HCV RNA PCR

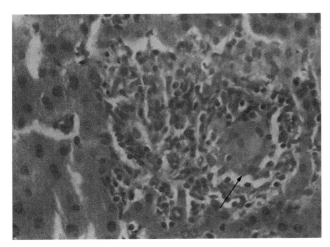

Fig. 31.1. A well-demarcated hepatic granuloma in zone 1 shows a giant cell (arrow), pale-staining epithelioid cells and a rim of lymphocytes. (H & E, ×160.)

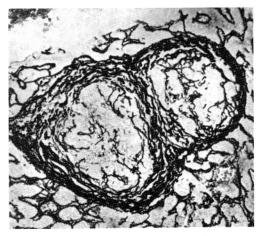

Fig. 31.3. Same section as in Fig. 31.2 stained to show reticulin formation around the granulomas. (Modified silver, ×90.)

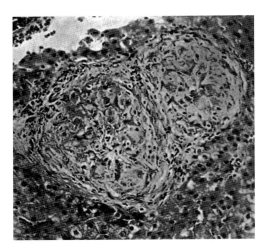

Fig. 31.2. Healing hepatic sarcoid. Two adjacent lesions are acquiring a structureless hyaline appearance and are surrounded by a connective tissue capsule. (H & E, ×90.)

capsule and healing is accompanied by hyaline change (Figs 31.2, 31.3).

There are some specific findings and subtypes of granulomas with suggestive diagnostic features:

• *Sarcoid-type granulomas* are small, well formed and discrete. Multinucleated giant cells may be present (see Fig. 31.1), and occasionally a central area of eosinophilic necrosis. Caseation is absent.

• *Necrotizing or caseating granulomas* are small to large, well formed with a necrotic centre. The histiocytic rim may have a palisade pattern and fibrosis is variable. They are associated with fungal infections and rarely with tuberculosis or Hodgkin's lymphoma.

• *Lipogranulomas* comprise poorly formed perivenular aggregates of histiocytes and macrophages, some containing fat. They are often associated with fatty liver. They are due to deposition of mineral oils used in the food industry.

• *Microgranulomas* consist only of a cluster of six or less histiocytes. They have many associations and probably represent a non-specific reaction to cell necrosis.

• *Fibrin-ring granulomas* are typical of Q fever, but are also seen as drug reactions (e.g. carbamazepine, allopurinol). They are also described with acute hepatitis A.

In addition to the routine haematoxylin and eosin and reticulin staining of liver biopsies to assess liver architecture, finding granulomas may prompt further specific staining, for example Ziehl–Neelsen and diastase–PAS for acid-fast bacilli and fungi. Positive findings with these are very helpful, but negative findings do not exclude the infections.

Clinical syndrome of hepatic granulomas

Granulomas are usually asymptomatic. The liver is palpable in only 20% of patients. Very rarely the picture is of active liver disease with marked functional disturbance and liver cell destruction and fibrosis on liver biopsy, or of the rare syndrome of 'granulomatous hepatitis'. Serum alkaline phosphatase elevations are the commonest biochemical abnormality and bilirubin levels usually normal. Serum angiotensin-converting enzyme is increased, a finding not specific for sarcoidosis.

Table 31.1 shows the investigations that are likely to establish the aetiology when granulomas have been found on biopsy; the precise diagnostic path will be modified by clinical acumen and epidemiological probabilities.

Specific causes and syndromes

Infections

Granulomas can occur with almost all types of infection. The most frequent are tuberculosis, brucellosis, toxoplasmosis, atypical mycobacteriosis, fungal diseases, syphilis, leishmaniasis and the infestations, schistosomiasis and toxocariasis (Table 31.2). In many instances, the granulomas are ill formed.

Mycobacteria

Miliary dissemination accompanies the primary complex of *Mycobacterium tuberculosis* and is also common with chronic adult tuberculosis. Liver biopsies in patients with tuberculosis have shown positive results in about 25%—providing a useful diagnostic tool in tuberculous meningitis when other methods have failed, and in miliary tuberculosis at the stage of an indeterminate pyrexia. In such cases Ziehl–Neelsen stains should be performed, an unfixed portion of the biopsy cultured for tubercle bacilli and PCR analysis for mycobacterial

Table 31.2. Hepatic granulomas associated with infections

Mycobacteria	*M. tuberculosis*
	M. avium-intracellulare
	Leprosy
Bacteria	*Brucella*
Spirochaetes	*T. pallidum*
Fungi	Histoplasmosis
	Coccidioidomycosis
	Blastomycosis
Protozoa	Toxoplasmosis
Helminths	Schistosomiasis
	Toxocara canis
	Fasciola hepatica
	Ascaris lumbricades
Rickettsiae	Q fever
Viruses	Hepatitis A
	Hepatitis C
	Cytomegalovirus

DNA has been advocated. Importantly, the Ziehl–Neelsen technique is insensitive—although specific— and a negative result does not rule out mycobacterial infection.

In western practice, the diagnostic distinction is often from sarcoidosis. The granulomas may be indistinguishable. Acid-fast bacilli are often difficult to find in mycobacteria-affected livers. Destruction of the reticulin framework, irregularity of the contour with a particularly dense cuff of lymphocytes and less numerous lesions with a tendency to coalesce all suggest tuberculosis.

Rarely, fulminant liver failure can result from tuberculosis. Granulomas are found after BCG vaccination, especially in the immunosuppressed.

Leprosy

Hepatic granulomas indistinguishable from those of sarcoidosis may be found in 62% of patients with lepromatous leprosy compared with the tuberculoid form, when only 21% are positive. *Mycobacterium leprae* bacilli are sometimes present.

Other bacteria

Brucella abortus infection may be complicated by granulomas. Hepatic tenderness and mild elevations of transaminases and alkaline phosphatase may be found in the acute stage. Histology shows a non-specific reactive hepatitis. Granulomas resemble those of sarcoidosis although they tend to be smaller and less demarcated (Fig. 31.4). Healing results in scarring. Necrotizing microgranulomas may be found in the bone marrow.

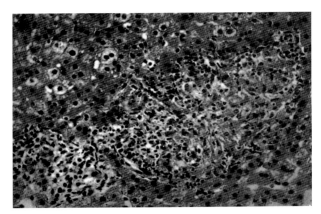

Fig. 31.4. Brucellosis. Granulomas in the liver; the smaller is little more than a collection of round cells. (H & E, ×170.)

Spirochaetes

In the secondary septicaemic stage of *syphilis*, spirochaetes invade the liver with production of miliary granulomas.

Fungal infections

In *histoplasmosis* the liver is second only to the spleen in frequency of involvement. In the granulomatous form, the lesions are histologically identical with those of sarcoidosis, except for the presence of intracellular fungus in the Kupffer cells. Liver biopsy can be used for diagnosis, both staining for *Histoplasma capsulatum* and by culture. Histoplasmosis leads to discrete hepatic calcification.

Coccidioidomycosis and *blastomycosis* also produce sarcoid-like granulomas and the organisms may be demonstrated.

Protozoa

Toxoplasmosis may be associated with granulomas, usually without giant cells [30].

Helminths

The hepatic granulomatous reaction to the *Schistosoma* ovum is of delayed hypersensitivity type, related to antigen released by the egg. Eggs or their remnants are seen in 94% of liver biopsies. The remnants of eggs are of diagnostic importance.

Toxocara canis is spread by cats and dogs. The second stage can infect the liver of man forming granulomas.

With *Fasciola hepatica* the clinical picture in the acute stage is of cholangitis with fever, right upper quadrant pain and hepatomegaly. Eosinophilia and raised serum alkaline phosphatase are noted. Hepatic granulomas and ova in the liver may occasionally be seen.

Ascariasis is particularly common in the Far East, India and South Africa. Ova of the round worm *Ascaris lumbricoides* reach the liver by retrograde passage up the bile ducts. The adult worm may lodge in the common bile duct, producing partial bile duct obstruction and secondary cholangitic abscesses.

Rickettsia

Q fever has predominantly pulmonary manifestations but, occasionally, hepatitis may be prominent and clinically may mimic anicteric viral hepatitis. The granulomas have a characteristic ring of fibrinoid necrosis surrounded by lymphocytes and histiocytes, with a clear space in the centre of the granuloma giving a doughnut appearance.

Viruses

Hepatitis A. In liver biopsies during the acute hepatitis, occasionally fibrin-ring granulomas may be found.

Hepatitis C. Epithelioid granulomas are in approximately 10% of surgical transplant liver specimens from patients with hepatitis C-related cirrhosis, less commonly in needle biopsies [31]. Hepatitis B does not do this.

Cytomegalovirus. Acute infection produces a mononucleosis syndrome. Transient well-formed hepatic granulomas may be associated.

Hepatic granulomas in the patient with AIDS (see Chapter 22)

In HIV-AIDS, liver granulomas are frequent and have multiple causes (Table 31.3) [32,33], and these vary geographically and with the concurrent use of antiretroviral agents. Liver biopsy is particularly helpful in showing *M. tuberculosis* or *M. avium-intracellulare*. The granulomas tend to be poorly formed without lymphocyte cupping, giant cells or central caseation. Acid-fast bacilli are present in large numbers in clusters of foamy histiocytes or within Kupffer cells. *Cytomegalovirus* and *Herpes simplex* infections may also be associated with hepatic granulomas.

Fungal infections may disseminate and initiate granuloma formation. They include *Cryptococcus neoformans*, histoplasmosis, coccidiomycosis and *Candida albicans*.

Granulomas may also be related to drug therapy. Trimethoprim–sulfamethoxazole is a common offender, causing granulomatous hepatitis and jaundice. In patients with HIV undergoing treatment there are, of course, many potential drug effects on the liver [34,35].

Table 31.3. Hepatic granulomas in patients with AIDS

Infections	*Mycobacterium avium-intracellulare*
	Mycobacterium tuberculosis
	Cytomegalovirus
	Histoplasmosis
	Toxoplasmosis
	Cryptococcosis
Neoplasms	Hodgkin's and non-Hodgkin's lymphoma
Drugs	Sulfonamides
	Antibiotics
	Antifungals
	Isoniazid

Sarcoidosis

Sarcoidosis is a disease of unknown aetiology, characterized by granulomatous lesions involving most organs. Involvement of lungs, lymph nodes, eyes, skin and the neurological system may be associated with well-recognized clinical features, although this is not always so. The liver is frequently affected, although granulomas are often asymptomatic.

Hepatic histology

Classical sarcoid granulomas are repetitively monotonous, all being at the same stage of development; though small they may coalesce. As the granuloma heals, reticulin fibres are deposited and it is replaced or surrounded by a fibrous reaction (Fig. 31.2). Eventually, the granuloma may disappear or only be seen as a nodule of collagen (Fig. 31.3) or an acellular mass of hyaline material with a fibrous capsule.

Since the hepatic lesions are focal, and fibrosis is restricted to healing lesions, sarcoidosis does not produce the diffuse fibrosis and nodular regeneration of cirrhosis. An association with jaundice and hepatic failure is very rare.

Clinical features

Overt liver disease is rare. The liver is palpable in only 20% of patients. Occasionally, there is active liver disease with marked hepatic functional abnormalities and liver cell destruction, and fibrosis on liver biopsy [36]. Typically, however, the evidence of hepatic involvement arises not from the clinical picture but from the result of liver biopsy. This shows typical features in about 60% of patients with sarcoid manifestations elsewhere [37,38]. Liver biopsy is indicated as a diagnostic approach when another more accessible tissue, such as lymph gland or skin, is not appropriate.

Biochemical changes—an elevated alkaline phosphatase is the most characteristic liver function test abnormality. Serum angiotensin-converting enzyme is increased but not diagnostic.

CT scanning shows discrete upper abdominal lymph node enlargement in about 60% of patients with sarcoidosis. Hepatic CT changes are found only in 38% of those with known hepatic involvement with multiple, small low-attenuation areas on contrast-enhanced scans.

MRI shows multiple, diffuse, densely packed islands of isointense or slightly hyperintense parenchyma on proton density images and corresponding foci of hypointensity on T_2-weighted images—contrasting with the hyperintense T_2-weighted images characteristic of metastatic or inflammatory disease.

Treatment

In most cases the hepatic involvement does not require treatment—and in any case the response to corticosteroid therapy is poor with little improvement in liver function tests [39]. Improvement seems to be limited to those with mild disease where such improvement in biochemical tests is of doubtful clinical significance. Associated symptoms of sarcoidosis elsewhere in the body, and systemic symptoms such as fatigue, may necessitate treatment.

If there is significant liver disease the following clinical patterns are recognized [40]:

Portal hypertension. Young, black people of either sex, appear more susceptible to this manifestation. Portal hypertension is presinusoidal due to portal (zone 1) granulomas. Sinusoidal block may be superimposed due to fibrosis [41]. Rarely, oesophageal bleeding is a real problem. These patients tolerate shunts well. Corticosteroids do not prevent the portal hypertension.

Budd–Chiari syndrome. Sarcoidosis has been reported in association with hepatic vein occlusion [42].

Cholestasis. Rarely patients with sarcoidosis, usually male and black, show features of chronic intrahepatic cholestasis. They present with fever, malaise, weight loss, jaundice and usually pruritus. Serum alkaline phosphatase levels are very high and transaminases increased about two to five times. Hepatosplenomegaly is usual. Liver biopsy usually shows granulomas. Portal areas show damaged or even absence of bile ducts [43] (Fig. 31.5). Sequential liver biopsies show relentless progression of the fibrosis and bile duct loss. The prognosis is poor. The patients usually die within 2–18 years from the onset. Corticosteroids are not helpful. Ursodeoxycholic acid may be used to control pruritus. Liver transplantation may be necessary. However,

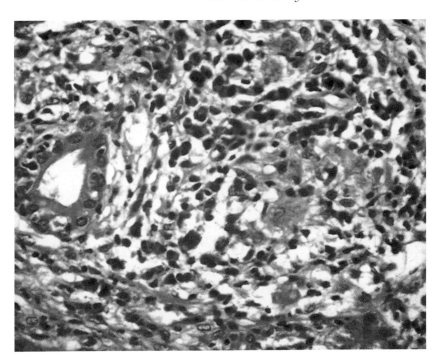

Fig. 31.5. Chronic cholestasis in sarcoidosis. A damaged bile duct is surrounded by an inflammatory infiltrate including lymphocytes. (H & E, ×160.)

post-transplant multiple hepatic granulomas can recur, but without clinical deterioration [44]. The condition may resemble and even be indistinguishable from PBC [45].

Extrahepatic cholestasis [46] due to bile duct inflammation or portal hilar lymphadenopathy, and diffuse stricturing resembling primary sclerosing cholangitis, or indeed an overlap syndrome, may also occur [47].

'Granulomatous hepatitis'

Hepatic granulomas may be associated with a prolonged, febrile syndrome [48,49]. Some patients are eventually diagnosed as having an infection, such as tuberculosis, histoplasmosis or Q fever, or a lymphoma. Those that defy diagnosis are labelled 'granulomatous hepatitis'. The sufferer is often a middle-aged or elderly male. The granulomas are not widespread. Biochemical tests of liver function are moderately impaired with increases in serum alkaline phosphatase, and slight increases in serum transaminases and globulins. Serum bilirubin is normal. The condition may subside spontaneously or necessitate short- or long-term prednisolone treatment. The ultimate prognosis is excellent [48,50]. Those not responding to, or unwilling to take, corticosteroids may benefit from azathioprine or low-dose, oral pulse methotrexate.

Granulomatous drug reactions (see Chapter 24)

Drugs are rare causes of hepatic granulomas, but identification of a granuloma in a liver biopsy should always raise the possibility that it is drug related and not the underlying disease. Typically such granulomas are part of a general hypersensitivity reaction, developing 10 days to 4 months after starting the drug. They may be associated with fever, rash, lymphadenopathy and arthritis.

Serum biochemistry shows increases in alkaline phosphatase and γ-GT. Transaminases may be modestly increased. A rise in serum bilirubin is unusual with a simple granulomatous reaction.

Liver histology shows predominant granulomas. Caseation is absent. Tissue eosinophilia is found in about 70%. Fatty change, portal zone inflammation and bile duct injury are occasionally present. The lesion heals without concentric fibrosis. Such findings with cholestasis should always suggest a drug reaction.

Prognosis is usually excellent with recovery within 6 weeks of withdrawing the drug. Rarely, severe reactions may lead to consideration of corticosteroid therapy.

An enormous number of drugs may be implicated. Drugs that can cause a predominantly granulomatous reaction are listed in Table 31.4. Allopurinol, carbamazepine, glibenclamide and sulphonamides are the most common culprits. Recently, tumour necrosis factor receptor blockers have been added to the list [51]. They are all rare reactions but can be fatal. In all, the histological picture is mixed granulomatous, hepatocellular, cholangitic and vasculitic elements. Carbamazepine and allopurinol are associated with fibrin-ring granulomas [52].

Table 31.4. Important causes of granulomatous drug reactions

Allopurinol
Carbamazepine
Diltiazem
Glibenclamide
Hydralazine
Quinidine/quinine
Sulfonamides

Industrial causes

Beryllium poisoning leads to pulmonary granulomas. Hepatic involvement consists of miliary sarcoid-like granulomas. Pulmonary and hepatic granulomas may be due to inhalation of *cement* and *mica dust*, and to *copper* in vineyard sprayers.

Other conditions with hepatic granulomas

In the early stages of PBC the liver may show widespread hepatic granulomas with a histological picture indistinguishable from sarcoidosis. *Whipple's disease*, due to *Trophyrema whippelii* may be accompanied by hepatic granulomas with bacillary inclusions.

Non-specific reticuloendothelial proliferations: 'reactive hepatitis'

Focal accumulations of mononuclear and epithelioid cells are found in many diseases—perhaps most frequent in viral infections, including infectious mononucleosis, during the recovery phase of viral hepatitis when they contain iron, and in influenza. Occasionally, they are noted in pyogenic infections and septicaemias where polymorphonuclear leucocytes are also present. Their distinction from small sarcoid granulomas may be difficult. If such an accumulation of cells is found in a liver biopsy section, the whole block should be sectioned serially to identify typical granulomas.

Generalized proliferation of Kupffer cells is another frequent finding occurring in infections and in malignant disease.

The liver in diabetes mellitus

Clinical features

Type 1 diabetes

There are usually no clinical features referable to the liver. Occasionally, however, the liver is greatly enlarged, firm and with a smooth, tender edge, and this may fluctuate dramatically. Some of the nausea, abdominal pain and vomiting of diabetic ketosis may be due to this. Hepatomegaly is present in around 10% of well-controlled diabetics and in 60% of uncontrolled diabetics. The enlargement is due to increased glycogen. Insulin therapy in the presence of a very high blood sugar level augments the glycogen content of the liver and, in the initial stages of treatment, hepatomegaly may increase.

Type 2 diabetes

The liver may be enlarged with a firm, smooth, non-tender edge. Enlargement is due to steatosis; the rising incidence of non-alcoholic steatosis and steatohepatitis is well recognized, and Type 2 diabetes is a key feature of the metabolic syndrome that predisposes to non-alcoholic steatohepatitis (NASH) and non-alcoholic fatty liver disease (NAFLD).

Biochemistry

In well-controlled diabetics, routine tests are usually normal. Acidosis may produce mild changes including hyperglobulinaemia and a slightly raised serum bilirubin level, returning to normal with diabetic control. Eighty per cent of diabetics with fatty liver have abnormal serum biochemical tests—such as transaminases, alkaline phosphatase and γ-GT. Hepatomegaly, whether due to increased amounts of glycogen in type 1 diabetes or to fatty change in type 2, does not correlate with the results of the liver function tests.

Sulphonylurea therapy can be complicated by cholestatic or granulomatous liver disease.

Hepatic histology

In Type 1 diabetes, histopathology shows normal or increased glycogen in the livers of severe untreated diabetes. *Glycogenic infiltration of the liver cell nuclei* (Fig. 31.6) appears as vacuolization.

The histological appearances in Type 2 diabetes are those of NAFLD and NASH, the latter leading to fibrosis and cirrhosis.

Liver and thyroid

The liver plays an important part in the transport, storage, activation and metabolism of thyroid hormones [53]. It synthesizes the proteins which transport thyroxine (T_4) in the circulation. The liver contains 10–30% of the body's exchangeable T_4, excluding the thyroid, and is the major site for conversion of T_4 to the biologically active tri-iodothyronine (T_3). The liver also removes reverse T_3, the biological inactive product of T_4. Finally around 25% of the daily T_4 secreted by the thyroid is

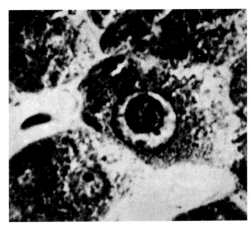

Fig. 31.6. Glycogen infiltration of a hepatic nucleus. Cells contain much glycogen. (Best's carmine for glycogen, ×1150.)

metabolized by oxidative deamination, or excreted into bile after glucuronidation and sulphation. There is also enterohepatic circulation of unmetabolized T_4 excreted in bile.

Despite all these hepatic contributions to the handling of thyroid hormones, most patients with liver disease are clinically euthyroid, although standard function tests may give misleading results. Serum total T_4 may be raised or decreased in association with varying levels of thyroid hormone binding proteins. The free T_4 index is usually normal. A low T_4 variant of 'sick euthyroid syndrome' is reported in 30% of cirrhotic patients and is associated with reduced short- and long-term survival. In *alcoholic liver disease* raised serum levels of thyrotrophin (TSH) and free T_4 are associated with normal or low T_3 values. In *primary biliary cirrhosis* and *autoimmune hepatitis* T_4-binding globulins are increased but free hormone concentrations are reduced, probably because of decreased thyroid function associated with the high incidence of thyroiditis in these patients.

However hypo- and hyperthyroidism may be associated with liver disease, and influence the severity of liver injury [54].

Thyrotoxicosis

Minor abnormalities of liver function are seen in hyperthyroidism, typically a slight increase in alkaline phosphatase returning to normal after treatment [55,56]. However, jaundice in thyrotoxic patients may be due to heart failure. In addition, thyrotoxicosis may cause severe cholestasis in patients without heart failure [57]. Thyrotoxicosis may also aggravate an underlying defect in serum bilirubin metabolism, such as Gilbert's syndrome, by decreasing bilirubin UDP–glucuronosyl transferase activity.

Myxoedema

Ascites without congestive heart failure occurs rarely in patients with myxoedema and has been attributed to centrizonal congestion and fibrosis [58]. The pathogenesis is unknown. It disappears on giving thyroxine. There is a high ascitic protein content, more than 25 g/L.

Jaundice may be related to neonatal thyroid deficiency.

Liver and adrenal

Undiagnosed Addison's disease can be associated with mild elevation of transaminase levels [59]. These return to normal after treatment with corticosteroids.

Liver and growth hormone

The liver and kidney degrade growth hormone. Basal and stimulated growth hormone concentrations are elevated in cirrhotic patients and correlate with the degree of liver dysfunction. These increased levels may contribute to insulin resistance and glucose intolerance in cirrhosis. Acromegaly does not develop despite the chronic elevation of growth hormone in cirrhosis, however in acromegaly the liver enlarges in line with other viscera.

Amyloidosis

Amyloidosis describes a group of conditions linked by a common feature, the extracellular deposition of a protein in an abnormal fibrillar form. It is called amyloid because the waxy infiltration of organs resembles starch (Latin: *amylum*) in its staining. It may be hereditary or acquired, systemic or localized, an incidental finding or cause death. Clinical features develop because of the disruption of normal function in kidney, heart and other organs by the deposition of amyloid fibrils.

Classification of the amyloidoses is based on the protein involved (Table 31.5). Those of particular interest to the hepatologist are AL and AA because of the clinical features, and ATTR because of the role of liver transplantation. Other proteins responsible for amyloidosis include apolipoprotein A1 (AApoA1) and lysozyme (ALys). The common biochemical feature is that the proteins involved can exist in two stable structures, a normal soluble form and an abnormal fibril. Fibrils form by autoaggregation. This is related to overproduction of the soluble form, but why some individuals develop amyloid and others do not is unclear. All amyloid fibrils share a similar core ultrastructure and many physicochemical properties. All amyloid deposits contain the normal plasma protein serum amyloid P (SAP) component, and this is the basis for radiolabelled

Table 31.5. Classification of amyloidosis

Type*	Fibril	Syndrome
AA	Serum amyloid A	Reactive (secondary) amyloid
		acquired (e.g. rheumatoid)
		hereditary (FMF)
AL	Monoclonal immunoglobulin light chain	Primary amyloid
		myeloma associated
		no association
ATTR	Transthyretin (TTR)	Familial amyloidotic polyneuropathy

FMF, familial Mediterranean fever.
*Other types: Aβ$_2$M (renal failure dialysis), Aβ (Alzheimer's disease), A1APP (diabetes/ insulinoma).

SAP scanning used in specialist centres to show the distribution and amount of amyloid.

In collected series, AL amyloid is the most common type. In a UK study of 484 patients with systemic amyloidosis, AL accounted for 37%, AA 28%, hereditary 20% and dialysis-related 14%. Forty-seven other patients had localized amyloid syndromes [60]. In an American study, 86% had AL [61].

Clinical features

AL amyloid (formerly primary amyloid) is caused by deposition of fibrils from all or part of a monoclonal immunoglobulin light chain, more commonly lambda than kappa, which usually can be detected in serum or urine. Most patients have a subtle monoclonal gammopathy. Multiple myeloma is diagnosed in only 10–20% of cases. In about 15% of patients a gammopathy cannot be demonstrated. The common clinical presentations are nephrotic syndrome, cardiomyopathy, carpal tunnel syndrome and a sensory–motor neuropathy. Hepatomegaly is found in 25%. Intestinal involvement includes motility disturbances and malabsorption. Macroglossia or periorbital purpura suggest AL amyloidosis.

AA amyloid (formerly secondary amyloid) is caused by fibrils of AA protein derived from the circulating acute phase reactant serum amyloid A (SAA) by proteolytic cleavage. SAA is synthesized by hepatocytes, transcriptionally regulated by cytokines, and is an apolipoprotein. Elevated SAA is a prerequisite for the development of AA amyloidosis, but not every patient with elevated SAA will develop the disease. Juvenile and adult rheumatoid arthritis are the commonest underlying inflammatory conditions, although chronic sepsis, tuberculosis, Crohn's disease and malignant neoplasms may be responsible. Presentation is usually with proteinuria, nephrotic syndrome or renal failure, which is the cause of death in half of cases. The spleen is affected early and may be enlarged. Liver involvement, seen in around 25% of patients, is a sign of extensive disease.

The autosomal recessive disorder *familial Mediterranean fever* (FMF), characterized by acute attacks of fever with sterile peritonitis, pleurisy or synovitis, predisposes to AA amyloid [62]. FMF primarily affects non-Ashkenazi Jewish, Armenian, Turkish and Middle-eastern Arab populations. The abnormality reflects mutations in a neutrophil protein called pyrin or marenostrin, but diagnosis remains clinical rather than by genotype [63]. Family studies have identified rare instances with autosomal dominant inheritance. The usual manifestation of amyloidosis in FMF is renal, progressing to end-stage disease. Liver, spleen and gastrointestinal tract may be involved.

Familial amyloidotic polyneuropathy (FAP) is caused by the deposition of variant transthyretin (TTR) [64]. Normal TTR is mainly produced by the liver and transports thyroid hormones and vitamin A. Over 60 mutations have been found in the *TTR* gene. FAP is characterized by progressive peripheral and autonomic neuropathy as a mutant TTR is deposited in nerves, and spleen, heart, eyes, thyroid and adrenals. The liver is generally spared (see domino transplantation below).

Other forms of hereditary systemic amyloidosis are extremely rare—amongst them apolipoprotein A-I, apolipoprotein A-II, fibrinogen α chain and lysozyme amyloidosis are most often associated with clinical liver involvement.

Hepatic involvement

Using SAP scintigraphy, identifying sites of amyloid deposition and importantly allowing quantification, hepatic amyloidosis was shown in 54% of patients with AL amyloid and 18% of those with AA [60]. Hepatic amyloid was only detected in one of 53 patients with FAP. SAP scintigraphy correlates with hepatic histology when there are parenchymal or stromal amyloid deposits but not with diffuse vascular deposits. A major advantage of the availability of SAP scanning is that it can be used to quantify the load of amyloid deposition and monitor response to therapy, as it is now clear that with appropriate therapy in some cases the burden of amyloid deposition can be reversed.

On clinical examination, hepatomegaly in a patient with amyloidosis suggests hepatic involvement [65,66], although occasionally the liver may not be enlarged. An enlarged spleen infiltrated with amyloid may be found. The serum alkaline phosphatase may be raised, but levels overlap between patients (both AA and AL) with and without liver involvement.

If available, hepatic histology in systemic amyloidosis may show vascular deposition and variable interstitial amyloid, but the pattern is not diagnostically helpful [67]. The amyloid is shown as homogeneous, amorphous, eosinophilic material. It stains with alkaline alcoholic Congo red or methyl violet (Fig. 31.7). Polarization microscopy of Congo red stained sections shows apple-green birefringent fibrils. The amyloid is deposited between the columns of liver cells and the sinusoidal wall in the space of Disse. The liver cells are not themselves involved but are compressed to a variable extent. The midzone and portal areas are most heavily infiltrated. Occasionally, in AL amyloid the amyloid is found only in the portal tracts in the walls of hepatic arterioles. Electron microscopy confirms fibrils 10 nm long that do not branch.

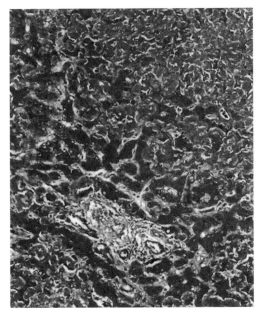

Fig. 31.7. Amyloid is shown as amorphous dark staining material between the liver cells and sinusoids. (Methyl violet, ×40.)

However, percutaneous liver biopsy causes haemorrhage in 4–5% of patients with amyloid [68]. Whether the historical reports of a significant risk of fracturing the waxy liver with amyloid are relevant with current techniques is unclear, but liver biopsy is not the preferred diagnostic path.

Clinical features of hepatic involvement

Hepatocellular failure is rare as is portal hypertension, which when present is of the sinusoidal type and has a poor prognosis [69,70]. Severe intrahepatic cholestasis may rarely complicate AL amyloidosis, presumably due to interference with bile passage into canaliculi and small bile ducts—the prognosis is poor [71].

Diagnostic approach

Clinical suspicion of amyloidosis leads to consideration of the best site of biopsy (see below) to obtain tissue for appropriate staining, and a search for evidence of the cause. This may be suggested by a history of chronic inflammation (AA) or a family history (FAP). To identify AL amyloidosis, immunoelectrophoresis of serum and urine for monoclonal protein, and bone marrow biopsy with immunohistochemical staining of plasma cells for light chains, are required. In FAP, isoelectric focusing of serum will show bands of variant and wild-type transthyretin, and genomic DNA analysis may show a mutant *TTR* gene.

Although biopsy of the affected tissue (heart, kidney) is likely to be diagnostic, it is generally safer to sample other areas—subcutaneous abdominal fat pad, rectal mucosa and labial salivary gland give a positive result in up to 75–80% of cases. As commented above, liver biopsy is best avoided.

^{123}I-*SAP scintigraphy* is a specific and sensitive method for detecting and monitoring amyloidosis during treatment of the underlying cause, but is a specialized tool with restricted availability.

Prognosis

This varies according to the type of amyloidosis, the degree of organ involvement and the response to therapy of the underlying condition. Patients with AL amyloidosis have a mean survival of 1–2 years—perhaps longer with intensive chemotherapy. Survival is not affected by liver involvement, though it is by symptomatic heart disease (median survival 6 months).

The prognosis for AA amyloidosis is affected by the underlying chronic disease. The 5-year survival in those with liver deposits is reduced compared with those without liver involvement (43 vs. 72%). Survival is significantly improved when serum amyloid A level can be maintained in the reference range (<10 mg/L) [72].

Patients with FAP may survive for up to 15 years. Patients with transthyretin mutations associated with a younger age at disease onset have a more rapid progression of neurological and cardiac disease and a shorter survival [64].

Treatment

AA amyloid is treated by controlling the underlying disease—by eradicating infections such as tuberculosis, occasionally by surgery to remove an infectious focus, or by intensive anti-inflammatory/ immunosuppressive and in some instances anticytokine (TNF-α, IL-β or IL-6 blockade) therapy. Prophylactic colchicine prevents the development of amyloidosis in FMF. There is currently no specific treatment aimed at the amyloid deposits but there are emerging strategies using small molecules that interact with the fibril component of the deposits or deplete amyloid P component.

Treating AL amyloid remains difficult. Melphalan combined with prednisone only has a 30% response rate with a mean survival of 18 months, but newer strategies with thalidomide and cyclophosphamide improve outcome in some. Higher-dose chemotherapy with peripheral blood stem cell support also improves outcome in patients fit enough to tolerate the treatment. Such treatment also improves liver function.

Liver transplantation is the definitive treatment for FAP with a 75% 5-year survival [73,74]. Liver transplantation results in disappearance of the variant TTR from plasma, and some regression of neurological disease. Recovery from autonomic neuropathy is greater than from peripheral neuropathy. Furthermore, the explanted liver from patients with FAP can be transplanted into selected recipients (domino transplantation), on the basis that these livers may be structurally and functionally normal apart from the production of variant transthyretin, having only been removed to arrest the build-up of further amyloid and clinical progression of polyneuropathy. Follow-up of recipients of FAP livers has shown the anticipated propensity for the development of neuropathy within 8–10 years, so recipient selection (ideally older) is important.

Porphyrias

Porphyrias are clinical syndromes caused by defects in the pathway of biosynthesis of haem (Fig. 31.8). Porphyrins accumulate as they are not converted to haem, and this may reflect a number of specific enzyme defects in the metabolic pathway. In addition, the lack of haem production results in increased activity of a key porphyrin synthesizing enzyme δ-aminolaevulinic acid (ALA)-synthetase, due to loss of normal regulatory negative feedback. Haem is an important component of

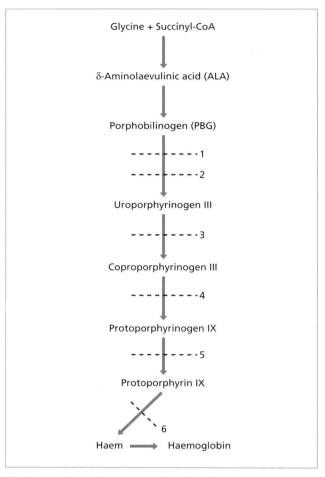

Fig. 31.8. Porphyria and the biosynthesis of porphyrins. Numbers indicate site of enzyme defect leading to:
1 Acute intermittent porphyria
2 Congenital erythropoietic porphyria
3 Porphyria cutanea tarda and hepatoerythropoietic porphyria
4 Hereditary coproporphyria
5 Variegate porphyria
6 Erythropoietic protoporphyria (see text for enzyme deficiency responsible).

both haemoglobin and enzymes such as the cytochrome P450 oxidase system so porphyrin production is most pronounced in hepatic cells and erythrocytes, giving one broad classification of porphyrias as hepatic or erythropoietic (Table 31.6).

There are two broad clinical patterns [75]:
• *Neurological*, due to accumulation of early precursors in the pathway (ALA/ porphobilinogen (PBG)) with the acute attacks including abdominal pain, peripheral neuropathy, autonomic dysfunction, tachycardia, hypertension, hyponatraemia and psychosis.
• *Cutaneous*, in particular photosensitivity due to accumulation of substrates later in the pathway.

Table 31.6. Classifications of porphyria

Acute	
neuroporphyria	*Acute intermittent porphyria*
neurocutaneous	*Hereditary coproporphyria*
	Variegate porphyria
Non-acute (cutaneous)	*Porphyria cutanea tarda*
	Erythropoietic protoporphyria
	Congenital erythropoietic
	porphyria

Hepatic in italic; erythropoietic in roman.

Some types of porphyria give both neurological and cutaneous features.

Most porphyrias are inherited as autosomal dominant conditions, but there is low penetrance. The majority of carriers have latent porphyria, and attacks may then be precipitated by drugs, hormonal factors and endogenous metabolic changes—but in perhaps 80% of carriers there are never any manifestations.

Differentiation between the various porphyrias depends upon analysis of porphyrin metabolites in urine, faeces and erythrocytes. These diagnostic tests may only yield definitive results during acute attacks [75].

Hepatic porphyrias

The acute hepatic porphyrias are *acute intermittent porphyria*, *hereditary coproporphyria*, *variegate porphyria* and the very rare *5-ALA dehydratase* porphyria [76]. A prevalence of 5 per 100 000 has been estimated but there are wide geographic variations reflecting founder effects (e.g. South African white people). Acute hepatic porphyrias are marked by neuropsychiatric attacks with vomiting, abdominal colic, constipation, hypertension and peripheral neuropathy, typically lasting several days. During these attacks, large amounts of the porphyrin precursors, PBG and ALA, are excreted in the urine. All hepatic porphyrias are exacerbated by countless enzyme-inducing drugs including barbiturates, sulfonamides, oestrogens, oral contraceptives, griseofulvin, chloroquine and possibly alcohol [77]. Hormones are important inducers and women develop attacks in pregnancy and premenstrually.

A clinical picture similar to acute hepatic porphyria can occur in severe lead poisoning when ALA dehydratase is markedly reduced.

Acute intermittent porphyria

The basic deficiency is in hepatic PBG deaminase. Acute attacks are as described above; photosensitivity is absent. In acute attacks the urine darkens on standing. Diagnosis may depend on a high index of suspicion on first presentation. The key investigation is the documentation of increased porphobilinogen in urine in the acute attack. Between attacks, or after haem therapy, the levels may not be abnormal.

If mild, acute attacks may respond adequately to glucose loading, but infusions of haematin or haem arginate, which repress or inhibit hepatic ALA synthetase, are now recommended for all but the mildest attacks—despite a non-rigorous evidence base. Intensive care may be warranted, particularly if the neuropathy affects respiratory function.

Long-term management involves avoidance of precipitating factors, particularly medications. General anaesthesia can be performed safely in known patients with appropriate choice of drugs; the danger is in the unknown [78]. Suppression of menstruation may be appropriate (e.g. by LH/RH antagonists) in women with repeated monthly attacks. Rarely, orthotopic liver transplantation has been performed and cures the metabolic defect [79].

The risk of hepatocellular carcinoma is increased over 30-fold in acute hepatic porphyrias, not merely reflecting confounding factors such as alcoholism or HBV/HCV infection [80].

Hereditary coproporphyria [81]

The deficiency is in coproporphyrinogen oxidase. Attacks may be neurological or cutaneous with lesions as in porphyria cutanea tarda (see below). Faecal and urinary coproporphyrin are increased with a corresponding increase in protoporphyrin. Acute attacks are treated as for acute intermittent porphyria.

Variegate porphyria

The defect is in protoporphyrinogen oxidase. This variant is frequently encountered in South Africa and New England. The features are intermediate between acute intermittent porphyria and hereditary coproporphyria. Protoporphyrin and porphyrins may be increased in the stool between attacks. Biliary porphyrin estimation may be diagnostic in the asymptomatic patient. Acute attacks are treated as for acute intermittent porphyria.

Porphyria cutanea tarda

The fourth type of hepatic porphyria, *porphyria cutanea tarda*, may be associated with hepatocellular disease. It is not exacerbated by barbiturates and acute neurological attacks are not seen. It is the commonest porphyria and is usually latent and the patient symptom free [82]. It is due to a reduction in uroporphyrinogen decarboxylase (URO-D) activity. Two forms are described: familial

(20% of patients), with point mutations in the URO-D gene, and sporadic, where there is a URO-D defect restricted to the liver perhaps due to an inhibitor rather than mutation. In both types a background of liver iron overload appears necessary for clinical expression and there is usually evidence of liver dysfunction.

When symptomatic the condition is characterized by photosensitive skin, blistering and scarring, pigmentation and hypertrichosis. Uroporphyrin is increased in the urine. Sensitivity to drugs such as barbiturates is absent, but exposure to alcohol and oestrogens may precipitate attacks.

Deterioration of liver function from any cause may exacerbate symptoms, as when the liver is healthy, the porphyrin is excreted harmlessly into the bile; when the liver is diseased, porphyrins are diverted into the blood—coincidentally increasing urine excretion—and initiating cutaneous symptoms, particularly in response to light. The porphyrin itself may also be hepatotoxic.

Liver biopsy usually shows an abnormality, most frequently siderosis, mild steatosis, focal necrosis and portal fibrosis with some inflammation [83]. Less than 15% have cirrhosis. The excess hepatic iron is highly significant as venesection has a good therapeutic effect, presumably related to iron removal [82]. The iron excess often reflects carriage of the C282Y mutation in the *HFE* (haemochromatosis) gene, being over 40% (homozygosity plus heterozygosity) in one study [84], but may also reflect alcohol intake and in some cases HCV infection. A high prevalence of hepatitis C is often reported in porphyria cutanea tarda, but it varies greatly (8–80%) between different countries. The incidence of hepatocellular carcinoma is increased; this appears to be related to the presence of chronic liver disease (HCV, alcoholic or haemochromatotic) than a direct aetiological association of the metabolic defect [85].

Erythropoietic porphyrias

The erythropoietic porphyrias are *erythropoietic protoporphyria* (dominant) and *congenital erythropoietic porphyria* (autosomal recessive) and *hepatoerythropoietic porphyria* (autosomal recessive).

Erythropoietic protoporphyria

The enzyme ferrochelatase is deficient. Inheritance is dominant with variable penetrance [86]. Protoporphyrin is increased in tissues and urine. The major manifestation is skin photosensitivity. Liver biopsies show focal deposits of pigment containing 'Maltese-cross' protoporphyrin crystals by fluorescence. Electron microscopy shows abnormalities of nuclei, endoplasmic reticulum and membranes, despite normal light microscopy.

The spectrum of liver involvement ranges from normal liver function (20%) to mild abnormalities of liver function tests, to chronic liver disease and cirrhosis (5–10%) [87]. Complications include gallstones containing protoporphyrin. In end-stage protoporphyric liver disease, neurotoxicity has been reported.

Liver transplantation has been successful for severe liver disease [87] although precautions should be taken to reduce the risk of cutaneous reactions during surgery. The metabolic defect, residing in bone marrow, is not corrected in this way so there may be recurrent liver damage. Since the red cell is the source of protoporphyrin, bone marrow transplantation is a potential therapeutic approach [88].

The rarest but most serious picture is rapidly progressing photosensitivity, cholestasis and haemolysis. There is severe upper abdominal pain and splenomegaly with rapid deterioration. Emergency treatment includes haematin infusion and red cell transfusions to reduce porphyrin and red cell production. Plasmapheresis or albumin dialysis may reduce free protoporphyrin. The enterohepatic circulation of protoporphyrin may be blocked by oral cholestyramine or charcoal. Liver transplantation may be the only ultimate option.

Congenital erythropoietic porphyria

The enzyme uroporphyrinogen III cosynthase is deficient [89]. The major clinical problem in this rare type is photosensitivity. Neurological symptoms do not occur. The liver may be enlarged and contain excess iron.

Hepatoerythropoietic porphyria

This very rare type, presenting within the first year of life with skin disease, is due to homozygous deficiency of URO-D. It is marked by hepatosplenomegaly and cirrhosis. Liver biopsies fluoresce but there is no iron excess. The acute presentation may be preceded by acute viral hepatitis.

Secondary coproporphyrias

Heavy metal intoxication, especially with lead, causes porphyria with ALA and coproporphyrin in the urine. Erythrocyte protoporphyrins are increased. Coproporphyrinuria may also be seen with sideroblastic anaemia, various liver diseases, Dubin–Johnson syndrome and as a complication of drug therapy.

Non-metastatic complications of malignancy

Renal cell carcinomas may be associated with abnormal liver function tests; whilst in part this may reflect production of variant alkaline phosphatase by the neoplasm, increased release of alkaline phosphatase and γ-GT from the liver may occur as a paraneoplastic effect mediated by cytokines released from the tumour [90,91]. Lymphomas may induce hepatic granulomas and abnormal liver biochemistry in the absence of liver infiltration.

Bone-marrow/ stem cell transplantation; graft-versus-host disease

Graft-versus-host disease (GVHD) reflects the targeting of donor immune cells to host histocompatibility antigens, and the poorer the HLA-match at transplantation the higher the incidence of the condition. It most commonly affects the skin, but thereafter liver and gut are the key target organs. In acute GVHD (within first 100 days post-transplant, generally at about 30–60 days) there is skin involvement in 80%, gut involvement (watery or bloody diarrhoea and pain) in 50% and liver involvement—predominantly cholestasis also in 50%. Whilst liver biopsy may reveal characteristic findings (endothelialitis, portal tract lymphocytic involvement and bile duct damage) [92], patients are often profoundly cytopenic at the time rendering biopsy inadvisable. The differential is wide, because of other potential causes of cholestasis such as sinusoidal obstruction syndrome (formerly called veno-occlusive disease) from pretransplant conditioning, drugs, sepsis and viral infection; evidence of skin and gut involvement (the characteristic maculopapular rash, particularly on palms and soles, and/or positive findings on gastrointestinal endoscopic biopsies) is therefore helpful. Treatment is by immunosuppression—corticosteroids as first line, with treatments such as extracorporeal photophoresis (harvesting white cells, light-irradiating them after incubation with a sensitizer and returning the treated population to the patient) and cytokine blockade now establishing a role [93]. Response rates vary with severity, with complete remission in less than 50% of cases. In chronic GVHD, cholestasis and progressive bile-duct damage are characteristic, and the response to immunosuppression poor. Infection due to high level immunosuppression is the major risk in these patients.

References

1 Seaman WE, Ishak KG, Plotz PH. Aspirin induced hepatotoxicity in patients with systemic lupus erythematosus. *Ann. Intern. Med.* 1974; **80**: 1–8.

2 Matsumoto T, Yoshimine T, Shimouchi K *et al.* The liver in systemic lupus erythematosus: pathologic analysis of 52 cases and review of the Japanese Autopsy Registry Data. *Hum. Pathol.* 1992; **23**: 1151–1158.

3 Matsumoto T, Kobayashi S, Shimizu H *et al.* The liver in collagen diseases: pathologic study of 160 cases with particular reference to hepatic arteritis, primary biliary cirrhosis, autoimmune hepatitis and nodular regenerative hyperplasia of the liver. *Liver* 2000; **20**: 366–731.

4 Keshavarzian A, Rentsch R, Hodgson HJ. Clinical implications of liver biopsy findings in collagen-vascular disorders. *J. Clin. Gastroenterol.* 1993; **17**: 219–226.

5 Sekiya M, Sekigawa I, Hishikawa T *et al.* Nodular regenerative hyperplasia of the liver in systemic lupus erythematosus. The relationship with anticardiolipin antibody and lupus anticoagulant. *Scand. J. Rheumatol.* 1997; **26**: 215–217.

6 Wanless IR. Micronodular transformation (nodular regenerative hyperplasia) of the liver: a report of 64 cases among 2500 autopsies and a new classification of benign hepatocellular nodules. *Hepatology* 1990; **11**: 787–797.

7 Reshamwala PA, Keliner DE, Heller T. Nodular regenerative hyperplasia: not all nodules are created equal. *Hepatology* 2006; **44**: 7–14.

8 Irving KS, Sen D, Tahir H *et al.* A comparison of autoimmune liver disease in juvenile and adult populations with systemic lupus erythematosus-a retrospective review of cases. *Rheumatology (Oxford)* 2007; **46**: 1171–1173.

9 Murdaca G, Colombo BM, Sprecacenere B *et al.* Autoimmune intrahepatic cholangiopathy associated with antiphospholipid antibody syndrome. *Eur. J. Gastroenterol. Hepatol.* 2007; **19**: 910–912.

10 Mor F, Beigel A, Inbar M *et al.* Hepatic infarction in a patient with the lupus anticoagulant. *Arthritis Rheum.* 1989; **32**: 491–495.

11 Thompson PW, Houghton BJ, Clifford C *et al.* The source and significance of raised serum enzymes in rheumatoid arthritis. *Q. J. Med.* 1990; **76**: 869–879.

12 Campion G, Maddison PJ, Goulding N *et al.* The Felty syndrome: a case-matched study of clinical manifestations and outcome, serologic features, and immunogenetic associations. *Medicine (Baltimore)* 1990; **69**: 69–80.

13 Rosenstein ED, Kramer N. Felty's and pseudo-Felty's syndromes. *Semin. Arthritis Rheum.* 1991; **21**: 129–142.

14 Laine L, Goldkind L, Curtis SP *et al.* How common is diclofenac-associated liver injury? Analysis of 17,289 arthritis patients in a long-term prospective clinical trial. *Am. J. Gastroenterol.* 2009; **104**: 356–362.

15 Favreau M, Tannenbaum H, Lough J. Hepatic toxicity associated with gold therapy. *Ann. Intern. Med.* 1977; **87**: 717–719.

16 Thiéfin G, Morelet A, Heurgué A *et al.* Infliximab-induced hepatitis: absence of cross-toxicity with etanercept. *Joint Bone Spine* 2008; **75**: 737–739.

17 Salliot C, van der Heijde D. Long term safety of Methotrexate monotherapy in rheumatoid arthritis patients: A systematic literature research. *Ann. Rheum. Dis.* 2009; **68**: 1100–1104.

18 Routsias JG, Tzioufas AG. Sjögren's syndrome—study of autoantigens and autoantibodies. *Clin. Rev. Allergy Immunol.* 2007; **32**: 238–251.

19 Hatzis GS, Fragoulis GE, Karatzaferis A *et al.* Prevalence and longterm course of primary biliary cirrhosis in primary Sjögren's syndrome. *J. Rheumatol.* 2008; **35**: 2012–2016.

20 Montaño-Loza AJ, Crispín-Acuña JC, Remes-Troche JM *et al.* Abnormal hepatic biochemistries and clinical liver disease in patients with primary Sjögren's syndrome. *Ann. Hepatol.* 2007; **6**: 150–155.

21 Nardi N, Brito-Zerón P, Ramos-Casals M *et al.* Circulating auto-antibodies against nuclear and non-nuclear antigens

in primary Sjögren's syndrome: prevalence and clinical significance in 335 patients. *Clin. Rheumatol.* 2006; **25**: 341–346.

22 Ramos-Casals M, Loustaud-Ratti V, De Vita S *et al*; SS-HCV Study Group. Sjögren syndrome associated with hepatitis C virus: a multicenter analysis of 137 cases. *Medicine (Baltimore)*. 2005; **84**: 81–89.

23 Powell FC, Schroeter AL, Dickinson ER. Primary biliary cirrhosis and the CREST syndrome. *Q. J. Med.* 1987; **62**: 75–82.

24 Ebert EC, Hagspiel KD, Nagar M *et al*. Gastrointestinal involvement in polyarteritis nodosa. *Clin. Gastroenterol. Hepatol.* 2008; **6**: 960–966.

25 Bailey M, Chapin W, Licht H *et al*. The effects of vasculitis on the gastrointestinal tract and liver. *Gastroenterol. Clin. N. Am.* 1998; **27**: 747–782.

26 Gaya DR, Thorburn D, Oien KA *et al*. Hepatic granulomas: a 10 year single centre experience. *J. Clin. Pathol.* 2003; **56**: 850–853.

27 Denk H, Scheuer PJ, Baptista A *et al*. Guidelines for the diagnosis and interpretation of hepatic granulomas. *Histopathology* 1994; **25**: 209–218.

28 Kleiner DE. Granulomas in the liver. *Semin. Diagn. Pathol.* 2006; **23**: 161–169.

29 Drebber U, Kasper HU, Ratering J *et al*. Hepatic granulomas: histological and molecular pathological approach to differential diagnosis–a study of 442 cases. *Liver Int.* 2008; **28**: 828–34.

30 Ortego TJ, Robey B, Morrison D *et al*. Toxoplasma chorioretinitis and hepatic granulomas. *Am. J. Gastroenterol.* 1990; **85**: 1418–1420.

31 Ozaras R, Tahan V, Mert A *et al*. The prevalence of hepatic granulomas in chronic hepatitis C. *J. Clin. Gastroenterol.* 2004; **38**: 449–452.

32 Amarapurkar AD, Sangle NA. Histological spectrum of liver in HIV–autopsy study. *Ann. Hepatol.* 2005; **4**: 47–51.

33 Lefkowitch JH. The liver in AIDS. *Semin. Liver Dis.* 1997; **17**: 335–344.

34 Roca B. Adverse drug reactions to antiretroviral medication. *Front. Biosci.* 2009; **14**: 1785–1792.

35 Gupta NK, Lewis JH. Review article: The use of potentially hepatotoxic drugs in patients with liver disease. *Aliment. Pharmacol. Ther.* 2008; **28**: 1021–1041.

36 Blich M, Edoute Y. Clinical manifestations of sarcoid liver disease. *J. Clin. Gastroenterol. Hepatol.* 2004; **19**: 732–737.

37 Devaney K, Goodman ZD, Epstein MS *et al*. Hepatic sarcoidosis clinicopathologic feature in 100 patients. *Am. J. Surg. Pathol.* 1993; **17**: 1272–1280.

38 Ayyala US, Padilla ML. Diagnosis and treatment of hepatic sarcoidosis. *Curr. Treat. Options Gastroenterol.* 2006; **9**: 475–483.

39 Johns CJ, Michele TM. The clinical management of sarcoidosis. A 50-year experience at the Johns Hopkins Hospital. *Medicine (Baltimore)* 1999; **78**: 65–111.

40 Ebert EC, Kierson M, Hagspiel KD. Gastrointestinal and hepatic manifestations of sarcoidosis. *Am. J. Gastroenterol.* 2008; **103**: 3184–3192.

41 Valla D, Pessegueiro-Miranda H, Degott C *et al*. Hepatic sarcoidosis with portal hypertension. A report of seven cases with a review of the literature. *Q. J. Med.* 1987; **63**: 531–544.

42 Russi EW, Bansky G, Pfaltz M *et al*. Budd Chiari syndrome in sarcoidosis. *Am. J. Gastroenterol.* 1986; **81**: 71–75.

43 Nakanuma Y, Kouda W, Harada K *et al*. Hepatic sarcoidosis with vanishing bile duct syndrome, cirrhosis, and portal phlebosclerosis. Report of an autopsy case. *J. Clin. Gastroenterol.* 2001; **32**: 181–184.

44 Fidler HM, Hadziyannis SJ, Dhillon AP *et al*. Recurrent hepatic sarcoidosis following liver transplantation. *Transplant. Proc.* 1997; **29**: 2509–2510.

45 Stanca CM, Fiel MI, Allina J *et al*. Liver failure in an antimitochondrial antibody-positive patient with sarcoidosis: primary biliary cirrhosis or hepatic sarcoidosis? *Semin. Liver Dis.* 2005; **25**: 364–370.

46 Rezeig MA, Fashir BM. Biliary tract obstruction due to sarcoidosis: a case report. *Am. J. Gastroenterol.* 1996; **92**: 527–528.

47 Ilan Y, Rappaport I, Feigin R *et al*. Primary sclerosing cholangitis in sarcoidosis. *J. Clin. Gastroenterol.* 1999; **16**: 326–328.

48 Sartin JS, Walker RC. Granulomatous hepatitis: a retrospective review of 88 cases. *Mayo Clin. Proc.* 1991; **66**: 914–918.

49 Simon HB, Wolff SM. Granulomatous hepatitis and prolonged fever of unknown origin: a study of 13 patients. *Medicine (Baltimore)* 1973; **52**: 1–21.

50 Zoutman DE, Ralph ED, Frei JV. Granulomatous hepatitis and fever of unknown origin. An 11-year experience of 23 cases with three years' follow-up. *J. Clin. Gastroenterol.* 1991; **13**: 69–75.

51 Farah M, Al Rashidi A, Owen DA *et al*. Granulomatous hepatitis associated with etanercept therapy. *J. Rheumatol.* 2008; **35**: 349–351.

52 Vanderstigel M, Zafrani ES, Lejonc JL *et al*. Allopurinol hypersensitivity syndrome as a cause of hepatic fibrin-ring granulomas. *Gastroenterology* 1986; **9**: 188–190.

53 Malik R, Hodgson H. The relationship between the thyroid gland and the liver. *Q. J. Med.* 2002; **95**: 559–569.

54 Oren R, Dotan I, Papa M *et al*. Inhibition of experimentally induced cirrhosis in rats by hypothyroidism. *Hepatology* 1996; **24**: 419–423.

55 Babb RR. Associations between diseases of the thyroid and the liver. *Am. J. Gastroenterol.* 1984; **79**: 421–423.

56 Huang MJ, Liaw YF. Clinical associations between thyroid and liver diseases. *J. Gastroenterol. Hepatol.* 1995; **10**: 344–350.

57 Barnes SC, Wicking JM, Johnston JD. Graves' disease presenting with cholestatic jaundice. *Ann. Clin. Biochem.* 1999; **36**: 677–679.

58 De Castro F, Bonacini M, Walden JM *et al*. Myxedema ascites: report of two cases and review of the literature. *J. Clin. Gastroenterol.* 1991; **13**: 411–414.

59 Boulton R, Hamilton MI, Dhillon AP *et al*. Subclinical Addison's disease: a cause of persistent abnormalities in transaminase values. *Gastroenterology* 1995; **109**: 1324–1327.

60 Lovat LB, Persey MR, Madhoo S *et al*. The liver in systemic amyloidosis: insights from ^{123}I serum amyloid P component scintigraphy in 484 patients. *Gut* 1998; **42**: 727–734.

61 Kyle RA, Gertz MA. Primary systemic amyloidosis: clinical and laboratory features in 474 cases. *Semin. Hematol.* 1995; **32**: 45–59.

62 Bodar EJ, Drenth JP, van der Meer JW *et al*. Dysregulation of innate immunity: hereditary periodic fever syndromes. *Br. J. Haematol.* 2009; **144**: 279–302.

63 Booth DR, Gillmore JD, Lachmann HJ *et al.* The genetic basis of autosomal dominant familial Mediterranean fever. *Q. J. Med.* 2000; **93**: 217–221.

64 Ando Y, Nakamura M, Araki S. Transthyretin-related familial amyloidotic polyneuropathy. *Arch. Neurol.* 2005; **62**: 1057–1062.

65 Gertz MA, Kyle RA. Hepatic amyloidosis: clinical appraisal in 77 patients. *Hepatology* 1997; **25**: 118–121.

66 Gillmore JD, Lovat LB, Hawkins PN. Amyloidosis and the liver. *J. Hepatol.* 1999; **30**: 17–33.

67 Comenzo RL. Amyloidosis. *Current Treat. Options Oncol.* 2006; **7**: 225–236.

68 Harrison RF, Hawkins PN, Roche WR *et al.* 'Fragile' liver and massive hepatic haemorrhage due to hereditary amyloidosis. *Gut* 1996; **38**: 151–152.

69 Ebert EC, Nagar M. Gastrointestinal manifestations of amyloidosis. *Am. J. Gastroenterol.* 2008; **103**: 776–787.

70 Petre S, Shah IA, Gilani N. Review article: gastrointestinal amyloidosis — clinical features, diagnosis and therapy. *Aliment. Pharmacol. Ther.* 2008 1; **27**: 1006–1016.

71 Faa G, Van Eyken P, De Vos R *et al.* Light chain deposition disease of the liver associated with AL-type amyloidosis and severe cholestasis. *J. Hepatol.* 1991; **12**: 75–82.

72 Gillmore JD, Lovat LB, Persey MR *et al.* Amyloid load and clinical outcome in AA amyloidosis in relation to circulating concentration of serum amyloid A protein. *Lancet* 2001; **358**: 24–29.

73 Stangou AJ, Hawkins PN. Liver transplantation in transthyretin-related familial amyloid polyneuropathy. *Curr. Opin. Neurol.* 2004; **17**: 615–620.

74 Monteiro E, Freire A, Barroso E. Familial amyloid polyneuropathy and liver transplantation. *J. Hepatol.* 2004; **41**: 188–194.

75 Anderson KE, Bloomer JR, Bonkovsky HL *et al.* Recommendations for the diagnosis and treatment of the acute porphyrias. *Ann. Intern. Med.* 2005; **142**: 439–450.

76 Sassa S. Modern diagnosis and management of the porphyrias. *Br. J. Haematol.* 2006; **135**: 281–292.

77 Thunell S, Pomp E, Brun A. Guide to drug porphyrogenicity prediction and drug prescription in the acute porphyrias. *Br. J. Clin. Pharmacol.* 2007; **64**: 668–679.

78 Dover SB, Plenderleith L, Moore MR *et al.* Safety of general anaesthesia and surgery in acute hepatic porphyria. *Gut* 1994; **35**: 1112–1115.

79 Seth AK, Badminton MN, Mirza D *et al.* Liver transplantation for porphyria: who, when, and how? *Liver Transpl.* 2007; **13**: 1219–1227.

80 Andant C, Puy H, Bogard C *et al.* Hepatocellular carcinoma in patients with acute hepatic porphyria: frequency of occurrence and related factors. *J. Hepatol.* 2000; **32**: 933–939.

81 Martásek P. Hereditary coproporphyria. *Semin. Liver Dis.* 1998; **18**: 25–32.

82 Sarkany RP. The management of porphyria cutanea tarda. *Clin. Exp. Dermatol.* 2001; **26**: 225–232.

83 Siersema PD, Rademakers LHPM, Cleton MI *et al.* The difference in liver pathology between sporadic and familial forms of porphyria cutanea tarda: the role of iron. *J. Hepatol.* 1995; **25**: 259–267.

84 Roberts AG, Whatley SD, Morgan RR *et al.* Increased frequency of the haemochromatosis Cys282Tyr mutation in sporadic porphyria cutanea tarda. *Lancet* 1997; **349**: 321–323.

85 Gisbert JP, García-Buey L, Alonso A *et al.* Hepatocellular carcinoma risk in patients with porphyria cutanea tarda. *Eur. J. Gastroenterol. Hepatol.* 2004; **16**: 689–692.

86 Gouya L, Puy H, Lamoril J *et al.* Inheritance in erythropoietic protoporphyria: a common wild-type ferrochelatase allelic variant with low expression accounts for clinical manifestations. *Blood* 1999; **93**: 2105–2110.

87 Anstey AV, Hift RJ. Liver disease in erythropoietic protoporphyria: insights and implications for management. *Gut* 2007; **56**: 1009–1018.

88 Wahlin S, Harper P. The role for BMT in erythropoietic protoporphyria. *Bone Marrow Transpl.* 2009; **45**: 393–394.

89 Desnick RJ, Glass IA, Xu W *et al.* Molecular genetics of congenital erythropoetic porphyria. *Semin. Liver Dis.* 1998; **18**: 77–84.

90 Chuang YC, Lin AT, Chen KK *et al.* Paraneoplastic elevation of serum alkaline phosphatase in renal cell carcinoma: incidence and implication on prognosis. *J. Urol.* 1997; **158**: 1684–1687.

91 Blay JY, Rossi JF, Wijdenes J *et al.* Role of interleukin-6 in the paraneoplastic inflammatory syndrome associated with renal-cell carcinoma. *Int. J. Cancer.* 1997; **72**: 424–430.

92 McDonald GB. Advances in prevention and treatment of hepatic disorders following hematopoietic cell transplantation. *Best Pract. Res. Clin. Haematol.* 2006; **19**: 341–352.

93 Ferrara JLM, Levine JE, Reddy P *et al.* Graft versus host disease. *Lancet* 2009; **373**: 1550–1561.

CHAPTER 32
The Liver in Infections

Christopher C. Kibbler

Centre for Medical Microbiology, University College London, and Department of Medical Microbiology, Royal Free Hampstead NHS Trust, London, UK

Learning points

- The management of bacterial infections, including liver abscesses, requires careful choice of antibiotics. The increasing incidence of resistance means that every attempt should be made to isolate the micro-organism(s) responsible. The need for less familiar antibiotics in many cases should prompt discussion with infectious disease physicians and microbiologists when treating all but the most straight forward infections.

- In the UK and Europe, the majority of fungal infections of the liver are opportunistic. In the USA and rest of the world, the liver may be affected by endemic fungi.

- The outcome of hydatid disease has been transformed by the use of the PAIR technique (percutaneous puncture, aspirate, inject 25% alcohol, re-aspirate), which has largely superseded surgery.

- Schistosomiasis is cured in up to 90% of cases if treated early in the course of the disease with praziquantel.

Introduction

The liver may be affected either directly or indirectly by many agents of infection. The consequences of bacterial, fungal and parasitic infections will be considered in this chapter, while viral infections are dealt with in Chapters 17 to 21. The liver conditions related to HIV infection are described in Chapter 22.

Jaundice of infections

Bacterial pneumonia

Jaundice is an unusual complication of pneumonia. It is, however, still frequent in Africans, where it may be related partly to haemolysis in those deficient in glucose-6-phosphate dehydrogenase [1]. The jaundice has cholestatic and hepatocellular elements, reflected in elevated serum transaminases and alkaline phosphatase levels, which are usually mild.

Liver biopsy shows non-specific changes; electron microscopy shows cholestasis. There is also evidence of toxic liver injury. Increased numbers of hepatic stellate cells are seen during the acute stage.

Bacteraemia and septic shock

Liver function abnormalities, including modest increases in serum alkaline phosphatase, transaminases and bile salts, are not uncommon in patients with severe infections, bacteraemia, toxic shock and endotoxaemia [2,3]. In two-thirds, jaundice is a feature and, if it persists, carries a bad prognosis.

Hepatic histology shows non-specific hepatitis, including midzonal and peripheral necrosis. Cholestasis may be marked and in severe cases is shown as inspissated bile within dilated and proliferated portal and periportal bile ductules [4]. Cultures of the liver are sterile.

The causes are multifactorial. Hepatic hypoperfusion plays a part. The cholangiolar lesions might be related to interference with canalicular exchange of water and electrolytes, to endotoxaemia, to staphylococcal exotoxin [5] or to interference with the peribiliary vascular plexus as a result of shock [2]. TNF-α may mediate endotoxin-induced cholestasis [6]. Endotoxin interferes with bile acid transport, down-regulating basolateral uptake and canalicular export systems [7] (see Chapter 11).

The syndrome of jaundice associated with extrahepatic infection is functional and reversible upon control of the infection.

Pyogenic liver abscess

Over the past 50 years there has been a marked change in the aetiology of pyogenic liver abscess [8]. Abscesses

---

secondary to biliary disease, particularly malignant, continue to increase. Because of the greater number of immunosuppressed patients, the proportion with abscesses from opportunistic infections has risen.

There is earlier diagnosis because of the routine availability of scanning for suspected liver disease.

Aetiology

Underlying biliary disease is the most frequent cause, being present in approximately 40–50% of cases [8–10]. Septic cholangitis can complicate any form of biliary obstruction, especially if partial. More cases are related to surgical, endoscopic or radiological treatment of hepatobiliary disease despite the use of prophylactic antibiotics. Biliary stenting for malignant biliary and pancreatic disease is a particular association. Abscess may occur in sclerosing cholangitis and congenital biliary anomalies, especially Caroli's disease.

Portal pyaemia may follow pelvic or gastrointestinal infection, resulting in portal pylephlebitis or septic emboli. It can follow appendicitis, empyema of the gallbladder, diverticulitis, regional enteritis [11], *Yersinia* ileitis [12], perforated gastric or colonic ulcers, leaking anastomoses, pancreatitis [13] or infected haemorrhoids.

Neonatal umbilical sepsis may spread to the portal vein with subsequent liver abscesses.

Injury to the *hepatic arterial system* may lead to liver abscesses. This can follow cholecystectomy. In liver transplant patients, abscesses may develop 2 weeks postoperatively associated with technical complications, particularly hepatic arterial thrombosis. Abscesses may follow local treatment of liver tumours by transhepatic chemoembolization or percutaneous tumour injections [14]. They may also follow therapeutic hepatic arterial catheterization to treat colonic cancer metastases [15].

Increase in the incidence of liver abscesses may also be related to the number of severely *immunosuppressed patients*. These include those post-transplant, and those with leukaemia receiving chemotherapy [16].

Traumatic causes include penetrating wounds or blunt trauma from road traffic accidents.

A solitary liver abscess may follow *direct spread* from an adjacent septic focus such as a perinephric abscess.

Diabetes is present in up to 40% of cases and is more commonly associated with abscesses due to *Klebsiella pneumoniae* [8,17].

About one half of abscesses are *cryptogenic*. This is especially so in the elderly.

Infecting agents

The causative bacteria (Table 32.1) depend upon the source of initial infection. Those causing abscesses asso-

Table 32.1. Organisms isolated from pyogenic liver abscesses

Aerobes
  Escherichia coli
  Klebsiella pneumoniae and other species
  Enterobacter spp.
  Pseudomonas spp.
  Staphylococcus aureus
  Streptococci:
    Group D
    α-haemolytic
    Microaerophilic
  Enterococcus spp.
  Yersinia enterocolitica
  Listeria monocytogenes
  Salmonella spp.
  Gardnerella vaginalis
Anaerobes
  Bacteroides fragilis
  Bacteroides spp.
  Fusobacterium spp.
  Clostridium perfringens
  Clostridium septicum
  Peptococcus spp.
  Actinomyces spp.
Yeasts

ciated with biliary disease and intra-abdominal sepsis are derived from the gut and include *Escherichia coli*, *Streptococcus faecalis*, *Klebsiella pneumoniae* and *Proteus vulgaris*. Such abscesses are frequently polymicrobial and often include anaerobes. Liver abscesses associated with biliary stents may contain resistant *Klebsiella*, *Enterobacter* and *Pseudomonas* species.

Systemic bacteraemia usually causes single-organism abscesses, which are often multiple. Organisms include the *Streptococcus milleri* group, which are microaerophilic organisms, *Staphylococcus aureus* and *Klebsiella pneumoniae* [10].

Rare causes include *Yersinia enterocolitica* [12] and *Brucella* species.

The abscess may be sterile, but this is usually due to previous antibiotic therapy or to inadequate, particularly anaerobic, culture techniques.

Pathology

The enlarged liver may contain multiple yellow abscesses, of variable size, or a single abscess encased in fibrous tissue and usually found in the right lobe. With pylephlebitis, the portal vein and its branches contain pus and blood clots. There may be perihepatitis or adhesion formation. A chronic liver abscess may persist for as long as 2 years before death or diagnosis. In biliary-associated cases, multiple foci correspond to the intrahepatic bile duct system.

Small pyaemic abscesses may also be found in lung, kidney, brain or spleen. Direct extension from the liver may lead to subphrenic or pleuropulmonary suppuration. Extension to the peritoneum or rupture of a sinus pointing under the skin are rare. A small amount of ascites may be present.

Histologically, areas remote from the abscess show portal zone infection and surrounding disintegrating hepatocytes being infiltrated by polymorphs.

Clinical features

Features such as diabetes, biliary disease, malignancy or immunosuppressive states are important comorbidities.

Presentation is with abdominal pain and fever with features of a space-occupying lesion in the liver.

The onset may be insidious and diagnosis delayed for at least 1 month. A single abscess is often insidious and cryptogenic, especially in the elderly. Multiple abscesses are more acute and the cause is more often identified. Subdiaphragmatic irritation or pleuropulmonary spread leads to right shoulder tip pain and to an irritable cough. The liver is enlarged and tender and the pain is accentuated by percussion over the lower ribs.

Jaundice is late unless there is biliary disease. However, it is more common than with amoebic abscess.

Recovery may be followed by portal hypertension due to thrombosis of the portal vein.

A neutrophil leucocytosis is usual and C-reactive protein and serum alkaline phosphatase are usually raised.

Blood cultures may grow the causative organism or organisms [18].

Localization of the abscess

Ultrasound distinguishes a solid from a fluid-filled lesion (Fig. 32.1). *Computed tomography (CT) scanning* is particularly valuable (Fig. 32.2) although false negatives can be due to lesions near the dome of the liver and to microabscesses. Multiple small abscesses may aggregate, suggesting the beginning of coalescence into single larger abscesses (*cluster sign*) [19].

Magnetic resonance imaging (MRI) shows a lesion with sharp borders, hypointense on T_1-weighting, and hyperintense on a T_2-weighted image. Appearances are not specific or diagnostic of a biliary or haematogenous origin [20].

MR or endoscopic cholangiography may be used to diagnose cholangitic abscesses.

Aspirated material is positive on culture in 70–90% [18]. It should be cultured aerobically, anaerobically and in a carbon dioxide-enriched atmosphere for the *Streptococcus milleri* group. Organisms in culture-negative pus may be identifiable using 16S PCR and sequencing of the

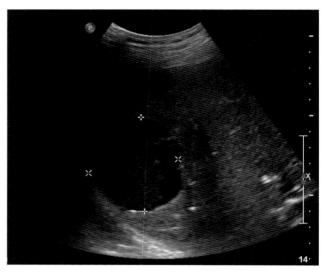

Fig. 32.1. Ultrasound of a pyogenic liver abscess shows a low-density lesion containing echogenic material which is pus and necrotic tissue. Acoustic enhancement beyond the lesion is characteristic.

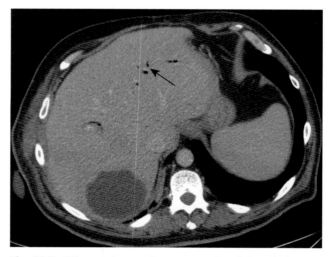

Fig. 32.2. CT scan shows a low attenuation defect in the right lobe of the liver. Note gas in bile ducts (arrow).

product. Rarely, aseptic abscesses occur in patients with inflammatory bowel disease (usually in association with splenic abscesses) and these appear to be non-infective in origin [21].

Treatment

Management has been revolutionized by the widespread use of imaging, especially ultrasound, allowing localization and easy aspiration for both diagnostic and therapeutic purposes (Fig. 32.3). The majority of abscesses can be managed by systemic antibiotics and aspiration, which may need to be repeated [22].

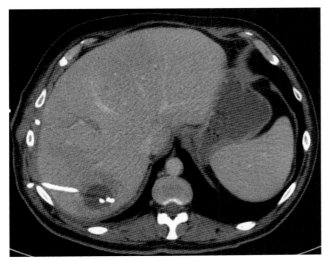

Fig. 32.3. Same patient as in Fig. 32.2 after directed puncture and drainage. The abscess is smaller and with antibiotic treatment resolved.

Intravenous antibiotics are rarely effective alone. Drainage is indicated if signs of sepsis persist. Open surgical drainage is rarely indicated [23]. However, solitary left-sided abscess may require surgical drainage, especially in children [24].

With multiple abscesses, the largest is aspirated and the smaller lesions usually resolve with antibiotics. Occasionally, percutaneous drainage of each is necessary.

Every attempt should be made to make a microbiological diagnosis as this will influence the choice of antimicrobial therapy. Polymicrobial infections may require combination therapy, although antimicrobials such as co-amoxiclav and piperacillin/ tazobactam are often suitable. The increasing incidence of infections caused by resistant Gram-negative organisms means that therapeutic decisions are difficult and these cases should be managed in conjunction with a microbiologist or infectious diseases physician. Therapy is likely to be required for at least 3 weeks. Intravenous therapy for 2 weeks, followed by 4 weeks of oral treatment has been shown to be effective [25,26].

Biliary obstruction must be relieved, usually by endoscopic retrograde cholangiopancreatography (ERCP), papillotomy and stone removal. If necessary, a biliary stent is inserted (Chapter 12). Even with eventual cure, fever may continue for 1–2 weeks [18].

The aseptic abscesses discussed above usually respond to corticosteroid therapy, although relapse occurs.

Prognosis

Needle aspiration and antibiotic therapy have lowered the mortality in recent years [16,26]. The prognosis is better for a unilocular abscess in the right lobe where survival is around 90%. The outcome for multiple abscesses, especially if biliary in origin, is very poor. The prognosis is worsened by delay in diagnosis, associated disease, particularly malignancy [27], hyperbilirubinaemia, hypoalbuminaemia, pleural effusion and older age [28].

Hepatic amoebiasis

Three species of *Entamoeba* are known to infect humans: *E. histolytica*, *E. dispar* and *E. moshkovskii* [29]. *Entamoeba histolytica* is responsible for significant invasive disease, whereas *E. dispar* has a roughly tenfold greater prevalence. The epidemiology and pathogenicity of *E. moshkovskii* is still poorly understood [29]. Commercial faecal antigen detection assays, using monoclonal antibodies, are available to distinguish *E. histolytica* from the other microscopically identical species.

Entamoeba histolytica exists in a vegetative form and as cysts, which survive outside the body, often for several months, and are highly infectious. The cystic form passes unharmed through the stomach and small intestine and excysts into the vegetative, trophozoite form in the colon. Here, after a variable period of time, which may be many years, it invades the mucosa, forming typical flask-shaped ulcers. Only 10% of those harbouring the parasite develop invasive amoebiasis.

Amoebae are carried to the liver in the portal venous system. Rarely, they pass through the hepatic sinusoids into the systemic circulation with the production of abscesses in lungs and brain.

Amoebae multiply and block small intrahepatic portal radicles with consequent focal infarction of liver cells. They produce a number of proteolytic enzymes which destroy the liver parenchyma. The resultant inflammation and necrosis leads to recruitment of neutrophils and the formation of microabscesses which coalesce. The lesions produced are usually single (in more than 60% of cases) and of variable size.

The amoebic abscess is usually about the size of an orange. The most frequent site is in the right lobe, often superoanteriorly, just below the diaphragm. The centre consists of a large necrotic area which has liquefied into thick, reddish-brown pus. This has been likened to anchovy or chocolate sauce. It is produced by lysis of liver cells. Fragments of liver tissue may be recognized in it. Initially, the abscess has no well-defined wall, but merely shreds of shaggy, necrotic liver tissue.

Histologically, the necrotic areas consist of degenerate liver cells, leucocytes, red blood cells, connective tissue strands and debris. Amoebae may be identified in the abscess wall. Hepatocyte death is by apoptosis, with evidence of activation of both extrinsic and intrinsic pathways [30].

Small lesions heal with scars, but larger abscesses show a chronic wall of connective tissue of varying age.

The lesion is focal and liver away from the abscess or microabscesses is normal.

Secondary bacterial infection of the abscess occurs in about 20%. The pus then becomes green or yellow and foul smelling.

Epidemiology

Colonic amoebae have a worldwide distribution, but hepatic amoebiasis is a disease of the tropics and subtropics. Endemic areas are Africa, south-east Asia, Mexico, Venezuela and Colombia. The majority of abscess cases occur in young adult males.

In temperate climates, symptomless carriers of toxic strains are often found without colonic ulcers. They are frequent commensals in men who have sex with men, although invasive disease is being increasing described in this population in the Far East [31,32].

In the tropics a new arrival is heavily exposed, especially when sanitation is poor. Locals are less prone, presumably because of partial immunity induced by repeated contact.

The latent period between the intestinal infection and hepatic involvement has not been explained.

Clinical features

A history of travel or residence in tropical or subtropical areas is usually elicited. Amoebic dysentery is associated in only 10% and cysts in the stool in only 15%. Past history of dysentery is rare. Hepatic amoebiasis has been recorded as long as 30 years after the primary infection. Multiple abscesses are frequent in such areas as Mexico and Taiwan.

The onset is usually *subacute* with symptoms lasting up to 6 months. Rarely, it may be *acute* with rigors and sweating and a duration of less than 10 days. Fever is variously intermittent, remittent or even absent unless an abscess becomes secondarily infected; it rarely exceeds 40°C. Deep abscesses may present simply as fever without signs referable to the liver.

Jaundice is unusual and, if present, mild. Bile duct compression is rare.

The patient looks ill, with a peculiar sallowness of the skin, like faded suntan.

Pain in the liver area may commence as a dull ache, later becoming sharp and stabbing. If the abscess is near the diaphragm, there may be referred shoulder pain accentuated by deep breathing or coughing. Alcohol makes the pain worse, as do postural changes. The patient tends to lean to the left side; this opens up the right intercostal spaces and diminishes the tension on the liver capsule. The pain increases at night.

A swelling may be visible in the epigastrium or bulging the intercostal spaces. Hepatic tenderness is virtually constant. It may be elicited over a palpable liver edge or by percussion over the lower right chest wall. The spleen is not enlarged.

The lungs may show consolidation of the right lower zone, consolidation or an effusion. Pleural fluid may be blood stained.

Examination of faeces.   Cysts and vegetative forms are rare.

Serological tests

There are a number of test formats for detecting anti-*Entamoeba* antibodies, the commonest being enzyme immunoassay (EIA) and fluorescent antibody assays. IgG antibodies remain positive for some time after clinical cure. Amoebic abscess is unlikely if these tests are negative [33].

Biochemical tests

In chronic cases, serum alkaline phosphatase values are usually about twice normal. Increases in transaminases are found only in those who are acutely ill or with severe complications. A rise in serum bilirubin is unusual except in those with superinfection or rupture into the peritoneum.

Radiological features

Chest X-ray may show a high right diaphragm, obliteration of the costophrenic and cardiophrenic angles by adhesions, pleural effusion or right basal pneumonia. A right lateral abscess may cause widening of the intercostal spaces. The liver shadow may be enlarged with a raised immobile right diaphragm. The abscess commonly causes a bulge in the anteromedial part of the right diaphragm.

An abscess in the left lobe of the liver may produce a crescentic deformity of the lesser curve of the stomach.

Ultrasound scan is the most useful for large abscesses and for follow-up. *CT* shows the abscess with a somewhat irregular edge and low attenuation (Fig. 32.4). It is more sensitive than ultrasound for small abscesses. It may show extrahepatic involvement, for instance in the lung [34].

MRI can also be used for diagnosis and to follow treatment [35]. Liquefaction of the cavity may be shown as early as 4 days after starting treatment [35].

Diagnostic criteria

Diagnostic criteria are:
• History of exposure in an endemic area
• An enlarged, tender liver in a young male

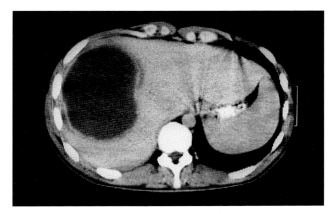

Fig. 32.4. CT scan of the liver in a 21year old man with fever and right upper quadrant pain. Ultrasound scan had not shown a definite abnormality, presumably due to the echogenicity of the pus being close to normal liver. The CT shows a large space-occupying lesion from which 1 litre of pus was drained. This was an infected amoebic abscess.

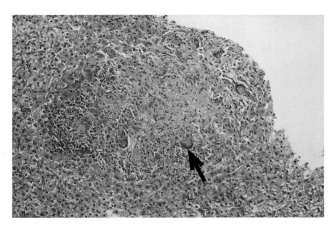

Fig. 32.5. Miliary tuberculosis: a caseating granuloma contains lymphocytes, epithelial cells and numerous giant cells (arrow). There is central caseation.

• Response to metronidazole
• Leucocytosis without anaemia in those with a short history, and less marked leucocytosis and anaemia with a long history
• Suggestive posteroanterior and lateral chest X-ray
• Scanning showing a filling defect
• A positive amoebic fluorescent antibody test.

Complications

Rupture into the lungs or pleura causes empyema, hepatobronchial fistula or pulmonary abscess. The patient coughs up pus, develops pneumonitis or lung abscess or a pleural effusion.

Rupture into the pericardium is a complication of amoebic abscess in the left lobe.

Intraperitoneal rupture results in acute peritonitis. If the patient survives the initial event, long-term results are good. Abscesses of the left lobe may perforate into the lesser sac.

Rupture into the portal vein, bile ducts or gastrointestinal tract is rare.

Secondary infection is suspected if prostration is particularly great, and fever and leucocytosis high. Aspiration reveals yellowish, often fetid, pus and culture reveals the causative organism.

Treatment

Metronidazole, 750mg three times a day for 5–10 days, has a 95% success rate. The time to defervescence is 3–5 days [18]. Failures may be related to the persistence of intestinal amoebiasis, drug resistance or inadequate absorption.

The time taken for the abscess to disappear depends on its size and varies from 10 to 300 days [36].

Aspiration is rarely necessary even with very large abscesses [37]. It should be done under ultrasound or CT guidance. A tense abscess in the left lobe that is likely to rupture into the peritoneum demands aspiration. Other indications are failure to respond after 4–5 days' treatment and secondary bacterial infection [29]. The mortality from amoebic liver abscess should be zero [18].

A course of oral amoebocide, such as diloxanide furoate, should be given to cover amoebae persisting in the gut.

Tuberculosis of the liver

Abdominal tuberculosis is more common in immigrants from developing countries and also increasingly in patients with AIDS [38].

The liver may be involved as part of miliary tuberculosis or as local tuberculosis where evidence of extrahepatic disease is not obvious. Rarely, hepatic tuberculosis can cause fulminant liver failure [39].

The basic lesion is the *granuloma*, which is very frequent in the liver in both pulmonary and extrapulmonary tuberculosis (Fig. 32.5). The lesions usually heal without scarring but sometimes with focal fibrosis and calcification.

Pseudotumoral hepatic *tuberculomas* are rare [40]. There may be no evidence of extrahepatic tuberculosis [41]. The tuberculomas may be multiple, consisting of a white, irregular, caseous abscess surrounded by a fibrous capsule (Fig. 32.6). The distinction from Hodgkin's disease, secondary carcinoma or actinomycosis by naked-eye appearance may be difficult. Occasionally, the necrotic area calcifies.

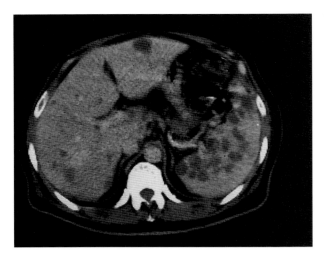

Fig. 32.6. Hepatosplenic tuberculosis. CT scan showing scattered filling defects in the liver and spleen. Aspirate showed acid-fast bacilli and the culture was positive.

Tuberculous cholangitis is extremely rare, resulting from spread of caseous material from the portal tracts into the bile ducts.

Biliary stricture is a rare complication [42].

Tuberculous pylephlebitis results from rupture of caseous material. It is usually rapidly fatal although chronic portal hypertension can result [43].

Tuberculous glands at the hilum may lead rarely to biliary obstruction.

Clinical features

These may be few or absent. The condition may present as a pyrexia of unknown origin, together with the typical features of tuberculosis: night sweats and weight loss. Jaundice may appear in overwhelming miliary tuberculosis, particularly in the racially susceptible. Rarely, multiple caseating granulomas lead to massive hepatosplenomegaly and death in liver failure [39].

Biochemical tests

Serum globulin is increased so that the albumin/globulin ratio is reduced. Alkaline phosphatase is disproportionately elevated [41].

Diagnosis

Initial diagnosis may be difficult, with few features pointing to hepatic involvement in many cases. Tuberculomas in liver and spleen are difficult to differentiate from lymphoma. Liver biopsy is essential. The indications are unexplained fever and weight loss with hepatomegaly or hepatosplenomegaly. A portion of the biopsy should be stained for acid-fast bacilli and cul-

tured. Positives are obtained in about 50%. The diagnosis may be expedited by the use of PCR. The patient may have other supportive evidence of tuberculosis, such as a positive tuberculin or interferon-γ release test, although these are insufficient to distinguish active tuberculosis from latent disease [44].

A *plain X-ray* of the abdomen may reveal hepatic calcification. This may be multiple and confluent in tuberculoma, discrete and scattered and of uniform size, or large and chalky adjoining a stricture in the common bile duct [45].

CT may show a lobulated mass or multiple filling defects in liver and spleen (Fig. 32.6).

Extrahepatic features of tuberculosis may not be obvious.

Treatment is that for extrapulmonary tuberculosis, with four agents for the first 2 months (usually rifampicin, isoniazid, pyrazinamide and ethambutol) followed by two agents for at least a further 4 months [46].

The effect on the liver of tuberculosis elsewhere

Amyloidosis may complicate chronic tuberculosis. Fatty change is due to wasting and toxaemia. Drug jaundice may follow therapy, especially with isoniazid, rifampicin and pyrazinamide, and may result in fulminant hepatic failure.

Other mycobacteria

Atypical mycobacteria can produce a granulomatous hepatitis, particularly as part of the AIDS syndrome (see Chapter 22). *Mycobacterium scrofulaceum* can cause a granulomatous hepatitis, characterized by a rise in alkaline phosphatase, tiredness and low-grade fever. Isolation of the organism requires liver biopsy culture [47]. Treatment is usually with non-standard regimens and depends upon susceptibility results.

Hepatic actinomycosis

Hepatic involvement due to *Actinomyces* species is usually a sequel to intestinal actinomycosis, especially of the caecum and appendix, occurring in 15% of cases of abdominal actinomycosis [48]. It spreads by direct extension or, more often, via the portal vein, but can be primary. Large greyish-white masses, superficially resembling malignant metastases, soften and form collections of pus, separated by fibrous tissue bands, simulating a honeycomb. The liver becomes adherent to adjacent viscera and to the abdominal wall, with the formation of sinuses. These lesions contain the characteristic 'sulphur granules', which consist of branching, Gram-positive filaments with eosinophilic, clubbed ends. It should be noted that the infection is mixed (particularly with other anaerobes) in more than 30% of cases [49].

Clinical features

The patient is often toxic, febrile, sweating, wasted and anaemic. There is local, sometimes irregular, enlargement of the liver with tenderness of one or both lobes. The overlying skin may have the livid, dusky hue seen over a taut abscess that is about to rupture. Multiple, irregular sinus tracks develop. Similar sinuses may develop from the ileocaecal site or from the chest wall if there is pleuropulmonary extension.

Diagnosis

The diagnosis should be suspected in patients developing sinus tracts, and the organism can be isolated from the pus. If actinomycosis is suspected before this stage, percutaneous liver biopsy may reveal sulphur granules with typical organisms [50].

Early presentation is as pyrexia, hepatosplenomegaly and anaemia. It may be months before multiple abscesses are detected, often by ultrasound, CT [51] or MRI [52]. Anaerobic blood cultures may be positive.

Treatment

Intravenous penicillin in high doses is the mainstay of treatment. Alternative agents are doxycycline and clindamycin. Therapy is usually needed for at least 4 weeks and continuation with oral therapy after this time may be appropriate [49]. However, additional, or alternative agents may be needed to cover other bacteria in those with mixed infections, at least for the initial period. Surgical resection may be necessary [53].

Syphilis of the liver

Congenital

The fetal liver is heavily infected by any transplacental infection. It is firm, enlarged and swarming with spirochaetes. Initially, there is a diffuse hepatitis, but gradually fibrous tissue is laid down between the liver cells and in the portal zones, and this leads to a true pericellular cirrhosis.

Since hepatic involvement is but an incident in a widespread spirochaetal septicaemia, the clinical features are seldom those of the liver disease. The fetus may be stillborn or die soon after birth. If the infant survives, other manifestations of congenital syphilis are obvious, apart from the hepatosplenomegaly and mild jaundice. In recent years, syphilis is a rare cause of neonatal jaundice.

In older children who have survived without this florid neonatal picture, the hepatic lesion may be a gumma.

Diagnosis can be confirmed by blood serology, which is always positive.

Secondary

In the secondary septicaemic stage, spirochaetes produce miliary granulomas [54].

Fifty per cent of sufferers have raised serum enzyme levels [55], although clinical hepatitis is rare. However, sometimes the picture is of severe cholestatic jaundice [56].

Serology is positive with raised reagin (VDRL or RPR assays) and syphilis-specific antibody titres. Serum alkaline phosphatase levels are high. The M1 cardiolipin fluorescent antimitochondrial antibody is positive and becomes normal with recovery [56].

Liver biopsy shows non-specific changes with moderate infiltration with polymorphs and lymphocytes, and some hepatocellular disarray, but cholestasis is absent or mild except in the severely cholestatic patients [56]. Portal-to-central zone necrosis can be seen (Fig. 32.7). Spirochaetes are sometimes detected in the liver biopsy if special stains are used.

Tertiary

Gummas may be single or multiple. They are usually in the right lobe. They consist of a caseous mass with a fibrous capsule. Healing is followed by deep scars and coarse lobulation (*hepar lobatum*).

Hepatic gummas are usually diagnosed incidentally, by ultrasound or CT, at surgery or at autopsy. Ultrasound-guided biopsy of a nodule shows aseptic necrosis, granulomas and spirochaetes [57]. Serology is positive. Antibiotic treatment is successful.

Treatment

All cases of syphilis should be managed in conjunction with a genitourinary physician. First-line treatment remains penicillin in the form of benzathine or procaine penicillin (or benzylpenicillin in the case of congenital syphilis). Alternative agents include other beta-lactams, doxycycline and macrolides [58].

Jaundice complicating penicillin treatment

Rarely, the patient shows an idiosyncrasy to penicillin. Jaundice, chills and fever, often with a rash (*erythema of Milan*), occur about 9 days after starting therapy. This is part of the Herxheimer reaction. The mechanism of the jaundice is unclear.

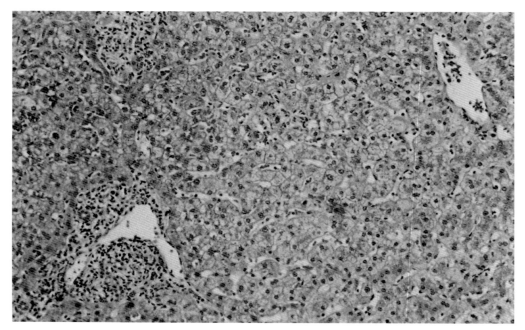

Fig. 32.7. Liver in secondary syphilis. Mononuclear cell infiltration can be seen in portal zones and in the sinusoids. (H & E, ×160.)

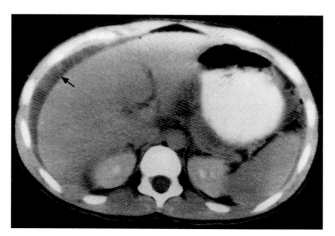

Fig. 32.8. CT in chlamydial perihepatitis shows 'violin string' adhesions between liver and anterior abdominal wall (arrowed) and ascites.

Perihepatitis

This upper abdominal peritonitis is associated with genital infections, particularly those due to *Chlamydia trachomatis* and less often, *Neisseria gonorrhoeae* [59]. It affects young, sexually active women and simulates biliary tract disease. Diagnosis is by laparoscopy. The liver surface shows white plaques, tiny haemorrhagic spots and 'violin string' adhesions.

CT may also show 'violin string' adhesions (Fig. 32.8) [60]. Treatment is as for pelvic inflammatory disease, usually with a combination of a third-generation cephalosporin and doxycycline [61].

Leptospirosis

Pathogenic *Leptospira* related to human disease can be classified by DNA typing into 250 serovars belonging to 24 serogroups [62]. The disease due to *Leptospira icterohaemorrhagiae* was described by Weil in 1886 [63]. It is a severe infection spread by the urine of infected rats. The whole group of leptospiral infections should be designated leptospirosis.

Weil's disease

Mode of infection

Living *Leptospira* are continually excreted in the urine of infected rats and survive for months in pools, canals, flood water or damp soil. The patient is infected by contaminated water or by direct occupational contact with infected rats. Those affected include participants in water sports, agricultural and sewer workers and fish cutters. Cities in Europe, South and Central America and Asia (such as the favelas of Brazil), where rat populations are expanding, provide a source of infection [64]. The disease is most prevalent in late summer and autumn in temperate regions.

Pathology

Histopathological changes are slight in relation to the marked functional impairment of kidneys and liver. The damage is at a subcellular level. Non-esterified fatty acids from the cell wall of the spirochaetes have been

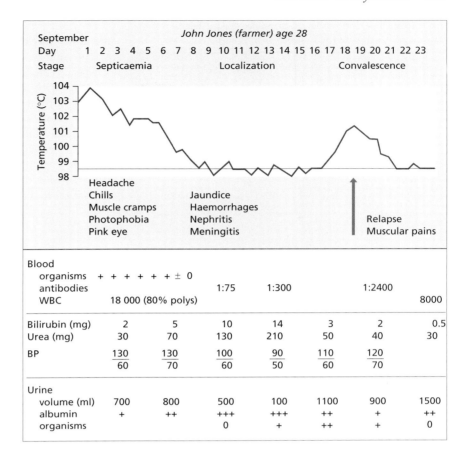

Fig. 32.9. The clinical course of a patient with Weil's disease.

suggested to play an important role in the development of acute tubular necrosis, and outer membrane protein extracts have been shown to stimulate a proinflammatory cytokine response via TLR2 receptors in the renal tubules [65]. Plasma tumour necrosis factor-α (TNF-α) levels have been related to the severity of organ involvement [66].

Liver necrosis is minimal and focal [67]. Zone 3 necrosis is absent. Active hepatocellular regeneration, shown by mitoses and nuclear polyploidy, is out of proportion to cell damage. Swollen Kupffer cells contain leptospiral debris. Leucocyte infiltration and bile thrombi are prominent in the deeply jaundiced. Cirrhosis is not a sequel.

The kidneys shows tubular necrosis and interstitial nephritis.

Skeletal muscle shows punctate haemorrhages and focal necrosis.

The heart may show haemorrhages in all layers.

Haemorrhage into tissues, especially skin and lungs, is due to capillary injury and thrombocytopenia.

Jaundice is related to hepatocyte dysfunction magnified by renal failure impairing urinary bilirubin excretion. Tissue haemorrhages and haemolysis increase the bilirubin load on the liver. Hypotension with diminished hepatic blood flow contributes.

Clinical features (Fig. 32.9)

The clinical picture is not pathognomonic and the disease is heavily under-diagnosed. It is more often anicteric than icteric. The incubation period is 2–14 days [68]. The course may be divided into three stages: the first or septicaemic phase lasts for about 7 days, the second or toxic stage for a similar period, and the third or convalescent period begins in the third week.

The first or febrile stage is marked by the presence of the spirochaete in the circulating blood.

The onset is abrupt, with prostration, high fever and even rigors. The temperature rises rapidly to 39.5–40.5°C and falls by lysis within 3–10 days.

Abdominal pain, nausea and vomiting may simulate an acute abdominal emergency, and severe muscular pains, especially in the back or calves, are common.

Central nervous system involvement is shown by severe headache, mental confusion and sometimes meningism. The cerebrospinal fluid confirms meningeal involvement. If jaundice is present, there is xanthochromia.

The eyes show a characteristic suffusion.

In those with severe disease, bleeding may occur from nose, gut or lung, with skin petechiae or ecchymoses.

Table 32.2. The differential diagnosis of Weil's disease from viral hepatitis during the first week of illness

	Weil's disease	Viral hepatitis
Onset	Sudden	Gradual
Headache	Constant	Occasional
Muscle pains	Severe	Mild
Conjunctival injection	Present	Absent
Prostration	Great	Mild
Disorientation	Common	Rare
Haemorrhagic diathesis	Common	Rare
Nausea and vomiting	Present	Present
Abdominal discomfort	Common	Common
Bronchitis	Common	Rare
Albuminuria	Present	Absent
Leucocyte count	Polymorph leucocytosis	Leucopenia with lymphocytosis

Pneumonitis with cough, sore throat and rhonchi occurs in 40% of sufferers and in some cases this may progress to haemorrhagic pulmonary disease (severe pulmonary haemorrhage syndrome) or adult respiratory distress syndrome (ARDS).

Jaundice appears between the fourth and seventh day in 80% of patients. It is a grave sign, for the disease is never fatal in the absence of icterus. The liver is enlarged, but not the spleen.

The urine shows albumin and bile pigment. The stools are well coloured.

There is a leucocytosis of $10–30 \times 10^9$/L with a relative increase in polymorphs. Thrombocytopenia may be profound and other clotting abnormalities may be present, such as a prolonged prothrombin time [69].

The second or icteric stage in the second week is characterized by a normal temperature but without clinical improvement. This is the stage of deepening jaundice, with increasing renal and myocardial failure. Albuminuria persists, there is a rising blood urea, and oliguria may proceed to anuria. Death may be due to renal failure. A markedly elevated creatinine phosphokinase level reflects myositis.

Severe prostration is accompanied by a low blood pressure and a dilated heart. There may be transient cardiac dysrhythmias and electrocardiograms may show a prolonged P–R or Q–T interval, with T-wave changes. Death may be due to circulatory failure.

During this stage, the *Leptospira* can be found in the urine, and rising antibody titres demonstrated in the serum.

The third or convalescent stage starts at the beginning of the third week. Clinical improvement is shown by a brightening of the mental state, fading of the jaundice, a rise in blood pressure and an increased urinary volume, with a drop in the blood urea concentration. Albuminuria is slow to disappear.

Temperature may rise during the third week (Fig. 32.9), associated with muscle pains. Such relapses occur in 20% of cases.

There is great variation in the clinical course ranging from a mild illness, clinically indistinguishable from influenza, to a prostrating, fatal disease with anuria.

Diagnosis

Before the appearance of antibodies, PCR demonstration of *Leptospira* is the best method of diagnosis [70].

Rising titres of antibodies are sought by Dot-enzyme-linked immunosorbent assay (ELISA) [71] or immunofluorescence [72]. The microscopic agglutination test is considered the gold standard assay and is usually performed by reference laboratories [73].

Leptospira may be cultured from blood during the first 10 days. Urine cultures are positive during the second week and persist for several months. Culture is laborious and less sensitive than molecular methods, but allows serovar identification, that is serological typing using serum-containing antibodies against different antigens.

Liver function tests are non-contributory.

Differential diagnosis

In the early stages, Weil's disease may be confused with septicaemic bacterial infections or typhus fever. When jaundice is evident acute viral hepatitis must be excluded (Table 32.2). Important distinguishing points are the sudden-onset, increased polymorph count and albuminuria of Weil's disease.

Spirochaetal jaundice would be diagnosed more often if blood samples for antibodies were taken from patients with obscure icterus and fever.

Prognosis

Mortality varies from less than 1% to more than 20% [73]. This depends on the depth of jaundice, renal and myocardial involvement, and the extent of haemorrhages. Death is usually due to renal failure. The mortality is negligible in non-icteric patients, and is lower in those under 30 years old. Since many mild infections are probably unrecognized, the overall mortality may be considerably less.

Although transient relapses in the third and fourth weeks are common, final recovery is complete.

Prevention

Protective clothing should be provided for workers in industries with a high incidence of Weil's disease, and adequate measures taken to control rodents. Bathing in stagnant water should be avoided.

Treatment

Early, mild leptospirosis may be treated by doxycycline (100 mg by mouth) twice daily for 1 week. More seriously ill patients, particularly with vomiting, may be treated with high-dose benzylpenicillin or cephalosporins for 1 week [74,75]. Aminoglycosides and macrolides have also been successfully used [73].

Prognosis is improving with earlier diagnosis, attention to fluid and electrolyte balance, renal dialysis, antibiotics and circulatory support.

Other types of leptospirosis

In general, these infections are less severe than those due to *L. icterohaemorrhagiae*. *L. canicola* infection, for example, is characterized by headache, meningitis and conjunctival infection. Albuminuria is only found in 40%, and jaundice in only 18% of patients. The frequent presentation is that of 'benign aseptic meningitis'. The disease affects young adults who have usually been in close contact with an infected dog. Fatalities in humans are virtually unknown.

Diagnosis is confirmed in a similar way to Weil's disease. The spinal fluid shows a lymphocytic picture in most cases.

Relapsing fever

This arthropod-borne infection is caused by spirochaetes of the genus *Borrelia*. *Borrelia recurrentis* is the cause of louse-borne relapsing fever, now only found in Ethiopia and surrounding countries, whereas tick-borne relapsing fever is caused by at least 15 different *Borrelia* species around the world and is reported in North and South America, Africa, Asia and Europe.

The *Borrelia* multiply in the liver, invading liver cells and causing focal necrosis. Just before the crisis the *Borrelia* roll up and are ingested by reticuloendothelial cells. Surviving *Borrelia* remain in the liver, spleen, brain and bone marrow until the next relapse [76]. Subsequent immune 'escape' is due to *vmp* antigenic variation [77].

Clinical features [78]

The incubation period is 4–14 days. The onset is acute with chills, a continuous high temperature, headache, muscle pains and profound prostration. The patient is flushed, sometimes with injected conjunctivae, and epistaxes. In severe attacks, tender hepatosplenomegaly and jaundice develop. The jaundice is similar to that of Weil's disease. Sometimes a rash develops on the trunk. There may be bronchitis.

These symptoms continue for 4–9 days and then the temperature falls, often with collapse of the patient. This may be fatal, but more usually the symptoms and signs then rapidly abate, the patient remains afebrile for about 1 week, when there is a relapse. There may be a second or even a third milder relapse before the disease ends.

Diagnosis

Spirochaetes can rarely be found in thick blood films and molecular methods are increasingly being used [79]. Agglutination and complement fixation tests are available [76]. Organisms may be identified by lymph node aspiration, or from the insect bite site.

Treatment

Tetracyclines and streptomycin are more effective than penicillin. Erythromycin and ceftriaxone are also effective [77]. Mortality is 2–5% without treatment.

Lyme disease

This is due to a tick-borne spirochaete, *Borrelia burgdorferi*. It has been reported to cause hepatitis with numerous liver cell mitoses [80] and also granulomatous hepatitis [81]. Mild liver function test abnormalities are frequent in the early erythema migrans stage, but these resolve with antibiotic treatment [82]. Lyme disease does not seem to cause permanent hepatic sequelae.

Rickettsial infections

Q fever

This disease usually has predominantly pulmonary manifestations. Although frank jaundice is uncommon, hepatomegaly and elevated aminotransferases are common and clinical features may mimic anicteric viral hepatitis [83,84,85].

The liver shows a granulomatous hepatitis. Portal areas contain abundant lymphocytes and the limiting plate is destroyed. Kupffer cells are hypertrophied. The granulomas have a characteristic ring of fibrinoid necrosis surrounded by lymphocytes and histiocytes. In the centre of the granuloma is a clear space giving a 'doughnut' appearance (Fig. 32.10). The diagnosis is made by showing a rising titre of antibodies to *Coxiella burnetii* 2–3 weeks after the infection. Indirect

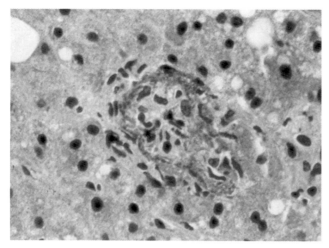

Fig. 32.10. Liver biopsy in Q fever showing a granuloma with fibrin rings having a clear centre. (Martius scarlet blue, ×350.)

immunofluorescence is the reference method for antibody detection, but ELISA and complement fixation tests are also used.

Treatment of the acute disease is with doxycycline, macrolides or fluoroquinolones.

Rocky mountain spotted fever

Jaundice and rises in serum enzymes sometimes occur. Liver histology shows portal zone inflammation with large mononuclear cells. Hepatocellular necrosis is inconspicuous but erythrophagocytosis is marked. Rickettsiae may be demonstrated in the portal zones by immunofluorescence microscopy [86].

Diagnosis is by means of serology, usually with the indirect immunofluorescent test, and PCR assays appear less sensitive for blood samples. Treatment is with tetracyclines or chloramphenicol [87].

Infection with *Bartonella henselae*

This is a bacterium related to the rickettsia and is the cause of cat scratch disease. It also causes peliosis hepatis, the hepatic form of bacillary angiomatosis, a proliferative vascular condition. The disease is characterized by hepatic nodules, biopsy of which reveals neovascular proliferative lesions containing the organism [88]. The infection is typically seen in the AIDS population or other immunosuppressed patients such as organ transplant recipients or those with malignances. The condition typically presents with fever, weight loss, abdominal pain, hepatosplenomegaly and occasionally jaundice.

CT shows focal hepatic defects and mediastinal and periportal lymphadenopathy. The disease may be diagnosed by the detection of antibodies by immunofluorescent assay (IFA).

The recommended treatment is with doxycycline plus either erythromycin or rifampicin. Alternative agents include clarithromycin and ciprofloxacin [89].

Fungal infections

Opportunistic fungal infections

These usually affect the immunocompromised, including sufferers from AIDS, acute leukaemia [90], cancer [91] and following transplantation.

The liver may be involved in disseminated infection, together with other organs, particularly kidney, spleen, heart, lungs and brain. Fever with a raised serum transaminase or alkaline phosphatase indicates needle liver biopsy.

Ultrasound shows multiple hypoechoic areas throughout the liver and spleen, often with a target (bull's eye) configuration [92]. *CT* shows multiple, non-enhancing, low-attenuation lesions [90]. The scanning appearances are not diagnostic.

The histological picture is usually granulomatous and a fungal aetiology may be identified by appropriate stains and cultures, so allowing selection of appropriate antifungal treatment [93,94].

The liver is affected in up to three-quarters of those with disseminated *Candida albicans* infection who come to autopsy [94]. Hepatic granulomas and microabscesses are the commonest histological lesions. *Candida* can be demonstrated in the liver on microscopy but are difficult to culture in this disease [95]. Two forms of disseminated candidiasis are described: acute (ADC) and chronic (CDC). Acute disease is usually characterized by an accompanying rash and CDC is typically seen in a patient undergoing an allogenic haematopoietic stem cell transplant on engraftment. The treatment for either form is with fluconazole. Alternative agents include lipid-associated amphotericin B, a different triazole, for example voriconazole, or an echinocandin, such as caspofungin.

Disseminated aspergillosis may affect the severely immunocompromised patient, usually following an initial respiratory tract infection [96]. Mortality in some of these patient groups is greater than 50% [97]. Treatment is with an extended spectrum triazole, such as voriconazole, lipid associated amphotericin B, or an echinocandin [98].

Hepatic cryptococcosis usually affects the immunocompromised but sometimes it may be seen in the otherwise apparently normal host. Liver biopsy shows granulomas with yeast-like (usually encapsulated) organisms. The picture may resemble sclerosing cholangitis when bile is positive for the fungus. Treatment is usually with a formulation of amphotericin B plus flucytosine, at least initially, followed by fluconazole.

Pathogenic/endemic fungal infections

These infections can occur in the apparently normal host who has been exposed where the disease is endemic. Some patients may suffer onset of disease following latent infection acquired previously in an endemic area. Diagnosis may be made on culture of the causative organism from affected tissue or by means of serology.

Histoplasmosis may disseminate from a primary lung infection and cause a granulomatous infection of the liver. Other affected organs include the adrenals, kidneys and spleen. The organism may be detected in blood cultures and there is a specific urinary antigen assay. Treatment is with itraconazole or an amphotericin B formulation and adrenal support may be necessary in the initial phases [99].

Disseminated coccidioidomycosis may involve the liver in the severely immunocompromised [100].

Blastomyces dermatitidis may cause cholangitis in the elderly or immunocompromised [101].

These latter two diseases are treated with itraconazole or amphotericin B.

Schistosomiasis (bilharzia)

Hepatic schistosomiasis is usually a complication of the intestinal disease, since emboli of *Schistosoma* ova reach the liver from the intestines via the mesenteric veins. *S. mansoni* and *S. japonicum* affect the liver. *S. haematobium* typically involves the bladder and urinary tract but can sometimes involve the liver.

Schistosomiasis affects more than 200 million people in 74 countries. *S. japonicum* is prevalent in Japan, China, Indonesia and the Philippines. *S. mansoni* is found in Africa, the Middle East, the Caribbean and Brazil [102].

Pathogenesis

Eggs, excreted in the faeces, hatch out in water to release free-swimming embryos which enter appropriate snails and develop into fork-tailed cercariae. These re-enter human skin in contact with infected water, provoking an IgE-mediated dermatitis. They burrow down to the capillary bed, whence there is widespread haematogenous dissemination. Those reaching the mesenteric capillaries enter the intrahepatic portal system, where they grow rapidly. Katayama syndrome is the immune-complex-mediated reaction to early egg deposition.

The extent and severity of chronic liver disease correlates with the intensity and duration of egg production and hence with the number of eggs excreted. Adult male and female worms can exist for about 5 years, producing 300–3000 eggs daily in portal venules. If liver disease is advanced, faecal egg counts may fall because of senescence of adult worms or previous therapy.

S. japonicum is more pathogenic than *S. mansoni* (each adult worm pair produces 10 times as many eggs) and produces hepatosplenic schistosomiasis more often and faster.

In the liver, the ova penetrate and obstruct the portal branches and are deposited either in the large radicles, producing the coarser type of bilharzial hepatic fibrosis, or in the small portal tracts, producing the fine diffuse form.

The granulomatous reaction to the *Schistosoma* ovum is of delayed hypersensitivity type, related to antigen released by the egg. Th2-type helper lymphocytes play an important role in granuloma formation , producing IL-4 and IL-13, which determine the size of granulomas and initiate the fibrotic process [103].

Portal fibrosis is related to the adult worm load. The classic, clay-pipestem cirrhosis is due to fibrotic bands originating from the granulomas. Fibrosis may be slowly reversible with treatment.

Wide, irregular, thin-walled arteriolar spaces are found in 85% of cases in the thickened portal tracts. These angiomatoids are useful in distinguishing the bilharzial liver from other forms of hepatic fibrosis. Remnants of ova are also diagnostic. There is little or no bile duct proliferation. Nodular regeneration and disturbance of the hepatic architecture is not sufficient to justify the term 'cirrhosis'.

In areas where schistosomiasis, hepatitis virus B and C coexist, a mixed picture of schistosomal fibrosis with cirrhosis may be seen.

Splenic enlargement is mainly due to portal venous hypertension and reticuloendothelial hyperplasia. Very few ova are found in the spleen. Portal–systemic collateral channels are numerous.

There are associated bilharzial lesions in the intestines and elsewhere. Fifty per cent of patients with rectal schistosomiasis have granulomas in the liver.

Clinical features

Schistosomiasis shows three stages. Itching follows the entry of the cercariae through the skin. This is followed by a stage of fever, urticaria and eosinophilia. Finally, the third stage of deposition of ova results in intestinal, urinary and hepatic involvement.

Initially, the liver and spleen are firm, smooth and easily palpable. This is followed by hepatic fibrosis and eventually portal hypertension which may appear years after the original infection. Oesophageal varices develop. Bleeding episodes are recurrent but rarely fatal.

The liver shrinks in size and the spleen becomes much larger. Dilated abdominal wall veins and a venous hum over the liver are indications of the portal venous obstruction. Ascites and oedema may develop. The blood shows leucopenia and anaemia. The faeces at this stage contain few, if any, parasites.

Patients tolerate blood loss well and hepatic encephalopathy is unusual. Hepatocellular function remains good although there is a large portosystemic collateral circulation.

Aspiration liver biopsy (Fig. 32.11). Eggs or their remnants are seen in 94% of livers from those with faecal eggs. Remnants of ova may be seen but appearances are not usually diagnostic and the liver biopsy mainly excludes other types of liver disease.

Diagnostic tests

Detection of ova in urine, stool or rectal mucosal biopsy (rectal 'snip') is still the accepted method of diagnosing active infection (Fig. 32.12). Bleeding may be a complication of rectal biopsy in those with portal hypertension. *Serological antibody tests* indicate past exposure and antibodies may persist after parasitological cure.

Detection of circulating schistosomal antigen indicates active disease. An ELISA for detecting circulating soluble egg antigens in serum correlates with egg output [104,105].

CT shows dense bands following the portal vein to the liver edge; these enhance with contrast [106,107].

Ultrasound shows greatly thickened portal veins (Fig. 32.13). It may be used to grade fibrosis [108]. Liver, spleen, periportal and pancreatic lymph nodes are diffusely enlarged without evidence of portal hypertension.

Colour Doppler shows an increase in blood flow velocity in the portal and superior mesenteric varices and the development of collaterals [109].

Portal hypertension

This is presinusoidal and related to the portal granulomas. As the portal venous blood flow falls, hepatic arterial blood flow increases so that total hepatic blood flow is not significantly reduced. Retrograde flow develops in the portal vein [110].

At the stage of haemorrhage from varices the granulomatous reaction may have subsided and the picture is predominantly that of fibrosis.

Biochemical changes

Serum alkaline phosphatase may be raised. Hypoalbuminaemia can be related to poor nutrition and to the effects of repeated gastrointestinal haemorrhages. Serum transaminases are virtually normal.

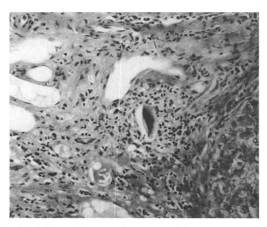

Fig. 32.11. Bilharzial liver. An ovum of *S. mansoni* has lodged in a portal tract which shows a granulomatous reaction. (H & E, ×64.)

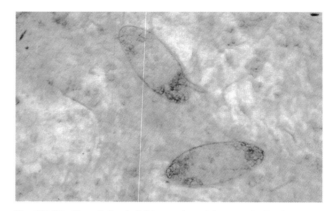

Fig. 32.12. Rectal ('snip') biopsy in schistosomiasis. A 'squash' preparation in glycerol reveals the ova of *S. mansoni*.

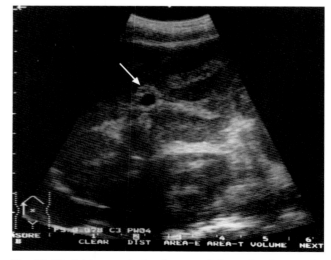

Fig. 32.13. Schistosomiasis: ultrasound shows bright portal tracts and a portal vein with a greatly thickened wall (arrow).

Disease association

The prognosis is worsened by concomitant hepatitis B or hepatitis C infection.

When associated with an immunosuppressed state, granuloma formation is reduced.

Treatment

Chemotherapy aims to relieve symptoms and prevent further deposition of the eggs which will produce further fibrosis. If egg excretion is stopped, the life cycle of the parasite is blocked. Chemotherapy reduces community transmission of disease.

Praziquantel has high therapeutic activity against all species of *Schistosoma* and is the mainstay of treatment. It is safe and non-toxic in a single dose of 40–75 mg/kg orally. The drug paralyses the worm which migrates in the blood stream to the liver where it is attacked by phagocytes, granulocytes and cell-mediated immune cells. It decreases messenger RNA levels of the major proteins associated with fibrosis [111]. Cure rates of 60–90% are obtained and patients who continue to excrete eggs are usually cured by a second course of treatment [105].

Metrifonate is an organophosphate compound, effective only in *S. haematobium* infection. It is given orally and has negligible toxicity. However, it is not currently available.

Oxamniquine 20 mg/kg per day for 3 days is effective only against *S. mansoni*. South American strains are less sensitive than North or South African and larger doses may be required. It is expensive and well tolerated. Side effects include dizziness, drowsiness and headache.

Artemether is effective in acute schistosomiasis and may be useful in transmission control.

Disease control

This is by health education and reducing contamination of water. Attacks on the snails are limited by cost, the need to repeat over long periods and the effects on fish.

Mass treatment by drugs such as praziquantel is limited by cost. Artemether has been used to reduce new infections during the transmission season and can be used for specific populations (such as flood relief workers) in areas where the disease is endemic [112].

Vaccines

Schistosomal antigens have been identified and used as the basis of vaccines, but so far none has progressed beyond phase II trials [103].

Bleeding oesophageal varices

A single bleed is rarely fatal although bleeding is the primary cause of death in these patients. It is usually controlled by sclerotherapy or variceal banding and reduced by propranolol prophylaxis (Chapter 9). Distal splenorenal shunt is preferred over total shunts. Gastro-oesophageal devascularization with splenectomy may be the procedure of choice [110] as it has a low mortality and encephalopathy rate. Transjugular intrahepatic portosystemic shunt (TIPS) may be a satisfactory alternative, but post-shunt jaundice is enhanced.

Malaria [113]

Although the liver is involved in malaria and severely ill patients may become jaundiced, there is no direct or specific liver pathology. In the *erythrocytic stage*, the parasite is engulfed by reticuloendothelial cells. The liver suffers from the general effects of the toxaemia and pyrexia [114].

In the *pre-erythrocytic* (exoerythrocytic) stage, schizogony takes place in the liver without obvious effect on its function. The hepatocyte is invaded by the sporozoite through the formation of the parasitophorous vacuole. The nucleus divides many times and, at last (in about 6–12 days), a spherical or irregular body containing thousands of ripe merozoites is formed. This schizont bursts and the merozoites are discharged into the sinusoids and invade erythrocytes. In quartan or benign tertian malaria, a few merozoites return to the liver cells to initiate the exoerythrocytic or relapse cycle. In malignant tertian, this does not happen and there are no true relapses. The tissue stage of human malaria is confined to the liver cells. The infection of both liver cells and erythrocytes appears to be governed by Haem-oxygenase-1, which is up-regulated during initial invasion. Absence or down-regulation results in proinflammatory cytokine release and termination of infection [115].

Pathology

The liver shows sinusoidal dilatation and congestion, portal infiltration and Kupffer cells proliferation. Focal, non-specific granulomas may be seen in the sinusoids. Brown 'malarial' pigment (iron and haemofuscin) is seen in Kupffer cells. Malarial parasites are not shown. Hepatocyte damage is slight with nuclei of variable size and shape and increased mitoses.

In *P. falciparum* malaria sinusoids may contain parasitized, clumped erythrocytes.

Reaction to the malarial parasite is reticuloendothelial, with minor effects on the liver cells and no fibrosis. The high incidence of cirrhosis in malarial areas is due to other factors.

Clinical features

There are usually no specific hepatic features. Occasionally, in acute malignant malaria, there may be mild jaundice, hepatomegaly and tenderness over the liver.

Hepatic function

Increases in serum bilirubin are rarely above 50 μmol/L (3 mg/dL). Serum transaminases increase slightly and serum globulin concentrations rise.

Kala-azar (visceral leishmaniasis)

Visceral leishmaniasis is primarily a reticuloendothelial disease, involving lymph nodes, liver, spleen and bone marrow. Periportal cellular infiltrations and macrophage accumulations are scattered throughout the liver and within them the Leishman–Donovan bodies may be identified (Fig. 32.14). Mature granuloma formation seems to correlate with resolving infection in the liver [116]. Some portal zone fibrosis has been seen in some cases [117]. The picture is similar in the American, Mediterranean and Oriental types.

Kala-azar presents with fever, splenomegaly, a firm, tender liver, pancytopenia, anaemia and very high serum globulins. The disease may be self resolving but usually runs a chronic course without treatment. Death in advanced disease usually occurs as a result of bacterial sepsis. HIV coinfection is common in endemic areas and relapse after full treatment occurs in more than 50% of such cases. The disease has occurred in liver transplant recipients, but appears uncommon, occurring at a rate of 1 in 800 in patients from an endemic area of Spain [118].

Diagnosis is usually by means of microscopic identification of amastigotes in tissue aspirates or biopsies. Aspiration of the bone marrow is positive in more than 50%. The *Leishmania* direct agglutination antibody test is positive in more than 70% of cases, although sensitivity is much reduced in HIV coinfected cases. Treatment choices lie between pentavalent antimony compounds and liposomal amphotericin B [119]. Miltefosine is an orally active drug which appears to have efficacy approaching that of amphotericin B [120]. Paromomycin is another alternative drug [121].

Hydatid disease

Hydatid disease is due to the larval or cyst stage of infection by the tapeworm, *Echinococcus granulosus*, which lives in dogs. Humans, sheep and cattle are intermediate hosts. There are three other species of *Echinococcus*: *E. multilocularis*, *E. vogeli* and *E. oligarthrus*. The latter two cause cystic disease in South America, whereas *E. granulosus* is the commonest form of disease in the UK and the Northern Hemisphere.

Biology (Fig. 32.15)

Humans are infected by the excreta of dogs, often during childhood. The dog is infected by eating the viscera of sheep, which contain hydatid cysts. Scolices, contained in the cysts, adhere to the small intestine of the dog and become adult worms which attach to the intestinal wall. Each worm sheds 500 ova into the bowel. The infected faeces of the dog contaminate grass and farmland, and the contained ova are ingested by sheep, pigs, camels or humans. The ova adhere to the coats of dogs, so people are infected by handling dogs, as well as by eating contaminated vegetables.

The ova have chitinous envelopes which are dissolved by gastric juice. The liberated ovum burrows through the intestinal mucosa and is carried by the portal vein to the liver, where it develops into an adult cyst. Seventy per cent of hydatid cysts form in the liver. A few ova may pass through the liver and heart, and are held up in the lungs, causing pulmonary cysts. Others may reach the general circulation causing spleen, brain and bone cysts.

Development of the hepatic cyst (Fig. 32.16)

The adult cyst develops slowly from the ovum and provokes a cellular response in which three zones can be distinguished: a peripheral zone of fibroblasts, an intermediate layer of endothelial cells and an inner zone of round cells and eosinophils. The peripheral zone, derived from the host tissues, becomes the *adventitia* or ectocyst, a thick layer which may calcify. The intermediate and inner zones become hyalinized (the *laminated layer*). Finally, the cyst becomes lined with the *germinal layer*, which gives rise to pedunculated nodes of multiplying cells which project into the lumen of the cyst as *brood capsules*. Scolices develop from the brood capsules and eventually indent it. The attachment of the brood capsules to the germinal layer becomes progressively thinner until the capsule bursts, releasing the scolices into the cyst fluid. These fall to the bottom and are termed *hydatid sand*. Cysts may rupture, or become secondarily infected.

Daughter and even grand-daughter cysts develop by fragmentation of the germinal layer. The majority of cysts in adult patients are thus multilocular. The cyst fluid is a transudate of serum. It contains protein and is antigenic. If released into the circulation, eosinophilia or anaphylaxis may result.

Endemic regions

The disease is common in sheep-raising countries, where dogs have access to infected offal. These include South Australia, New Zealand, Africa, South America,

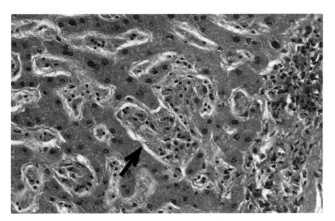

Fig. 32.14. Kala-azar. Liver biopsy shows enlarged Kupffer cells (arrow) distending the sinusoids. These contain Leishman–Donovan bodies. (H & E, ×100.)

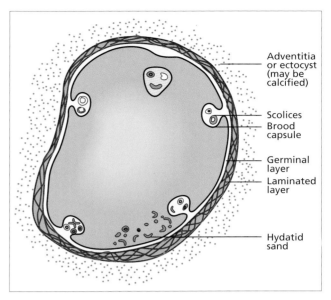

Fig. 32.16. The basic constitution of a hydatid cyst.

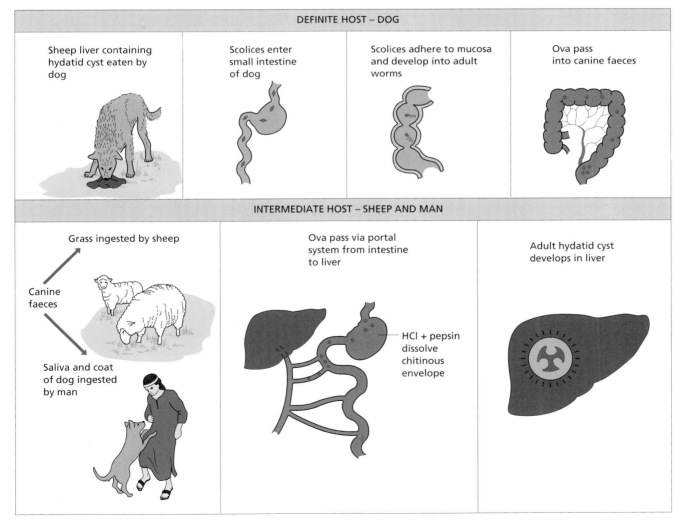

DEFINITE HOST – DOG

Sheep liver containing hydatid cyst eaten by dog

Scolices enter small intestine of dog

Scolices adhere to mucosa and develop into adult worms

Ova pass into canine faeces

INTERMEDIATE HOST – SHEEP AND MAN

Grass ingested by sheep

Canine faeces

Saliva and coat of dog ingested by man

Ova pass via portal system from intestine to liver

HCl + pepsin dissolve chitinous envelope

Adult hydatid cyst develops in liver

Fig. 32.15. The life cycle of the hydatid parasite.

southern Europe, especially Cyprus, Greece and Spain, and the Middle and Far East. The disease is rare in Britain, apart from some areas in Wales.

Clinical features

These depend on the site, the stage and whether the cyst is alive or dead. The rest of the liver hypertrophies and hepatomegaly results.

The *uncomplicated hydatid cyst* may be silent and found incidentally. Only 10–20% of hydatid cysts are diagnosed in individuals under 16 years of age. The disease should be suspected if a rounded smooth swelling, continuous with the liver, is found in a patient who is not obviously ill. The only complaints may be a dull ache in the right upper quadrant and sometimes a feeling of abdominal distension. The tension in the cyst is high and fluctuation is never marked.

Complications

Rupture. Intraperitoneal rupture is frequent and leads to multiple cysts throughout the peritoneal cavity with intestinal obstruction and gross abdominal distension.

The pressure in the cyst greatly exceeds that in bile and rupture into bile ducts is frequent. This may lead to cure or to cholestatic jaundice with recurrent cholangitis.

Colonic rupture leads to elimination per rectum and to secondary infection.

The cysts may adhere to the diaphragm, rupture into the lungs and result in expectoration of daughter cysts. Pressure on and rupture into the hepatic veins leads to the Budd–Chiari syndrome. Secondary involvement of the lungs may follow.

Infection. Secondary invasion by pyogenic organisms follows rupture into biliary passages, giving the picture of a pyogenic abscess; the parasite dies. Occasionally, the entire cyst content undergoes aseptic necrosis and again the parasite dies. This amorphous yellow debris must be distinguished from the pus of secondary infection.

Other organs. Cysts can occur in lung, kidney, spleen, brain or bone, but mass infestation is rare; the liver is usually the only organ involved. If a hydatid cyst is found elsewhere, there is always concomitant infestation of the liver.

Hydatid allergy. Cyst fluid contains a number of foreign proteins including proteases and cyclophilins which sensitize the host. This may lead to severe anaphylactic shock but more commonly to recurrent urticaria or 'hives'. Most such patients have specific IgE immunoglobulins [122].

Membranous glomerulonephritis. This is seen occasionally and may be related to glomerular deposits of hydatid antigens [123,124].

Diagnosis

Serological tests

Hydatid fluid contains specific antigens, leakage of which sensitizes the patient with the production of antibodies.

ELISA gives positive results in about 85% [125].

Results may be negative for all tests if the cyst has never leaked, if it contains no scolices or if the parasite is dead.

Eosinophilia of greater than 7% is found in about 30% of patients.

Imaging

Radiology usually shows a raised, poorly moving right diaphragm and hepatomegaly. Calcium may be laid down in the ectocyst as a distinct round or oval opacity (Fig. 32.17) or merely as shreds.

Floating bodies indicate the presence of free-moving daughter cysts. Infected gas-containing cysts may show a fluid level.

Hepatic cysts may displace the stomach or hepatic flexure of the colon. Characteristic radiological changes may be seen in the lungs, spleen, kidney or bone.

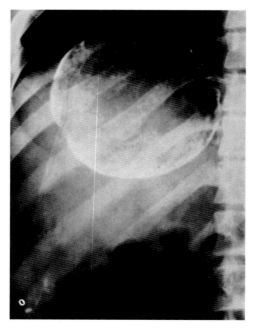

Fig. 32.17. X-ray of the abdomen shows a calcified hydatid cyst in the liver.

Ultrasound or *CT scanning* demonstrates single or multiple cysts which may be uni- or multiloculated, and thin or thick walled (Figs 32.18, 32.19). Ultrasound and CT are highly sensitive for diagnosis: 97.7% for ultrasound and 100% for CT.

Ultrasound changes have provided the basis for typing of cysts (Table 32.3)[126]. The more recent WHO classification is into active, transitional and inactive cysts [127]. Based on the appearance of the cyst, its wall and contents, typing is CL (cystic lesion) or CE 1 to 5 (Cystic Echinococcosis). Infected and degenerate cysts are poorly define [128].WHO typing by ultrasound is intended to reflect the natural history of hydatid disease, and aid its study.

MRI may show a characteristic intense rim, daughter cysts and detachment of the membranes [129]. Intrahepatic and extrahepatic rupture can be defined.

ERCP may show cysts in the bile ducts (Figs 32.20, 32.21).

Prognosis

The uncomplicated hepatic hydatid cyst carries a reasonably good prognosis. The risk of complications is, however, always present. Intraperitoneal or intrapleural rupture is grave, but rupture into the biliary tree is not so serious because spontaneous cure may follow the biliary colic. Infection is controlled by antibiotics.

Table 32.3. Classification of ultrasound appearances in hydatid disease as described by Gharbi *et al* [126]

Type	Description
I	Purely cystic
II	Detached membrane
III	Undulating in cyst cavity
	Multiseptate cyst
IV	Heterogenous complex mass (dead parasite)
	Calcified mass (eggshell) (dead parasite)

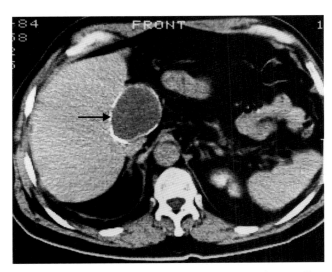

Fig. 32.18. CT scan shows calcified hydatid cyst (arrowed) in the quadrate lobe of the liver (contrast-enhanced scan).

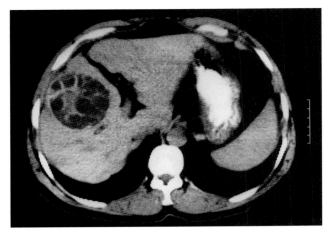

Fig. 32.19. CT scan. Hydatid cyst in right lobe of liver containing multiple septae produced by daughter cysts (contrast-enhanced scan).

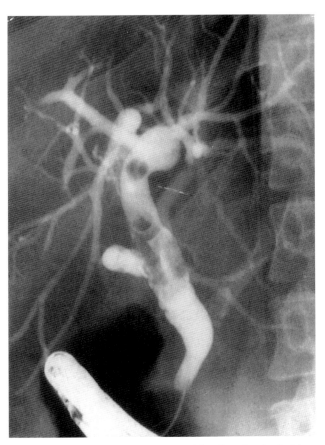

Fig. 32.20. Endoscopic cholangiography showing hydatid cysts in the common bile duct.

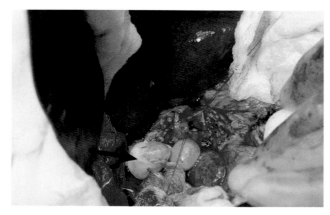

Fig. 32.21. Four glistening hydatid cysts (arrow) were removed surgically from the common bile duct of the patient shown in Fig. 32.20.

Table 32.4. Treatment of hydatid liver cysts [133]

Percutaneous puncture
Aspirate
Inject 95% alcohol
Re-aspirate

Treatment

Dogs should be denied access to infected offal and hands must be washed after handling dogs [130]. Dogs in affected areas must be regularly de-wormed.

Medical treatment

Mebendazole perfuses through the cyst membrane and interferes with microtubular function. However, it is poorly absorbed.

Albendazole is better absorbed and cyst levels equal that achieved in plasma. It is more effective than mebendazole. Approximately one-third of patients will respond to albendazole or albendazole plus praziqantel.

Medical therapy cannot be regarded as definitive. Albendazole can be given in a 6 to 24-month course for those unsuitable for surgery, with disseminated disease or with rupture. About 30% of cysts disappear, 30–50% degenerate or become smaller and 20–40% of cysts are unchanged [131,132].

Percutaneous drainage

Ultrasound-guided percutaneous drainage is as effective as surgery [133,134]. The 'PAIR' routine is used (Table 32.4) [133]. Sclerosing solutions such as 95% ethanol or hypertonic saline may induce sclerosing cholangitis in patients with a biliary communication. The presence of a communication contra-indicates PAIR [132,135]. If used, this approach is usually combined with albendazole treatment to prevent the risk of secondary seeding and reduce allergic reactions. Albendazole is continued for 1 month postprocedure.

Surgery

The object is to remove the cyst completely, without soiling and infecting the peritoneum and with complete obliteration of the resulting dead space. Complete removal of the cyst with its adventitia is ideal to avoid spillage. The usual operation is cystectomy with removal of the germinal and laminated layers and preservation of the host-derived ectocyst [136]. Surgical pericystectomy includes removal of the pericyst. The mortality for these operations is very low and the morbidity rate is 23.7% [136]. Relapse rates are up to 25%.

Hemihepatectomy or segmentectomy are occasionally performed. Cholangitis is treated by biliary drainage, usually by ERCP, papillotomy and cyst removal. Surgical biliary drainage may be necessary. The technical problem is great.

Rupture into the peritoneal cavity

The cyst contents are removed from the peritoneal cavity as far as possible by sucking and swabbing. The scolices, however, usually settle down in the peritoneal cavity and form daughter cysts so that recurrence is almost inevitable.

Urgent surgery has a substantial morbidity and mortality [137]. Chemotherapy is essential in combination with this.

Echinococcus multilocularis (alveolar echinococcosis)

This is found in the northern hemisphere. Rodents are intermediate hosts and foxes are definitive hosts. The larvae grow indefinitely and produce liver necrosis and a major granulomatous reaction. The disease behaves like a locally malignant tumour. Diagnosis is typically by means of radiology, biopsy and serology, using specific antigens. The *Echinococcus* invades liver and biliary tissue, hepatic veins, inferior vena cava and diaphragm. Chemotherapy is effective but not curative [138]. It is fatal unless completely removed by surgery, although it is frequently inoperable because of its late presentation [139]. Albendazole and mebendazole have been shown to suppress the disease for many years with a 16 to 20-year survival rate of approximately 70% [132]. Hepatic transplant may be necessary [140].

Ascariasis

Ascaris infection, a soil borne disease, is particularly common in the Far East, India and South Africa, but may be found elsewhere in subtropical regions. The roundworm *Ascaris lumbricoides* typically inhabits the jejunum, but may migrate through the Ampulla of Vater into the bile ducts. Ova arrive in the liver via the bile ducts. Here they provoke an immunological reaction and eggs, giant cells and granulomas are surrounded by a dense eosinophil infiltrate (Fig. 32.22). The adult worm is 15–30 cm long and occasionally may lodge in the common bile duct producing partial bile duct obstruction, and secondary cholangitic abscesses [141]. The *Ascaris* may be a nucleus for intrahepatic gallstones [142]. Biliary colic is a complication.

A *plain abdominal X-ray* may show calcified worms.

Clinical presentation is as acute cholecystitis, acute cholangitis, biliary colic, acute pancreatitis and, rarely, hepatic abscess [141].

Ultrasound shows long linear echogenic structures or strips which characteristically move. It can be used to monitor migration of the worms. It cannot diagnose duodenal ascariasis.

ERCP shows the *Ascaris* as a linear filling defect (Fig. 32.23). Worms can be seen moving into and out of the biliary tree from the duodenum [143].

Treatment is by ERCP with endoscopic worm extraction with or without sphincterotomy [144]. Failures need surgical treatment.

Single-dose treatment with albendazole, mebendazole or pyrantel pamoate will usually kill *Ascaris* [145] but it may remain in the bile ducts. Re-invasion is common.

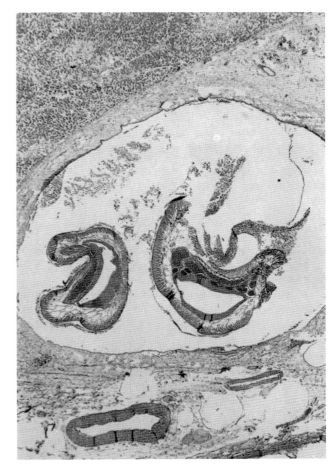

Fig. 32.22. Section shows a dead *Ascaris* in an intrahepatic blood vessel in a portal zone. There is surrounding fibrous tissue reaction. (H & E, ×40.)

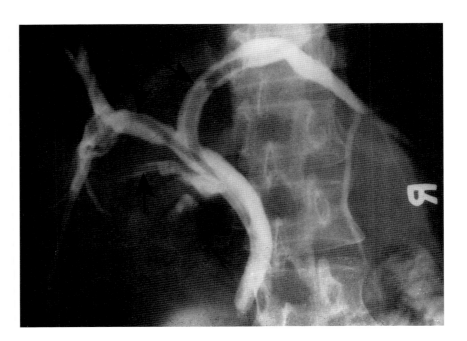

Fig. 32.23. Ascariasis: endoscopic cholangiography shows linear filling defects in the bile ducts due to *Ascaris* worms (arrows).

Strongyloides stercoralis

This soil-transmitted intestinal nematode is common in tropical countries, but also in temperate parts of the world, such as the Appalachian region of the USA. It is usually asymptomatic but can cause biliary obstruction due to biliary stenosis [146]. Hyperinfestation syndrome has also been reported in patients undergoing liver transplantation [147].

Diagnosis is usually made by detection of larvae in the stools, but antibody assays are also available.

Thiabendazole is effective treatment but is associated with hepatotoxicity. Alternatives are ivermectin and albendazole [148].

Trichinosis

This disease is caused by eating raw, infected pork and occasionally other wild animals, such as bears, with subsequent dissemination of *Trichinella* larvae throughout the body. Severity of disease correlates with the numbers of ingested larvae and characteristically has an acute phase with fever and gastrointestinal symptoms followed by a chronic phase with myalgia and muscle tenderness, where the parasite resides within the striated muscle cells and may persist for up to 40 years. Clinical features referable to the liver are unusual.

Hepatic histology may show invasion of hepatic sinusoids by *Trichinella* larvae and fatty change [149].

Diagnosis. This is difficult unless in an epidemic. The European Centre for Disease Control has produced a case definition based upon clinical features, laboratory evidence including eosinophilia and elevated muscle enzymes and epidemiological links to infected meat [150]. Antibodies may be detected by ELISA but, although sensitive, cross reactions occur with other infectious disease agents. Muscle pain and tenderness may warrant muscle biopsy and allow the diagnosis to be made.

Treatment. Efficacy relates to the timing of treatment after initial infection. Treatment is unsatisfactory in later disease. Albendazole and mebendazole are effective in the acute phase and corticosteroids may help alleviate symptoms [151].

Toxocara canis (visceral larva migrans)

This parasite is spread by cats and dogs and primarily causes disease in children. Following ingestion of eggs (or occasionally encapsulated larvae in animal organs) the liberated larvae migrate in the portal circulation into the liver. There they move slowly through the tissues (visceral lava migans) producing a trail of eosinophilic infiltration, granulomas and eosinophilic abscesses [152,153]. Hepatomegaly, recurrent pneumonia, eosinophilia and hypergammaglobulinaemia are associated findings. The serum ELISA antibody test is positive in the majority of cases. Imaging of the liver may show ill-defined, multiple nodules up to 1.5 cm in diameter [153].

Most cases are aymptomatic and the disease may be identified during investigation of eosinophilia or liver lesions. Treatment for severe disease or end-organ disease, such as ophthalmic or neurotoxocariasis, is with albendazole or diethyl carbamazine.

Liver flukes

Metacercaria in freshwater fish or on water plants are consumed and larvae develop in the duodenum and eventually reach the bile ducts. During the migratory phase they cause fever and eosinophilia. When they reach the biliary passages they may cause obstruction with complicating suppurative cholangitis.

There are three main genera of fluke: *Clonorchis*, *Opisthorchis* and *Fasciola* and it is estimated that 780 million people are at risk of infection with these worldwide.

Clonorchiasis and opisthorchiasis

These diseases are similar and caused by similar flukes, although differing in geographical location. *Clonorchis sinensis* is found mainly in north-east China, southern Korea, Japan, Taiwan, northern Vietnam and eastern Russia. Species of *Opisthorcis* cause infection in Laos, Thailand, Vietnam and Cambodia, and in Russia, Ukraine and Kazakhstan [154].

Disease can present years after the patient has left their country of origin as the biliary flukes may persist for decades. Metacercaria are ingested with improperly cooked or raw, fresh-water fish. The cyst wall is destroyed by trypsin in the duodenum and the larvae migrate from the duodenum through the ampulla of Vater into the peripheral intrahepatic bile ducts where they mature to adult worms. In uncomplicated cases, the changes are confined to the bile duct walls with abundant adenomatous formation; fibrosis increases with time [155]. Cholangiocarcinoma is a serious complication [156].

Clinical manifestations depend on the number of flukes, the period of infestation and the complications. With heavy infestation, the patient suffers weakness, epigastric discomfort, weight loss and diarrhoea. Jaundice is due to obstruction of the intrahepatic biliary tree by worms or inflammation. Infection leads to fever, chills and abdominal pain. Cholangiocarcinoma is marked by progressive jaundice and pruritus.

Diagnosis is based on finding ova in the stool or aspirated bile. Laboratory findings include eosinophilia and an increased serum alkaline phosphatase. Serological tests are available and are sensitive, but cannot distinguish between active and past infection.

Ultrasound, CT and *MRI* changes are based on flukes within dilated ducts and periductal changes without evidence of extrahepatic biliary obstruction [157].

ERCP shows filamentous filling defects in the bile ducts which have blunted tips. The defects are of uniform size and change in position [157].

The *therapeutic response* to praziquantel is greater than 80% [154]. The bile ducts may be cleared of stones by endoscopic or percutaneous techniques, or surgery [158,159].

Fascioliasis

The two causative species of this fluke are found mostly in the Americas (mainly Peru and Bolivia), Europe (including Britain), Asia, western Pacific and North Africa. The encysted metacercariae from the intermediate host snails survive on herbage and patients are usually infected by eating uncooked contaminated vegetables and salads.

The clinical picture in the acute stage is of cholangitis with fever, right upper quadrant pain and hepatomegaly. Eosinophilia and a raised serum alkaline phosphatase are usually present. The picture may simulate choledocholithiasis.

CT shows peripheral filling defects, sometimes crescentic, in the liver due to the migrating fluke (Fig. 32.24) [160].

ERCP shows several irregular linear or rounded filling defects in the bile ducts or segmental stenosis, with an inflammatory pattern [157]. Worms can be aspirated.

Liver biopsy shows infiltration of the portal zones with histiocytes, eosinophils and polymorphs. Hepatic granulomas and ova in the liver may occasionally be seen.

Diagnosis is suspected by finding the clinical picture of biliary tract disease with eosinophilia. It is confirmed by finding ova in the faeces. These, however, may not be detected until 12 weeks after the infection when parasites have attained sexual maturity. They disappear later.

The diagnosis may be confirmed by ELISA detection of circulating antibodies to *Fasciola hepatica* excretory–secretory antigens although this does not distinguish between current and past infection [161,162].

Treatment is by triclabendazole for both phases and single-dose cure rates of over 90% have been reported for acute-phase infection. Alternatives include praziquantel and bithionol.

Recurrent pyogenic cholangitis

This is a common disease in south-east Asia, although declining in incidence The initial cause is uncertain, but may be infection with *Clonorchis*, enteric microorganisms or malnutrition. Biliary stone and stricture formation follow recurrent bacterial infections. Other long-term sequelae include secondary biliary cirrhosis and cholangiocarcinoma. Treatment is by antibiotics and, as necessary, biliary drainage—either endoscopic, percutaneous or surgical. Transplantation may be necessary in certain cases [163].

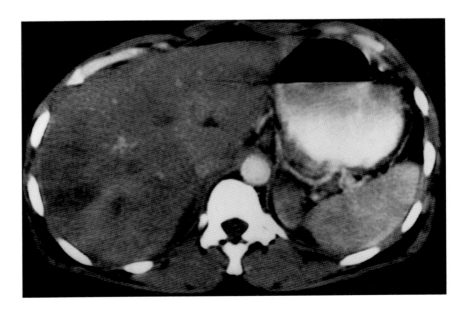

Fig. 32.24. *Fasciola hepatica.* CT in the migratory stage showing multiple, sometimes linear, filling defects at the periphery of the liver. Larvae have penetrated the gut wall, traversed the peritoneal cavity, and invaded the hepatic parenchyma. They eventually enter the bile ducts. (Courtesy of P.A. McCormick.)

References

1 Tugwell P, Williams AO. Jaundice associated with lobar pneumonia. *Q. J. Med.* 1977; **46**: 97–118.

2 Gourley GR, Chesney PJ, Davis JP et al. Acute cholestasis in patients with toxic-shock syndrome. *Gastroenterology* 1981; **81**: 928–931.

3 Sikuler E, Guetta V, Keynan A et al. Abnormalities in bilirubin and liver enzyme levels in adult patients with bacteremia. *Arch. Intern. Med.* 1989; **149**: 2246–2248.

4 Lefkowitch JH. Bile ductular cholestasis: an ominous histopathologic sign related to sepsis and 'cholangitis lenta'. *Hum. Pathol.* 1982; **13**: 19–24.

5 Quale JM, Mandel LJ, Bergasa NV et al. Clinical significance and pathogenesis of hyperbilirubinemia associated with *Staphylococcus aureus* septicemia. *Am. J. Med.* 1988; **85**: 615–618.

6 Whiting JF, Green RM, Rosenbluth AB et al. Tumor necrosis factor-alpha decreases hepatocyte bile salt uptake and mediates endotoxin-induced cholestasis. *Hepatology* 1995; **22**: 1273–1278.

7 Fuchs M, Sanyal AJ. Sepsis and cholestasis. *Clin. Liver Dis.* 2008; **12**: 151–172.

8 Huang CJ, Pitt HA, Lipsett PA et al. Pyogenic hepatic abscess. Changing trends over 42 years. *Ann. Surg.* 1996; **223**: 600–607.

9 Rahimian J, Wilson T, Oram V et al. Pyogenic liver abscess: recent trends in etiology and mortality. *Clin. Infect. Dis.* 2004; **39**: 1654–1659.

10 Meddings L, Myers RP, Hubbard J et al. A population-based study of pyogenic liver abscesses in the United States: incidence, mortality, and temporal trends. *Am. J. Gastroenterol.* 2010; **105**: 117–124.

11 Vakil N, Hayne G, Sharma A et al. Liver abscess in Crohn's disease. *Am. J. Gastroenterol.* 1994; **89**: 1090–1095.

12 Khanna R, Levendoglu H. Liver abscess due to *Yersinia enterocolitica*: case report and review of the literature. *Dig. Dis. Sci.* 1989; **34**: 636–639.

13 Ammann R, Münch R, Largiadèr F et al. Pancreatic and hepatic abscesses: a late complication in 10 patients with chronic pancreatitis. *Gastroenterology* 1992; **103**: 560–565.

14 De Baere T, Roche A, Amenabar JM et al. Liver abscess formation after local treatment of liver tumours. *Hepatology* 1996; **23**: 1436–1440.

15 Wong E, Khadori N, Carrasco CH et al. Infectious complications of hepatic artery catheterization procedures in patients with cancer. *Rev. Infect. Dis.* 1991; **13**: 583–586.

16 Branum GD, Tyson GS, Branum MA et al. Hepatic abscess. Changes in aetiology, diagnosis, and management. *Ann. Surg.* 1990; **212**: 655–662.

17 Yang CC, Chen CY, Lin XZ et al. Pyogenic liver abscess in Taiwan: emphasis on gas-forming liver abscess in diabetics. *Am. J. Gastroenterol.* 1993; **88**: 1911–1915.

18 Barnes PF, DeCock KM, Reynolds TN et al. A comparison of amebic and pyogenic abscesses of the liver. *Medicine (Baltimore)* 1987; **66**: 472–483.

19 Jeffrey RB Jr, Tolentino CS, Chang FC et al. CT of small pyogenic hepatic abscesses: the cluster sign. *Am. J. Roentgenol.* 1988; **151**: 487–489.

20 Méndez RJ, Schiebler ML, Outwater EK et al. Hepatic abscesses: MR imaging findings. *Radiology* 1994; **190**: 431–436.

21 André M, Aumaître, O Papo T et al. Disseminated aseptic abscesses associated with Crohn's disease: a new entity? *Dig. Dis. Sci.* 1998; **43**: 420–428.

22 Ch Yu S, Hg Lo R, Kan PS et al. Pyogenic liver abscess: treatment with needle aspiration. *Clin. Radiol.* 1997; **52**: 912–916.

23 Chung YF, Tan YM, Lui HF et al. Management of pyogenic liver abscesses—percutaneous or open drainage? *Singapore Med. J.* 2007; **48**: 1158–1165.

24 Moore SW, Millar AJ, Cywes S. Conservative initial treatment for liver abscesses in children. *Br. J. Surg.* 1994; **81**: 872–874.

25 Giorgio A, Tarantino L, Mariniello N et al. Pyogenic liver abscesses: 13 years of experience in percutaneous needle aspiration with US guidance. *Radiology* 1995; **195**: 122–124.

26 Mohsen AH, Green ST, Read RC et al. Liver abscess in adult: ten years experience in a UK centre. *Q. J. Med.* 2002; **95**: 797–802.

27 Yeh TS, Jan YY, Jeng LB et al. Pyogenic liver abscesses in patients with malignant disease: a report of 52 cases treated at a single institution. *Arch. Surg.* 1998; **133**: 242–245.

28 Lee K-T, Sheen P-C, Chen J-S et al. Pyogenic liver abscess: multivariate analysis of risk factors. *World J. Surg.* 1991; **15**: 372–376.

29 Pritt BS, Clark CG. Amebiasis. *Mayo Clin. Proc.* 2008; **83**: 1154–1159.

30 Santi-Rocca J, Rigothier MC, Guillén N. Host-microbe interactions and defense mechanisms in the development of amoebic liver abscesses. *Clin. Microbiol. Rev.* 2009; **22**: 65–75.

31 Goldmeier D, Sargeaunt PG, Price AB et al. Is *Entamoeba histolytica* in homosexual men a pathogen? *Lancet* 1986; **i**: 641–644.

32 Stark D, van Hal SJ, Matthews G et al. Invasive amebiasis in men who have sex with men, Australia. *Emerg. Infect. Dis.* 2008; **14**: 1141–1143.

33 Stanley SL Jr, Jackson TF, Foster L et al. Longitudinal study of the antibody response to recombinant *Entamoeba histolytica* antigens in patients with amoebic liver abscess. *Am. J. Trop. Med. Hyg.* 1998; **58**: 414–416.

34 Radin DR, Ralls PW, Colletti PM et al. CT of amebic liver abscess. *Am. J. Roentgenol.* 1988; **150**: 1297–1301.

35 Elizondo G, Weissleder R, Stark DD et al. Amebic liver abscess: diagnosis and treatment evaluation with MR imaging. *Radiology* 1987; **165**: 795–800.

36 Simjee AE, Patel A, Gathiram V et al. Serial ultrasound in amoebic liver abscess. *Clin. Radiol.* 1985; **36**: 61–68.

37 Chavez-Tapia NC, Hernandez-Calleros J, Tellez-Avila FI et al. Image-guided percutaneous procedure plus metronidazole versus metronidazole alone for uncomplicated amoebic liver abscess. *Cochrane Database Syst. Rev.* 2009; **1**: CD004886.

38 Guth AA, Kim U. The reappearance of abdominal tuberculosis. *Surg. Gynecol. Obstet.* 1991; **172**; 432–436.

39 Hussain W, Mutimer D, Harrison R et al. Fulminant hepatic failure caused by tuberculosis. *Gut* 1995; **36**: 792–794.

40 Achem SR, Kolts BE, Grisnik J et al. Pseudotumoral hepatic tuberculosis. Atypical presentation and comprehensive review of the literature. *J. Clin. Gastroenterol.* 1992; **14**: 72–77.

41 Chien R-N, Lin P-Y, Liaw Y-F. Hepatic tuberculosis: comparison of miliary and local form. *Infection* 1995; **23**: 5–8.

42 Fan ST, Ng IOL, Choi TK *et al.* Tuberculosis of the bile duct: a rare cause of biliary stricture. *Am. J. Gastroenterol.* 1989; **84**: 413–414.

43 Ruttenberg D, Graham S, Burns D *et al.* Abdominal tuberculosis—a cause of portal vein thrombosis and portal hypertension. *Dig. Dis. Sci.* 1991; **36**: 112–115.

44 Nyendak MR, Lewinsohn DA, Lewinsohn DM. New diagnostic methods for tuberculosis. *Curr. Opin. Infect. Dis.* 2009; **22**: 174–182.

45 Maglinte DD, Alvarez SZ, Ng AC *et al.* Patterns of calcifications and cholangiographic findings in hepatobiliary tuberculosis. *Gastrointest. Radiol.* 1988; **13**: 331–335.

46 World Health Organization. *Treatment of Tuberculosis: Guidelines*, 4th edn, 2009 WHO/HTM/TB/2009.420.

47 Patel KM. Granulomatous hepatitis due to *Mycobacterium scrofulaceum*: report of a case. *Gastroenterology* 1981; **81**: 156–158.

48 Wong JJ, Kinney TB, Miller FJ *et al.* Hepatic actinomycotic abscesses: diagnosis and management. *Am. J. Roentgenol.* 2006; **186**: 174–176.

49 Sharma M, Briski LE, Khatib R. Hepatic actinomycosis: an overview of salient features and outcome of therapy. *Scand. J. Infect. Dis.* 2002; **34**: 386–391.

50 Bhatt BD, Zuckerman MJ, Ho H *et al.* Multiple actinomycotic abscesses of the liver. *Am. J. Gastroenterol.* 1990; **85**: 309–310.

51 Mongiardo N, De Rienzo B, Zanchetta G *et al.* Primary hepatic actinomycosis. *J. Infect.* 1986; **12**: 65–69.

52 Nazarian LN, Spencer JA, Mitchell DG. Multiple actinomycotic liver abscesses: MRI appearances with aetiology suggested by abdominal radiography. Case report. *Clin. Imaging* 1994; **18**: 119–122.

53 Kasano Y, Tanimura H, Yamaue H *et al.* Hepatic actinomycosis infiltrating the diaphragm and right lung. *Am. J. Gastroenterol.* 1996; **91**: 2418–2420.

54 Case Records of the Massachusetts General Hospital. Case 27, 1983. *N. Engl. J. Med.* 1983; **309**: 35–43.

55 Schlossberg D. Syphilitic hepatitis: a case report and review of the literature. *Am. J. Gastroenterol.* 1987; **82**: 552–553.

56 Comer GM, Mukherjee S, Sachdev RK *et al.* Cardiolipin-fluorescent (M1) antimitochondrial antibody and cholestatic hepatitis in secondary syphilis. *Dig. Dis. Sci.* 1989; **34**: 1298–1302.

57 Maincent G, Labadie H, Fabre M *et al.* Tertiary hepatic syphilis. A treatable cause of multinodular liver. *Dig. Dis. Sci.* 1997; **42**: 447–450.

58 Kingston M, French P, Goh B *et al*; Syphilis Guidelines Revision Group 2008, Clinical Effectiveness Group. UK National Guidelines on the Management of Syphilis 2008. *Int. J. STD AIDS* 2008; **19**: 729–740.

59 Simson JN. Chlamydial perihepatitis (Curtis–Fitz Hugh syndrome) after hydrotubation. *Br. Med. J.* 1984; **289**: 544–545.

60 Haight JB, Ockner SA. *Chlamydia trachomatis* perihepatitis with ascites. *Am. J. Gastroenterol.* 1988; **83**: 323–325.

61 Trigg BG, Kerndt PR, Aynalem G. Sexually transmitted infections and pelvic inflammatory disease in women. *Med. Clin. N. Am.* 2008; **92**: 1083–1113.

62 Levett PN. Leptospirosis. *Clin. Microbiol. Rev.* 2001; **14**: 296–326.

63 Weil A. Über eine eigenthumliche mit Milztumour, Icterus and Nephritis einhergehene, acute Infektionskrankheit. *Dtsch. Arch. Klin. Med.* 1886; **39**: 209.

64 Vinetz JM, Glass GE, Flexner CE *et al.* Sporadic urban leptospirosis. *Ann. Intern. Med.* 1996; **125**: 794–798.

65 Cerqueira TB, Athanazio DA, Spichler AS *et al.* Renal involvement in leptospirosis–new insights into pathophysiology and treatment. *Braz. J. Infect. Dis.* 2008; **12**: 248–252.

66 Tajiki H, Salomao R. Association of plasma levels of tumour necrosis factor alpha with severity of disease and mortality among patients with leptospirosis. *Clin. Infect. Dis.* 1996; **23**: 1177–1178.

67 Arean VM. The pathologic anatomy and pathogenesis of fatal human leptospirosis (Weil's disease). *Am. J. Pathol.* 1962; **40**: 393–423.

68 Kobayashi Y. Clinical observation and treatment of leptospirosis. *J. Infect. Chemother.* 2001; **7**: 59–68.

69 Wagenaar JF, Goris MG, Sakundarno MS *et al.* What role do coagulation disorders play in the pathogenesis of leptospirosis? *Trop. Med. Int. Health* 2007; **12**: 111–122.

70 Brown PD, Gravekamp C, Carrington DG *et al.* Evaluation of the polymerase chain reaction for early diagnosis of leptospirosis. *J. Med. Microbiol.* 1995; **43**: 110–114.

71 Ribeiro MA, Souza CC, Almeida SH *et al.* Dot-ELISA for human leptospirosis employing immunodominant antigen. *J. Trop. Med. Hyg.* 1995; **98**: 452–456.

72 Appassakij H, Silpapojakul K, Wansit R *et al.* Evaluation of the immunofluorescent antibody test for the diagnosis of human leptospirosis. *Am. J. Trop. Med. Hyg.* 1995; **52**; 340–343.

73 Palaniappan RU, Ramanujam S, Chang YF. Leptospirosis: pathogenesis, immunity, and diagnosis. *Curr. Opin. Infect. Dis.* 2007; **20**: 284–292.

74 Watt G, Padre LP, Tuazon ML *et al.* Placebo-controlled trial of intravenous penicillin for severe and late leptospirosis. *Lancet* 1988; **i**: 433–435.

75 Griffith ME, Hospenthal DR, Murray CK. Antimicrobial therapy of leptospirosis. *Curr. Opin. Infect. Dis.* 2006 ; **19**: 533–537.

76 Felsenfeld O, Wolf RH. Immunoglobulins and antibodies in *Borrelia turicatae* infections. *Acta Trop.* 1969; **26**: 156–166.

77 Rebaudet S, Parola P. Epidemiology of relapsing fever borreliosis in Europe. *FEMS Immunol. Med. Microbiol.* 2006; **48**: 11–15.

78 Bryceson AD, Parry EHO, Perine PL *et al.* Louse-born relapsing fever: a clinical and laboratory study of 62 cases in Ethiopia and a reconsideration of the literature. *Q. J. Med.* 1970; **39**: 129–170.

79 Brahim H, Perrier-Gros-Claude JD, Postic D *et al.* Identifying relapsing fever Borrelia, Senegal. *Emerg. Infect. Dis.* 2005; **11**: 474–475.

80 Goellner MH, Agger WA, Burgess JH *et al.* Hepatitis due to recurrent Lyme disease. *Ann. Intern. Med.* 1988; **108**: 707–708.

81 Zanchi AC, Gingold AR, Theise ND *et al.* Necrotizing granulomatous hepatitis as an unusual manifestation of Lyme disease. *Dig. Dis. Sci.* 2007; **52**: 2629–2632.

82 Horowitz HW, Dworkin B, Forseter G *et al.* Liver function in early Lyme disease. *Hepatology* 1996; **23**: 1412–1417.

83 Dupont HL, Hornick RB, Levin HS *et al.* Q fever hepatitis. *Ann. Intern. Med.* 1971; **74**: 198–206.

84 Tissot-Dupont H, Raoult D, Brouquil P *et al.* Epidemiologic features and clinical presentation of acute Q fever in hospitalized patients: 323 French cases. *Am. J. Med.* 1992; **93**: 427–434.

85 Parker NR, Barralet JH, Bell AM. Q fever. *Lancet* 2006; **367**: 679–688.

86 Adams JS, Walker DH. The liver in rocky mountain spotted fever. *Am. J. Clin. Pathol.* 1981; **75**: 156–161.

87 Dantas-Torres F. Rocky Mountain spotted fever. *Lancet Infect. Dis.* 2007; **7**: 724–732.

88 Tompkins LS. Of cats, humans and *Bartonella. N. Engl. J. Med.* 1997; **337**: 1916–1917.

89 Maguiña C, Guerra H, Ventosilla P. Bartonellosis. *Clin. Dermatol.* 2009; **27**: 271–280.

90 Friedman E, Blahut RJ, Bender MD. Hepatic abscesses and fungemia from *Torulopsis glabrata*. Successful treatment with percutaneous drainage and amphotericin B. *J. Clin. Gastroenterol.* 1987; **9**: 711–715.

91 Thaler M, Pastakia FB, Shawker TH *et al.* Hepatic candidiasis in cancer patients: the evolving picture of the syndrome. *Ann. Intern. Med.* 1988; **108**: 88–100.

92 Pastakia B, Shawker TH, Thaler M *et al.* Hepatosplenic candidiasis: wheels within wheels. *Radiology* 1988; **166**: 417–421.

93 Korinek JK, Guarda LA, Bolivar R *et al. Trichosporon* hepatitis. *Gastroenterology* 1983; **85**: 732–734.

94 Lewis JH, Patel HR, Zimmerman HJ. The spectrum of hepatic candidiasis. *Hepatology* 1982; **2**: 479–487.

95 Gordon SC, Watts JC, Veneri RJ *et al.* Focal hepatic candidiasis with perihepatic adhesions: laparoscopic and immunohistologic diagnosis. *Gastroenterology* 1990; **98**: 214–217.

96 Park GR, Drummond GB, Lamb D *et al.* Disseminated aspergillosis occurring in patients with respiratory, renal and hepatic failure. *Lancet* 1982; **i**: 179–183.

97 Lin SJ, Schranz J, Teutsch SM. Aspergillosis case-fatality rate: systematic review of the literature. *Clin. Infect. Dis.* 2001; **32**: 358–366.

98 Walsh TJ, Anaissie EJ, Denning DW *et al*; Infectious Diseases Society of America. Treatment of aspergillosis: clinical practice guidelines of the Infectious Diseases Society of America. *Clin. Infect. Dis.* 2008; **46**: 327–360.

99 Wheat LJ, Freifeld AG, Kleiman MB *et al*; Infectious Diseases Society of America. Clinical practice guidelines for the management of patients with histoplasmosis: 2007 update by the Infectious Diseases Society of America. *Clin. Infect. Dis.* 2007; **45**: 807–825.

100 Howard PF, Smith JW. Diagnosis of disseminated coccidioidomycosis. *Arch. Intern. Med.* 1983; **143**: 1335–1338.

101 Ryan ME, Kirchner JP, Sell T *et al.* Cholangitis due to *Blastomyces dermatitidis. Gastroenterology* 1989; **96**: 1346–1349.

102 El-Garem AA. Schistosomiasis. *Digestion* 1998; **59**: 589–605.

103 Burke ML, Jones MK, Gobert GN *et al.* Immunopathogenesis of human schistosomiasis. *Parasite Immunol.* 2009; **31**: 163–176.

104 Van Etten L, Folman CC, Eggelte TA *et al.* Rapid diagnosis of schistosomiasis by antigen detection in urine with a reagent strip. *J. Clin. Microbiol.* 1994; **32**: 2404–2406.

105 Ross AG, Bartley PB, Sleigh AC *et al.* Schistosomiasis. *N. Engl. J. Med.* 2002; **346**: 1212–1220.

106 Fataar S, Bassiony H, Satyanath S. CT of hepatic schistosomiasis mansoni. *Am. J. Roentgenol.* 1985; **145**: 63–66.

107 Manzella A, Ohtomo K, Monzawa S *et al.* Schistosomiasis of the liver. *Abdom. Imaging.* 2008; **33**: 144–150.

108 Abdel-Wahab MF, Esmat G, Farrag A *et al.* Grading of hepatic schistosomiasis by the use of ultrasonography. *Am. J. Trop. Med. Hyg.* 1992; **46**: 403–408.

109 Salama ZA, El Dorry AK, Soliman MT *et al.* Doppler sonography of the portal circulation in cases with portal hypertension. *Med. J. Cairo Univ.* 1997; **65**: 347.

110 Alves CA, Alves AR, Abreu IO *et al.* Hepatic artery hypertrophy and sinusoidal hypertension in advanced schistosomiasis. *Gastroenterology* 1977; **72**: 126–128.

111 Kresina TF, Qing HE, Degli Esposti S *et al.* Gene expression of transferring growth factor beta 1 and extra-cellular matrix proteins in murine *Schistosoma mansoni* infection. *Gastroenterology* 1994; **107**: 773–780.

112 Xiao S, Tanner M, N'Goran EK *et al.* Recent investigations of artemether, a novel agent for the prevention of schistosomiasis japonica, mansoni and haematobia. *Acta Trop.* 2002; **82**: 175–181.

113 Cook GC. Malaria in the liver. *Postgrad. Med. J.* 1994; **70**: 780–784.

114 Hollingdale MR. Malaria and the liver. *Hepatology* 1985; **5**: 327–335.

115 Silvie O, Mota MM, Matuschewski K *et al.* Interactions of the malaria parasite and its mammalian host. *Curr. Opin. Microbiol.* 2008; **11**: 352–359.

116 Stanley AC, Engwerda CR. Balancing immunity and pathology in visceral leishmaniasis. *Immunol. Cell Biol.* 2007; **85**: 138–147.

117 Da Silva JR, De Paola D. Hepatic lesions in American kala-azar: a needle-biopsy study. *Ann. Trop. Med. Parasitol.* 1961; **55**: 249–255.

118 Campos-Varela I, Len O, Castells L *et al.* Visceral leishmaniasis among liver transplant recipients: an overview. *Liver Transpl.* 2008; **14**: 1816–1819.

119 Piscopo TV, Mallia Azzopardi C. Leishmaniasis. *Postgrad. Med. J.* 2007; **83**: 649–657.

120 Sundar S, Jha TK, Thakur CP *et al.* Oral miltefosine for Indian visceral leishmaniasis. *N. Engl. J. Med.* 2002; **347**: 1739–1746.

121 Jha TK, Olliaro P, Thakur CP *et al.* Randomized controlled trial of aminosidine (paromomycin) v. sodium stibogluconate for treating visceral leishmaniasis in North Bihar, India. *Br. Med. J.* 1998; **316**: 1200–1205.

122 Vuitton DA. Echinococcosis and allergy. *Clin. Rev. Allergy Immunol.* 2004; **26**: 93–104.

123 Sánchez Ibarrola A, Sobrini B, Guisantes J *et al.* Membranous glomerulonephritis secondary to hydatid disease. *Am. J. Med.* 1981; **70**: 311–315.

124 Gelman R, Brook G, Green J *et al.* Minimal change glomerulonephritis associated with hydatid disease. *Clin. Nephrol.* 2000; **53**: 152–155.

125 Babba H, Messedi A, Masmoudi S *et al.* Diagnosis of human hydatidosis: comparison between imaging and six serologic techniques. *Am. J. Trop. Med. Hyg.* 1994; **50**: 64–68.

126 Gharbi HA, Hassine W, Brauner MW *et al.* Ultrasound examination of the hydatic liver. *Radiology* 1981; **139**: 459–463.

127 WHO Informal Working Group. International classification of ultrasound images in cystic echinococcosis for application in clinical and field epidemiological settings. *Acta Tropica* 2003; **85**: 253–261.

128 Turgut AT, Akhan O, Bhatt S *et al.* Sonographic spectrum of hydatid disease. *Ultrasound Q.* 2008; **24**: 17–29.

129 Marani SA, Canossi GC, Nicoli FA *et al.* Hydatid disease: MR imaging study. *Radiology* 1990; **175**: 701–706.

130 Gemmell MA, Lawson JR, Roberts MG. Control of echinococcosis/hydatidosis: present status of worldwide progress. *Bull. WHO* 1986; **64**: 333–339.

131 Nahmias J, Goldsmith R, Soibalman M *et al.* Three to 7 years follow-up after albendazole treatment of 68 patients with cystic echinococcosis (hydatid disease). *Ann. Trop. Med. Parasitol.* 1994; **88**: 295–304.

132 Moro P, Schantz PM. Echinococcosis: a review. *Int. J. Infect. Dis.* 2009; **13**: 125–133.

133 Filice C, Pirola F, Brunetti E *et al.* A new therapeutic approach for hydatid liver cysts. Aspiration and alcohol injection under sonographic guidance. *Gastroenterology* 1990; **98**: 1366–1368.

134 Khuroo MS, Wani NA, Javid G *et al.* Percutaneous drainage compared with surgery for hepatic hydatid cysts. *N. Engl. J. Med.* 1997; **337**: 881–887.

135 Teres J, Gomez-Moli J, Bruguera M *et al.* Sclerosing cholangitis after surgical treatment of hepatic echinococcal cysts: report of three cases. *Am. J. Surg.* 1984; **148**: 694–697.

136 Ezer A, Nursal TZ, Moray G *et al.* Surgical treatment of liver hydatid cysts. *HPB (Oxford)* 2006; **8**: 38–42.

137 Schaefer JW, Khan MY. Echinococcosis (hydatid disease): lessons from experience with 59 patients. *Rev. Infect. Dis.* 1991; **13**: 243–247.

138 Ammann RW, Ilitsch N, Marincek B *et al.* Effect of chemotherapy on the larval mass and the long-term course of alveolar echinococcosis. *Hepatology* 1994; **19**: 735–742.

139 Wilson JF, Rausch RL, Wilson FR *et al.* Alveolar hydatid disease. Review of the surgical experience in 42 cases of active disease among Alaskan Eskimos. *Ann. Surg.* 1995; **221**: 315–323.

140 Bresson-Hadni S, Franza A, Miguet JP *et al.* Orthotopic liver transplantation for incurable alveolar echinococcosis of the liver: report of 17 cases. *Hepatology* 1991; **13**: 1061–1070.

141 Khuroo MS, Zargar SA, Mahajan R. Hepatobiliary and pancreatic ascariasis in India. *Lancet* 1990; **335**: 1503–1506.

142 Shulman A. Non-Western patterns of biliary stones and the role of ascariasis. *Radiology* 1987; **162**: 425–430.

143 Kamath PS, Joseph DC, Chandran R *et al.* Biliary ascariasis: ultrasonography, endoscopic retrograde cholangiopancreatography, and biliary drainage. *Gastroenterology* 1986; **91**: 730–732.

144 Manialawi MS, Khattar NY, Helmy MM *et al.* Endoscopic diagnosis and extraction of biliary *Ascaris. Endoscopy* 1986; **18**: 204–205.

145 Keiser J, Utzinger J. Efficacy of current drugs against soil-transmitted helminth infections: systematic review and meta-analysis. *JAMA* 2008; **299**: 1937–1948.

146 Delarocque Astagneau E, Hadengue A, Degottc C *et al.* Biliary obstruction resulting from Strongyloides stercoralis infection: report of a case. *Gut* 1994; **35**: 705–706.

147 Vilela EG, Clemente WT, Mira RR *et al.* Strongyloides stercoralis hyperinfection syndrome after liver transplantation: case report and literature review. *Transpl. Infect. Dis.* 2009; **11**: 132–136.

148 Segarra-Newnham M. Manifestations, diagnosis, and treatment of Strongyloides stercoralis infection. *Ann. Pharmacother.* 2007; **41**: 1992–2001.

149 Guattery JM, Milne J, House RK. Observations on hepatic and renal dysfunction in trichinosis. Anatomic changes in these organs occurring in cases of trichinosis. *Am. J. Med.* 1956; **21**: 567–582.

150 Dupouy-Camet J, Bruschi F. Management and diagnosis of human trichinellosis. In: Dupouy-Camet J, Murrell KD, eds. *FAO/WHO/OIE Guidelines for the Surveillance, Management, Prevention and Control of Trichinellosis.* Paris, France: World Organisation for Animal Health Press, 2007, p. 37–68.

151 Gottstein B, Pozio E, Nöckler K. Epidemiology, diagnosis, treatment, and control of trichinellosis. *Clin. Microbiol. Rev.* 2009; **22**: 127–145.

152 Zinkham WH. Visceral larva migrans. *Am. J. Dis. Child.* 1978; **132**: 627–633.

153 Lim JH. Toxocariasis of the liver: visceral larva migrans. *Abdom. Imaging.* 2008; **33**: 151–156.

154 Marcos LA, Terashima A, Gotuzzo E. Update on hepatobiliary flukes fascioliasis, opisthorchiasis and clonorchiasis. *Curr. Opin. Infect. Dis.* 2008; **21**: 523–530.

155 Hou PC, Pang LSC. *Clonorchis sinensis* infestation in man in Hong Kong. *J. Pathol. Bact.* 1964; **87**: 245–250.

156 Ona FV, Dytoc JNT. Clonorchis-associated cholangiocarcinoma: a report of two cases with unusual manifestations. *Gastroenterology* 1991; **101**: 831–839.

157 Lim JH, Mairiang E, Ahn GH. Biliary parasitic diseases including clonorchiasis, opisthorchiasis and fascioliasis. *Abdom. Imaging.* 2008; **33**: 157–165.

158 Jan YY, Chen MF. Percutaneous trans-hepatic cholangioscopic lithotomy for hepatolithiasis: long-term results. *Gastrointest. Endosc.* 1995; **42**: 1–5.

159 Jan YY, Chen MF, Wang CS *et al.* Surgical treatment of hepatolithiasis: long-term result. *Surgery* 1996; **120**: 509–514.

160 Pagola Serrano MA, Vega A, Ortega E *et al.* Computed tomography of hepatic fascioliasis. *J. Comp. Assist. Tomogr.* 1987; **11**: 269–272.

161 Cordova M, Herrera P, Nopo L *et al. Fasciola hepatica* cysteine proteinases: immunodominant antigens in human fascioliasis. *Am. J. Trop. Med. Hyg.* 1997; **57**: 660–666.

162 Espino AM, Marcet R, Finlay CM. Detection of circulating excretory secretory antigens in human fascioliasis by sandwich enzyme-linked immunosorbent assay. *J. Clin. Microbiol.* 1990; **28**: 2637–2640.

163 Nguyen T, Powell A, Daugherty T. Recurrent pyogenic cholangitis. *Dig. Dis. Sci.* 2010; **55**: 8–10.

CHAPTER 33
Space-Occupying Lesions: the Diagnostic Approach

Neil H. Davies & Dominic Yu
Department of Radiology, Royal Free Hospital, London, UK

Learning points

- This chapter describes the strengths and weaknesses of the different imaging modalities in the investigation of focal liver lesions.

- Each imaging modality should not be interpreted in isolation but rather as complementary to each other.

- A multidisciplinary team approach with accurate clinical information is vital in selecting the correct imaging algorithm.

- Broad imaging algorithms have been given but are not set in stone and local availability and expertise should always be taken into account.

Ultrasound

Ultrasound refers to high-frequency sound waves, which are above the audible range in humans, that is above a frequency of 20 kilohertz. However, for medical imaging purposes it refers to much higher frequencies of between 2 and 18 megahertz. The choice of transducer defines the frequency available, and each particular transducer represents a trade off between spatial resolution and depth of imaging. In imaging the liver, probes with frequencies between 2.5 and 7.5 megahertz are usually employed.

The addition of Doppler allows identification of flow within the vessels of the liver. The Doppler effect relies on the principle that the velocity and direction of flow in a vessel can be derived from the difference between the frequency of the ultrasound signal emitted from the transducer and that reflected back (echo) from the vessel.

Modern ultrasound machines are extremely sophisticated but relatively inexpensive when compared to CT and MRI, with small 'lap-top' style machines now

allowing scanning in the out-patient department or on the ward.

Dilated bile ducts, gallbladder disease, hepatic tumours and some diffuse hepatic abnormalities are usually demonstrated with relative ease.

Ultrasound of the liver is difficult in patients who are overweight, or who have excessive bowel gas, those with a high liver lying entirely covered by the rib margin and in patients in the immediate postoperative period who have dressings and painful scars.

A normal ultrasound shows the liver to have mixed echogenicity. Portal and hepatic veins, inferior vena cava and aorta are shown. The normal intrahepatic bile ducts are thin and run parallel to large portal vein branches. The right and left hepatic ducts are 1–3 mm in diameter and the common bile duct 2–7 mm in diameter. Ultrasound remains the investigation of choice for the gallbladder where wall thickness, polyps and stones can be depicted more accurately than with any other modality.

With Doppler there are unique signals in the hepatic veins, hepatic artery and portal vein. This technique may aid diagnosis in suspected hepatic vein outflow block (Budd–Chiari syndrome) [1,2], hepatic artery thrombosis (after liver transplantation) and portal vein thrombosis [3]. In portal hypertension the direction of portal flow and the patency of portosystemic shunts can be seen. Flattening of the Doppler waveform in the hepatic veins suggests the presence of cirrhosis [4]. Regular monitoring of flow through transjugular intrahepatic portosystemic shunts (TIPS) by Doppler ultrasound is useful in detecting shunt dysfunction before clinical signs of shunt dysfunction occur [5].

Focal hepatic lesions are better detected by ultrasound than diffuse liver disease. Lesions of 1 cm or more in diameter can be seen easily. Simple cysts have smooth walls and echo-free contents with no impedance to the

Sherlock's Diseases of the Liver and Biliary System, Twelfth Edition. Edited by James S. Dooley, Anna S.F. Lok, Andrew K. Burroughs, E. Jenny Heathcote.
© 2011 by Blackwell Publishing Ltd. Published 2011 by Blackwell Publishing Ltd.

transmission of sound waves. The appearance is diagnostic and, with small cysts, more accurate than CT. Hydatid cysts produce a characteristic appearance with the contained daughter cysts. Cavernous haemangiomata, the commonest liver neoplasm, is usually hyperechoic often with no impedance to transmission of sound waves. Such a lesion is usually less than 3 cm in diameter, detected incidentally in a patient with normal liver function tests and generally needs no further investigation. Lesions greater than 3 cm, where the appearances are not classical, or where metastases (especially hypervascular) are suspected, need further confirmation by dynamic enhanced CT or MRI. Malignant masses (primary or secondary carcinoma) produce a range of appearances on ultrasound, including a hyper- or hypoechoic pattern, and can be well circumscribed or infiltrative. Appearances highly suggestive of metastases include the bull's eye appearance (a hyperechoic rim surrounding a hypoechoic centre). Necrotic tumours may mimic abscesses or cysts.

Guided biopsy of a suspicious nodule may be required to establish the precise pathology but should only be performed following discussion of the potential options for treatment. If curative therapeutic attempts are planned, including surgery, biopsy is often contraindicated [6]. This is to avoid the risk of seeding, particularly when dealing with hepatocellular carcinoma [7].

Diffuse hepatic disease may be detected by ultrasound as may anatomical anomalies. In cirrhosis the edge of the liver is often irregular, the hepatic echo pattern coarse (i.e. increased irregular echogenicity) and there may be splenomegaly and ascites [8].

A fatty liver appears diffusely echogenic on ultrasound. However, accurate quantification of fat is not possible, partly because of the variation in echo pattern between normal individuals. In about 20% of patients with fatty liver, the liver appears normal, presumably because the fat is too finely dispersed.

A relatively recent development in ultrasound has been the use of contrast agents. These consist of gas-filled bubbles (usually less than 8 μm), stabilized by a thin shell. The contrast medium is administered as a single rapid bolus injection into an antecubital vein, followed by 5–10 mL of 0.9% saline solution to flush the line. Ultrasound scanning is started immediately with the benefit of the contrast lasting 4–5 minutes. Modern machines use specific imaging programmes, such as harmonic imaging to enhance the effect of microbubbles, and also to prolong the time window within which imaging is optimized.

Using contrast-enhanced ultrasound allows the operator to distinguish the different phases of hepatic blood flow in exactly the same way as contrast-enhanced CT or MR. Contrast-enhanced ultrasound provides more information for the characterization of lesions than either conventional or colour Doppler ultrasound [9]. For example contrast-enhanced ultrasound has a 94% sensitivity and a 93% specificity in the diagnosis of hepatocellular carcinoma [10]. Accuracy in characterizing haemangiomas is approximately equal to that of MR imaging, even for small lesions [11]. Contrast-enhanced ultrasound has a sensitivity of 77% and a specificity of 93% in the diagnosis of metastases [12]. This modality is more sensitive than conventional ultrasound in detecting liver metastases and almost as sensitive as CT or MR imaging. Low-mechanical-index contrast-specific ultrasound techniques, allow dynamic real-time evaluation of both the macrocirculation and microcirculation in hepatic lesions. Lesion enhancement patterns are usually typical for a given lesion, thereby maximizing the ability to characterize liver tumours and pseudotumours and allowing a definitive diagnosis in most cases. The enhancement patterns do not have a close correlation with the baseline ultrasound appearances. Nevertheless, because of the use of harmonic technologies at low emission frequencies, there is some loss of spatial resolution and overall image quality, typically resulting in a grainy appearance. Moreover, the depth at which the lesion resides affects the detectability of vascularity as poor signal arises from deep-seated lesions [13]. **Liver** attenuation (e.g. in patients with steatosis or chronic **liver** disease) further reduces the sensitivity of contrast-enhanced ultrasound.

Computed tomography

Multidetector computed tomography (MDCT), involving a continuous spiral exposure with X rays, is made with multiple rows of detectors and can be completed during a single breath-hold. Images can be reconstructed in any plane. The great advantage of this method is that the scan can be completed while there is peak concentration of contrast medium in the blood vessels of interest, and multiple phases can be obtained. The detail is superior to single-detector spiral CT, particularly for small blood vessels. Tumour detection is improved. Computer reconstruction allows three-dimensional images, which show the relationship of blood vessels to tumours, and, with intravenous cholangiographic medium, the biliary tree [14]. Pregnancy is a relative contraindication to the use of CT scanning.

The CT scan demonstrates detailed anatomy across the whole abdomen at the level of the image slice. Negative oral contrast (water) is usually given to help identify stomach and duodenum, although some institutions still use positive oral contrast. Enhancement by intravenous contrast medium, given as a bolus, demonstrates blood vessels, followed by the hepatic parenchyma [15]. There is renal excretion of contrast. Intravenous cholangiography as a source of contrast is very occasionally used to delineate the biliary system but is restricted to patients with normal liver function tests. CT gives good visualization of adjacent organs, particularly kidneys, pancreas, spleen and retroperitoneal lymph nodes.

CT demonstrates focal hepatic lesions and some diffuse conditions. Advantages over ultrasound are that it is less operator dependent. MDCT allows easy multiplanar reconstruction and manipulation of the images on the workstation. It is more reproducible; obese patients are well suited for CT. Pain, postoperative scars and dressings are no hindrance. CT-guided biopsy and aspiration are accurate. The disadvantages of CT are cost, the exposure to radiation, contrast-induced nephropathy and lack of portability—the patient must be brought to the scanner.

The liver appears homogeneous with an attenuation value (in Hounsfield units) similar to kidney and spleen. Portal vein branches are seen at the hilum. Intravenous enhancement is necessary to confidently differentiate these from dilated bile ducts. Hepatic veins are usually seen. Enhanced CT shows the portal vein and can be used to check its patency. Invading tumour or obstructing thrombus may be seen. Cavernomatous transformation can be recognized with two or more enhancing vessels in place of the obstructed portal vein. Doppler ultrasound, however, remains a complementary technique to demonstrate abnormalities of the portal vein, especially its direction of flow.

In Budd–Chiari syndrome there may be a patchy pattern of hepatic enhancement ('pseudotumour' appearance) which may wrongly be interpreted as tumour within the liver [16]. The caudate lobe is enlarged. Concomitant thromboses in the portal vein and vena cava can be identified.

An enhanced CT demonstrates the splenic vein and in portal hypertension the collaterals around the spleen and retroperitoneum. Spontaneous and surgical shunts can be demonstrated.

Normal bile ducts, both intra- and extrahepatic, are difficult to see. In the gallbladder, calcified stones can be demonstrated. However, ultrasound rather than CT is the technique of choice to search for gallbladder stones.

The shape of the liver, any anatomical abnormalities or lobe atrophy are seen. Liver volume can be calculated from the slices taken so as to measure the volume of potential liver remnant before resection, whether for cancer or live donation for liver transplantation. Tumour volume can also be calculated.

CT demonstrates diffuse liver disease due to cirrhosis, fat and iron. A nodular, uneven edge to the liver, which may be shrunken, suggests cirrhosis. Ascites and splenomegaly support this diagnosis. CT is of particular value in suspected cirrhosis when clotting deficiencies preclude routine percutaneous liver biopsy.

Fatty liver shows a lower attenuation value than normal. Even in an unenhanced scan, the blood vessels stand out with a higher attenuation value than the liver parenchyma.

In iron overload, hepatic density is increased on CT, and the unenhanced liver is brighter than the spleen or kidney [17]. Liver with a high copper content usually has a normal attenuation value.

Space-occupying lesions of 1 cm and more in diameter can be easily detected by CT. Both unenhanced and enhanced scans should be performed. Thus a filling defect on an unenhanced scan may be rendered isodense by intravenous contrast injection and missed. Conversely, an area isodense with normal liver on the unenhanced scan may only be seen after enhancement. It is important that the imaging sequence is set up optimally, to catch both the arterial and portal venous phases of enhancement.

Benign lesions (often detected by chance) include simple cysts and cavernous haemangiomas. Simple cysts can usually be confidently identified because of the low attenuation value of the centre, equivalent to water. Smaller cysts, however, may suffer from a partial volume effect (i.e. an artificially high attenuation value because of averaging with the surrounding block of normal tissue). Ultrasound may be necessary to confirm the small cyst.

Cavernous haemangioma appears as a low attenuation area on an unenhanced scan which subsequently fills in with contrast from the periphery (Fig. 33.1). In cases where CT appearance is equivocal and there is doubt about the precise nature of the lesion, an MRI scan may be necessary.

CT scans can detect solid lesions greater than 1 cm in diameter due to primary or secondary malignant tumour. They usually have a lower attenuation value than normal liver which remains during enhancement. Calcification is present in some metastases such as from colon (especially mucinous primary ones and after chemotherapy). Hepatocellular carcinoma is hyperattenuating on arterial phase and hypoattenuating (washout) on portal venous phase when compared to the surrounding liver. However, detection of small hepatocellular carcinomas in a multinodular cirrhotic liver on CT is not as sensitive as MRI. Injection of iodized oil (lipiodol) into the hepatic artery followed by unenhanced CT 2 weeks later may be used to detect small lesions but has been abandoned due to improved CT and MRI imaging.

Abscesses usually show a lower attenuation than normal liver. Aspiration/drainage under CT guidance is possible as with ultrasound. Hydatid cysts, particularly those that are old and inactive, may have a calcified rim. Daughter cysts can be seen in active disease [18].

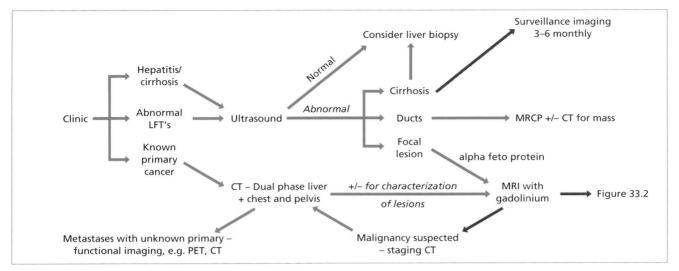

Fig. 33.1. Algorithm 1: a guide to imaging for the clinician in clinic dealing with the most common liver-related presentations. αFP, α-fetoprotein; LFTs, liver function tests; MRCP, magnetic resonance cholangiopancreatography; PET, positron emission tomography.

Enhanced CT is a valuable aid in abdominal trauma The size of any laceration or contusion can be seen, and the severity and extent of a haemoperitoneum evaluated. False aneurysms of the hepatic artery should be searched for.

An important function of CT, more so than ultrasound, is to define the anatomy for the surgeon considering hepatic resection or transplantation [19]. The segmental position of the lesion and its relationship to vessels can be identified accurately.

Magnetic resonance imaging

Magnetic resonance imaging (MRI) uses forcible alignment of hydrogen protons in a strong magnetic field, followed by short pulses of radiofrequency energy to deflect the protons. The subsequent release of energy as the protons realign is detected by receiver coils and used to create the image. The technique is safe with certain exceptions. Patients with cardiac pacemakers and internal magnetic material (clips, metallic foreign bodies) should not undergo MRI. Pregnancy is a relative contraindication and should be avoided, particularly in the first trimester. In addition, it is difficult to scan and monitor the ventilated patient.

Several types of measurement of tissue can be made, but those most commonly employed are the T_1 and T_2 relaxation times. The T_1 relaxation time is the time taken for hydrogen protons to realign within the external magnetic field after a radiofrequency pulse. The T_2 relaxation time describes the rate at which the axes of the protons move out of phase with each other because of the differing electromagnetic influence of adjacent protons. Tissues respond differently to the MRI process and scans can therefore characterize fluid, subacute and chronic haematoma, fat (Fig. 33.2), and vessels. Heavily T_2-weighted scans can be used to visualize the bile and pancreatic ducts without the need for contrast material; this is magnetic resonance cholangiopancreatography (MRCP).

On T_1-weighted scans the normal liver appears grey and homogeneous, with a signal greater than the spleen. On T_2-weighted scans the hepatic signal is less than that from spleen. Normal blood vessels usually appear black with T_1-weighted scans because the energy emanated during the radiofrequency pulse has passed out of the slice with blood flow by the time the return signal is recorded.

Although vessels and focal abnormalities can be identified on non-enhanced images, accurate assessment of the liver vasculature and characterization of defined lesions requires the use of contrast agents. There are three main categories used in liver imaging [20]:
• extracellular fluid agents
• hepatobiliary-specific agents
• reticuloendothelial agents.
The extracellular agents are the most commonly used and are composed of gadolinium chelated onto an organic compound. They predominantly act by shortening the T_1 relaxation times, resulting in increased signal on T_1-weighted images. They rely mainly on differential blood flow for lesion detection/ characterization and are considered safe at the low doses used for MRI scanning. At high doses they are nephrotoxic and there is a small risk of nephrogenic systemic fibrosis in patients with severe renal impairment [21].

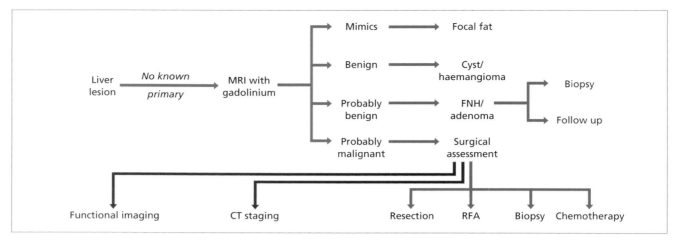

Fig. 33.2. Algorithm 2: the possible outcomes following an MRI scan of a focal liver lesion. FNH, focal nodular hyperplasia; RFA, radiofrequency ablation.

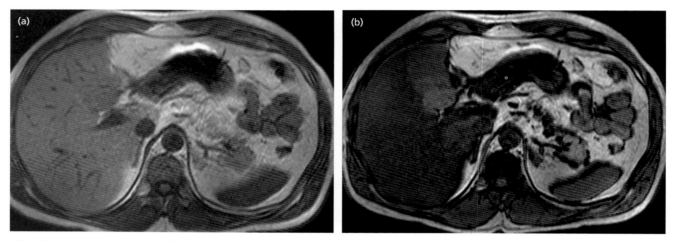

Fig. 33.3. Focal fatty sparing. T_1-weighted MRI in-phase image (a) and out-of-phase image (b) showing significant signal dropout of the liver on the out-of-phase image, indicating steatosis with relative sparing of segment IV.

The hepatobiliary-specific agents are also based on gadolinium (a previous manganese based compound is no longer available) and in the initial phase of imaging have similar properties to the extracellular agents. Subsequent uptake by hepatocytes allows for delayed imaging, which does not have to be precisely timed, offering potential advantages over the extracellular agents. Varying degrees of biliary excretion also allow delayed imaging of the bile ducts.

One of the specific benefits of these agents is the ability to distinguish between the two benign hepatocellular lesions; focal nodular hyperplasia and adenoma (Figs 33.3, 33.4). Focal nodular hyperplasia maintains its enhancement on the delayed images, whilst adenomas lose signal on the delayed scan [22,23]. This distinction can be much more difficult with standard enhanced MRI. It is important to realize that it may not be possible

to distinguish benign from well-differentiated malignant hepatocellular lesions, even with these agents, as opposed to the pattern of poorly differentiated hepatocellular carcinoma (Fig. 33.5).

The reticuloendothelial agents currently in use comprise the superparamagnetic iron oxide (SPIO) particles. These are preferentially phagocytosed by the Kupffer cells within the liver and cause dyshomogeneity in the local magnetic field, which manifests as T_2 signal loss. Normal liver tissue therefore accumulates SPIO, appearing as low signal compared to liver tumours as they are usually deficient in Kupffer cells.

Some centres claim improved detection of metastases using reticuloendothelial agents [24], whilst others recommend using them in combination with the extracellular gadolinium-based agents for improved detection of hepatocellular carcinoma. Currently, they are not

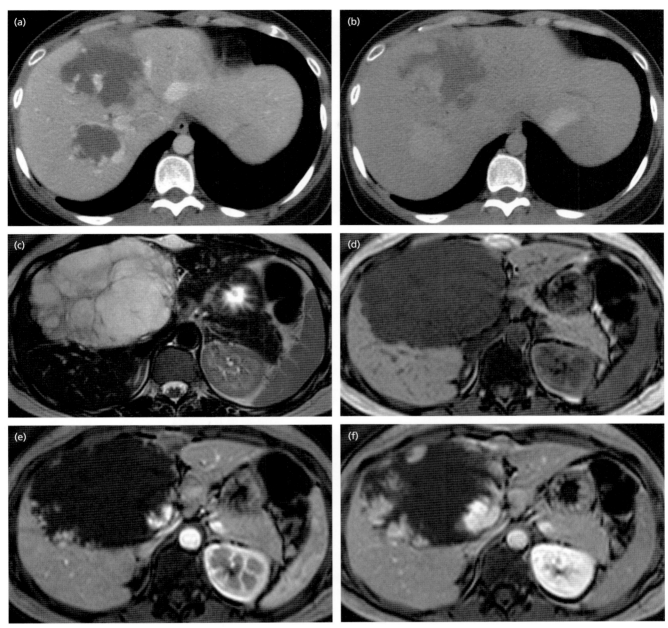

Fig. 33.4. Haemangioma. Portal venous phase CT (a) showing two focal lesions with peripheral enhancement, which on the delayed phase CT (b) demonstrated complete in-filling of the segment VII lesion but incomplete in-filling of the segment VIII, consistent with a haemangioma. MRI images showing a haemangioma which has a lobulated contour and exhibits high signal on T_2-weighted imaging (c), intermediate signal on T_1-weighted imaging (d), peripheral enhancement on arterial phase (e) and centripedal in-filling on portal venous phase imaging (f).

widely used, perhaps due to expense or patient intolerance (despite a slow infusion, 4% of patients experience severe low back pain).

Increasingly, MRI is playing an important role in the characterization of focal liver lesions. Advances in field gradient technology, multichannel surface coils, faster pulse sequences and contrast agents will allow faster and more reproducible imaging. Indeed, many centres already use diffusion-weighted imaging (DWI) to image the liver [25]. This technique relies on the diffusion of water molecules between tissues. In highly cellular tissues, such as tumours, the diffusion of water protons is restricted relative to the adjacent normal liver, allowing improved detection of lesions. This may have important applications in assessing treatment response and detecting liver fibrosis and cirrhosis. The use of apparent

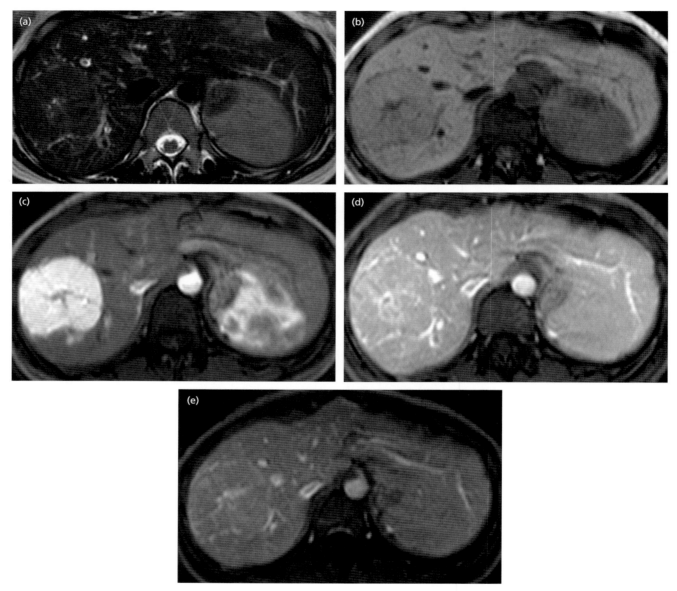

Fig. 33.5. Focal nodular hyperplasia (FNH). MRI images demonstrating a typical FNH in segment VIII of the liver. T$_2$-weighted imaging (a) shows a focal lesion in segment VIII which is of slightly higher signal (hyperintense) compared to surrounding liver with a small higher-signal central scar, but on T$_1$-weighted imaging (b) the lesion is slightly hypointense with a small lower-signal central scar. The lesion exhibits vivid enhancement on the arterial phase (c) with a non-enhancing central scar, becoming isointense on the portal venous phase (d) with enhancement of the central scar on the delayed phase (e).

diffusion coefficient (ADC), as an objective measure of DWI, has shown promising results in distinguishing benign from malignant lesions. ADC may have a role in combination with contrast agents in improving contrast-to-noise ratios, and hence further improving the detection of lesions.

MRI machines with higher magnetic field strengths (3 tesla and higher) currently increase the number of imaging artefacts within the liver, but may play a greater role in the future [26].

Radioisotope scanning

^{99m}Tc-labelled sulphur colloid is taken up by reticuloendothelial cells. Introduced in the 1960s, it was used to detect hepatic tumours, but could not differentiate between cysts and tissue. Lesions 4 cm in diameter are usually demonstrated, but sensitivity falls below this size. Reduced patchy hepatic uptake with increased activity from bone marrow and spleen denotes chronic liver disease. Ultrasound has replaced isotope scanning for the detection of space-occupying lesions. Isotope scanning has also been replaced in other situations, such as Budd–Chiari syndrome where the characteristic findings (preferential uptake by the caudate lobe) are not reliable enough to be of routine clinical value.

[67]Gallium citrate is taken up by liver tumours and by inflammatory processes, for example abscesses, but again the newer techniques, ultrasound and CT, are more appropriate for the majority of patients and centres. Gallium scanning retains a role in the complex patient with chronic sepsis of unknown origin when a focus of increased radioactivity may suggest an inflammatory collection.

[99m]Tc-labelled iminodiacetic acid (IDA) derivatives have a role in the imaging of the biliary tract to assess biliary excretion.

[99m]Tc-labelled red blood cells was used to establish the diagnosis of cavernous haemangioma. It is now completely replaced by CT and MRI for imaging of haemangiomata.

^{111}In-DTPA octreotide binds to somatostatin receptors, which are expressed on neuroendocrine tumours. Scintigraphy with this agent will demonstrate over 90%

of carcinoid tumours [27]. Its particular value is in showing 'unexpected' lesions in extrahepatic locations and in lymph nodes, not shown by MRI and CT.

Single photon emission computed tomography (SPECT) is a nuclear medicine technique using gamma rays. It provides three-dimensional information and can be displayed in multiplanar reconstruction, thus lesion localization is superior to the use of conventional gamma cameras.

Positron emission tomography

Positron emission tomography (PET) is based upon the principle that a positron emitted from a radioactive substance combines with an electron to form two photons travelling in opposite directions and that these can be localized by confidence detection. Positron-emitting radionuclides (synthesized in a cyclotron) include ^{15}O, ^{13}N, ^{11}C and ^{18}F, and these can be used to study regional blood flow and metabolism. This technique has been used to study hepatic blood flow. Because of increased glucose utilization in malignant tissue, PET scanning with 2[^{18}F]-fluoro-2-deoxy-D-glucose (F-18 FDG) can

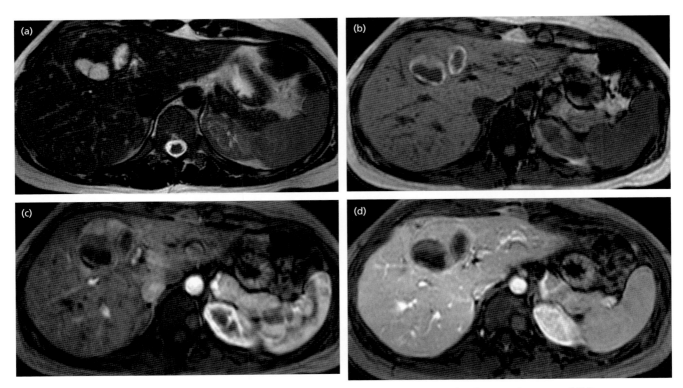

Fig. 33.6. Hepatic adenoma with haemorrhage. T$_2$-weighted MRI image (a) showing a heterogeneous signal lesion in segment IVa, with an isointense area anteriorly and two hyperintense areas posteriorly with hypointense rims. On T$_1$-weighted imaging (b), the anterior area is again isointense but the two posterior areas are hyperintense peripherally and hypointense centrally. The anterior area exhibits hyperintensity on arterial phase (c), which becomes isointense on portal venous phase (d) while the posterior areas do not enhance after gadolinium consistent with an adenoma with haemorrhage posteriorly.

detect carcinomas. This method has only a 55% sensitivity in detecting hepatocellular carcinoma, compared with 90% for CT [28]. Poorly differentiated tumours have greater activity than well-differentiated types. PET scanning may demonstrate distant metastases from the primary tumour not seen by CT. This is a useful function in the management of patients with recurrent colorectal carcinoma [29]. Gallium-68 Dotatate PET has recently been shown to be more sensitive in detecting low grade neuroendocrine tumour than F-18 FDG PET [30]. PET/CT combines the functional assessment of lesions with the anatomical details of unenhanced CT, and thus can provide more accurate localization of lesions.

MR spectroscopy

MR spectroscopy allows non-invasive evaluation of biochemical changes in tissue *in vivo*. Changes in molecules involved in selected areas of cellular metabolism can be detected. The technique currently remains experimental, but has been applied to patients with liver disease [31]. Phosphorus-31 spectroscopy shows an increase in phospholipid membrane precursors (phosphomonoester or PME peak) and a decrease in phospholipid membrane degradation products and endoplasmic reticulum (phosphodiester or PDE peak). These changes correlate with severity of liver disease and may reflect

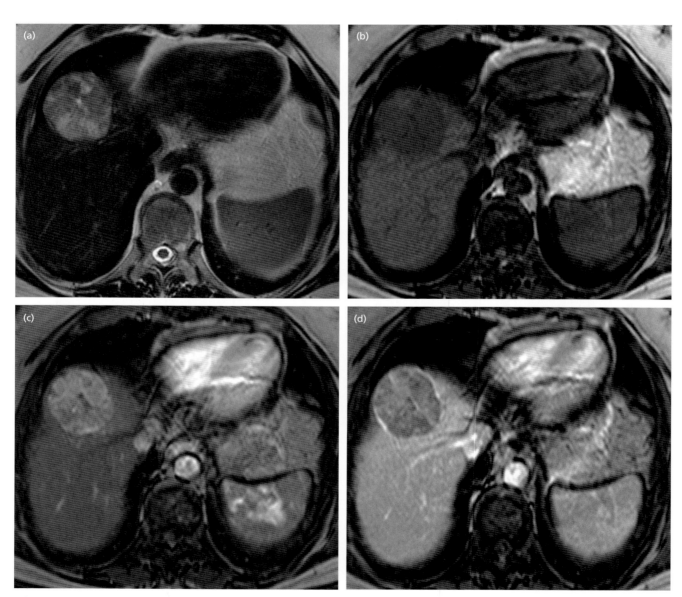

Fig. 33.7. Hepatocellular carcinoma. T_2-weighted MRI image (a) showing a heterogeneous hyperintense lesion, which is hypointense on T_1-weighted imaging (b), exhibits vivid arterial enhancement (c) and becomes hypointense on portal venous phase (washout) (d), consistent with hepatocellular carcinoma.

increased turnover of cell membranes as the liver regenerates. Clinical application of the technique remains elusive, but a role in acute liver failure and assessment of donor liver tissue is possible.

Conclusions and choice of imaging technique

The choice of technique for hepatobiliary imaging depends upon the patient's problem that has to be solved and the availability of the appropriate apparatus, operator and interpreter. Strict diagnostic algorithms cannot be formulated that will be appropriate to all units. Radioisotope scanning has been largely superseded by ultrasound, CT and MRI, which are better in detecting lesions and characterizing them. With an experienced ultrasonographer, this technique is the initial examination of choice for the majority of patients with suspected hepatobiliary disease. Equivocal results can be further studied by CT or MRI as necessary.

CT and MRI characterize most hepatic lesions better than ultrasound, but are more costly and less widely available. In some centres, CT replaces ultrasound as the primary procedure, often more out of availability and convenience (for the clinician) than specific need.

Algorithms, as given in Figs 33.6 and 33.7, have been formulated to try to give some general radiological guidelines that the clinician can use in everyday practice.

References

1 Bolondi L, Gaiani S, Li Bassi S *et al.* Diagnosis of Budd–Chiari syndrome by pulsed Doppler ultrasound. *Gastroenterology* 1991; **100**: 1324–1331.

2 Cura M, Haskal Z, Lopera J. Diagnostic and interventional radiology for Budd-Chiari syndrome. *RadioGraphics* 2009; **29**: 669–681.

3 Zwiebel WJ. Sonographic diagnosis of hepatic vascular disorders. *Semin. Ultrasound CT MR* 1995; **16**: 34–48.

4 Colli A, Cocciolo M, Riva C *et al.* Abnormalities of Doppler waveform of hepatic veins in patients with chronic liver disease: correlation with histological findings. *Am. J. Roentgenol.* 1994; **162**: 833–837.

5 Mancuso A, Fung K, Mela M *et al.* TIPS for acute and chronic Budd-Chiari syndrome: a single-centre experience. *J. Hepatol.* 2003; **38**: 751–754.

6 Stigliano R, Marelli L, Yu D *et al.* Seeding following percutaneous diagnostic and therapeutic approaches for hepatocellular carcinoma. What is the risk and the outcome? Seeding risk for percutaneous approach of HCC. *Cancer Treat. Rev.* 2007; **33**: 437–447.

7 Perkins JD. Seeding risk following percutaneous approach to hepatocellular carcinoma. *Liver Transpl.* 2007; **13**: 1603.

8 Aubé C, Oberti F, Korali N *et al.* Ultrasonographic diagnosis of hepatic fibrosis or cirrhosis. *J. Hepatol.* 1999; **30**: 472–478.

9 Solbiati L, Tonolini M, Cova L *et al.* The role of contrast-enhanced ultrasound in the detection of focal liver lesions. *Eur. Radiol.* 2001; **11** (Suppl. 3): 15–26.

10 Kim TK, Choi BI, Han JK *et al.* Hepatic tumors: contrast agent–enhancement patterns with pulse-inversion harmonic US. *Radiology* 2000; **216**: 411–417.

11 Strobel D, Raeker S, Martus P *et al.* Phase inversion harmonic imaging versus contrast-enhanced power Doppler sonography for the characterization of focal liver lesions. *Int. J. Cardiol* 2003; **18**: 63–72.

12 von Herbay A, Vogt C, Haussinger D. Late-phase pulse-inversion sonography using the contrast agent Levovist: differentiation between benign and malignant focal lesions of the liver. *AJR Am. J. Roentgenol.* 2002; **179**: 1273–1279.

13 Bauer A, Solbiati L, Wessman N. Ultrasound imaging with SonoVue: low mechanical index real-time imaging. *Acad. Radiol.* 2002; **9** (Suppl. 1): 282–284.

14 Kitami M, Takase K, Murakami G *et al.* Types and frequencies of biliary tract variations associated with a major portal venous anomaly: analysis with multi–detector row CT cholangiography. *Radiology* 2006; **238**: 156–166.

15 Torabi M, Hosseinzadeh K, Federle MP. CT of nonneoplastic hepatic vascular and perfusion disorders. *RadioGraphics* 2008; **28**: 1967–1982.

16 Brancatelli G, Vilgrain V, Federle MP *et al.* Budd-Chiari syndrome: spectrum of imaging findings. *AJR Am. J. Roentgenol.* 2007; **188**: W168–W176.

17 Baron RL, Peterson MS. Screening the cirrhotic liver for hepatocellular carcinoma with ct and mr imaging: opportunities and pitfalls. *Radiographics* 2001; **21**: S117–S132.

18 Mortelé KJ, Ros PR. Cystic focal liver lesions in the adult: differential ct and mr imaging features. *RadioGraphics* 2001; **21**: 895–910.

19 Deshpande RR, Heaton ND, Rela R. Surgical anatomy of segmental liver transplantation. *Br. J. Surg.* 2002; **89**: 1078–1088.

20 Seale MK, Catalano OA, Saini S *et al.* Hepatobiliary-specific MR contrast agents: role in imaging the liver and biliary tree. *Radiographics* 2009; **29**: 1725–1748.

21 Cowper SE. Nephrogenic systemic fibrosis: an overview. *J. Am. Coll. Radiol.* 2008; **5**: 23–28.

22 Hammerstingl R, Huppertz A, Breuer J *et al.* Diagnostic efficacy of gadoxetic acid (primovist)-enhanced MRI and spiral CT for a therapeutic strategy: comparison with intraoperative and histopathologic findings in focal liver lesions. *Eur. Radiol.* 2008; **18**: 457–467.

23 Huppertz A, Haraida S, Kraus A *et al.* Enhancement of focal liver lesions at gadoxetic acid–enhanced MR imaging: correlation with histopathologic findings and spiral CT—initial observations. *Radiology* 2005; **234**: 468–478.

24 Kim YK, Lee JM, Kim CS *et al.* Detection of liver metastases: gadobenate dimeglumine-enhanced three-dimensional dynamic phases and one-hour delayed phase MR imaging versus superparamagnetic iron oxide-enhanced MR imaging. *Eur. Radiol.* 2005; **15**: 220–228.

25 Taouli B, Koh DM. Diffusion-weighted MR imaging of the liver. *Radiology* 2010; **254**: 47–66.

26 Ramalho M, Altun E, Herédia V *et al.* Liver MR imaging: 1.5T versus 3T. *Magn. Reson. Imaging Clin. N. Am.* 2007; **15**: 321–347.

27 Caplin ME, Buscombe JR, Hilson AJ *et al.* Carcinoid tumour. *Lancet* 1998; **352**: 799–805.

28 Khan MA, Combs CS, Brunt EM *et al.* Positron emission tomography in the evaluation of hepatocellular carcinoma. *J. Hepatol.* 2000; **32**: 792–797.

29 Huebner RH, Park KC, Shepherd JE *et al.* A meta-analysis of the literature for whole-body FDG PET detection of recurrent colorectal cancer. *J. Nucl. Med.* 2000; **41**: 1177–1189.

30 Putzer D, Gabriel M, Kendler D *et al.* Comparison of (68)Ga-DOTA-Tyr(3)-octreotide and (18)F-fluoro-L -dihydroxyphenylalanine positron emission tomography in neuroendocrine tumor patients. *Q. J. Nucl. Med. Mol. Imaging* 2010; **54**: 68–75.

31 Taylor-Robinson SD. Applications of magnetic resonance spectroscopy to chronic liver disease. *Clin. Med.* 2001; **1**: 54–60.

CHAPTER 34
Benign Liver Tumours

Ian R. Wanless

Queen Elizabeth II Health Sciences Centre, Dalhousie University, Halifax, NS, Canada

Learning points

- Sensitive imaging techniques reveal a wide variety of focal variations that include benign neoplasms, regenerative nodules and pseudolesions.

- The most frequent focal benign lesions are haemangioma, focally fatty change, simple cyst and focal nodular hyperplasia. Hepatocellular adenoma is less frequent but of greater clinical significance.

- Hypervascular lesions are often malignant. Many benign lesions may also be hypervascular, largely in response to degeneration and shunt formation. Focal nodular hyperplasia is always hypervascular but always benign.

- Some benign lesions require ablation therapy because of a significant risk for malignant transformation. This is especially true of hepatocellular adenomas that occur in men.

The increased use of imaging techniques has led to the frequent identification of focal lesions in the liver, many of which are benign. A classification of benign focal liver lesions is shown in Table 34.1. In this classification, lesions are divided into those of hepatocellular, biliary or stromal origin. The entities listed conform to the nomenclature proposed in the fourth edition of the *World Health Organization Classification of Tumours of the Digestive System* [1]. This is a good general source for more information.

Benign focal liver tumours may be either neoplastic proliferations or hyperplastic expansions occurring in response to injury (regenerative nodules) [2]. Thus tumour refers to a space occupying lesion that is not necessarily neoplastic in nature. Pseudotumours are local variations, such as focal fatty change, inflammatory pseudotumour or regional parenchymal extinction (confluent hepatic fibrosis), which may be mistaken for a proliferation on imaging studies.

Diagnosis of focal liver lesions

Most focal liver lesions are defined by their histological appearance. In recent years, the quality of imaging techniques has improved so that, when combined with the clinical context, a presumptive diagnosis can often be made [3,4]. Clinical follow-up may add comfort that the presumptive diagnosis is correct. However, the best course of action is often to perform a liver biopsy. This usually provides a rapid and definitive diagnosis while minimizing patient anxiety and expediting the onset of therapy. Simultaneous biopsies of lesion and background are recommended, guided by ultrasound control. This will establish the context and ensure that the lesion has been sampled. Sampling error is the usual cause of failure to obtain a biopsy diagnosis. Fine-needle aspiration obtains very small fragments of tissue which are sufficient for diagnosis of extreme lesions such as moderate-to-poorly-differentiated carcinomas. However, early malignant lesions measuring less than 2 cm diameter are generally well-differentiated with subtle deviations from normality. For these small lesions, needle biopsy is recommended.

Hepatocellular tumours

Hepatocellular adenoma

Hepatocellular adenoma is a benign neoplasm composed of hepatocytes. Adenomas are multiple in up to a third of cases. Adenomatosis is defined arbitrarily as the presence of at least 10 lesions in the liver [5]. Recent advances allow adenomas to be subclassified into four types based on immunohistochemical and molecular features [6,7]. These types have distinct risk factors and histological appearances.

Sherlock's Diseases of the Liver and Biliary System, Twelfth Edition. Edited by James S. Dooley, Anna S.F. Lok, Andrew K. Burroughs, E. Jenny Heathcote.
© 2011 by Blackwell Publishing Ltd. Published 2011 by Blackwell Publishing Ltd.

Table 34.1. Benign liver tumours and pseudotumours

Hepatocellular lesions

   Hepatocellular adenoma

   Dysplastic nodule

   Focal nodular hyperplasia and other regenerative nodules

   Arterialized regenerative nodules

   Nodular regenerative hyperplasia

   Focal fatty change and focal fatty sparing

Biliary and cystic lesions

   Bile duct adenoma (peribiliary gland hamartoma)

   Mucinous cystic neoplasm (formerly biliary cystadenoma)

   Serous cystic neoplasm (formerly microcystic adenoma)

   Intraductal papillary neoplasm (formerly 'biliary papillomatosis')

   Biliary adenofibroma

   Bile duct hamartoma (von Meyenburg complex)

   Simple cyst and polycystic disease

   Cystic dilation of peribiliary glands

   Ciliated hepatic foregut cyst

Mesenchymal lesions

   Cavernous haemangioma

   Infantile haemangioma (formerly infantile haemangioendothelioma)

   Peliosis hepatis

   Lymphangioma and lymphangiomatosis

   Angiomyolipoma

   Epithelioid haemangioendothelioma

   Solitary fibrous tumour

   Mesenchymal hamartoma

   Regional parenchymal extinction

   Inflammatory pseudotumour

   Other mesenchymal tumours

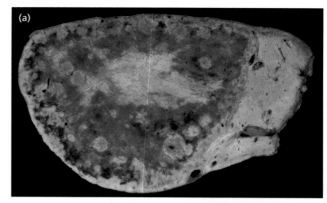

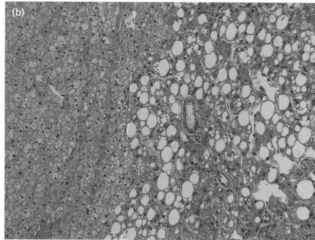

Fig. 34.1. Hepatocellular adenoma in a patient with glycogen storage disease. (a) Macroscopic appearance of a large, 15-cm adenoma in a non-cirrhotic liver. The cut surface shows variegation related to congestion without a central scar. (b) The microscopic appearance shows widened plates of nearly normal hepatocytes supplied by unaccompanied arteries. The tumour cells contain fat droplets. At left is background liver showing increased cytoplasmic glycogen, typical of glycogen storage disease.

Histology

In general, hepatocellular adenoma has uniform, well-organized trabecula one to two cells in width (Fig. 34.1) which are supplied by arteries, usually unaccompanied by other portal tract structures. Mitoses are almost never seen. Central fibrosis is uncommon but may develop in response to haemorrhage and necrosis. The background liver is usually normal although steatosis or features of glycogen-storage disease may be seen.

The four types of adenoma are: hepatocyte nuclear factor-1α (HNF-1α) inactivated, β-catenin activated, inflammatory and unclassified. HNF-1α-inactivated adenomas show steatosis, absence of significant inflammation and decreased staining for liver fatty acid binding protein. In β-catenin-activated adenoma, nuclear atypia and pseudoglandular differentiation are frequent and tumour cells stain for glutamine synthetase and β-catenin. The inflammatory type often has ductular differentiation adjacent to the arterial supply, inflammatory infiltration, sinusoidal dilatation (accounting for an earlier designation as 'telangiectatic adenoma') and staining with serum amyloid A protein and C-reactive protein.

Clinical features

Women are affected more than men, usually within the childbearing years. The patient may present with a right upper quadrant mass. Hepatic tenderness and abdominal pain are associated with intratumoural haemorrhage; this may be followed by rupture and intraperitoneal haemorrhage. Serum biochemical tests may be normal. In the presence of tumour necrosis, transaminases and alkaline phosphatase may be elevated. Serum α-fetoprotein is normal. Progression to hepatocellular carcinoma occurs in up to 8% of all patients with adenoma [8–10]. The risk of malignant transformation in men is 40–50%.

Most patients have a recognizable risk factor, especially long-standing exposure to oral contraceptives in approximately 90% of cases. Other risk factors include anabolic steroid or danazol use and glycogen storage disease (type 1 and 3). HNF-1α-inactivated adenomas occur almost exclusively in women and are associated with maturity-onset diabetes of the young type 3 (MODY3) diabetes. Most cases of adenomatosis are of this type. β-catenin-activated adenomas are often associated with glycogenosis, male hormone administration and male gender, and increased risk of malignant transformation. Inflammatory adenoma is often associated with elevated serum C-reactive protein, elevated erythrocyte sedimentation rate and, rarely, with fever and anaemia. This type has an increased risk of haemorrhage; malignant transformation may occur.

Diagnosis

The differential diagnosis is usually that of focal nodular hyperplasia (FNH) because of the similar demographic profiles. Clinical imaging techniques can distinguish these two lesions in the majority of cases. Contrast-enhanced ultrasonography is particularly effective in this differential [4]. Magnetic resonance imaging is especially useful to detect steatosis or haemorrhage [9].

Malignant transformation of adenoma can be suspected if there is a nodule-in-nodule imaging pattern or there is rapid clinical growth; most cases with malignant change are found in lesions greater than 8 cm diameter. Serum α-fetoprotein is usually not elevated in these cases.

Histologically, FNH almost always has some evidence of ductular proliferation. Central degenerative changes may cause adenoma to mimic FNH clinically and histologically. The pattern of glutamine synthetase staining differs in FNH and adenoma. Hepatocellular carcinoma is suggested by wide or irregular plates and mitotic figures. A histologically low-grade hepatocellular nodule in a cirrhotic liver is unlikely to be an adenoma; in this context the lesion is more likely to be a dysplastic nodule, well-differentiated hepatocellular carcinoma or arterialized regenerative nodule.

Management

Adenoma is a usually a stimulated lesion. Thus, hormones and other stimuli must be stopped. In many cases the lesions will regress. Control of glycogen storage disease may also allow regression. Surgical excision should be considered for lesions that are symptomatic or measure greater than 5 cm diameter. Adenomas in men should always be excised because of the high risk of malignant transformation [9,10]. The risk of haemorrhagic complication in pregnancy appears to be low but enlargement may occur [9]. Bleeding adenomas may be controlled by arterial embolization, decreasing the morbidity of subsequent excision [11]. When lesions are multiple, complete excision may not be possible; however, this is not an indication for transplantation [9].

Dysplastic nodule

Dysplastic nodules are early neoplastic precursors of hepatocellular carcinoma [2,12]. They are asymptomatic anomalies, less than 2 cm in diameter, found in cirrhotic livers during imaging or macroscopic examination. The serum α-fetoprotein level is usually less than 200 ng/mL. Malignant transformation occurs in 50% of biopsy proven high-grade dysplastic nodules followed for 2 years [13]. Malignant transformation is suggested by imaging features of hypervascularity, increasing size or nodule-in-nodule configuration.

By definition, dysplastic nodules show histological atypia that is insufficient for the diagnosis of hepatocellular carcinoma (Fig. 34.2). The atypical changes are part of a gradual spectrum so that histological diagnosis is difficult. The immunohistochemical profile is useful to detect the transition to malignancy [14].

The differential diagnosis of space-occupying lesions in cirrhotic livers includes dysplastic nodule, hepatocellular carcinoma, cholangiocarcinoma, haemangioma, simple cyst, metastasis, arterialized regenerative nodule and regional parenchymal extinction.

Dysplastic nodules are not histologically uniform. Thus, needle biopsy diagnosis is susceptible to sampling error and complete excision is necessary to exclude focal carcinoma. Nevertheless, biopsy can be definitive and is useful to expedite therapy. In selected patients, it may be appropriate to treat the lesion with alcohol- or radiofrequency ablation immediately following the biopsy. Ablation without prior biopsy is not recommended.

Focal nodular hyperplasia

Focal nodular hyperplasia (FNH) is a benign nodule composed of hepatocytes with a characteristic appearance on imaging and histology. FNH is the second most frequent benign liver nodule (after haemangioma), occurring in 0.8% of the adult population [15] with a 10:1 female to male ratio. Although women usually present in their reproductive years and the majority have taken oral contraceptives, a pathogenic role of

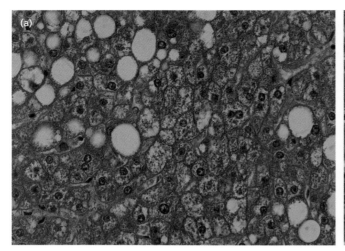

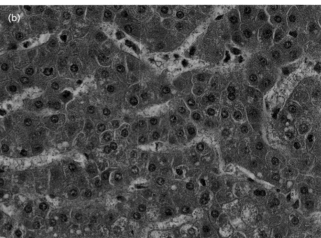

Fig. 34.2. Dysplastic nodule (a) and well-differentiated hepatocellular carcinoma (b), both from the same liver. The dysplastic nodule shows low N/C ratio and plates one to two cells in thickness. The carcinoma shows increased N/C ratio with plates two to four cells in thickness.

hormones has not been proven [10,16]. Most lesions are asymptomatic and discovered incidentally. Large lesions may present with pain or an abdominal mass.

Most lesions are less than 2 cm in diameter but may be as large as 10 cm or more (Fig. 34.3). Lesions are multiple in a third of patients. Pedunculated lesions are not rare. Histologically, the lesion consists of normal hepatocytes with regions of fibrous tissue containing large arteries and proliferating bile ducts. The background liver is usually normal, although hepatic haemangioma is found in 20% of cases.

FNH is thought to be a hyperplastic response to an artery-to-portal vein shunt [17]. Although usually cryptogenic, FNH may be initiated by local trauma or other cause of venous injury in an otherwise normal liver [18]. Classical FNH and other arterialized regenerative nodules can occur with abnormalities such as portal vein agenesis, portal vein thrombosis, patent ductus venosus, hepatic vein thrombosis and hereditary haemorrhagic telangiectasia [19]. Molecular studies have usually demonstrated a polyclonal pattern, as would be expected in a reactive lesion [20,21].

Interpretation of small biopsies is occasionally difficult using routine stains. However, the recent introduction of the glutamine synthetase stain allows for much improved diagnostic accuracy (Fig. 34.3c).

Diagnosis

A confident diagnosis can be made by imaging when there is a hypervascular mass supplied with a single central artery and centrifugal blood flow [4]. These features are most easily identified on contrast enhanced ultrasonography (CEUS). A central scar is seen in 60%

of lesions on imaging. In its absence, confusion with hepatocellular adenoma or hepatocellular carcinoma may occur. Liver biopsy is not usually necessary but is very useful when diagnosis is in doubt, especially when CEUS is not available or a central scar is not identified.

Clinical behaviour and management

FNH is a static lesion; if there is growth, an alternate diagnosis should be entertained [22,23]. Rupture and malignant transformation have been reported only rarely and need to be confirmed. FNH should be treated conservatively without surgery. However, exceptions may be considered when the diagnosis is not certain or if the lesion is large, pedunculated or symptomatic. The presence of FNH is not a contraindication to hormone therapy or pregnancy.

Arterialized regenerative nodule

This category of nodules includes FNH but also similar lesions that lack some of the classical features of FNH. These lesions have been reported with various designations including incomplete FNH, pre-FNH, FNH-like nodules in cirrhosis, regenerative nodules in Budd–Chiari syndrome, nodular hyperplasia in hereditary haemorrhagic telangiectasia, hyperplasia adjacent to metastatic tumour (peritumoural hyperplasia) and large regenerative nodule in nodular regenerative hyperplasia (NRH). Their common characteristics are benign hepatocytes, arterialized (CD34 positive) sinusoids, and hypervascularity on various imaging modalities. This category is useful when a lesion has not been fully char-

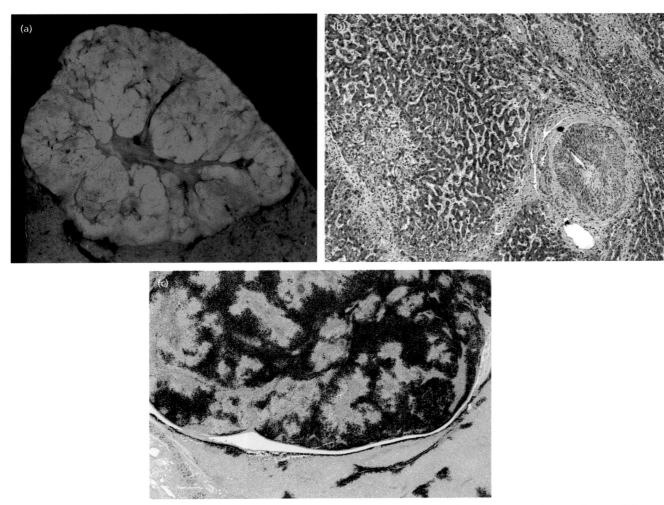

Fig. 34.3. Focal nodular hyperplasia. (a) Cut section of a 6-cm lesion showing fibrous septation and central scar. (b) Microscopic view. The lesion is composed of benign-appearing hepatocytes supplied by altered portal tracts. Note a thick-walled dystrophic vessel (right) and proliferating bile ducts (left). (c) Focal nodular hyperplasia at low magnification stained to show glutamine synthetase. This enzyme is strongly expressed near hepatic veins but not in periarterial regions, giving the classic map-like pattern. Outside the lesion (bottom) a normal, perivenous staining pattern is seen.

acterized or when some features of FNH are lacking on histological examination.

Nodular regenerative hyperplasia

This condition is defined histologically by the presence of micronodules 1–2 mm in diameter delineated by regions of atrophy and without fibrous septa [24,25].

NRH is a non-specific response to irregular obliteration of small portal veins. This obliteration is usually caused by local portal tract inflammation of any cause, especially with systemic arteritis (rheumatoid arthritis, polyarteritis nodosa, systemic lupus erythematosus, systemic sclerosis), portal vein thrombosis (myeloproliferative diseases, hypercoagulable states), neoplastic infiltration (especially lymphoma), early stage primary biliary cirrhosis and toxic injury (e.g. methotrexate, azathiooprine, oxaliplatin) [26]. NRH and non-cirrhotic portal hypertension rarely occurs after liver transplantation. These events are explained in many cases by portal vein thrombosis or anastomotic stricture [27].

The lesions may be asymptomatic or associated with portal hypertension. Patients with portal hypertension present with splenomegaly and varices, and less often with ascites [28]. The liver is enlarged if there is underlying myeloproliferative disease. Hepatic vein wedge pressure may be moderately elevated. Liver function is normal but alkaline phosphatase is commonly elevated. Portocaval shunting procedures are well tolerated.

Imaging usually shows minimal, non-specific changes. There may be features of arterialization and collateral drainage. Occasionally, livers with NRH contain larger nodules that are visible on imaging studies. These are usually coexistent arterialized regenerative nodules [29]. However, the possibility of hepatocellular or metastatic carcinoma should be considered.

Liver biopsy is useful when the clinical situation demands exclusion of cirrhosis. A needle biopsy less than 2 cm in length may not be sufficient to exclude macronodular cirrhosis and incomplete septal cirrhosis.

Focal fatty change and focal fatty sparing

Regional variation in amount of liver cell fat can produce entities called pseudolesions or pseudotumours, usually discovered during imaging [30–32]. Focal fatty change generally occurs near the hilum, possibly as a response to insulin delivery from a pancreatic vein into the peribiliary plexus [33]. The reverse effect of focal fatty sparing in an otherwise fatty liver can occur when a region near the hilum is perfused with low-insulin blood from a pyloric vein [34]. Because focal fatty sparing can only occur in the presence of fatty liver disease, most of these patients have alcoholism or obesity.

Focal fatty change also occurs under the hepatic capsule in patients receiving insulin into the peritoneal cavity as part of peritoneal dialysis therapy [35]. This was the original observation leading to the discovery that hyperinsulinaemia is the key to non-alcoholic steatohepatitis.

Biliary and cystic lesions

Bile duct adenoma

This is a subcapsular nodule composed of small uniform duct-like glands [36]. It has been suggested that this lesion is a hamartoma arising from peribiliary gland elements [37]. The lesion is commonly mistaken for metastatic carcinoma. The absence of atypia and glandular variation helps make the diagnosis. A variant with clear cell morphology closely mimics renal cell carcinoma [38].

Mucinous cystic neoplasm (formerly biliary cystadenoma)

This rare neoplasm is composed of a multiloculated cyst lined by mucin-secreting, tall columnar epithelium. The subepithelial stroma has an 'ovarian-like' appearance [39]. Patients are almost always female. When a large duct is involved, the lesion may occlude the common bile duct and cause jaundice [40]. The background liver may show effects of biliary obstruction. The tumour must be distinguished from polycystic disease, simple cyst and eccinococcal cyst. Whenever mucinous cystic

neoplasm is suspected, complete resection is strongly recommended, as malignancy can only be excluded by extensive histological examination [41]. Fenestration is contraindicated.

Intraductal papillary neoplasm (formerly 'biliary papillomatosis')

Low-grade neoplasia of the biliary tree may be associated with papillary growth and mucus hypersecretion [42,43]. The lesions often produce large amounts of thick mucin causing biliary obstruction without an obvious tumour mass. Although these lesions may be stable for many years, there is an increased risk of malignant degeneration. Carcinoma can be excluded only by resection and detailed sampling of the duct wall [44]. Biliary intraepithelial neoplasia (BILIN, formerly 'dysplasia and carcinoma *in situ*') may be found in regions without obvious mass lesions [43].

Biliary adenofibroma

This rare lesion forms a large fibrous mass containing complex tubulocystic cavities lined by biliary epithelium. The tumour resembles a huge von Meyenburg complex [45,46].

Bile duct hamartoma (von Meyenburg complex)

Bile duct hamartoma is a malformation comprised of irregular and dilated bile ducts in a fibrous matrix [47]. They are most often encountered at surgery as small, flat or depressed dark spots on the capsular surface. Most lesions are microscopic in size. When the lesions are large or multiple they are associated with polycystic kidney disease or polycystic liver disease. Small, solitary lesions occur in the elderly and in cirrhotic livers as an acquired degenerative lesion.

Simple cyst and polycystic disease

Simple cyst (solitary non-parasitic cyst) is a solitary unilocular lesion, possibly developmental, post-traumatic or postinflammatory in origin. The lesions are usually found in women [48] or children [49]. The lining is comprised of cuboidal or flattened biliary epithelium with a hypocellular fibrous stroma. If treated by fenestration, biopsy of the wall is recommended to exclude mucinous cystic neoplasm [50]. The differential diagnosis includes eccinococcal cyst in which a laminated PASD-positive fibrous capsule lines the cavities.

In polycystic disease, histologically similar lesions are present in large numbers [51]. The lesions may be confined to liver but usually involve both liver and kidneys [52]. Although the main clinical problem is related to renal involvement or massive hepatomegaly, obstructive jaundice or portal hypertension rarely occur [53].

Cystic dilation of peribiliary glands

Cystic dilatation of the peribiliary glands may be found in patients with polycystic liver disease, solitary cyst or in severe chronic liver disease including cirrhosis, portal vein thrombosis and hepatocellular carcinoma [54]. Marked dilatation of these cysts may be associated with biliary obstruction near the bifurcation [55].

Ciliated hepatic foregut cyst

This is a rare solitary cystic lesion occurring at all ages [56]. They may present with pain or be discovered as incidental findings. The cavity measures 1–4 cm in diameter and is lined by ciliated columnar cells, goblet cells and a few endocrine cells. Squamous carcinoma may develop within the lesions.

Mesenchymal tumours

Cavernous haemangioma

Cavernous haemangioma is the most prevalent focal mass lesion in the liver, occurring in 5–10% of the population (Fig. 34.4). Small lesions are asymptomatic. Large or multiple lesions may be associated with pain, mass effect, congestive heart failure or consumption coagulopathy, especially in children [57,58]. A vascular bruit may be heard. Lesions may enlarge in pregnancy and during medication with oral contraceptives, but rupture is rare and malignant transformation does not occur.

Imaging techniques can usually confirm the diagnosis without biopsy [59–61]. If the lesion thromboses, the high vascularity of the organizing thrombus may be

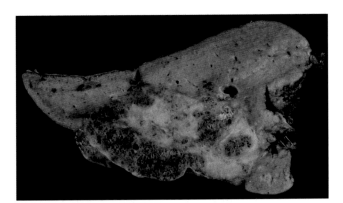

Fig. 34.4. Haemangioma. Cut section of a 4-cm lesion showing focal sclerosis secondary to organized thrombosis. Sclerotic regions are hypervascular, a feature causing confusion with hepatocellular carcinoma.

mistaken for hepatocellular carcinoma [62]. Biopsies are often composed of several small fragments of connective tissue with endothelialized surfaces. This minimal tissue may be diagnostic if the lesion is considered.

Peliosis hepatis

Peliosis hepatis may also form large, blood-filled cavities but the walls do not have the well-developed structure seen in haemangioma [63]. A history of anabolic steroid therapy would favour a diagnosis of peliosis.

Angiomyolipoma

This is a rare tumour that occurs in women more than men (5:1) with a mean age in the fifth decade [64]. Tuberous sclerosis may be associated in 10%. Lesions may be incidental findings or present with mass effect; rupture is rare. The lesions are usually solitary with a heterogeneous hypoechoic pattern on ultrasonography. CT shows hypervascularity and often low-density fatty areas [65].

Most lesions have a mixed histological appearance with areas that are predominantly lipomatous, myomatous, angiomatous, trabecular or oncocytic. Tumour cells stain for KIT (CD117), melanocytic markers (e.g. HMB-45, MART-1) and smooth muscle actin, but are cytokeratin negative [64,66]. Mitoses are not seen. The lesions are often misdiagnosed histologically as hepatocellular carcinoma, adenoma, sarcoma or leiomyoma. Biopsy is usually diagnostic if appropriate immunohistochemical stains are performed.

Epithelioid haemangioendothelioma

This rare tumour presents as multiple masses in the liver [67–69]. There is a female predominance (60%) often with a history of oral contraceptive use. The course is variable with metastases in up to half of patients. This malignant tumour is included here because long-term survival, even with metastases, is not uncommon.

The tumour is composed of endothelial cells that typically contain intracytoplasmic lumina. These cells are positive for endothelial markers such as CD34 and podoplanin [70]. The stroma contains inflammatory cells and dense fibrosis. The background liver is not cirrhotic.

Mesenchymal hamartoma

Mesenchymal hamartoma is a benign mass lesion that usually presents before the age of 2 but rarely is discovered in adults [71–73]. The tumour is characterized by marked lymphoedema of portal tracts with cystic degeneration. The histological appearance may not be specific, with some lesions being a malformation and others being neoplasms.

Other mesenchymal tumours

Lipoma and *myelolipoma* rarely occur in the liver and are diagnosed by similar criteria to the lesion in other sites [74]. *Ectopic adrenal gland* rarely occurs attached to or beneath the capsule of the right lobe. *Pseudolipoma* is a necrotic appendix epiploica that has sloughed from the colon and become attached to the hepatic capsule [75].

Leiomyoma is rarely found in liver. Immunosuppressed individuals are at risk for development of Epstein–Barr virus-associated leiomyoma and leiomyosarcoma in liver and elsewhere. *Gastrointestinal stromal tumours* may metastasize to liver even if they are histologically 'benign' [76].

Regional parenchymal extinction

Large regions of parenchyma that suffer obstruction of a large hepatic vein or bile duct may undergo collapse and resorption [77]. These lesions vary in their size and location and have been reported as confluent hepatic fibrosis, segmental atrophy, atrophy of the left lobe and potato liver. Although often idiopathic, these lesions may be seen in cirrhosis of any cause, sarcoidosis, tertiary syphilis and after treatment of hepatic neoplasms.

Inflammatory pseudotumour

Inflammatory pseudotumour is a localized region of parenchymal extinction occurring in a non-cirrhotic liver. Most lesions are idiopathic and associated with a low-grade febrile illness. The lesion contains fibrous tissue with small lymphocytes, plasma cells, and eosinophils. There is invariably obstruction of medium-sized veins. Because of the non-specific histological appearance, several different entities have been reported under this name. Some lesions appear to be a response to fungal infection, tuberculosis or other bacterial infection, Epstein–Barr virus infection [78], parasitic infestation, biliary obstruction [79,80] or bile leak. Some lesions are rich in IgG4-positive plasma cells [81] and may be associated with autoimmune pancreatitis [82].

The differential diagnosis includes inflammatory myofibroblastic tumour [80], lymphoma, follicular dendritic cell tumour [78], abscess and regressed malignant tumours after therapy.

Most cases of inflammatory pseudotumour are diagnosed after resection. Biopsy is seldom definitive. However, a lesion with consistent features in appropriate clinical setting may be followed without therapy. Some lesions will regress spontaneously [83,84].

References

1 Bosman FT, Carneiro F, Hruban RH, Theise ND, eds. *World Health Organization Classification of Tumours of the Digestive System*, 4th ed. Lyon: IARC Press, 2010.
2 International Working Party. Terminology of nodular hepatocellular lesions. *Hepatology* 1995; **22**: 983–993.
3 Forner A, Vilana R, Ayuso C *et al*. Diagnosis of hepatic nodules 20 mm or smaller in cirrhosis: Prospective validation of the noninvasive diagnostic criteria for hepatocellular carcinoma. *Hepatology* 2008; **47**: 97–104.
4 Kim TK, Jang HJ, Burns PN *et al*. Focal nodular hyperplasia and hepatic adenoma: differentiation with low-mechanical-index contrast-enhanced sonography. *AJR Am. J. Roentgenol.* 2008; **190**: 58–66.
5 Vetelainen R, Erdogan D, de Graaf W *et al*. Liver adenomatosis: re-evaluation of aetiology and management. *Liver Int.* 2008; **28**: 499–508.
6 Bioulac-Sage P, Rebouissou S, Thomas C *et al*. Hepatocellular adenoma subtype classification using molecular markers and immunohistochemistry. *Hepatology* 2007; **46**: 740–748.
7 Bioulac-Sage P, Laumonier H, Couchy G *et al*. Hepatocellular adenoma management and phenotypic classification: the Bordeaux experience. *Hepatology* 2009; **50**: 481–489.
8 Micchelli ST, Vivekanandan P, Boitnott JK *et al*. Malignant transformation of hepatic adenomas. *Mod. Pathol.* 2008; **21**: 491–497.
9 Dokmak S, Paradis V, Vilgrain V *et al*. A single-center surgical experience of 122 patients with single and multiple hepatocellular adenomas. *Gastroenterology* 2009; **137**: 1698–1705.
10 Zucman-Rossi J, Jeannot E, Nhieu JT *et al*. Genotype-phenotype correlation in hepatocellular adenoma: new classification and relationship with HCC. *Hepatology* 2006; **43**: 515–524.
11 Stoot JH, van der Linden E, Terpstra OT *et al*. Life-saving therapy for haemorrhaging liver adenomas using selective arterial embolization. *Br. J. Surg.* 2007; **94**: 1249–1253.
12 International Consensus Group for Hepatocellular Neoplasia. Pathologic diagnosis of early hepatocellular carcinoma: a report of the international consensus group for hepatocellular neoplasia. *Hepatology* 2009; **49**: 658–664.
13 Borzio M, Fargion S, Borzio F *et al*. Impact of large regenerative, low grade and high grade dysplastic nodules in hepatocellular carcinoma development. *J. Hepatol.* 2003; **39**: 208–214.
14 Di Tommaso L, Destro A, Seok JY *et al*. The application of markers (HSP70 GPC3 and GS) in liver biopsies is useful for detection of hepatocellular carcinoma. *J. Hepatol.* 2009; **50**: 746–754.
15 Wanless IR, Albrecht S, Bilbao J *et al*. Multiple focal nodular hyperplasia of the liver associated with vascular malformations of various organs and neoplasia of the brain: a new syndrome. *Mod. Pathol.* 1989; **2**: 456–462.
16 Mathieu D, Kobeiter H, Maison P *et al*. Oral contraceptive use and focal nodular hyperplasia of the liver. *Gastroenterology* 2000; **118**: 560–564.
17 Wanless IR, Sapp H, Guindi M *et al*. The pathogenesis of focal nodular hyperplasia: an hypothesis based on histologic review of 20 lesions including 3 occurring in early biliary cirrhosis. *Hepatology* 2006; **44**: 491A.

18 Wanless IR. Epithelioid hemangioendothelioma, multiple focal nodular hyperplasias, and cavernous hemangiomas of the liver. *Arch. Pathol. Lab. Med.* 2000; **124**: 1105–1107.

19 Wanless IR, Mawdsley C, Adams R. On the pathogenesis of focal nodular hyperplasia of the liver. *Hepatology* 1985; **5**: 1194–1200.

20 Paradis V, Laurent A, Flejou JF *et al.* Evidence for the polyclonal nature of focal nodular hyperplasia of the liver by the study of X-chromosome inactivation. *Hepatology* 1997; **26**: 891–895.

21 Bioulac-Sage P, Rebouissou S, Sa Cunha A *et al.* Clinical, morphologic, and molecular features defining so-called telangiectatic focal nodular hyperplasias of the liver. *Gastroenterology* 2005; **128**: 1211–1218.

22 Ohmoto K, Honda T, Hirokawa M *et al.* Spontaneous regression of focal nodular hyperplasia of the liver. *J. Gastroenterol.* 2002; **37**: 849–853.

23 Kuo YH, Wang JH, Lu SN *et al.* Natural course of hepatic focal nodular hyperplasia: a long-term follow-up study with sonography. *J. Clin. Ultrasound.* 2009; **37**: 132–137.

24 Wanless IR. Micronodular transformation (nodular regenerative hyperplasia) of the liver: a report of 64 cases among 2500 autopsies and a new classification of benign hepatocellular nodules. *Hepatology* 1990; **11**: 787–797.

25 Reshamwala PA, Kleiner DE, Heller T. Nodular regenerative hyperplasia: not all nodules are created equal. *Hepatology* 2006; **44**: 7–14.

26 Rubbia-Brandt L, Lauwers GY, Wang H *et al.* Sinusoidal obstruction syndrome and nodular regenerative hyperplasia are frequent oxaliplatin-associated liver lesions and partially prevented by bevacizumab in patients with hepatic colorectal metastasis. *Histopathology* 2010; **56**: 430–439.

27 Devarbhavi H, Abraham S, Kamath PS. Significance of nodular regenerative hyperplasia occurring de novo following liver transplantation. *Liver Transpl.* 2007; **13**: 1552–1556.

28 Morris JM, Oien KA, McMahon M *et al.* Nodular regenerative hyperplasia of the liver: survival and associated features in a UK case series. *Eur. J. Gastroenterol. Hepatol.* 2010; **22**: 1001–1005.

29 Ames JT, Federle MP, Chopra K. Distinguishing clinical and imaging features of nodular regenerative hyperplasia and large regenerative nodules of the liver. *Clin. Radiol.* 2009; **64**: 1190–1195.

30 Koseoglu K, Ozsunar Y, Taskin F *et al.* Pseudolesions of left liver lobe during helical CT examinations: prevalence and comparison between unenhanced and biphasic CT findings. *Eur. J. Radiol.* 2005; **54**: 388–392.

31 Yoshimitsu K, Honda H, Kuroiwa T *et al.* Unusual hemodynamics and pseudolesions of the noncirrhotic liver at CT. *Radiographics* 2001; **21**: S81–96.

32 Kobayashi S, Matsui O, Gabata T. Pseudolesion in segment IV of the liver adjacent to the falciform ligament caused by drainage of the paraumbilical vein: demonstration by power Doppler ultrasound. *Br. J. Radiol.* 2001; **74**: 273–276.

33 Battaglia DM, Wanless IR, Brady AP *et al.* Intrahepatic sequestered segment of liver presenting as focal fatty change. *Am. J. Gastroenterol.* 1995; **90**: 2238–2239.

34 Matsui O, Takahashi S, Kadoya M *et al.* Pseudolesion in segment IV of the liver at CT during arterial portography: correlation with aberrant gastric venous drainage. *Radiology* 1994; **193**: 31–35.

35 Wanless IR, Bargman JM, Oreopoulos DG *et al.* Subcapsular steatonecrosis in response to peritoneal insulin delivery: a clue to the pathogenesis of steatonecrosis in obesity. *Mod. Pathol.* 1989; **2**: 69–74.

36 Allaire GS, Rabin L, Ishak KG *et al.* Bile duct adenoma. A study of 152 cases. *Am. J. Surg. Pathol.* 1988; **12**: 708–715.

37 Bhathal PS, Hughes NR, Goodman ZD. The so-called bile duct adenoma is a peribiliary gland hamartoma. *Am. J. Surg. Pathol.* 1996; **20**: 858–864.

38 Albores-Saavedra J, Hoang MP, Murakata LA *et al.* Atypical bile duct adenoma, clear cell type: a previously undescribed tumor of the liver. *Am. J. Surg. Pathol.* 2001; **25**: 956–960.

39 Devaney K, Goodman ZD, Ishak KG. Hepatobiliary cystadenoma and cystadenocarcinoma. A light microscopic and immunohistochemical study of 70 patients. *Am. J. Surg. Pathol.* 1994; **18**: 1078–1091.

40 Ray S, Khamrui S, Mridha AR *et al.* Extrahepatic biliary cystadenoma: an unusual cause of recurrent cholangitis. *Am. J. Surg.* 2010; **199**: e3–4.

41 Delis SG, Touloumis Z, Bakoyiannis A *et al.* Intrahepatic biliary cystadenoma: a need for radical resection. *Eur. J. Gastroenterol. Hepatol.* 2008; **20**: 10–14.

42 Nakanuma Y, Sasaki M, Ishikawa A *et al.* Biliary papillary neoplasm of the liver. *Histol. Histopathol.* 2002; **17**: 851–861.

43 Zen Y, Adsay NV, Bardadin K *et al.* Biliary intraepithelial neoplasia: an international interobserver agreement study and proposal for diagnostic criteria. *Mod. Pathol.* 2007; **20**: 701–709.

44 Imvrios G, Papanikolaou V, Lalountas M *et al.* Papillomatosis of intra- and extrahepatic biliary tree: Successful treatment with liver transplantation. *Liver Transpl.* 2007; **13**: 1045–1048.

45 Tsui WM, Loo KT, Chow LT *et al.* Biliary adenofibroma. A heretofore unrecognized benign biliary tumor of the liver. *Am. J. Surg. Pathol.* 1993; **17**: 186–192.

46 Varnholt H, Vauthey JN, Dal Cin P *et al.* Biliary adenofibroma: a rare neoplasm of bile duct origin with an indolent behavior. *Am. J. Surg. Pathol.* 2003; **27**: 693–698.

47 Redston MS, Wanless IR. The hepatic von Meyenburg complex: prevalence and association with hepatic and renal cysts among 2843 autopsies [corrected]. *Mod. Pathol.* 1996; **9**: 233–237.

48 Regev A, Reddy KR, Berho M *et al.* Large cystic lesions of the liver in adults: a 15-year experience in a tertiary center. *J. Am. Coll. Surg.* 2001; **193**: 36–45.

49 Rogers TN, Woodley H, Ramsden W *et al.* Solitary liver cysts in children: not always so simple. *J. Pediatr. Surg.* 2007; **42**: 333–339.

50 Tan YM, Ooi LL, Soo KC *et al.* Does laparoscopic fenestration provide long-term alleviation for symptomatic cystic disease of the liver? *ANZ J. Surg.* 2002; **72**: 743–745.

51 Everson GT, Helmke SM, Doctor B. Advances in management of polycystic liver disease. *Expert Rev. Gastroenterol. Hepatol.* 2008; **2**: 563–576.

52 van Keimpema L, de Koning DB, van Hoek B *et al.* Patients with isolated polycystic liver disease referred to liver centres: clinical characterization of 137 cases. *Liver Int.* 2010, in press.

53 van Keimpema L, Hockerstedt K. Treatment of polycystic liver disease. *Br. J. Surg.* 2009; **96**: 1379–1380.

54 Terada T, Nakanuma Y. Pathological observations of intrahepatic peribiliary glands in 1,000 consecutive autopsy

livers. III. Survey of necroinflammation and cystic dilatation. *Hepatology* 1990; **12**: 1229–1233.

55 Wanless IR, Zahradnik J, Heathcote EJ. Hepatic cysts of periductal gland origin presenting as obstructive jaundice. *Gastroenterology* 1987; **93**: 894–898.

56 Sharma S, Dean AG, Corn A *et al*. Ciliated hepatic foregut cyst: an increasingly diagnosed condition. *Hepatobiliary Pancreat. Dis. Int.* 2008; **7**: 581–589.

57 Wananukul S, Voramethkul W, Nuchprayoon I *et al*. Diffuse neonatal hemangiomatosis: report of 5 cases. *J. Med. Assoc. Thai.* 2006; **89**: 1297–1303.

58 Kim JD, Chang UI, Yang JM. Clinical challenges and images in GI. Diffuse hepatic hemangiomatosis involving the entire liver. *Gastroenterology* 2008; **134**: 1830, 2197.

59 Wen YL, Kudo M, Zheng RQ *et al*. Characterization of hepatic tumors: value of contrast-enhanced coded phase-inversion harmonic angio. *AJR Am. J. Roentgenol.* 2004; **182**: 1019–1026.

60 Burns PN, Wilson SR. Focal liver masses: enhancement patterns on contrast-enhanced images–concordance of US scans with CT scans and MR images. *Radiology* 2007; **242**: 162–174.

61 Kamaya A, Maturen KE, Tye GA *et al*. Hypervascular liver lesions. *Semin. Ultrasound CT MR* 2009; **30**: 387–407.

62 Vilgrain V, Boulos L, Vullierme MP *et al*. Imaging of atypical hemangiomas of the liver with pathologic correlation. *Radiographics* 2000; **20**: 379–397.

63 Wanless IR. Vascular disorders. In: Burt AD, Portmann BC, Ferrell L, eds. *MacSween's Pathology of the Liver*, 5th edn. Edinburgh: Churchill-Livingstone-Elsevier, 2007, p. 613–648.

64 Tsui WM, Colombari R, Portmann BC *et al*. Hepatic angiomyolipoma: a clinicopathologic study of 30 cases and delineation of unusual morphologic variants. *Am. J. Surg. Pathol.* 1999; **23**: 34–48.

65 Li T, Wang L, Yu HH *et al*. Hepatic angiomyolipoma: a retrospective study of 25 cases. *Surg. Today.* 2008; **38**: 529–535.

66 Makhlouf HR, Remotti HE, Ishak KG. Expression of KIT (CD117) in angiomyolipoma. *Am. J. Surg. Pathol.* 2002; **26**: 493–497.

67 Woodall CE, Scoggins CR, Lewis AM *et al*. Hepatic malignant epithelioid hemangioendothelioma: a case report and review of the literature. *Am. Surg.* 2008; **74**: 64–68.

68 Bonaccorsi-Riani E, Lerut JP. Liver transplantation and vascular tumours. *Transpl. Int.* 2010; **23**: 686–691.

69 Lin J, Ji Y. CT and MRI diagnosis of hepatic epithelioid hemangioendothelioma. *Hepatobiliary Pancreat. Dis. Int.* 2010; **9**: 154–158.

70 Fujii T, Zen Y, Sato Y *et al*. Podoplanin is a useful diagnostic marker for epithelioid hemangioendothelioma of the liver. *Mod. Pathol.* 2008; **21**: 125–130.

71 Cook JR, Pfeifer JD, Dehner LP. Mesenchymal hamartoma of the liver in the adult: association with distinct clinical features and histological changes. *Hum. Pathol.* 2002; **33**: 893–898.

72 Yesim G, Gupse T, Zafer U *et al*. Mesenchymal hamartoma of the liver in adulthood: immunohistochemical profiles, clinical and histopathological features in two patients. *J. Hepatobiliary Pancreat. Surg.* 2005; **12**: 502–507.

73 Chang HJ, Jin SY, Park C *et al*. Mesenchymal hamartomas of the liver: comparison of clinicopathologic features between cystic and solid forms. *J. Korean Med. Sci.* 2006; **21**: 63–68.

74 Savoye-Collet C, Goria O, Scotte M *et al*. MR imaging of hepatic myelolipoma. *AJR Am. J. Roentgenol.* 2000; **174**: 574–575.

75 Sasaki M, Harada K, Nakanuma Y *et al*. Pseudolipoma of Glisson's capsule. Report of six cases and review of the literature. *J. Clin. Gastroenterol.* 1994; **19**: 75–78.

76 Chourmouzi D, Sinakos E, Papalavrentios L *et al*. Gastrointestinal stromal tumors: a pictorial review. *J. Gastrointestin. Liver Dis.* 2009; **18**: 379–383.

77 Wanless IR, Wong F, Blendis LM *et al*. Hepatic and portal vein thrombosis in cirrhosis: possible role in development of parenchymal extinction and portal hypertension. *Hepatology* 1995; **21**: 1238–1247.

78 Bai LY, Kwang WK, Chiang IP *et al*. Follicular dendritic cell tumor of the liver associated with Epstein-Barr virus. *Jpn J. Clin. Oncol.* 2006; **36**: 249–253.

79 Xing X, Li H, Liu WG. Hepatic segmentectomy for treatment of hepatic tuberculous pseudotumor. *Hepatobiliary Pancreat. Dis. Int.* 2005; **4**: 565–568.

80 Yamamoto H, Yamaguchi H, Aishima S *et al*. Inflammatory myofibroblastic tumor versus IgG4-related sclerosing disease and inflammatory pseudotumor: a comparative clinicopathologic study. *Am. J. Surg. Pathol.* 2009; **33**: 1330–1340.

81 Zen Y, Fujii T, Sato Y *et al*. Pathological classification of hepatic inflammatory pseudotumor with respect to IgG4-related disease. *Mod. Pathol.* 2007; **20**: 884–894.

82 Kanno A, Satoh K, Kimura K *et al*. Autoimmune pancreatitis with hepatic inflammatory pseudotumor. *Pancreas* 2005; **31**: 420–423.

83 Tsou YK, Lin CJ, Liu NJ *et al*. Inflammatory pseudotumor of the liver: report of eight cases, including three unusual cases, and a literature review. *J. Gastroenterol. Hepatol.* 2007; **22**: 2143–2147.

84 Yamaguchi J, Sakamoto Y, Sano T *et al*. Spontaneous regression of inflammatory pseudotumor of the liver: report of three cases. *Surg. Today.* 2007; **37**: 525–529.

CHAPTER 35
Primary Malignant Neoplasms of the Liver

Morris Sherman

University of Toronto and University Health Network, Toronto, Ontario, Canada

Learning points

- Patients at risk for hepatocellular carcinoma should undergo surveillance with ultrasonography at 6-monthly intervals.

- Lesions detected at screening must be aggressively investigated because treatment of early hepatocellular carcinoma has a high cure rate.

- Liver transplantation is the best treatment option for suitable patients with hepatocellular carcinoma; however, this option is seldom available.

- Cholangiocarcinoma remains a cancer with a poor prognosis; however, a small number of patients will be cured by aggressive therapy followed by transplantation.

Hepatocellular carcinoma

Epidemiology

Hepatocellular carcinoma (HCC) is the fifth most common cancer in the world and the third most common cause of cancer death [1–6]. The incidence of HCC varies in different countries, mainly depending on the prevalence of chronic liver disease, particularly chronic viral hepatitis. The proportion of cases of HCC attributable to hepatitis B or hepatitis C varies in different geographic area, with most cases occurring in China, South-East Asia, Philippines and in Sub-Saharan Africa. The aetiological agent of HCC is known in more than 90% of cases. Thus, for example, in South East Asia, hepatitis B is the most common underlying cause, whereas in Japan and Southern Europe it is chronic hepatitis C. The highest incidence of HCC is in Asia, accounting for about 76% of all cases worldwide [6]. Table 35.1 shows some of the age-adjusted incidence ratios in different parts of the world. The most common risk factor and predisposing condition worldwide is chronic infection with the hepatitis B virus (HBV), which accounts for 52.3% of all HCC [6].

Beasley et al. [7], in a seminal prospective study, showed the relative risk (RR) of HCC to be about 100 in HBV carriers versus non-carriers. The yearly incidence of HCC in the HBV surface antigen (HBsAg) positive group was 0.5%, increasing to 1% by age 70. In HBV carriers with cirrhosis, the RR was 961 compared to uninfected controls, with an incidence of HCC of 2.5% per year. Sakuma et al. in a similar study in Japan [8] found a RR of 50 for HCC associated with HBsAg carrier status in male railway workers, with an incidence of 0.4% per year.

However, the incidence of HCC in HBV carriers varies widely [9–12]. Villeneuve et al. [9] found no tumours in a cohort infected with HBV and followed for 16 years. McMahon et al. [10] reported an annual incidence of HCC of 0.26% in a study of HBV-infected individuals in Alaska and Sherman et al. [11] reported 0.46% in Canada. In an Italian cohort of hepatitis B carriers with cirrhosis, the incidence was about 2% per year [12].

A similar association between chronic hepatitis C (HCV) and HCC has also been demonstrated, with RRs varying considerably [13–15]. In chronic hepatitis C, cirrhosis is with few exceptions a necessary precondition for the development of HCC. HCC is between 20 and 200 times more common in hepatitis C cirrhosis than in the non-infected, with an incidence ranging from 1.3% per year to about 5% per year [13–15]. HCV is the second most common cause of HCC, accounting for 20% of all HCC [6].

Cirrhosis is the most important additional risk factor for HCC; the annual risk of developing HCC is between 1% and 6% [16–22]. The risk of HCC is higher if cirrhosis is due to viral infection, compared to non-viral causes [21,22], but remains high in patients with cirrhosis due to genetic haemochromatosis [23] and primary biliary cirrhosis [24], but less so when due to alcohol, α1-antitrypsin deficiency and some rare metabolic diseases

Sherlock's Diseases of the Liver and Biliary System, Twelfth Edition. Edited by James S. Dooley, Anna S.F. Lok, Andrew K. Burroughs, E. Jenny Heathcote.
© 2011 by Blackwell Publishing Ltd. Published 2011 by Blackwell Publishing Ltd.

Table 35.1. Age-adjusted incidence rates for hepatocellular carcinoma in different parts of the world

Geographic region	Age-adjusted incidence rate per 100 000/year
China	30
Africa	16
Northern Europe	5
Southern Europe	5
North America	12

Table 35.2. Liver diseases associated with the development of hepatocellular carcinoma

Non-cirrhotic	Cirrhotic
Hepatitis B	Hepatitis B
Hepatitis C	Hepatitis C
Hereditary tyrosinaemia	Alcoholic cirrhosis
Hepatic adenoma	Non-alcoholic fatty liver disease
	Primary biliary cirrhosis
	Autoimmune hepatitis
	Genetic haemochromatosis
	α_1-antitrypsin deficiency

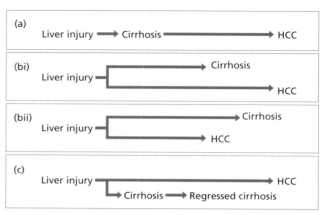

Fig. 35.1. Hypothetical relationship between cirrhosis and HCC. (a) Cirrhosis is a necessary precondition for HCC. Therefore HCC develops after cirrhosis. (b) Cirrhosis and HCC are separate outcomes of the same disease process (hepatic inflammation, necrosis and regeneration). In most cases cirrhosis develops before HCC (bi). Some times, HCC develops in livers not yet cirrhotic (bii). (c) Special case for some hepatitis B patients in whom HCC develops after disease inactivation and regression of cirrhosis.

(Table 35.2). Coinfection with hepatitis B and hepatitis C greatly increases the risk of HCC [17] as does the presence of two concomitant liver diseases. Diabetes may be an independent risk factor for HCC.

Increasing age and male sex are also independent risk factors for HCC in the presence of cirrhosis [22], and also in HBsAg carriers shown by Beasley *et al.* [7], and in surveillance studies of HBV-positive individuals [10,25], in whom this is likely to be due to a function of longer duration of infection, although an effect of age per se cannot be excluded. In Alaska, HCC was detected at a rate of 0.2% per year in asymptomatic HBsAg-positive male carriers less than 20 years old, increasing to 1.1% in males over 50 years old at the start of screening [10].

The peak incidence of HCC occurs at different ages in different parts of the world. In Asia, the incidence increases progressively until age 70 years [7], whereas in Africa the peak incidence is about 55 years [6]. In the highest-risk areas, where HBV is the major cause of HCC there is a relatively greater incidence in children and young adults.

Exposure to aflatoxin increases the risk of HCC in patients with chronic hepatitis B, but to date there are no studies in diseases other than hepatitis B [26].

The incidence of HCC has risen in Japan, Israel, Canada, Australia, Italy and Spain, as well as in the USA and France [1–5]. More recent data suggest that HCC rates may have stabilized in some countries in Europe

or may be falling in some areas, for example Japan [27,28]. In the USA, the incidence has increased twofold, mainly as a result of hepatitis C but with a contribution from hepatitis B [1]. These changes are closely tied to the epidemiology of viral hepatitis in these countries.

Cirrhosis is an almost invariable precursor to HCC, except in chronic hepatitis B. This has led to the concept that cirrhosis is a preneoplastic lesion or that cirrhosis is a common pathway by which different liver diseases result in HCC. An alternative hypothesis is that cirrhosis and HCC are independent consequences of the same process, with HCC taking longer to develop than cirrhosis (Fig. 35.1). The common factor linking all liver diseases with HCC would be the presence of repeated or persistent low-grade necrosis or cell injury, followed by regeneration, predisposing to an increased possibility of oncogenic mutations developing in actively dividing cells in damaged liver tissue [29].

Pathology

Dysplasia

The development of HCC is a process that takes place over many years. However, most of the changes occur at a genetic level, and these have no morphological counterpart. Several nodular anatomical lesions have been identified, which have an increased prevalence in livers containing hepatocellular carcinoma. Therefore, these lesions, which include cirrhotic nodules, dysplastic foci and dysplastic nodules, have been considered as possible precursor lesions for malignancy [30,31].

A dysplastic focus is a recognizable cluster of hepatocytes that is different from the surrounding liver. The cells within the focus differ from those of adjacent hepatocytes with respect to cytoplasmic staining, nuclear size, nuclear atypia and often hepatitis B surface antigen deposition. Dysplastic lesions are called foci if smaller than 1 mm in diameter and nodules if at least 1 mm in diameter.

Dysplastic nodules occur in a quarter of explanted cirrhotic livers, often coexisting with hepatocellular carcinoma [32]. These are commonly detected by ultrasound examination as nodules larger than the background cirrhotic nodules. Grossly dysplastic nodules often bulge above the cut surface and have a soft texture. Lesions may be either more bile-stained or paler than surrounding liver (due to fat). Necrosis and haemorrhage are not seen.

Histologically, low-grade and high-grade dysplastic nodules represent parts of a spectrum. Low-grade dysplastic nodules are comprised of hepatocytes that are minimally abnormal. They often have a fibrous surrounding scar, and are thus usually distinct from the surrounding cirrhotic liver. There may be increased cell density but there is no cytological atypia, except that the cells might be larger than non-nodular hepatocytes (large-cell dysplasia) [33]. High-grade lesions have more atypia and may be difficult to distinguish from carcinoma. High-grade dysplastic nodules may also have a nodular appearance, either vaguely nodular or with a more distinct margin. However, they do not have a true capsule. The cytoplasm may be eosinophilic or contain fat. There is some cellular atypia, in that the cells are usually small, and may show some minor changes in the nucleocytoplasmic ratio, or some nuclear pleiomorphism, but not enough to identify the lesion as malignant. There may be increased cell density and an irregular trabecular pattern. Unpaired arteries are frequently present in small numbers and portal tracts are present [34]. The liver cell plates are one to two cells wide (Fig. 35.2).

Small-cell dysplasia has characteristics that suggest the condition may be a true precursor to HCC [35]. Firstly, there may be expression of proliferation markers such as proliferating cell nuclear antigen (PCNA), increased labelling index of silver staining of the nucleolar organizing region (AgNOR) and expression of Ki-67 [36], which is often highly expressed [37,38]. Secondly, transitions have been described between small-cell dysplasia and HCC, with the so-called nodule-in-nodule appearance [34,37], which is the appearance of a small focus of HCC within a larger dysplastic nodule. Based on a number of studies, the lesions can be ranked in ascending order of intensity of proliferation. Large cirrhotic nodules show least evidence of proliferation, similar to that seen in smaller cirrhotic nodules. Lesions showing large-cell dysplasia also have low proliferation indices and are not preneoplastic, and small-cell dysplasia shows proliferation markers similar to HCC.

Very early HCC

Japanese pathologists have described what is probably the earliest discernable lesion of HCC, the so-called vaguely nodular lesion, which has ill-defined margins. This is also known as very early HCC [38,39], and has a somewhat vague outline on ultrasound. The cells show varying grades of dysplasia (Fig. 35.3) and more than 40% of the lesions contain fat. There may be invasion of the portal space by hepatocytes, but vascular invasion is absent. The pathology of these 'very early HCC' lesions has been defined in resected specimens, and therefore their natural history is unknown. However, small foci of typical HCC within the vaguely nodular lesions have been described, suggesting that these lesions are precursors of typical HCC. Table 35.3 indicates the differences between very early HCC and well-differentiated HCC. Very early HCC is probably the earliest morphological manifestation of malignancy. Histological examination shows the acinar cords being occupied by dysplastic hepatocytes. In resected specimens, a clear margin can often be seen within the cords, where normal hepatocytes are replaced by abnormal hepatocytes (Fig. 35.3). The first malignant cells start to destroy the normal architecture of the liver and also start to acquire their own arterial blood supply, as demonstrated by the appearance of a few unpaired arterioles. Portal tracts may still be present, but may be reduced in number, resulting in an overall reduced blood supply. Thus on dynamic imaging studies these lesions may be hypovascular, rather than the typical hypervascularity that characterizes well-differentiated HCC. The abnormal hepatocytes frequently contain fat and may show some degree of dysplasia, with altered nucleocytoplasmic ratios. In resected specimens, hepatocytes can be seen invading the portal tract (stromal invasion). The lesions may stain positively with CD34, a marker of vascular endothelium, indicating neoangiogenesis. They may also stain positively for glypican 3, a marker of early HCC [40]. Since all these studies have been performed with resected specimens it is not possible to say for certain that these lesions would have gone on to become clearly malignant. However, stromal invasion of the portal tract suggests at least some malignant potential [41]. In addition, follow-up of these lesions using ultrasound has demonstrated that some have become clearly defined malignancies.

Progressed HCC

Progressed HCC encompasses all histological variants of HCC apart from very early HCC. Progressed HCC

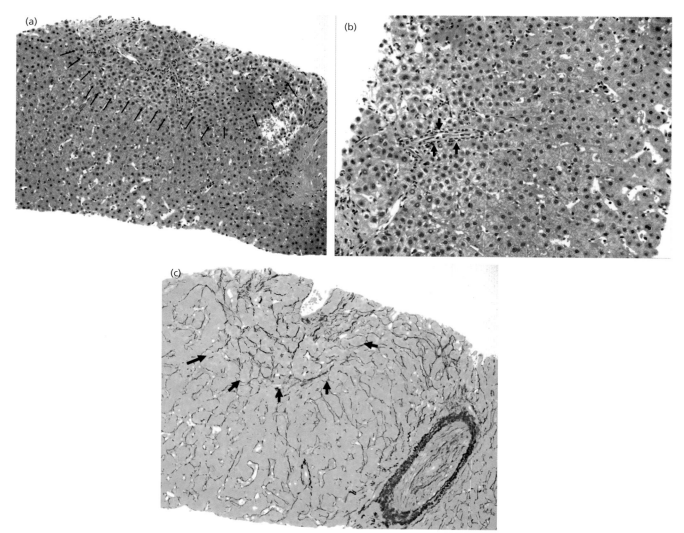

Fig. 35.2. High-grade dysplasia. (a) Lesion showing the boundary between normal liver and dysplastic nodule (arrows). (b) There is a single unpaired artery (arrow). Note the smaller (dysplastic) cells surrounding the artery compared to the cells are the other end of the biopsy, which are normal. The dysplastic cells replace the normal cells in the liver chords, which are intact. (c) The reticulin stain confirms that the chord structure is intact (arrows). (Courtesy of Dr. M Guindi)

can be categorized as well-differentiated, moderately differentiated and poorly differentiated, according to the presence or absence of cord-like structure, pseudoacinar formation and cellular morphology. Well-differentiated HCC consists of plates of cords of cells lined by endothelium. The cords may be many cells thick. The cells are hepatocyte-like but have vesicular nuclei, nuclear pleomorphism and finely granular cytoplasm. Bile canaliculi may be seen. There is usually little or no fibrous stroma. Moderately differentiated tumours contain glandular structures, called pseudoacini, which may be bile stained. In poorly differentiated tumours the plate structure may be absent. The cells may be very large, with multiple bizarre nuclei. The most poorly differentiated tumours may be difficult to distinguish from other adenocarcinomas.

Pathogenesis

Although the relationship between chronic liver disease and HCC is clear, not much else is known about the pathogenesis of HCC. In the case of viral hepatitis, presumably, repeated episodes of necrosis and regeneration result in an increased DNA mutation rate and a decreased rate of repair of these mutations. Over time, sufficient specific mutations accumulate that lead to the development of HCC. However, in diseases such as haemochromatosis and α1-antitrypsin deficiency, in which necrosis is not a major feature, it is more difficult to understand how HCC might develop. One theory is that cells affected by an accumulation of iron or α1-antitrypsin globules are injured, but not dead [29]. They nonetheless give off regenerative signals to neighbouring cells which

Table 35.3. Characteristics of small nodular lesions in a cirrhotic liver

	Low-grade dysplastic nodule	High-grade dysplastic nodule	Very early HCC	Progressed HCC
Pathological features				
Gross appearance			Vaguely nodular	Distinctly nodular
Cellular morphology	Large-cell dysplasia	Small-cell dysplasia	Well-differentiated HCC	Moderately differentiated HCC
Portal tracts	Normal to slightly reduced	Reduced	Occasional to absent	Absent
Unpaired arteries	None	Occasional	Moderate number	Abundant
Mitoses	None	None	None/ occasional	Present
Stromal invasion	None	None	+/–	+/–
Vascularity on imaging				
Arterial phase	Isointense/ hypointense	Isointense/ hypointense	Isointense/ hypointense/ rarely hyperintense	Hyperintense
Venous phase	Isointense	Isointense	Isointense/ hypointense	Hypointense

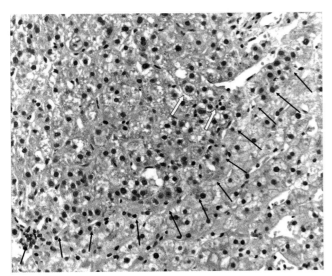

Fig. 35.3. Very early HCC. The interface between normal liver tissue and the very early HCC is outlined (black arrows). The cells of the HCC are dysplastic, but the presence of mitosis (white arrows) makes this likely to be HCC rather than high-grade dysplasia. (Courtesy of Dr. M Guindi)

consequently divide and would thus be subject to the same risk of mutations as in viral hepatitis.

HCC is a very vascular cancer. New growth of arterial vessels occurs early in pathogenesis. This implies a role for angiogenic factors, such as VEGF and its receptor. Many HCCs have high levels of VEGF expression [42,43], and high levels of VEGF, whether in tissue or in serum, may be correlated with poor outcome [42,43].

Microarray studies using gene chips have elucidated the pattern of gene expression in HCC [44–51]. There are at least three major patterns. Approximately one-third of tumours have abnormalities in proliferative signals related to the tyrosine kinase receptor pathway. These include EGFR, IGF-IR, RAS, and RAF/MAP-K pathways, as well as PI3K-Akt-mTOR pathways [44]. Another one-third of HCC have cell proliferation driven by activation of the Wnt/β-catenin pathway, mostly as a result of mutations in the β-catenin gene [46]. Yet another subset of HCCs has changes in genes involved in interferon signalling [44]. These results suggest that HCC is not a homogeneous disease, but that there are at least three, and maybe more, pathogenetic pathways that might lead to the phenotypic expression of HCC. The implication is that these different pathways may have different outcomes, both when treated and if left untreated. A separate gene signature has been associated with early recurrence of HCC after treatment [46,47]. Similarly, other gene signatures, associated with a poor prognosis, have been identified [45]. Proliferative and antiapoptotic genes are over-expressed in HCC with a poor prognosis.

Microarray analyses have also been applied to gene expression in normal liver, cirrhotic nodules, dysplastic nodules, early HCC and well-differentiated HCC [48–51]. These studies showed a differential pattern of gene expression between all the stages of disease. The studies confirmed that the usual biomarkers used for HCC surveillance (α-fetoprotein (AFP), glycosylated AFP (AFP-L3) and des gamma carboxyprothrombin (DCP)), are not expressed in early HCC. Glypican-3 in contrast, is expressed in early HCC but not in dysplastic nodules. This is the basis for the use of this marker as a histological stain to aid identification of early HCC.

Genome-wide microarray analysis has also identified a gene signature from tissue surrounding the malignant nodule that predicted late recurrence of HCC (more than 2 years after resection) [52]. This analysis also identified an expression pattern that predicted poor outcomes. There was some overlap between these two sets of markers, suggesting that in part the poor outcomes were related to recurrence. Late recurrence is thought to represent newly developed HCC, rather than recurrence from a previously treated HCC. That a gene signature can predict the onset of recurrent disease distant in time and location from the original tumour suggests the existence of a 'field defect', that is the whole liver may be abnormal, 'preneoplastic' and consisting of a single clone of cells. This also raises the possibility that in future biopsy of a cirrhotic liver might predict who is at risk for HCC and who is not.

Despite all these advances, the sum of genetic changes required to produce HCC remains uncertain.

Clinical presentation

Symptomatic presentation

If patients present with symptoms the cancer is advanced, and cure is unlikely. Patients presenting with symptoms may have any combination of jaundice, ascites or variceal bleeding; encephalopathy is rare. These symptoms may also develop as HCC progresses, in patients in whom previous treatment for HCC has failed. Thus it is important in all patients who present with these features to image the liver. Rupture of an HCC or bleeding into an HCC both cause severe abdominal pain. In addition, rupture may be associated with hypotension and shock. Finally, the first presentation of HCC may be with weight loss and other constitutional symptoms that are common to many cancers.

HCC has the unusual distinction of frequently producing paraneoplastic syndromes. These include hypoglycaemia, related to the production of an insulin-like peptide [53], hypercalcaemia [54], thrombocytosis [55] and hypercoagulability with venous thrombosis. New onset of any of these conditions in a patient with liver disease requires imaging of the liver.

Asymptomatic presentation

More patients are being diagnosed at early stages of disease, before the onset of symptoms, due to more frequent imaging of the abdomen, usually by ultrasound, liberally used for a variety of abdominal complaints unrelated to liver disease. In addition, many patients known to be at risk for HCC are being diagnosed by the deliberate institution of surveillance programmes.

Differential diagnosis

The differential diagnosis depends on the presentation. Patients with known chronic liver disease presenting with liver failure may not have HCC, and should be evaluated for other complications such as renal failure or infection, or other factors that may have precipitated

symptoms. Patients presenting with rupture of an HCC should be evaluated as for any acute abdomen. Patients with liver disease presenting with cancer symptoms may have other intra-abdominal or haematological cancers. However, patients who present without symptoms who have a mass in the liver need to have HCC distinguished from benign lesions such as haemangioma, focal nodular hyperplasia, hepatic adenoma, metastases or other primary liver cancers. In most cases radiology is sufficient for diagnosis, but in some cases, as discussed later, a biopsy is needed.

Surveillance

The purpose of surveillance is to detect HCC early, at a stage where treatment responses are more durable and cure is more frequently possible. There is a single randomized controlled trial from China that compares survival in a screened versus unscreened population, in patients with chronic hepatitis B and offered only resection as treatment [56]. Despite several methodological flaws, such as a poor compliance, this study demonstrated a 37% decrease in HCC mortality in the screened group. It is not certain that these results can be directly applied to HCC related to other causes, or in other areas of the world. In particular, the likelihood of resection in patients with hepatitis C and HCC detected by surveillance is lower, because advanced cirrhosis is more frequent. Nonetheless, these data strongly suggest that surveillance is effective for enhancing survival.

In the absence of experimental data, cost–efficacy analyses have been used to evaluate whether HCC surveillance is effective. These confirm that surveillance of HCC in patients with cirrhosis due to hepatitis C or other causes is effective and cost effective [57–61]. Table 35.4 summarizes these studies. The results have also defined the HCC incidence rates at which surveillance becomes effective (providing more than 3 months increased life expectancy) and cost-effective. Therefore surveillance for HCC should be standard care for all patients with cirrhosis, and in hepatitis B for patients over age 40 for men and over age 50 for women [62]. Patients with a first-degree relative with HCC, patients coinfected with hepatitis B and HIV are at high risk, and should undergo surveillance when diagnosed. African men seem to acquire HCC at a younger age and should also start surveillance at an earlier age.

Surveillance using biomarkers

α-fetoprotein (AFP) [63,64], des gamma carboxyprothrombin (DCP) [65–67] and the AFP-L3/AFP ratio [66,67] have been proposed as surveillance tests for HCC. AFP-L3 is a glycosylated form of AFP which is produced in higher concentration by HCC than by

Table 35.4. Cost–efficacy analyses of hepatocellular carcinoma surveillance

	Population	Comparisons	Incremental longevity	Incremental cost–utility ratio
Sarasin 1996 [58]	Cirrhosis, Child A	AFP+US vs. no surveillance	0.25–0.75 life years gained (best candidates)	$26000–$55000
Arguedas 2003 [59]	Hepatitis C cirrhosis, Child A	No surveillance vs. AFP vs. AFP+US vs. AFP+CT vs. AFP+MRI	~0.25 life years gained	US+AFP $22575 AFP+CT $14675 AFP+MRI $101143
Lin 2004 [61]	Hepatitis C cirrhosis, Child A	AFP plus CT or US every 6 or 12 months vs. no surveillance		12 month surveillance $23043–$51750 6 month surveillance $80840–$96727
Patel 2005 [60]	Hepatitis C cirrhosis, Child A	AFP + US every 6 months vs. no surveillance	1–4 years	$50400–$58400
Thompson Coon 2008 [57]	Hepatitis C cirrhosis Hepatitis B cirrhosis Alcoholic cirrhosis	AFP ± US every 6 or 12 months	50% reduction in HCC-related mortality	£20000–£60000

All cost efficacy analyses are only as good as the assumptions that are used to create the model. In the case of HCC surveillance, a lack of data means that there are many questionable assumption which can be faulted. The studies by Arguedas *et al.* [59] and Lin *et al.* [61] use data on the performance characteristics of CT scanning from studies in which the technique is used for diagnosis. There are no studies in which the performance characteristics of CT scanning have been determined when used as a surveillance test. The sensitivity and specificity are likely to be less good when used for surveillance. In the study by Thomson Coon *et al.* they assume that the sensitivity of AFP is not affected by tumour size. AFP increases as tumour size increases in those who are AFP-positive. AFP is more likely to be elevated in advanced disease, which disqualifies it as a useful marker for early disease. The analysis by Patel *et al.* [60] assumes that ultrasound cannot find lesions smaller than 2cm. However, this is not the case, since in surveillance programmes up to 60% of HCCs are detected smaller than 2cm. AFP, α-fetoprotein.

normal liver. However, all these markers are more likely to be elevated in patients with advanced HCC than in patients with early disease [68,69]. Several studies have shown that AFP is both insufficiently sensitive or specific to be used as a surveillance test [11,63]. The other markers are less well studied, but the initial results are not promising. Therefore these tests should not be used for HCC surveillance [62].

Surveillance by ultrasonography

Ultrasonography is the surveillance test of choice for HCC [62]. Despite the presence of cirrhosis, ultrasonography can identify nodules that are either HCC or dysplastic nodules that may become HCC. Most cirrhotic nodules are smaller than 1cm, although larger nodules are not uncommon. Therefore, any nodule that is larger than 1cm or that enlarges over time is suspicious for HCC and warrants investigation using the recall algorithms presented in Fig. 35.4.

Surveillance interval

The surveillance interval depends on the growth rate of the tumour and on the size at which outcome changes.

HCC doubling time ranges on average from 4 to 12 months [70,71]. The prognosis of HCC starts to decline once the HCC is larger than about 2cm in diameter [72,73]. Thus ideally, the surveillance interval should be set so that lesions will be detected before they reach 2cm in diameter. The ideal surveillance interval is not known. Several studies have suggested that there is no difference in outcome with 6 versus 12-monthly surveillance [74,75]. However, more recent data suggest that survival is better following a 6-monthly surveillance interval [76]. Thus, the recommendation is to provide surveillance every 6 months [62].

Diagnosis

The tests used to diagnose HCC include radiology, biopsy and AFP serology. Which tests should be used depends on the clinical context. Imaging, either with CT scan or MRI, is always required to determine the extent of disease. In the setting of a patient with known hepatitis B or cirrhosis of other aetiology when a mass is found incidentally during surveillance by ultrasound, the likelihood of it being HCC depends on its size. The larger the lesion, the more likely it is HCC.

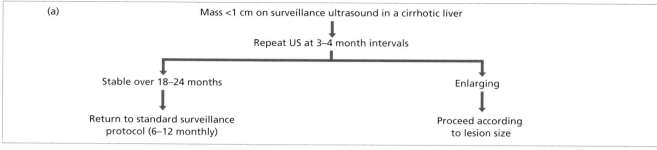

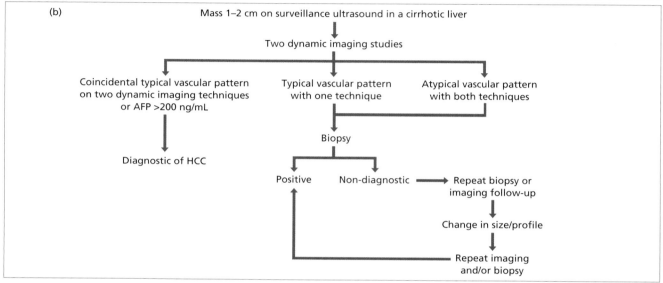

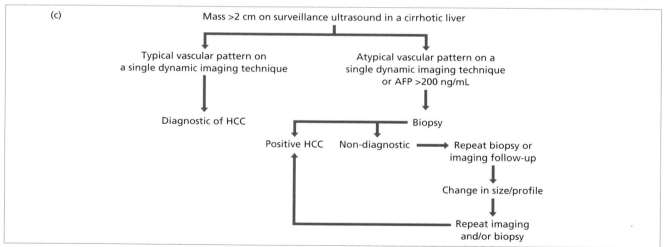

Fig. 35.4. Diagnostic algorithms for HCC at different sizes. These algorithms were developed for patients with cirrhosis but apply equally well to non-cirrhotic patients with chronic hepatitis B or C. However, they do not apply to patients with no underlying liver disease, in whom all small (<3 cm) lesions suspicious for HCC should undergo biopsy. (a) Diagnostic algorithm for lesions smaller than 1 cm. These have a low likelihood of being HCC so the algorithm suggests only monitoring. (b) Diagnostic algorithm for lesions between 1 and 2 cm in diameter. The likelihood of these being HCC is higher than for lesions smaller than 1 cm. However, radiology can be difficult to interpret at this size lesion; therefore the recommendation is that two diagnostic radiological imaging tests are required for a positive radiological diagnosis. (c) Diagnostic algorithm for lesions larger than 2 cm. Typical radiological appearances are highly specific, so if present no biopsy is necessary. AFP, α-fetoprotein.

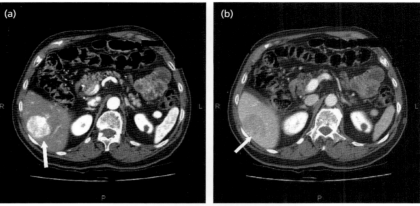

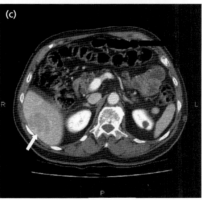

Fig. 35.5. Triphasic CT scan of HCC. (a) The arterial phase is identified by the aorta, which is very bright. The HCC in the liver is brighter than the surrounding liver (arrow). (b) In the venous phase (identified by a weaker signal in the aorta) the HCC is less bright than the surrounding liver (washout) (arrow). (c) In the delayed phase, the HCC remains less bright than the surrounding liver.

The radiological features of HCC are highly specific [77,78]. However, the smaller the lesion, the less likely that that typical features will be found. HCC exhibits hypervascularity on the arterial phase of a dynamic study (CT, MRI or contrast ultrasound), and 'washout' during the venous phase. The physiological basis for these appearances is as follows. During the arterial phase the portal venous blood in the liver dilutes the contrast agent, which is in the arterial blood. The tumour is fed by only arterial blood so that the contrast is undiluted. Therefore the tumour contains a higher concentration of contrast agent, and appears brighter than the surrounding liver. During the venous phase the portal blood now contains contrast, whereas the arterial blood feeding the tumour no longer contains contrast. Thus the liver will be brighter than the lesion, or, in the terminology used, the lesion exhibits 'washout' of contrast (Fig. 35.5). Other vascular tumours tend to have a dual arterial and venous blood supply, so they may enhance more than the liver in the arterial phase—they do not 'washout'. This has led to the development of diagnostic algorithms, which define the role of radiology and tumour biopsy (Fig. 35.5)[62].

If the AFP is greater than 200 ng/mL in the setting of a mass in a cirrhotic liver, the likelihood of HCC is greater than 90%, and biopsy is not required [79].

A new lesion detected with surveillance ultrasound is an indication for additional investigation. The strategy of waiting to see whether the lesion will grow and then treat as malignancy runs the risk of delaying treatment until the lesion reaches a size where the likelihood of complete eradication of tumour decreases [80]. For example, if a lesion is detected at 1 cm, then 6 months later it may be larger than 2 cm, and less likely to be completely eradicated.

Lesions less than 1 cm in diameter on ultrasound in a cirrhotic liver have a low likelihood of being HCC [81]. Even if CT or MRI show arterial vascularization, the vascularized areas may not correspond to HCC foci [82,83]. However, the possibility remains high that minute hepatic nodules detected by ultrasonography may become malignant over time [84]. Therefore these nodules need to be regularly followed-up every few months in order to detect growth suggestive of malignant transformation (Fig. 35.4a). Lack of growth over a period of more than 1–2 years suggests that the lesion is not HCC.

Lesions between 1 and 2 cm have an indeterminate likelihood of being HCC. The AASLD guidelines [62] recommended that the diagnosis of HCC can be made without biopsy in patients with chronic liver disease and cirrhosis who have a mass between 1 and 2 cm if the mass shows characteristic radiological features on at least two dynamic imaging techniques (Fig. 35.4b). Lesions showing typical features on both techniques should be treated as HCC since the positive predictive value of the clinical and radiological findings exceeds 95% [77,78]. If the two techniques give discordant results (one typical and one atypical) or if both techniques give atypical results, a biopsy is required to confirm the diagnosis. If the lesion is larger than 2 cm, only a single dynamic radiological study is necessary to confirm the diagnosis if the findings are typical of HCC (Fig. 35.4c). If the appearances are not typical, a biopsy should be done. It is important to note that although a positive biopsy is diagnostic, a negative biopsy can never be taken as proof that an HCC does not exist. In these small lesions, placement of the biopsy needle is difficult and sampling errors are common. Pathological interpreta-

tion of the earliest changes of HCC is also difficult and the difference between dysplasia and HCC may be subtle and easily missed. Thus, a negative biopsy requires either a second biopsy or more frequent follow-up with ultrasound. If the lesion either enlarges or changes appearance, the diagnostic work-up must be repeated.

Very early HCC is hypovascular on imaging, and has 'atypical' imaging (Fig. 35.6); these lesions should be biopsied. Cholangiocarcinoma is vascular in the arterial phase but does not washout, so a biopsy would be indicated.

Role of liver biopsy

Liver biopsy to diagnose HCC remains a controversial issue. Biopsy carries a median risk of tumour seeding of

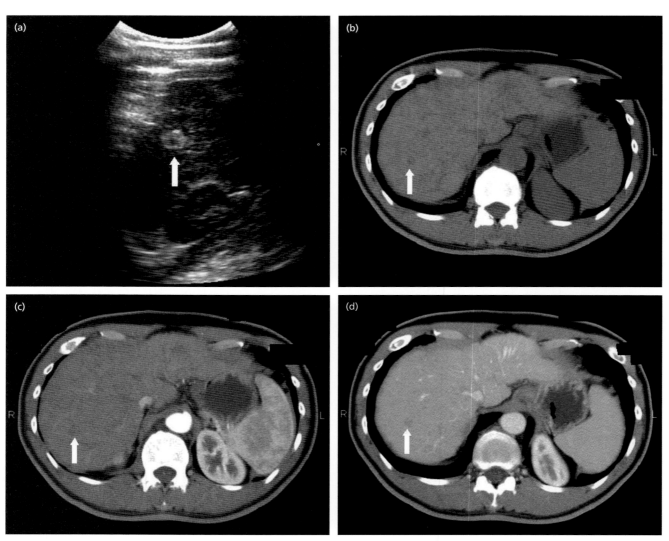

Fig. 35.6. Very early HCC on ultrasound and triphasic CT scan. Note that the lesion is hypoattenuating (less bright) in the non-contrast phase because of fat in the lesion. In the

arterial and venous phases it remains hypoattenuating indicating that it is relatively hypovascular compared to the surrounding liver.

2.29% (0–11%) [85] so if resection or transplantation is contemplated, tumour seeding converts a curable situation to an incurable one. The risk of tumour seeding from biopsy of small lesions is less well characterized but when the lesion is small, seeding is reduced if ablative therapy is used after biopsy (median risk is 1.5% for percutaneous ethanol injection (PEI) or radiofrequency ablation (RFA)) [85]. Biopsy is indicated when radiology is unable to confirm a diagnosis. The biopsy has to be performed under ultrasound guidance, and should be with as large a needle as is safe to use. This ensures a larger specimen, increasing the diagnostic accuracy. A core biopsy is required. A fine-needle aspirate cannot distinguish well-differentiated HCC from normal hepatocytes, as architectural features are used to distinguish a well-differentiated HCC from normal tissue, such as thickened cords, trabecular pattern, etc. These features cannot be assessed in fine-needle aspirate specimens [85].

Staging of HCC

There are many staging systems for HCC; none are universally accepted. In Europe and North America, the Tumour Node Metastasis (TNM), Barcelona Cancer of the Liver Clinic (BCLC) [86] (Fig. 35.7) and Model for End Stage Liver disease (MELD) [87] or Cancer of the Liver Italian Program (CLIP) [88] systems are in common use. TNM is the classical cancer staging system, but is of less value for HCC because it does not capture liver function. Since Child–Pugh status is one of the best predictors of outcome of HCC, this is a major omission. An

attempt to correct this is the sT or simplified TNM [89]. This includes an assessment of fibrosis. TNM also includes vascular invasion, including microvascular invasion, as a prognostic criterion. This information is not usually available prior to resection or transplantation, again limiting the usefulness of this staging system. MELD was not designed as an HCC staging system, and should not be used as such. The BCLC staging system was developed to separate out clinical stages of HCC that have distinctly different outcomes. It includes measures of liver function and performance status, both significant predictors of outcome. The BCLC staging system also has the advantage that it links different clinical stages to treatments that are appropriate to that stage. The CLIP score was developed using classical methodology, but suffers from being insensitive to prognosis associated with small HCC. Tumour size does not change the CLIP score until the lesion occupies 50% of the liver.

The Chinese University Prognostic Index (CUPI) [90] was developed primarily in patients with hepatitis B, where as the CLIP and BCLC were developed primarily in hepatitis C. CUPI has not gained wide acceptance. Finally, in Japan, several additional staging systems have been developed, which are not used elsewhere. The discussion of treatment that follows is based mainly on use of the BCLC system.

The prognosis of HCC is largely dependent on the stage at presentation, and on the underlying liver disease. Child–Pugh stage is a major determinant of outcome, confirmed in a systematic review of outcomes in HCC [91]. Other important predictors of outcome are

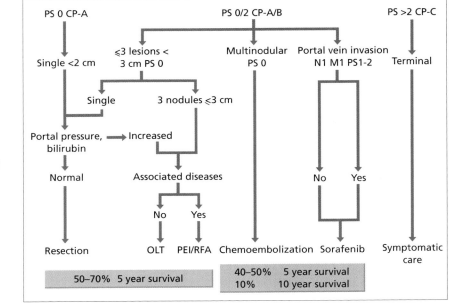

Fig. 35.7. The Barcelona Cancer of the Liver Clinic (BCLC) scheme for staging of liver cancer and the treatment strategies that are recommended for each stage. The expected survival from the categories of treatment is shown below. PS, performance score; CP, Child–Pugh class; N, node; M, metastases; OLT, orthotopic liver transplant; PEI, percutaneous ethanol injection; RFA, radiofrequency ablation.

tumour stage (irrespective of staging system), age, tumour burden and vascular invasion and performance status. An elevated AFP is a predictor of poor outcome. Figure 35.7 gives approximate expected 5-year survival for patients with HCC classified by the BCLC staging system [86].

Treatment

Preamble

There are a large number of therapeutic techniques that have been used for HCC. These include liver resection, liver transplantation, hepatic artery ligation, hepatic artery embolization, chemoembolization, internal radiotherapy, external beam radiotherapy, various chemotherapy regimens, local ablation with heat (radiofrequency or microwaves), cold (cryotherapy), corrosive substances such as ethanol, acetic acid or hot saline, and more recently targeted agents such as raf-kinase or VEGF inhibitors. The level of evidence for most of the therapeutic options is limited to phase 1 or 2 cohort studies. As a result, treatment of HCC is not adequately standardized. There are few randomized controlled trials of HCC therapy, most of which are limited to the treatment of advanced disease. There are no studies that compare treatments considered effective for early stage disease (surgical resection, transplantation, percutaneous ablation) to no treatment or best supportive care, nor are such studies ever likely to be performed.

Resection

This is the treatment of choice for HCC in patients without cirrhosis, who account for just 5% of the cases in Western countries, and for about 40% in Asia. These patients will tolerate major resections with low risk of morbidity. Resection in patients with cirrhosis carries increased risks of hepatic decompensation with right lobectomy being more risky than left lobectomy. In properly selected patients, the postoperative mortality should be no higher than 1–2%, and in many centres it is lower. The 5-year survival after resection should exceed 50 to 70% [92,93].

There are several predictors of outcome after liver resection. Best outcomes are associated with good liver function, that is Child's A cirrhosis. Normal bilirubin concentration and the absence of clinically significant portal hypertension as measured by hepatic vein pressure gradient (<10 mmHg) or detected clinically, are the best predictors of excellent outcomes after surgery, with minimal risk for postoperative liver failure [94]. Patients with significant portal hypertension may develop postoperative decompensation (mostly ascites), and have a

5-year survival of less than 50%. Survival of patients with both portal hypertension and elevated bilirubin is less than 30% at 5 years. Other methods to assess liver function have been used, such as indocyanine green (ICG) retention, used in Japan; ICG retention greater than 15% at 15 min suggests inadequate liver function and is a contraindication to resection [95]. Safe resection in patients with more advanced liver disease, for example Child–Pugh B [96], is possible, and some patients do well, but over-all survival is not as good as for patients with better liver function. Patients with more advanced disease might be better served by transplantation or, if the lesion is small, by RFA. Similarly, resection has been performed in patients with macrovascular invasion [96,97]. Again the overall survival is less good than in patients who do not have this complication. Whether overall survival is improved in these patients compared to either no treatment, or the currently indicated treatments for these patients, namely sorafenib (see below), is not known.

Most groups restrict resection to patients with a single tumour in a suitable anatomical location for resection. The size of the tumour is not a clear-cut limiting factor. Although the risk of vascular invasion and dissemination increases with size, some tumours may grow as a large single mass with no evidence of vascular invasion. In these, surgery may be safely performed and the risk of recurrence is not significantly increased as compared to smaller tumours.

The most powerful predictors of postoperative recurrence are the presence of microvascular invasion and/or additional tumour sites [98–101]. There is no form of therapy confirmed by more than one group to reduce the risk of recurrence.

Some surgeons use the size of the contralateral lobe as a factor in determining whether a lesion is resectable, as surgery becomes hazardous if the lobe that is to be left behind is too small. Safer resection can potentially result from portal vein embolization of the lobe to be removed [102], as the lobe to be left behind hypertrophies in response to the embolization. Failure to achieve hypertrophy then becomes a contraindication to resection. However, no randomized studies have proven its value.

Liver transplantation

Excellent results can be achieved in patients who have a solitary HCC less than 5 cm or who have up to three nodules all smaller than 3 cm [103,104], known as the Milan criteria [103], with an average survival of 70% at 5 years and less than a 15% recurrence rate. Therefore, early HCC is a clear indication for liver transplantation.

As with resection, the most powerful predictors of recurrence after transplantation in the absence of extrahepatic spread are macro- or microscopic vascular invasion and poorly differentiated tumours.

There have been attempts to extend these criteria, based on the observation that some patients with more advanced disease than staged with the Milan criteria can be successfully transplanted with no recurrence of HCC. However, when these listing criteria are expanded, the outcome is less good. Thus, the issue is what level of survival after transplantation is still acceptable, given the scarcity of organs. In the absence of microvascular invasion, the two most important factors are the size of the largest lesion and number of lesions with greater importance for the largest size. An analysis of a large database suggested that as long as the number of lesions and size of the largest lesion, in cm, was equal to or less than 7 there was about 70% 5-year survival, without microvascular invasion, as compared to the 80% 5-year survival for those transplanted within Milan criteria [105]. These data require validation before being widely implemented.

Using conventional listing criteria, one can expect a drop-out rate of about 25% due to tumour progression at 1 year depending on the size of the donor pool and waiting time. This translates into a 60% survival rate for transplantation, based on an intention-to-treat analysis of patients from the time placed on a transplant waiting list [106].

Patients listed for transplantation are often treated with transarterial chemoembolization (TACE) or RFA to prevent progression of the cancer to exceed listing criteria. Similarly, these therapies have also been used to down-stage tumours to fit listing criteria [107,108]. Whether these procedures enhance survival or reduce post-transplant recurrence rates is not established, but recurrence rates appear higher than in patients transplanted with HCCs that were within Milan criteria at all times. The selection of patients with HCC for liver transplantation is influenced by the size of the donor pool, as survival outcomes should be similar for other aetiologies of liver disease to ensure similar benefit from a scarce resource.

Living donor orthotopic liver transplant

After the first successful attempt [109], more than 3000 living donor operations have been performed worldwide in adults using the right hepatic lobe from the donor. Overall survival rates can be similar to those for cadaveric liver transplantation [110,111]. Decision analysis taking into account the risk of drop-out while waiting (4% per month), the expected survival of the recipient (70% at 5 years) and the risk for the donor (1:200 or 1:250 mortality) indicates that living donor donation is a cost-effective approach if the waiting time exceeds 7 months [112].

Local ablation

This is the best treatment option for patients with early stage HCC who are not suitable for resection or transplantation. Destruction of tumour cells can be achieved by the injection of chemical substances (ethanol, acetic acid, hot saline) or by heating or freezing (radiofrequency, microwave, laser, cryotherapy). The efficacy of percutaneous ablation is assessed by dynamic imaging 1 month after therapy. Absence of contrast uptake within the tumour reflects necrosis, while the persistence of contrast uptake indicates viable tumour.

Percutaneous ablation is usually performed under ultrasound guidance, either percutaneously or laparoscopically. Ethanol injection is highly effective for small HCC and has a low rate of adverse effects [113,114]. It can achieve complete necrosis in 90–100% of HCC less than 2 cm, but only in 70% of tumours between 2 and 3 cm and only 50% in HCC between 3 and 5 cm [113,114]. Long-term studies indicate that Child–Pugh A patients with successful tumour necrosis may achieve a 50% survival at 5 years. This compares well with the outcome of resection [115].

Radiofrequency ablation (RFA) is a more efficient option. The insertion electrodes that deliver heat around the tip can induce a wide region of tumour necrosis (Fig. 35.8). The efficacy of RFA in tumours below 2 cm is similar to PEI [116], but results in better survival with fewer sessions for larger tumours [117,118]. The currently available needles are most effective for tumours that are up to about 4 cm in diameter. However, the ability to completely ablate the lesion decreases as the lesion exceeds 2 cm in size [119]. Meta-analysis confirms the superiority of RFA over PEI for lesions more than 2 cm [117]. The main drawback of radiofrequency is its higher cost and the higher rate of adverse events (pleural effusion, peritoneal bleeding) that can affect up to almost 10% of treated patients. There is a 0.5% mortality. Subcapsular location and poor tumour differentiation have been associated with increased risk of peritoneal seeding [120], and thus this type of tumour may not be suitable for RFA. Proximity of the tumour to a large blood vessel decreases the efficacy of RFA because of a heat sink effect from blood flowing in the vessel.

An emerging indication is to perform RFA for lesions smaller than 2 cm in size instead of resection [116]. This is based on studies that show a 5-year local recurrence rate of less than 2% for these small lesions.

Embolic therapy

Transarterial chemoembolization (TACE) requires the advancement of the catheter into the hepatic artery and then to lobar and segmental branches, injection of chemotherapy, followed by obstruction of arterial flow by

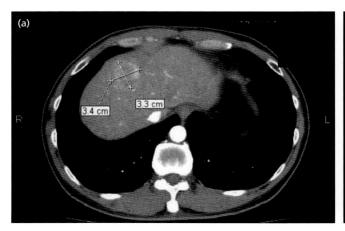

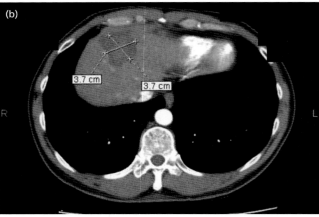

Fig. 35.8. CT scan of a small HCC before and after treatment by radiofrequency ablation. The ablation zone (indicted by the crossed lines) is larger than the original tumour and no longer enhances, but it is avascular (no contrast flowing through the area), indicating necrosis.

embolization. The more distal the catheter placement, the more treatment is delivered to the tumour, and the less the injury to the surrounding liver. Transarterial embolization (TAE) is a similar procedure without the use of chemotherapy. Many centres suspend the chemotherapy agent in lipiodol, an oily contrast agent used for lymphographic studies. Lipiodol is partly retained within the tumour, but whether this increases the exposure of the neoplastic cells to chemotherapy has not been shown (Fig. 35.9) [121]. Several chemotherapeutic agents have been used for TACE, but the most common are doxorubicin or cisplatin. TACE has been shown in two well-designed randomized controlled trials and in a meta-analysis to improve survival compared to best supportive care [122,123]. An earlier randomized controlled trial of TACE versus no therapy included patients with more advanced disease and failed to show any survival advantage to chemoembolization [124]; this has been interpreted to show that patients with more advanced liver disease do not do well with TACE. Thus, many centres only use TACE for patients who have Child's A cirrhosis, although some have included patients with a Child–Pugh score of 7 (Child B). However, the benefit for patients with this severity of liver disease has not been shown conclusively. The efficacy of TACE is limited by hepatic function, as described, but also by the presence of portal vein thrombosis, whether due to tumour or not. Complete portal vein thrombosis is a contraindication to TACE as there is risk of inducing ischaemic necrosis of that segment, which can be fatal. TACE can be performed with acceptable toxicity in patients with branch portal vein occlusion. However, as thrombosis due to vascular invasion in itself adversely affects prognosis it cannot be assumed that TACE enhances survival.

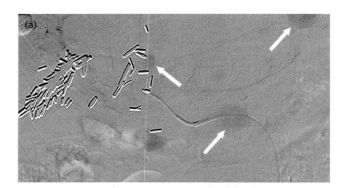

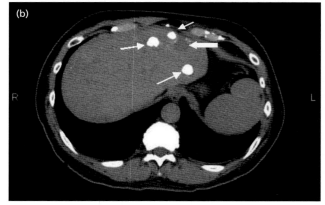

Fig. 35.9. CT scan of an HCC after treatment by chemoembolization. (a) Angiogram performed for transarterial chemoembolization. Note three vascular tumours (arrows). (b) Precontrast phase CT scan showing dense lipiodol uptake in the treated lesions (thin arrows). Note also that there is a prior left hepatic lobectomy with surgical clips present. There is also a previous radiofrequency ablation zone (thick arrow), with some lipiodol staining at the periphery, indicating residual disease after the radiofrequency ablation.

The side effects of TACE are the same as for systemic administration of chemotherapy, but also includes the postembolization syndrome. The chemotherapy may cause nausea, vomiting, bone marrow depression, alopecia and renal failure. The postembolization syndrome is seen in up to 50% of patients and consists of fever, abdominal pain and a moderate degree of ileus and is usually self limited and lasts less than 48 hours. A minority of patients may develop severe infectious complications such as hepatic abscess or cholecystitis.

The transarterial procedure has not been standardized; different chemotherapeutic agents, in different doses, and different embolic agents are used, for example gelfoam pellets, gelfoam powder, metallic coils or polyvinyl alcohol, and different schedules for repeated sessions [125]. More recently, a new technique has been employed to deliver TACE using drug-eluting resin beads. These have been compared to standard TACE in a randomized controlled trial; no differences between the two groups in outcome was reported, but there was much improved toxicity with the beads [126].

TAE has not been as well studied. Although there are randomized controlled trials comparing TAE and TACE [127,128] that suggest no difference in outcome these are of poor quality, and cannot be taken to indicate that the two treatments are equivalent. TAE has been compared to no treatment in a single trial [122] which did not show a statistically significant difference, although that trial was stopped before the appropriate sample size had been reached. On balance, therefore, TAE in Child's A cirrhosis remains of unproven benefit.

Medical therapy

Systemic chemotherapy with any of the available agents has only marginal antitumour activity, minimal impact on survival and is associated with significant decrease in quality of life [129,130]. Octreotide administration is ineffective [131]. Administration of interferon has also failed to show any activity [132].

The only medical therapy that has been shown to enhance survival in HCC is sorafenib, a multikinase inhibitor. This is an oral agent that blocks several pathways in the cancer cell, including angiogenesis through the VEGF pathway and proliferation via RAF-MEK-ERK pathway. There have been two randomized controlled trials, identical in design, comparing sorafenib to placebo in patients with advanced HCC, that is BCLC stage C [133,134]. Both studies demonstrated a survival advantage of about 2 months, with a 30% reduction in the risk of dying over a period of about 1 year. Patients included in these studies had Child's A cirrhosis. The survival benefit of sorafenib with more severe cirrhosis has not been demonstrated. Sorafenib is associated with several important side effects. These include skin rashes, including hand–foot syndrome, a blistering desquamating rash, diarrhoea, fatigue and hypertension. Current studies are evaluating sorafenib in combination with established therapies and with newer agents, in which more than a 2-month survival benefit may be shown.

Other therapies

Many therapies have not been assessed in randomized controlled trials (Table 35.5). Most important of these is intra-arterial radiotherapy using ^{90}Yttrium attached to either microscopic glass or resin beads. These are injected via the hepatic artery or a branch that feeds the tumour. Objective responses have been demonstrated in terms of reduction of tumour size and induction of necrosis. However, neither of these two methods has been tested against any other form of therapy, so it is unknown whether there is a survival advantage [135]. These are procedures that are complex to perform, and require an additional procedure to ensure that intrahepatic shunts do not divert the beads to the lung. However, these procedures can be used in patients with portal vein invasion, without fear of ischemic necrosis of liver, and for large lesions unsuitable for TACE [135].

Hepatic artery infusion of chemotherapy is popular in Japan. This involves placing a subcutaneous injection port attached to a catheter in the hepatic artery, and providing regular (daily or weekly) infusion of a chemotherapeutic drug. This procedure can result in decrease in tumour size, but has only been evaluated in small, poorly designed, phase 2 trials. There are as many regimens used as there have been studies. No survival advantage has ever been described, and in some cases the reported survival was no better than expected for similar untreated patients. This form of treatment is therefore not recommended [125].

Summary

Hepatocellular carcinoma in the early 21st century can be considered a potentially curable disease in many patients with the availability of life-prolonging treatment. However, to achieve this, certain facilities and procedures have to be in place. Patients at risk of developing HCC have to undergo rigorous surveillance using the best available method, namely ultrasonography. Lesions identified on ultrasonography have to be aggressively investigated, including, if necessary, more than one biopsy. If a diagnosis of HCC has been confirmed and if the lesion is single and 2 cm or less in diameter, use of the appropriate treatment may often led to cure. If the cancer is not curable, an appreciable improvement in survival can be obtained. The next decade holds the promise of identifying molecular markers of the biological behaviour of HCC and of the presence of tumour

Table 35.5. Ineffective or incompletely tested therapies that are used to treat HCC

Treatment modality	Likely or definitely ineffective	Incompletely tested
Hepatic artery infusion of chemotherapy	×	×
Hepatic artery ligation		×
Intrahepatic ^{131}I lipiodol		×
^{99}Yttrium-labelled glass beads or resin		×
Tamoxifen	×	
Octreotide (long-acting somatostatin)	×	
Conformal radiotherapy		×
Combined TACE and RFA		×
Resection with thrombectomy for portal vein invasion		×
TACE or TAE in patients with Child's B cirrhosis	×	×
TACE or TAE in patients with vascular invasion	×	×
Down-staging prior to liver transplantation with TACE or RFA		×
Bridging therapy with TACE or RFA prior to liver transplant		×

These are therapies that show tumour response (tumour shrinkage) but for which no survival advantage has been demonstrated compared to either supportive care or alternative therapies that might be suitable for the same patient (incompletely tested). Some procedures are not completely tested but are likely to be ineffective.
RFA, radiofrequency ablation; TACE, transarterial chemoembolization; TAE, transarterial embolization.

itself. Advances in understanding of the biology of HCC will result in more and more small-molecule inhibitors of tumour metabolism, hopefully to be used together, to continuously control neoplastic activity and growth, much like the suppression of HIV and hepatitis B replication today.

Cholangiocarcinoma

Cholangiocarcinoma (CCA) is a neoplasm of the epithelium of the intra- or extrahepatic biliary tree. It is likely that the mechanisms underlying the development of intra- versus extrahepatic CCA are different because intrahepatic CCA is increasing in incidence, whereas the incidence of extrahepatic CCA is falling or stable [136]. This section will deal only with intrahepatic CCA.

Epidemiology

Intrahepatic CCA is a disease of the six and seventh decades, and has a slight male predominance. It accounts for about 3% of all gastrointestinal cancers and is the second most frequent primary cancer of the liver. In many parts of the world the incidence of this disease is increasing [137–139]. The cause of this increase is not really understood, but a number of risk factors are known. These include infection with liver flukes, in particular *Opisthorchus viverrini* and *Clonorchis sinensis* [140], which are endemic in parts of South East Asia, such as parts of Thailand where this tumour is very common. Other risk factors include sclerosing cholangitis [141], Caroli's disease or other causes of hepatolithiasis, hepatitis C, exposure to Thorotrast or dioxins and biliary enteric procedures. In addition, more recently, data have emerged suggesting that cirrhosis is also a risk factor for intrahepatic CCA [138,142], although the magnitude of risk is not nearly as high as for HCC. However, most patients do not have identifiable risk factors.

Pathogenesis

Not much is known about the pathogenesis of CCA. Chronic inflammation and cholestasis play an important role, particularly in conditions such as sclerosing cholangitis, hepatolithiasis and infections with flukes. As with many other cancers, inflammatory cytokines probably play a role, as does generation of nitric oxides and subsequently reactive oxygen species, which may induce DNA breaks and impair mismatch repair of damaged DNA. Altered regulation of a number of oncogenes and genes involved in cell cycling has been identified, such as p53 and k-ras; however, the frequency with which these alterations occur is by no means universal, sometimes occurring in only a small percentage of CCAs. Interleukin 6 (IL-6), an inflammatory cytokine seems to have a more definitive role in the pathogenesis of CCA. IL-6 is important in the pathogenesis of many cancers. CCA cells produce high levels of IL-6 [143,144]. This in turn produces down-stream antiapoptotic effects, increased telomerase activity, allowing cells to evade senescence, and activation of kinases that stimulate cell division. EGFR, ErbB-2 and hepatocyte growth factor are also activated in CCA.

Clinical presentation and diagnosis

Intrahepatic CCA is usually clinically silent until late in the course of the disease. The disease is rare in individu-

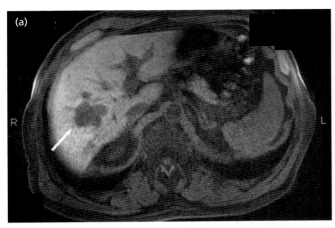

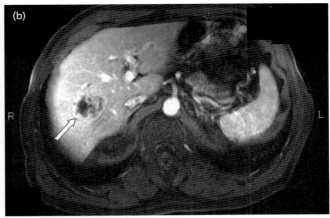

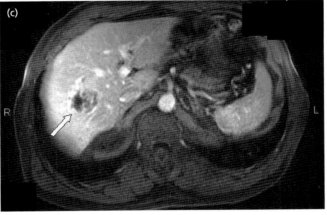

Fig. 35.10. Radiographic appearance of cholangiocarcinoma. (a) Precontrast MRI. The tumour is indicated by the arrow. (b) Arterial phase MRI of the same lesion. There is some enhancement at the periphery of the lesion but the central area is necrotic. (c) Venous phase MRI of the same lesion. The appearances are the same as in the arterial phase (no washout).

als under age 40. The most common presentation is with symptoms of a liver mass or cancer symptoms, such as pain, night sweats, anorexia and weight loss, and a decreased performance status.

Serological markers such as CEA, CA19-9 and CA125 are frequently elevated, but are not specific for CCA [145]. In the presence of a liver mass, an elevated CA19-9 has a sensitivity of about 80% and a specificity of nearly 100% for the diagnosis of CCA. However, in patients with primary sclerosing cholangitis (PSC) the sensitivity and specificity are less good. MRI is the radiological examination of choice, once a liver mass suspicious for CCA has been documented (Fig. 35.10). This provides information about the location and extent of the lesion, and the presence of intrahepatic metastases. Endoscopic retrograde cholangiopancreatography (ERCP) is of little value for intrahepatic CCA. Endoscopic ultrasound is the most useful test for evaluating lymph node spread, and also will allow fine needle biopsy of the nodes. Positron emission tomography (PET) scanning has also been used. Intrahepatic CCA is staged using the TNM system.

Management

Despite advances in treatment the prognosis of intrahepatic CCA remains poor. Surgical resection remains the only curative therapy, but is seldom feasible because of the late presentation of the cancer. However, for those patients who are good candidates for resection (localized disease confined to the liver, no vascular invasion), and whose resection results in clear margins there is a survival rate of between 22 and 44% [146,147]. The results of liver transplantation are poor (up to 18% 5-year survival) [148] so intrahepatic CCA is not an indication for liver transplantation. A protocol involving brachytherapy and extensive staging procedures to ensure nonextrahepatic spread (including laparotomy) has resulted in better survival after liver transplantation.

Radiotherapy has been tried, with conflicting results. There are no controlled trials, making it difficult to evaluate the potential role for radiotherapy.

Palliative therapy for CCA includes 5-fluorouracil and gemcitabine [149]. Combination of these agents with other chemotherapeutic agents has only been partly evaluated. There are insufficient data to support the use of any combination therapy.

Other malignant neoplasms of the liver

Fibrolamellar hepatocellular carcinoma

This is a variant of HCC that occurs largely in younger patients without any of the usual HCC risk factors. It is characterized by the scirrhous nature of the tumour, but is of hepatocyte origin [150]. More than 90% of cases occur in patients younger than 25 years of age [151]. The male:female ratio is about equal or with slight female predominance. The absence of risk factors means that this cancer is usually only diagnosed when symptomatic. The prognosis of fibrolamellar HCC is better than for HCC, perhaps because of the absence of underlying liver disease [151].

Cholangiolocellular carcinoma

Cholangiolocellular carcinoma is a neoplasm that is thought to arise from the cells lining the ducts of Hering. Characterization of tumours using markers of hepatic and biliary progenitor cells indicates that the cell of origin of cholangiolocellular carcinoma is the hepatic progenitor cell [152].

Patients with this rare tumour (about 1% of all liver malignancies) often have the same risk factors as for HCC, such as chronic viral hepatitis, haemochromatosis or α1-antrypsin deficiency, but these risk factors may be absent in about half the patients. The cells are mostly arranged in gland-like structures, and are small and uniform in appearance. Treatment is as for HCC.

Angiosarcoma

This is the most common sarcoma arising in the liver, but it is nonetheless a very rare tumour. However, it is the only primary liver cancer for which a causal association with an exposure to toxins is documented. These are thorium dioxide (Thorotrast) [153], a radioactive substance once used as a radiographic contrast dye, vinyl chloride monomer (VCM) [154] and exposure to arsenic (used in the past in the wine industry) [155]. Today, Thorotrast is no longer used, and in the industrialized nations exposure to VCM monomer is tightly controlled, so that no VCM-associated cases have been described in workers exposed after about 1976. Spontaneous angiosarcoma occurs, usually in the sixth or seventh decades of life.

There are changes in the liver that precede the development of angiosarcoma in VCM-exposed individuals. These include hepatocyte hyperplasia, sinusoidal dilata-tion, endothelial cell enlargement and nuclear pleiomorphism and polychromasia [156].

This tumour presents late and is almost universally fatal within 6 months of presentation.

Malignant epithelioid haemangioendothelioma

This is a cancer of vascular origin. Only about 430 patients have been documented in the literature [157]. The outcome is highly variable, and in many patients this is a low-grade malignancy. This cancer can also occur in organs other than the liver, such as lung and kidney. The clinical presentation is variable, ranging from asymptomatic patients to advanced liver failure or cancer symptoms. There are no specific radiological findings, but often the appearances are similar to those seen with metastases to the liver. The cancer can be treated by resection, although results are often disappointing. Liver transplantation has been used, even in patients with extrahepatic disease; survival at 5 years is 70% or more [158].

Other sarcomas

Almost all possible types of sarcoma have been reported as primary liver tumours. These include embryonal sarcoma, rhabdomyosarcoma, leiomyosarcoma, fibrosarcoma, etc. A standardized management of these lesions is not available, partly because of the rarity of these lesions but also because they are aggressive tumours with a very poor prognosis whatever treatment used.

References

1 El-Serag H, Mason AC. Rising incidence of hepatocellular carcinoma in the United states. *N. Eng. J. Med.* 1999; **340**: 745–750.
2 Okuda K, Fujimoto I, Hanai A *et al.* Changing incidence of hepatocellular carcinoma in *Japan. Cancer Res.* 1987; **47**: 4967–4972.
3 Taylor-Robinson SD, Foster GR *et al.* Increase in primary liver cancer in the UK 1979–1974. *Lancet* 1997; **350**: 1142–1143.
4 Deuffic S, Poynard T, Buffat L *et al.* Trends in primary liver cancer. *Lancet* 1998; **351**: 214–215.
5 Stroffolini T, Andreone P, Andriulli A *et al.* Characteristics of hepatocellular carcinoma in Italy. *J. Hepatol.* 1998; **29**: 944–952.
6 Bosch FX, Ribes J, Cléries R *et al.* Epidemiology of hepatocellular carcinoma. *Clin. Liver Dis.* 2005; **9**: 191–211.
7 Beasley RP, Hwang LY, Lin CC *et al.* Hepatocellular carcinoma and hepatitis B virus. A prospective study of 22 707 men in Taiwan. *Lancet* 1981; **2**: 1129–1133.
8 Sakuma K, Saitoh N, Kasai M *et al.* Relative risks of death due to liver disease among Japanese male adults having various statuses for hepatitis B s and e antigen/antibody in serum: a prospective study. *Hepatology* 1988; **8**: 1642–1646.

9 Villeneuve JP, Desrochers M, Infante-Rivard C *et al*. A long-term follow-up study of asymptomatic hepatitis B surface antigen-positive carriers in Montreal. *Gastroenterology* 1994 **106**: 1000–1005.

10 McMahon B J, Alberts S R, Wainwright R B *et al*. Hepatitis B-related sequelae. Prospective study of 1400 hepatitis B surface antigen-positive Alaska native carriers. *Arch. Intern. Med*. 1990; **150**: 1051–1054.

11 Sherman M, Peltekian K M, Lee C. Screening for hepatocellular carcinoma in chronic carriers of Hepatitis B virus: Incidence and prevalence of hepatocellular carcinoma in a North American urban population. *Hepatology* 1995; **22**: 432–438.

12 Fattovich G, Giustina G, Schalm SW *et al*. Occurrence of hepatocellular carcinoma and decompensation in western European patients with cirrhosis type B. The EUROHEP Study Group on Hepatitis B Virus and Cirrhosis. *Hepatology* 1995; **21**: 77–82.

13 Fattovich G, Giustina G, Degos F *et al*. Morbidity and mortality in compensated cirrhosis type C: a retrospective follow-up study of 384 patients. *Gastroenterology* 1997; **2**: 463–472.

14 Bruix J, Barrera J M, Calvert X *et al*. Prevalence of antibodies to hepatitis C virus in Spanish patients with hepatocellular carcinoma and hepatitis cirrhosis. *Lancet* 1989; **ii**: 1004–1006.

15 Niederau C, Lange S, Heintges T *et al*. Prognosis of chronic hepatitis C: results of a large, prospective cohort study. *Hepatology* 1998; **28**: 1687–1695.

16 Ikeda K, Saitoh S, Koida I *et al*. A multivariate analysis of risk factors for hepatocellular carcinoma: A prospective observation of 795 patients with viral and alcoholic cirrhosis. *Hepatology* 1993; **18**: 47–53.

17 Benvegnu L, Fattovich G, Noventa F *et al*. Concurrent hepatitis B and C virus infection and risk of hepatocellular carcinoma in cirrhosis. A prospective study. *Cancer* 1994; **74**: 2442–2448.

18 Cottone M, Turri M, Caltagirone M *et al*. Screening for hepatocellular carcinoma in patients with Childs A cirrhosis: an 8 year prospective study by ultrasound and alphafetoprotein. *J. Hepatol*. 1994; **21**: 1029–1034.

19 Borzio M, Bruno S, Roncalli M *et al*. Liver cell dysplasia is a major risk factor for hepatocellular carcinoma in cirrhosis. A prospective study. *Gastroenterology* 1995; **108**: 812–817.

20 Pateron D, Ganne N, Trinchet JC *et al*. Prospective study of screening for hepatocellular carcinoma in Caucasian patients with cirrhosis. *J. Hepatol*. 1994; **20**: 65–71.

21 Colombo M, De Franchis R, Del Ninno E *et al*. Hepatocellular carcinoma in Italian patients with cirrhosis. *Lancet* 1991; **325**: 675–680.

22 Zaman SN, Melia WM, Johnson RD *et al*. Risk factors in development of hepatocellular carcinoma in cirrhosis: Prospective study of 613 patients. *Lancet* 1985; **1**: 1357–1360.

23 Fargion S, Fracanzani AL, Piperno A *et al*. Prognostic factors for hepatocellular carcinoma in genetic haemochromatosis. *Hepatology* 1994; **20**: 1426–1431.

24 Caballeria L, Pares A, Castells A *et al*. Hepatocellular carcinoma in primary biliary cirrhosis: similar incidence to that in hepatitis C virus-related cirrhosis. *Am. J. Gastroenterol*. 2001; **96**: 1160–1163.

25 Fattovich G, Brollo L, Giustina G *et al*. Natural history and prognostic factors for chronic hepatitis type B. *Gut* 1991; **32**: 294–298.

26 Ross RK, Yuan JM, Yu MC *et al*. Urinary aflatoxin biomarkers and risk of hepatocellular carcinoma. *Lancet* 1992; **339**: 943–946.

27 Umemura T, Ichijo T, Yoshizawa K *et al*. Epidemiology of hepatocellular carcinoma in Japan. *J. Gastroenterol*. 2009; **44** (Suppl. 19): 102–107.

28 Bosetti C, Levi F, Boffetta P *et al*. Trends in mortality from hepatocellular carcinoma in Europe, 1980–2004. *Hepatology* 2008; **48**: 137–145.

29 Rudnick DA, Perlmutter DH. Alpha-1-antitrypsin deficiency: a new paradigm for hepatocellular carcinoma in genetic liver disease. *Hepatology* 2005; **42**: 514–521.

30 International Working Party. Terminology of nodular hepatocellular lesions. *Hepatology* 1995; **22**: 983–993.

31 International Consensus Group for Hepatocellular Neoplasia. Pathologic diagnosis of early hepatocellular carcinoma: a report of the international consensus group for hepatocellular neoplasia. *Hepatology* 2009; **49**: 658–664.

32 Hytiroglou P, Theise ND, Schwartz M *et al*. Macroregenerative nodules in a series of adult cirrhotic liver explants: issues of classification and nomenclature. *Hepatology* 1995; **21**: 703–708.

33 Roncalli M, Roz E, Coggi G *et al*. The vascular profile of regenerative and dysplastic nodules of the cirrhotic liver: implications for diagnosis and classification. *Hepatology* 1999; **30**: 1174–1178.

34 Arakawa M, Kage M, Sugihara S *et al*. Emergence of malignant lesions within an adenomatous hyperplastic nodule in a cirrhotic liver. Observations in five cases. *Gastroenterology* 1986; **91**: 198–208.

35 Tiniakos DG, Brunt EM. Proliferating cell nuclear antigen and Ki-67 labeling in hepatocellular nodules: a comparative study. *Liver* 1999; **19**: 58–68.

36 Dutta U, Kench J, Byth K *et al*. Hepatocellular proliferation and development of hepatocellular carcinoma: a case-control study in chronic hepatitis C. *Hum. Pathol*. 1998; **29**: 1279–1284.

37 Borzio M, Trere D, Borzio F *et al*. Hepatocyte proliferation rate is a powerful parameter for predicting hepatocellular carcinoma development in liver cirrhosis. *Mol. Pathol*. 1998; **510**: 96–101.

38 Kojiro M. Focus on dysplastic nodules and early hepatocellular carcinoma: an Eastern point of view. *Liver Transpl*. 2004; **10** (2 Suppl. 1): S3–S8.

39 Nakashima T, Kojiro M. *Hepatocellular Carcinoma*. Tokyo: Springer Verlag, 1987.

40 Libbrecht L, Severi T, Cassiman D *et al*. Glypican-3 expression distinguishes small hepatocellular carcinomas from cirrhosis, dysplastic nodules, and focal nodular hyperplasia-like nodules. *Am. J. Surg. Pathol*. 2006; **30**: 1405–1411.

41 Kojiro M, Roskams T. Early hepatocellular carcinoma and dysplastic nodules. *Sem. Liver Dis*. 2005; **25**: 133–142.

42 Kanda M, Nomoto S, Nishikawa Y *et al*. Correlations of the expression of vascular endothelial growth factor B and its isoforms in hepatocellular carcinoma with clinico-pathological parameters. *J. Surg. Oncol*. 2008 1; **98**: 190–196.

43 Schoenleber SJ, Kurtz DM, Talwalkar JA *et al.* Prognostic role of vascular endothelial growth factor in hepatocellular carcinoma: systematic review and meta-analysis. *Br. J. Cancer* 2009; **100**: 1385–1392.

44 Breuhahn K, Vreden S, Haddad R *et al.* Molecular profiling of human hepatocellular carcinoma defines mutually exclusive interferon regulation and insulin-like growth factor II overexpression. *Cancer Res.* 2004; **64**: 6058–6064.

45 Lee JS, Chu IS, Heo J *et al.* Classification and prediction of survival in hepatocellular carcinoma by gene expression profiling. *Hepatology* 2004; **40**: 667–676.

46 Okabe H, Satoh S, Kato T *et al.* Genome-wide analysis of gene expression in human hepatocellular carcinomas using cDNA microarray: identification of genes involved in viral carcinogenesis and tumor progression. *Cancer Res.* 2001; **61**: 2129–2137.

47 Iizuka N, Oka M, Yamada-Okabe H *et al.* Oligonucleotide microarray for prediction of early intrahepatic recurrence of hepatocellular carcinoma after curative resection. *Lancet* 2003; **361**: 923–929.

48 Llovet JM, Chen Y, Wurmbach E *et al.* A molecular signature to discriminate dysplastic nodules from early hepatocellular carcinoma in HCV cirrhosis. *Gastroenterology* 2006; **131**: 1758–1767.

49 Nam SW, Lee JH, Noh JH *et al.* Comparative analysis of expression profiling of early-stage carcinogenesis using nodule-in-nodule-type hepatocellular carcinoma. *Eur. J. Gastroenterol. Hepatol.* 2006; **18**: 239–247.

50 Wurmbach E, Chen YB, Khitrov G *et al.* Genome-wide molecular profiles of HCV-induced dysplasia and hepatocellular carcinoma. *Hepatology* 2007; **45**: 938–947.

51 Nam SW, Park JY, Ramasamy A *et al.* Molecular changes from dysplastic nodule to hepatocellular carcinoma through gene expression profiling. *Hepatology* 2005; **42**: 809–818.

52 Hoshida Y, Villanueva A, Kobayashi M *et al.* Gene expression in fixed tissues and outcome in hepatocellular carcinoma. *N. Engl. J. Med.* 2008; **359**: 1995–2004.

53 Wing JR, Panz VR, Joffe BI *et al.* Hypoglycemia in hepatocellular carcinoma: failure of short-term growth hormone administration to reduce enhanced glucose requirements. *Metabolism* 1991; **40**: 508–512.

54 Mahoney EJ, Monchik JM, Donatini G *et al.* .Life-threatening hypercalcemia from a hepatocellular carcinoma secreting intact parathyroid hormone: localization by sestamibi single-photon emission computed tomographic imaging. *Endocr. Pract.* 2006; **12**: 302–306.

55 Ryu T, Nishimura S, Miura H *et al.* Thrombopoietin-producing hepatocellular carcinoma. *Intern. Med.* 2003; **42**: 730–734.

56 Zhang BH, Yang BH, Tang ZY. Randomized controlled trial of screening for hepatocellular carcinoma. *J. Cancer Res. Clin. Oncol.* 2004; **130**: 417–422.

57 Thompson Coon J, Rogers G, Hewson P *et al.* Surveillance of cirrhosis for hepatocellular carcinoma: a cost-utility analysis. *Br. J. Cancer* 2008; **98**: 1166–1175.

58 Sarasin FP, Giostra E, Hadengue A. Cost-effectiveness of screening for detection of small hepatocellular carcinoma in western patients with Child-Pugh class A cirrhosis. *Am. J. Med.* 1996; **101**: 422–434.

59 Arguedas MR, Chen VK, Eloubeidi MA *et al.* Screening for hepatocellular carcinoma in patients with hepatitis C cir-

rhosis: a cost-utility analysis. *Am. J. Gastroenterol.* 2003; **98**: 679–690.

60 Patel D, Terrault NA, Yao FY *et al.* Cost-effectiveness of hepatocellular carcinoma surveillance in patients with hepatitis C virus-related cirrhosis. *Clin. Gastroenterol. Hepatol.* 2005; **3**: 75–84.

61 Lin OS, Keeffe EB, Sanders GD *et al.* Cost-effectiveness of screening for hepatocellular carcinoma in patients with cirrhosis due to chronic hepatitis C. *Aliment. Pharmacol. Ther.* 2004; **19**: 1159–1172.

62 Bruix J, Sherman M. Management of hepatocellular carcinoma. *Hepatology* 2005; **42**: 1208–1236.

63 Trevisani F, D'Intino PE, Morselli-Labate AM *et al.* Serum alpha-fetoprotein for diagnosis of hepatocellular carcinoma in patients with chronic liver disease: influence of HBsAg and anti-HCV status. *J. Hepatol.* 2001; **34**: 570–575.

64 Pateron D, Ganne N, Trinchet JC *et al.* Prospective study of screening for hepatocellular carcinoma in Caucasian patients with cirrhosis. *J. Hepatol.* 1994; **20**: 65 –71.

65 Marrero JA, Su GL, Wei W *et al.* Des-gamma carboxyprothrombin can differentiate hepatocellular carcinoma from nonmalignant chronic liver disease in American patients. *Hepatology* 2003; **37**: 1114–1121.

66 Durazo FA, Blatt LM, Corey WG *et al.* Des-gamma-carboxyprothrombin, alpha-fetoprotein and AFP-L3 in patients with chronic hepatitis, cirrhosis and hepatocellular carcinoma. *J. Gastroenterol. Hepatol.* 2008; **23**: 1541–1548.

67 Sterling RK, Jeffers L, Gordon F *et al.* Utility of Lens culinaris agglutinin-reactive fraction of alpha-fetoprotein and des-gamma-carboxy prothrombin, alone or in combination, as biomarkers for hepatocellular carcinoma. *Clin. Gastroenterol. Hepatol.* 2009; **7**: 104–113.

68 Miyaaki H, Nakashima O, Kurogi M *et al.* Lens culinaris agglutinin-reactive alpha-fetoprotein and protein induced by vitamin K absence II are potential indicators of a poor prognosis: a histopathological study of surgically resected hepatocellular carcinoma. *J. Gastroenterol.* 2007; **42**: 962–968.

69 Carr BI, Kanke F, Wise M *et al.* Clinical evaluation of lens culinaris agglutinin-reactive alpha-fetoprotein and des-gamma-carboxy prothrombin in histologically proven hepatocellular carcinoma in the United States. *Dig. Dis. Sci.* 2007; **52**: 776–782.

70 Taouli B, Goh JS, Lu Y *et al.* Growth rate of hepatocellular carcinoma: evaluation with serial computed tomography or magnetic resonance imaging. *J. Comput. Assist. Tomogr.* 2005; **29**: 425–429.

71 O'Malley ME, Takayama Y, Sherman M. Outcome of small (10-20 mm) arterial phase-enhancing nodules seen on triphasic liver CT in patients with cirrhosis or chronic liver disease. *Am. J. Gastroenterol.* 2005; **100**: 1523–1528.

72 Sala M, Llovet JM, Vilana R *et al*; Barcelona Clínic Liver Cancer Group. Initial response to percutaneous ablation predicts survival in patients with hepatocellular carcinoma. *Hepatology* 2004; **40**: 1352–1360.

73 Nathan H, Schulick RD, Choti MA *et al.* Predictors of survival after resection of early hepatocellular carcinoma. *Ann. Surg.* 2009; **249**: 799–805.

74 Trevisani F, De NS, Rapaccini G *et al.* Semiannual and annual surveillance of cirrhotic patients for hepatocellular carcinoma: effects on cancer stage and patient survival

(Italian experience). *Am. J. Gastroenterol.* 2002; **97**: 734–744.

75 Santagostino E, Colombo M, Rivi M *et al.* A 6-month versus a 12-month surveillance for hepatocellular carcinoma in 559 hemophiliacs infected with the hepatitis C virus. *Blood* 2003; **102**: 78–82.

76 Kim DY, Han KH, Ahn SH *et al.* Semiannual surveillance for hepatocellular carcinoma improved patient survival compared to annual surveillance (Korean experience). *Hepatology* 2007; **46** (Suppl. 1) 403A.

77 Nicolau C, Vilana R, Catalá V *et al.* Importance of evaluating all vascular phases on contrast-enhanced sonography in the differentiation of benign from malignant focal liver lesions. *AJR Am. J. Roentgenol.* 2006; **186**: 158–167.

78 Iannaccone R, Laghi A, Catalano C *et al.* Hepatocellular carcinoma: role of unenhanced and delayed phase multidetector row helical CT in patients with cirrhosis. *Radiology* 2005; **234**: 460–467.

79 Torzilli G, Minagawa M, Takayama T *et al.* Accurate preoperative evaluation of liver mass lesions without fine-needle biopsy. *Hepatology* 1999; **30**: 889–893.

80 Bremner KE, Bayoumi AM, Sherman M *et al.* Management of solitary 1 cm to 2 cm liver nodules in patients with compensated cirrhosis: a decision analysis. *Can. J. Gastroenterol.* 2007; **21**: 491–500.

81 Burrel M, Llovet JM, Ayuso C *et al.* MRI angiography is superior to helical CT for detection of HCC prior to liver transplantation: An explant correlation. *Hepatology* 2003; **38**: 1034–1042.

82 Jeong YY, Mitchell DG, Kamishima T. Small (<20 mm) enhancing hepatic nodules seen on arterial phase MR imaging of the cirrhotic liver: clinical implications. *AJR Am. J. Roentgenol.* 2002; **178**: 1327–1334.

83 Fracanzani AL, Burdick L, Borzio M *et al.* Contrast-enhanced doppler ultrasonography in the diagnosis of hepatocellular carcinoma and premalignant lesions in patients with cirrhosis. *Hepatology* 2001; **34**: 1109–1112.

84 Takayama T, Makuuchi M, Hirohashi S *et al.* Malignant transformation of adenomatous hyperplasia to hepatocellular carcinoma. *Lancet* 1990; **336**: 1150–1153.

85 Stigliano R, Marelli L, Yu D *et al.* Seeding following percutaneous diagnostic and therapeutic approaches for hepatocellular carcinoma. What is the risk and the outcome? Seeding risk for percutaneous approach of HCC. *Cancer Treat. Rev.* 2007; **33**: 437–447.

86 Llovet JM, Brú C, Bruix J. Prognosis of hepatocellular carcinoma: the BCLC staging classification. *Semin. Liver Dis.* 1999; **19**: 329–338.

87 Sharma P, Harper AM, Hernandez JL *et al.* Reduced priority MELD score for hepatocellular carcinoma does not adversely impact candidate survival awaiting liver transplantation. *Am. J. Transplant.* 2006; **6**: 1957–1962.

88 The Cancer of the Liver Italian Program (CLIP) investigators. A new prognostic system for hepatocellular carcinoma: a retrospective study of 435 patients. *Hepatology* 1998; **28**: 751–755.

89 Vauthey JN, Lauwers GY, Esnaola NF *et al.* Simplified staging for hepatocellular carcinoma. *J. Clin. Oncol.* 2002; **20**: 1527–1536.

90 Leung TW, Tang AM, Zee B *et al.* Construction of the Chinese University Prognostic Index for hepatocellular carcinoma and comparison with the TNM staging system, the Okuda staging system, and the Cancer of the Liver Italian Program staging system: a study based on 926 patients. *Cancer* 2002; **94**: 1760–1769.

91 Tandon P, Garcia-Tsao G. Prognostic indicators in hepatocellular carcinoma: a systematic review of 72 studies. *Liver Int.* 2009; **29**: 502–510.

92 Fong Y, Sun RL, Jarnagin W *et al.* An analysis of 412 cases of hepatocellular carcinoma at a Western center. *Ann. Surg.* 1999; **229**: 790–799.

93 Grazi GL, Ercolani G, Pierangeli F *et al.* Improved results of liver resection for hepatocellular carcinoma on cirrhosis give the procedure added value. *Ann. Surg.* 2001; **234**: 71–78.

94 Bruix J, Castells A, Bosch J *et al.* Surgical resection of hepatocellular carcinoma in cirrhotic patients: prognostic value of preoperative portal pressure. *Gastroenterology* 1996; **111**: 1018–1022.

95 Ishikawa M, Yogita S, Miyake H *et al.* Clarification of risk factors for hepatectomy in patients with hepatocellular carcinoma. *Hepatogastroenterology* 2002; **49**: 1625–1631.

96 Ishizawa T, Hasegawa K, Aoki T *et al.* Neither multiple tumors nor portal hypertension are surgical contraindications for hepatocellular carcinoma. *Gastroenterology* 2008; **134**: 1908–1916.

97 Le Treut YP, Hardwigsen J, Ananian P *et al.* Resection of hepatocellular carcinoma with tumor thrombus in the major vasculature. A European case-control series. *J. Gastrointest. Surg.* 2006; **10**: 855–862.

98 Okada S, Shimada K, Yamamoto J *et al.* Predictive factors for postoperative recurrence of hepatocellular carcinoma. *Gastroenterology* 1994; **106**: 1618–1624.

99 Shirabe K, Kanematsu T, Matsumata T *et al.* Factors linked to early recurrence of small hepatocellular carcinoma after hepatectomy: univariate and multivariate analyses. *Hepatology* 1991; **14**: 802–805.

100 Adachi E, Maeda T, Matsumata T *et al.* Risk factors for intrahepatic recurrence in human small hepatocellular carcinoma. *Gastroenterology* 1995; **108**: 768–775.

101 Poon RT, Fan ST, Lo CM *et al.* Intrahepatic recurrence after curative resection of hepatocellular carcinoma: long-term results of treatment and prognostic factors. *Ann. Surg.* 1999; **229**: 216–222.

102 Palavecino M, Chun YS, Madoff DC *et al.* Major hepatic resection for hepatocellular carcinoma with or without portal vein embolization: Perioperative outcome and survival. *Surgery* 2009; **145**: 399–405.

103 Mazzaferro V, Regalia E, Doci R *et al.* Liver transplantation for the treatment of small hepatocellular carcinomas in patients with cirrhosis. *N. Engl. J. Med.* 1996; **334**: 693–699.

104 Figueras J, Jaurrieta E, Valls C *et al.* Survival after liver transplantation in cirrhotic patients with and without hepatocellular carcinoma: a comparative study. *Hepatology* 1997; **25**: 1485–1489.

105 Mazzaferro V, Llovet JM, Miceli R *et al*; Metroticket Investigator Study Group. Predicting survival after liver transplantation in patients with hepatocellular carcinoma beyond the Milan criteria: a retrospective, exploratory analysis. *Lancet Oncol.* 2009; **10**: 35–43.

106 Fuster J, Bruix J. Intention-to-treat analysis of surgical treatment for early hepatocellular carcinoma: resection versus transplantation. *Hepatology* 1999; **30**: 1434–1440.

107 Heckman JT, Devera MB, Marsh JW *et al.* Bridging locoregional therapy for hepatocellular carcinoma prior

to liver transplantation. *Ann. Surg. Oncol.* 2008; **15**: 3169–3177.

108 Graziadei IW, Sandmueller H, Waldenberger P *et al.* Chemoembolization followed by liver transplantation for hepatocellular carcinoma impedes tumor progression while on the waiting list and leads to excellent outcome. *Liver Transpl.* 2003; **9**: 557–563.

109 Strong RW, Lynch SV, Ong TH *et al.* Successful liver transplantation from a living donor to her son. *N. Engl. J. Med.* 1990; **322**: 1505–1507.

110 Kawasaki S. Living-donor liver transplantation for hepatocellular carcinoma. *Hepatogastroenterology* 2002; **49**: 53–55.

111 Gondolesi GE, Roayaie S, Munoz L *et al.* Adult living donor liver transplantation for patients with hepatocellular carcinoma: extending UNOS priority criteria. *Ann. Surg.* 2004; **239**: 142–149.

112 Sarasin FP, Majno PE, Llovet JM *et al.* Living donor liver transplantation for early hepatocellular carcinoma: A life-expectancy and cost-effectiveness perspective. *Hepatology* 2001; **33**: 1073–1079.

113 Livraghi T, Bolondi L, Lazzaroni S *et al.* Percutaneous ethanol injection in the treatment of hepatocellular carcinoma in cirrhosis. A study on 207 patients. *Cancer* 1992; **69**: 925–929.

114 Vilana R, Bruix J, Bru C *et al.* Tumor size determines the efficacy of percutaneous ethanol injection for the treatment of small hepatocellular carcinoma. *Hepatology* 1992; **16**: 353–357.

115 Huang GT, Lee PH, Tsang YM *et al.* Percutaneous ethanol injection versus surgical resection for the treatment of small hepatocellular carcinoma: a prospective study. *Ann. Surg.* 2005; **242**: 36–42.

116 Livraghi T, Meloni F, Di Stasi M *et al.* Sustained complete response and complications rates after radiofrequency ablation of very early hepatocellular carcinoma in cirrhosis: Is resection still the treatment of choice? *Hepatology* 2008; **47**: 82–89.

117 Germani G, Pleguezuelo M, Curusamy K *et al.* Clinical outcomes of radiogrequncy ablation, percutaneous alcohol, and acetic acid injection for hepatocellular carcinoma. *J. Hepatol.* 2010; **52**: 380–388.

118 Lencioni RA, Allgaier HP, Cioni D *et al.* Small hepatocellular carcinoma in cirrhosis: randomized comparison of radio-frequency thermal ablation versus percutaneous ethanol injection. *Radiology* 2003; **228**: 235–240.

119 Lin SM, Lin CJ, Lin CC *et al.* Radiofrequency ablation improves prognosis compared with ethanol injection for hepatocellular carcinoma < or = 4 cm. *Gastroenterology* 2004; **127**: 1714–1723.

120 Livraghi T, Solbiati L, Meloni MF *et al.* Treatment of focal liver tumors with percutaneous radio-frequency ablation: complications encountered in a multicenter study. *Radiology* 2003; **226**: 441–451.

121 Pleguezuelo M, Marelli L, Missier M *et al.* TACE versus TAE as therapy for hepatocellular carcinoma. *Expert Rev. Anti Cancer Ther.* 2008; **8**: 1623–1644.

122 Llovet JM, Real MI, Montanya X *et al.* Arterial embolization, chemoembolization versus symptomatic treatment in patients with unresectable hepatocellular carcinoma: a randomized controlled trial. *Lancet* 2002; **359**: 1734–1739.

123 Lo CM, Ngan H, Tso WK *et al.* Randomized controlled trial of transarterial lipiodol chemoembolization for unresect-

able hepatocellular carcinoma. *Hepatology* 2002; **35**: 1164–1171.

124 GETCH. A comparison of lipiodol chemoembolization and conservative treatment for unresectable hepatocellular carcinoma. Groupe d'Etude et de Traitement du Carcinome Hepatocellulaire. *N. Engl. J. Med.* 1995; **332**: 1256–1261.

125 Lammer J, Malagari K, Vogl T *et al*; On Behalf of the PRECISION V Investigators. Prospective Randomized Study of Doxorubicin-Eluting-Bead Embolization in the Treatment of Hepatocellular Carcinoma: Results of the PRECISION V Study. *Cardiovasc. Intervent. Radiol.* 2009; **33**: 41–52.

126 Chang JM, Tzeng WS, Pan HB *et al.* Transcatheter arterial embolization with or without cisplatin treatment of hepatocellular carcinoma. A randomized controlled study. *Cancer* 1994; **74**: 2449–2453.

127 Kawai S, Okamura J, Ogawa M *et al.* Prospective and randomized clinical trial for the treatment of hepatocellular carcinoma—a comparison of lipiodol-transcatheter arterial embolization with and without adriamycin (first cooperative study). The Cooperative Study Group for Liver Cancer Treatment of Japan. *Cancer Chemother. Pharmacol.* 1992; **31** (Suppl.): S1–6.

128 Marelli L, Stigliano R, Triantos C *et al.* Transarterial therapy for hepatocellular carcinoma—which technique is more effective. *Cardiovasc. Intervent. Radiol.* 2007; **30**: 6–25.

129 Gish RG, Porta C, Lazar L *et al.* Phase III randomized controlled trial comparing the survival of patients with unresectable hepatocellular carcinoma treated with nolatrexed or doxorubicin. *J. Clin. Oncol.* 2007; **25**: 3069–3075.

130 Yeo W, Mok TS, Zee B *et al.* A randomized phase III study of doxorubicin versus cisplatin/interferon alpha-2b/doxorubicin/fluorouracil (PIAF) combination chemotherapy for unresectable hepatocellular carcinoma. *J. Natl. Cancer Inst.* 2005; **97**: 1532–1538.

131 Becker G, Allgaier HP, Olschewski M *et al*; HECTOR Study Group. Long-acting octreotide versus placebo for treatment of advanced HCC: a randomized controlled double-blind study. *Hepatology* 2007; **45**: 9–15.

132 Llovet JM, Sala M, Castells L *et al.* Randomized controlled trial of interferon treatment for advanced hepatocellular carcinoma. *Hepatology* 2000; **31**: 54–58.

133 Llovet JM, Ricci S, Mazzaferro V *et al*; SHARP Investigators Study Group. Sorafenib in advanced hepatocellular carcinoma. *N. Engl. J. Med.* 2008; **359**: 378–390.

134 Cheng AL, Kang YK, Chen Z *et al.* Efficacy and safety of sorafenib in patients in the Asia-Pacific region with advanced hepatocellular carcinoma: a phase III randomised, double-blind, placebo-controlled trial. *Lancet Oncol.* 2009; **10**: 25–34.

135 Salem R, Lewandowski RJ, Mulcahy MF *et al.* Radioembolisation for Hepatocellular Carcinoma using Yitrium 90 microspheres: a comprehensive report of long term outcomes. *Gastroenterology* 2010; **138**: 52–64.

136 Patel T. Worldwide trends in mortality from biliary tract malignancies. *BMC Cancer* 2002; **2**: 1353–1357.

137 Shaib YH, El-Serag HB, Davila JA *et al.* Risk factors of intrahepatic cholangiocarcinoma in the United States: a case-control study. *Gastroenterology* 2005; **128**: 620–626.

138 Taylor-Robinson SD, Toledano MB, Arora S *et al.* Increase inmortality rates from intrahepatic cholangiocarcinoma in England and Wales 1968-1998. *Gut* 2001; **48**: 816–20.

139 Parkin DM, Srivatanakul P, Khlat M *et al*. Liver cancer in Thailand I: a case-control study of cholangiocarcinoma. *Int. J. Cancer* 1991; **48**: 323–28.

140 Chalasani N, Baluyut A, Ismail A *et al*. Cholangiocarcinoma in patients with primary sclerosing cholangitis: a multi-center casecontrol study. *Hepatology* 2000; **31**: 7–11.

141 Sorensen HT, Friis S, Olsen JH *et al*. Risk of liver and other types of cancer in patients with cirrhosis: a nationwide cohort study in Denmark. *Hepatology* 1998; **28**: 921–25.

142 Boberg KM, Schrumpf E, Bergquist A *et al*. Cholangiocarcinoma in primary sclerosing cholangitis: K-ras mutations and Tp53 dysfunction are implicated in the neoplastic development. *J. Hepatol.* 2000; **32**: 374–380.

143 Goydos JS, Brumfield AM, Frezza E *et al*. Marked elevation of serum interleukin-6 in patients with cholangiocarcinoma: validation of utility as a clinical marker. *Ann. Surg.* 1998; **227**: 398–404.

144 Yokomuro S, Tsuji H, Lunz JG 3rd *et al*. Growth control of human biliary epithelial cells by interleukin 6, hepatocyte growth factor, transforming growth factor beta1, and activin A: comparison of a cholangiocarcinoma cell line with primary cultures of non-neoplastic biliary epithelial cells. *Hepatology* 2000; **32**: 26–35.

145 Nehls O, Gregor M, Klump B. Serum and bile markers for cholangiocarcinoma. *Semin. Liver Dis.* 2004; **24**: 139–154.

146 Madariaga JR, Iwatsuki S, Todo S *et al*. Liver resection for hilar and peripheral cholangiocarcinomas: a study of 62 cases. *Ann. Surg.* 1998; **227**: 70–79.

147 Ohtsuka M, Ito H, Kimura F *et al*. Results of surgical treatment for intrahepatic cholangiocarcinoma and clinico-pathological factors influencing survival. *Br. J. Surg.* 2002; **89**: 1525–1531.

148 Meyer CG, Penn I, James L. Liver transplantation for cholangiocarcinoma: results in 207 patients. *Transplantation* 2000; **69**: 1633–1637.

149 Alberts SR, Gores GJ, Kim GP *et al*. Treatment options for hepatobiliary and pancreatic cancer. *Mayo Clin. Proc.* 2007; **82**: 628–637.

150 Craig JR, Peters RL, Edmondson HA *et al*. Fibrolamellar carcinoma of the liver: a tumor of adolescents and young adults with distinctive clinico-pathologic features. *Cancer* 1980; **46**: 372–379.

151 El-Serag HB, Davila JA. Is fibrolamellar carcinoma different from hepatocellular carcinoma? A US population-based study. *Hepatology* 2004; **39**: 798–803.

152 Komuta M, Spee B, Vander Borght S *et al*. Clinicopathological study on cholangiolocellular carcinoma suggesting hepatic progenitor cell origin. *Hepatology* 2008; **47**: 1544–1556.

153 Kato I, Kido C. Increased risk of death in thorotrast-exposed patients during the late follow-up period. *Jpn J. Cancer Res.* 1987; **78**: 1187–1192.

154 Ward E, Boffetta P, Andersen A *et al*. Update of the follow-up of mortality and cancer incidence among European workers employed in the vinyl chloride industry. *Epidemiology* 2001; **12**: 710–718.

155 Falk H, Herbert J, Crowley S *et al*. Epidemiology of hepatic angiosarcoma in the United States: 1964–1974. *Environ. Health Perspect.* 1981; **41**: 107–113.

156 Popper H, Maltoni C, Selikoff IJ. Vinyl chloride-induced hepatic lesions in man and rodents. A comparison. *Liver* 1981; **1**: 7–20

157 Uchimura K, Nakamuta M, Osoegawa M *et al*. Hepatic epithelioid hemangioendothelioma. *J. Clin. Gastroenterol.* 2001; **32**: 431–434.

158 Lerut JP, Orlando G, Adam R *et al*. The place of liver transplantation in the treatment of hepatic epitheloid haemangioendothelioma: report of the European Liver Transplant Registry. *Ann. Surg.* 2007; **246**: 949–957.

CHAPTER 36
Hepatic Transplantation

Andrew K. Burroughs & James O'Beirne
Royal Free Sheila Sherlock Liver Centre, Royal Free Hospital, London, UK

Learning points

- Policies for liver organ allocation to prioritize recipients are based on medical urgency, medical utility or transplant benefit.

- There is an increasing use of donors with suboptimal characteristics, and also use of split livers and live donors to cope with donor shortage. Non-heart-beating donors are increasingly used.

- The best outcomes are with primary biliary cirrhosis and hepatitis B related cirrhosis (disease recurrence can be completely prevented by antiviral therapy). The worst outcomes are with hepatocellular carcinoma, hepatitis C related cirrhosis and primary sclerosing cholangitis.

- Recurrent hepatitis C remains a major problem, but new antiviral therapy may significantly increase sustained viral response rates, both before and after liver transplantation. This will lead to better outcomes.

- Acute cellular rejection is not a major determinant of outcome after liver transplantation. The major cause of early death remains infection.

- Late complications and causes of death include complications associated with cardiovascular morbidity, cancer, including lymphoproliferative disease and disease recurrence, particularly hepatitis C.

In 1955, Welch performed the first transplantation of the liver in dogs [1]. In 1963, Starzl and his group carried out the first successful hepatic transplant in man [2], but it took 4 years for a recipient to survive 1 year.

The number of liver transplants has escalated and, in 2010, over 15 000 patients were transplanted in the USA, Europe and China. Elective liver transplantation in low-risk patients has over a 90% 1-year survival. Improved results are related to more careful patient selection, to better surgical techniques and postoperative care, and to reduced chronic rejection. Better use of immunosuppression has contributed. There remains a donor shortage despite extending criteria for acceptance of donor organs and performing live donor procedures in adults using donor right lobes. Recurrent disease is now a major cause of mortality.

Selection of patients (Tables 36.1, 36.2)

The patient selected for transplant should suffer from irreversible, progressive disease for which there is no acceptable alternative therapy. The patient and the family must understand the magnitude of the undertaking and be prepared to face the difficult early postoperative period and life-long immunosuppression, increased risks of cancer and recurrent disease.

Demand has exceeded supply of donor organs. The time spent awaiting transplant and deaths occurring before it can be performed have increased. The waiting time for low-risk patients is over 6–12 months in many countries. Although in general this may be longer for those of blood group B and AB, group O recipients may have the longest waiting time because group O is the universal donor type. Depending on the system of organ distribution, such livers can be given to recipients having any ABO group. Whole donor livers suitable for children are particularly rare and this has led to the split-liver technique (see Fig. 36.5), with use of the left lobe.

The equitable distribution of the available donor livers is difficult. Results (and costs) are much better if the patient is low risk (ambulatory) compared with high risk (in intensive care), and if the donor liver has optimal characteristics. Decisions are usually made by a multi-disciplinary panel taking into account the wishes of the patient and their family.

There are three possible policies for liver organ allocation to prioritize recipients: medical urgency, utility and transplant benefit [3]. Medical urgency is based on the severity of cirrhosis. In the USA and in seven European countries (Eurotransplant zone), the Model for End-stage Liver Disease (MELD) is used [4]. MELD is a score

Sherlock's Diseases of the Liver and Biliary System, Twelfth Edition. Edited by James S. Dooley, Anna S.F. Lok, Andrew K. Burroughs, E. Jenny Heathcote.
© 2011 by Blackwell Publishing Ltd. Published 2011 by Blackwell Publishing Ltd.

Table 36.1. Transplant listing criteria in the UK

Superurgent listing (patients have first priority for receiving cadaveric liver grafts)

Paracetamol (acetaminophen) poisoning:

Category 1: pH <7.25 more than 24h after overdose and after fluid resuscitation

Category 2: prothrombin time >100s or INR >6.5 and serum creatinine >300 μmol/L or anuria, and grade 3–4 encephalopathy

Category 3: serum lactate more than 24h after overdose >3.5 mmol/L on admission or >3.0 mmol/L after fluid resuscitation

Category 4: 2 of the 3 criteria from category 2 with clinical deterioration e.g. increased intracranial pressure, FiO$_2$ >50%, increasing requirement inotropes, in the absence of sepsis

Seronegative hepatitis, hepatitis A or B, idiosyncratic drug reaction

Category 5: prothrombin time >100s or INR >6.5 and any grade of encephalopathy

Category 6: any grade encephalopathy and any 3 from the following: idiosyncratic drug reaction or seronegative hepatitis; age >40 years; jaundice to encephalopathy >7 days; serum bilirubin >300 μmol/L; prothrombin time >50s or INR >3.5

Category 7: acute presentation Wilson's disease or Budd–Chiari syndrome with any grade of encephalopathy

Category 8: hepatic artery thrombosis day 0 to 21 after liver transplantation

Category 9: early graft dysfunction days 0 to 7 with aspartate transaminase >10000 U/L, INR >3.0, serum lactate 3 mmol/L, absence of bile secretion

Category 10: live liver donor who develops severe liver failure within 4 weeks of donor operation

Elective listing (all must have a projected 5-year survival after liver transplantation of ≥50%)

Estimated 1-year mortality without liver transplantation >9% using UKELD score >49 points* (calculator at NHS Blood and Transplant, www.nhsbt.nhs.uk)

Hepatocellular carcinoma: diagnosed radiologically by two concordant imaging techniques. Based on CT a single lesion ≤5 cm maximum diameter or ≤3 lesions each ≤3 cm diameter, each† without macrovascular invasion nor metastases

Variant syndromes: diuretic resistant ascites, hepatopulmonary syndrome, chronic hepatic encephalopathy, persistent/intractable itching, familial amyloidosis, primary hyperlipidaemia, polycystic liver disease, recurrent cholangitis

*Patients with alcoholic liver disease, past intravenous drug abuse and current methadone users assessed as per separate UK guidelines.
†Currently extended criteria being piloted.

based on serum bilirubin, creatinine and INR (Table 36.2). There are several limitations of the MELD score, including interlaboratory variations in measuring serum creatinine [5,6], gender differences in creatinine values [7] and variations in INR [8].

Despite more objectively measured variables than in the Child–Pugh system, which includes ascites and encephalopathy, and a greater spread of scores (up to 40 with MELD compared to between 5 and 15 with the Child–Pugh score), the MELD system does not have better prediction for survival than Child–Pugh score for cirrhosis in general [9], nor for mortality within 3 months on a transplant waiting list [10]. Indeed, known adverse prognostic factors in cirrhosis and/or heavily influencing quality of life, such as chronic encephalopathy, resistant ascites, recurrent cholangitis, difficult-to-treat variceal bleeding and low serum sodium, are not taken into account. Neither are metabolic conditions. These conditions are part of the 'MELD exceptions', assessed

by special Regional Review Boards. Serum sodium is incorporated into the United Kingdom End Stage Liver Disease Score (UKELD), which determines minimal listing criteria [11]. MELD does not correlate with quality of life [12]. However, the diagnosis of hepatocellular carcinoma is catered for in the MELD allocation system by giving more points to these patients. The introduction of MELD in the USA has resulted in fewer new waiting list registrations, higher transplantation rates without increase in mortality after liver transplantation and a reduction of mortality on the waiting list [13], because time waiting on a list was removed as a major criterion. However, where the original allocation system did not have this policy, the introduction of MELD has led to a deterioration of outcomes after transplantation [14].

The second alternative for an allocation system can be based on utility, which considers outcome after liver transplantation as well as death on the waiting list. The MELD system ensures a sickest first principle, but if this

Table 36.2. Transplant listing criteria in USA

Status 1A and 1B patients have first priority for receiving cadaveric liver grafts
These patients and those with MELD score >25 are re-certified every 7 days
Status 1A 18 years or older with:
    fulminant hepatic failure (onset encephalopathy <8 weeks of jaundice)
      and ventricular dependence, renal support and INR >2.0
      or acute decompensation due to Wilson's disease
    primary non-function or hepatic artery thrombosis (HAT)* within ≤7 days or liver graft implantation
      and aspartate transaminase >3000 U/L and either INR >2.5, or acidosis
      or anhepatic following graft removal
Status 1B age less than 18 years
    chronic liver disease requiring ICU care with one of the following:
      (i) ventilator dependence
      (ii) gastrointestinal bleeding with >30 mL/kg red cells ≤24 h
      (iii) renal support
      (iv) Glasgow coma score <10 within previous 48 h
    and calculated MELD or PELD >25 points
All others†
    Based on increasing MELD/PELD scores

$$MELD = 0.957 \times \log_e(\text{creatinine [mg/dL]}) + 0.378 \times \log_e(\text{total bilirubin [mg/dL]}) + 1.120 \times \log_e(\text{INR}) + 0.643$$

$$PELD = 0.436 \,(\text{age} < 1 \text{ year} = 1, \text{ older} = 0) - 0.687 \times \log_e(\text{albumin [g/dL]}) + 0.480 \times \log_e(\text{total bilirubin [mg/dL]}) + 1.837 \times \log_e(\text{INR} + 0.667 \,(\text{growth-failure} = 1)$$

*If HAT ≤14 days not meeting above criteria are listed with the highest MELD score of 40.
†Hepatocellular carcinoma—a single lesion 2 cm diameter or more is given extra points
Regional Review Boards review exceptions to MELD.

by chance is combined with poor donor quality, the outcome is poor with less than a 50% chance of 1-year survival [15]. This can be considered an unacceptable outcome for the use of a scarce resource. The MELD system is a poor predictor of post-transplant survival [16]. Utility systems are becoming more important as the quality of donor organs is not improving, indeed it is worsening with increased use of suboptimal grafts (extended criteria grafts) [17]. Donor age is the most important risk factor [18,19], and also influences the severity of hepatitis C recurrence and increases the rate of fibrosis [20]. Utility models depend on validated models for outcome after liver transplantation. Only a few are available [18]. In the UK (Table 36.1), an estimated survival of 50% at 5 years is needed for selection onto the waiting list, with at least a 9% chance of dying within a year without transplantation [11].

Transplant benefit models represent the balance between waiting list and outcomes after liver transplant, that is the greatest difference between the two is the yard stick for prioritization. A virtual model has suggested most of the avoidable deaths occur on the waiting list [21]. However, the extent of survival benefit needs to be set by consensus, or according to the number of available donor organs. Thus, although survival benefit for HCV-related cirrhosis recipients with a MELD score between 9 and 20 is worse than those with alcoholic cirrhosis, it does not make clinical sense to wait for a MELD score of 30 (when there is no difference) before prioritizing for transplantation [22].

Candidates: outcome (Table 36.3)

The major indications for liver transplantation in the USA and Europe are HCV-related cirrhosis, alcoholic cirrhosis and hepatocellular carcinoma (Fig. 36.1). More patients with acute and subacute hepatic failure are being included and fewer with chronic hepatitis B because of effective antiviral therapy (Table 36.4).

Cirrhosis

All patients with end-stage cirrhosis should be considered for liver transplantation. Selection of the right time is difficult. The patient must not be moribund, so that the transplant will fail, or be capable of leading a relatively normal life for a long period, so that transplant is unnecessary. In non-cholestatic cirrhosis, transplantation

Table 36.3. Possible candidates for hepatic transplantation

Cirrhosis
  Cryptogenic/ NASH-associated cirrhosis
  Autoimmune
  Virus B (HBV DNA negative or under effective antiviral therapy)
  Virus D
  Virus C
  Alcoholic (Chapter 25)
Cholestatic liver disease
  Primary biliary cirrhosis
  Biliary atresia
  Primary sclerosing cholangitis
  Secondary sclerosing cholangitis
  Graft-versus-host disease
  Chronic hepatic rejection
  Cholestatic sarcoidosis (Chapter 31)
  Chronic drug reactions (rare)
Primary metabolic disease (see Table 36.5)
Acute liver failure (Chapter 5)
Malignant disease (Chapter 35)
  Hepatocellular carcinoma
  Epithelioid haemangioendothelioma
  Hepatoblastoma
  Hepatic metastatic neuroendocrine tumours
Miscellaneous
  Budd–Chiari syndrome (Chapter 9)
  Short-bowel syndrome

NASH, non-alcoholic steatohepatitis.

Table 36.4. Percentage survival of 47 651 patients transplanted between January 1988 and June 2006 according to diagnosis of cirrhosis, acute liver failure and cancer

	Survival (%)			
Diagnosis	1 year	3 years	5 years	10 years
Cirrhosis	83	76	71	60
Acute liver failure	68	63	61	55
Cancer	78	62	53	40

Data from European Liver Transplant Registry, 2008.

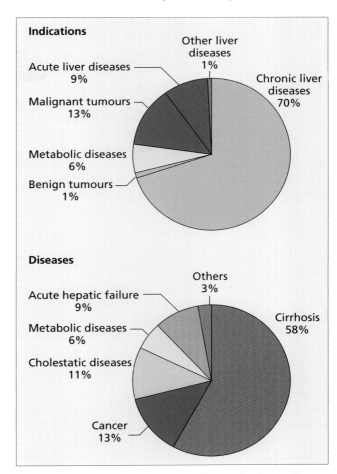

Fig. 36.1. Primary indications and diseases leading to liver transplantation in Europe between January 1988 and June 2006 (European Liver Transplant Registry).

should be considered if prothrombin time is more than 5 s prolonged, or the serum albumin concentration is less than 30 g/L, as well as resistant ascites, chronic encephalopathy and previous spontaneous bacterial peritonitis, resolved or ongoing renal impairment or intractable variceal bleeding. In cholestatic cirrhosis an additional consideration is a serum bilirubin more than 100 μmol/L. The cost of transplant is little different from that of long-term medical and surgical management of complications such as bleeding, coma and ascites.

The patients are poor operative risks if there is severely impaired blood coagulation and portal hypertension, so that blood loss is great. The technical difficulties are greater when cirrhosis is present, particularly when the liver is small and difficult to remove, or with previous abdominal surgery or extensive portal vein thrombosis. Survival at 1 year is much the same for all forms of cirrhosis, but long-term survival is dictated by disease recurrence.

Autoimmune chronic hepatitis

Post-transplant 5-year survival is 91% and graft survival 83% [23]. Despite triple immunosuppression, 33% develop recurrent chronic hepatitis of autoimmune type often related to insufficient immunosuppression. It mostly responds to changes in immunosuppression and is unrelated to the HLA status of the donor, but is associated with DR3 or DR4 in the recipient [24]. However, graft failure may occur [24].

Chronic viral hepatitis (Chapter 37)

Hepatic transplantation performed for *acute* fulminant viral hepatitis (A, B, D and most cases of E) is not followed by graft re-infection as the viral levels are very low. In the chronic situation, however, graft re-infection is very common, unless antiviral therapy is given as for hepatitis B, and currently is almost universal for HCV-related cirrhosis, unless there has been a sustained virological response before liver transplantation. Chronic hepatitis E has been described after liver transplantation.

Hepatitis B

Without antiviral therapy, post-transplant recurrence is usual and is related to viral replication in extrahepatic sites, particularly monocytes. A severe *fibrosing cholestatic hepatitis* may develop with ballooning of hepatocytes and ground-glass change [25]. This may be related to high cytoplasmic expression of viral antigens in the presence of immunosuppression [25]. HBV may sometimes be cytopathic.

Antiviral therapy in HBV DNA-positive patients selected for transplantation usually consists of dual therapy, lamivudine and tenofovir, or entecavir and tenofovir, which should be maintained after transplantation. If only lamivudine is available, hepatitis B immunoglobulin should be used intraoperatively, postoperatively on a daily basis, and then maintained lifelong [26]. Initial titres of anti-HBs should be above 100 IU/L. However, despite hepatitis B-specific immunoglobulin with lamivudine, break-through mutants can occur, causing recurrent hepatitis [27], which then should be treated by adding tenofovir.

Immunoglobulin can be weaned down and stopped if HBV DNA was negative before liver transplantation, but validated schedules are not available. Adequate compliance, with patient education, must be ensured to prevent the development of viral escape mutants. Laboratory facilities to detect viral resistance must be available.

Hepatitis B infection can now be controlled completely, maintaining or rapidly resulting in HBV DNA negativity in serum, so that HBV DNA negativity or appropriately falling HBV DNA titres in patients requiring an urgent liver transplant is sufficient to list for transplantation. Currently, hepatitis B cirrhosis without hepatocellular carcinoma has the best survival after liver transplantation, comparable to primary biliary cirrhosis.

HBV vaccination, following discontinuation of HBIG, may be associated with the development of protective serum titres of anti-HBs [28], but this is rare. More immunogenic vaccines may make this strategy viable.

Hepatitis delta

Without antiviral therapy for hepatitis B, transplantation is almost always followed by infection of the graft. HDV RNA and HDAg can be detected in the new liver and HDV RNA in the serum [29]. Hepatitis only develops if there is concomitant or superinfection with HBV, so that suppression of hepatitis B as described above prevents disease recurrence.

Hepatitis C virus

Hepatitis C is the commonest indication for liver transplantation in most centres in the USA and Europe. All patients who are positive for HCV by PCR pretransplant will remain positive, and 97% will develop recurrent hepatitis C post-transplant (Fig. 36.2). Infection of the graft can come from infected mononuclear cells which contain negative-strand viral RNA—the replicative intermediate of the viral genome. The overall 5-year survival of patients with HCV is less than that with other liver diseases [30] and 10-year survival is significantly worse [31].

Treatment for recurrence is not very effective with pegylated interferon and ribavirin [32]. Use of low-dose tapering steroids and azathioprine may slow down the rate of fibrosis [33].

Neonatal hepatitis

This disease of unknown aetiology is associated with jaundice, giant cell hepatitis and rarely liver failure necessitating liver transplant, which is curative [34].

Alcoholic liver disease

In Northern Europe, these patients provide the largest number of candidates for transplant. The selection and the results obtained are discussed in Chapter 25. Transplant benefit evaluation of survival is better than HCV-related cirrhosis with moderate severity of cirrhosis [22].

Cholestatic liver disease

End-stage biliary disease, usually involving the small intrahepatic bile ducts, is an excellent indication for hepatic transplantation (Fig. 36.3). Hepatocellular function is usually preserved until late and the timing of the transplant is easy. In every case the liver shows an advanced biliary cirrhosis, often combined with loss of bile ducts (*disappearing bile duct syndrome*).

Primary biliary cirrhosis (Chapter 15)

One-year patient survival is over 90% [35]. Recurrence can occur, but there are only few reports of subsequent graft failure.

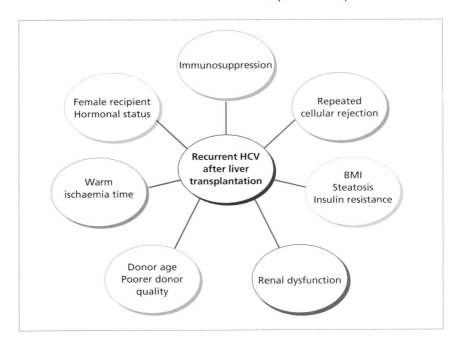

Fig. 36.2. Factors associated with recurrent HCV hepatitis after liver transplantation. BMI, body mass index.

Extrahepatic biliary atresia (Chapter 29)

This indication comprises 35–67% of paediatric liver transplants and is always indicated if infants are diagnosed after 3 months. Calculated 1-year survival is 75%. Results are excellent and long-term survivors have good physical and mental development, although re-transplant and post-transplant surgery is often necessary.

A previous Kasai procedure increases the operative difficulty and the morbidity.

Alagille's syndrome

Transplant is required only in very severe sufferers [36]. Associated cardiopulmonary disease may be fatal and careful preoperative assessment is necessary.

Primary sclerosing cholangitis (Chapter 16)

Sepsis and previous biliary surgery provide technical problems. Nevertheless, the results for transplantation are good, 1-year survival being 70% and 5-year survival 57%. Disease recurrence is frequent [37]. Colectomy pre-transplant is associated with less recurrence [37]. Cholangiocarcinoma is a complication that greatly reduces long-term survival. Inflammatory bowel disease must be monitored closely with annual surveillance colonoscopies. It can worsen after liver transplantation despite immunosuppressive drugs [38].

Other end-stage cholestatic diseases

Hepatic transplantation has been performed for graft-versus-host cirrhosis in a bone marrow recipient. Other

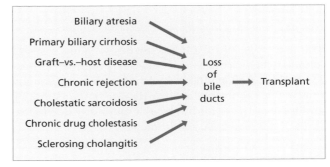

Fig. 36.3. Diseases with disappearing bile ducts treated by liver transplantation.

rare indications include cholestatic sarcoidosis (Chapter 31) and chronic drug reactions.

Primary metabolic disease

Liver homografts retain their original metabolic specificity. Consequently, liver transplantation is used for patients with inborn errors that result from defects in hepatic metabolism. Patients suffering from these conditions are good candidates. Selection depends on the prognosis and the likelihood of the later complication of primary liver tumours.

Liver transplantation for metabolic disorders is divided into those performed for *end-stage liver disease* or premalignant change and those performed for major *extrahepatic features*, in some cases associated with concomitant kidney transplantation (Table 36.5). Overall survival is over 85% at 5 years.

Table 36.5. Liver transplantation for metabolic disorders

End-stage disease or premalignant change
  α1-Antitrypsin deficiency
  Genetic haemochromatosis
  Wilson's disease
  Tyrosinaemia
  Galactosaemia
  Glycogen storage diseases
  Protoporphyria
  Neonatal haemochromatosis
  β-thalassaemia
  Cystic fibrosis
  Byler's disease
Major extrahepatic features
  Primary oxaluria type 1
  Homozygous hypercholesterolaemia
  Crigler–Najjar syndrome
  Primary coagulation disorders (factor VIII, IX, protein C)
  Urea cycle defects
  Mitochondrial respiratory chain defects
  Familial amyloidotic polyneuropathy

End-stage liver disease

Non-alcoholic fatty liver disease associated cirrhosis

The end stage of NAFLD is cirrhosis. Many cases of 'cryptogenic' cirrhosis are due to progressive non-alcoholic steatohepatitis. This is the fourth most common indication. Recurrence of liver disease is frequent [39], and there is excess cardiovascular morbidity due to features of the metabolic syndrome [40].

α_1-Antitrypsin deficiency

This is the most common metabolic disease leading to liver transplantation. Macronodular cirrhosis will develop in about 15% before the age of 20 years. Hepatocellular carcinoma is a complication. The plasma α_1-antitrypsin deficiency is corrected and the lung disease stabilizes after the transplant. Advanced pulmonary disease is a contraindication unless both lungs and liver are transplanted.

Genetic haemochromatosis (Chapter 26)

This is an uncommon indication for transplantation. Survival is lower than for other indications, because of infection and cardiac problems. Clear-cut recurrence of hepatic iron has not been reported but follow-ups are short [41].

Wilson's disease (Chapter 27)

Liver transplants have to be considered in patients presenting with fulminant hepatitis, in young cirrhotic patients with severe hepatic decompensation who have failed to improve after 3 months' adequate D-penicillamine treatment, and in effectively treated patients who have developed severe hepatic decompensation following discontinuance of penicillamine.

The overall survival is 72% increasing to 90% when the indication is fulminant Wilson's disease [42].

Neurological complications show significant improvement only if associated with liver disease [43].

Glycogen storage diseases (Chapter 29)

Liver transplantation has been successfully performed for types I and IV, with survival and continued growth into adult life.

Galactosaemia (Chapter 29)

A few patients diagnosed late develop advanced cirrhosis in childhood and early adult life and are candidates for transplantation.

Protoporphyria

This can lead to end-stage cirrhosis and so be an indication for liver transplantation [44]. Postoperatively, the high level of protoporphyrin in erythrocytes and faeces persists and the disease is not cured.

Tyrosinaemia

Hepatic transplantation is curative and should be considered early before the development of hepatocellular carcinoma [45].

β-Thalassaemia

Combined heart and liver transplantation has been reported for end-stage, iron-induced organ failure in an adult with homozygous β-thalassaemia [46].

Cystic fibrosis (Chapter 29)

Hepatic transplantation is indicated for predominant liver involvement. Combined liver–lung transplant is often necessary. The 3-year survival of young patients with end-stage respiratory failure complicated by cirrhosis is 70% [47].

Byler's disease

Byler's disease (progressive familial intrahepatic cholestasis type 1) results in death from cirrhosis or heart failure. The low serum apolipoprotein A_1 concentration is corrected by transplant performed for cirrhosis [48].

Correction of extrahepatic features

Oxaluria

Primary oxaluria type I, due to deficiency of hepatic peroxisomal alanine-glyoxylate aminotransferase, is corrected by simultaneous hepatic and renal transplantation [49]. Cardiac dysfunction reverses. The hepatic transplantation should preferably be done before renal damage has developed.

Homozygous hypercholesterolaemia

Liver transplant produces an 80% decrease in serum lipids. Cardiac transplant or coronary bypass are also usually necessary [50].

Crigler–Najjar syndrome

Liver transplant is indicated to prevent neurological sequelae when the serum bilirubin level is very high and cannot be controlled by phototherapy.

Primary coagulation disorders

The usual indication is HCV cirrhosis. Transplant cures the haemophilia but the effects of HIV infection and recurrent viral hepatitis remain post-transplant complications [51].

Urea cycle enzyme deficiencies

Transplantation has been performed for ornithine transcarbamylase deficiency as urea cycle enzymes are predominantly located in the liver [52]. The decision concerning the need for transplantation is difficult as some urea cycle disorders allow a normal lifestyle.

Mitochondrial respiratory chain defects

These may cause liver disease in neonates associated with hypoglycaemia and postprandial hyperlacticacidaemia. They have been treated by liver transplant.

Primary familial amyloidosis

Transplant, often by the domino technique, should be performed before the onset of significant polyneuropathy and before autonomic bladder and rectal dysfunction. Neurological improvement is variable [53].

Acute liver failure (Chapter 5)

Indications include fulminant viral hepatitis, Wilson's disease, acute fatty liver of pregnancy, drug overdose (for instance, paracetamol (acetaminophen)) and drug-related hepatitis [54].

Malignant disease (Chapter 35)

Hepatic transplantation has been disappointing in patients with liver tumours despite preoperative attempts at identifying extrahepatic spread. Patients with cancer have a low operative mortality, but the worst long-term survival. Recurrence is frequent; carcinomatosis is the usual cause of death.

Hepatocellular carcinoma (Chapter 35)

Patients with a single tumour 5 cm in diameter or less, and, if multifocal, only three tumours less than 3 cm in diameter [55] each, without macrovascular invasion have the lowest recurrence rate with a survival rate of over 70%. Vascular invasion, whether undetected macroscopically, or microscopic on examination of histological material, increases the recurrence rate and mortality [55,56]. Expansion of staging criteria is practiced in several centres, as well as down-staging with locoregional therapy with a period of observation to document control of tumour growth.

Fibrolamellar carcinoma

The tumour is localized to the liver and cirrhosis is absent. This may be the best type of tumour for transplantation, and in certain cases transplantation is performed with localized and treatable metastases.

Epithelioid haemangioendothelioma

This presents as multiple focal lesions in both lobes of an otherwise normal liver. The course is unpredictable and recurrence is likely in 50%. Metastatic spread does not always contraindicate surgery and this does not correlate with survival. It can be successfully treated by liver transplantation [57].

Hepatoblastoma

Transplantation results in a 50% survival at 24–70 months. Microscopic vascular invasion and anaplastic epithelium with extrahepatic spread are bad signs.

Neuroendocrine tumours

When resection is not possible, worthwhile palliation can result from hepatic transplantation [58], especially if the primary tumour can be resected.

712   *Chapter 36*

Abdominal cluster operations for right upper quadrant malignancy

Most of the organs derived from the embryonic foregut are removed including liver, duodenum, pancreas, stomach and intestine. With powerful immunosuppression, donor lymphoreticular cells circulate without causing clinical graft-versus-host disease and become those of the recipient without causing rejection [59]. The procedure is very radical and only few have survived without recurrent tumour.

Cholangiocarcinoma

Tumour recurrence is usual and 3-year survival is poor, being zero in some series, unless a preoperative regime of brachytherapy and chemotherapy with pretransplant staging laparotomy is instituted [60]. In most centres, patients with cholangiocarcinoma are not accepted as transplant candidates.

Budd–Chiari syndrome (Chapter 9)

Hepatic transplantation is used in those who are too ill to perform decompressive shunting by TIPS, and where previous portal–systemic shunts have failed [61]. The 5-year survival is over 70% [61]. Recurrence of thrombosis is a risk, especially in those who have an underlying coagulopathy, and life-long anticoagulation is necessary.

Absolute and relative contraindications
(Table 36.6)

Absolute

These include uncorrectable cardiopulmonary disease, ongoing infection, metastatic malignancy and severe brain damage.

Transplant should not be done if the patient cannot comprehend the magnitude of the undertaking and the exceptional physical and psychological commitment required [62].

Relative (higher risk)

Patients are at higher risk if they have advanced liver disease and are being treated in an intensive care unit and particularly if they are ventilation-dependent.

Children do particularly well but technical difficulties increase below the age of 2 years.

Risk increases with a body weight of more than 100 kg.

Multiorgan transplant adds to the risk.

Table 36.6. Absolute and relative contraindications to liver transplantation

Absolute

Psychological, physical and social inability to tolerate the procedure

Active sepsis

Metastatic malignancy (except hepatic neuroendocrine tumours)

Cholangiocarcinoma (except trial protocols with neoadjuvant therapy and staging laparotomy)

AIDS

Advanced cardiopulmonary disease

Relative (higher risk)

Age more than 65 or less than 2 years

Prior-portacaval shunt

Prior complex hepatobiliary surgery

Portal vein thrombosis

Re-transplant

Multiorgan transplants

Obesity

HIV

Serum creatine more than 1.7 mg/dL (150 μmol/L)

Chronic renal failure (requires combined liver/ kidney transplantation)

Cytomegalovirus mismatch

Advanced liver disease

A pretransplant serum creatinine level exceeding 1.7 mg/dL is the most accurate predictor of post-transplant death [63].

CMV mismatch (recipient negative, donor positive) adds to the risk.

Portal vein thrombosis makes the transplant more difficult and survival is reduced. However, the operation is usually possible [64]. An anastomosis is made between the donor portal vein and the recipient confluence of superior mesenteric vein and splenic vein, or a venous graft from the donor is used. Rarely, portacaval hemitransposition is performed [65].

Previous surgical portacaval shunts make the operation more difficult and a distal splenorenal shunt creates least problems. TIPS for variceal bleeding is the most satisfactory preliminary to transplantation [66]. Careful positioning of the stent is important, avoiding an excessive length down the portal vein, or protrusion into the vena cava.

Previous complex surgery in the upper abdomen also makes the transplant technically very difficult.

Re-transplantation

The average re-transplantation rate is about 10%. Over half are due to primary non-function and hepatic arterial thrombosis, the remainder for chronic rejection and recurrent disease.

In Europe, primary transplant is associated with an 80% survival at 1 year. This is reduced to less than 50% for re-transplantation [18].

General preparation of the patient

The usual clinical, biochemical and serological investigation of any patient with liver disease is detailed.

Blood group, antibodies to cytomegalovirus and hepatitis C are measured and markers of hepatitis B infection noted. An assessment of renal function, preferably with radioisotope techniques of glomerular filtration rate measurement, should be made.

In patients with malignant disease, metastases must be sought by all possible techniques.

Cardiopulmonary assessment should be thorough, including the presence and severity of hepatopulmonary syndrome and severe pulmonary hypertension.

Imaging. Splanchnic vasculature and particularly the hepatic artery and portal vein must be visualized as a guide to surgery. Doppler ultrasound is routine. The hepatic arterial tree is also shown in contrast-enhanced helical CT [67]. MRI may be used as an alternative, or together with CT to exclude vascular abnormalities and silent malignancy [67].

The bile ducts are visualized by MRI cholangiography [68] or, if cholangiocarcinoma is suspected, by endoscopic retrograde cholangiopancreatography (ERCP) and endoscopic ultrasound (EUS).

The pretransplant medical 'work-up' takes about 5 days. It includes psychiatric counselling, nutritional assessment [69] and confirmation of the diagnosis. The patient may wait many months for a suitable donor liver and, during this period, intensive psychosocial support and close medical supervision is necessary.

Donor selection and operation

Donation may be *informed with consent* from the family, the clinician ensuring that the family have been consulted, or *presumed consent* including the patient having specifically indicated their wish to donate. Mandated consent requires a written confirmation during life to donate when one dies, which overcomes the reservations of relatives. In Spain, with the highest donation transplantation rate in Europe there is the custom of informed consent, with a very well-resourced programme of trained co-ordinators. Better education, support and advice is needed for all clinical staff who have contact with potential donors.

Donor shortage has encouraged the use of livers formerly regarded as unsatisfactory. These include livers from donors with abnormal liver tests, elderly donors, those with prolonged ICU stay receiving inotropes, or with moderate steatosis which was formerly an exclusion criterion [17]. Use of these marginal livers does not seem to have increased graft loss. There is an increasing use of controlled non-heart-beating donors [70].

Donors are considered between 2 months and 75–80 years of age, victims of brain injury that has resulted in brain death. For heart-beating donors, cardiovascular and respiratory functions are sustained by mechanical ventilation. The recovery of livers and other vital organs from heart-beating cadavers minimizes the ischaemia that occurs at normal body temperatures and is a major contribution to graft success.

Transplant across A, B and O blood groups may be followed by severe rejection and biliary complications. It should be avoided unless necessitated by an emergency situation [71], when appropriate adsorption and transfusion protocols should be used.

HLA matching is not practiced and indeed there is some evidence that selected HLA class II mismatches may be advantageous, particularly in preventing the vanishing bile duct syndrome [72].

Hepatitis B and C viral markers, CMV antibodies and HIV testing should be done.

The donor operation is as follows. The hepatic structures are dissected and the liver is precooled through the portal vein with Ringer's lactate and 1000 mL of University of Wisconsin (UW) or other preservation solution perfused through the aorta and portal vein. A cannula in the distal inferior vena cava provides a vent for venous outflow. After removal, the cold liver is further flushed with an additional 1000 mL UW or other preservation solution through the hepatic artery and portal vein and stored in this solution in a plastic bag on ice in a portable cooler. This routine has extended the preservation time to at least 18 h so that the recipient operation may be semielective and not performed at unsocial hours. However, with non-heart-beating donors, and others with suboptimal quality, transplantation is performed with the shortest possible cold ischaemic time. Most centres now have designated multiorgan retrieval teams.

If possible, and particularly for elective procedures, the size of the donor liver should be matched to that of the recipient. This is based on a body weight within 10 kg of the recipient. Occasionally, a small-sized liver is transplanted into a larger patient. The donor liver

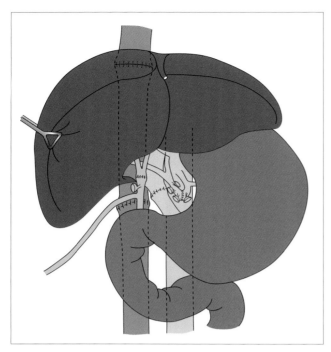

Fig. 36.4. Completed orthotopic liver transplantation. Biliary tract reconstruction is by duct-to-duct anastomosis.

increases in size at the rate of about 70 mL/day until it achieves the volume expected for the recipient's size, age and sex [73].

The recipient operation (Fig. 36.4)

The average operative time is 8 h. Blood loss is variable, volumes being minimal or massive, but a proportion of transplants do not require any blood to be transfused. Cell savers have proven useful when high blood loss is anticipated; the blood is aspirated from the abdominal cavity, washed repeatedly, re-suspended and infused.

The hilar structures and vena cava above and below the liver are dissected. The various vessels are cross-clamped and divided to allow removal of the liver. The recipient vena cava can be left *in situ* to allow a piggy back technique in which single anastomosis is performed between the allograft supra hepatic inferior vena cava and the confluence of the hepatic veins.

During the implantation of the new liver, it is necessary to occlude the splanchnic and vena caval circulations. During this anhepatic phase, veno-venous bypass may be used to prevent pooling in the lower part of the body and splanchnic congestion allowing greater haemodynamic stability. The cannulae are placed in the inferior vena cava (via the femoral vein) and the portal vein, and run to the subclavian vein.

Once all vascular anastomoses are completed, the preservation fluid is flushed out of the graft before opening the blood supply to the liver. Portal vein thrombosis must be excluded. Hepatic arterial anomalies are frequent, and vessel grafts from the donor should be available for arterial reconstructions.

The usual order of anastomoses is: (a) suprahepatic vena cava; (b) intrahepatic vena cava; (c) portal vein; (d) hepatic artery; and (e) biliary system. The bile duct is usually reconstructed by direct anastomosis with external bile drainage through a T-tube in selected cases. If the recipient bile duct is diseased or absent, end-to-side Roux-en-Y choledochojejunostomy is chosen. Haemostasis is essential before closing the abdomen; perihepatic drains are placed.

Segmental (split) liver transplantation

Because of the difficulty in obtaining small donor livers for young children, segments of adult cadaveric livers have been used (Fig. 36.5, Table 36.7). Two viable grafts can be obtained from a single donor liver [74]; with experience, results are nearly as satisfactory or similar to full liver grafts (93% 1-year survival) [75]. There are more complications, including increased intraoperative blood loss and biliary problems [76].

Cadaveric split liver grafts are also being used in the adult [77,78]. The split may be done *ex vivo* on the bench. Alternatively, the split may be done *in situ* with similar results for graft survival (85%) and patient survival (90%). Two grafts of optimal quality are obtained [79]. In children it has reduced the need for live donors [80].

Live-related transplantation

This was introduced because of the shortage of small cadaveric grafts for children. The liver is obtained from a live-related donor [81]. This technique was used originally largely in children, often with biliary atresia [82], but this has been reduced due to the use of cadaveric split livers. The lack of cadaveric liver grafts also contributed to the development of live liver donation in some countries, such as Japan.

There are important ethical considerations concerning the donor, who is usually a relative, and must give free and informed consent. There must be a patient advocate, a doctor who has no connection with the transplant team. The transplant has the advantage of being an elective operation. Ischaemia time is shortened and there is less re-perfusion injury. Living-related donation has been extended to the adult, using right lobe grafts for patients with well compensated cirrhosis and mild portal hypertension, and in acute liver failure when a cadaveric donor is not available at short notice.

There is a recognized but small risk to the live donor of left hepatectomy to provide a paediatric graft. Operative stay averages 11 days and the blood loss is

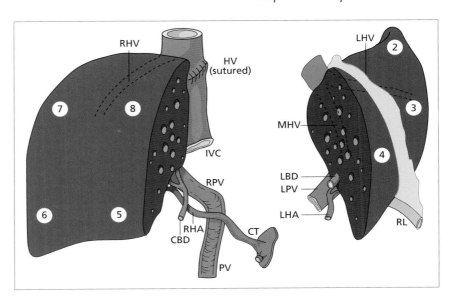

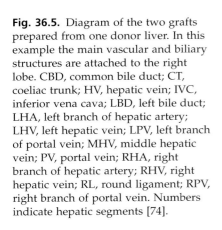

Fig. 36.5. Diagram of the two grafts prepared from one donor liver. In this example the main vascular and biliary structures are attached to the right lobe. CBD, common bile duct; CT, coeliac trunk; HV, hepatic vein; IVC, inferior vena cava; LBD, left bile duct; LHA, left branch of hepatic artery; LHV, left hepatic vein; LPV, left branch of portal vein; MHV, middle hepatic vein; PV, portal vein; RHA, right branch of hepatic artery; RHV, right hepatic vein; RL, round ligament; RPV, right branch of portal vein. Numbers indicate hepatic segments [74].

Table 36.7. Strategies to overcome shortage of heart-beating, brain-stem-dead liver donors

Better clinician and public education
Presumed consent
Split livers
Live-related donors
Partial auxiliary grafts
Non-heart-beating donors
Hepatocyte transplantation

only about 200–300 mL. Rarely, the donor may have operative and postoperative complications such as injury to the bile duct. There have been at least two reported deaths [83].

The required size of a donation is much greater for an adult than for a child. The critical limit of graft size is unknown, but is probably around 50% of the predicted liver volume, although it may be as low as 25%. This has led to the use of right lobe grafts [84]. However, the mortality for a right lobe is much higher, about 1 : 250. Problems are increased with postoperative cholestasis and biliary complications [85], and 'small for size' syndrome, which is related to increased flow from the portal vein through a reduced liver mass. Combined kidney–right hepatic lobe transplants from a living donor are performed [86]. The patient suffered transient hepatic impairment.

Auxiliary liver transplantation

Healthy liver tissue is introduced leaving the native liver *in situ* [87]. It may be indicated in acute liver failure where there is a chance that the patient's own liver will regenerate [88]. It may also be used in the treatment of some metabolic defects [89].

A reduced size graft is usually used. The left lobe of the donor liver is excised and the right lobe anastomosed to the portal vein, inferior vena cava and aorta of the recipient. The donor liver hypertrophies and the recipient's own liver atrophies.

Complications, particularly portal vein thrombosis and primary graft non-function, are increased.

Auxiliary liver transplantation offers the possibility of a life time free of immunosuppressive therapy. This is discontinued when the host liver has recovered. In time the auxiliary is likely to atrophy and should probably be removed.

Domino liver transplantation

Structurally normal livers are removed to control a metabolic defect such as familial amyloid polyneuropathy [90]. Such a liver may be offered for transplant to a recipient who has given full consent. The consequences of the metabolic defect will be delayed for between 10 and 20 years [53]. Transplanted liver grafts have been successfully reused [91].

Hepatocyte transplantation

Transplantation of human hepatocytes is being developed to treat metabolic liver disease where a supply of normally functioning liver cells can correct a genetic deficiency [92]. However, the recipient may require long-term immunosuppression. Transplanted hepatocytes may be used to replace a missing or inactive enzyme, as in the Crigler–Najjar syndrome [93], glycogen storage disease type 1a [94] and urea cycle disorders

[95], or to inactivate a disease-inducing gene or over-express a normal gene [96]. However, hepatocyte transplantation still has many challenges [97].

Xenotransplantation

Several non-human livers have been transplanted into humans. There are eight accounts of such transplants from pig, baboon or chimpanzee. No recipient has lived longer than 72h [98]. The main limitation is immunological, including hyperacute and delayed xenograft rejection and T-cell-dependent xenograft rejection. Various control strategies are under investigation [99] but the problems will be difficult to overcome.

Human infections, particularly viruses (especially porcine endogenous retroviruses) may be introduced with the xenotransplant. There are ethical difficulties in accepting xenotransplantation [99].

Liver transplantation in paediatrics

The mean age is about 3 years, but successful transplant can be performed in infants within the first year of life [100]. The scarcity of paediatric donors necessitates adult reduced-liver or split-liver donations.

Post-transplant, growth is good and the quality of life excellent.

The small size of the vessels and bile ducts poses technical problems. Pretransplant anatomy should be identified by CT or, preferably, MRI. Hepatic artery thrombosis occurs in at least 17% [101]. Re-transplants are frequent. Biliary complications are also common.

One-year survival is generally better than in adults and is 10% higher long term. Infections are frequent, particularly varicella, Epstein–Barr, mycobacteria, *Candida* and CMV.

Immunosuppression

There have been major advances in both scientific understanding and the therapy of rejection. Multiple therapy is usually given and the choice varies between centres and is nowadays tailored to both the individual patient and to the underlying disease. Most immunosuppressive regimens include a calcineurin inhibitor—that is ciclosporin or tacrolimus. These are given with corticosteroids and/or azathioprine or mycopenalate mofetil. IL2 receptor blockers allow a delay and/or a reduced dose of tacrolimus or ciclosporin to minimize renal toxicity of these drugs. Some centres do not use a calcineurin inhibitor initially but use azathioprine and methylprednisolone, introducing ciclosporin or tacrolimus only when renal function is adequate. This policy has not been evaluated versus IL2 receptor blockers.

Hepatitis C

The course of recurrent HCV hepatitis is variable. A histological defined acute hepatitis (lobular hepatitis) often without alanine transaminase flares, occurs in some between 1 and 4 months after transplant and is associated with more rapid worsening of recurrent HCV (estimates vary between 25 and 45%). Chronic hepatitis develops in up to 90%, but can be very mild and very slowly progressive. However, approximately 50% have more severe hepatitis and about 30% develop cirrhosis within 5 years of transplantation. A severe form of recurrence called fibrosing cholestatic hepatitis [102] occurs in up to 6%, and is usually fatal unless re-transplantation is undertaken. Once cirrhosis is diagnosed histologically, decompensation occurs [103].

Factors affecting severity of recurrence are high viral load pretransplant [104], increasing donor age [20] and donor female gender [105], liver steatosis, warm ischaemic time, recipient age, immune system, viral coinfection, immunosuppression, alcohol, cannabis use and histological acute hepatitis. Influence of quasispecies and genotype are controversial.

Use of azathioprine [33,106] and low-dose steroids maintained beyond 6 months are associated with less severe recurrence [33]. More immunopotent regimens, particularly use of repeated boluses of corticosteroids [107] and antilymphocyte preparations, are associated with more severe recurrence, although interaction with other risk factors is not well evaluated [108]. Antiviral therapy, particularly for genotype 1 HCV is far less effective than in the non-transplant situation [32], but if a sustained virological response is achieved, this improves prognosis. There is a small increased risk of chronic rejection and *de novo* autoimmune hepatitis with use of interferon. Maintenance of antiviral therapy often requires use of growth factors to maintain haemoglobin and platelet counts.

Ciclosporin side effects include nephrotoxicity, but the glomerular filtration usually stabilizes after a few months. Nephrotoxicity is enhanced by drugs such as the aminoglycosides. Electrolyte disturbances include hyperkalaemia, uric acidaemia and a fall in serum magnesium. Other complications include hypertension, weight gain, hirsutism, gingival hypertrophy and diabetes mellitus. Lymphoproliferative diseases can be seen long term. Cholestasis can develop. Neurotoxicity is shown by mood alterations, seizures, tremor and headaches.

Ciclosporin and tacrolimus can interact with other drugs leading to changing blood levels (Table 36.8).

Ciclosporin has a narrow therapeutic index and its use has to be monitored carefully. Trough blood levels are taken, at first frequently and then at regular intervals. Blood levels 2 hours after dosing may improve the side-effect profile.

Table 36.8. Interaction between ciclosporin (and tacrolimus) and other drugs

Increase levels
  Erythromycin/ clarithromycin
  Ketoconazole/ fluconazole
  Corticosteroids
  Metoclopramide
  Verapamil, nifedipine, diltiazem
Decrease levels
  Octreotide
  Carbamaezepine
  Phenobarbitone
  Phenytoin
  Rifampicin
  Septrin (Bactrim)
  Omeprazole
  Caspofungin
  Isoniazid
Interaction leading to enhanced neurotoxicity
  Aciclovir
  Aminoglycosides
  Amiodrone
  Amphotericin B
  Angiotensin converting enzyme inhibitors
  Erythromycin/ clarithomycin/ azithromycin
  Fibrates
  H₂ antagonists
  Vancomycin
  Omeprazole/ lansoprazole
  Grapefruit juice

Tacrolimus (FK 506) is more powerful than ciclosporin in inhibiting IL2 synthesis and controlling rejection. It has been used to salvage patients with repeated liver rejection [109]. It is better than ciclosporin in terms of patient and graft survival [110, 111], and there is less chronic rejection. Side effects include nephrotoxicity, diabetes, diarrhoea, nausea and vomiting, but less hypertension than with ciclosporin. Neurological complications (tremors and headache) are as common with tacrolimus as with ciclosporin.

Azathioprine side effects include myelosuppression, cholestasis, peliosis hepatis, perisinusoidal fibrosis and nodular regenerative hyperplasia.

Both *mycophenolate mofetil* and *sirolimus* are non-nephrotoxic. *Sirolimus* inhibits B- and T-cell activity by inhibition of IL2 pathways [112]. Mycophenalate can be used in combination with calcineurin inhibitors, and sirolimus with reduced tacrolimus doses, or alone.

Previously, *antilymphocyte globulin* and *T-cell antibodies* were given to prevent acute rejection. They have been replaced by *specific monoclonal antibodies* directed against the IL2 receptor [113]. These receptors are expressed only by activated lymphocytes and the monoclonal antibodies are given early to reduce acute rejection. *Basiliximab* remains in commercial use.

The difficulties in balancing the risks of too much immunosuppression, which increases infections and risk of malignancy, with too little immunosuppression, which increases graft rejection, are still a major issue in liver transplantation. The tendency over past decades has been to reduce maintenance immunosuppression without increased loss of grafts. An unanswered question is the role of induction, particularly with antilymphocyte preparations.

Tolerance

Donor cells have been identified in the blood of recipients of liver transplantation. This *chimerism* could influence the host immune system with development of tolerance to donor tissues. A donor liver may be spontaneously accepted more often than other organs [114]. This opens up the possibility of stopping immunosuppressive therapy. However, this is rarely possible. After a successful 5-year survival of a primary graft, between 15 and 30% of patients may be able to stop immunotherapy in the subsequent 3 years. The other two-thirds developed graft abnormalities [115]; chimerism was not associated with tolerance. Factors suggesting the successful withdrawal of immunosuppression were transplantation for a non-immunological condition, poor MHC mismatch and a low incidence of early acute rejection [113]. However, currently these patients cannot be predicted sufficiently well to plan withdrawal of immunosuppression.

Operational, or 'almost' tolerance, denoted prope (near) tolerance [116], requires a short window after transplant during which there is immunological engagement between the graft and the host. This suggests over-immunosuppression in this period will prevent tolerance.

Postoperative course

This is not always without complications, particularly in the adult. Further surgery such as for control of bleeding, biliary reconstruction or draining abscesses may be necessary. Temporary renal support is needed in about 5–10% of cases.

Re-transplantation is required in 5–10% of patients. The main indications are primary graft failure, hepatic arterial thrombosis, chronic rejection and recurrent disease. Renal support may be required. Results are not so satisfactory as for the first transplant.

Factors determining an adverse result include poor pretransplant nutrition, Child's grade C status, a raised serum creatinine level and severe coagulation abnormalities. Poor results are also related to the amount of blood products required during surgery, the need for renal support post-transplant and repeated rejection.

The operation is easier in those without cirrhosis and portal hypertension, and the perioperative mortality is considerably less.

The causes of death are surgical technical complications, bacterial sepsis (either immediate or late), biliary leaks and hepatic rejection, with or without infections, often related to over immunosuppression.

The patient usually spends about 2–3 weeks in hospital and is usually fully rehabilitated by 6 months.

Quality of life is usually excellent in the majority of patients with return to normal at home and work. Drug ingestion and monitoring are a burden. Social functioning improves in most [117]. The patient's age, duration of disability before transplant and type of job significantly affect the post-transplant employment status. Those with recurrent disease, for instance HCV, have a worse quality of life than those without recurrent disease [118].

More than 87% of paediatric survivors are fully rehabilitated with normal growth, both physical and psychosexual.

Post-transplantation complications
(Table 36.9)

The three major problems are:
1 primary graft non-function (days 1–3);
2 rejection (from 5–10 days); and
3 infections (days 3–14 and after).

Primary non-function has no exact definition but is characterized by worsening liver function, particularly coagulation, acidosis, little bile secretion (if a T-tube is in place) and renal dysfunction (Fig. 36.6). Specialist investigations must be available [119]. These include CT [120], MRI, magnetic resonance cholangiopancreatography (MRCP) and Doppler imaging, HIDA scanning, angiography [121] and percutaneous and endoscopic cholangiography.

Technical complications

Surgical complications are most frequent in children with small vessels and bile ducts.

Routine Doppler ultrasonography is used for detection of hepatic arterial, hepatic venous, portal venous or inferior vena caval stenosis or thrombosis.

CT or MRI, or ultrasound is used to evaluate hepatic parenchymal abnormalities, perihepatic collections and biliary dilatation.

Cholangiography through the T-tube or MRCP is used to define biliary abnormalities. HIDA scanning or cholangiography may be used to show biliary leaks.

Guided needle placement allows aspiration of fluid collections.

Table 36.9. Complications of liver transplantation

Weeks	Complications
1	Primary graft non-function
	Hepatic artery thrombosis
	Bile leaks
	Renal
	Pulmonary
	Central nervous system
1–4	Cellular rejection
	Cholestasis
	Hepatic artery thrombosis
5–12	CMV hepatitis
	Cellular rejection
	Biliary complications
	Hepatic artery thrombosis
	Hepatitis C
12–26	Cellular rejection
	Biliary complications
	Hepatitis C
	EBV hepatitis
	Drug-related hepatitis
>26	Ductopenic rejection (rare)
	EBV hepatitis
	Portal vein thrombosis
	Disease recurrence (HBV in the absence of adequate antiviral drugs, HCV, tumours)
	Post-transplant lymphoproliferative disorder

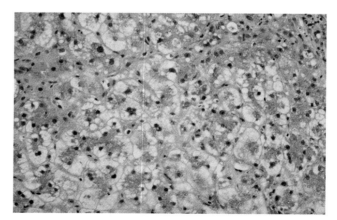

Fig. 36.6. Graft ischaemia 2 days after liver transplantation. Hepatocytes are swollen with loss of cytoplasm. (H & E,×380.)

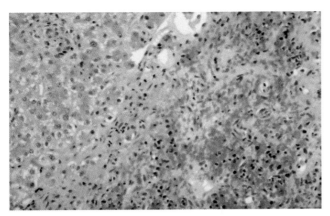

Fig. 36.7. Hepatic infarction, 3 days post-transplant, due to hepatic artery thrombosis. An area of necrotic, infarcted hepatocytes with haemorrhage adjoins normal liver tissue. (H & E,×150.)

Subcapsular hepatic necrosis. This is related to disproportionate size between donor and recipient. It can be visualized by CT scanning and usually resolves spontaneously [122].

Bleeding. This is more likely if the removal of a diseased liver has left a raw area on the diaphragm, or if there have been adhesions from previous surgery or infection, or with split liver lobes. Treatment is by transfusion and re-operation if necessary.

Vascular complications

Hepatic artery thrombosis is most frequent in children [101]. It may be acute, usually presenting within the first 30 days, marked by clinical deterioration, fever and bacteraemia, a rise in enzymes, coagulopathy and acidosis, and hepatic necrosis (Fig. 36.7). Alternatively it may be silent, presenting several weeks later with biliary complications [123] including leaks and strictures, and recurrent bacteraemia and abscesses.

Doppler ultrasound is diagnostic, although triple-phase helical CT may be necessary to show intrahepatic branch occlusion. The findings may be confirmed by angiography. Re-transplantation is the usual treatment.

Hepatic arterial stenosis usually develops at the anastomotic site. If diagnosed early in the postoperative period it may be corrected surgically. Later, balloon angioplasty may be successful.

Portal vein thrombosis is uncommon in adults. It presents as graft dysfunction and massive ascites. Urgent revascularization is essential. If not corrected, re-transplant is necessary. It may be silent, presenting as variceal bleeding weeks to months after the transplant.

Hepatic vein occlusion is common in patients who have had liver transplantation for the Budd–Chiari syndrome.

Table 36.10. Biliary complications of liver transplantation

Leaks
    Early (0–2 weeks) anastomotic
    Late (4 months) after T-tube removal
Strictures
    Anastomotic (6–12 months)
    Non-anastomotic/ intrahepatic (3 months)

Occasionally, there is stricturing of the suprahepatic–caval anastomosis and this can be treated by balloon dilatation. It is more common with the 'piggy back' technique for inferior vena cava reconstruction.

Biliary tract complications

Bile secretion recovers spontaneously over a 10–12-day period and is strongly dependent upon bile salt secretion. The incidence of complication is 6–34% of all transplants, usually during the first 3 months (Table 36.10) [124,125]. The management requires a multidisciplinary approach involving transplant surgeons, endoscopists and interventional radiologists. The majority of biliary complications can be resolved endoscopically [126], but it is important not to delay surgical intervention for a permanent biliary repair.

Bile leaks may be early (first 30 days) related to the bile duct anastomosis or late (about 4 months) after T-tube removal. Abdominal pain and peritoneal signs may be masked by immunosuppression. Early leaks are diagnosed by ERCP or percutaneous cholangiography. HIDA scanning may be useful. They are usually treated by the endoscopic insertion of a stent or nasobiliary drain.

Extrahepatic anastomotic strictures present after about 5 months as intermittent fever and fluctuating serum biochemical abnormalities. There is a wide differential diagnosis including rejection and sepsis. They are diagnosed by MRI cholangiography [68], ERCP or percutaneous cholangiopancreatography and treated by balloon dilatation and/or insertion of plastic stents [124,126]. Hepatic arterial patency must be established. They are more common with split grafts whether from cadaveric or live donors.

Non-anastomotic or *'ischaemic-type' biliary strictures* develop in 2–19% [127] after several months. They develop in the donor common hepatic duct, with variable extension into the main intrahepatic ducts. On cholangiography, the wall of the duct may appear irregular and hazy, presumably reflecting areas of necrosis and oedema. Attempts are made to treat them by balloon dilatation and stenting. Hepaticojejunostomy is sometimes possible. Re-transplant may be necessary.

They are associated with multifactorial damage to the hepatic arterial plexus around bile ducts. Factors include prolonged cold ischaemia time, hepatic arterial thrombosis, ABO blood group incompatibility, rejection, foam cell arteriopathy and a positive lymphocytotoxic cross-match. Peribiliary arteriolar endothelial damage contributes to segmental microvascular thrombosis and hence to multiple segmental biliary ischaemic strictures. They are more common with non-heart-beating donors.

Biliary stones, sludge and casts can develop any time following transplant. Obstruction, particularly biliary stricture, may be important. Foreign bodies such as T-tubes and stents may serve as a nidus for stone formation. Ciclosporin is lithogenic.

Treatment is by endoscopic sphincterotomy and stone extraction with nasobiliary irrigation if necessary.

Renal failure

Oliguria is virtually constant post-transplant, but in some renal dysfunction and failure is more serious. The causes include pre-existing kidney disease, intraoperative or postoperative hypotension and shock, sepsis, suboptimal donor quality, primary non-function, acute hepatic arterial thrombosis, nephrotoxic antibiotics and ciclosporin or tacrolimus. Renal failure may accompany severe graft rejection or overwhelming infection. Long-term renal dysfunction is frequent. Early reduction of glomerular filtration rate, such as less than 60 mL/min at 3 months, is strongly associated with subsequent renal failure, which may require kidney transplantation [128].

Pulmonary complications

In infants, and rarely in adults [129], death *during* liver transplantation may be related to platelet aggregates in small lung vessels. Intravascular catheters, platelet infusions and cell debris from the liver may contribute.

In the ICU, pulmonary infiltrates are most frequently due to pulmonary oedema and pneumonia. Other causes are atelectasis and respiratory distress syndrome [130]. In the first 30 days, pneumonia is usually due to methicillin-resistant *Staphylococcus aureus*, *Pseudomonas* and less frequently aspergillosis. After 4 weeks, pneumonia due to CMV and *Pneumocystis* is seen.

In one report, 87% of patients with pneumonia required ventilation and 40% were bacteraemic. Pyrexia, leucocytosis, poor oxygenation and cultures of the bronchial secretions indicate pneumonia and demand antibiotic therapy. The overall mortality for those having pulmonary infiltrates in the ICU is 28% [130].

Pleural effusion is virtually constant and in about 18% aspiration is necessary.

A post-transplant hyperdynamic syndrome tends to normalize with time.

The hepatopulmonary syndrome (Chapter 7) is usually corrected by liver transplant but only after a difficult post-transplant course with prolonged hypoxaemia, mechanical ventilation and intensive care [131]. Pulmonary hypertension usually requires continued therapy for some weeks, but improves after liver transplantation.

Non-specific cholestasis

This is frequently seen in the first few days, with the serum bilirubin peaking at 14–21 days. Liver biopsy suggests extrahepatic biliary obstruction but cholangiography is normal. Factors involved include mild preservation injury, sepsis, haemorrhage and renal failure. If infection is controlled, liver and kidney function usually recover but a prolonged stay in the ICU is usually necessary.

Rejection

Immunologically, the liver is a privileged organ with regard to transplantation, having a higher resistance to immunological attack than other organs. The liver cell probably carries fewer surface antigens. Nevertheless, episodes of rejection, of varying severity, are virtually constant.

Cellular rejection is initiated through the presentation of donor HLA antigens by antigen-presenting cells to host helper T cells in the graft. These helper T cells secrete IL2 which activates other T cells. The accumulation of activated T cells in the graft leads to T-cell-mediated cytotoxicity and a generalized inflammatory response.

Hyperacute rejection is very rare and is due to presensitization to donor antigens. Acute (cellular) rejection is fully reversible, but chronic (ductopenic) is not. Repeated cellular rejection is associated with chronic rejection. The differential diagnosis of rejection from opportunistic infections is difficult and liver biopsy is essential. Increased immunosuppression to combat rejection favours infection.

Acute cellular rejection

Depending on the type of induction and maintenance immunosuppression, up to 60 to 80% of patients will have at least one episode of rejection, which may not be significant clinically, usually 5–10 days post-transplant and within the first 6 weeks [132]. Acute rejection does not have an adverse effect on patient or graft survival [132]. There is little need to give higher immunosuppression during the first few days. Sometimes, the patient feels ill, there is mild pyrexia and tachycardia, and the liver may enlarge and be tender. Serum bilirubin,

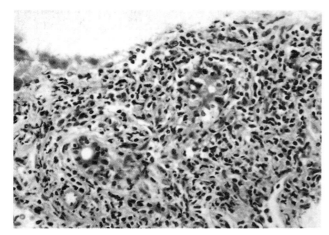

Fig. 36.8. Acute rejection: a damaged bile duct infiltrated with lymphocytes is seen in a densely cellular portal tract. (H & E,×100.)

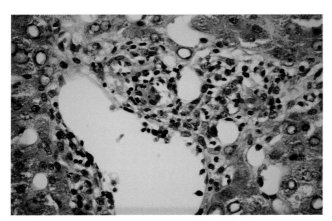

Fig. 36.9. Acute cellular rejection 8 days post-transplant. Liver biopsy shows portal zone infiltration with mononuclear cells and endothelialitis of cells lining the portal vein. (H & E,×100.)

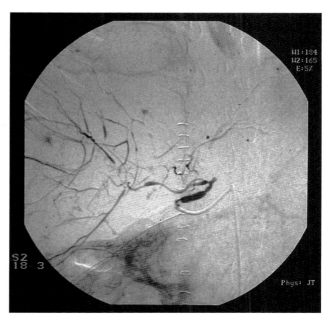

Fig. 36.10. Hepatic arteriogram in acute cellular rejection shows separation of intrahepatic arterial tree with marked narrowing.

transaminases and prothrombin time increase. The liver enzyme changes lack specificity and a liver biopsy is essential to confirm the diagnosis. Peripheral blood eosinophilia is common [133].

Rejection is diagnosed histologically by the classical triad of portal inflammation, bile duct damage (Fig. 36.8) and subendothelial inflammation of portal and terminal hepatic veins (endothelialitis) (Fig. 36.9). Eosinophils may be conspicuous [134], and hepatocellular necrosis may be seen. Zone 3 changes may also be another feature of cellular rejection [135].

Rejection may be graded into mild, moderate and severe (Table 36.11) [134,136]. An infiltrate containing eosinophils is a specific feature of cellular rejection [134]. Hepatic arteriography shows separation and narrowing of hepatic arteries (Fig. 36.10). In 85%, treatment is successful by increasing immunosuppression. Boluses of

high-dose methylprednisolone are given, for example 1 g intravenously daily for 3 days. Those who are steroid-resistant can be given antilymphocyte preparations. Tacrolimus rescue may also be tried. Those failing to respond to these measures often proceed to ductopenic rejection. Re-transplant may be needed if the rejection continues.

Chronic ductopenic rejection

Bile ducts are progressively damaged and ultimately disappear [137]. The mechanism seems to be immunological with aberrant expression of HLA class II antigens on bile ducts. Donor–recipient HLA class I mismatch with class I antigen expression on bile ducts is contributory.

The incidence of chronic rejection has decreased from 20 to 15% in the 1980s to less than 5% currently [138]. The precise reasons for this are not clearly understood.

Ductopenic rejection is defined as loss of interlobular and septal bile ducts in 50% of portal tracts. Duct loss is calculated from the ratio of the number of hepatic arteries to bile ducts within a portal tract (normal greater than 0.7). Preferably, 20 portal tracts should be studied [139]. Foam cell obliterative arteriopathy increases the bile duct damage. Ductopenic rejection may be graded histologically into mild, moderate and severe (Table 36.11) [138].

Bile duct epithelium is penetrated by mononuclear cells, resulting in focal necrosis and rupture of the

Table 36.11. NIDDK-LTD nomenclature and grading of liver allograft rejection [136]

Acute rejection*		Chronic (ductopenic) rejection†	
Grade	Histopathological findings	Grade	Histopathological findings
A0 (none)	No rejection	B1 (early or mild)	Bile duct loss, without centrilobular cholestasis, perivenular sclerosis or hepatocellular ballooning or necrosis and drop-out
A1 (mild)	Rejection infiltration in some, but not most, of the triads, confined within the portal spaces		
A2 (moderate)	Rejection infiltrate involving most or all of the triads, with or without spill-over into lobule No evidence of centrilobular hepatocyte necrosis or drop-out	B2 (intermediate/ moderate)	Bile duct loss, with one of the following four findings: centrilobular cholestasis, perivenular sclerosis, hepatocellular ballooning, necrosis and drop-out
A3 (severe)	Infiltrate in some or all of the triads, with or without spill-over into the lobule, with or without inflammatory cell linkage of the triads, associated with moderate–severe lobular inflammation and lobular necrosis and drop-out	B3 (late or severe)	Bile duct loss, with at least two of the following four findings: centrilobular cholestasis, perivenular sclerosis, hepatocellular ballooning, or centrilobular necrosis and drop-out

*The diagnosis of acute rejection is based on the presence of at least two of the following three findings: (a) predominantly mononuclear but mixed portal inflammation; (b) bile duct inflammation/ damage; and (c) subendothelial localization of mononuclear cells in the portal and central veins. Similar grading with the addition of infiltrate containing eosinophils, which are also a specific feature of cellular rejection was developed at the Royal Free Hospital [134]. Thereafter, the severity of rejection is graded on the above findings.
†Bile duct loss in >50% of triads must be present for the diagnosis.

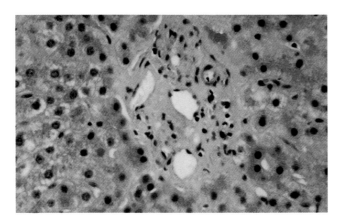

Fig. 36.11. Chronic ductopenic rejection. Bile ducts have disappeared from the portal tract which contains only a hepatic arterial branch, a portal vein and no inflammation. (H & E,×380.)

epithelium. Eventually, bile ducts disappear and portal inflammation subsides (Fig. 36.11). Larger arteries (not seen in a needle biopsy) show subintimal foam cells, intimal sclerosis and hyperplasia. Centrizonal necrosis and cholestasis develop and eventually biliary cirrhosis.

Ductopenic rejection usually follows early cellular rejection, with bile duct degeneration and then ductope-nia. The onset is usually within the first 3 months but can be sooner. Cholestasis is progressive. It has an inflammatory phase [140], during which it may respond to increased immunosuppression with tacrolimus and steroids.

Hepatic arterial occlusions may be a feature of chronic rejection (Fig. 36.12), leading to bile duct stricturing shown by cholangiography. CMV cholangitis can also lead to the sclerosing cholangitis picture.

Features indicating that irreversible graft damage has occurred, include absence of the features of acute rejection, bile duct loss in 80% of portal tracts, severe central-to-central bridging, perivenular fibrosis and loss of small portal arterioles in 30% of portal tracts [138].

Infections

Over 50% will experience an infection in the post-transplant period [141]. This may be primary, reactivation or related to opportunistic organisms (Fig. 36.13). It is important to note the degree of immunosuppression and history of any previous infection [142].

Bacterial

These are seen during the first 2 months and are usually related to technical complications. They include pneu-

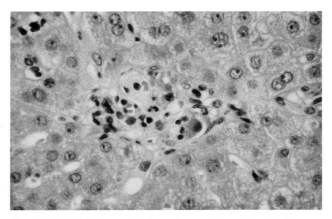

Fig. 36.14. CMV hepatitis 4 weeks post-transplant. A focus of inflammation shows hepatocytes containing inclusion bodies. (H & E,×160.)

fused blood or donor liver), or it may be a secondary reactivation. The single most important risk factor is a positive donor with CMV antibodies.

Infection is increased in those having a re-transplant or with hepatic artery thrombosis and a prolonged ICU stay. It is associated with reduced survival [143].

Infection presents within 90 days post-transplant, the peak being at 28–38 days. It continues for months in those with poor graft function who require heavy immunosuppression. CMV is the most common cause of hepatitis in the liver allograft patient. However, with the use of monitoring CMV DNA in serum, early treatment of infection is usually possible, preventing CMV disease.

The picture of CMV disease is of a mononucleosis-like syndrome with fever and increased transaminases. The lungs are particularly involved in the severely affected. Chronic infection is associated with cholestatic hepatitis and the vanishing bile duct syndrome.

'Pizza pie' retinitis and gastroenteritis are other features.

Liver biopsy shows clusters of polymorphs and lymphocytes with CMV intranuclear inclusions (Fig. 36.14). Bile duct atypia and endothelialitis are absent. Immunostaining, using a monoclonal antibody against an early CMV antigen, confirms diagnosis (Fig. 36.15) [144].

Routine prophylaxis for CMV with oral valganciclovir is effective [145] and is used in some centres but preemptive strategies, based on regular CMV DNA monitoring in blood, result in similar outcomes [146]. Immunosuppression should be reduced with either CMV infection or disease. Most infections respond to oral valganciclovir, but intravenous therapy may be needed.

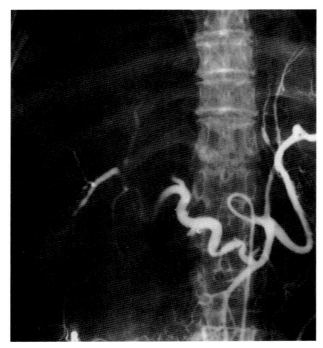

Fig. 36.12. Chronic rejection: coeliac angiogram shows pruning of the intrahepatic arterial tree. Filling did not improve later in the series of films.

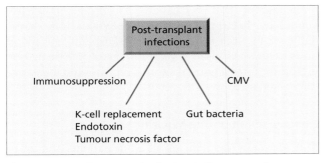

Fig. 36.13. Mechanisms of infection in liver transplant recipients.

monia, wound sepsis, liver abscess and biliary sepsis. They may be related to invasive procedures and vascular lines. They are usually of endogenous origin and selective bowel decontamination is used prophylactically by some centres.

Early deaths in transplant patients are almost always due to sepsis, but there is a life-long risk of infections. This is reduced by early withdrawal of corticosteroid suppression and minimizing maintenance immunosuppression.

Cytomegalovirus

This infection is common, but symptomatic disease is less common. It may be primary (coming from the trans-

Herpes simplex virus

This infection is usually related to immunosuppression-induced reactivation and very rarely is a primary

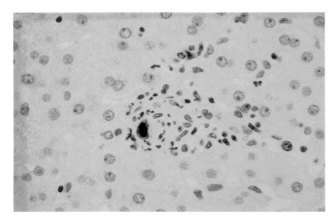

Fig. 36.15. Immunoperoxidase staining (×160) confirms the presence of CMV as a brown intranuclear deposit.

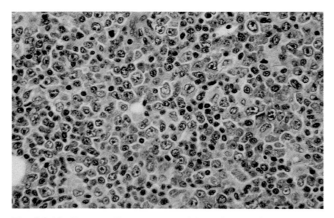

Fig. 36.16. Epstein–Barr-associated lymphoproliferative syndrome in a child aged 3 years, at 6 months post-transplant. A lymph node from the porta hepatis showing sheets of lymphocytes replacing the normal lymph gland architecture. (H & E,×300.)

infection. Liver biopsy shows confluent areas of necrosis with surrounding viral inclusions. This infection has virtually disappeared with prophylactic aciclovir.

Epstein–Barr virus

This is most frequent in children as a primary infection. It causes a mononucleosis–hepatitis picture (Fig. 36.16). It is often asymptomatic. The diagnosis is made serologically (see Chapter 21). High titres of EBV DNA are associated with lymphoproliferative disorder.

Hepatitis E virus

About 60% of patients with evidence of an acute hepatitis E infection develop chronic hepatitis. Cirrhosis has been described; severe reduction in immunosuppression can clear HEV [147].

Adenovirus

These infections are seen in children. They are usually mild, but fatal hepatitis can develop. There is no recognized treatment, except reduction of immunosuppression.

Varicella

This can complicate transplants in children, rarely in adults. It is treated with intravenous valganciclovir.

Nocardia

This infection usually affects the chest but skin and cerebral lesions may also occur.

Fungal infections

Aspergillosis has a high mortality with increases in serum bilirubin and renal failure. Brain abscess may be a complication. It may be treated by liposomal amphotericin or capsofungin.

Pneumocystis pneumonia

This presents in the first 6 months. It is diagnosed by bronchoscopy and bronchoalveolar lavage. It is prevented by Bactrim (Septrin) prophylaxis, one tablet daily for the first 6 months post-transplant, but many units only practice selective prophylaxis. It is treated by high-dose intravenous Bactrim (Septrin) and pentamidine aerosols.

De novo **autoimmune hepatitis**

This occurs in less than 2% of adult patients and up to 5% of children who have a liver transplant [148]. It can also occur in patients treated with interferon and ribavirin preparations for recurrent HCV hepatitis. Patients usually respond to conventional therapy for autoimmune hepatitis.

Malignancies

Six to twenty per cent of organ transplant recipients will develop cancer, usually within 5 years from transplantation [149]. Many are related to immunosuppression. Malignancies include skin cancers, epithelial cancers, lymphoproliferative diseases, Kaposi's sarcoma [150], the latter particularly in patients of Mediterranean origin. Yearly cancer surveillance is essential for all patients post-transplant and routine PAP smears and mammograms should be done. Patients with inflammatory bowel disease should have yearly surveillance colonoscopies.

Lymphoproliferative disorders

These complicate all solid organ transplants, the incidence being 1.8–4%. The tumour is usually a non-Hodgkin's B-cell lymphoma. It affects children more than adults. There is a strong association with Epstein–Barr infection. The tumour presents 3–72 months post-transplant in lymph nodes or in the allograft itself. One-third of cases respond to reducing or stopping immunosuppression. Rituximab and systemic chemotherapy are useful in another third, but in another third the outcome is fatal [150].

Drug-related toxicity and interactions

This must always be considered in any reaction, whether hepatitic or cholestatic. Causative drugs include azathioprine, ciclosporin, tacrolimus, antibiotics, antihypertensives and antidepressants. Interactions due to cytochrome P450 occur with macrolide antibiotics, antifungals and amiodarone. Sirolimus potentiates neurotoxicity of calcineurin inhibitors and tacrolimus use results in higher levels of mycophenalate metabolites.

Disease recurrence

If antiviral therapy is not used, hepatitis B appears at 2–12 months and may lead to cirrhosis and liver failure within 1–3 years (see hepatitis B section above). Recurrent hepatitis C is seen at any time after the first 4 weeks. Hepatitis E may recur.

Hepatocellular carcinoma recurs in the graft or as metastases, particularly in the lung, usually within the first 2 years.

Budd–Chiari syndrome may re-appear quite soon after transplantation if anticoagulation is not well controlled. Primary biliary cirrhosis, primary sclerosing cholangitis, autoimmune hepatitis and non-alcoholic steatohepatitis may all recur, usually several years after transplant.

Central nervous system toxicity and complications

Several central nervous system changes can follow liver transplantation [151]. Half the patients show fits, children being more susceptible than adults. Ciclosporin-associated fits are controlled by phenytoin but this induces (accelerates) ciclosporin metabolism. Tacrolimus can also cause neurotoxicity. Calcineurin inhibitors should be withdrawn.

Central pontine myelinolysis is related to sudden alterations in serum electrolytes, perhaps in combination with ciclosporin. CT scan shows white-matter lucencies.

Ciclosporin is bound to lipoprotein fractions in the blood. Patients with low serum cholesterol values are at particular risk of central nervous system toxicity after transplantation.

Cerebral infarction is related to perioperative hypotension, or air/ microthrombus embolism.

Cerebral abscess is seen, although rarely.

Headaches in the first few weeks can persist. Calcineurin inhibitors have been incriminated [150]; they may result in migraine [152]. Reduction in dose usually abolishes these.

Tremor is a common side effect of immunosuppressants, including corticosteroids, tacrolimus and ciclosporin. It is usually mild and responds to reduction or cessation of medication.

A second transplant is associated with a greater risk of mental abnormalities, seizures and focal motor defects.

Bone disease

Patients having liver transplants usually have some previous degree of hepatic osteodystrophy. The bones deteriorate post-transplant and vertebral collapse can occur within the first year. The cause is multifactorial and includes cholestasis, ciclosporin, corticosteroid therapy and bed rest [153]. Recovery takes place with time. Appropriate monitoring with bone density scans and prophylaxis with hormone replacement therapy if indicated, calcium and vitamin D supplementation and diphosphonates should be used.

Ectopic soft-tissue calcification [154]

This is rare; it can develop diffusely and is associated with respiratory insufficiency and bone fractures. It is secondary to hypocalcaemia due to citrate infused in fresh frozen plasma, and, in addition, renal failure and secondary hyperparathyroidism. Tissue injury and administration of exogenous calcium lead to the soft-tissue calcium deposition.

Metabolic syndrome

As well as features of the metabolic syndrome being prevalent before liver transplantation in many patients [155], due to the general increase in the population [156], and specifically increased in non-alcoholic steatohepatitis (NASH)-associated cirrhosis, they are also increasingly common after liver transplantation. Metabolic syndrome has been described in about 50% of transplanted patients within 6 months of liver transplantation in the USA [157]. Cardiovascular disease accounts for 20 to 40% of non-liver-related deaths after transplantation [155,158]. Diabetes, hypertension and renal insufficiency individually are associated with a twofold increased risk of mortality after transplant [159]. Hyperlipidaemia is seen in over 50% of patients [160], and is exacerbated by mTOR inhibitors such as sirolimus.

Metabolic syndrome is a risk factor for progression of recurrent HCV [161]. Viral eradication leads to increased serum lipids by improving hepatic steatosis [162].

Hypertension can be present in up to 77% of recipients, diabetes in up to 22%, obesity in up to 40%, renal dysfunction in up to 50% and hyperlipidaemia in up to 66% [163]. Specific therapy and early diagnosis is needed [163].

Steroid minimization, or steroid avoidance and early steroid withdrawal, as well as minimizing calcineurin inhibitors should be a therapeutic goal in liver transplant recipients [163,164], as it reduces conditions such as diabetes associated with metabolic syndrome, and renal dysfunction.

Pregnancy after liver transplantation

See Chapter 30.

Conclusion

Hepatic transplantation is a tremendous undertaking that does not begin or end with the surgery. The patient and family need psychiatric and social support. There must be a national organization to procure and increased the supply of organs. The survivor requires life-long medical and surgical supervision, together with costly drugs, both immunosuppressive and antiviral agents.

Attending physicians in referring hospital and in general practice [163,165,166] must keep in touch with the transplant centre. They should be aware of possible late complications, particularly infections, chronic rejection, biliary complications and lymphoproliferative and other malignancies. Appropriate influenza and other vaccinations as well as standard screening procedures for malignancy, including for the skin, should be instituted.

References

1 Welch CS. A note on transplantation of the whole liver in dogs. *Transpl. Bull.* 1955; **2**: 54.
2 Starzl TE, Marchioro TL, von Kaulla KN *et al.* Homotransplantation of the liver in humans. *Surg. Gynecol. Obstet.* 1963; **117**: 659–676.
3 Cholongitas E, Germani G, Burroughs AK. Prioritization for liver transplantation. *Nat. Rev. Gastroenterol. Hepatol.* 2010, in press.
4 Wiesner R, Edwards E, Freeman E *et al.* Model for end stage liver disease [MELD] and allocation of donor livers. *Gastroenterology* 2003; **124**: 191–196.
5 Cholongitas E, Marelli L, Kerry A *et al.* Different methods of creatinine measurement significantly affect MELD scores. *Liver Transpl.* 2007; **13**: 523–529.

6 Goulding C, Cholongitas E, Nair D *et al.* Assessment of reproducibility of creatinine measurement and MELD scoring in four liver transplant units in the UK. *Nephrol. Dial. Transpl.* 2010; **25**: 960–966.
7 Cholongitas E, Marelli M, Kerry A *et al.* Female liver transplant recipients with the same GFR as male recipients have lower MELD scores – a systematic bias. *Am. J. Transpl.* 2007; **7**: 685–692.
8 Trotter JF, Brimhall B, Arjal R *et al.* Specific laboratory methodologies achieve higher model for end stage liver disease (MELD) scores for patients listed for liver transplantation. *Liver Transpl.* 2004; **10**: 995–1000.
9 Cholongitas E, Papatheodoridis GV, Vangeli M *et al.* Systematic review: The model for end stage liver disease—should it replace Child-Pugh classification for assessing prognosis in cirrhosis. *Aliment. Pharmacol. Ther.* 2005; **22**: 1079–1089.
10 Cholongitas E, Marelli L, Shusang V *et al.* A systematic review of the performance of the model for end stage liver disease [MELD] in the setting of liver transplantation. *Liver Transpl.* 2006; **12**: 1049–1061.
11 Neuberger J, Gimson A, Davies M *et al.* Selection of patients for liver transplantation and allocation of donated livers in the UK. *Gut* 2008; **57**: 252–257.
12 Saab S, Ibrahim AB, Shpaner A *et al.* MELD fails to measure quality of life in liver transplant candidates. *Liver Transpl.* 2005; **11**: 218–223.
13 Freeman R, Wiesner R, Edwards E. Results of the first year of the new liver allocation plan. *Liver Transpl.* 2004; **10**: 7–13.
14 Weismuller TJ, Negum A, Becker T *et al.* The introduction of MELD based organ allocation impacts 3 month survival after liver transplantation by influencing pre-transplant patient characteristics. *Transpl. Int.* 2009; **22**: 970–978.
15 Ioannou GN. Development and validation of a model predicting graft survival after liver transplantation. *Liver Transpl.* 2006; **12**: 1594–1606.
16 Jacob M, Copley LP, Lewsey JD *et al.* Pre-transplant MELD score and post liver transplantation survival in the UK and Ireland. *Liver Transpl.* 2004; **10**: 903–907.
17 Feng S, Goodrich NP, Bragg-Gresham JL *et al.* Characteristics associated with liver graft failure: the concept of a donor risk index. *Am. J. Transpl.* 2006; **6**: 783–790.
18 Burroughs AK, Sabin CA, Rolles K *et al.* 3 month and 12 month mortality after first liver transplant in adults in Europe: predictive models for outcome. *Lancet* 2006; **367**: 225–232.
19 Halldorson JB, Bakthavatsalam R, Fix O *et al.* D-MELD. A simple predictor of post liver transplant mortality for optimization of donor/recipient matching. *Am. J. Transpl.* 2009; **9**: 318–326.
20 Berenguer M, Prieto M, San Juan F *et al.* Contribution of donor age to the recent decrease in patients survival among HCV infected liver transplant recipients. *Hepatology* 2002; **36**: 202–210.
21 Shaubel DE, Guidinger MK, Biggins SW *et al.* Survival benefit based deceased donor liver allocation. *Am. J. Transpl.* 2009; **9**: 970–981.
22 Lucey MR, Shaubel DE, Guidinger MK *et al.* Effect of alcoholic liver disease and hepatitis C infection on waiting list and post transplant mortality and transplant survival benefit. *Hepatology* 2009; **50**: 400–406.

23 Ratziu V, Samuel D, Sebagh M *et al*. Long-term follow-up after liver transplantation for autoimmune hepatitis: evidence of recurrence of primary disease. *J. Hepatol.* 1999; **30**: 131–141.

24 Gonzalez-Koch A, Czaja AJ, Carpenter HA *et al*. Recurrent autoimmune hepatitis after orthotopic liver transplantation. *Liver Transpl.* 2001; **4**: 302–310.

25 Davies SE, Portmann BC, O'Grady JG *et al*. Hepatic histological findings after transplantation for chronic hepatitis B virus infection, including a unique pattern of fibrosing cholestatic hepatitis. *Hepatology* 1991; **13**: 150–157.

26 Rosenau J, Bahl MJ, Tillmann HL *et al*. Lamivudine and low-dose hepatitis B immune globulin for prophylaxis of hepatitis B reinfection after liver transplantation—possible role of mutations in the YMDD motif prior to transplantation as a risk factor for reinfection. *J. Hepatol.* 2001; **34**: 895–902.

27 Mutimer D, Pillay D, Dragon E *et al*. High pretreatment serum hepatitis B virus titre predicts failure of lamivudine prophylaxis and graft re-infection after liver transplantation. *J. Hepatol.* 1999; **30**: 715–721.

28 Sanchez-Fueyo A, Rimola A, Grande L *et al*. Hepatitis B immunoglobulin discontinuation followed by hepatitis B virus vaccination: a new strategy in the prophylaxis of hepatitis B virus recurrence after liver transplantation. *Hepatology* 2000; **31**: 496–501.

29 Zignego AL, Dubois F, Samuel D *et al*. Serum hepatitis delta virus RNA in patients with delta hepatitis and in liver graft recipients. *J. Hepatol.* 1990; **11**: 102–110.

30 Feray C, Caccamo L, Alexander GJM *et al*. European Collaborative study on factors influencing outcome after liver transplantation for hepatitis C. *Gastroenterology* 1999; **117**: 619–625.

31 Forman LM, Lewis JB, Berlin JA *et al*. The association between hepatitis C infection and survival after orthotopic liver transplantation. *Gastroenterology* 2002; **122**: 889–896.

32 Xirouchakis E, Triantos C, Manousou P *et al*. Systematic review of pegylated interferon and ribavirin post liver transplantation. *J. Viral. Hep.* 2008; **15**: 699–709.

33 Manousou P, Samonakis D, Cholongitas E *et al*. outcome of recurrent hepatitis virus C infection after liver transplantation in a randomized trial of tacrolimus monotherapy versus triple therapy. *Liver Transpl.* 2009; **15**: 1783–1791.

34 Adrian-Casavilla F, Reyes J, Tzakis A *et al*. Liver transplantation for neonatal hepatitis as compared to the other two leading indications for liver transplantation in children. *J. Hepatol.* 1994; **21**: 1035–1039.

35 Kim WR, Wiesner RH, Therneau TM *et al*. Optimal timing of liver transplantation for primary biliary cirrhosis. *Hepatology* 1998; **28**: 33–98.

36 Cardona J, Houssin D, Gauthier F *et al*. Liver transplantation in children with Alagille syndrome—a study of 12 cases. *Transplantation* 1995; **60**: 339–342.

37 Cholongitas E Shusang V, Papatheodoridis G *et al*. Risk factors for recurrence of primary sclerosing cholangitis after liver transplantation. *Liver Transpl.* 2008; **134**: 138–142.

38 Papatheodoridis G, Hamilton M, Mistry P *et al*. Ulcerative colitis has an aggressive course after orthotopic liver transplantation for primary sclerosing cholangitis. *Gut* 1998; **43**: 539–544.

39 Ong JP, Reddy V, Gramlich TL *et al*. Cryptogenic cirrhosis and risk of recurrence of nonalcoholic fatty liver disease after liver transplantation. *Gastroenterology* 2000; **118**: A973.

40 Angulo P. Non-alcoholic fatty liver disease and liver transplantation. *Liver Transpl.* 2006; **12**: 253–234.

41 Kowdey KV, Brandhagen DJ, Gish RG *et al*. Survival after Liver Transplantation in patients with hepatic iron overload. The National Hemochromatosis Transplant Registry. *Liver Transpl.* 2006; **126**: 494–503.

42 Schilsky ML, Scheinberg IH, Sternlieb I. Liver transplantation for Wilson's disease: indications and outcome. *Hepatology* 1994; **19**: 583–587.

43 Eghtesad B, Nezakatgoo N, Geraci LC *et al*. Liver transplantation for Wilson's disease: a single centre experience. *Liver Transpl. Surg.* 1999; **5**: 467–474.

44 Herbert A, Corbin D, Williams A *et al*. Erythropoietic protoporphyria: unusual skin and neurological problems after liver transplantation. *Gastroenterology* 1991; **100**: 1753–1757.

45 Mieles LA, Esquivel CO, Van Thiel DH *et al*. Liver transplantation for tyrosinemia: a review of 10 cases from the University of Pittsburgh. *Dig. Dis. Sci.* 1990; **38**: 153–157.

46 Olivieri NF, Liu PP, Sher GD *et al*. Brief report: combined liver and heart transplantation for end-stage iron-induced organ failure in an adult with homozygous beta-thalassaemia. *N. Engl. J. Med.* 1994; **330**: 1125–1127.

47 Couetil JP, Soubrane O, Houssin DP *et al*. Combined heart–lung–liver, double lung–liver and isolated liver transplantation for cystic fibrosis in children. *Transpl. Int.* 1997; **10**: 33–39.

48 Burdelski M, Rodeck B, Latta A *et al*. Treatment of inherited metabolic disorders by liver transplantation. *J. Inherit. Metab. Dis.* 1991; **14**: 604–618.

49 Watts RW, Morgan SH, Danpure CJ *et al*. Combined hepatic and renal transplantation in primary hyperoxaluria type I: clinical report of nine cases. *Am. J. Med.* 1991; **90**: 179–188.

50 Revell SP, Noble-Jamieson G, Johnston P *et al*. Liver transplantation for homozygous familial hypercholesterolaemia. *Arch. Dis. Child.* 1995; **73**: 456–458.

51 Gordon FH, Mistry PK, Sabin CA *et al*. Outcome of orthotopic liver transplantation in patients with haemophilia. *Gut* 1998; **42**: 744–749.

52 Todo S, Starzl ET, Tzakis A. Orthotopic liver transplantation for urea cycle enzyme deficiency. *Hepatology* 1992; **15**: 419–422.

53 Perdigoto R, Furtado AL, Furtado E *et al*. The Coimbra University Hospital experience in liver transplantation in patients with familial amyloidotic polyneuropathy. *Transpl. Proc.* 2003; **35**: 1125.

54 Bismuth H, Samuel D, Castaing D *et al*. Orthotopic liver transplantation in fulminant and subfulminant hepatitis—the Paul Brousse experience. *Ann. Surg.* 1995; **222**: 109–119.

55 Mazzaferro V, Llovet JM, Miceli R *et al*; Metroticket Investigator Study Group. Predicting survival after liver transplantation in patients with hepatocellular carcinoma beyond the Milan criteria: a retrospective, exploratory analysis. *Lancet Oncol.* 2009; **10**: 35–43.

56 Marelli L, Grasso A, Pleguezuelo M *et al*. Tumour size and differentiation in predicting recurrence of hepatocellular carcinoma after liver transplantation: external validation

of a new prognostic score. *Ann. Surg. Oncol.* 2008; **15**: 3503–3511.

57 Lerut JP, Orlando G, Adam R *et al.* The place of liver transplantation in the treatment of hepatic epitheloid haemangioendothelioma: report of the European Liver Transplant Registry. *Ann. Surg.* 2007; **246**: 949–957.

58 Olausson M, Friman S, Cahlin C *et al.* Indications and results of liver transplantation in patients with neuroendocrine tumours. *World J. Surg.* 2002; **26**: 998–1004.

59 Starzl TE, Todo S, Tzakis A *et al.* The many faces of multivisceral transplantation. *Surg. Gynecol. Obstet.* 1991; **172**: 338–344.

60 Rea DJ, Heimbach JK, Rosen CB *et al.* Liver Transplantation with neoadjuvant chemoradiation is more effective than resection for hilater cholangiocarcinoma. *Ann. Surg.* 2005; **242**: 451–461.

61 Mentha G, Giostra E, Majno PE *et al.* Liver Transplantation for Budd-Chiari syndrome: a European study on 248 patients from 51 centres. *J. Hepatol.* 2006; **44**: 250–258.

62 Maddrey WC, ed. *Transplantation of the Liver*, 2nd edn. Norwalk: Appleton & Lange, 1994.

63 Gonwa TA, McBride MA, Anderson K *et al.* Continued influence of pre-operative renal function on outcome of orthotopic liver transplant (OLTX) in the US: where will MELD lead us. *Am. J. Transpl.* 2006; **6**: 2651–2659.

64 Stieber AC, Zetti G, Todo S *et al.* The spectrum of portal vein thrombosis in liver transplantation. *Ann. Surg.* 1991; **213**: 199–206.

65 Gerunda GE, Merenda R, Neri D *et al.* Cavoportal hemitransposition: a successful way to overcome the problem of total portosplenomesenteric thrombosis in liver transplantation. *Liver Transpl.* 2002; **8**: 72–75.

66 Guerrini GP, Pleguezuelo M, Maimone S *et al.* Impact of tips pre liver transplantation for the outcome post-transplantation. *Am. J. Transpl.* 2009; **9**: 192–200.

67 Nghiem HV. Imaging of hepatic transplantation. *Radiol. Clin. North Am.* 1998; **36**: 429–443.

68 Fulcher AS, Turner MA. Orthotopic liver transplantation: evaluation with MR cholangiography. *Radiology* 1999; **211**: 715–722.

69 Gunsar F, Raimondo ML, Jones S *et al.* Nutritional status and prognosis in cirrhotic patients. *Alim. Pharmacol. Ther.* 2006; **15**: 563–572.

70 Deshpande R, Heaton N. Can non-heart beating donors replace cadaveric heart beating liver donors. *J. Hepatol.* 2006; **45**: 499–503.

71 Gugenheim J, Samuel D, Reynes M *et al.* Liver transplantation across ABO blood group barriers. *Lancet* 1990; **336**: 519–523.

72 Neuberger JM, Adams DH. Is HLA matching important for liver transplantation? *J. Hepatol.* 1990; **11**: 1–4.

73 Van Thiel DH, Gavaler JS, Kam I *et al.* Rapid growth of an intact human liver transplanted into a recipient larger than the donor. *Gastroenterology* 1987; **93**: 1414–1419.

74 Emond JC, Whitington PF, Thistlethwaite JR *et al.* Transplantation of two patients with one liver: analysis of a preliminary experience with 'split-liver' grafting. *Ann. Surg.* 1990; **212**: 14–22.

75 Rogiers X, Malago M, Gawad K *et al.* In situ splitting of cadaveric livers. The ultimate expansion of a limited donor pool. *Ann. Surg.* 1996; **224**: 331–339.

76 Bismuth H, Houssin D. Reduced sized orthotopic liver grafts in hepatic transplantation in children. *Surgery* 1984; **95**: 367–370.

77 Busuttil RW, Goss JA. Split liver transplantation. *Ann. Surg.* 1999; **229**: 313–321.

78 Azoulay D, Castaing D, Adam R *et al.* Split-liver transplantation for two adult recipients: feasibility and long term outcomes. *Ann. Surg.* 2001; **233**: 565–574.

79 Toso C, Ris F, Menthe G *et al.* Potential impact of in situ liver splitting on the number of available grafts. *Transplantation* 2002; **74**: 222–226.

80 Gridelli B, Spada M, Petz W *et al.* Split liver transplantation eliminates the need for living donor liver transplantation in children with end stage liver cholestatic disease. *Transplantation* 2003; **75**: 1197–1203.

81 Jurim O, Shackleton CR, McDiarmid SV *et al.* Living-donor liver transplantation at UCLA. *Am. J. Surg.* 1995; **169**: 529–532.

82 Broelsch CE, Whitington PF, Emond JC *et al.* Liver transplantation in children from living related donors. Surgical techniques and results. *Ann. Surg.* 1991; **214**: 428–437.

83 Grewal HP, Thistlethwaite JR, Loss GE *et al.* Complications in 100 living-liver donors. *Ann. Surg.* 1998; **228**: 214–219.

84 Wachs ME, Bak TE, Karrer FM *et al.* Adult living donor liver transplantation using a right hepatic lobe. *Transplantation* 1998; **68**: 1313–1316.

85 Ghobrial RM, Saab S, lassman C *et al.* Donor and recipients outcomes in right lobe living donor liver transplantation. *Liver Transpl.* 2002; **8**: 901–909.

86 Marujo WC, Barros MFA, Cory RA *et al.* Successful combined kidney–liver right lobe transplant from a living donor. *Lancet* 1999; **353**: 641.

87 Moritz MJ, Jarrell BE, Munoz SJ *et al.* Regeneration of the native liver after heterotopic liver transplantation for fulminant hepatic failure. *Transplantation* 1993; **55**: 952–954.

88 Van Hoek B, de Boer J, Boudjema K *et al.* Auxiliary vs. orthotopic liver transplantation for acute liver failure. *J. Hepatol.* 1999; **30**: 699–705.

89 Rela M, Muesian P, Volea-Melendez H *et al.* Auxiliary partial orthotopic liver transplantation for Crigler–Najjar syndrome type 1. *Ann. Surg.* 1999; **229**: 565–569.

90 Dyer PA, Bobrow M. Domino hepatic transplantation using the liver from a patient with familial amyloid polyneuropathy. *Transplantation* 1999; **67**: 1202.

91 Moreno GE, Gomez R, Gonzalez P *et al.* Reuse of liver grafts after early death of the first recipient. *World J. Surg.* 1996; **20**: 309–312.

92 Gupta S. Hepatocyte transplantation: emerging insights into mechanisms of liver re-population and their relevance to potential therapies. *J. Hepatol.* 1999; **30**: 162–170.

93 Fox IJ, Chowdhury JR, Kaufman SS *et al.* Treatment of the Crigler-Najjar syndrome type 1 with hepatocyte transplantation. *N. Engl. J. Med.* 1998; **338**: 1422–1426.

94 Muraca M, Gerunda G, Neri D *et al.* Hepatocyte transplantation as a treatment for glycogen storage disease type 1a. *Lancet* 2002; **359**: 317–318.

95 Horslen SP, McCowan TC, Goertzen TC *et al.* Isolated hepatocyte transplantation in an infant with a severe urea cycle disorder. *Pediatrics* 2003; **111**: 1262–1267.

96 Chowdhury JR. Prospects of liver cell transplantation and liver-directed gene therapy. *Semin. Liver Dis.* 1999; **19**: 1–6.

97 Soltys KA, Sotu-Gutierrex A, Nagaya M *et al.* Barriers to the successful treatment of liver disease by hepatocyte transplantation. *J. Hepatol.* 2010; **53**: 769–774.

98 Lambrigts D, Sachs DH, Cooper DK. Discordant organ xenotransplantation in primates: world experience and current status. *Transplantation* 1998; **68**: 547–561.

99 Schneider MKJ, Seebach JD. Xenotransplantation literature update: November 2009—January 2010 *Xenotransplantation* 2010; **17**: 166–170.

100 Beath SV, Brook GD, Kelly DA *et al.* Successful liver transplantation in babies under 1 year. *Br. Med. J.* 1993; **307**: 825–828.

101 Tan KC, Yandza T, de Hemptinne B *et al.* Hepatic artery thrombosis in paediatric liver transplantation. *J. Pediatr. Surg.* 1988; **23**: 927–930.

102 Schluger LK, Sheiner PA, Thung SN *et al.* Severe recurrent cholestatic hepatitis C following orthotopic liver transplantation. *Hepatology* 1996; **23**: 971–976.

103 Kalambokis G, Manousou P, Samonakis D *et al.* Clinical outcome of HCV-related graft cirrhosis and prognostic value of hepatic venous pressure gradient. *Transpl. Int.* 2009; **22**: 172–181.

104 Charlton M, Seaberg E, Wiesner R *et al.* Predictors of patient and graft survival following liver transplantation for hepatitis C. *Hepatology* 1998; **28**: 823–830.

105 Belli LS, Burroughs AK, Burra P *et al.* Liver transplantation for HCV cirrhosis: improved survival in recent years and increased severity of recurrent disease in female recipients: results of a long term retrospective study. *Liver Transpl.* 2007; **13**: 733–740.

106 Germani G, Pleguezuelo M, Villamil F *et al.* Azathioprine in liver transplantatioin: A re-evaluation of its use and a comparison with mycophenalate mofetil. *Am. J. Transpl.* 2009; **9**: 1725–1731.

107 Sheiner PA, Schwartz ME, Mor E *et al.* Severe or multiple rejection episodes are associated with early recurrence of hepatitis C after orthotopic liver transplantation. *Hepatology* 1995; **21**: 30–34.

108 Samonakis D, Germani G, Burroughs AK. Immunosuppression and liver transplantation for hepatitis C infection. *J. Hepatol.* 2010, in press.

109 Starzl TE, Todo S, Fung J *et al.* FK 506 for liver, kidney and pancreas transplantation. *Lancet* 1989; **ii**: 1000–1004.

110 Grady JG, Burroughs AK, Hardy P *et al* and the UK and ROFI Liver Transplant Study Group. Tacrolimus versus microemulsified ciclosporin in liver transplantation: the TMC randomized controlled trial. *Lancet* 2002; **360**: 1119–1125.

111 O'Grady J, Hardy P, Burroughs AK *et al* UK and Ireland Transplant Study group. Randomized controlled tiral of tacrolimus versus microemulsified cyclosporine (TMC) in liver transplantation: post study surveillance to three years. *Am. J. Transpl.* 2007; **7**: 137–141.

112 Watson CJ, Friend PJ, Jamieson NY *et al.* Sirolimus: a potent new immunosuppressant for liver transplantation. *Transplantation* 1999; **67**: 505–509.

113 Geissler EK, Schitt JH. Immunosuppression for liver transplantation. *Gut* 2009; **58**: 452–463.

114 Riordan SM, Williams R. Tolerance after liver transplantation: does it exist and can immunosuppression be withdrawn? *J. Hepatol.* 1999; **31**: 1106–1119.

115 Mazariegos GV, Reyes J, Marino IR *et al.* Weaning of immunosuppression in liver transplant recipients. *Transplantation* 1997; **63**: 243–249.

116 Calne R. Prope tolerance: A step in the search for tolerance in the clinic. *World J. Surg.* 2000; **24**: 793–796.

117 Hunt CM, Camargo CA, Dominitz JA *et al.* Effect of postoperative complications on health and employment after liver transplantation. *Clin. Transplant.* 1998; **12**: 99–103.

118 Singh N, Gayowski T, Wagener MM *et al.* Quality of life, functional status and depression in male liver transplant recipients with recurrent viral hepatitis C. *Transplantation* 1999; **67**: 69–72.

119 Holbert BL, Campbell WL, Skolnick ML. Evaluation of transplanted liver and postoperative complications. *Radiol. Clin. North Am.* 1995; **33**: 521–540.

120 Dupuy D, Costello P, Lewis D *et al.* Abdominal CT findings after liver transplantation in 66 patients. *Am. J. Roentgenol.* 1991; **156**: 1167–1170.

121 Orons PD, Zajko AB. Angiography and interventional procedures in liver transplantation. *Radiol. Clin. North Am.* 1995; **33**: 541–558.

122 Abecassis J-P, Pariente D, Hazebroucq V *et al.* Subcapsular hepatic necrosis in liver transplantation: CT appearance. *Am. J. Roentgenol.* 1991; **156**: 981–983.

123 Gunsar F, Rolando N, Pastacaldi S *et al.* Late hepatic artery thrombosis after liver orthotopic liver transplantation. *Liver Transpl.* 2003; **9**: 605–611.

124 Tung BY, Kimmey MB. Biliary complications of orthotopic liver transplantation. *Dig. Dis.* 1999; **17**: 133–144.

125 Mazariegos GV, Molmenti EP, Kramer DJ. Early complications after orthotopic liver transplantation. *Surg. Clin. North Am.* 1999; **79**: 109–129.

126 Taibibian JH, Asham E, Goldstein L *et al.* Endoscopic treatment with multiple stents for post liver transplantation non-anastomotic biliary strictures. *Gastrointest. Endosc.* 2009; **69**: 1236–1243.

127 Fisher A, Miller CM. Ischemic-type biliary strictures in liver allografts—the Achilles heel revisited. *Hepatology* 1995; **21**: 589–591.

128 Sanchez EQ, Melton LD, Chinnakotta S *et al.* Predicting renal failure after liver transplantation from measured glomerular filtration rate: review of up to 15 years of follow up. *Transplantation* 2010; **89**: 232–235.

129 Sankey EA, Crow J, Mallett S *et al.* Pulmonary platelet aggregates: an under recognised cause of sudden intra-operative death in adults undergoing liver transplantation. *J. Clin. Path.* 1993; **46**: 222–222.

130 Singh N, Gayowski T, Wagener MM. Pulmonary infiltrates in liver transplant recipients in the intensive care unit. *Transplantation* 1999; **67**: 1138–1144.

131 Krowka MJ. Hepatopulmonary syndrome: what are we learning from interventional radiology, liver transplantation and other disorders? *Gastroenterology* 1995; **109**: 1009–1013.

132 Wiesner RH, Demetris AJ, Belle SH *et al.* Acute hepatic allograft rejection: incidence, risk factors, and impact on outcome. *Hepatology* 1998; **28**: 638–645.

133 Nagral A, Quaglia A, Sabin C *et al.* Blood and graft eosinophils in acute cellular rejection of liver allografts. *Transpl. Proc.* 2001; **33**: 2588–2593.

134 Datta Gupta S, Hudson M, Burroughs AK *et al*. Grading of cellular rejection after orthotopic liver transplantation. *Hepatology* 1995; **21**: 46–57.

135 Hubscher SG. Central perivenulitis: a common and potentially important finding in later post-transplant liver biopsies. *Liver Transpl*. 2008; **14**: 596–600.

136 Demetris AJ, Seaberg EC, Batts KP *et al*. Reliability and predictive value of the National Institute of Diabetes and Digestive and Kidney Diseases liver transplantation database. Nomenclature and grading system for cellular rejection of liver allografts. *Hepatology* 1995; **21**: 408–416.

137 Wiesner RH, Ludwig J, Vanhoek B *et al*. Current concepts in cell-mediated hepatic allograft rejection leading to ductopenia and liver failure. *Hepatology* 1991; **14**: 721–729.

138 International Panel. Update of the International Banff schema for liver allograft rejection: working recommendations for the histopathologic staging and reporting of chronic rejection. *Hepatology* 2000; **31**: 792.

139 International Working Party. Terminology of hepatic allograft rejection. *Hepatology* 1995; **22**: 648.

140 Quaglia AF, Del Vecchio Blanco G *et al*. Development of ductopenic lvier allograft rejection includes a hepatitic phase prior to duct loss. *J. Hepatol.* 2000; **33**: 773–780.

141 Hadley S, Samore MH, Lewis WD *et al*. Major infectious complications after orthotopic liver transplantation and comparison of outcomes in patients receiving cyclosporin or FK 506 as primary immunosuppression. *Transplantation* 1995; **59**: 851–859.

142 Wade JJ, Rolando N, Hayllar K *et al*. Bacterial and fungal infections after liver transplantation: an analysis of 284 patients. *Hepatology* 1995; **21**: 1328–1336.

143 Falagas ME, Paya C, Ruthazer R *et al*. Significance of cytomegalovirus for long-term survival after orthotopic liver transplantation. *Transplantation* 1998; **66**: 1020–1028.

144 Paya CV, Holley KE, Wiesner RH *et al*. Early diagnosis of cytomegalovirus hepatitis in liver transplant recipients: role of immunostaining, DNA hybridization and culture of hepatic tissue. *Hepatology* 1990; **12**: 119–126.

145 Gane E, Slaiba F, Valdecasas GJC *et al*. Randomized trial of efficacy and safety of oral ganciclovir in the prevention of cytomegalovirus disease in liver-transplant recipients. *Lancet* 1997; **350**: 1729–1733.

146 Emery VC, Hassan-Walker AF, Burroughs AK *et al*. Human cytomegalovirus (HCMV) replication dynamics in *HCMV* naïve and experienced immunocompromised hosts. *J. Infect. Dis.* 2002; **185**: 1723–1728.

147 Kamar N, Abravanel F, Selves J *et al*. Influence of immunosuppressive therapy on the natural history of genotype hepatitis E virus infection after organ transplantation. *Transplantation* 2010; **89**: 353–360.

148 Kerkar N, Hadzic N, Davies ET *et al*. De novo autoimmune hepatitis after liver transplantation. *Lancet* 1998; **353**: 409–413.

149 Tan-Shalaby J, Tempero M. Malignancies after liver transplantation: a comparative review. *Semin. Liver Dis.* 1995; **15**: 156–164.

150 Kremers WK, Devarbhavi HC, Wiesner RH *et al*. Post transplant lymphoprofliferative disorders following liver transplantation: incidence, risk factors and survival. *Am. J. Transpl.*2006; **6**: 1017–1024.

151 Bronster DJ, Emre S, Mor E *et al*. Neurologic complications of orthotopic liver transplantation. *Mt Sinai J. Med.* 1994; **61**: 63–69.

152 Steiger MJ, Farrah T, Rolles K *et al*. Cyclosporin associated headache. *J. Neurol. Neurosurg. Psychiatry* 1994; **57**: 1258–1259.

153 Rodino MA, Shane E. Osteoporosis after organ transplantation. *Am. J. Med.* 1998; **104**: 459–469.

154 Munoz SJ, Nagelberg SB, Green PJ *et al*. Ectopic soft tissue calcium deposition following liver transplantation. *Hepatology* 1988; **8**: 476–483.

155 Laryea M, Watt KD, Molinari M *et al*. Metabolic syndrome in liver transplant recipients: prevalence and association with cardiovascular events. *Liver Transpl.* 2007; **13**: 1109–1114.

156 Ford E, Giles W, Dietz W. Prevalence of the metabolic syndrome among US adults. Findings from the Third National Health and Nutrition Examination Survey. *JAMA* 2002; **287**: 356–359.

157 Watt KDS, Charlton MR. Metabolic syndrome and liver transplantation: a review and guide to management. *J. Hepatol.* 2010; **53**: 199–206.

158 Johnston S, Morris JK, Cramb R *et al*. Cardiovascular morbidity and mortality after orthotopic liver transplantation. *Transplantation* 2002; **73**: 901–906.

159 Watt KD, Pedersen RA, Kremers WK *et al*. Evolution and causes and risk factors for mortality post transplant: results of the NIDDK long term follow up study. *Am. J. Transpl.* 2010; **10**: 1420–1426.

160 Pfitzmann R, Nussler NC, Hippler-Benscheidt M *et al*. Long term results after liver transplantation. *Transpl. Int.* 2008; **21**: 234–246.

161 Hanouneh IA, Feldstein AE, McCullough AJ *et al*. The significance of metabolic syndrome in the setting of recurrent hepatitis C after liver transplantation. *Liver Transpl.* 2008; **14**: 1287–1293.

162 Corey KE, Kane E, Munroe C *et al*. Hepatitis C virus infection and its clearance alter circulating lipids: implications for long term follow up. *Hepatology* 2009; **50**: 1030–1037.

163 Mells G, Neuberger J. Long term care of the Liver Allograft recipient. *Sem. Liver Dis.* 2009; **29**: 102–120.

164 Cholongitas E, Shusang V, Germani G *et al*. Long term follow up of immunosuppressive monotherapy in liver transplantation: tacrolimus and microemulsified cyclosporine. *Clin. Transpl.* 2010, in press.

165 Hasley PB, Arnold RM. Primary care of the Transplant Patients. *Am. J. Med.* 2010; **123**: 205–212.

166 McGuire BM, Rosenthal P, Brown CC *et al*. Long term management of the Liver Transplant Patient: Recommendations for the Primary Care Doctor. *Am. J. Transpl.*2009; **9**: 1988–2003.

CHAPTER 37
Liver Transplantation in Patients with Hepatitis B, C or HIV Infection

Norah Terrault

Division of Gastroenterology, University of California San Francisco, CA, USA

Learning points

- With prophylactic therapies, such as hepatitis B immune globulin and nucleos(t)ide analogues, recurrent HBV infection can be prevented in the vast majority of transplant recipients with HBV.

- In patients with recurrent HBV infection, long-term suppression of HBV DNA with nucleos(t)ide analogues is necessary to prevent disease progression and graft loss from recurrent disease.

- Recurrent HCV is universal in patients who are viraemic at the time of transplantation as no prophylactic therapies are available.

- Older donor age, acute rejection requiring treatment and cytomegalovirus infection are well-recognized risks for recurrent cirrhosis in HCV patients.

- Eradication of HCV with treatment is the only means of preventing graft loss due to recurrent disease but antiviral therapy with peginterferon and ribavirin is effective in less than 50% of patients overall.

- HIV is not a contraindication for liver transplantation, but outcomes of HCV–HIV coinfected patients are inferior to those with HCV monoinfection.

Introduction

In most liver transplant programmes in North America and Europe, hepatitis C virus (HCV) infection is the most frequent indication for transplantation and hepatitis B virus (HBV) accounts for 10% or less of transplants performed. In Asia, HBV infection is the most frequent indication. The proportion of patients with liver cancer as the primary indication for liver transplantation (LT) has increased in recent years [1], reflecting an increasing incidence of hepatocellular carcinoma (HCC) among patients with chronic viral hepatitis and improved access to transplantation provided by the institution of Model of End-stage Liver Disease (MELD) exception points for HCC (Fig. 37.1).

Recurrent HCV infection is universal after transplantation in viraemic recipients [2]. Recurrent HBV infection occurs in 80% of patients in the absence of prophylactic therapies and, in the absence of specific therapeutic interventions, graft losses due to recurrent disease are frequent [3,4]. Therapeutic strategies for HBV have evolved over the past decade to the point that prevention of recurrent infection is now the norm for HBV patients undergoing LT. In contrast, for patients with HCV infection, therapies to prevent infection are not available and treatment of recurrent hepatitis after transplantation is only modestly effective.

HIV infection was previously regarded as a contraindication for liver transplantation. This is no longer the case due, in large part, to advances in antiretroviral therapy and prevention of opportunistic infections. With the increased longevity of HIV-infected patients, deaths due to the complications of end-stage liver disease have emerged as a major cause of mortality [5,6]. End-stage liver disease secondary to HCV and HBV are the most frequent indications for LT in HIV-infected individuals.

Hepatitis B and liver transplantation

Historically, HBV-related liver disease was considered a relative contraindication for liver transplantation (LT) due of high rates of HBV recurrence, accelerated disease progression and patient survival rates of only 50% at 5 years [4]. Advances in HBV therapies in the mid-late 1990s improved outcomes dramatically (Fig. 37.2). With use of hepatitis B immune globulin (HBIG) and nucleos(t)ide analogues, recurrent infection can be prevented in the majority of patients. The current 5-year survival rates for patients transplanted for HBV are

Sherlock's Diseases of the Liver and Biliary System, Twelfth Edition. Edited by James S. Dooley, Anna S.F. Lok, Andrew K. Burroughs, E. Jenny Heathcote.
© 2011 by Blackwell Publishing Ltd. Published 2011 by Blackwell Publishing Ltd.

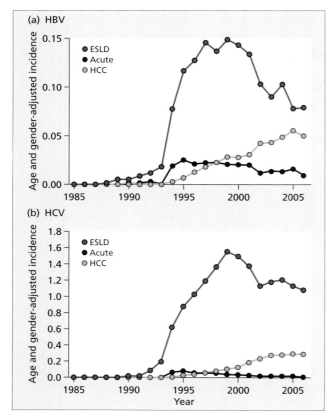

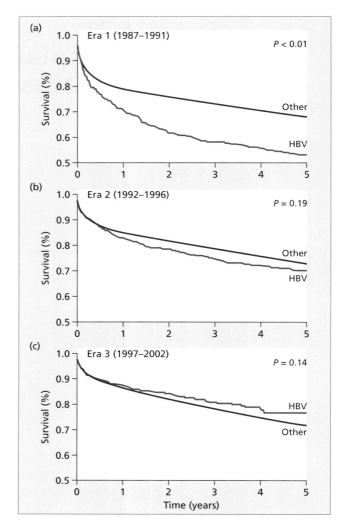

Fig. 37.1. Incidence rates for Organ Procurement and Transplantation Network waiting-list registration between 1985 and 2005 by underlying disease (fulminant hepatitis, hepatocellular carcinoma (HCC) and end-stage liver disease (ESLD)) for HBV (a) and HCV (b). Since 1999, the proportion of patients with HBV wait-listed for liver transplantation due to ESLD has declined by 47% (a) whereas the proportion of patients with HCV wait-listed for ESLD has declined by 30% (b). The increases in patients wait-listed for HCC has increased for both HBV and HCV, reflecting the institution of Model of End-stage Liver Disease (MELD) in 2002 and the increasing burden of HCC in those with chronic viral hepatitis. Source [1].

Fig. 37.2. Patient survival of US adult liver transplant recipients with HBV versus other indications in three different eras: Era 1 (1987–1991), Era 2 (1992–1996) and Era 3 (1997–2002). Survival was significantly improved in Eras 2 and 3 compared to Era 1. Source [7].

approximately 80% [7]. Moreover, the widespread use of antiviral therapy for decompensated cirrhosis has resulted in fewer patients requiring LT for decompensated cirrhosis [1]. The primary indication for LT in HBV patients in most countries is HCC [1,8].

Natural history and factors affecting disease recurrence

In the absence of prophylactic therapies, the risk of HBV reinfection after LT is approximately 80% overall, and related largely to the level of HBV replication at the time of transplantation [3]. Patients with fulminant hepatitis B, delta coinfection and hepatitis B e antigen (HBeAg)-

negative chronic HBV have lower rates of recurrence than patients with HBeAg-positive chronic HBV. Recurrent infection has an accelerated course post-LT with cirrhosis developing within the first 3 years in the majority [3,4]. Both enhanced HBV replication and reduced host immune responses presumably contribute to the rapid disease progression. Additionally, there is a unique fibrosing cholestatic hepatitis variant, first described in HBV-infected transplant recipients in the early 1990s, characterized by high intrahepatic levels of HBV DNA, hepatocyte ballooning with cholestasis and a paucity of inflammatory cells [9]. Prior to the availability of effective antivirals, this represented the most severe and uniformly fatal form of recurrent HBV infection.

Table 37.1. Antiviral therapy in HBV-infected patients on the waiting list

Patient profile	First-choice antiviral	Antiviral alternatives	Considerations
Treatment-naive	Entecavir Tenofovir	Lamivudine Telbivudine Adefovir	Combination therapy is not necessary if use drug with low risk of resistance, such as tenofovir or entecavir If cost is an issue, lamivudine, adefovir monotherapy can be considered but only in patients with low HBV DNA level and short time to LT (<6 months)
Lamivudine-resistant	Tenofovir (change or add) Emtricitabine and tenofovir	Add adefovir	Unclear if combination therapy superior to tenofovir alone Combination therapy may minimize risk of resistance to second drug Time to undetectable HBV DNA level may be longer with adefovir than tenofovir or tenofovir plus emtricitabine Cross-resistance expected with entecavir and telbivudine
Adefovir-resistant	Add entecavir Add lamivudine	Tenofovir	Combination therapy may minimize risk of resistance Only a subset with adefovir-resistant HBV respond to tenofovir alone
Entecavir-resistant	Tenofovir (change or add)	Add adefovir	Unclear if combination therapy superior to tenofovir Combination therapy may minimize risk of resistance Cross-resistance expected with lamivudine and telbivudine

In the current era of prophylactic therapy, recurrent infection is infrequently seen. The factors associated with failure of prophylactic therapy are pre-LT HBV DNA levels and presence of drug-resistant HBV [10,11]. Additionally, two recent studies found HCC recurrence post-LT to be a significant risk factor for recurrent HBV infection [12,13], hypothesized to be due to micrometastatic HCC cells repopulating the new liver graft and inducing recurrence of both HBV infection and HCC after LT.

Low levels of HBV DNA in liver and peripheral blood mononuclear cells (PBMCs) has been reported in serum HBsAg-negative transplant recipients on long-term prophylactic therapy [14,15]. Clinically evident disease is absent. The clinical relevance of this low-level virus is unclear but these extrahepatic reservoirs may be a source of graft reinfection, supporting the need for lifelong prophylaxis.

Treatment of patients with HBV on the waiting list

The goals of therapy in patients on the waiting list are the achievement of a low or undetectable HBV DNA level and avoidance of drug resistance. Treatment is long term and the choice of nucleos(t)ide analogue(s) used depends primarily on prior drug experience (Table 37.1). In treatment-naïve patients, the preferred drugs are those with potent antiviral activity and low risk of resistance, such as entecavir or tenofovir. Since all nucleos(t)ide analogues are renally cleared, doses need to be adjusted to renal function. Nephrotoxicity has been described with tenofovir and close monitoring for this complication is recommended. Interferon is con-

traindicated in patients with decompensated cirrhosis and not recommended in those with compensated cirrhosis since safer oral alternatives are available. Inhibition of viral replication prior to LT reduces the risk of reinfection of the graft post-LT. Achievement of sustained viral suppression pre-LT is associated with stabilization of liver disease, delay in need for LT and improved pre-LT survival [16,17]. Patients with HBV DNA levels above 10 000 IU/mL at time of LT and those with drug-resistant HBV pre-LT have a higher risk of recurrent HBV despite prophylaxis [11]. Since virological breakthrough in patients with underlying cirrhosis can result in worsening of liver function and even death from rapidly progressive liver failure, close monitoring for the development of resistance is important. If salvage therapy is initiated early after virological breakthrough is identified, clinical outcomes are not affected [18,19]. For those patients failing to achieve an undetectable HBV DNA level with single-drug therapy or who have drug resistance, combination antiviral treatment is recommended [20].

Preventing HBV recurrence post-transplantation

Preventive therapy begins from the time of transplantation and continues life long. The combination of HBIG and one or more nucleos(t)ide analogues is a highly effective prophylactic therapy [21]. HBV recurrence is reported in 10% or less of patients receiving combination HBIG and lamivudine with up to 5 years' follow-up [10,22]. The published literature on the efficacy and safety of other nucleos(t)ide analogues such as entecavir and tenofovir in combination with HBIG are sparse, but

Table 37.2. Prevention strategies for HBV in liver transplant recipients*

Risk group	HBV DNA level at time of liver transplant	Anhepatic phase	Postoperative early (first week)	Postoperative first year	Beyond first year
Low	Undetectable	HBIG 5000–10 000 IU	Antiviral(s) *plus* low-dose HBIG	Antiviral(s) *plus* low-dose HBIG *or* Antiviral(s) *plus* short-duration HBIG	Antiviral(s) *plus* low-dose HBIG *or* Combination antivirals without HBIG
High	Detectable *or* Drug-resistant	HBIG 5000–10 000 IU	Antiviral(s) *plus* higher-dose HBIG (target anti-HBs titres approximately 500 U/L)	Antiviral(s) *plus* HBIG (target anti-HBs approximately 200 U/L)	Antiviral(s) *plus* low-dose HBIG *or* Combination antivirals without HBIG may be an option (but data lacking as to whether as efficacious as antivirals plus HBIG)

*Approach suggested by the author based upon available retrospective data.
HBIG, hepatitis B immune globulin.

are predicted to be effective (possibly more effective because of lower risk of resistance). The doses of HBIG given vary greatly from centre to centre. Early protocols using HBIG alone provided doses of 5000–10 000 IU monthly to maintain anti-HBs titres of above 500 IU/L during the first week post-LT, above 250 IU/L during weeks 2–12 post-LT, and above 100 IU/L after week 12, as these levels best predict success of prophylaxis [23]. Lower doses of HBIG can be used when combined with nucleos(t)ide analogues, especially if patients have an undetectable HBV DNA level at time of LT. The Australasian Liver Transplant Study Group used intramuscular HBIG dosed at 400 to 800 IU daily for the first week, weekly for the first month, and then monthly thereafter in combination with lamivudine. In this study, more than 50% of patients had undetectable HBV DNA at the time of LT and 96% success in preventing recurrent HBV at 5 years was reported [10].

Factors associated with failure of prophylaxis include pre-LT HBV DNA levels and history of drug-resistant HBV. Prophylactic strategies should be tailored to the replication status of the patient at the time of transplantation and history of drug resistance (Table 37.2). HBIG use is limited by cost and the need for parenteral administration. Prophylactic regimens using lower doses of HBIG, less frequently administrated and/or given by the intramuscular route are preferable to minimize exposure to human blood products and increase convenience. Protocols using limited-duration HBIG or replacement of HBIG by another nucleos(t)ide analogue with complementary resistance profile have been associated with low rates of recurrence with 2–4 years' follow-up [24–26]. Combined nucleoside and nucleotide analogue therapy may also be an alternative, especially after the first year when risk of recurrence is low [26].

Anti-HBc positive donors

Anti-HBc positive donors are routinely utilized in many transplant programmes, especially in countries where HBV is endemic [27]. These organs are a recognized source of '*de novo*' HBV in transplant recipients and the risk of post-LT infection correlates with the antibody status of the recipient [28,29]. Recipients lacking both anti-HBs and anti-HBc have a 60–70% risk of HBV infection, those with anti-HBc or anti-HBs alone have a risk of 10–20%, and those with anti-HBc and anti-HBs have the lowest risk, 0–5% [28]. When possible, anti-HBc-positive organs are best used in HBV-infected transplant recipients, as prophylaxis is already provided. In HBsAg-negative recipients, prophylactic therapy is recommended to prevent *de novo* infection [29].

A recent survey of LT programmes in the USA, Canada, Europe and Asia found that nucleos(t)ide analogues given for an indefinite duration was the most common prophylactic approach, with lamivudine used by the majority [30]. Approximately 60% of LT programmes also used HBIG for variable periods post-LT, and whether HBIG added to nucleos(t)ide analogues therapy reduces the risk of prophylaxis failure is unknown. The least costly form of prophylaxis is lamivudine monotherapy. Antivirals with a lower rate of resistance, such as tenofovir or entecavir, may be considered although the risk of virological breakthrough in this setting is predicted to be very low [28].

Management of recurrent HBV in liver transplant recipients

HBV recurrence after liver transplantation is usually the result of failed prophylaxis, either due to non-compliance or the emergence of drug-resistant HBV. Recurrence of HBV infection has been traditionally defined by reappearance of HBsAg in serum. However, with use of sensitive PCR assays, recurrence may be first manifested as reappearance of HBV DNA in serum in the absence of HBsAg. Serological evidence of recurrence is accompanied by elevated levels of HBV DNA in serum followed by clinical evidence (elevated alanine aminotransferase (ALT) levels and hepatitis on biopsy) of recurrent disease.

To minimize fibrosis progression and graft loss due to recurrent disease, life-long control of viral replication is essential post-LT. The availability of safe and effective antivirals has allowed the majority of patients with recurrent HBV infection to survive without graft loss from recurrent disease. There is no role for HBIG once serum HBsAg becomes persistently detectable. The choice of antivirals is guided by prior antiviral history and drug resistance profiles. Lamivudine, adefovir or telbivudine are not recommended as a single-drug therapy due to the high risk of resistance but may be used as part of a combination regimen. In patients with drug-resistant HBV, a nucleoside analogue (lamivudine, telbivudine, entecavir, emtricitabine) combined with a nucleotide analogue (adefovir or tenofovir) offers the best option for long-term suppression [20]. Regardless of the therapy chosen, close monitoring for initial response and subsequent virological breakthrough is essential to prevent disease progression and flares of hepatitis. Patients with a suboptimal response to a specific drug therapy, warrant a change of drug(s), with add-on therapy generally recommended over sequential, single-drug therapy.

Retransplantation

Retransplantation for graft failure due to recurrent disease is infrequent in the current era of HBV therapeutics. Retransplantation is not contraindicated in patients with recurrent HBV disease and outcomes are expected to be good, if effective prophylactic therapy can be provided [31,32]. Since most patients who require retransplantation have failed prior antiviral therapies, testing for drug resistance mutations prior to transplantation will help select an effective antiviral therapy. In this higher-risk group, combination prophylaxis of antivirals and HBIG is recommended.

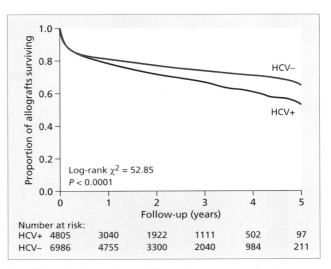

Fig. 37.3. Graft survival of US adult liver transplant recipients with and without HCV. Anti-HCV-positive transplant recipients had a significantly lower rate of survival than transplant recipient without HCV with 1, 3 and 5-year survival rates of 76.9%, 66.4% and 56.8% compared to 80.1%, 73.3% and 67.7% respectively ($P < 0.001$). Source [33].

Hepatitis C and liver transplantation

HCV is the most common indication for LT in the USA and Europe, with a growing proportion undergoing LT for the primary indication of HCC [1]. Graft survival is reduced in HCV-infected transplant recipients compared with non-HCV patients, with a 23% increased risk of death at 5 years post-LT [33] (Fig. 37.3). In the European Liver Transplant Database, the patient survival rate for HCV patients is 66% at 5 years and 54% at 10 years (personal communication V. Karam, European Liver Transplant Registry, March 2009). Recurrent HCV disease is the most common cause of graft loss.

Natural history and factors associated with severe recurrent disease

Recurrence of hepatitis C typically presents with elevated liver tests or histological findings of hepatitis within the first year post-LT [34]. HCV RNA levels are, on average, approximately $1-\log_{10}$ IU/mL higher post-LT compared to pre-LT. HCV RNA levels correlate poorly with disease severity [35]. Chronic hepatitis (Fig. 37.4) evolves to cirrhosis at a variable rate but more rapidly than in non-transplant patients. The cholestatic variant of hepatitis C is the most severe presentation of HCV recurrence, and is frequently associated with high HCV viral levels and the rapid development of graft failure (Fig. 37.5) [36]. Several donor, recipient and

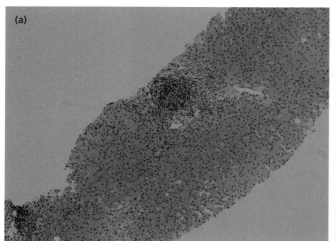

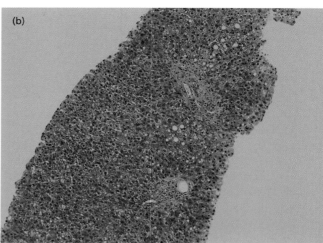

Fig. 37.4. Photomicrographs of recurrent chronic HCV disease. (a) Photomicrograph showing a mild portal-based lymphocytic infiltrate and mild interface activity. The bile ducts are intact. (H&E stain) (b) Early fibrosis surrounding portal tracts with a few short fibrous septa. (Trichrome stain) Courtesy of Dr Vivian Tan, University of California San Francisco.

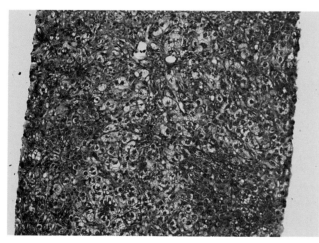

Fig. 37.5. Photomicrograph of cholestatic variant of recurrent hepatitis. This trichrome stain highlights the centrilobular hepatocellular ballooning with pericellular fibrosis and minimal portal or lobular inflammation. Courtesy of Dr Vivian Tan, University of California San Francisco.

transplant-related factors have been associated with poor post-transplant outcomes (Table 37.3). Potentially modifiable factors include donor age, prolonged cold ischaemia time, cytomegalovirus (CMV) infection, acute rejection requiring treatment and post-transplant insulin-resistance or diabetes.

Older donors are associated with a higher rate of graft loss but HCV-infected patients are affected more than non-HCV patients. The risk of graft loss in HCV-infected recipients with donors aged between 41 and 50, 51 and 60, and over 60 years of age are 67% (HR = 1.67, 95% CI:

1.34–2.09), 86% (HR = 1.86, 95% CI: 1.48–2.34) and 221% higher (HR 2.21, 95% CI: 1.73–2.81) respectively, than those recipients with donor under age 40 years [37]. The increase in graft loss reflects the heightened rate of progression to cirrhosis in those with older donors [38–40]. A recent consensus conference on use of extended criteria donors, recommended that 'elderly donors' not be utilized in HCV-infected patients [41].

There is a strong positive association between treated acute rejection (≥1 episode) and risk of recurrent cirrhosis [42]. In recognition of this association, experts recommend a conservative approach to treatment of rejection, with avoidance of corticosteroid boluses and lymphocyte-depleting drugs when possible [43]. The goal is to provide sufficient immunosuppression to prevent moderate to severe rejection while simultaneously avoiding excessive immunosuppression.

Prolonged cold ischaemia time (≥12 hours) [44,45] is associated with higher rates of graft loss and risk of developing severe fibrosis. Prolonged warm ischaemia time (≥90 minutes) has been linked with worse outcomes in one study [46]. CMV infection, though an infrequent post-transplant complication, is a strong risk factor for more severe fibrosis in patients with HCV infection [47–50]. CMV may affect HCV disease progression via its immunomodulatory effects and cytokine-mediated profibrogenic effects. Post-LT diabetes, insulin resistance and steatosis have been variably associated with a higher risk of advanced fibrosis and probably reflect overlapping metabolic risks [51–53]. Both CMV infection and post-LT diabetes are factors that are potentially modifiable. Since HCV-infected transplant recipients have a higher prevalence of *de novo* post-transplant

Table 37.3. Factors associated with higher risk of recurrent cirrhosis in HCV patients

Category	Specifics	Strength of association
Recipient-related	HIV coinfection	+++
	African-American race	+
	Female gender	+
Donor-related	Older donor age	+++
	Longer cold ischaemia time	+++
	Longer warm ischaemia time	+
HCV-related	HCV genotype 1	+/–
	High HCV viral load pre-liver transplantation	+
Transplant-related	Treated acute rejection	+++
	Cytomegalovirus infection	+++
	Insulin-resistance/ diabetes	+++
	Steatosis	+

diabetes compared to non-HCV patients [54–56], immunosuppressive regimens with less diabetogenic potential may reduce the risk of both diabetes and fibrosis progression.

Initial studies suggested post-LT outcomes for living donor recipients with HCV are worse compared to deceased donor liver transplant recipients with HCV [57–59]. Subsequently, studies showed similar graft and patient survival once centres had experience with living donor liver transplantation [60]. Additionally, there are no significant differences in the time to development of HCV recurrence, severity of HCV recurrence or fibrosis progression rates between living versus deceased donor recipients with follow-up periods up to 2 years [61–64].

Anti-HCV-positive donors

Overall patient and graft survival are not affected by use of anti-HCV-positive donors [65–68]. One study reported significantly worse survival with older (>50 years of age) anti-HCV-positive donors compared to older anti-HCV-negative donors, though this finding requires confirmation [65]. In a detailed virological study of 14 patients with genotype 1 who received HCV-infected genotype 1 livers, an approximately equal proportion of patients had persistence of the recipient strain versus superinfection and takeover of the donor strain post-transplantation [69]. The rate of histological disease progression appears to be comparable in patients receiving an anti-HCV-positive versus anti-HCV-negative donor, with one study finding a longer disease-free survival when the donor strain dominated post-LT [70]. Additional recommendations regarding use of anti-HCV-positive donors include informed consent of recipients regarding potential risks and the use of liver biopsy

to exclude donor organs with any evidence of fibrosis or more than minimal inflammation [41,66].

Overview of management of HCV infection in transplant recipients

Approach to immunosuppression

Despite many studies, there are few definitive recommendations that can be made regarding the 'best' immunosuppression for HCV-infected patients. Areas of controversy include the type of calcineurin inhibitor (ciclosporin versus tacrolimus), type of antiproliferative drug (azathioprine versus mycophenolate mofetil), and the risk–benefit of corticosteroids. Since acute rejection requiring treatment with corticosteroid boluses and lymphocyte-depleting drugs is associated with a higher risk of severe post-transplant HCV disease, the goal of immunosuppression is to provide sufficient immunosuppression to avoid acute rejection that requires treatment with these drugs.

Ciclosporin has anti-HCV effects *in vitro* [71]. However, studies have not firmly established a benefit of ciclosporin over tacrolimus in HCV-infected transplant recipients. A systematic review of five studies (366 patients total) found no statistically significant difference in graft survival (RR = 0.86; 95% CI: 0.61–1.21) between tacrolimus versus ciclosporin-based immunosuppression but the quality of the studies was insufficient to evaluate the relationship between type of calcineurin inhibitor and risk of recurrent cirrhosis [72].

Retrospective studies also suggest azathioprine may be better for HCV-infected patients than mycophenolate mofetil, even though mycophenolate mofetil shares some mechanisms of action to ribavirin (inhibition of

Table 37.4. Antiviral treatment options for HCV-infected liver transplant recipients

Treatment option	Timing	Target population	Drug used and management tips
Pretransplant	Initiated prior to transplantation with goal of achieving negative HCV RNA before surgery	Selective use only Target patients with low MELD and favorable response characteristics	Graduated increase in peginterferon and ribavirin doses may improve tolerability Adjust ribavirin dose to renal function Growth factors recommended for management of cytopenias
Early post-transplant therapy	Pre-emptive: within first 8 weeks Early: typically 2–6 months post-liver transplant	Selective use only Consider in those who are clinically stable and predicted to be at high risk for progressive disease Cholestatic hepatitis	Combination therapy using peginterferon and ribavirin is treatment of choice SVR rates similar or lower than therapy delayed until histological disease present Slows disease progression compared to untreated controls
Delayed post-transplant therapy	Initiated for progressive or severe histological or biochemical disease	Significant or progressive HCV disease Stage ≥2 (scale of 4) Grade 3 or 4 (scale of 4)	Combination therapy with peginterferon and ribavirin is treatment of choice Adjust ribavirin dose to renal function Growth factors recommended for management of cytopenias SVR best predicted by early virological responses and genotype Risk of rejection and 'autoimmune-like hepatitis'; monitor immunosuppression carefully

MELD, Model of End-stage Liver Disease; SVR, sustained viral response.

inosine 5′-monophosphate dehydrogenase). A recent systematic review concluded data were insufficient to recommend one antiproliferative drug over the other [73]. In the prospective HCV-3 study, there were no differences in HCV disease severity after 2 years in patients receiving tacrolimus, mycophenolate mofetil and prednisone for immunosuppression compared to those receiving tacrolimus and prednisone [74].

The strongest link between lymphocyte-depleting agents and risk of recurrent cirrhosis is within the context of treating acute rejection. Interleukin-receptor antagonists are not a risk factor [74], except alemtuzumab, which has been associated severe recurrent HCV [75]. Finally, while corticosteroid boluses for treatment of acute rejection are associated with a higher risk of cirrhosis, there are conflicting data on the risks of maintenance corticosteroids. There is no difference in severity of HCV disease in patients receiving steroid-free immunosuppression compared to corticosteroid-containing immunosuppression [68].

Pretransplant treatment of HCV-infected patients on the waiting list (Table 37.4)

Achievement of a sustained virological response prior to LT eliminates the risk of recurrent HCV after LT, while achievement of an undetectable HCV RNA level on treatment reduces the risk of recurrence [76,77]. This provides the rationale for considering antiviral therapy pretransplant. Overall, however, response rates are low, with sustained viral response (SVR) seen in 13% with genotype 1 and 50% with genotype 2/3 HCV [76,78,79]. On treatment virological responses are more frequent, occurring in 30% of patients with genotype 1 and 83% with genotype 2/3 [76,77,80,81]. Non-1 genotype, early virological response and adherence to therapy predict response to treatment [76,82].

Treatment of patients on the waiting list should be selective, limited to those with mildly decompensated disease (MELD less than 20) and with favourable baseline characteristics (genotype 2 or 3 and/or low viral load). Treatment of patients with advanced decompensation (Child–Pugh class B+ or C; MELD ≥20) is contraindicated due to an unacceptably high risk of complications [81]. Even in patients with mildly decompensated disease, treatment is discontinued in up to 30% due to adverse events. Thus, risk and benefit need to be considered carefully and such treatment should be undertaken only in experienced transplant centres.

Post-transplant prophylactic and pre-emptive antiviral therapy (Table 37.4)

Prophylactic hepatitis C antibody therapy has been evaluated as a strategy to prevent infection in HCV-infected patients, but was found to be ineffective [83,84]. Therefore, although hepatitis C immune globulin (HCIG) has orphan drug approval in Europe, there is no established role for its use in LT recipients.

Pre-emptive antiviral therapy is started within the first few weeks post-transplantation, when histological injury is minimal or absent. Treatment is applicable only to patients without post-transplant complications who are well enough to tolerate antiviral therapy and treatment discontinuations due to adverse events are frequent, even with careful selection of patients [85]. The rationale of pre-emptive treatment is similar to that of treating acute infection, in which early exposure to antiviral therapy is associated with enhanced SVR rates. However, studies of post-LT pre-emptive antiviral therapy report low SVR rates (16% median, range 8% to 39%) [85–89]. A trend towards reduced histological severity in patients receiving pre-emptive therapy compared to untreated controls, even in the absence of a virological response, suggests early treatment may slow disease progression [88–92]. However, based upon the low SVR rate, this therapeutic strategy is not generally recommended and pre-emptive therapy should be used selectively in those at risk for rapidly progressive disease.

Post-transplant antiviral therapy for recurrent disease (Table 37.4)

The primary goal of post-LT antiviral therapy is viral eradication. Antiviral therapy is typically started once recurrent and progressive histological disease is present. Sustained viral clearance is associated with fibrosis stabilization or regression [93,94] and improved graft survival [95,96] (Fig. 37.6). Overall, approximately 30–40% of transplant recipients treated with peginterferon and

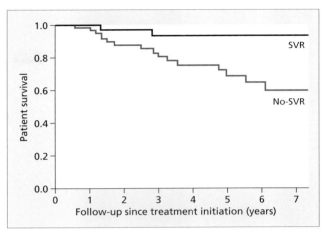

Fig. 37.6. Survival following initiation of antiviral therapy. Survival is significantly improved by achievement of a sustained virological response (SVR). Source [96].

ribavirin will achieve SVR [97,98]. Biochemical responses are seen in at least half of those treated. Histological improvements are primarily, but not exclusively, seen in responders [99,100]. The baseline factors associated most consistently with SVR include non-1 genotype, low pretreatment HCV viral load and absence of prior antiviral therapy. Ciclosporin rather than tacrolimus-based immunosuppression has been associated with higher SVR rates in some studies [101,102]. As in the non-transplant setting, early virological responses are highly predictive of SVR and non-SVR. Failure to achieve a decline in HCV RNA during the first 3 months of treatment is highly predictive of non-SVR [103–107]. Achievement of an undetectable HCV RNA at week 4 of treatment predicts an 80% or greater likelihood of SVR with 48 weeks treatment [105].

Dose reductions are reported in up to 50% of patients [108]. Discontinuation of treatment due to adverse effects is more frequent than that reported in the non-transplant setting. In the systematic review of peginterferon and ribavirin therapy in transplant recipients, the pooled estimate of the treatment discontinuation rate was 26% (95% CI 20–32%) [97]. Cytopenias, mood disturbances and acute rejection are the most common reasons for dose reduction or discontinuation. It has been recommended that the target dose of ribavirin be adjusted to creatinine clearance. Use of growth factors to manage cytopenias is advocated by experts, and although tolerability may be improved, there is no convincing evidence that growth factor use improves SVR rates [97,109].

Since interferon has immune modulatory properties, immunological complications of interferon-based therapy include acute rejection, chronic rejection and autoimmune-like hepatitis (also called plasma-cell hepatitis) (Fig. 37.7) [89,106,110–113]. These complications

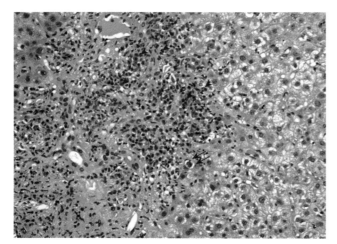

Fig. 37.7. Photomicrograph of plasma-cell hepatitis, also called *de novo* autoimmune hepatitis. A portal-based mononuclear inflammatory infiltrate is present with a prominent component of plasma cells (arrowheads). Interface hepatitis, in which the inflammation extends from the portal tract into the lobules and is associated with hepatocyte injury, is a typical feature. The necrotic hepatocytes form acidophilic bodies (double arrows). Courtesy of Barbara McKenna, University of Michigan.

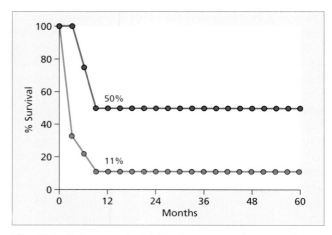

Fig. 37.8. Patient survival following retransplantation for recurrent HCV. Patients requiring retransplantation within the first year (orange line) have significantly lower survival than those requiring retransplantation after the first year (blue line) ($P = 0.05$). Source [123].

are rare, can occur during or shortly after completion of antiviral therapy and, in some studies, are associated with recent lowering of immunosuppression or subtherapeutic blood levels of calcineurin inhibitors. Management of these immunological complications includes discontinuation of antiviral therapy and amplification of immunosuppression. However, graft losses can occur related to progressive chronic rejection or autoimmune-like hepatitis, even when these measures are undertaken.

Retransplantation

Outcomes with retransplantation are lower than first transplantation, regardless of aetiology of disease, but some studies report worse survival among HCV-infected compared to non-HCV patients [114–117]. The 1-year graft survival following retransplantation for HCV varies from 40 to 70% [117–122], probably reflecting the selection criteria used by different centres. Factors most consistently associated with reduced survival after retransplantation are preoperative serum bilirubin and serum creatinine, recipient age, donor age and poor preoperative clinical condition [118–120]. Retransplantation done for early severe recurrent disease, including cholestatic hepatitis, is associated with poor outcomes if retransplantation occurs within the first year [123] (Fig. 37.8). In a multicenter study evaluating HCV-infected patients considered for retransplantation due to recurrent disease, 50% were not listed and the

most common reasons for not listing were recurrent HCV within 6 months (22%), fibrosing cholestatic hepatitis (19%) and renal dysfunction (9%) [122]. While no universal criteria are used to determine who is offered retransplantation for recurrent HCV cirrhosis, current wisdom suggests retransplantation needs to occur before multiorgan failure or marked debilitation, probably with a MELD in the low-to-mid 20s [124] and with avoidance of extended criteria donors.

HIV and liver transplantation

Historically, the presence of HIV infection was an absolute contraindication to liver transplantation. In the past decade, this has changed as management of HIV infection has improved and patients with HIV are surviving longer. Commonly used criteria for selection of HIV-infected patients for LT include a CD4 count above 100 cells/mm^3, an undetectable HIV viral load or HIV infection predicted to be suppressible with antiretroviral therapy and an absence of opportunistic infections [125–127]. Among HIV-infected persons, chronic viral hepatitis (HBV and HCV) is the most frequent indication for transplantation. Early referral is important to minimize deaths without transplantation [128,129]. In HCV–HIV coinfected patients, progression from first decompensation to death is more rapid than in HCV monoinfected patients [130]. In HBV–HIV coinfected patients, survival to transplantation is related to severity of disease at presentation and whether uncontrolled drug-resistant HBV infection is present [129].

Important aspects of post-transplantation care of HIV patients include the management of drug interactions (antiretrovirals and immunosuppressants) and drug toxicities, and the prevention and/or treatment of recur-

Table 37.5. Survival of HCV–HIV coinfected liver transplant recipients*

Author, year	N	Country	Patient survival (%)			
			1 year	2 years	3 years	5 years
Vennarecci, 2007 [138]	12†	Italy	83	58	58	–
Duclos-Vallee, 2008 [135]	35	France	–	73	–	51
de Vera, 2006 [137]	27	USA	67	–	56	33
Miro, 2007‡ [139]	60	Spain	87	70	64	–
Terrault, 2009‡ [136]	81	USA	71	–	59	–

*Includes only studies with ≥10 transplant recipients.
†Survival for entire cohort of which 11/12 were HCV positive.
‡Abstract form only.

rent viral hepatitis. Interactions between antiretroviral drugs and calcineurin inhibitors and sirolimus are well recognized [131,132]. Patients on protease-inhibitor regimens require significantly reduced doses of ciclosporin, tacrolimus and sirolimus to avoid toxicity. Conversely, efavirenz-containing regimens enhance cytochrome P450 activity and the dose of calcineurin inhibitors needs to be increased to maintain target levels. Additionally, hepatotoxicity related to antiretroviral drugs may be a potential cause of liver test abnormalities or abnormal histology in transplant recipients.

HBV and HIV coinfected liver transplant recipients

Short and immediate-term survival are excellent in HBV–HIV coinfected patients. In the two largest series of HBV–HIV coinfected transplant recipients, the survival rates were 80% and 100% with follow-up of approximately 3 years, which was not significantly different from HBV monoinfected patients [133,134]. Importantly, there are no reported deaths from recurrent HBV disease. The success of transplantation in HBV–HIV coinfected patients stems largely from the availability of highly effective prophylactic HBV therapies. Combination HBV prophylaxis using HBIG plus nucleos(t)ide analogues is recommended. Since tenofovir, lamivudine and emtricitabine are part of antiretroviral regimens and have HBV activity, drug interruptions due to antiretroviral intolerance or lack of efficacy requires that alternative HBV therapy be given. In these situations, HBIG monotherapy, especially if the duration of antiretroviral therapy interruption is short term, is an option. Alternatively, HBIG combined with an anti-HBV drug that does not have HIV activity, such as adefovir or telbivudine, can be used.

HCV–HIV liver transplant recipients

Reported post-transplant outcomes of HCV–HIV coinfected patients are poorer than non-HCV-infected, HIV-infected transplant recipients and HCV monoinfected transplant recipients. HCV–HIV coinfected transplant recipients have a 1-year survival of 67–87% and a 3-year post-transplantation survival of 56–64% (Table 37.5). The factor most consistently associated with reduced survival post-LT is a high pretransplant MELD score. Other factors identified in some but not all studies include older donor age, body mass index less than 21 kg/m², treated acute rejection and intolerance of antiretroviral therapy post-transplant [135–137].

Patients who are HCV RNA positive pretransplantation develop recurrent disease, though spontaneous clearance of virus has been described. In studies comparing the onset of hepatitis and rate of progression to cirrhosis, coinfected transplant recipients have an accelerated pace compared to HCV-monoinfected patients [135]. The risk of graft loss due to recurrent disease is 27–54% after just 3–5 years. As in HCV-monoinfected patients, the only effective means of preventing disease progression is to eradicate HCV. Treatment with peginterferon and ribavirin has low efficacy, with reported SVR rates of 11–27% [125].

Pending the availability of more efficacious antiviral therapies for recurrent HCV infection, the best approach for improving survival in HCV–HIV coinfected patients is optimization of donor, recipient and post-transplant factors to minimize risk of progressive disease. Early antiviral therapy can be considered in stable patients.

References

1 Kim WR, Terrault NA, Pedersen RA *et al*. Trends in waitlist registration for liver transplantation for viral hepatitis in the US. *Gastroenterology* 2009; **137**: 1680–1686.
2 Everhart J, Wei Y, Eng H *et al*. Recurrent and new hepatitis C virus infection after liver transplantation. *Hepatology* 1999; **29**: 1220–1226.
3 Samuel D, Muller R, Alexander G *et al*. Liver transplantation in European patients with the hepatitis B surface antigen. *N. Engl. J. Med.* 1993; **329**: 1842–1847.

4 Todo S, Demetris A, Van Thiel D *et al.* Orthotopic liver transplantation for patients with hepatitis B virus-related liver disease. *Hepatology* 1991; **13**: 619–626.

5 Thio C, Seaberg E, Skolasky RJ *et al.* HIV-1, hepatitis B virus, and risk of liver-related mortality in the Multicenter Cohort Study (MACS). *Lancet* 2002; **360**: 1921–1926.

6 Weber R, Sabin CA, Friis-Moller N *et al.* Liver-related deaths in persons infected with the human immunodeficiency virus: the D: A: D study. *Arch. Intern. Med.* 2006; **166**: 1632–1641.

7 Kim W, Poterucha J, Kremers W *et al.* Outcome of liver transplantation for hepatitis B in the United States. *Liver Transpl.* 2004; **10**: 968–974.

8 Yuen MF, Hou JL, Chutaputti A. Hepatocellular carcinoma in the Asia pacific region. *J. Gastroenterol. Hepatol.* 2009; **24**: 346–353.

9 Davies S, Portmann B, O'Grady J *et al.* Hepatic histological findings after transplantation for chronic hepatitis B virus infection, including a unique pattern of fibrosing cholestatic hepatitis. *Hepatology* 1991; **13**: 150–157.

10 Gane EJ, Angus PW, Strasser S *et al.* Lamivudine plus low-dose hepatitis B immunoglobulin to prevent recurrent hepatitis B following liver transplantation. *Gastroenterology* 2007; **132**: 931–937.

11 Marzano A, Gaia S, Ghisetti V *et al.* Viral load at the time of liver transplantation and risk of hepatitis B virus recurrence. *Liver Transpl.* 2005; **11**: 402–409.

12 Faria LC, Gigou M, Roque-Afonso AM *et al.* Hepatocellular carcinoma is associated with an increased risk of hepatitis B virus recurrence after liver transplantation. *Gastroenterology* 2008; **134**: 1890–1899.

13 Kiyici M, Yilmaz M, Akyildiz M *et al.* Association between hepatitis B and hepatocellular carcinoma recurrence in patients undergoing liver transplantation. *Transpl. Proc.* 2008; **40**: 1511–1517.

14 Roche B, Feray C, Gigou M *et al.* HBV DNA persistence 10 years after liver transplantation despite successful anti-HBS passive immunoprophylaxis. *Hepatology* 2003; **38**: 86–95.

15 Terrault N, Zhou S, Combs C *et al.* Prophylaxis in liver transplant recipients using a fixed dosing schedule of hepatitis B immunoglobulin. *Hepatology* 1996; **24**: 1327–1333.

16 Schiff E, Lai CL, Hadziyannis S *et al.* Adefovir dipivoxil for wait-listed and post-liver transplantation patients with lamivudine-resistant hepatitis B: final long-term results. *Liver Transpl.* 2007; **13**: 349–360.

17 Yao FY, Terrault NA, Freise C *et al.* Lamivudine treatment is beneficial in patients with severely decompensated cirrhosis and actively replicating hepatitis B infection awaiting liver transplantation: a comparative study using a matched, untreated cohort. *Hepatology* 2001; **34**: 411–416.

18 Osborn MK, Han SH, Regev A *et al.* Outcomes of patients with hepatitis B who developed antiviral resistance while on the liver transplant waiting list. *Clin. Gastroenterol. Hepatol.* 2007; **5**: 1454–1461.

19 Lampertico P, Vigano M, Manenti E *et al.* Adefovir rapidly suppresses hepatitis B in HBeAg-negative patients developing genotypic resistance to lamivudine. *Hepatology* 2005; **42**: 1414–149.

20 Lok AS, McMahon BJ. Chronic hepatitis B. *Hepatology* 2007; **45**: 507–539.

21 Terrault N, Roche B, Samuel D. Management of the hepatitis B virus in the liver transplantation setting: a European and an American perspective. *Liver Transpl.* 2005; **11**: 716–732.

22 Yao F, Osorio R, Roberts J *et al.* Intramuscular hepatitis B immune globulin combined with lamivudine for prophylaxis against hepatitis B recurrence after liver transplantation. *Liver Transpl. Surg.* 1999; **5**: 6.

23 McGory R, Ishitani M, Oliveira W *et al.* Improved outcome of orthotopic liver transplantation for chronic hepatitis B cirrhosis with aggressive passive immunization. *Transplantation* 1996; **61**: 1358–1364.

24 Buti M, Mas A, Prieto M *et al.* Five year follow-up of a randomized study comparing lamivudine vs. lamivudine + HBIG in the prevention of HBV recurrence after liver transplantation. *Hepatology* 2005; **42**: A491.

25 Wong SN, Chu CJ, Wai CT *et al.* Low risk of hepatitis B virus recurrence after withdrawal of long-term hepatitis B immunoglobulin in patients receiving maintenance nucleos(t)ide analogue therapy. *Liver Transpl.* 2007; **13**: 374–381.

26 Angus PW, Patterson SJ, Strasser SI *et al.* A randomized study of adefovir dipivoxil in place of HBIG in combination with lamivudine as post-liver transplantation hepatitis B prophylaxis. *Hepatology* 2008; **48**: 1460–1466.

27 Celebi Kobak A, Karasu Z, Kilic M *et al.* Living donor liver transplantation from hepatitis B core antibody positive donors. *Transpl. Proc.* 2007; **39**: 1488–1490.

28 Dickson RC, Everhart JE, Lake JR *et al.* Transmission of hepatitis B by transplantation of livers from donors positive for antibody to hepatitis B core antigen. The National Institute of Diabetes and Digestive and Kidney Diseases Liver Transplantation Database. *Gastroenterology* 1997; **113**: 1668–1674.

29 Munoz S. Use of hepatitis B core antibody-positive donors for liver transplantation. *Liver Transpl.* 2002; **8** (10 Suppl. 1): S82–86.

30 Perrillo R. Hepatitis B virus prevention strategies for antibody to hepatitis B core antigen-positive liver donation: a survey of North American, European, and Asian-Pacific transplant programs. *Liver Transpl.* 2009; **15**: 223–232.

31 Roche B, Samuel D, Feray C *et al.* Retransplantation of the liver for recurrent hepatitis B virus infection: the Paul Brousse experience. *Liver Transpl. Surg.* 1999; **5**: 166–174.

32 Ishitani M, McGory R, Dickson R *et al.* Retransplantation of patients with severe posttransplant hepatitis B in the first allograft. *Transplantation* 1997; **64**: 410–414.

33 Forman LM, Lewis JD, Berlin JA *et al.* The association between hepatitis C infection and survival after orthotopic liver transplantation. *Gastroenterology* 2002; **122**: 889–896.

34 Shiffman M, Contos M, Luketic V *et al.* Biochemical and histological evaluation of recurrent hepatitis C following orthotopic liver transplantation. *Transplantation* 1994; **57**: 526–532.

35 Chazouilleres O, Kim M, Combs C *et al.* Quantitation of hepatitis C virus RNA in liver transplant recipients. *Gastroenterology* 1994; **106**: 994–999.

36 Taga S, Washington M, Terrault N *et al.* Cholestatic hepatitis C in liver allografts. *Liver Transpl. Surg* 1998; **4**: 304–310.

37 Lake JR, Shorr JS, Steffen BJ *et al.* Differential effects of donor age in liver transplant recipients infected with hep-

atitis B, hepatitis C and without viral hepatitis. *Am. J. Transpl.* 2005; **5**: 549–557.

38 Neumann U, Berg T, Bahra M *et al.* Fibrosis progression after liver transplantation in patients with recurrent hepatitis C. *J. Hepatol.* 2004; **41**: 830–836.

39 Burak KW, Kremers WK, Batts KP *et al.* Impact of cytomegalovirus infection, year of transplantation, and donor age on outcomes after liver transplantation for hepatitis C. *Liver Transpl.* 2002; **8**: 362–369.

40 Berenguer M, Prieto M, San Juan F *et al.* Contribution of donor age to the recent decrease in patient survival among HCV-infected liver transplant recipients. *Hepatology* 2002; **36**: 202–210.

41 Durand F, Renz JF, Alkofer B *et al.* Report of the Paris consensus meeting on expanded criteria donors in liver transplantation. *Liver Transpl.* 2008; **14**: 1694–1707.

42 Prieto M, Berenguer M, Rayon J *et al.* High incidence of allograft cirrhosis in hepatitis C virus genotype 1b infection following transplantation: relationship with rejection episodes. *Hepatology* 1999; **29**: 250–256.

43 Wiesner R, Sorrell M, Villamil F, International Liver Transplantation Society Expert Panel. Report of the first International Liver Transplantation Society expert panel consensus conference on liver transplantation and hepatitis C. *Liver Transpl.* 2003; **9**: S1–9.

44 Feng S, Goodrich NP, Bragg-Gresham JL *et al.* Characteristics associated with liver graft failure: the concept of a donor risk index. *Am. J. Transpl.* 2006; **6**: 783–790.

45 Briceno J, Marchal T, Padillo J *et al.* Influence of marginal donors on liver preservation injury. *Transplantation* 2002; **74**: 522–526.

46 Baron PW, Sindram D, Higdon D *et al.* Prolonged rewarming time during allograft implantation predisposes to recurrent hepatitis C infection after liver transplantation. *Liver Transpl.* 2000; **6**: 407–412.

47 Razonable RR, Burak KW, van Cruijsen H *et al.* The pathogenesis of hepatitis C virus is influenced by cytomegalovirus. *Clin. Infect. Dis.* 2002; **35**: 974–981.

48 Rosen HR, Chou S, Corless CL *et al.* Cytomegalovirus viremia: risk factor for allograft cirrhosis after liver transplantation for hepatitis C. *Transplantation* 1997; **64**: 721–726.

49 Chopra KB, Demetris AJ, Blakolmer K *et al.* Progression of liver fibrosis in patients with chronic hepatitis C after orthotopic liver transplantation. *Transplantation* 2003; **76**: 1487–1491.

50 Humar A, Kumar D, Raboud J *et al.* Interactions between cytomegalovirus, human herpesvirus-6, and the recurrence of hepatitis C after liver transplantation. *Am. J. Transpl.* 2002; **2**: 461–466.

51 Veldt BJ, Poterucha JJ, Watt KD *et al.* Insulin resistance, serum adipokines and risk of fibrosis progression in patients transplanted for hepatitis C. *Am. J. Transpl.* 2009; **9**: 1406–1413.

52 Foxton MR, Quaglia A, Muiesan P *et al.* The impact of diabetes mellitus on fibrosis progression in patients transplanted for hepatitis C. *Am. J. Transpl.* 2006; **6**: 1922–1929.

53 Yilmaz N, Shiffman ML, Stravitz RT *et al.* A prospective evaluation of fibrosis progression in patients with recurrent hepatitis C virus following liver transplantation. *Liver Transpl.* 2007; **13**: 975–983.

54 Khalili M, Lim JW, Bass N *et al.* New onset diabetes mellitus after liver transplantation: the critical role of hepatitis C infection. *Liver Transpl.* 2004; **10**: 349–355.

55 Baid S, Cosimi AB, Farrell ML *et al.* Posttransplant diabetes mellitus in liver transplant recipients: risk factors, temporal relationship with hepatitis C virus allograft hepatitis, and impact on mortality. *Transplantation* 2001; **72**: 1066–1072.

56 Bigam DL, Pennington JJ, Carpentier A *et al.* Hepatitis C-related cirrhosis: a predictor of diabetes after liver transplantation. *Hepatology* 2000; **32**: 87–90.

57 Garcia-Retortillo M, Forns X, Llovet J *et al.* Hepatitis C recurrence is more severe after living donor compared to cadaveric liver transplantation. *Hepatology* 2004; **40**: 699–707.

58 Thuluvath P, Yoo H. Graft and patient survival after adult live donor liver transplantation compared to a matched cohort who received a deceased donor transplantation. *Liver Transpl.* 2004; **10**: 1263–1268.

59 Gaglio P, Malireddy S, Levitt B *et al.* Increased risk of cholestatic hepatitis C in recipients of grafts from living versus cadaveric liver donors. *Liver Transpl.* 2003; **9**: 1028–1035.

60 Terrault NA, Shiffman ML, Lok AS *et al.* Outcomes in hepatitis C virus-infected recipients of living donor vs. deceased donor liver transplantation. *Liver Transpl.* 2007; **13**: 122–129.

61 Humar A, Beissel J, Crotteau S *et al.* Whole liver versus split liver versus living donor in the adult recipient: an analysis of outcomes by graft type. *Transplantation* 2008; **85**: 1420–1424.

62 Selzner N, Girgrah N, Lilly L *et al.* The difference in the fibrosis progression of recurrent hepatitis C after live donor liver transplantation versus deceased donor liver transplantation is attributable to the difference in donor age. *Liver Transpl.* 2008; **14**: 1778–1786.

63 Shiffman M, Stravitz R, Contos M *et al.* Histologic recurrence of chronic hepatitis C virus in patients after living donor and deceased donor liver transplantation. *Liver Transpl.* 2004; **10**: 1248–1255.

64 Schmeding M, Neumann UP, Puhl G *et al.* Hepatitis C recurrence and fibrosis progression are not increased after living donor liver transplantation: a single-center study of 289 patients. *Liver Transpl.* 2007; **13**: 687–692.

65 Khapra AP, Agarwal K, Fiel MI *et al.* Impact of donor age on survival and fibrosis progression in patients with hepatitis C undergoing liver transplantation using HCV+ allografts. *Liver Transpl.* 2006; **12**: 1496–1503.

66 Arenas JI, Vargas HE, Rakela J. The use of hepatitis C-infected grafts in liver transplantation. *Liver Transpl.* 2003; **9**: S48–51.

67 Marroquin CE, Marino G, Kuo PC *et al.* Transplantation of hepatitis C-positive livers in hepatitis C-positive patients is equivalent to transplanting hepatitis C-negative livers. *Liver Transpl.* 2001; **7**: 762–768.

68 Velidedeoglu E, Desai NM, Campos L *et al.* Effect of donor hepatitis C on liver graft survival. *Transpl. Proc.* 2001; **33**: 3795–3796.

69 Laskus T, Wang LF, Rakela J *et al.* Dynamic behavior of hepatitis C virus in chronically infected patients receiving liver graft from infected donors. *Virology* 1996; **220**: 171–176.

70 Vargas HE, Laskus T, Wang LF *et al*. Outcome of liver transplantation in hepatitis C virus-infected patients who received hepatitis C virus-infected grafts. *Gastroenterology* 1999; **117**: 149–153.

71 Watashi K, Hijikata M, Hosaka M *et al*. Cyclosporin A suppresses replication of hepatitis C virus genome in cultured hepatocytes. *Hepatology* 2003; **38**: 1282–1288.

72 Berenguer M, Royuela A, Zamora J. Immunosuppression with calcineurin inhibitors with respect to the outcome of HCV recurrence after liver transplantation: Results of a meta-analysis. *Liver Transpl.* 2007; **13**: 21–29.

73 Germani G, Pleguezuelo M, Villamil F *et al*. Azathioprine in liver transplantation: a reevaluation of its use and a comparison with mycophenolate mofetil. *Am. J. Transpl.* 2009; **9**: 1725–1731.

74 Klintmalm GB, Washburn WK, Rudich SM *et al*. Corticosteroid-free immunosuppression with daclizumab in HCV(+) liver transplant recipients: 1-year interim results of the HCV-3 study. *Liver Transpl.* 2007; **13**: 1521–1531.

75 Marcos A, Eghtesad B, Fung JJ *et al*. Use of alemtuzumab and tacrolimus monotherapy for cadaveric liver transplantation: with particular reference to hepatitis C virus. *Transplantation* 2004; **78**: 966–971.

76 Everson GT, Trotter J, Forman L *et al*. Treatment of advanced hepatitis C with a low accelerating dosage regimen of antiviral therapy. *Hepatology* 2005; **42**: 255–262.

77 Forns X, Navasa M, Rodes J. Treatment of HCV infection in patients with advanced cirrhosis. *Hepatology* 2004; **40**: 498.

78 Tekin F, Gunsar F, Karasu Z *et al*. Safety, tolerability, and efficacy of pegylated-interferon alfa-2a plus ribavirin in HCV-related decompensated cirrhotics. *Aliment. Pharmacol. Ther.* 2008; **27**: 1081–1085.

79 Iacobellis A, Siciliano M, Perri F *et al*. Peginterferon alfa-2b and ribavirin in patients with hepatitis C virus and decompensated cirrhosis: a controlled study. *J. Hepatol.* 2007; **46**: 206–212.

80 Thomas RM, Brems JJ, Guzman-Hartman G *et al*. Infection with chronic hepatitis C virus and liver transplantation: a role for interferon therapy before transplantation. *Liver Transpl.* 2003; **9**: 905–915.

81 Crippin JS, McCashland T, Terrault N *et al*. A pilot study of the tolerability and efficacy of antiviral therapy in hepatitis C virus-infected patients awaiting liver transplantation. *Liver Transpl.* 2002; **8**: 350–355.

82 Carrion JA, Martinez-Bauer E, Crespo G *et al*. Antiviral therapy increases the risk of bacterial infections in HCV-infected cirrhotic patients awaiting liver transplantation: A retrospective study. *J. Hepatol.* 2009; **50**: 719–728.

83 Davis GL, Nelson DR, Terrault N *et al*. A randomized, open-label study to evaluate the safety and pharmacokinetics of human hepatitis C immune globulin (Civacir) in liver transplant recipients. *Liver Transpl.* 2005; **11**: 941–949.

84 Schiano TD, Charlton M, Younossi Z *et al*. Monoclonal antibody HCV-AbXTL68 in patients undergoing liver transplantation for HCV: results of a phase 2 randomized study. *Liver Transpl.* 2006; **12**: 1381–1389.

85 Shergill AK, Khalili M, Straley S *et al*. Applicability, tolerability and efficacy of preemptive antiviral therapy in hepatitis C-infected patients undergoing liver transplantation. *Am. J. Transpl.* 2005; **5**: 118–124.

86 Reddy R, Fried M, Dixon R *et al*. Interferon alfa-2b and ribavirin vs. placebo in early treatment in patients transplanted for hepatitis C end-stage liver disease: results of a multicenter randomized trial. *Gastroenterology* 2002; **122**: 199.

87 Mazzaferro V, Tagger A, Schiavo M *et al*. Prevention of recurrent hepatitis C after liver transplantation with early interferon and ribavirin treatment. *Transpl. Proc.* 2001; **33**: 1355–1357.

88 Sugawara Y, Makuuchi M, Matsui Y *et al*. Preemptive therapy for hepatitis C virus after living-donor liver transplantation. *Transplantation* 2004; **78**: 1308–1311.

89 Chalasani N, Manzarbeitia C, Ferenci P *et al*. Peginterferon alfa-2a for hepatitis C after liver transplantation: two randomized, controlled trials. *Hepatology* 2005; **41**: 289–298.

90 Singh N, Gayowski T, Wannstedt CF *et al*. Interferon-alpha for prophylaxis of recurrent viral hepatitis C in liver transplant recipients: a prospective, randomized, controlled trial. *Transplantation* 1998; **65**: 82–86.

91 Sheiner P, Boros P, Klion F *et al*. The efficacy of prophylactic interferon alfa-2b in preventing recurrent hepatitis C after liver transplantation. *Hepatology* 1998; **28**: 831–838.

92 Kuo A, Lan B, Feng S *et al*. Long-term histologic effects of preemptive antiviral therapy in ?liver transplant recipients with hepatitis C virus infection. *Liver Transpl.* 2008; **14**: 1491–1497.

93 Bizollon T, Ahmed S, Radenne S *et al*. Long term histological improvement and clearance of intrahepatic hepatitis C virus RNA following sustained response to interferon-ribavirin combination therapy in liver transplanted patients with hepatitis C virus recurrence. *Gut* 2003; **52**: 283–287.

94 Abdelmalek M, Firpi R, Soldevila-Pico C *et al*. Sustained viral response to interferon and ribavirin in liver transplant recipients with recurrent hepatitis C. *Liver Transpl.* 2004; **10**: 199–207.

95 Picciotto FP, Tritto G, Lanza AG *et al*. Sustained virological response to antiviral therapy reduces mortality in HCV reinfection after liver transplantation. *J. Hepatol.* 2007; **46**: 459–465.

96 Berenguer M, Palau A, Aguilera V *et al*. Clinical benefits of antiviral therapy in patients with recurrent hepatitis C following liver transplantation. *Am. J. Transpl.* 2008; **8**: 679–687.

97 Berenguer M. Systematic review of the treatment of established recurrent hepatitis C with pegylated interferon in combination with ribavirin. *J. Hepatol.* 2008; **49**: 274–287.

98 Xirouchakis E, Triantos C, Manousou P *et al*. Pegylated-interferon and ribavirin in liver transplant candidates and recipients with HCV cirrhosis: systematic review and meta-analysis of prospective controlled studies. *J. Viral Hepat.* 2008; **15**: 699–709.

99 Berenguer M, Palau A, Fernandez A *et al*. Efficacy, predictors of response, and potential risks associated with antiviral therapy in liver transplant recipients with recurrent hepatitis C. *Liver Transpl.* 2006; **12**: 1067–1076.

100 Carrion JA, Navasa M, Garcia-Retortillo M *et al*. Efficacy of antiviral therapy on hepatitis C recurrence after liver transplantation: a randomized controlled study. *Gastroenterology* 2007; **132**: 1746–1756.

101 Cescon M, Grazi GL, Cucchetti A *et al*. Predictors of sustained virological response after antiviral treatment for hepatitis C recurrence following liver transplantation. *Liver Transpl.* 2009; **15**: 782–789.

102 Bizollon T, Pradat P, Mabrut JY *et al*. Histological benefit of retreatment by pegylated interferon alfa-2b and ribavirin in patients with recurrent hepatitis C virus infection posttransplantation. *Am. J. Transpl.* 2007; **7**: 448–453.

103 Oton E, Barcena R, Moreno-Planas JM *et al*. Hepatitis C recurrence after liver transplantation: viral and histologic response to full-dose peg-interferon and ribavirin. *Am. J. Transpl.* 2006; **6**: 2348–2355.

104 Lodato F, Berardi S, Gramenzi A *et al*. Peg-interferon alfa-2b and ribavirin for the treatment of genotype 1 hepatitis C recurrence after liver transplantation. *Aliment. Pharmacol. Ther.* 2008; **28**: 450–457.

105 Hanouneh IA, Miller C, Aucejo F *et al*. Recurrent hepatitis C after liver transplantation: on-treatment prediction of response to peginterferon/ribavirin therapy. *Liver Transpl.* 2008; **14**: 53–58.

106 Sharma P, Marrero JA, Fontana RJ *et al*. Sustained virologic response to therapy of recurrent hepatitis C after liver transplantation is related to early virologic response and dose adherence. *Liver Transpl.* 2007; **13**: 1100–1108.

107 Roche B, Sebagh M, Canfora ML *et al*. Hepatitis C virus therapy in liver transplant recipients: response predictors, effect on fibrosis progression, and importance of the initial stage of fibrosis. *Liver Transpl.* 2008; **14**: 1766–1777.

108 Terrault NA. Hepatitis C therapy before and after liver transplantation. *Liver Transpl.* 2008; **14** (Suppl. 2): S58–66.

109 Wang CS, Ko HH, Yoshida EM *et al*. Interferon-based combination anti-viral therapy for hepatitis C virus after liver transplantation: a review and quantitative analysis. *Am. J. Transpl.* 2006; **6**: 1586–1599.

110 Berardi S, Lodato F, Gramenzi A *et al*. High incidence of allograft dysfunction in liver transplanted patients treated with pegylated-interferon alpha-2b and ribavirin for hepatitis C recurrence: possible de novo autoimmune hepatitis? *Gut* 2007; **56**: 237–242.

111 Kontorinis N, Agarwal K, Elhajj N *et al*. Pegylated interferon-induced immune-mediated hepatitis post-liver transplantation. *Liver Transpl.* 2006; **12**: 827–830.

112 Cholongitas E, Samonakis D, Patch D *et al*. Induction of autoimmune hepatitis by pegylated interferon in a liver transplant patient with recurrent hepatitis C virus. *Transplantation* 2006; **81**: 488–490.

113 Samuel D, Bizollon T, Feray C *et al*. Interferon-alpha 2b plus ribavirin in patients with chronic hepatitis C after liver transplantation: a randomized study. *Gastroenterology* 2003; **124**: 642–650.

114 Pelletier SJ, Schaubel DE, Punch JD *et al*. Hepatitis C is a risk factor for death after liver retransplantation. *Liver Transpl.* 2005; **11**: 434–440.

115 Rosen H, Prieto M, Casanovas-Taltavull T *et al*. Validation and refinement of survival models for liver retransplantation. *Hepatology* 2003; **38**: 460–469.

116 Ghabril M, Dickson R, Wiesner R. Improving outcomes of liver retransplantation: an analysis of trends and the impact of Hepatitis C infection. *Am. J. Transpl.* 2008; **8**: 404–411.

117 Neff GW, O'Brien CB, Nery J *et al*. Factors that identify survival after liver retransplantation for allograft failure caused by recurrent hepatitis C infection. *Liver Transpl.* 2004; **10**: 1497–1503.

118 Ghobrial RM, Farmer DG, Baquerizo A *et al*. Orthotopic liver transplantation for hepatitis C: outcome, effect of immunosuppression, and causes of retransplantation during an 8-year single-center experience. *Ann. Surg.* 1999; **229**: 824–831.

119 Testa G, Crippin JS, Netto GJ *et al*. Liver transplantation for hepatitis C: recurrence and disease progression in 300 patients. *Liver Transpl.* 2000; **6**: 553–561.

120 Facciuto M, Heidt D, Guarrera J *et al*. Retransplantation for late liver graft failure: predictors of mortality. *Liver Transpl.* 2000; **6**: 174–179.

121 Ghabril M, Dickson RC, Machicao VI *et al*. Liver retransplantation of patients with hepatitis C infection is associated with acceptable patient and graft survival. *Liver Transpl.* 2007; **13**: 1717–1727.

122 McCashland T, Watt K, Lyden E *et al*. Retransplantation for hepatitis C: results of a U.S. multicenter retransplant study. *Liver Transpl.* 2007; **13**: 1246–1253.

123 Ercolani G, Grazi GL, Ravaioli M *et al*. Histological recurrent hepatitis C after liver transplantation: Outcome and role of retransplantation. *Liver Transpl.* 2006; **12**: 1104–1111.

124 Burton JR, Jr., Sonnenberg A, Rosen HR. Retransplantation for recurrent hepatitis C in the MELD era: maximizing utility. *Liver Transpl.* 2004; **10** (10 Suppl. 2): S59–64.

125 Samuel D, Weber R, Stock P *et al*. Are HIV-infected patients candidates for liver transplantation? *J. Hepatol.* 2008; **48**: 697–707.

126 Roland ME, Barin B, Carlson L *et al*. HIV-infected liver and kidney transplant recipients: 1- and 3-year outcomes. *Am. J. Transpl.* 2007; **8**: 355–365.

127 Miro JM, Aguero F, Laguno M *et al*. Liver transplantation in HIV/hepatitis co-infection. *J. HIV Ther.* 2007; **12**: 24–35.

128 Ragni MV, Eghtesad B, Schlesinger KW *et al*. Pretransplant survival is shorter in HIV-positive than HIV-negative subjects with end-stage liver disease. *Liver Transpl.* 2005; **11**: 1425–1430.

129 Terrault NA, Carter JT, Carlson L *et al*. Outcome of patients with hepatitis B virus and human immunodeficiency virus infections referred for liver transplantation. *Liver Transpl.* 2006; **12**: 801–807.

130 Pineda JA, Romero-Gomez M, Diaz-Garcia F *et al*. HIV coinfection shortens the survival of patients with hepatitis C virus-related decompensated cirrhosis. *Hepatology* 2005; **41**: 779–789.

131 Frassetto LA, Browne M, Cheng A *et al*. Immunosuppressant pharmacokinetics and dosing modifications in HIV-1 infected liver and kidney transplant recipients. *Am. J. Transpl.* 2007; **7**: 2816–2820.

132 Teicher E, Vincent I, Bonhomme-Faivre L *et al*. Effect of highly active antiretroviral therapy on tacrolimus pharmacokinetics in hepatitis C virus and HIV co-infected liver transplant recipients in the ANRS HC-08 Study. *Clin. Pharmacokinet.* 2007; **46**: 941–952.

133 Tateo M, Roque-Afonso AM, Antonini TM *et al*. Long-term follow-up of liver transplanted HIV/hepatitis B virus coinfected patients: perfect control of hepatitis B virus replication and absence of mitochondrial toxicity. *AIDS* 2009; **23**: 1069–1076.

134 Coffin C, Stock P, Berg C *et al*. Virologic and clinical outcomes of hepatitis B virus infection in HIV-HBV coinfected transplant recipients. *Am. J. Transpl.* 2010; **10**: 1268–1275.

135 Duclos-Vallee JC, Feray C, Sebagh M *et al*. Survival and recurrence of hepatitis C after liver transplantation in patients coinfected with human immunodeficiency virus and hepatitis C virus. *Hepatology* 2008; **47**: 407–417.

136 Terrault N, Barin B, Schiano T *et al*. Survival and risk of severe hepatitis C virus recurrence in liver transplant recipients coinfected with human immunodeficiency virus and HCV. *Hepatology* 2009: **50** (Suppl. 4); 396A.

137 de Vera ME, Dvorchik I, Tom K *et al*. Survival of liver transplant patients coinfected with HIV and HCV is adversely impacted by recurrent hepatitis C. *Am. J. Transpl.* 2006; **6**: 2983–2993.

138 Vennarecci G, Ettorre GM, Antonini M *et al*. Liver transplantation in HIV-positive patients. *Transpl. Proc.* 2007; **39**: 1936–1938.

139 Miró J, Montejo M, Castells L *et al*. Prognostic factors of mortality in HCV-HIV-coinfected liver transplant recipients from the FIPSE OLT-HIV-05—GESIDA 45-05 cohort study (2002-06). 15th Conference on Retroviruses and Opportunistic Infections, 2008, Boston, MA (abstract).

Index

Note: Page numbers in *italic* refer to figures and/or tables

Sherlock's Diseases of the Liver and Biliary System, Twelfth Edition. Edited by
James S. Dooley, Anna S.F. Lok, Andrew K. Burroughs, E. Jenny Heathcote.
© 2011 by Blackwell Publishing Ltd. Published 2011 by Blackwell Publishing Ltd.

vasopressin
  in ascites formation 222–3
  for treatment of variceal bleeding 182, *182*
venesection 528
venography *see* angiography
venous hum 162
venous stars 112
very low density lipoprotein (VLDL) 26, 27, 552
vinyl chloride 177, 698
viramidine 423
visceral larva migrans (*T. canis*) 619, 654
vitamin A 177, *242*, 243
vitamin B$_{12}$ 49
vitamin D *242*, 243, 244
vitamin E *242*, 243
vitamin K 50–1, *242*
  therapy 52, 243
VLDL (very low density lipoprotein) 26, 27, 552
Von Gierke's disease (GSD IA) 590, 710
von Meyenberg complex (hamartoma) 319, *320*, 676

W
wedged hepatic venous pressure (WHVP) 170, *179*
weight loss
  in NAFLD 559
  surgery 560
weight-loss products 498, 499

Weil's disease
  clinical features 641–2, *641*
  diagnosis 642, *642*
  mode of infection 640
  pathology 640–1
  prognosis 642
  treatment 643
Wernicke's encephalopathy 130
West Haven criteria (mental status) *124*
Whipple's disease 622
Whipple's operation (pancreatoduodenectomy) 300, 306–7
white blood cells *see* leucocytes
white matter lesions 131
Wilson's disease 534–43
  biochemistry 76, 539, 587
  in children 537, 587–8
    non-Wilson's-related cirrhosis 588
  clinical features 537–9, 587
    with ALF 74, 76, 86, 537–8, *538*
    autoimmune-hepatitis-like 462, 538, *538*
    by age of onset *537*
    neuropsychiatric 130–1, 539
  copper and 534, *535*, 539, *540*, 541
  diagnosis 540
  histopathology 536, *536*, 537, 588
  molecular genetics 534–6, *535*, 539
  in pregnancy 542, 611
  prognosis 542–3
  screening 538, 540
  treatment 86, 540–2, *541*, 588, 611
    liver transplantation 542, 710
Wolman's disease 593

women
  alcoholic liver disease 510–11
  drug-related liver injury in 483–4
  gallstones 265

X
X-rays
  amoebiasis 637
  ascites 215
  cholecystitis 269
  hydatid cysts 650, *650*
  in jaundice 247
  liver size 7
  portal vein 163, *164*
  tuberculosis 638
xanthogranulomatous cholecystitis 278
xanthoma *242*, 243
  in PBC 332
xanthomatosis 63
xenobiotics, in PBC 336

Y
yellow fever virus (YFV) 430–1

Z
Zellweger's syndrome 247, 579
zidovudine 442
Zieve's syndrome 49
zinc
  hepatic encephalopathy 143
  Wilson's disease 542, 611